CRAM

Rehabilitation
of the Patient with
Respiratory
Disease

Rehabilitation
of the Patient with
Respiratory
Disease

Editors

Neil S. Cherniack, M.D.
Professor of Medicine and Physiology
University of Medicine and Dentistry of
*   New Jersey—New Jersey Medical School*
Newark, New Jersey

Murray D. Altose, M.D.
Professor of Medicine
Case Western Reserve University
Chief of Staff
Veterans Administration Medical Center
Cleveland, Ohio

and

Ikuo Homma, M.D.
Chairman and Professor of Physiology
Second Department of Physiology
Showa University School of Medicine
Tokyo, Japan

McGraw-Hill
Health Professions Division
New York St. Louis San Francisco Auckland Bogotá Caracas Lisbon London Madrid
Mexico City Milan Montreal New Delhi San Juan Singapore Sydney Tokyo Toronto

McGraw-Hill

A Division of The McGraw·Hill Companies

1234567890 KGPKGP 998

ISBN 0-07-011649-0

This book was set in Palatino by Bi-Comp, Inc. The editors were Joseph Hefta and Steven Melvin; the production supervisor was Catherine Saggese.

In memory of a very talented writer and painter, Charles Dunn, who created our cover illustration and who died quite unexpectedly.

Quebecor Printing/Kingsport was the printer and binder.

Cataloging-in-Publication data is on file for this title at the Library of Congress.

CONTENTS

CONTRIBUTORS

Numbers in brackets refer to chapters written or cowritten by the contributor

Loutfi S. Aboussouan, M.D. [47]
Assistant Professor of Medicine, Division of Pulmonary and Critical Care Medicine, Wayne State University, Detroit, Michigan

Mitsuru Adachi, M.D. [8]
Professor of Medicine, Showa University School of Medicine, Tokyo, Japan

Nancy L. Adams, Ph.D. [21]
Clinical Neuropsychologist, General Mental Health Services, Cleveland Veterans Administration Hospital, Cleveland, Ohio

Murray D. Altose, M.D. [1, 39]
Professor of Medicine, Case Western Reserve University, Cleveland, Ohio; and Chief of Staff, VA Medical Center, Cleveland, Ohio

John R. Bach, M.D., F.C.C.P., F.A.A.P.M.R. [36]
Professor of Physical Medicine and Rehabilitation, University of Medicine and Dentistry of New Jersey (UMDNJ)-New Jersey Medical School, Newark, New Jersey; Codirector of the Jerry Lewis Muscular Dystrophy Association Clinic, UMDNJ-New Jersey Medical School, Newark, New Jersey; Director, Center for Ventilatory Management Alternatives, University Hospital, Newark, New Jersey; and Kessler Institute for Rehabilitation, West Orange, New Jersey

Ahmed Bahammam, M.D., M.R.C.P. [46]
Physician, Section of Respiratory Diseases, University of Manitoba, Winnipeg, Manitoba, Canada

Klaus Ballanyi, M.D., Prof. Dr. Rer. Nat. [5]
Zentrum Physiology and Pathophysiology, University of Gottingen, Gottingen, Germany

Janet Barry, P.T.R. [57, 58, 59]
Physical Therapist, Physical Medicine and Rehabilitation, The Cleveland Clinic Foundation, Cleveland, Ohio

Robert C. Basner, M.D. [14]
Associate Professor of Medicine, Department of Medicine, Section of Respiratory and Critical Care Medicine, University of Illinois at Chicago College of Medicine, Chicago, Illinois; and Director, Center for Sleep and Ventilatory Disorders, University of Illinois Hospital, Chicago, Illinois

Leonard Bielory, M.D. [24]
Associate Professor of Medicine and Pediatrics, UMDNJ–New Jersey Medical School, Newark, New Jersey; and Allergy and Immunology, UMDNJ-Doctors Office Center, Newark, New Jersey

Gisella Borzone, M.D., Ph.D. [42]
Assistant Professor, Department of Respiratory Diseases, Division of Medicine, Pontificia Universidad Catolica de Chile, Santiago, Chile

Sidney S. Braman, M.D. [49]
Professor of Medicine, Brown University; and Director, Pulmonary and Critical Care Medicine, Rhode Island Hospital, Providence, Rhode Island

Matthew Brenner, M.D. [51]
Clinical Professor of Surgery, University of California, Los Angeles, School of Medicine, University of California, Los Angeles, Los Angeles, California

Robert Brown, M.D., C.M. [45]
Chief, Pulmonary and Critical Care Section, Department of Medicine, Brockton/West Roxbury Veterans Affairs Medical Center, West Roxbury, Massachusetts; and Associate Professor of Medicine, Harvard Medical School, Boston, Massachusetts

Gale Browning, M.D. [57, 58, 59]
Director, Rehabilitation Unit, The Cleveland Clinic Foundation, Cleveland, Ohio

Bartolome R. Celli, M.D. [9]
Professor of Medicine, Tufts University, Boston, Massachusetts; and Chief, Pulmonary Critical Care, St. Elizabeth's Medical Center, Boston, Massachusetts

E. Paul Cherniack, M.D. [37, 54]
Geriatrics and Extended Care Service, Bronx VA Medical Center, Bronx, New York; and Assistant Professor of Geriatrics, Department of Geriatrics and Adult Development, Mount Sinai School of Medicine, New York, New York

Neil S. Cherniack, M.D. [1, 13, 39]
Director of Research and Clinical Affairs, and Professor of Medicine and Physiology, University of Medicine and Dentistry New Jersey, New Jersey Medical School, Newark, New Jersey

Noreen M. Clark, Ph.D. [55]
Dean and Marshall H. Becker Professor of Public Health, School of Public Health, University of Michigan, Ann Arbor, Michigan

Francis C. Cordova, M.D. [33]
Assistant Professor of Medicine, Division of Pulmonary Disease and Critical Care Medicine, Department of Medicine, Temple University School of Medicine, Philadelphia, Pennsylvania

Jerome A. Dempsey, Ph.D. [7]
John Robert Sutton Professor of Preventive Medicine, Department of Preventive Medicine, The John Rankin Laboratory of Pulmonary Medicine, University of Wisconsin-Madison Medical School, Madison, Wisconsin

André de Troyer, M.D. [3]
Professor of Medicine, Chest Service, Erasme University Hospital; and Director, Laboratory of Cardiorespiratory Physiology, Brussels School of Medicine, Brussels, Belgium

Lisa L. Dever, M.D. [27]
Chief, Infectious Diseases Clinic, VA New Jersey Health Care System, East Orange, New Jersey; and Assistant Professor of Medicine, UMDNJ-New Jersey Medical School, Newark, New Jersey

Rajiv Dhand, M.D. [31]
Associate Professor of Medicine, Division of Pulmonary and Critical Care Medicine, Loyola University of Chicago Stritch School of Medicine, and Edward Hines Jr. Veterans Affairs Hospital, Maywood, Illinois

Anthony F. DiMarco, M.D. [32]
Professor of Medicine, Case Western Reserve University, Division of Pulmonary and Critical Care Medicine, MetroHealth Medical Center, Cleveland, Ohio

Charles Dunn [62]
Author, Artist, and Lecturer, Brooklyn, New York

Kathleen Ellstrom, R.N., Ph.D. [38]
Division of Pulmonary and Critical Care Medicine, Department of Medicine, University of California, Los Angeles, School of Medicine, Los Angeles, California

Stanley B. Fiel, M.D. [48]
Professor of Medicine, Pulmonary and Critical Care Division, Medical College of Pennsylvania, Philadelphia, Pennsylvania

Richard Fischel, M.D., Ph.D. [51]
Assistant Clinical Professor of Surgery, Department of Thoracic Surgery, Chapman Medical Center, Orange, California; Cedars-Sinai Medical Center, Los Angeles, California; and Department of Radiology, Lakewood Regional Medical Center, Lakewood, California

Bernard Gardner, M.D. [52]
Professor of Surgery, UMDNJ–New Jersey Medical School, Newark, New Jersey

Arthur F. Gelb, M.D. [51]
Clinical Professor of Medicine, Pulmonary and Critical Care Division, UCLA School of Medicine, Los Angeles, California; and Medical Director of Respiratory Services, Lakewood Regional Medical Center, Lakewood, California

Audrey G. Gift, Ph.D., R.N., F.A.A.N. [22]
Professor, Associate Dean for Research; and Doctoral Program, Michigan State University College of Nursing, East Lansing, Michigan

Craig A. Harms, M.D. [7]
John Rankin Laboratory of Pulmonary Medicine, Department of Preventive Medicine, University of Wisconsin-Madison, Madison, Wisconsin

Nicholas S. Hill, M.D. [49]
Professor of Medicine, Brown University, Providence, Rhode Island; Director, Critical Care Medicine, Rhode Island Hospital, Providence, Rhode Island

Ikuo Homma, M.D., Ph. D. [29, 30]
Professor and Chairman, Second Department of Physiology, Showa University School of Medicine, Tokyo, Japan

David W. Hudgel, M.D. [20]
Professor of Medicine, Sleep Disorders Medicine and Allergy, Pulmonary and Critical Care Medicine, Department of Medicine, Case Western Reserve University; and MetroHealth Medical Center, Cleveland, Ohio

Norman Hymowitz, M.D. [28]
Professor of Clinical Psychiatry, Department of Psychiatry, UMDNJ-New Jersey Medical School, Newark, New Jersey

Akinori Iwasaki, M.D. [43]
Professor, Second Department of Surgery, Second Department of Internal Medicine, School of Medicine, Fukuoka University, Nanakuma, Fukuoka, Japan

Waldemar G. Johanson, Jr., M.D., M.P.H. [27]
Professor and Chairman, Department of Medicine, UMDNJ-New Jersey Medical School, Newark, New Jersey

Bruce D. Johnson, M.D. [34]
Senior Associate Consultant, Division of Cardiovascular Diseases, Mayo Clinic and Foundation, Rochester, Minnesota

Paul W. Jones, M.D. [60]
Professor of Respiratory Medicine, Division of Physiological Medicine, St. George's Hospital Medical School, London, United Kingdom

Richard E. Kanner, M.D. [23]
Professor of Medicine, Division of Respiratory, Critical Care and Occupational Pulmonary Medicine, Department of Internal Medicine, University of Utah Health Sciences Center, Salt Lake City, Utah

Steven G. Kelsen, M.D. [33]
Professor of Medicine and Physiology, Director, Division of Pulmonary Medicine and Critical Care Medicine, Temple University Hospital, Philadelphia, Pennsylvania

Talmadge E. King, Jr., M.D. [10]
Senior Faculty Member, Department of Medicine, National Jewish Center for Immunology and Respiratory Medicine, Denver, Colorado; and Vice Chairman for Clinical Affairs and Professor of Medicine, Pulmonary and Critical Care Division, Department of Medicine, University of Colorado Health Sciences Center, Denver, Colorado

Eric C. Kleerup, M.D. [38]
Division of Pulmonary and Critical Care Medicine, Department of Medicine, University of California, Los Angeles, School of Medicine, Los Angeles, California

Mordechai R. Kramer, M.D. [35]
Senior Lecturer in Internal Medicine, Pulmonary Department, Hadassah Medical Center, Jerusalem, Israel

Meir Kryger, M.D., F.R.C.P.C. [46]
Professor of Medicine, Section of Respiratory Diseases, University of Manitoba, Winnipeg, Manitoba, Canada; and Director, Sleep Disorders Centre

Franco Laghi, M.D. [12]
Assistant Professor, Division of Pulmonary and Critical Care Medicine, Edward Hines Jr. Veterans Administration Hospital, and Loyola University of Chicago Stritch School of Medicine, Maywood, Illinois

Peter M. Lalley, M.D., Prof. Ph.D. [5]
Zentrum Physiology and Pathophysiology, University of Gottingen, Gottingen, Germany

Marc H. Lavietes, M.D. [15, 25]
Associate Professor of Medicine, Director, Pulmonary Function Laboratory, New Jersey Medical School, Newark, New Jersey

Sanford Levine, M.D. [34]
Professor of Medicine, Pulmonary and Critical Care Section, Philadelphia VA Medical Center, Philadelphia, Pennsylvania

Richard Levinson, M.D. [61]
Author, Physician, and Artist, Scottsdale Medical Pavilion, Scottsdale, Arizona

Nathan Levitan, M.D. [50]
Medical Director, Clinical Cancer Programs for the Ireland Cancer Center; and University Hospital Health Systems, Cleveland, Ohio

Steven L. Lieberman, M.D. [45]
Director, Medical Intensive Care Unit, Pulmonary and Critical Care Section, Department of Medicine, Brockton/West Roxbury Veterans Affairs Medical Center, West Roxbury, Massachusetts; and Instructor of Medicine, Harvard Medical School, Boston, Massachusetts

Theodore G. Liou, M.D. [23]
Assistant Professor of Medicine, Division of Respiratory, Critical Care and Occupational Pulmonary Medicine, Department of Internal Medicine, University of Utah Health Sciences Center, Salt Lake City, Utah

Carmen Lisboa, M.D. [42]
Professor, Department of Respiratory Diseases, Division of Medicine, Pontificia Universidad Catolica de Chile, Santiago, Chile

Melvin Lopata, M.D. [17]
Vice-Chairman, Department of Medicine, University of Illinois College of Medicine, Chicago, Illinois

Harold L. Manning, M.D. [16]
Section of Pulmonary and Critical Care Medicine, Dartmouth-Hitchcock Medical Center, Dartmouth Medical School, Lebanon, New Hampshire

Matthew G. Marin, M.D. [25]
Professor of Medicine, Director, Pulmonary and Critical Care Medicine, New Jersey Medical School, Newark, New Jersey

Lawrence Martin, M.D. [18]
Chief, Division of Pulmonary and Critical Care Medicine, Mt. Sinai Medical Center, Cleveland, Ohio

Kevin McCully, Ph.D. [34]
Research Associate Professor of Medicine, Division of Geriatrics, MCP-Hahnemann Medical School, Philadelphia, Pennsylvania

Robert J. McKenna, Jr., M.D. [51]
Clinical Professor of Surgery, UCLA School of Medicine, Los Angeles, California; Department of Thoracic Surgery, Chapman Medical Center, Orange, California, Cedars-Sinai Medical Center, Los Angeles, California; and Department of Radiology, Lakewood Regional Medical Center, Lakewood, California

Sushmita Mikkilineni, M.D. [53]
Assistant Professor of Pediatrics, University of Medicine and Dentistry of New Jersey-Robert Wood Johnson Medical School, New Brunswick, New Jersey

Kenji Minoguchi, M.D., Ph.D. [8]
Professor of Medicine, Showa University, School of Medicine, Tokyo, Japan

Yoshimi Miyamoto [2]
Department of Engineering, University of Yamagata, Yamagata-ken, Japan

Hugo D. Montenegro, M.D. [26]
Professor of Medicine, Respiratory Diagnostic Center, Division of Pulmonary and Critical Care Medicine, University Hospitals of Cleveland, Cleveland, Ohio

Georgia L. Narsavage, Ph.D., R.N., C.S. [22]
Associate Professor, Associate Dean, University of Scranton College of Professional Studies, Scranton, Pennsylvania

Taitan Nguyen, B.S.E. [34]
Research Associate, Pulmonary and Critical Care Section, Philadelphia VA Medical Center, Philadelphia, Pennsylvania

Faryle Nothwehr, M.A., M.P.H. [55]
School of Public Health, University of Michigan, Ann Arbor, Michigan

Pam O'Dell-Rossi, M.P.A., O.T.R./L. [57, 58, 59]
Occupational Therapist, Physical Medicine and Rehabilitation, The Cleveland Clinic Foundation, Cleveland, Ohio

Arie Oliven, M.D. [44]
Professor of Medicine, Technion Faculty of Medicine, Haifa, Israel

Ergün Önal, M.D. [14]
Professor of Medicine, Department of Medicine, Section of Respiratory and Critical Care Medicine, University of Illinois at Chicago College of Medicine, Chicago, Illinois; and VA West Side Medical Center, Chicago, Illinois

John Oppenheimer, M.D. [24]
Clinical Assistant Professor of Medicine, UMDNJ–New Jersey Medical School, Newark, New Jersey

Doug Orens, M.B.A., R.R.T. [56]
Manager, Respiratory Therapy Section, Pulmonary and Critical Care Department, Cleveland Clinic Foundation, Cleveland, Ohio

Jonathan B. Orens, M.D. [41]
Assistant Professor of Medicine, Division of Pulmonary and Critical Care Medicine, Department of Medicine, University of Maryland School of Medicine, Baltimore, Maryland

Ralph J. Panos, M.D. [10]
Associate Professor of Medicine, Pulmonary Division, Department of Medicine, Northwestern University Medical School, Chicago, Illinois

Mieczyslaw Pokorski, M.D., Ph.D. [6]
Department of Neurophysiology, Medical Research Center, Polish Academy of Sciences, Warsaw, Poland

Gary W. Raff, M.D. [52]
Research Fellow, Department of Cardiothoracic Surgery, Children's Hospital, Philadelphia, Pennsylvania

Jeffrey P. Renston, M.D. [32]
Assistant Professor of Medicine, Case Western Reserve University, MetroHealth Center, Cleveland, Ohio

Diethelm W. Richter, M.D. [5]
Professor, Zentrum Physiology and Pathophysiology, University of Gottingen, Gottingen, Germany

Lewis J. Rubin, M.D. [41]
Professor of Medicine and Physiology, Division of Pulmonary and Critical Care Medicine, Department of Medicine, University of Maryland School of Medicine, Baltimore, Maryland

Vinod Sahgal, M.D. [4, 56, 57, 58, 59]
Chairman, Department of Physical Medicine and Rehabilitation, Cleveland Clinic Foundation, Cleveland, Ohio; and Professor, Department of Physical Medicine and Rehabilitation, Ohio State University, University Medical Center, Cleveland, Ohio

Mark J. Schein, M.D. [51]
Clinical Assistant Professor of Radiology, USC School of Medicine, Los Angeles, California; and Department of Radiology, Lakewood Regional Medical Center, Lakewood, California

Deborah Schneider, C.R.R.N., R.N. [56]
Director, Patient Care Services, Neurology, Neurosurgery, and Rehabilitation, Cleveland Clinic Foundation, Cleveland, Ohio

Richard M. Schwartzstein, M.D. [16]
Clinical Director, Division of Pulmonary and Critical Care Medicine, Beth Israel Deaconess Medical Center, Harvard Medical School, Boston, Massachusetts

Takayuki Shirakusa, M.D. [43]
Professor of Surgery, Second Department of Surgery, Second Department of Internal Medicine, School of Medicine, Fukuoka University, Nanakuma, Fukuoka, Japan

John M. Shneerson, D.M., F.R.C. P. [11]
Director of Respiratory Support and Sleep Centre, Papworth Hospital, Cambridge, England

Peggy M. Simon, M.D. [40]
Associate Professor of Medicine and Physiology, Dartmouth-Hitchcock Medical Center, Lebanon, New Hampshire

Suzanne C. Smeltzer, R.N., Ed.D. [15]
Associate Professor, College of Nursing, Villanova University, Villanova, Pennsylvania

James K. Stoller, M.D. [47]
Assistant Clinical Professor, Case Western Reserve University, Cleveland, Ohio; and Head, Section of Respiratory Therapy, Department of Pulmonary and Critical Care Medicine, The Cleveland Clinic Foundation, Cleveland, Ohio

Gerald Supinski, M.D. [19]
Associate Professor of Medicine, Case Western Reserve University, Cleveland, Ohio; and Pulmonary Disease Division, Metropolitan General Hospital, Cleveland, Ohio

Donald P. Tashkin, M.D. [38]
Professor of Medicine, Division of Pulmonary and Critical Care Medicine, Department of Medicine, University of California, Los Angeles, School of Medicine, Los Angeles, California

Sevgi Tetik, M.D. [4]
The Cleveland Clinic Foundation, Cleveland, Ohio

Martin J. Tobin, M.D. [12, 31]
Professor of Medicine, Director, Division of Pulmonary and Critical Care Medicine, Loyola University of Chicago Stritch School of Medicine, and Edward Hines Jr. Veterans Affairs Hospital, Maywood, Illinois

Hideo Toyoshima, M.D. [43]
Second Department of Surgery, Second Department of Internal Medicine, School of Medicine, Fukuoka University, Nanakuma, Fukuoka, Japan

Thomas J. Wetter, M.D. [7]
John Rankin Laboratory of Pulmonary Medicine, Department of Preventive Medicine, University of Wisconsin-Madison, Madison, Wisconsin

Minoru Yoshida, M.D. [43]
Second Department of Surgery, Second Department of Internal Medicine, School of Medicine, Fukuoka University, Nanakuma, Fukuoka, Japan

Noe Zamel, M.D. [51]
Professor of Medicine, Pulmonary Division, University of Toronto, Toronto, Ontario, Canada; and Faculty of Medicine, Toronto University, Toronto, Ontario, Canada

FOREWORD

The first "rehabilitation" institutions in the late 1940s were created for patients with severe pulmonary impairment secondary to tuberculosis or poliomyelitis neuromuscular respiratory paralysis. With increased incidence of poliomyelitis these institutions evolved into general rehabilitation facilities. Thus, pulmonary rehabilitation has been the cornerstone of the field of rehabilitation with perhaps the best documented clinical outcomes.

Members of the faculty of the University of Medicine and Dentistry's (UMDNJ) New Jersey Medical School have been at the forefront of many aspects of pulmonary rehabilitation since the 1970s. Dr. Cherniack has brought together members of the UMDNJ-New Jersey Medical School faculty with other internationally acclaimed experts in the field of pulmonary rehabilitation from four European countries, as well as from Asia and South America. This book is a comprehensive, balanced critical review of the current evaluation and management techniques used for patients with pulmonary impairment, written from the dual perspectives of the pulmonary specialist and the rehabilitation physician. It addresses the complete spectrum of respiratory impairment from asthma to emphysema, from spinal cord injury and neuromuscular disease to stroke. Pathophysiology is dicussed in detail with a special emphasis on respiratory muscle function, brain and nervous system dysfunction, and sleep disordered breathing. Each disease is discussed with respect to prevention, drug therapy, physical therapy, and behavioral and psychosocial approaches. The wide scope of this book is suggested by the chapter devoted to art therapy in pulmonary rehabilitation and considerations from the viewpoints of pediatricians and geriatricians. This work brings together a body of knowledge that should be of interest to internists, surgeons, physiatrists, psychologists, sociologists, therapists, nurses, residents, and medical students who want a complete view of the effective measures available to treat major pulmonary impairment.

Joel A. DeLisa, M.D., M.S.
Professor and Chairman
Department of Physical Medicine and Rehabilitation
President, Kessler Medical Rehabilitation Research and
Education Corporation

PREFACE

The tools and techniques available to pulmonary physicians have become increasingly effective but more complex. These include the following: improved types of ventilators have greatly enhanced the ability to sustain patients with respiratory failure. Giant steps have been taken in the treatment of lung infections. There has been an information explosion with regard to lung inury and the pathophysiology of the tracheobronchial tree. New and extremely fruitful areas of research in respiratory muscle structure, function, and biochemistry have increased our recognition of their impact on major lung diseases enormously. The importance of normal sleep has been established. Effective methods of smoking cessation, a vital step in many patients with respiratory disease, have been developed.

Despite these major advances, however, few respiratory diseases are completely cured or quickly reversed by drugs alone. Many cause permanent damage or incapacitate patients for sufficiently long times, so that steps must be taken to maintain function while the respiratory disease is being treated. Moreover, injury to the nervous system or disease of the immune system, muscles, or cardiovascular system can have serious adverse consequences for breathing so that therapeutic measures are necessary to maintain respiratory function. Fortunately, since the days of poliomyelitis, there has been steady and substantial progress made in rehabilitation medicine and in the use of physical and behavioral techniques to restore respiratory function.

This seems to be a particularly opportune time to bring together experts from pulmonary and rehabilitative medicine to produce a comprehensive survey of rehabilitation methods in patients with respiratory disease.

The first part of this book deals with the physiology and pathophysiology of a broad spectrum of lung disease with special emphasis placed on the respiratory muscles, regulation of breathing and sleep pathophysiology, areas in which much recent basic and clinical research has focused.

The second part of the book concentrates on the assessment and treatment of patients with these diseases as well as on methods of disease prevention such as smoking cessation techniques. Neuropsychological and physical techniques of evaluating patients are discussed as are the theoretical benefits and practical use of specific modalities of treatment such as exercise, respiratory muscle training, and electrical stimulation of the respiratory muscles. In the final sections, rehabilitative methods that are useful in each specific pulmonary disease are surveyed with chapters especially focused on pediatric and geriatric patients. Recent treatment advances including lung reduction surgery and noninvasive ventilation are discussed in detail. Thus, the use of rehabilitative medicine in the major respiratory disease are reviewed in separate chapters from various points of view.

The editors and contributors to this book come from many different countries and we have made a conscious effort to present pulmonary rehabilitation from the perspective of physicians from different disciplines around the world. The book can either be read as a survey of respiratory rehabilitation or used as a reference by health science students, physicians, and other health care givers.

We have enjoyed assembling this book and wish to particularly thank the editors of McGraw-Hill for their encouragement and advice. We would also like to thank Charles Dunn for the cover illustration and Stella Rogers for her tireless efforts in answering contributors' questions, encouraging them to meet deadlines, and assembling the chapters. Finally, I would like to thank the coeditors and all the contributors for their hard work in making this volume possible.

To Sandy, Emily, Evan, Andy, Patty, Maggie, YZ, Ariella, Madeline, and Luke

PART I

PHYSIOLOGIC FOUNDATIONS

Chapter 1

LUNG AND CHEST WALL MECHANICS

MURRAY D. ALTOSE

NEIL S. CHERNIACK

The ventilatory apparatus consists of the lungs and the surrounding chest wall, which includes the rib cage, intercostal muscles, and diaphragm. During breathing the lungs and chest wall from a mechanical standpoint can be regarded as elements of a pump operating in series so that the elastic and resistive characteristics of both are additive as far as breathing is concerned. At the end of a normal expiration, the respiratory muscles are at rest. The volume of air in the lungs at the resting end-expiratory position is determined by the balance between the elastic recoil forces of the lung, which at end-expiration favor collapse and the elastic properties of the chest wall, which at end-expiration favor expansion. These opposing forces produce a subatmospheric pressure of about 5 cmH$_2$O in the potential space between the visceral and parietal pleura.[1,2]

The elastic recoil of the lungs is measured from the transpulmonary pressure, the difference between alveolar pressure (PA), and pleural pressure (Ppl), under static conditions when airflow is arrested (Fig. 1-1). Similarly, when the respiratory muscles are relaxed, the elastic recoil of the chest wall is measured from the difference between pleural pressure and the pressure at the external surface of the chest.

Chest expansion produced by inspiratory muscle contraction causes the pleural pressure as well as alveolar pressure to become subatmospheric, causing air to flow into the lung from the atmosphere. The difference between alveolar pressure and the pressure at the airway opening or mouth (Pm), divided by the rate of airflow (V̇), is a measure of the resistance (R) to flow in the tracheobronchial tree.[1-4]

Air moves into the lungs during inspiration until the alveolar pressure reaches atmospheric levels and the pressure gradient between the alveoli and the airway opening is eliminated. At the end of the inspiration, lung volume and consequently the recoil pressure of the lung are greater than those at the end of preceding expiration. The change in transpulmonary pressure for a given change in volume is a measure of lung elastance or stiffness. Compliance, the reciprocal of elastance, is more commonly used in describing lung elastic properties.[1-4]

At end-inspiration, the inspiratory muscles relax and the elastic recoil of the lung is released. This causes the alveolar pressure to exceed the pressure at the nose and the mouth so that air flows out of the lungs. During quiet breathing expiration occurs passively. At high levels of ventilation, as with exercise, the expiratory muscles of the rib cage and abdomen help push air out, shortening expiratory time.

Lung volumes can be subdivided into a number of compartments. The volume of air in the lungs at the normal, resting end-expiratory position is termed the *functional residual capacity (FRC)* (Fig. 1-2). This is the volume at which the outward recoil of the chest is of the same magnitude as the inward recoil of the lung. The maximum volume of air that can be pulled into the lungs from functional residual capacity is termed the *inspiratory capacity (IC)*. The inspiratory capacity is made up of the tidal volume plus the inspiratory reserve volume. The volume of air in the lungs at the end of a maximum inspiration is the *total lung capacity (TLC)*. This volume is determined by inspiratory muscle strength and the elastic recoil of the lung and the chest wall. The vital capacity is the maximum volume of air that can be exhaled after a maximum inspiration. The maximum volume of air that can be forcibly exhaled from functional residual capacity is the *expiratory reserve volume (ERV)*. The volume of air remaining in the lungs after such a maximum expiratory effort is the residual volume. This volume depends on expiratory muscle strength, airway closure at low lung volumes and by the reduced chest wall compliance at small lung volumes. Airway closure is more important in setting residual volume in the elderly than in the young.[5,6]

The elastic recoil of the chest wall is such that the chest, were it unopposed by the lungs, would enlarge to about 70 percent of the total lung capacity. This volume is the equilibrium or resting position of the chest wall, where the pressure gradient across the chest wall (the difference between the pleural pressure and the pressure at the body surface) is zero. If the volume of gas in the lungs is increased even more to expand the thorax, the chest wall, like the lung, would tend to recoil inward. At volumes less than 70 percent of the total lung capacity, the recoil of the chest is directed outward and is opposite to that of the lung. As residual volume is approached, the compliance of the chest wall falls to very low levels. The stiffness of the chest wall at low lung volumes is one of the major determinants of residual volume.[1-4]

The recoil of the lung is determined from the difference between PA and Ppl. Also, the recoil of the chest wall (when the respiratory muscles are completely at rest) is determined from the difference between Ppl and the pressure at the surface of the body (Pbs). Therefore the recoil of the entire respiratory system Prs can be expressed as the algebraic sum of the two:

$$\text{Prs} = (\text{PA} - \text{Ppl}) + (\text{Ppl} - \text{Pbs}) = \text{PA} - \text{Pbs}$$

where Prs is the sum of the two recoils. When the pressure at the surface of the chest is atmospheric[1-4] (i.e., Pbs = 0),

$$\text{Prs} = \text{PA}$$

Figure 1-3 shows typical expiratory static pressure-volume curves for a normal person, a patient with emphysema, and a patient with pulmonary fibrosis.[5] Pressure-volume relationships are conventionally measured during interruptions in

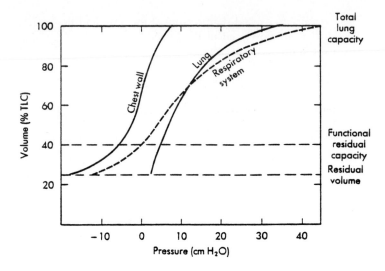

FIGURE 1-1 Pressure-volume relationships of the lung, chest wall, and combined system. At any lung volume the elastic recoil of the total respiratory lung-chest wall system is determined from the algebraic sum of the recoil pressures of the lung and chest wall. [Reprinted with permission from Cherniack NS, Altose MD, Kelsen SG: The respiratory system, in Berne RM, Levy MN (eds.): *Physiology.* St. Louis, Mosby, 1983.]

expiration following a full inspiration to total lung capacity. Because of the loss of lung elastic recoil in patients with emphysema, the pressure-volume curve of the lungs is shifted upward and to the left. The transpulmonary pressure at any given lung volume is reduced and the total lung capacity is enlarged. The increased stiffness of the lungs in pulmonary fibrosis results in a shift of the pressure-volume curve downward and to the right. The transpulmonary pressure at a given lung volume is elevated and total lung capacity is reduced.

Components of Lung Elastic Recoil

Lung elasticity depends on the physical properties of the lung tissues and the surface tension of the film lining the alveolar walls.[1,2] It arises from the elastin and collagen fibers in the alveolar walls surrounding bronchioles and pulmonary capillaries. Elastin fibers can be stretched to nearly double their initial length, but collagen fibers are poorly extensible and act primarily to limit further expansion at large lung volumes. Lung expansion during breathing seems to occur through an unfolding and geometrical rearrangement of fibers in the alveolar walls. Changes in the arrangement and physicochemical properties of the elastin and collagen fibers

in the lungs account for the increasing distensibility of the lungs with advancing age. Disease processes also alter elasticity (Fig. 1-3). Emphysema is characterized by a destruction of alveolar walls by proteases released by neutrophils and macrophages. This results in decreased elastic recoil and increased lung compliance. Naturally occurring antiproteases combat the process.[7,8] Conversely, pulmonary fibrosis decreases the distensibility of the lungs.

The surface forces acting at the air-liquid interface in the alveoli increase the pressure required to distend the lung and contribute considerably to the recoil pressure. Filling the lung with saline eliminates the air-liquid interface and abolishes surface forces without affecting the elasticity of the pulmonary tissues. At any given volume, the transpulmonary pressure of the liquid-distended lung is about half of that of the lung inflated with air. The contribution of surface forces to the elastic recoil of the lungs is greater at low than at high volumes.[9]

Surfactant is produced by the type II granular pneumocyte and consists of dipalmitoyl lecithin conjugated with protein. It has two important characteristics. The surface tension of surfactant is very low, which helps reduce surface forces. Second, as the surface area of the film is reduced, the surface tension decreases yet further.[10] This is critical in maintaining the stability of alveoli and prevents their collapse.

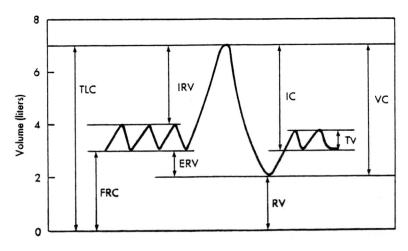

FIGURE 1-2 Lung volumes and subdivisions. [Reprinted with permission from Cherniack NS, Altose MD, Kelsen SG: The respiratory system, in Berne RM, Levy MN (eds.): *Physiology.* St. Louis, Mosby, 1983.]

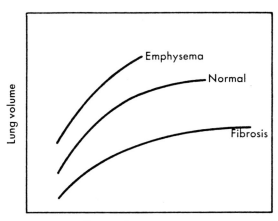

FIGURE 1-3 A comparison of lung volume-pressure relationships in a normal patient and patients with emphysema and pulmonary fibrosis. [Reprinted with permission from Cherniack NS, Altose MD, Kelsen SG: The respiratory system, in Berne RM, Levy MN (eds.): *Physiology.* St. Louis, Mosby, 1983.]

Alveolar stability is also enhanced by a process of interdependence. If disease or injury causes some alveoli to lose volume, tissue attachments of the collapsing region tend to prevent collapse. The reverse occurs in regions that tend to increase their size. This interdependence between adjacent parts of the lung acts as a homeostatic mechanism, minimizing atelectasis and gas trapping.[11]

Airway Resistance

The most common physiologic abnormality of the lung is airway obstruction and is the hallmark of asthma and bronchitis. When the gas flow through the airways is laminar, the resistance of the airways to the flow is inversely proportional to the fourth power of the radius, according to Poiseuille's law.[1-4] Airway resistance is the ratio of driving pressure divided by flow, and when flow is laminar, resistance is independent of the magnitude of the flow. However, when flow is turbulent, the resistance increases with increasing flow.

Two methods are commonly used to measure airway resistance: (1) lung resistance (RL) using the esophageal balloon and (2) airway resistance (Raw) using the body plethysmograph. Lung resistance includes both airway resistance and lung tissue viscous resistance. Total lung resistance is determined during spontaneous breathing. The transpulmonary pressure is determined and separated into the component required to overcome elastic forces and the component required to produce airflow. The pressure to produce airflow divided by the flow rate provides a measure of total lung resistance.[12] The ratio of the change in lung volume during the breath to the change in transpulmonary pressure from end-expiration to end-inspiration (points where airflow momentarily ceases) provides a measure of dynamic lung compliance. The body plethysmograph provides a very simple, quick and noninvasive method for measuring airway resistance, but this method does not account for lung tissue viscous resistance.

There are two major determinants of airway lumen size and therefore of airway resistance: elastic recoil of the lungs and the intrinsic geometry of the airways. The pressure surrounding intrathoracic airways (peribronchial pressure) approximates pleural pressure. As the lung expands and the pleural pressure becomes more subatmospheric, the peribronchial pressure follows. Because the airways are distensible, the increasing pressure gradient across the airway wall causes the airways to dilate. The greatest increase in airway caliber with changes in lung volume is between RV and FRC. With further increases in lung volume the airways lengthen but there is little further increase in airway cross-section. As a result, as shown in Fig. 1-4, there is a curvilinear relationship between airway resistance and lung volume. Airway conductance (Gaw) the reciprocal of resistance increases linearly with lung expansion. Specific airway conductance (S Gaw) is obtained by dividing airway conductance by lung volume.[13]

Determinants of Airway Caliber

Airway caliber is affected by the tone of the airway smooth muscles, thickening of the walls, airway secretion, foreign bodies, or external compression. The major sites of the resistance to airflow are in the nose, pharynx, and larynx. Airways less than 2 mm in diameter account for very little of the resistance of the entire airway. Substantial changes in the caliber of small peripheral airways may only negligibly affect overall airway resistance.[14]

The effects of changes in transmural pressure on airway caliber depend on their compliance. The trachea is almost completely surrounded by cartilaginous rings, which tend to prevent collapse even when the pressure surrounding the trachea is greater than intraluminal pressure. The bronchi are less well supported by incomplete cartilaginous rings and cartilaginous plates; the bronchioles lack any cartilaginous support, are much more compliant, and can be compressed when the extraluminal pressure exceeds that within the airways. All airways can be stiffened, although to differ-

FIGURE 1-4 Relationship between lung volume and airway resistance. [Reprinted with permission from Cherniack NS, Altose MD, Kelsen SG: The respiratory system, in Berne RM, Levy MN (eds.): *Physiology.* St. Louis, Mosby, 1983.]

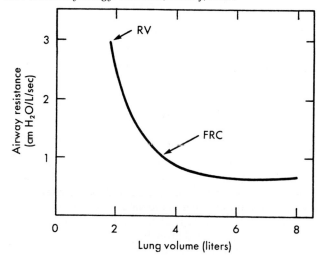

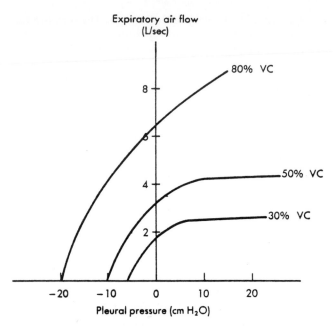

FIGURE 1-5 Isovolume pressure-flow curves. [Reprinted with permission from Cherniack NS, Altose MD, Kelsen SG: The respiratory system, in Berne RM, Levy MN (eds.): *Physiology.* St. Louis, Mosby, 1983.]

ent degrees, by contraction of the smooth muscle in their walls.

Control of Airway Smooth Muscle

Airway smooth muscle contraction is controlled by autonomic nervous activity, circulating hormones, and chemicals released by cells located in or near the tracheobronchial tree. Nerve fibers from three different systems (parasympathetic, synmpathetic, and nonadrenergic inhibitory) supply airway smooth muscle. Stimulation of parasympathetic nerve fibers, carried in the vagal trunks, causes release of acetylcholine, which contracts airway smooth muscle. In humans the parasympathetic activity is probably the most important of the neural influences on airway smooth muscle tone. Airway pollutants such as SO_2 incite coughing and bronchial narrowing by stimulating irritant receptors that are located in the airway submucosa and whose afferent fibers are carried in the vagi. The effects on the sympathetic nervous system in humans are unclear. The nonadrenergic inhibitory system acts to decrease the tone of smooth muscle. The neural mediator of this system may be a purine derivative. Failure of the nonadrenergic bronchodilator system may be one of the factors contributing to increased airway reactivity in asthmatics.

The responsiveness of airway smooth muscle can be evaluated clinically by measuring the changes in FEV_1 or airway resistance following the inhalation of graded doses of the parasympathomimetic agent, methacholine. Asthmatics and many patients with chronic obstructive pulmonary disease (COPD) show exaggerated broncho-constrictive responses to the inhalation of methacholine.

Determinants of Maximum Airflow

Maximum rates of airflow are critically dependent on lung volume. Figure 1-5 shows the relationship between rates of airflow and lung volume during maximal expiratory and inspiratory maneuvers. During a maximum forced expiratory maneuver, airflow rates reach a peak near total lung capacity and then progressively decline as lung volume falls toward residual volume.

Rates of airflow during expiratory maneuvers vary not only with lung volume, but also with effort and the mechanical properties of the lungs and airways.[15-17]

The relationship between expiratory flow rate and pleural pressures at a given lung volume (iso-volume pressure-flow curve) is shown in Fig. 1-6. A family of curves can be constructed, describing the relationship between pleural pressure and expiratory flow rates for different lung volumes. At large lung volumes, near total lung capacity, expiratory flow increases progressively with increasing effort and pleural pressure. In contrast, at lower lung volumes, expiratory airflow rates reach a maximum level at relatively low positive pleural pressures and thereafter, increasing effort produces no further increase in rates of airflow. These findings demonstrate that at large lung volumes expiratory airflow is effort-dependent while at lower lung volumes expiratory airflow is relatively independent of effort once a certain threshold has been reached.

A number of different theoreis have been proposed to explain the relative effort-independence of maximum expiratory airflow at low lung volumes.[15-18] The equal pressure-point theory suggests that as the pleural pressure becomes more and more positive at low lung volumes, it acts to com-

FIGURE 1-6 A maximum flow-volume loop. Lung volume is plotted on the horizontal axis; total lung capacity is shown on the extreme left and residual volume on the extreme right. Airflow during inspiration is directed down, whereas airflow during expiration is directed upward on the vertical axis. [Reprinted with permission from Cherniack NS, Altose MD, Kelsen SG: The respiratory system, in Berne RM, Levy MN (eds.): *Physiology.* St. Louis, Mosby, 1983.]

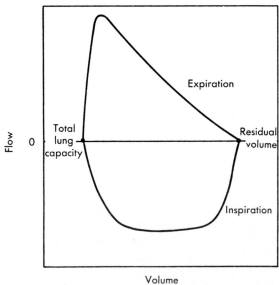

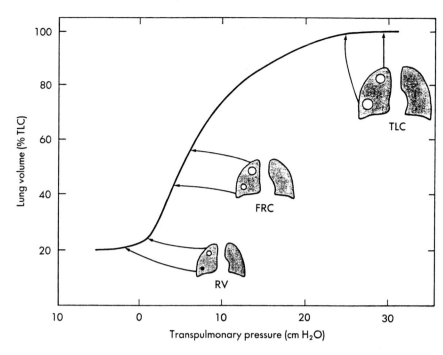

FIGURE 1-7 Regional distribution of lung volume. Because of the difference in pleural pressure from the apex to the base of the lung, the transpulmonary pressure of alveoli at the lung apex will differ from that of alveoli at the lung base. At a given lung volume, alveoli at the apex and at the base will fall on different locations of the same pressure-volume curve. [Reprinted with permission from Cherniack NS, Altose MD, Kelsen SG: The respiratory system, in Berne RM, Levy MN (eds.): *Physiology*. St. Louis, Mosby, 1983.]

press large downstream intrathoracic airways. This dynamic compression increases as the pleural pressure becomes more and more positive raising the resistance of the large intrathoracic airways and preventing flow rates from increasing any further. The equal pressure point theory also proposes that the driving pressure for maximum expiratory flow corresponds to the elastic recoil pressure of the lungs (PL) that maximum expiratory airflow in the effort-independent range is a function of the resistance of the airway upstream from the point where the intraluminal and extramural airway pressure equalize (Rus), according to the following equation:

$$Vmax = PL / Rus$$

Flow-volume curves also can be obtained during maximum inspiratory efforts. Normally, maximum inspiratory flow is a function of effort and airway resistance at all lung volumes. With certain abnormalities of the extrathoracic airways, maximum inspired flow can become effort-independent when the negative intrathoracic pressures act to constrict and narrow the extrathoracic airways.

Fluttering in the upper airways in the region of epiglottis for example may be seen in patients with obstructive sleep apnea and may give rise to rapid flow oscillations on the inspiratory and expiratory flow-volume curve.

Regional Distribution of Alveolar Volume and Ventilation

In the upright position there is a pleural pressure gradient of approximately 0.2 cmH$_2$O/cm of height from the top to the bottom of the lung. Because of the weight of the lung and the effects of gravity, pleural pressure is more subatmospheric at the apex of the lung, and it becomes progressively less negative toward the lung base. Consequently, the trans-

pulmonary pressure, that is, alveolar minus pleural pressure, is greater at the apex than at the base of the lung.

At any given overall lung volume, alveoli at the apex and at the base fall on different *locations* of the same pressure-volume curve by virtue of their differing transpulmonary pressures[19] (Fig. 1-7). Near total lung capacity, the pressure-volume curve is flat so that despite the differences in transpulmonary pressure, alveoli at the lung apex and base are uniformly expanded and are approximately the same size. At intermediate lung volumes where the pressure-volume curve is steep, alveoli at the lung apices are larger than those at the lung bases because of the regional differences in transpulmonary pressure. At low lung volumes near residual volume, the pleural pressure at the bottom of the lung may actually exceed the pressure inside the airways. The negative transmural airway pressure leads to closure of airways in the gravity-dependent zones of the lung base. Also, because of the regional difference in compliance, alveolar ventilation is greater in the bottom third than at the top third of the lungs. In the erect position, blood flow to the lung is also greater at the lung bases. The ratio of ventilation to perfusion is greater at the top than at the bottom of the lungs so that the partial pressure of oxygen in arterial blood (Pa$_{O_2}$) is higher at the apex than it is toward the lung basis.[20] During a slow inspiration from residual volume, the alveoli of the upper lung zones start to fill first, but units at the lung bases receive no ventilation until the transpulmonary pressure exceeds a critical level and the airways reopen. However, during an inspiration from functional residual capacity, ventilation to alveoli in the lung bases is greater than to alveoli at the apex of the lung because with given change in transpulmonary pressure, alveoli at the lung bases enlarge more than those at the lung apex. (Compliance is greater.)

The evenness of ventilation in the lungs and the volume at which the airways in the lung bases begin to close can be assessed by the single-breath nitrogen washout test. The

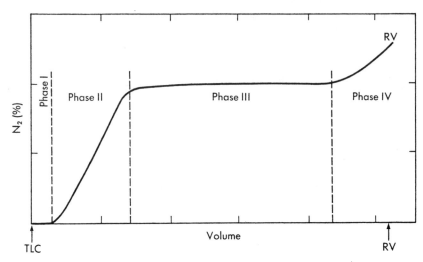

FIGURE 1-8 Single-breath nitrogen washout curve. Lung volume is plotted on the horizontal axis. The concentration of nitrogen in the exhaled air is plotted on the vertical axis. [Reprinted with permission from Cherniack NS, Altose MD, Kelsen SG: The respiratory system, in Berne RM, Levy MN (eds.): *Physiology*. St. Louis, Mosby, 1983.]

patient first takes a single full inspiration of 100% O_2 from residual volume to total lung capacity. The pattern of distribution of the inspired gas is such that at the end of the maximum inspiration of O_2 the concentration of nitrogen is lower in the alveoli of the lung bases than in the alveoli of the upper lung zones.

During the subsequent slow exhalation from total lung capacity to residual volume, the concentration of nitrogen in the exhaled air changes as shown in Fig. 1-8. The initial portion of the exhaled air consists only of O_2 that filled dead space (phase I). As the alveolar air that does contain nitrogen begins to be washed out, the concentration of nitrogen in the expired air rises steeply (phase II) to reach a plateau (phase III). If ventilation is distributed evenly and leaves all regions of the lung synchronously during expiration, phase III will be flat. The nonuniform distribution of ventilation results in a progressive rise in the nitrogen concentration as the volume of air expired increases. At low lung volumes, when the airways at the lung base close, only alveoli at the top of the lung continue to empty. Because the concentration of nitrogen in the alveoli of the upper lung zones is higher, there is an abrupt increase in the slope of the nitrogen–lung volume curve (phase IV). The volume at which this deflection occurs is known as the *closing volume*.[5,21]

Dynamic Pressure-Volume Relationships

The changes in lung volume and pleural pressure during a normal breathing cycle may be displayed in a pressure-volume diagram in which pressure and volume are determined by the elastic properties of the lung and the resistance of the airways (Fig. 1-9). The change in volume and pleural pressure from end-expiration to end-inspiration is the dynamic compliance.[22] Normally the dynamic compliance closely approximates the static compliance. It remains essentially unchanged even when breathing frequency is increased up to 60 breaths per minute. Since lung units consisting of airways and alveoli are arranged in parallel, the change in volume depends on the resistance and compliance of the respective airways and air spaces. When the products of resistance and compliance, that is, the time constants, are approximately the same, the volume changes produced by

a given pressure change are greater than when they are not. Unequal time constants make for uneven distribution of ventilation. Fenestrations in the lung tissue between alveoli (pores of Kohn) and between alveoli and respiratory bronchioles (canals of Lambert) allow air to reach alveoli even if the bronchioles that supply them directly are blocked. In healthy persons they help to minimize further the effects of unequal time constants within the lung.

Work of Breathing

The respiratory muscles perform mechanical work in overcoming the elastic recoil of the respiratory system and the resistance of the airways and tissues during breathing. Work (W) is defined as the product of pressure (P) and volume (V) according to the equation $W = P\, dV$.

The mechanical work used to overcome the elastic recoil

FIGURE 1-9 Dynamic pressure-volume relationships during a single breath. Pleural pressure is plotted on the horizontal axis, and lung volume is plotted on the vertical axis. Inspiration is designated by the solid line and expiration by the interrupted line. [Reprinted with permission from Cherniack NS, Altose MD, Kelsen SG: The respiratory system, in Berne RM, Levy MN (eds.): *Physiology*. St. Louis, Mosby, 1983.]

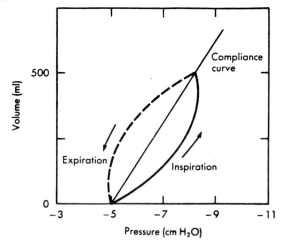

and to expand the lung is partially stored as potential energy. That energy is released during expiration and is used to overcome airway and tissue resistance. Accordingly, expiration is passive during quiet breathing. However, at high levels of ventilation and when airway resistance is increased, additional mechanical work is required during expiration to overcome these nonelastic forces.

Lung disease increases the work of breathing and energy expenditure of the respiratory muscle, but the relationship between work and energy expenditure is not linear.

The energy expenditure during breathing can be determined by measuring O_2 consumption at rest and at an increased level of ventilation produced by voluntary hyperventilation or by CO_2 breathing. The added O_2 uptake at the higher level of ventilation represents that used by the muscles of respiration. The O_2 cost of breathing is normally about 1 mL per liter of ventilation. Ordinarily it constitutes less than 5 percent of the total O_2 consumption of the body. At high levels of ventilation, however, the O_2 cost of breathing becomes progressively greater.[4]

At any given level of ventilation, the work of breathing depends on the breathing pattern. Large tidal volumes increase the elastic work of breathing, whereas rapid breathing frequencies increase the work against resistive forces. One idea is that tidal volume and breathing frequency during spontaneous breathing tend to assume values that minimize the work of breathing. Lung diseases can greatly increase the work of breathing. If work becomes sufficiently great, the respiratory control system can no longer maintain normal gas exchange and arterial P_{O_2} falls and P_{CO_2} rises.

The efficiency of the respiratory muscles is defined as the ratio of mechanical work to the energy expenditure, that is,

$$\text{Efficiency} = \frac{\text{mechanical work}}{\text{energy expenditure}}$$

The efficiency of the respiratory muscles is normally only about 5 to 10 percent, considerably less than the efficiency of limb skeletal muscle. In the presence of lung or chest wall disease, the respiratory muscles are even less efficient.

References

1. Radford EP Jr: Static mechanical properties of mammalian lungs, in Fenn WO, Rahn H (eds): *Handbook of Physiology*, vol 1, *Respiration*. Bethesda, MD, American Physiological Society, 1964; pp 429–449.
2. Rahn H, Otis AB, Chadwick LE, Fenn WO: The pressure-volume diagram of the thorax and lung. *Am J Physiol* 146:161, 1946.
3. Otis AB, Fenn WO, Rahn H: Mechanics of breathing in man. *J Appl Physiol* 2:592, 1950.
4. Campbell EJM, Agostoni E, Newsom Davis J: *The Respiratory Muscles: Mechanics and Neural Control*, 2d ed. Philadelphia, Saunders, 1970.
5. Gelb AF, Zamel N: Simplified diagnosis of small airway obstruction. *N Engl J Med* 288:395, 1973.
6. Hoeppner VH, Cooper DM, Zamel N, et al: Relationship between elastic recoil and closing volume in smokers and non-smokers. *Am Rev Respir Dis* 109:81, 1974.
7. Johanson, WG Jr, Pierce AK: Effects of elastase, collagenase and papain on structure and function of rat lungs in vitro. *J Clin Invest* 51:288, 1972.
8. Gibson GJ, Pride NB: Lung distensibility: The static pressure-volume curve of the lungs and its use in clinical assessment. *Br J Dis Chest* 70:143, 1976.
9. Clements JA, King RJ: Composition of the surface active material, in Crystal RG (ed): *The Biochemical Basis of Pulmonary Function*. New York, Marcel Dekker, 1976.
10. Clements JA, Tierney DF: Alveolar instability associated with altered surface tension, in Fenn WO, Rahn H (eds): *Handbook of Physiology*, sec 3, *Respiration*, vol III. Bethesda, MD, American Physiological Society, 1964.
11. Menkes H, Lindsay D, Wood L, et al: Interdependence of lung units in intact dog lungs. *J Appl Physiol* 32:681, 1972.
12. Mead J, Whittenberger JL: Physical properties of human lungs measured during spontaneous respiration. *J Appl Physiol* 5:779, 1953.
13. DuBois AB, Botelho SY, Comroe JH: A new method for measuring airway resistance in man using a body plethysmograph: Values in normal subjects and in patients with respiratory disease. *J Clin Invest* 35:327, 1956.
14. Macklem PT, Mead J: Resistance of central and peripheral airways measured by a retrograde catheter. *J Appl Physiol* 22:395, 1967.
15. Stubbs SE, Hyatt RE: Effect of increased lung recoil on maximal expiratory flow in normal subjects. *J Appl Physiol* 32:325, 1972.
16. Hyatt RE, Okeson GC, Rodarte JR: Influence of expiratory flow limitation on the pattern of lung emptying in normal man. *J Appl Physiol* 35:411, 1973.
17. Mead J, Turner JM, Macklem PT, Little LB: Significance of the relationship between lung recoil and maximum expiratory flow. *J Appl Physiol* 22:95, 1967.
18. Dawson SV, Elliott EA: Wave-speed limitation on expiratory flow—A unifying concept. *J Appl Physiol* 43:498, 1977.
19. Milic-Emili J, et al: Regional distribution of inspired gas in the lung. *J Appl Physiol* 21:749, 1966.
20. West JB (ed): *Bioengineering Aspects of the Lung. Lung Biology and Health Series*, vol 3. New York, Marcel Dekker, 1977.
21. McCarthy DS, Spencer R, Greene R, Milic-Emili J: Measurement of closing volume as a simple and sensitive test for early detection of small airway disease. *Am J Med* 52:747, 1972.
22. Woolcock AJ, Vincent NJ, Macklem PT: Frequency dependence of compliance as a test for obstruction in the small airways. *J Clin Invest* 48:1097, 1969.

Chapter 2
GAS EXCHANGE
YOSHIMI MIYAMOTO

Pressure, Flow, and Volume of Gases

FUNDAMENTAL LAWS RELATING TO GAS EXCHANGE

Most physiologists express pressure in terms of mmHg or Torr, although since pressure has a dimension of force per unit area, it is generally recommended to use the more logical units such as pascal (Pa) or kilopascal (kPa), that is, newtons (N) per square meter or 1000 N / m². In this chapter, however, we use mmHg because of its great popularity at present. Since 7.5 mmHg = 1 kPa, the standard atmospheric pressure at sea level 760 mmHg is equal to 101,325 Pa or 101.3 kPa.

The molecules of a gas are constantly moving in a random direction. Therefore, gas molecules in a closed chamber produce pressure by colliding with the wall of the chamber. If the volume of gas is compressed, the density of the molecules increases so that the probability of collisions becomes higher, resulting in a rise in pressure. *Boyle's (Mariotte's) law* states that at a constant temperature the volume of a given mass of gas varies reciprocally with its absolute pressure, that is, the product of volume V and absolute pressure P is constant. This means that if the pressure and volume of a gas changes from P_1 and V_1 to P_2 and V_2 without a change in temperature, then $P_1V_1 = P_2V_2$.

The volume of a gas at a constant pressure increases proportionally to the absolute temperature. If the volume of a gas at absolute temperature T_1 is V_1, and the volume of the same mass of gas is V_2 at temperature T_2, then $V_1/V_2 = T_1/T_2$. The same relation holds true between the pressure of a gas and its absolute temperature provided that the volume is constant. The velocity of gas molecules increases in proportion to the square root of the absolute temperature. When a gas in a container is heated, the gas molecules move more frequently which raises pressure if the volume of the gas is constant, or at a constant pressure the space between molecules must increase, that is, the volume must increase *Charle's (Gay-Lussac's) law*.

If a mixture of several gases is distributed uniformly in the same space, each gas behaves independently as if it alone were in that space. The pressure of each gas, that is, partial pressure or tension, depends on its own fractional concentration regardless of the fraction of other gases, and the total pressure of the mixture of gases is equal to the arithmetic sum of the partial pressures (*Dalton's law*). For example, dry air consists of 20.94% O_2, 0.04% CO_2, 79% N_2, and traces of inert gases such as argon. In standard barometric pressure at sea level, the partial pressures of these gases are 159.1, 0.3, and 600.4 mmHg, respectively. The sum of the partial pressures equals barometric pressure. When air is inhaled into the lung, it is immediately saturated by water vapor.

The partial pressure of water vapor in a gas in contact with a liquid phase is dependent on temperature and independent of barometric pressure; the warmer the liquid, the greater the vapor pressure. The saturated water vapor pressure at a body temperature of 37°C is 47 mmHg. A figure for fractional concentrations of O_2, CO_2, and N_2 in the alveolar air of a healthy person is 0.145, 0.056, and 0.798, respectively. Partial pressures of these gases are then approximately 103, 40.0, and 569 mmHg, respectively; this is obtained by multiplying the gas fractions by 713.

PARTIAL PRESSURE, GAS FLOW, AND CONDUCTANCE

Let us assume two closed chambers in each of which a given gas is distributed uniformly but in different concentrations, so that a partial pressure gradient of the gas exists between the two chambers. When the two chambers are connected by a tube, gas flows through the tube from the higher pressure compartment to the lower pressure compartment. The amount of gas transferred per unit time $\dot{V}$ is proportional to the partial pressure difference between the two chambers ΔP, and the proportional constant G is defined as the *conductance* of the tube.

$$\dot{V} = G \, \Delta P \qquad \text{Eq. (1)}$$

If $\dot{V}$ and ΔP are expressed, for example, in mL / min and mmHg, respectively, then G should have a unit of mL / min / mmHg or ml × mmHg / min. The reciprocal of G, which is called *resistance* (R = 1/G), is then given by the drop of partial pressure per unit transfer rate of gas.

$$R = \Delta P / \dot{V} \qquad \text{Eq. (2)}$$

The relation is the same as when electrons flow through a resistance R connected between two batteries with different potentials (Ohm's law: R = $\Delta e / i$, where Δe = potential difference between two batteries and i = current, i.e., number of electrons transferred per unit time).

Oxygen Flow from the Atmosphere to the Tissues

OXYGEN PARTIAL PRESSURE CASCADE IN THE RESPIRATORY SYSTEM

The respiratory gas exchange system can be subdivided into five major compartments: (1) inspired gas, (2) alveolar gas, (3) pulmonary capillary blood, (4) tissue capillary blood, and (5) tissues. These compartments are connected in series, and oxygen flows through them depending on the partial pressure gradient of each compartment. The connecting pathways between compartments can be regarded as conductances G or resistances R of this system (Fig. 2 1). Whenever oxygen flows along the pathways the initial partial pressure of oxygen in air loses its energy and the partial pressure drops, just as in the potential drop of an electric circuit in which resistances are connected in series. We breathe air with a P_{O_2} of 150 mmHg under the condition being saturated by water vapor. Assuming that the mean partial pressure of

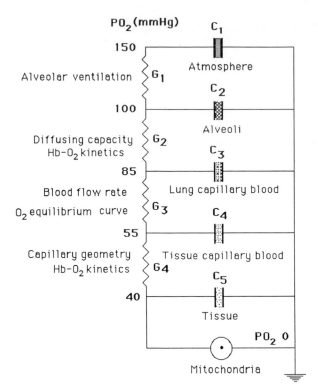

FIGURE 2-1 P_{O_2} cascade in the respiratory gas exchange system. The respiratory system can be subdivided into five major compartments. O_2 is stored in each compartment represented by capacitances C. A P_{O_2} gradient is established along the compartments according to the O_2 capacity of each. O_2 flows from the atmosphere to the tissues depending on the P_{O_2} gradient. [Adapted from Otis (1987).]

O_2 in the tissues is equal to the mixed venous P_{O_2} (= 40 mmHg), then the pressure drop from the atmosphere to the tissues is $150 - 40 = 110$ mmHg.

Each compartment has its own oxygen storage capacity. The physical property of the capacity differs in each compartment. The O_2 capacity of compartment 1 is regarded as infinite since it represents the atmospheric air. Since inspired oxygen is first stored in the alveoli, the O_2 capacity of compartment 2 may be represented by lung volume. The O_2 capacity of the pulmonary blood may be given by the product of the blood volume and the slope of the oxygen equilibrium curve representing the chemical reaction rate of hemoglobin with O_2. The concept of capacity is immaterial in the steady state of gas exchange, but is of great importance in the transient states because the rapidity of responses of any system consisting of a capacitance and a resistance is determined by the product of the resistance and the capacitance, that is, *time constant*. Let us consider that electric capacitor C is charged by a battery with a potential Eo through an electric resistor R. The potential across capacitor $E(t)$ increases exponentially as a function of time according to the following equation.

$$E(t) = Eo(1 - e^{-t/\tau}) \qquad \text{Eq. (3)}$$

where τ is the time constant of this system ($\tau = R \times C$). Conversely, when a capacitor already charged by Eo is discharged through a resistor R, the equation would be

$$E(t) = Eo \times e^{-t/\tau} \qquad \text{Eq. (4)}$$

The system will reach equilibrium after a period of time has elapsed: When $t = \tau$, E rises by 63 percent of Eo [Eq. (3)] or drops by 37 percent of Eo [Eq. (4)]. A state of practical equilibrium will be attained after a time corresponding to 6τ (99.75 percent equilibrium).

Conductance between Inspired Gas and Alveolar Gas

The amount of oxygen taken up from the alveolar gas by the body's metabolism over a given period of time is equal to the difference between the amount inspired and the amount expired in that time. Assuming that alveolar ventilation during inspiration and expiration is equal (actually, this does not occur, as described later) for simplicity, the oxygen uptake ($\dot{V}_{O_2}$) is expressed by the following equation adopting the conservation of mass principle.

$$\dot{V}_{O_2} = \dot{V}_A(F_{I_{O_2}} - F_{A_{O_2}}) \qquad \text{Eq. (5)}$$

where $\dot{V}_A$ is alveolar ventilation, $F_{I_{O_2}}$ is the O_2 fraction in inspired air, and $F_{A_{O_2}}$ is the O_2 fraction in the alveoli. Converting fractions in terms of partial pressures,

$$\dot{V}_{O_2} = \dot{V}_A \frac{P_{I_{O_2}} - P_{A_{O_2}}}{P_B - 47} \qquad \text{Eq. (6)}$$

On the other hand, conductance for oxygen between the inspired gas and alveolar gas (G_1 of Fig. 2-1) is defined as

$$G_1 = \frac{\dot{V}_{O_2}}{P_{I_{O_2}} - P_{A_{O_2}}} \qquad \text{Eq. (7)}$$

Substituting Eq. (6) into Eq. (7) we obtain

$$G_1 = \frac{\dot{V}_A}{P_B - 47} \qquad \text{Eq. (8)}$$

Eq. (8) states that G_1 is directly proportional to alveolar ventilation.

Alveolar ventilation is the effective ventilation according to gas exchange and is defined as the difference between total ventilation ($\dot{V}_E$) and dead space ventilation ($\dot{V}_D$).

$$\dot{V}_A = \dot{V}_E - \dot{V}_D = f(V_T - V_D) \qquad \text{Eq. (9)}$$

where f is breath frequency, V_T is tidal volume, and V_D is dead space volume consisting of the anatomic dead space (conductive airways) and the physiologic dead space (alveolar spaces without perfusion). It is apparent that $\dot{V}_A$, or the conductance between the atmosphere and the alveoli G_1, will decrease with increasing V_D. Typical figures of V_T and V_D for a healthy male at rest is 500 mL and 150 mL, respectively. Since f is approximately 12 breaths per minute, $\dot{V}_E$ and $\dot{V}_A$ are 6 L/min and 4.2 L/min, respectively. However, there would be innumerable combinations of tidal volume and breath frequency for a given alveolar ventilation. It is assumed that the respiratory control system chooses the optimum combination of f and V_T so that work related to breathing remains minimal.

GAS EXCHANGE AND ALVEOLAR VENTILATION

As we breathe air, gases in the lungs are only three species, that is, oxygen, carbon dioxide, and nitrogen. The difference between the amount of a given gas entering the alveoli per unit time during inspiration and the amount leaving the alveoli during expiration gives the amount of the gas absorbed or excreted by the body's metabolism. Assuming that these gases are dry, the net gas exchange for oxygen (O_2 uptake, $\dot{V}_{O_2}$), for carbon dioxide (CO_2 output, $\dot{V}_{CO_2}$), and for nitrogen exchange ($\dot{V}_{N_2}$) are as follows, respectively:

$$\dot{V}_{O_2} = F_{IO_2}\dot{V}_{AI} - F_{AO_2}\dot{V}_{AE} \qquad \text{Eq. (10)}$$

$$\dot{V}_{CO_2} = F_{ACO_2}\dot{V}_{AE} - F_{ICO_2}\dot{V}_{AI} \qquad \text{Eq. (11)}$$

$$\dot{V}_{N_2} = F_{IN_2}\dot{V}_{AI} - F_{AN_2}\dot{V}_{AE} \qquad \text{Eq. (12)}$$

where $\dot{V}_{AI}$ and $\dot{V}_{AE}$ represent alveolar ventilation during inspiration and expiration and F_I and F_A denote fractional concentrations of inspired and alveolar gases of each species, respectively.

The N_2 fractions of Eq. (12) can be replaced using O_2 and CO_2 fractions as follows:

$$F_{IN_2} = 1 - F_{IO_2} - F_{ICO_2} \qquad \text{Eq. (13)}$$

$$F_{EN_2} = 1 - F_{EO_2} - F_{ECO_2} \qquad \text{Eq. (14)}$$

Since the fraction of CO_2 in air is negligible, F_{ICO_2} of Eqs. (11) and (13) would be nil under normal circumstances.

Now let us take the difference between Eqs. (10) and (11), and substitute Eqs. (13) and (14) into the subtracted form.

$$\dot{V}_{O_2} - \dot{V}_{CO_2} = \dot{V}_{AI} - \dot{V}_{AE} - (F_{IN_2}\dot{V}_{AI} - F_{AN_2}\dot{V}_{AE}) \qquad \text{Eq. (15)}$$

Since no gas exchange occurs for N_2 in the steady states, then $\dot{V}_{N_2}$ of Eq. (12) is nil.

$$\dot{V}_{AI} = \frac{F_{AN_2}}{F_{IN_2}}\dot{V}_{AE} \qquad \text{Eq. (16)}$$

Substituting Eq. (16) in Eq. (15)

$$\dot{V}_{O_2} - \dot{V}_{CO_2} = \dot{V}_{AI} - \dot{V}_{AE} \qquad \text{Eq. (17)}$$

The terms on the left hand side of Eq. (17) can be written as

$$\dot{V}_{O_2} - \dot{V}_{CO_2} - (1 - R)\dot{V}_{O_2} \qquad \text{Eq. (18)}$$

Where

$$R = \frac{\dot{V}_{CO_2}}{\dot{V}_{O_2}} \qquad \text{Eq. (19)}$$

R represents the *respiratory gas exchange ratio*, which is defined as the ratio of the amount of carbon dioxide excreted from the body to the amount of oxygen taken up in the body over a given period of time.

Alveolar ventilation during inspiration is not identical to alveolar ventilation during expiration because of the difference between $\dot{V}_{O_2}$ and $\dot{V}_{CO_2}$. Assuming that the dead space volume is equal during inspiration and expiration, inspiratory minute ventilation ($\dot{V}_I$) is greater than expiratory minute ventilation ($\dot{V}_E$) by the difference $\dot{V}_{O_2} - \dot{V}_{CO_2}$. $\dot{V}_I$ and $\dot{V}_E$ are equal only when the gas exchange ratio (R) is in unity. In the steady state, R equals the *respiratory quotient* (RQ), being the ratio of the metabolic CO_2 production to the O_2 consumption in the tissues. Assuming that the typical figures of $\dot{V}_{O_2}$ and $\dot{V}_{CO_2}$ of a healthy person at rest at sea level are 250 mL/min and 200 mL/min, respectively, R is around 0.8. R increases beyond unity during severe exercise because CO_2 production increases to compensate for the metabolic acidosis accompanied by lactate production during anaerobic glucolysis (see Chap. 7).

We can obtain the gas exchange ratio directly by substituting Eqs. (10) and (11) in Eq. (19).

$$R = \frac{\dot{V}_{AE}F_{ACO_2}}{\dot{V}_{AI}F_{IO_2} - \dot{V}_{AE}F_{AO_2}} \qquad \text{Eq. (20)}$$

Substituting Eqs. (13) and (14) in Eq. (16)

$$\frac{\dot{V}_{AI}}{\dot{V}_{AE}} = \frac{1 - F_{AO_2} - F_{ACO_2}}{1 - F_{IO_2}} \qquad \text{Eq. (21)}$$

Substituting Eq. (21) in Eq. (20) to eliminate the terms of ventilation

$$R = \frac{F_{ACO_2}}{\left[\dfrac{1 - F_{AO_2} - F_{ACO_2}}{1 - F_{IO_2}}\right]F_{IO_2} - F_{AO_2}} \qquad \text{Eq. (22)}$$

Rearranging and solving for F_{AO_2}

$$F_{AO_2} = F_{IO_2} - F_{ACO_2}\left[F_{IO_2} + \frac{1 - F_{IO_2}}{R}\right] \qquad \text{Eq. (23)}$$

Converting to partial pressures

$$P_{AO_2} = P_{IO_2} - P_{ACO_2}\left[F_{IO_2} + \frac{1 - F_{IO_2}}{R}\right] \qquad \text{Eq. (24)}$$

The equation in parenthesis of Eq. (24) is a correcting factor for R. When $R = 1$, then the correcting factor is unity. Equation (24) is called the *alveolar ventilation equation*. Since we can measure P_{ACO_2} and R, P_{AO_2} can be calculated. A normal figure for a subject at rest breathing air at sea level, whose P_{ACO_2} and R are 40 mmHg and 0.8 mmHg, respectively, P_{AO_2} would be:

$$P_{AO_2} = 150\,\text{mmHg} - 40\,\text{mmHg}\left[0.21 + \frac{1 - 0.21}{0.8}\right]$$

$$= 102\,\text{mmHg}$$

We can derive alveolar P_{CO_2} directly from Eq. (11) assuming that $F_{I_{CO_2}} = 0$.

$$P_{A_{CO_2}} = (PB - 47)\frac{\dot{V}_{CO_2}}{\dot{V}_A} \qquad \text{Eq. (25)}$$

Equation (25) is the alveolar ventilation equation for CO_2 which states that alveolar P_{CO_2} is directly proportional to metabolic CO_2 production and is inversely related to alveolar ventilation. For practical use Eq. (25) is often expressed as

$$P_{A_{CO_2}} (\text{mmHg}) = 0.863 \frac{\dot{V}_{CO_2} (\text{mL}/\text{min})}{\dot{V}_A (\text{L}/\text{min})}$$

Since $\dot{V}_A$ is usually expressed in BTPS (body temperature and pressure saturated with water vapor), while $\dot{V}_{O_2}$ and $\dot{V}_{CO_2}$ are given in STPD [standard temperature (0°C), pressure, and dry], the right hand side of Eq. (25) must be multiplied by a correcting factor of 1.21. When $\dot{V}_{CO_2}$ and $\dot{V}_A$ are 200 mL/min and 4.2 L/min, respectively, then $P_{A_{CO_2}}$ is 41 mmHg.

Hyperventilation is defined as ventilation in excess of metabolic requirements. If $P_{A_{CO_2}}$ is less than normal, alveolar hyperventilation may occur. Conversely, if $P_{A_{CO_2}}$ is greater than normal, this may indicate alveolar hypoventilation. Alveolar ventilation can be altered by changes in either minute ventilation or dead space ventilation. Any increase in V_D will reduce $\dot{V}_A$ unless $\dot{V}_E$ increases accordingly.

DIFFUSING CAPACITY OF THE LUNG

Conductance for the oxygen flow from the alveoli to pulmonary capillary blood (G_2 of Fig. 1) is defined as

$$G_2 = \frac{\dot{V}_{O_2}}{P_{A_{O_2}} - P_{LC_{O_2}}} \qquad \text{Eq. (26)}$$

where $P_{LC_{O_2}}$ is the mean P_{O_2} of pulmonary capillary blood, whose P_{O_2} is minimal at the arterial side and maximal at the venous side of the pulmonary circulation system. The alveolar-blood conductance for oxygen flow is called the *diffusing capacity* of the lung (D_{LO_2}). Oxygen diffuses from the alveoli to the capillary blood across the barrier of the gas-blood interface and finally combines with hemoglobin (Hb) in the red cells. The diffusion barrier for O_2 from the alveoli to Hb consists of the alveolar and capillary membrane, the plasma layer surrounding the red cells, and the red cell membrane. Another barrier for the transportation of oxygen lies within the red cell interior. This includes the diffusion resistance of intracellular fluid filled with Hb and the kinetic resistance related to the chemical reaction of oxygen with Hb. Since oxygen molecules must move through both the resistances that are connected in series,

$$\frac{1}{D_{LO_2}} = \frac{1}{D_M} + \frac{1}{\theta V_C} \qquad \text{Eq. (27)}$$

where D_M is the membrane component of the diffusing capacity, θ is the reaction rate of O_2 with Hb, and V_C is the volume of the pulmonary capillary blood.

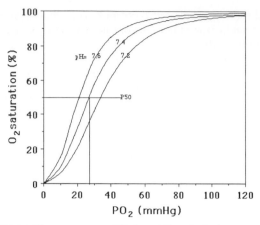

FIGURE 2-2 The oxygen equilibrium (dissociation) curves at different pH. The curve shifts left (the Hb affinity of O_2 increases) with an increase in pH and shifts right (the Hb affinity of O_2 decreases) with a decrease in pH, demonstrating the fixed-acid Bohr effect. P_{50} indicates the P_{O_2} at which Hb is saturated by 50%. The O_2 affinity of Hb decreases (the curve shifts right) with increasing P_{CO_2} (Bohr effect), elevates the temperature, and increases 2,3-DPG concentration in plasma, which increases with the reverse changes of these factors. [Based on equations presented by Severinghaus (1979).]

OXYGEN EQUILIBRIUM (DISSOCIATION) CURVE

Oxygen content in blood is subdivided into: (1) a dissolved component in plasma and (2) a chemically combined component with Hb in the red cells. The amount of a gas dissolved in plasma is directly proportional to the partial pressure of the gas (Henry's law). The solubility of any gas differs from one gas to another. For example, 100 mL of blood plasma (37°C) dissolves 0.003 mL of O_2 per 1 mmHg P_{O_2} gradient, while the solubility of CO_2 is 0.067 mL/100 mL plasma/mmHg. Therefore, the amount of dissolved O_2 in blood is given by the product of the partial pressure and the solubility for O_2. If P_{O_2} is 100 mmHg, the amount of dissolved O_2 in 100 mL plasma is $0.003 \times 100 = 0.3$ mL. In contrast, 1g of Hb is theoretically capable of combining 1.39 mL of O_2 chemically. In actuality, however, Hb can carry up to only 1.35 mL O_2/g even when fully saturated, because a small portion of Hb is converted into an abnormal form which cannot bind to oxygen. This type of Hb is called *methemoglobin* and its concentration is increased by smoking and inhalation of air containing carbon monoxide. The blood of a healthy adult usually contains 15 percent of Hb, meaning that the O_2 amount combined with 100 mL of blood would be $15 \times 1.35 = 20$ mL at maximum.

The relationship between the amount of O_2 combined chemically with Hb and P_{O_2} in blood is not linear as in dissolved O_2, but is an S-shaped curve which has a steeper slope between the lower range of P_{O_2} variation (from 10 to 50 mmHg) and a very flat slope for the higher range (from 70 to 100 mmHg). This particular shape of the O_2 equilibrium curve has two advantages: (1) in the lungs, the loading of O_2 by Hb is ensured even if arterial P_{O_2} decreases, and (2) in the tissues, the O_2 unloading from Hb is facilitated since a slight reduction in P_{O_2} dissociates a large amount of O_2 (Fig. 2-2).

The extent to which Hb combines with O_2 is usually expressed as the percentage saturation ratio of the O_2 actually combined with Hb to the maximum amount of O_2 combining with Hb (*oxygen capacity*). For a young, healthy adult O_2 capacity is 20.6 mL O_2 per 100 mg blood. Arterial blood is usually saturated by 97 percent under normal conditions.

The affinity of Hb to oxygen is quantitatively expressed by P_{O_2} at which Hb is saturated by 50 percent (P_{50}). When oxygen affinity increases, the equilibrium curve shifts to the left, thereby the P_{50} of Hb can be achieved at a lower P_{O_2}, while decreased O_2 affinity shifts to the right and increases the P_{50}.

Hydrogen ions (H^+) also bind to Hb. Therefore, an increase in H^+ (a decrease in pH) reduces the O_2 affinity of Hb and causes a shift to the right of the O_2 equilibrium curve (Fig. 2-2). Increased P_{CO_2} in blood also shifts the O_2 equilibrium curve to the right. The effects of CO_2 on O_2 affinity, that is, the *Bohr effect*, is in part due to the direct binding of CO_2 molecules to the α and β chains of Hb and to the hydration reaction of CO_2 producing H^+. The latter is called the fixed-acid Bohr effect. In the lungs, O_2 affinity increases as Hb releases CO_2, facilitating the loading of O_2, and conversely in the tissues, the affinity decreases as Hb combines with CO_2, which promotes O_2 release from the capillary blood to the tissues.

Increases in temperature also reduce the O_2 affinity and shift the O_2 equilibrium curve to the right. When temperature rises, the metabolic rate and O_2 demand of the tissues increase. The decreased affinity of Hb helps O_2 unloading from the tissue capillary blood to the tissues.

2,3-Diphosphoglycerate (2,3-DPG) is an intermediate metabolite produced in the red cells during anaerobic glycolysis and plays an important role in the regulation of the O_2 affinity of blood under various circumstances such as in gas exchange between maternal and fetal blood in the placenta or adaptation to high altitude.

P_{O_2} GRADIENT ALONG THE PULMONARY CAPILLARY

Let us consider the P_{O_2} change in pulmonary capillary blood from the pulmonary artery to the pulmonary vein. At the inlet of the capillary P_{O_2} is at a minimum and equal to that of the mixed venous blood, and at the outlet capillary P_{O_2} rises to the level of alveolar P_{O_2} if an equilibrium is achieved between the alveolar gas and the capillary blood. The mixed venous blood is charged by O_2 during the period of its travel from the arterial side to the venous side of the pulmonary circulation, which is normally about 0.75 s.

The P_{O_2} at any point along the lung capillary, $P_{LC_{O_2}}(t)$, rises exponentially starting from the mixed venous $P_{O_2}(P\overline{v})$ toward the arterial P_{O_2} which is at equilibrium with P_{O_2} in the alveoli (P_A).

$$\Delta P_{LC_{O_2}}(t) = (P_{LC} - P\overline{v}) = (P_A - P\overline{v})(1 - e^{-t/\tau}) \qquad \text{Eq. (28)}$$

The τ of the exponent is a time constant that determines the slope of the exponential rise of $P_{LC_{O_2}}(t)$ with time; the shorter the τ, the steeper the slope, and it is given by the product of resistance R and capacitance C of the O_2 charging system (Fig. 2-3). Since the conductance connecting the alveoli and the pulmonary capillary blood is given by the diffusing capacity of the lung, D_L, the resistance of the system is $1/D_L$.

The capacitance component of the lung may be represented

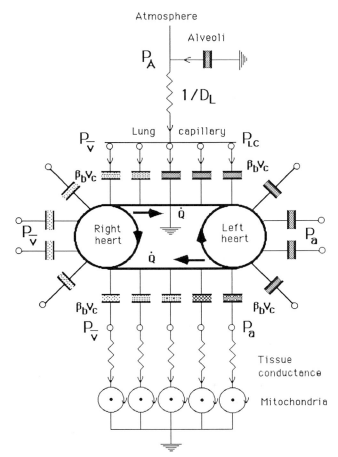

FIGURE 2-3 An electrical analog representing the loading of oxygen from the alveoli to the lung capillary blood and the unloading from the tissue capillary blood to the tissues. P_A = alveolar P_{O_2}, $P\overline{v}$ = mixed venous P_{O_2}, P_{LC} = end-lung capillary P_{O_2}, P_a = arterial P_{O_2}, βb = the slope of O_2 equilibrium curve, V_C = pulmonary capillary blood volume, D_L = lung diffusing capacity. [Adapted from Otis (1987) and Piiper and Sheid (1980).]

by the product of the pulmonary capillary blood volume V_C and the slope of the O_2 equilibrium curve $\beta b (= \Delta C / \Delta P)$. Since the slope of the equilibrium curve cannot be represented by any constant, this expression is valid only as a rough estimate of the O_2 diffusing system. Allowing that the total time in transit is small, the time the blood spends in the capillary is t', and $t' = V_C/\dot{Q}$, where $\dot{Q}$ is the pulmonary capillary blood flow. Replacing V_C by $\dot{Q}t'$, the capacitance of the system is $\beta b \dot{Q}t'$. The time constant of this system τ is then given by $\beta b \dot{Q}t'/D_L$. The P_{O_2} changes in the lung capillaries can be expressed in a normalized form as

$$\frac{P_{LC} - P\overline{v}}{P_A - P\overline{v}} = 1 - e^{-t/\tau} \qquad \text{Eq. (29)}$$

where

$$\tau = \frac{\beta b \dot{Q}t'}{D_L}$$

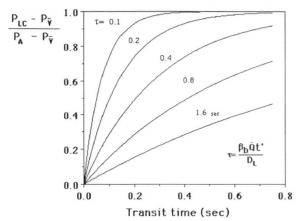

$$\frac{P_{LC} - P_{\bar{V}}}{P_A - P_{\bar{V}}}$$

$$\tau = \frac{\beta_b \dot{Q} t'}{D_L}$$

Transit time (sec)

FIGURE 2-4 Normalized changes in P_{O_2} in pulmonary capillary blood (P_{LC}) during a transit period of 0.75 s (t'). The zero and 1.0 points of the ordinate correspond to P_{O_2} levels of the mixed venous blood and the alveoli. The τ is the time constant for the equilibrium between the lung capillary blood and the alveolar gas. $P_{A_{O_2}}$ = alveolar P_{O_2}, $P_{\bar{V}_{O_2}}$ = mixed venous P_{O_2}, D_L = lung diffusing capacity, $\dot{Q}$ = cardiac output, and βb = the slope of O_2 equilibrium curve. [Adapted from Otis (1987).]

Figure 2-4 shows changes in normalized P_{LC} values when a small segment of blood passes along the pulmonary capillaries with a transit time t' of 0.75 s. The time constant for O_2 transfer from the alveoli to the pulmonary capillary blood is directly proportional to the cardiac output and inversely proportional to the diffusing capacity of the lungs. Therefore, under a constant D_L the time constant is solely dependent on $\dot{Q}$. In healthy lungs under normal conditions the D_L does not significantly affect the time constant. The time constant for O_2 equilibrium in a normal lung is less than 0.1 s. This means that the pulmonary capillary blood almost equilibrates with O_2 within one-third of the total transit time. In normoxic conditions O_2 transfer rate in the lung is therefore perfusion-limited. If the time required for the equilibrium is longer than the transit time of a red cell in the capillary, the gas transfer rate is limited by both perfusion and diffusion. When gas mixtures with a lower concentration of O_2 are inhaled, the time constant for equilibrium is prolonged because the slope of the dissociation curve available is now steep (a greater βb). This leads the O_2 transfer in the lung to become diffusion-limited.

MEASUREMENT OF DIFFUSING CAPACITY
The diffusing capacity of the lungs for oxygen is given by G_2 of Eq. (26), in which $\dot{V}_{O_2}$ is easily measurable, and $P_{A_{O_2}}$ can be estimated from the alveolar ventilation equation, but the determination of the mean capillary P_{O_2} is difficult although it is possible. If changes in P_{O_2} along the pulmonary capillary were represented by any exponential equations such as that given by Eq. (29), calculation for the $P_{LC_{O_2}}$ would not be so difficult if the P_{O_2} values of the mixed venous and arterial blood are known. However, since the exponent of Eq. (29) is not constant, construction of the $P_{LC_{O_2}}$ curve rising from the mixed venous level toward the end-capillary level must be calculated by a complicated numerical procedure called *Bohr's integration*.

The diffusing capacity of the lung can be measured far

more easily by breathing gas mixtures with a low concentration of carbon monoxide. CO has a much higher βb than $\dot{O}_2$ because its affinity to Hb is 250 times greater. The time constant for CO transfer in the lungs is about 30 s, making the equilibrium extremely slow. This gas is therefore diffusion-limited and hence is well suited for measuring the diffusion properties of the lungs.

In a manner similar to $D_{L_{O_2}}$, $D_{L_{CO}}$ is defined as

$$D_{L_{CO}} = \frac{\dot{V}_{CO}}{P_{A_{CO}} - P\overline{LC}_{CO}} \qquad \text{Eq. (30)}$$

Since no detectable CO is present in the environment, its mixed venous concentration can be ignored. Furthermore, because of its high affinity to Hb, any molecules of CO diffusing into blood from the alveoli bind immediately to Hb. As a result, the partial pressure of CO in the pulmonary capillary blood is essentially zero throughout its entire length so long as CO of a very low concentration (0.3 to 0.4%) is inhaled. Then, Eq. (30) becomes very simple.

$$D_{L_{CO}} = \frac{\dot{V}_{CO}}{P_{A_{CO}}} \qquad \text{Eq. (31)}$$

In the single breath method the subject fully inspires a gas mixture containing 0.35% CO, 21% O_2, and 5% helium in nitrogen, holds the breath for 10 s, then expires. Helium is used to estimate the lung volume which is necessary to calculate for the initial fraction of CO. An end-expiratory gas sample is collected for the CO fraction after the breath holding. $D_{L_{CO}}$ is then calculated by comparing the CO fractions in the alveolar gas at the beginning and the end of the breath holding period. The normal value of $D_{L_{CO}}$ for healthy adults is about 25 mL/min per mmHg at rest.

Graham's law states that the rates of diffusion of different gases under the same conditions are inversely proportional to the square root of the densities of these gases. On the other hand, the concentration of a dissolved gas in a liquid is given by the product of the solubility and partial pressure of the gas (Henry's law). Since the rate of diffusion is directly proportional to the concentration gradient, a gas with higher solubility diffuses more rapidly than gases with lower solubility unless other conditions are equal. Combining Graham's law and Henry's law, the relative rates of diffusion of two different gases, x and y, between a gas-liquid interface are expressed as follows.

$$\frac{\dot{V}_X}{\dot{V}_Y} = \frac{\alpha_x \sqrt{MW_y}}{\alpha_y \sqrt{MW_x}} \qquad \text{Eq. (32)}$$

where $\dot{V}$ is the volume of a gas diffusing the gas-liquid interface per unit time, α is the solubility of the gas in molar concentration per unit partial pressure, and MW is the molecular weight of the gas. For O_2 and CO diffusions through the alveolar membrane

$$\frac{D_{L_{O_2}}}{D_{L_{CO}}} = \frac{0.0244\sqrt{28}}{0.0185\sqrt{32}} = 1.23$$

Assuming that the normal value of $D_{L_{CO}}$ is 25 mL/min per mmHg, it can be converted to a $D_{L_{O_2}}$ of 31 mL/min per mmHg. The diffusing capacity increases markedly during exercise, because the area for diffusion increases as more pulmonary capillaries open.

OXYGEN FLOW FROM THE PULMONARY CAPILLARY BLOOD TO THE TISSUES

O_2 FLOW FROM THE PULMONARY CAPILLARY TO THE TISSUE CAPILLARY

Conductance for oxygen flow from the pulmonary capillary blood to the tissue capillary blood is defined as

$$G_3 = \frac{\dot{V}_{O_2}}{P\overline{LC}_{O_2} - P\overline{TC}_{O_2}} \qquad \text{Eq. (33)}$$

where $P\overline{TC}_{O_2}$ is the mean oxygen partial pressure in the tissue capillary blood. $\dot{V}_{O_2}$ is also expressed according to the Fick principle.

$$\dot{V}_{O_2} = (Ca_{O_2} - C\overline{v}_{O_2})\dot{Q} = (Pa_{O_2} - P\overline{v}_{O_2})\beta b\dot{Q} \quad \text{Eq. (34)}$$

where Ca_{O_2}, $C\overline{v}_{O_2}$, Pa_{O_2}, and $P\overline{v}_{O_2}$ are the oxygen concentrations and partial pressures in arterial and mixed venous blood, respectively, and βb is the mean slope of the O_2 equilibrium curve between the arterial and venous P_{O_2} range. Substituting Eq. (34) in Eq. (33), the conductance between the pulmonary to tissue capillary blood G_3 is given by

$$G_3 = \frac{(Pa_{O_2} - P\overline{v}_{O_2})\beta b\dot{Q}}{P\overline{LC}_{O_2} - P\overline{TC}_{O_2}} \qquad \text{Eq. (35)}$$

G_3 is directly dependent on βb and $\dot{Q}$ if other variables remain constant. Although βb is not easily altered since it is determined by the physical characteristics of blood, $\dot{Q}$ can increase severalfold during exercise and reduce conductance in response to increasing oxygen demands of the body.

O_2 FLOW FROM TISSUE CAPILLARY BLOOD TO THE TISSUES

The conductance between the tissue capillary blood to the tissues (G_4 of Fig. 2-1) is defined as the O_2 flow divided by the difference between the mean oxygen partial pressure in the tissue capillaries and that in the tissues ($P\overline{T}_{O_2}$).

$$G_4 = \frac{\dot{V}_{O_2}}{P\overline{TC}_{O_2} - P\overline{T}_{O_2}} \qquad \text{Eq. (36)}$$

The conductance G_4 depends on the kinetics of the oxygen unloading from the oxygenated Hb in the red cells. Unloading of oxygen from Hb is governed by the oxygen equilibrium curve, and hence is influenced by the Bohr effect, the concentration of 2,3-DPG, and the temperature of the tissue capillary blood. Once oxygen molecules leave Hb in the red cells they diffuse through the tissues to the mitochondria. Therefore, the conductance for O_2 diffusion in the tissues also depends on the geometric orientation of the capillaries, perfusion through each capillary, and distribution of the mitochondria in the tissues. Although O_2 diffuses in all directions from the capillary site where it is released, the major

direction of diffusion is likely to be in a radial direction perpendicular to the capillary axis. P_{O_2} in the tissues is highest at the region adjacent to the arterial end of the capillaries and lowest at the venous end and declines as the distance from the capillary lengthens. The mean tissue P_{O_2} differs from organ to organ, being relatively lower in the liver and the active skeletal muscles and higher in the heart and the kidneys. This is determined by the balance between the rate of O_2 delivery by perfusion and the rate of O_2 consumption by the mitochondria. Most tissues have a mean P_{O_2} ranging between 10 and 40 mmHg. The capillary geometry is primarily determined by the anatomic structure of the tissues but is continuously controlled via neural and humoral mechanisms so that adequate oxygen delivery to the tissues is ensured.

O_2 CONSUMPTION AND CO_2 PRODUCTION IN THE MITOCHONDRIA

In the mitochondria, oxygen is utilized to metabolize respiratory substrates such as carbohydrates, proteins, and fats and to produce energy in the form of adenosine triphosphate (ATP). Oxygen uptake ($\dot{V}_{O_2}$) and carbon dioxide production ($\dot{V}_{CO_2}$) are closely linked in aerobic metabolism. When carbohydrate is metabolized, the ratio $\dot{V}_{CO_2}/\dot{V}_{O_2}$, which is called the *respiratory quotient* (RQ), is 1.0. When fat and protein are metabolized, RQ is approximately 0.7 and 0.8, respectively. The RQ depends on the relative quantities of carbon, hydrogen, and oxygen molecules contained in each substrate. Thus, the RQ for the whole body varies according to the percentages of carbohydrate, fat, and protein being oxidized. At rest, the RQ of a healthy person is around 0.8. The mitochondria consume oxygen at a constant rate until tissue P_{O_2} is reduced to 1 mmHg or less.

Carbon Dioxide Flow from the Tissues to the Atmosphere

Carbon dioxide produced in the mitochondria diffuses into the tissue capillary blood, is transported via the venous circulation to the lung capillaries, is released in the alveoli according to the carbon dioxide equilibrium curve, and finally disperses into the atmosphere by ventilation. The transport system of CO_2 is the same as that for O_2, but the direction of the CO_2 flow and the partial pressure gradient to drive the flow is reversed. The highest P_{CO_2} is found in the tissue cells and the lowest at the arterial end of the tissue capillaries. Because the solubility for CO_2 is much higher than the solubility for O_2, the P_{CO_2} gradient along the tissue capillaries is smaller in comparison with the P_{O_2} gradient. On average the P_{CO_2} at the arterial end of the tissue capillaries is about 40 mmHg and rises to 46 mmHg at the venous end under normal conditions.

CARBON DIOXIDE IN BLOOD

CO_2 in blood is stored in three different forms (Fig. 2-5). Some dissolves physically in the plasma and the red cells and amounts to 6 percent of total arterial CO_2 content. Some CO_2 combines with the protein groups of plasma and Hb molecules in the red cells to form carbamino compounds (4 percent), but most CO_2 reacts with water in the red cells to form bicarbonate under the catalysis of carbonic anhydrase (90 percent).

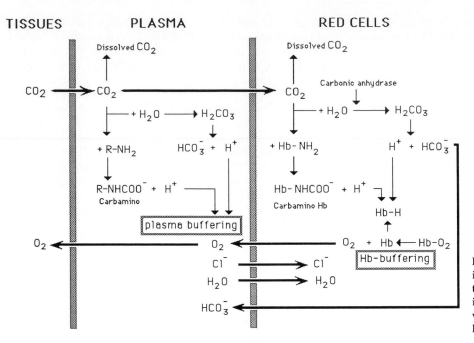

FIGURE 2-5 Movements of carbon dioxide from the tissues to the plasma and the red cells in the capillaries and chemical reactions in each compartment. A reverse process occurs in the lung capillary blood.

The solubility of CO_2 in blood is about 24 times greater than that of O_2. At body temperature the CO_2 content in blood is 0.067 mL/100 mL blood per a unit change of P_{CO_2}. Therefore, 100 mL of the arterial blood, of which P_{CO_2} is 40 mmHg, contains $0.067 \times 40 = 2.68$ mL of dissolved CO_2.

When CO_2 diffuses from the tissues into the tissue capillary blood, CO_2 molecules dissolve first in the plasma, and a small amount of dissolved CO_2 reacts with water to produce carbonic acid [Eq. (37)]. Since the equilibrium of the hydration reaction shifts to the left extremely, the concentration of CO_2 in plasma is about 1000 times greater than the concentration of H_2CO_3.

$$CO_2 + H_2O \rightleftharpoons H_2CO_3 \qquad \text{Eq. (37)}$$

H_2CO_3 dissociates further into $HCO_3^- + H^+$, and the H^+ ions bind to some protein groups of the plasma to neutralize the acidity (buffering). A part of the dissolved CO_2 reacts further with amino groups of plasma protein to form carbamino compounds [Eq. (38)]. H^+ ions released from the reaction are also buffered by the plasma protein buffering system.

$$R - NH_2 + CO_2 \rightleftharpoons R - NHCOO^- + H^+ \qquad \text{Eq. (38)}$$

Most CO_2 molecules that dissolve in the plasma continue to diffuse into the red cells in which some still remains in dissolved form. However, in the red cells the hydration process of CO_2 is accelerated and carbonic acid is formed at a rapid rate because the enzyme called *carbonic anhydrase* contained in the red cells now catalyzes this reaction. Carbonic acid dissociates into protons and bicarbonate. The H^+ ions are then buffered by amino groups of Hb. The efficiency of Hb as a buffer is enhanced when red cells are deoxygenated, that is, reduced Hb binds to more H^+ than oxygenated Hb does. This is because the binding of Hb to O_2 or H^+ is reciprocal. As Hb_{O_2} unloads more O_2 into the tissues, it reacts with more H^+ (Haldane effect). When HCO_3^- accumulates in the red cells, a concentration gradient of this anion is built up between the inside and outside of the red cells. Some HCO_3^- diffuses from the red cells into the plasma until equilibrium is achieved across the cell membrane. To maintain the electrical neutrality, simultaneous movements of equivalent cations should accompany bicarbonate efflux. However, since the red cell membrane is relatively impermeable to cations, chloride ions move into the red cells instead. The bicarbonate-chloride exchange is called *Hamburger shift (chloride shift)*. Since the CO_2 hydration and accompanying ion movements increase the osmolarity of the red cells, some water diffuses into the cells resulting in a slight swelling of the red cells in venous blood.

A part of the dissolved CO_2 in the red cells combines with some amino groups of Hb, forming carbamino compounds, and releases protons. The H^+ ions are also buffered by the protein groups of Hb. Although the carbamino shares only a small fraction of total CO_2 storage in blood, it contributes much to the CO_2 content difference between the arterial and venous blood, accounting for approximately 40 percent of total CO_2 output from the lungs.

In the pulmonary capillary blood the reverse process occurs. Chloride ions move from the red cells into the plasma, and bicarbonate ions enter from the plasma into the red cells. The Hb buffering system releases protons as the reduced Hb is oxygenated in the lung capillaries. The HCO_3^- combines with the H^+ to form H_2CO_3, which is then dehydrated to CO_2 and H_2O. The dehydration process is also accelerated by the catalysis of carbonic anhydrase. The CO_2 diffuses through the red cell membrane, plasma, and capillary-alveolar membrane according to the P_{CO_2} gradient and is finally released into the alveoli as a gas. The diffusion rate of CO_2 is 20 times more rapid than O_2 because of its high solubility in water, and hence, an equilibrium is achieved promptly between the P_{CO_2} in the pulmonary capillary blood and that in the alveolar air. Under normal circumstances, no detectable alveolar to arterial P_{CO_2} difference is present. Water moves from the red cells into the plasma to maintain osmotic equilibrium under the altered ion distribution across the cell

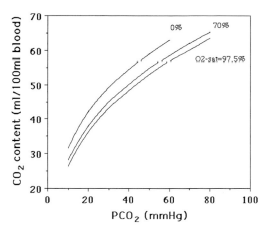

FIGURE 2-6 The carbon dioxide equilibrium (dissociation) curve. The affinity of Hb to CO_2 decreases as Hb is oxygenated (Haldane effect). [Based on numerical data of Comroe et al. (1962).]

membrane and results in a reduction in the volume of the erythrocytes in arterial blood.

The relationship between the CO_2 content and P_{CO_2} in blood is expressed by the *carbon dioxide equilibrium curve* (Fig. 2-6). Unlike the oxygen equilibrium curve, the CO_2 equilibrium curve is nearly linear over the physiologic range of P_{CO_2}. The CO_2 equilibrium curve shifts to the right when Hb is saturated with O_2. The reduced Hb can carry more CO_2 at a given P_{CO_2} than oxygenated Hb. This phenomenon is called the *Haldane effect*. The Haldane effect contributes to facilitate the unloading of CO_2 from the venous blood to the alveoli as the mixed venous blood is oxygenated, and it conversely facilitates to load CO_2 from the tissues as tissue capillary blood is deoxygenated.

ACID-BASE REGULATION

The body's respiratory metabolism produces carbon dioxide continuously. Assuming that the CO_2 output of a healthy adult is 200 mL/min at rest, this corresponds to about 9 mM/min since 1 mg molecular weight (1 mM) of CO_2 occupies 22.3 mL. So, total CO_2 output per day is at least 13,000 mM. The hydration reaction of CO_2 in the blood produces the same mEq of carbonic acid each day, while the excretion of nonvolatile fixed acids from the kidney is only 40 to 70 mEq per day. Therefore, the respiratory system plays a key role in the regulation of the acidity in the blood and extracellular fluid by eliminating gaseous CO_2 through the lungs.

As we have already seen, CO_2 molecules dissolved in blood are readily hydrated to carbonic acid by the catalysis of carbonic anhydrase, and carbonic acid is further dissociated into bicarbonate and hydrogen ions. The dissociation reaction of the carbonic acid at equilibrium can be written as

$$[H^+] = K \frac{[H_2CO_3]}{[HCO_3^-]} \qquad \text{Eq. (39)}$$

where K is an equilibrium constant and the brackets denote the molar concentration of each substance. Taking the logarithm of both sides of Eq. (39) and converting $[H^+]$ to pH ($pH = -\log[H^+]$) yields

$$pH = pK + \log \frac{[HCO_3^-]}{[H_2CO_3]} \qquad \text{Eq. (40)}$$

where $pK = -\log K$. This is called the *Henderson-Hasselbalch equation*. Since in the plasma the concentration of H_2CO_3 is only one thousandth of that of dissolved CO_2, and the hydration of CO_2 and subsequent dissociation of H_2CO_3 is actually a continuous reaction, $[H_2CO_3]$ of Eq. (40) may be replaced by $[CO_2]$.

$$pH = pK + \log \frac{[HCO_3^-]}{[CO_2]} \qquad \text{Eq. (41)}$$

The constant pK' is an apparent pK when $[HCO_3^-]$ is replaced by $[CO_2]$. At body temperature, pK' is 6.1. Since P_{CO_2} in the plasma is easily measurable as opposed to total CO_2 content, it is convenient to convert $[CO_2]$ into a product of solubility and P_{CO_2}. The solubility of CO_2 in the plasma is 0.067 mL/100 mL blood. However, in the analysis of the acid-base balance the concentration is usually expressed in mM/L rather than vol%. Since 1 mM/L CO_2 corresponds to 2.23 vol%, the solubility for CO_2 expressed in molar units ($\alpha\,CO_2$) is 0.067/2.23 = 0.03. Then,

$$pH = 6.1 + \log \frac{[HCO_3^-]}{[0.03 P_{CO_2}]} \qquad \text{Eq. (42)}$$

The Henderson-Hasselbalch equation states that plasma pH is determined by the concentration ratio, $[HCO_3^-]/[CO_2]$. The $[HCO_3^-]$ and P_{CO_2} of the arterial blood under normal conditions are 24 mM/L and 40 mmHg, respectively. Therefore, the normal pH value can be determined as

$$6.1 + \log 24/(0.03 \times 40) = 6.1 + \log 24/1.2 = 7.40$$

The ratio $[HCO_3^-]/[CO_2]$ is normally maintained at 20. The venous blood is in contact with the alveolar gas and CO_2 is excreted from the lungs into the atmosphere by ventilation, while CO_2 in the blood is continuously retained by the tissue metabolism. The CO_2 content and the acidity of the blood are thus determined as a function of ventilation controlled via a feedback loop regulating the gas exchange system. Increased P_{CO_2} and $[H^+]$ in the arterial blood stimulate the central and peripheral chemoreceptors in the respiratory controller, resulting in an enhancement of ventilation which leads to a drop in $[H^+]$ and P_{CO_2}. Conversely, decreased P_{CO_2} and $[H^+]$ induce a reverse process in the ventilation regulatory system to maintain the pH homeostasis of the blood. As a result, pH in the arterial blood deviates only slightly from 7.40 under various metabolic conditions.

When alveolar ventilation is abnormally low for a given CO_2 production, the arterial P_{CO_2} rises beyond the normal level (hypercapnia), the concentration of dissolved CO_2 increases, and pH drops, resulting in a condition called *respiratory acidosis*. If the arterial P_{CO_2} rises to 50 mmHg by hypoventilation, for example, $[CO_2]$ increases from 1.2 mM/L to 1.5 mM/L, reducing the ratio $[HCO_3^-]/[CO_2]$ to 16, and pH would drop from 7.40 to 7.30 if $[HCO_3^-]$ remains unchanged. However, the increased $[CO_2]$ shifts the hydration-dissociation equilibria toward the right, resulting in increases in both $[HCO_3^-]$ and $[H^+]$.

$$CO_2 + H_2O \rightleftharpoons H_2CO_3 \rightleftharpoons HCO_3^- + H^+ \qquad \text{Eq. (43)}$$

The increment of $[HCO_3^-]$ is not identical to the increment of $[H^+]$ because some H^+ ions are neutralized by the blood buffering system. As the concentration of bicarbonate increases, the actual ratio $[HCO_3^-]/[CO_2]$ becomes higher than 16, and pH remains at a slight reduction from its normal value. When the accumulation of CO_2 occurs in a slow process, renal compensation will occur. The renal tubular cells of the kidneys excrete H^+ in urine in a form of fixed acid, and instead, reabsorbs HCO_3^- into the blood. This process restores the ratio $[HCO_3^-]/[CO_2]$ to almost 20 and pH recovers to its normal value.

Conversely, when alveolar ventilation is abnormally high in relation to metabolic CO_2 production, arterial P_{CO_2} would be lower than normal. Hyperventilation and the resultant hypocapnia are induced as a result of various forms of excessive stimulation to the medullary respiratory center. When P_{CO_2} drops, $[HCO_3^-]$ in the plasma also drops because the decreased P_{CO_2} shifts the hydration-dissociation equilibria toward the left. However, since the ratio $[HCO_3^-]/[CO_2]$ is still greater than 20, pH rises and a condition called *respiratory alkalosis* occurs. The kidneys excrete the excess HCO_3^- in the urine; the ratio $[HCO_3^-]/[CO_2]$ recovers to 20 and pH returns to its normal value.

The concentration of bicarbonate is regulated primarily by the kidneys, while P_{CO_2} in the plasma is controlled by the gas exchange system of respiration. Therefore, the ratio $[HCO_3^-]/[CO_2]$ depends on the ratio of the lung function to the renal function.

When exercise exceeds a certain critical level, energy required for continuing the exercise is supplied partially via anaerobic glycolysis because of insufficient oxygen delivery to the muscles. The concentration of lactic acid in the blood increases and dissociates into lactate and H^+. The excess H^+ reacts with bicarbonate, resulting in a drop in the ratio $[HCO_3^-]/[CO_2]$ and pH. This condition is called *metabolic acidosis*. The increase in $[H^+]$ stimulates the respiratory center to drive ventilation so that the arterial P_{CO_2} drops secondarily. The ratio $[HCO_3^-]/[CO_2]$ and pH return to nearly normal. Metabolic acidosis occurs in various situations such as in the abnormal metabolism of fats, diabetic ketosis, or an excessive excretion of bicarbonate via the kidneys and the intestine under diseased conditions.

Alveolar Ventilation and Perfusion

THE VENTILATION TO PERFUSION RATIO

Oxygen taken up by ventilation diffuses into the pulmonary circulation and is delivered to the body tissues by systemic arterial circulation. Conversely, carbon dioxide produced in the tissues is transferred into the pulmonary circulation and is expelled into the atmosphere by ventilation. Therefore, the efficiency of the gas exchange between alveolar ventilation and pulmonary perfusion determines the gas compositions in the arterial blood.

Assuming that the lungs consist of a single homogeneous compartment with a constant ventilation and perfusion, oxygen taken up by the unit lung over a given period is given by the difference between the amount of O_2 inspired and the amount of O_2 expired during that time.

$$\dot{V}_{O_2} = \dot{V}_A(F_{I_{O_2}} - F_{A_{O_2}}) \qquad \text{Eq. (44)}$$

Oxygen transferred from the lungs to the body tissues is given by the Fick's principle as being the difference between the amount leaving the lungs and the amount returning to the lungs, where Ca and $C\bar{v}$ are concentrations of arterial and mixed venous blood, respectively, and $\dot{Q}_C$ is the pulmonary capillary blood flow.

$$\dot{V}_{O_2} = \dot{Q}_C(Ca_{O_2} - C\bar{v}_{O_2}) \qquad \text{Eq. (45)}$$

Combining both equations, the ratio of alveolar ventilation to pulmonary capillary blood flow $(\dot{V}_A/\dot{Q}_C)$ is expressed as a function of O_2 content in the blood and O_2 fraction in the alveoli.

$$\frac{\dot{V}_A}{\dot{Q}c} = \frac{(Ca_{O_2} - C\bar{v}_{O_2})}{(F_{I_{O_2}} - F_{A_{O_2}})} \qquad \text{Eq. (46)}$$

This equation shows that at given values of $F_{I_{CO_2}}$ and $C\bar{v}_{O_2}$ the arterial and alveolar compositions of O_2 are determined by the ratio of alveolar ventilation to pulmonary capillary blood flow, $\dot{V}_A/\dot{Q}c$, not by the absolute values of each.

Similarly, carbon dioxide compositions in the blood and the alveoli can be expressed by the same $\dot{V}_A/\dot{Q}c$ ratio. For air breathing,

$$\frac{\dot{V}_A}{\dot{Q}c} = \frac{(C\bar{v}_{CO_2} - Ca_{CO_2})}{F_{A_{CO_2}}} \qquad \text{Eq. (47)}$$

Since the gas exchange for O_2 and CO_2 occurs simultaneously, Eqs. (46) and (47) can be combined in the steady state.

$$\frac{\dot{V}_A}{\dot{Q}c} = \frac{(Ca_{O_2} - C\bar{v}_{O_2})}{(F_{I_{O_2}} - F_{A_{O_2}})} = \frac{(C\bar{v}_{CO_2} - Ca_{CO_2})}{F_{A_{CO_2}}} \qquad \text{Eq. (48)}$$

The gas fractions for O_2 and CO_2 in the alveoli can be converted into respective partial pressures, and the gas contents in the blood can also be expressed in terms of partial pressures referred to as the respective equilibrium curves for O_2 and CO_2. If we assume a complete equilibrium of O_2 and CO_2 diffusion between the alveolar gas and the end-capillary blood in the steady state, the $\dot{V}_A/\dot{Q}c$ can be given by the following equations, in which arterial and alveolar partial pressures are represented by common P_{O_2} and P_{CO_2}.

$$\frac{\dot{V}_A}{\dot{Q}c} = \frac{\beta b_{O_2}(P_{O_2} - P\bar{v}_{O_2})(P_B - 47)}{(P_{I_{O_2}} - P_{O_2})} \qquad \text{Eq. (49)}$$

$$= \frac{\beta b_{CO_2}(P\bar{v}_{CO_2} - P_{CO_2})(P_B - 47)}{P_{CO_2}}$$

where βb_{O_2} and βb_{CO_2} are slopes of the equilibrium curves for each gas. Numerical solution of Eq. (49) is difficult because the Bohr effect on βb_{O_2} and the Haldane effect on βb_{CO_2} should be incorporated. The graphic expression of this

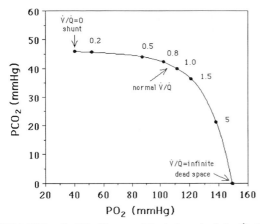

FIGURE 2-7 The O_2-CO_2 diagram. The left end of the $\dot{V}A/\dot{Q}c$ line indicates the point where there is no ventilation (P_{O_2} and P_{CO_2} equal to those of mixed venous blood). The right end of the line represents the point where there is no perfusion (P_{O_2} and P_{CO_2} equal to those of air saturated by water vapor). Normal $VA/\dot{Q}c$ is around 0.85. [Adapted from Comroe et al. (1962).]

function is called the O_2-CO_2 diagram (Fig. 2-7). The left end of the $\dot{V}A/\dot{Q}c$ line indicates the point where there is no ventilation ($\dot{V}A/\dot{Q}c = 0$), at which P_{O_2} and P_{CO_2} are equal to those of the mixed venous blood, that is, 40 and 46 mmHg, respectively. The right end of the line represents the point where there is no perfusion ($\dot{V}A/\dot{Q}c$ = infinite, P_{O_2} = 149 mmHg, and P_{CO_2} = 0). The O_2 saturation and CO_2 content in the arterial blood at each $\dot{V}A/\dot{Q}c$ can be included in the diagram if necessary. The O_2-CO_2 diagram is useful when analyzing the gas exchange characteristics of a lung unit under standard conditions.

UNEVEN DISTRIBUTION OF VENTILATION TO PERFUSION RATIO

The ventilation to perfusion ratio of a given unit of the lungs varies from region to region. Even in healthy lungs, there is always an uneven distribution of $\dot{V}A/\dot{Q}c$ to a certain extent. The $\dot{V}A/\dot{Q}c$ of the lungs in an upright position is higher near the top and lower near the bottom, mainly because of the hydrostatic effect of gravity on the pulmonary circulation. Assuming that the alveolar ventilation and the pulmonary capillary blood flow are 4.2 L/min and 5.0 L/min, respectively, the mean $\dot{V}A/\dot{Q}c$ for a healthy adult would be 0.85 at rest.

A simple two-compartment model can simulate the effects of regional $\dot{V}A/\dot{Q}c$ differences on the total gas exchange under various conditions. The model lung consists of two parallel compartments A and B which are commonly perfused by venous blood with a P_{O_2} of 40 mmHg (O_2 saturation = 75%) and a P_{CO_2} of 46 mmHg. First, a couple of $\dot{V}A$ and $\dot{Q}c$ are given to each compartment, then P_{O_2} and P_{CO_2} of each are determined by reading corresponding values of the $\dot{V}A/\dot{Q}c$ point along the O_2-CO_2 diagram. The O_2 saturation and the CO_2 content of the mixed arterial blood are determined by perfusion-weighted averages of the two compartments, and the P_{O_2} and P_{CO_2} of the mixed alveolar gas are determined by ventilation-weighted averages.

TABLE 2-1 Example of Venous-Admixture-Like Perfusion

Compartment	A	B	Combined
$\dot{V}A$(L/min)	2.0	0.5	2.5
$\dot{Q}c$(L/min)	2.5	2.5	5.0
$\dot{V}A/\dot{Q}c$	0.8	0.2	0.5
Pa_{O_2}(mmHg)	102	52	66
Sa_{O_2}(%)	97.5	84.0	90.8
PA_{O_2}(mmHg)	102	52	92

NOTE: Compartment A is normally ventilated and perfused, while B is normally perfused but poorly ventilated. In combined arterial blood Pa_{O_2} drops markedly, resulting in a total DA-a_{O_2} of 26 mmHg. (A and B are assumed to be perfused by venous blood with a P_{O_2} of 40 mmHg, S_{O_2} = 75%, and a P_{CO_2} of 46 mmHg.)

VENOUS-ADMIXTURE-LIKE PERFUSION

This type of $\dot{V}A/\dot{Q}c$ abnormality is summarized in Table 2-1. Compartment A is normally ventilated and perfused ($\dot{V}A/\dot{Q}c = 0.8$) and hence has a normal end-capillary P_{O_2} and a normal O_2 saturation. Compartment B is poorly ventilated while having a normal perfusion ($\dot{V}A/\dot{Q}c = 0.2$), resulting in a lower end-capillary P_{O_2} and a lower O_2 saturation. The alveolar gas of each unit is assumed to be in equilibrium with the respective end-capillary P_{O_2}. The S_{O_2} of the mixed arterial blood is halfway between those of compartment A and B since the perfusion for each compartment is equal in this case. Reflecting the blood leaving the poorly ventilated region (B), the saturation of the combined blood is slightly insufficient. The arterial P_{O_2} is determined from the combined arterial O_2 saturation to be 66 mmHg. On the other hand, since the ventilation of B is only a quarter of that of A, the ventilation-weighted P_{O_2} in the mixed alveolar gas is determined to be 92 mmHg. As a result, a large alveolar to arterial P_{O_2} difference (DA-a_{O_2}) appears. This type of $\dot{V}A/\dot{Q}c$ unevenness is similar to the admixture of venous blood to arterial blood (shunt), leading to hypoxia and slight hypercapnia.

Let us assume that the ventilation of A of the above model increases to compensate for the hypoventilation of B (Table 2-2). The $\dot{V}A/\dot{Q}c$ of A rises by 1.5 which results in an increase in PA_{O_2}. However, this does little to help improve the S_{O_2} of the mixed arterial blood, because the O_2 equilibrium curve is flat during the higher range of P_{O_2}. Hyperventilation in A, on the other hand, raises alveolar tension in proportion to the increment of ventilation, PA_{O_2} in the mixed alveolar gas increases, resulting in more increase in DA-a_{O_2}. On the other

TABLE 2-2 Compensation for the Venous-Admixture-Like Perfusion Given in Table 2-1

Compartment	A	B	Combined
$\dot{V}A$(L/min)	3.75	0.5	4.25
$\dot{Q}c$(L/min)	2.5	2.5	5.0
$\dot{V}A/\dot{Q}c$	1.5	0.2	0.85
Pa_{O_2}(mmHg)	121	52	66
Sa_{O_2}(%)	98.0	84.0	91.0
PA_{O_2}(mmHg)	121	52	113

NOTE: Ventilation in compartment A increases to keep total ventilation normal. However, the compensatory hyperventilation fails to improve the Pa_{O_2} of combined arterial blood, and the total DA-a_{O_2} remains at a high level of 47 mmHg. (A and B are assumed to be perfused by venous blood with a P_{O_2} of 40 mmHg, S_{O_2} = 75%, and a P_{CO_2} of 46 mmHg.)

TABLE 2-3 An Example of Dead-Space-Like Ventilation

Compartment	A	B	Combined
$\dot{V}_A$(L/min)	2.0	2.0	4.0
$\dot{Q}c$(L/min)	4.6	0.4	5.0
$\dot{V}_A/\dot{Q}c$	0.43	5.0	0.8
Pa_{O_2}(mmHg)	82	138	88
Sa_{O_2}(%)	96.0	98.6	96.2
PA_{O_2}(mmHg)	82	138	110

NOTE: Both compartments are ventilated normally, but compartment B is poorly perfused while compartment A is excessively perfused so that total blood flow is kept normal. The Pa_{O_2} of combined arterial blood drops to a certain extent, resulting in a moderate increase in D_A-a_{O_2}. (A and B are assumed to be perfused by venous blood with a P_{O_2} of 40 mmHg, $S_{O_2} = 75\%$, and a P_{CO_2} of 46 mmHg.)

TABLE 2-4 Compensation for the Dead-Space-Like Ventilation Given in Table 2-3

Compartment	A	B	Combined
$\dot{V}_A$(L/min)	4.0	2.0	6.0
$\dot{Q}c$(L/min)	4.6	0.4	5.0
$\dot{V}_A/\dot{Q}c$	0.87	5.0	1.2
Pa_{O_2}(mmHg)	107	138	110
Sa_{O_2}(%)	97.8	98.6	97.8
PA_{O_2}(mmHg)	107	138	117

NOTE: Ventilation of compartment A increases to match its elevated perfusion. This markedly improves the Pa_{O_2} of the combined arterial blood and the total D_A-a_{O_2}. (A and B are assumed to be perfused by venous blood with a P_{O_2} of 40 mmHg, $S_{O_2} = 75\%$, and a P_{CO_2} of 46 mmHg.)

hand, hypercapnia appearing in the venous-admixture-like perfusion can be eliminated by the compensatory hyperventilation of compartment A.

DEAD-SPACE-LIKE VENTILATION

If the perfusion for a compartment is poor, this compartment acts as a dead space (Table 2-3). Ventilation of the two compartments is maintained as normal, while perfusion for compartment B is limited, and instead, compartment A is excessively perfused to maintain total blood flow as normal. Thus, $\dot{V}_A/\dot{Q}c$ is low in A and extremely high in B. As a result, P_{O_2} in blood leaving compartment A is lower than normal, leading to a corresponding drop in S_{O_2}. Since compartment B is poorly ventilated it has a gas composition more like the gas in a physiologic dead space. Thus, alveolar P_{O_2} in B is extremely high and the end-capillary blood is fully saturated. P_{O_2} of the mixed alveolar gas maintains a normal value, but a slight reduction appears in the mixed arterial P_{O_2} because the contribution of blood leaving the low $\dot{V}_A/\dot{Q}c$ compartment (A) is dominant. This leads to a considerable increase in D_A-a_{O_2}.

Now, assume that hyperventilation takes place in compartment A to improve the hypoxic condition, leaving compartment B intact (Table 2-4). The alveolar and arterial P_{O_2} of compartment A increases significantly and hypoxemia in the mixed arterial blood recovers to normal. In contrast to the venous-admixture-like perfusion, compensatory hyperventilation occuring in the dead-space-like ventilation is effective in reducing the P_{O_2} difference between the mixed gas and blood.

The P_{CO_2} difference between the total alveolar gas and the total arterial blood is less significant than the P_{O_2} difference under the same circumstances, because of the less venous to arterial P_{CO_2} difference and the linear characteristics of the CO_2 equilibrium curve.

TRUE SHUNT

When a part of venous blood enters directly into the pulmonary vein or the systemic circulation without contacting alveolar gas, the arterial P_{O_2} drops in proportion to the amount of venous blood mixed. This is called *true venous admixture* or *shunt*. Even in healthy persons approximately 2.5 percent of the total pulmonary capillary blood flow mixes with arterial blood via the thebesian and the bronchial circulation. As a result, O_2 saturation of 97.5% in the end-capillary blood drops to 97.0% in the arterial blood. The amount of true venous admixture may increase in some heart diseases, leading to serious arterial hypoxemia.

Suggested Readings

Cherniack NS: *Respiration in Health and Disease*. Philadelphia, W.B. Saunders, 1972.

Comroe JH, Forster RE Jr, DuBois AB, et al: *The Lung: Clinical Physiology and Pulmonary Function Tests*. Chicago, Year Book Medical Publishers, 1962.

Hlastala MP, Berger AJ: *Physiology of Respiration*. New York, Oxford University Press, 1996.

Otis AB: An overview of gas exchange, in Farhi LE, Tenny SM (eds): *Handbook of Physiology*, Sec 3, *The Respiratory System*, vol IV, *Gas Exchange*. Bethesda, MD, American Physiological Soc, Chap. 1, 1987, pp 1–11.

Piiper J, Sheid P: Blood-gas equilibration in lungs, in West JB (ed): *Pulmonary Gas Exchange. Ventilation, Blood Flow, and Diffusion*, vol 1. New York Academic Press, 1980, pp 131–171.

Minies AH: *Respiratory Physiology*. New York, Raven Press, 1993.

Severinghaus JW: Simple, accurate equations for human blood O_2 dissociation computations. *J Appl Physiol* 46:599, 1979.

Chapter 3
RESPIRATORY MUSCLE FUNCTION
ANDRÉ DE TROYER

The mechanical action of any skeletal muscle is essentially determined by the anatomy of the muscle and by the structures it has to displace when it contracts. The respiratory muscles are structurally and functionally skeletal muscles, and their task is to displace the chest wall rhythmically to pump gas in and out of the lungs. This chapter, therefore, starts with a discussion of the basic mechanical structure of the chest wall. It next analyzes the actions of the muscles that displace the chest wall. For the sake of clarity, the functions of the diaphragm, the muscles of the rib cage, and the muscles of the abdominal wall are analyzed sequentially. However, since all these muscles normally work together in a coordinated manner, the most critical aspects of their mechanical interactions are also emphasized. Finally, some disorders are considered in which the respiratory displacements of the chest wall are abnormal due to a particular distribution of muscle weakness or chronic hyperinflation.

The Chest Wall

The chest wall can be thought of as consisting of two compartments, the rib cage and the abdomen, separated from each other by a thin musculotendinous structure, the diaphragm[1] (Fig. 3-1). These two compartments are mechanically arranged in parallel. Expansion of the lungs, therefore, can be accommodated by expansion of either the rib cage or the abdomen or both compartments simultaneously.

Although the rib cage is a complex structure, its displacements during breathing are essentially related to the motion of the ribs, and this motion occurs primarily through a rotation around the axes defined by the articulations of the ribs with the vertebral bodies and transverse processes,[2,3] as shown in Fig. 3-2. Indeed, each rib is fixed dorsally by these two vertebral joints, which together form a hinge. The axis of this hinge, however, is oriented laterally, dorsally, and caudally. In addition, the ribs are curved and slope caudally and ventrally from their costotransverse articulations such that their ventral ends and the costal cartilages are more caudal than their dorsal part. When the ribs are displaced in the cranial direction, therefore, their ventral ends move laterally and ventrally as well as cranially, the cartilages rotate cranially around the chondrosternal junctions, and the sternum is displaced ventrally. As a result, there is usually an increase in both the lateral and the dorsoventral diameter of the rib cage (see Fig. 3-2; see also Fig. 3-3). Conversely, an axial displacement of the ribs in the caudal direction is usually associated with a decrease in rib cage diameters. The muscles that elevate the ribs as their primary action therefore have an inspiratory effect on the rib cage, whereas the muscles that lower the ribs have an expiratory effect on the rib cage. It must be appreciated, however, that although the ribs

move predominantly by a rotation, there is some misfit at the surfaces of the costovertebral and chondrosternal joints. The long cartilages of ribs 8, 9, and 10 even articulate with one another by little synovial cavities rather than with the sternum. Hence the upper ribs tend to move as a unit with the sternum, but the lower ribs have some freedom to move independently.[4,5] Both in animals and in humans, deformations of the rib cage therefore may occur under the influence of muscle contraction.

The respiratory displacements of the abdominal compartment are more straightforward because if one neglects the 100 to 300 mL of abdominal gas volume, its contents are virtually incompressible. The abdomen thus behaves as a liquid-filled container, and any local inward displacement of its boundaries results in an equal outward displacement elsewhere. Furthermore, many of these boundaries, such as the spine dorsally, the pelvis caudally, and the iliac crests laterally, are virtually fixed, so the parts of the abdominal container that can be displaced are largely limited to the ventral abdominal wall and the diaphragm. When the diaphragm contracts during inspiration (see below), therefore, its descent usually results in an outward displacement of the ventral abdominal wall; conversely, when the abdominal muscles contract, they cause in general an inward displacement of the stomach wall, resulting in a cranial motion of the diaphragm into the thoracic cavity.

The Diaphragm

The diaphragm is anatomically unique among skeletal muscles in that its muscle fibers radiate from a central tendinous structure (the central tendon) to insert peripherally into skeletal structures. The crural (or vertebral) portion of the diaphragmatic muscle inserts on the ventrolateral aspect of the first three lumbar vertebrae and on the aponeurotic arcuate ligaments, and the costal portion inserts on the xiphoid process of the sternum and the upper margins of the lower six ribs. From their insertions, the costal fibers run cranially so that they are directly apposed to the inner aspect of the lower rib cage (see Fig. 3-1). In standing humans at rest, this so-called zone of apposition of the diaphragm to the rib cage[6] is about 6 to 7 cm in height in the midaxillary line and occupies 25 to 30 percent of the total internal surface area of the rib cage. Although the older literature has suggested the possibility of an intercostal motor innervation of some portions of the diaphragm, it is now clearly established that its only motor supply is through the phrenic nerves, which, in humans, originate in the third, fourth, and fifth cervical segments.

ACTIONS OF THE DIAPHRAGM

As the muscle fibers of the diaphragm are activated during inspiration, they develop tension and shorten. As a result, the axial length of the apposed diaphragm diminishes, and the dome of the diaphragm, which corresponds primarily to the central tendon, descends relative to the costal insertions of the muscle. The dome remains relatively constant in size and shape during breathing, but its descent has two effects. First, it expands the thoracic cavity along the craniocaudal axis. Hence pleural pressure falls, and depending on whether the airways are open or closed, lung volume increases or

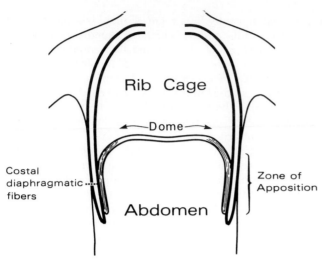

FIGURE 3-1 Frontal section of the chest wall at end-expiration. Note the cranial orientation of the costal diaphragmatic fibers and their apposition to the inner aspect of the lower rib cage (zone of apposition). [Reprinted, with permission, from A De Troyer and SH Loring: Actions of the respiratory muscles, in C Roussos (ed): *The Thorax*, 2d ed. New York, Marcel Dekker, 1995, pp 535–563.]

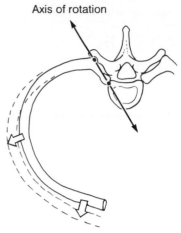

FIGURE 3-2 Diagram of a typical thoracic vertebra and a rib (viewed from above). The rib articulates both with the body and the transverse process of the vertebra (*closed circles*) and moves essentially through a rotation around the axis defined by these articulations. From these articulations, however, the rib slopes downward and ventrally. Therefore, when it becomes more horizontal in inspiration (*dotted line*), it causes an increase in both the anteroposterior and the transverse diameter of the rib cage (*open arrows*). [Reprinted, with permission, from A De Troyer: Mechanics of the chest wall muscles, in AD Miller, B Bishop, and AL Bianchi (eds): *Neural Control of the Respiratory Muscles*. Roca Raton, FL, CRC Press, 1996, pp 59–73.]

alveolar pressure falls. Second, it produces a caudal displacement of the abdominal visceral mass and an increase in abdominal pressure, which, in turn, pushes the ventral abdominal wall outward.

In addition, because the muscle fibers of the costal diaphragm insert onto the upper margins of the lower six ribs, they also apply a force on these ribs when they contract. This force, in fact, is equal to the force exerted on the central tendon and under normal circumstances is directed cranially due to the cranial orientation of the fibers (Fig. 3-3). It therefore has the effect of lifting the ribs and rotating them outward. The fall in pleural pressure and the increase in abdominal pressure induced by diaphragmatic contraction, however, act simultaneously on the rib cage, which probably explains why the action of the diaphragm on the rib cage has been controversial for so long.

ACTION OF THE DIAPHRAGM ON THE RIB CAGE

When the diaphragm in anesthetized dogs is activated selectively by electrical stimulation of the phrenic nerves, the upper ribs move caudally, and the cross-sectional area of the upper portion of the rib cage decreases.[7] In contrast, the lower ribs move cranially, and the cross-sectional area of the lower portion of the rib cage increases. When a bilateral pneumothorax is subsequently introduced so that the fall in pleural pressure is eliminated, isolated contraction of the diaphragm causes a greater expansion of the lower rib cage, but the dimensions of the upper rib cage now remain unchanged.[7] When contracting alone, the canine diaphragm thus has two opposing effects on the rib cage. On the one hand, it has an expiratory action on the upper rib cage, and the fact that this action is abolished by a pneumothorax indicates that it is due to the fall in pleural pressure. On the other hand, it also has an inspiratory action on the lower rib cage. Measurements of chest wall motion during phrenic

nerve pacing in patients with transection of the upper cervical cord[8,9] and during quiet breathing in patients who use their diaphragm exclusively because of a traumatic transection of the lower cervical cord[10,11] have shown that, as in the dog, the diaphragm in humans has both an expiratory action on the upper rib cage and an inspiratory action on the lower rib cage.

Theoretical and experimental work has confirmed that the inspiratory action of the diaphragm on the lower rib cage

FIGURE 3-3 Insertional component of diaphragmatic action. During inspiration, as the fibers of the costal diaphragm contract, they exert a force on the lower ribs (*arrow*). If the abdominal visceral mass opposes effectively the descent of the diaphragmatic dome (*open arrow*), this force is oriented cranially. As a result, the lower ribs are lifted and rotate outward. [Reprinted, with permission, from A De Troyer: Mechanics of the chest wall muscles, in AD Miller, B Bishop, AL Bianchi (eds): *Neural Control of the Respiratory Muscles*. Roca Raton, FL, CRC Press, 1996, pp 59–73.]

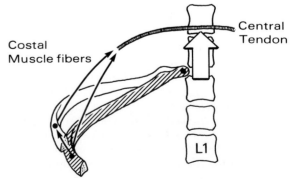

results in part from the force the muscle applies on the ribs by way of its insertions; this force is conventionally referred to as the *insertional force*.[12,13] This inspiratory action of the diaphragm, however, is also related to its apposition to the rib cage. The zone of apposition makes the lower rib cage, in effect, part of the abdominal container, and measurements in dogs and rabbits have established that during breathing the changes in pressure in the pleural recess between the apposed diaphragm and the rib cage are almost equal to the changes in abdominal pressure.[14] Pressure in this pleural recess rises rather than falls during inspiration, thus indicating that the rise in abdominal pressure is truly transmitted through the apposed diaphragm to expand the lower rib cage. This mechanism of diaphragmatic action has been called the *appositional force*.

Although the insertional and appositional forces make the normal diaphragm expand the lower rib cage, it should be appreciated that this action of the diaphragm is largely determined by the resistance provided by the abdominal contents to diaphragmatic descent (see Fig. 3-3). If this resistance is high (i.e., if abdominal compliance is low), the dome of the diaphragm descends less so that the zone of apposition remains significant throughout inspiration and the rise in abdominal pressure is greater. Therefore, for a given diaphragmatic contraction, the appositional force is greater and the expansion of the lower rib cage is increased. Conversely, if the resistance provided by the abdominal contents is small (if the abdomen is very compliant), the dome of the diaphragm descends more easily, the zone of apposition decreases more, and the rise in abdominal pressure is smaller. Consequently, the inspiratory action of the diaphragm on the rib cage is reduced. If the resistance provided by the abdominal contents were eliminated, not only would the zone of apposition disappear in the course of inspiration, but also the contracting diaphragmatic muscle fibers would become oriented transversely inward at their insertions onto the ribs. The insertional force would then have an expiratory rather than inspiratory action on the lower rib cage. Indeed, when a dog is eviscerated, the diaphragm causes a decrease rather than an increase in lower rib cage dimensions.[7,12,15]

INFLUENCE OF LUNG VOLUME

The balance between pleural pressure and the insertional and appositional forces of the diaphragm is also markedly affected by changes in lung volume. As lung volume decreases from functional residual capacity (FRC) to residual volume (RV), the zone of apposition increases, and the fraction of the rib cage exposed to pleural pressure decreases. As a result, the appositional force increases, and the effect of pleural pressure diminishes so that the inspiratory action of the diaphragm on the rib cage is enhanced. Conversely, as lung volume increases above FRC, the zone of apposition decreases, and a larger fraction of the rib cage becomes exposed to pleural pressure. The inspiratory action of the diaphragm on the rib cage is therefore diminished.[7,12,13] When lung volume approaches total lung capacity (TLC), the zone of apposition all but disappears, and the diaphragmatic muscle fibers become oriented transversely inward as well as cranially. As in the eviscerated animal, the insertional force of the diaphragm is then expiratory rather than inspiratory in direction.

The Muscles of the Rib Cage

THE INTERCOSTAL MUSCLES

The intercostal muscles are two thin layers of muscle occupying each of the intercostal spaces; they are termed *external* and *internal* because of their surface relations, the external being superficial to the internal. The external intercostals extend from the tubercles of the ribs dorsally to the costochondral junctions ventrally, and their fibers are oriented obliquely caudad and ventrally from the rib above to the rib below. In contrast, the internal intercostals extend from the angles of the ribs dorsally to the sternocostal junctions ventrally, and their fibers run obliquely caudad and dorsally from the rib above to the rib below. Thus, although the intercostal spaces in their lateral portion contain two layers of intercostal muscle running approximately at right angles to each other, they contain a single muscle layer in their ventral and dorsal portions. Ventrally, between the sternum and the chondrocostal junctions, the only fibers are those of the internal intercostal muscles. These latter, however, are particularly thick in this region of the rib cage, where they are conventionally called the *parasternal intercostals*. Dorsally, from the angle of the ribs to the vertebrae, the only fibers come from the external intercostal muscles, although they are duplicated by a spindle-shaped muscle running in each interspace from the tip of the transverse process of the vertebra cranially to the angle of the rib caudally; this muscle is the *levator costae*. All the intercostal muscles are innervated by the intercostal nerves.

ACTIONS ON THE RIBS

The actions of the intercostal muscles on the ribs are conventionally regarded according to the theory proposed by Hamberger in the mid-1700s.[16] This theory is based on geometric considerations and is illustrated in Fig. 3-4. When an intercostal muscle contracts in one interspace, it pulls the upper rib down and the lower rib up. However, since the fibers of the external intercostal slope obliquely caudad and ventrally from the rib above to the one below, their lower insertion is more distant from the center of rotation of the ribs (the vertebral articulations) than the upper one. When this muscle contracts, the torque acting on the lower rib is therefore greater than that acting on the upper rib, so its net effect is to raise the ribs. The orientation of the levator costae is similar to that of the external intercostal, and its action is also to raise the ribs. In contrast, the fibers of the internal intercostal run obliquely caudad and dorsally from the rib above to the one below. Therefore, their lower insertion is less distant from the center of rotation of the ribs than the upper one. As a result, when this muscle contracts, the torque acting on the lower rib is less than that acting on the upper rib, and its net effect is to lower the ribs. Hamberger finally concluded that although the parasternal intercostals are part of the internal intercostal layer, their action should be referred to the sternum rather than to the vertebral column. Their contraction, therefore, should raise the ribs.

Several of these conclusions have received direct experimental support. When the parasternal intercostal muscles in the dog are selectively activated by electrical stimulation, they produce a cranial displacement of the ribs into which they insert and an increase in lung volume.[17] Measurements

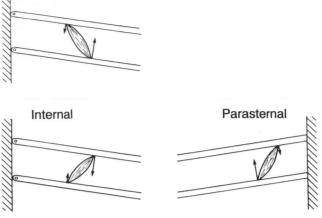

External

Internal **Parasternal**

FIGURE 3-4 Diagram illustrating the actions of the intercostal muscles on the ribs, as proposed by Hamberger.[16] The hatched area in the left panel represents the spine (dorsal view), and the hatched area in the lower right panel represents the sternum (ventral view). The two bars oriented obliquely represent two adjacent ribs. The external and internal intercostal muscles are depicted as single bundles, and the torques acting on the ribs during contraction of these muscles are represented by arrows. [Reprinted, with permission, from A De Troyer: Respiratory muscle function, in RAL Brewis, B Corrin, DM Geddes, and GJ Gibson (eds): *Respiratory Medicine*, 2d ed. London, WB Saunders, 1995, pp 125–133.]

of the changes in length of the canine parasternal intercostals in the different interspaces also have shown that, like the diaphragm, these muscles invariably shorten during passive inflation; they have, therefore, a clear-cut inspiratory mechanical advantage.[18,19] Stimulation of the levator costae in a single intercostal space similarly causes a cranial displacement of the rib into which it inserts.[20] However, when either the external or the internal interosseous intercostal muscle in a single interspace is selectively stimulated in the dog, there is a mutual approximation of the adjacent ribs, but the cranial displacement of the rib below is always greater than the caudal displacement of the rib above.[21,22] In addition, whereas the Hamberger mechanism would predict that inflation of the relaxed respiratory system above FRC produces shortening of all the external intercostals and lengthening of all the internal interosseous intercostals, measurements in dogs have shown that the changes in length of these muscles are variable and largely determined by the location of the muscles along the rostrocaudal axis of the rib cage. Thus, in the rostral interspaces these two sets of intercostal muscles tend to shorten during passive inflation, whereas in the caudal interspaces they both tend to lengthen.[23]

The Hamberger theory is thus incomplete, and the two major reasons for which this theory cannot entirely describe the actions of the intercostal muscles have been emphasized by Saumarez[24] and Wilson and De Troyer.[25] First, the Hamberger model is planar, whereas the real ribs are curved. As a result, the mechanical advantage of the external and internal intercostal muscles, as reflected by their changes in length during passive inflation, varies as a function of the position of the muscle fibers along the rib. Because of the curvature of the ribs, these changes in muscle length are greatest in

the dorsal region of the rib cage, decrease progressively as one moves around the cage, and are reversed as one approaches the sternum. The second reason is that the Hamberger theory is based on the idea that all the ribs rotate by equal amounts around parallel axes so that the distance between adjacent ribs remains constant. In fact, the radii of curvature of the different ribs are different, increasing from the top downward, and their rotational compliances are different as well.[19,25]

RESPIRATORY FUNCTION OF THE INTERCOSTAL MUSCLES

Regardless of the limitations of the Hamberger theory, a number of electromyographic studies in dogs,[17,26] cats,[27] and baboons[28] have clearly established that the parasternal intercostals are electrically active during the inspiratory phase of the breathing cycle (Fig. 3-5). Electromyographic recordings from intercostal muscles and nerves in these animals also have established that the external intercostal and levator costae muscles are active only during inspiration (see Fig. 3-5), whereas the internal interosseous intercostals are active only during expiration.[20,27–32] Of interest, the inspiratory activation of the external intercostals takes place predominantly in the dorsal region of the rostral interspaces,[27,29,32] where the muscles are thickest and have the greatest inspiratory mechanical advantage.[25] These features correspond to an inspiratory action on the rib cage, and indeed, when the diaphragm and parasternal intercostals in dogs are denervated so that the external intercostals and levator costae are the only muscles active during inspiration, the ribs move cranially.[20] Conversely, expiratory activation of the internal interosseous intercostals is predominant in the caudal interspaces,[32] where the muscles have a greater expiratory mechanical advantage.[25] This pattern corresponds to an expiratory action on the rib cage and the lung.[33]

Although the parasternal intercostals, the external intercostals in the rostral interspaces, and the levator costae contract together during inspiration and contribute to the inspiratory cranial displacement of the ribs, there is substantial evidence that in anesthetized animals the parasternal intercostals play a larger role than the external intercostals and levator costae during resting breathing. In anesthetized dogs and cats, the cranial motion of the ribs occurs together with a caudal displacement of the sternum.[4,17,34] This pattern of motion is due to the action of the parasternal intercostals.[17] Indeed, selective stimulation of these muscles causes the sternum to move caudally, whereas both the external intercostals and the levator costae displace the sternum cranially.[20,33] More important, when the canine parasternal intercostals are denervated in all interspaces, the inspiratory cranial motion of the ribs is reduced by 60 percent, yet the external intercostal and levator costae inspiratory activities are markedly increased.[35,36] Presumably these increases in inspiratory activity reduce the decrease in cranial rib motion resulting from the denervation of the parasternals. In contrast, when the canine external intercostals in all interspaces are severed and the parasternal intercostals are left intact, the inspiratory cranial displacement of the ribs decreases by only 10 percent, although the parasternal inspiratory activity is unchanged.[35]

Normal humans breathing at rest also have inspiratory activity in the parasternal intercostals and in the external

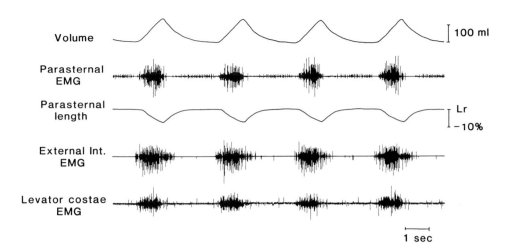

FIGURE 3-5 Pattern of electrical activation of the parasternal intercostal, external intercostal, and levator costae muscles in the baboon during resting breathing. The traces of lung volume (increase upward) and parasternal intercostal length (decrease downward) are also shown. Note that the three muscles (recorded in the third intercostal space) are active during inspiration; the parasternal intercostal also shortens in phase with inspiration.

intercostals of the most rostral interspaces.[37,38] Although it is difficult to compare the amounts of activity recorded in different muscles, activity in the human external intercostals also appears to be less consistent and to involve fewer motor units than activity in the parasternal intercostals.[37–39] This suggests that in humans as in quadrupeds, the contribution of the parasternal intercostals to resting breathing is greater than that of the external intercostals. In contrast to the parasternal intercostals, the external intercostals and levator costae are abundantly supplied with muscle spindles,[31,40] and they might therefore constitute a reserve, "load-compensating" system.[41]

NONRESPIRATORY FUNCTION OF THE INTERCOSTAL MUSCLES

The insertions and orientations of the external intercostals also suggest that contraction of these muscles on one side of the sternum would rotate the ribs in a transverse plane so that the upper ribs would move forward while the lower ribs would move backward (Fig. 3-6). In contrast, contraction of the internal intercostals on one side of the sternum would displace the upper ribs backward and the lower ribs forward. These muscles, therefore, would be ideally suited to twist the rib cage.

Measurements of the changes in length of these muscles during passive rotations of the thorax in anesthetized dogs have supported this idea.[23] When the animal's trunk was twisted to the left, the external intercostals on the right side of the chest and the internal interosseous intercostals on the left side shortened considerably. At the same time, the external intercostals on the left side and the internal intercostals on the right side lengthened. The opposite pattern was seen when the animal's trunk was passively rotated to the right, with a marked shortening of the right internal and left external intercostals and a lengthening of the left internals and right externals. Thus the length of these muscles changed in the way expected if they were producing the rotations, and indeed, electromyographic studies in normal humans have demonstrated recently that the external intercostals on the right side of the chest are active when the trunk is rotated to the left, whereas they are silent when the trunk is rotated to the right.[42] Conversely, the internal intercostals on the right side of the chest are active only when the trunk is

rotated to the right. Active use of these muscles during such postural movements is also consistent with their abundant supply of muscle spindles.

THE TRIANGULARIS STERNI

The *triangularis sterni*, also called the *transversus thoracis*, is a flat muscle that lies deep to the sternum and the parasternal intercostals. As shown in Fig. 3-7, its fibers originate from the dorsal aspect of the caudal half of the sternum and insert into the inner surface of the chondrocostal junctions of ribs 3 to 7. The muscle receives its motor supply from the intercostal nerves, and in the dog, its selective stimulation causes a caudal displacement of the ribs with a cranial motion of the sternum.[43]

FIGURE 3-6 Diagram illustrating the actions of the intercostal muscles during rotations of the trunk. Lateral view of an intercostal space on the right side of the chest. The two bars oriented obliquely represent two adjacent ribs. The external and internal intercostal muscles are depicted as single bundles, and the arrows indicate the component of tension vector acting along the ribs. [Reprinted, with permission, from A De Troyer: Mechanics of the chest wall muscles, in AD Miller, B Bishop, and AL Bianchi (eds): *Neural Control of the Respiratory Muscles.* Roca Raton, FL, CRC Press, 1996, pp 59–73.]

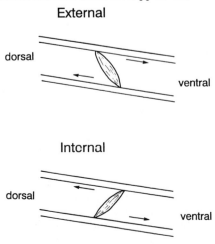

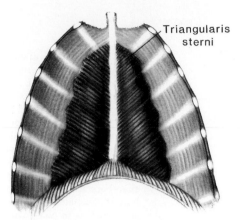

Triangularis
sterni

FIGURE 3-7 Dorsal aspect of the ventral wall of the rib cage in the dog, illustrating the insertions of the triangularis sterni muscle. Note that the rostral portion of the sternum and the first two ribs have been reflected; the triangularis sterni has no insertions there. [Reprinted, with permission, from A De Troyer and SH Loring: Actions of the respiratory muscles, in C Roussos (ed): *The Thorax*, 2d ed. New York, Marcel Dekker, 1995, pp 535–563.]

This muscle has an important respiratory function in mammalian quadrupeds. In the dog and the cat, it invariably contracts during the expiratory phase of the breathing cycle,[43,44] and in so doing it pulls the ribs caudally and deflates the rib cage below its neutral (resting) position.[43] Consequently, when the muscle relaxes at the end of expiration, there is a passive rib cage expansion and an increase in lung volume that precedes the onset of inspiratory muscle contraction. In these animals, the triangularis sterni thus shares the work of breathing with the inspiratory muscles and helps the parasternal intercostals produce the rhythmic inspiratory expansion of the rib cage.[43]

In contrast to quadrupeds, the triangularis sterni in normal humans is usually inactive during resting breathing.[45] However, it invariably contracts during voluntary or involuntary expiratory efforts such as coughing, laughing, and speech. Normal humans, in fact, cannot produce expiratory efforts without contracting the triangularis sterni. Presumably, the muscle then acts in concert with the internal interosseous intercostals to deflate the rib cage and increase pleural pressure.

THE SCALENES

The scalenes in humans comprise three muscle bundles that run from the transverse processes of the lower five cervical vertebrae to the upper surface of the first two ribs. When these muscles are selectively activated by electrical stimulation in dogs, they produce a marked cranial displacement of the ribs and sternum and cause an increase in the rib cage anteroposterior diameter. Although the scalenes traditionally have been considered as "accessory" muscles of inspiration, electromyographic studies with concentric needle electrodes have established that in normal humans they invariably contract in concert with the diaphragm and the parasternal intercostals during inspiration.[38,46,47]

There is no clinical setting that causes paralysis of all the inspiratory muscles without also affecting the scalenes.

Therefore, the isolated action of these muscles on the human rib cage cannot be defined precisely. Several observations, however, indicate that contraction of the scalenes is an important determinant of the motion of the sternum and the upper ribs during breathing. First, the sternum in resting humans moves cranially during inspiration. In contrast, in the dog, the scalenes are not active during breathing,[48] and the sternum moves caudally rather than cranially.[17] Second, when normal subjects attempt to inspire with the diaphragm alone, there is a marked, selective decrease in scalene activity associated with either less inspiratory increase or a paradoxical decrease in anteroposterior diameter of the upper rib cage.[47] Third, the inward inspiratory displacement of the upper rib cage characteristic of quadriplegia (see "Quadriplegia" below) is usually not observed when scalene function is preserved after lower cervical cord transection.[11] Since the scalenes are innervated from the lower five cervical segments, persistent inspiratory contraction is seen frequently in subjects with a transection at the C7 level or below. In such subjects, the anteroposterior diameter of the upper rib cage tends to remain constant or to increase slightly during inspiration.

THE STERNOCLEIDOMASTOIDS AND OTHER ACCESSORY MUSCLES OF INSPIRATION

Many additional muscles, such as the pectoralis minor, the trapezius, the erector spinae, the serrati, and the sternocleidomastoids, can elevate the ribs when they contract. These muscles, however, run between the shoulder girdle and the rib cage, between the spine and the shoulder girdle, or between the head and the rib cage. Therefore, they have primarily postural functions. In healthy individuals, they contract only during increased inspiratory efforts and, in contrast to the scalenes, are thus real "accessory" muscles of inspiration.

Of all these muscles, only the sternocleidomastoids have been studied thoroughly. These descend from the mastoid process to the ventral surface of the manubrium sterni and the medial third of the clavicle, and their action in humans has been inferred from measurements of chest wall motion in patients with transection of the upper cervical cord. Indeed, in such patients, the diaphragm and the intercostal, scalene, and abdominal muscles are paralyzed, but the sternocleidomastoids (the motor innervation of which largely depends on the eleventh cranial nerve) are spared and contract forcefully during unassisted inspiration.[5,8] When breathing spontaneously, these patients show a marked inspiratory cranial displacement of the sternum and a large inspiratory expansion of the upper rib cage, particularly in its anteroposterior diameter. These patients, however, also have an inspiratory decrease in the transverse diameter of the lower rib cage[5,8] (Fig. 3-8).

The Abdominal Muscles

The four abdominal muscles that have a significant respiratory function in humans constitute the ventrolateral wall of the abdomen. The *rectus abdominis* is the most ventral of these muscles. It originates from the ventral aspect of the sternum and the fifth, sixth, and seventh costal cartilages, and it runs caudally along the whole length of the abdominal wall to insert into the pubis. This muscle is enclosed in a sheath

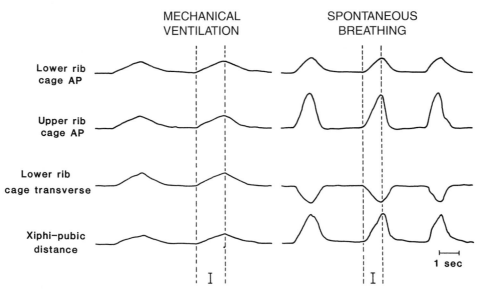

MECHANICAL VENTILATION

SPONTANEOUS BREATHING

Lower rib cage AP

Upper rib cage AP

Lower rib cage transverse

Xiphi–pubic distance

1 sec

FIGURE 3-8 Pattern of rib cage motion during mechanical ventilation (*left*) and during spontaneous breathing (*right*) in a quadriplegic subject with a traumatic transection of the upper cervical cord (C1). Each panel shows, from top to bottom, the respiratory changes in anteroposterior (AP) diameter of the lower rib cage, the changes in AP diameter of the upper rib cage, the changes in transverse diameter of the lower rib cage, and the changes in xiphipubic distance. Upward deflections correspond to an increase in diameter or an increase in xiphipubic distance (i.e., a cranial displacement of the sternum). *I* indicates the duration of inspiration. Note that during mechanical ventilation, all rib cage diameters and the xiphipubic distance increase in phase. During spontaneous inspiration, however, the xiphipubic distance and the upper rib cage AP diameter increase more than the lower rib cage AP diameter, and the lower rib cage transverse diameter decreases. [Reprinted, with permission, from A De Troyer: Mechanics of the chest wall muscles, in AD Miller, B Bishop, and AL Bianchi (eds): *Neural Control of the Respiratory Muscles*. Roca Raton, FL, CRC Press, 1996, pp 59–73.]

formed by the aponeuroses of the other three muscles. The most superficial of these is the *external oblique,* which originates by fleshy digitations from the external surface of the lower eight ribs, well above the costal margin, and directly covers the lower ribs and intercostal muscles. Its fibers radiate caudally to the iliac crest and inguinal ligament and medially to the linea alba. The *internal oblique* lies deep to the external oblique. Its fibers arise from the iliac crest and inguinal ligament, and they diverge to insert on the costal margin and an aponeurosis contributing to the rectus sheath down to the pubis. The *transversus abdominis* is the deepest of the muscles of the lateral abdominal wall. It arises from the inner surface of the lower six ribs, where it interdigitates with the costal insertions of the diaphragm. From this origin and from the lumbar fascia, the iliac crest, and the inguinal ligament, its fibers run circumferentially around the abdominal visceral mass and terminate ventrally in the rectus sheath.

ACTIONS OF THE ABDOMINAL MUSCLES

These four muscles have important functions as flexors (rectus abdominis) and rotators (external oblique, internal oblique) of the trunk, but as respiratory muscles, they have two principal actions. First, as they contract, they pull the abdominal wall inward and produce an increase in abdominal pressure. This causes the diaphragm to move cranially into the thoracic cavity, and this motion, in turn, results in an increase in pleural pressure and a decrease in lung volume. Second, these four muscles displace the rib cage due to their insertions on the ribs. These insertions would suggest that

the action of all abdominal muscles is to pull the lower ribs caudally and to deflate the cage, another expiratory action. Measurements of rib cage motion during electrical stimulation of the four abdominal muscles in dogs have shown, however, that the rise in abdominal pressure produced by these muscles also confers to them an inspiratory action on the rib cage.[49,50] Indeed, the zone of apposition of the diaphragm to the rib cage (see Fig. 3-1) allows the rise in abdominal pressure to be transmitted to the lower rib cage. In addition, by forcing the diaphragm cranially and stretching it, the rise in abdominal pressure causes passive diaphragmatic tension. This passive tension tends to raise the lower ribs and to expand the lower rib cage in the same way as does an active diaphragmatic contraction (insertional force of the diaphragm).

The action of the abdominal muscles on the rib cage is thus determined by the balance between the insertional, expiratory force of the muscles and the inspiratory force related to the rise in abdominal pressure. Isolated contraction of the external oblique in humans produces a small caudal displacement of the sternum and a large decrease in the rib cage transverse diameter, but the rectus abdominis, while causing a marked caudal displacement of the sternum and a large decrease in the anteroposterior diameter of the rib cage, also produces a small increase in the rib cage transverse diameter.[51] The isolated actions of the internal oblique and transversus abdominis muscles on the human rib cage are not known, but the anatomic arrangement of the transversus suggests that among the abdominal muscles, this muscle has the smallest insertional, expiratory action on the ribs and the greatest effect on abdominal pressure. Therefore, isolated contraction

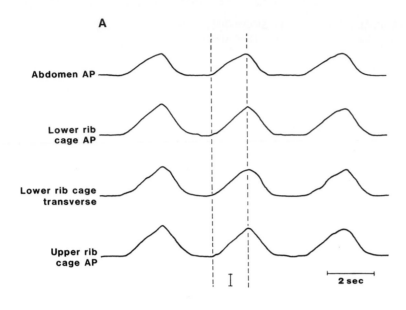

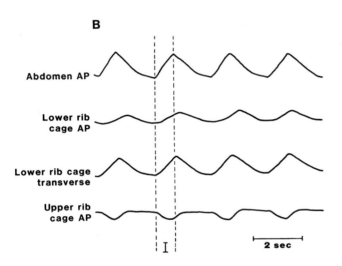

FIGURE 3-9 Pattern of chest wall motion in a healthy subject (*A*) and a C5 quadriplegic patient (*B*) breathing at rest in the seated posture. The respiratory changes in anteroposterior (AP) diameter of the abdomen, lower rib cage, and upper rib cage are shown, as well as the changes in transverse diameter of the lower rib cage. Same conventions as in Fig. 3–8. [Reprinted, with permission, from A De Troyer and M Estenne: The respiratory system in neuromuscular disorders, in C Roussos (ed): *The Thorax,* 2d ed. New York, Marcel Dekker, 1995, pp 2177–2212.]

of the transversus should produce little or no expiratory rib cage displacement.

RESPIRATORY FUNCTION OF THE ABDOMINAL MUSCLES

Irrespective of their actions on the rib cage, the abdominal muscles are primarily expiratory muscles through their action on the diaphragm and the lung, and they play important roles in activities such as coughing and speaking. However, when they contract rhythmically in phase with expiration and reduce lung volume below the neutral position of the respiratory system, their relaxation at end-expiration may promote a passive descent of the diaphragm and induce an increase in lung volume before the onset of inspiratory muscle contraction. The abdominal muscles therefore also may be considered as accessory muscles of inspiration.

This inspiratory action of the abdominal muscles takes place all the time in quadrupeds, and in dogs placed in the head-up or the prone position, the relaxation of the abdominal muscles at end-expiration accounts for up to 40 to 60 percent of the tidal volume.[52,53] Adult humans do not utilize such a breathing strategy at rest. However, phasic expiratory contraction of the abdominal muscles occurs in healthy subjects whenever the demand placed on the inspiratory muscles is abnormally increased, such as during exercise or during CO_2-induced hyperpnea. It is noteworthy that in these conditions, the transversus muscle is recruited well before activity can be recorded from either the rectus or the external oblique.[54,55] In view of the actions of these muscles, this differential recruitment also supports the idea that the effect of the abdominal muscles on abdominal pressure is more important to the act of breathing than their action on the rib cage.

There is a second mechanism by which the abdominal muscles can assist inspiration. Most normal human subjects, when adopting the standing posture, develop tonic abdominal muscle activity unrelated to the phases of the breathing cycle,[56] and studies in patients with transection of the upper cervical cord, in whom bilateral pacing of the phrenic nerves allows the degree of diaphragmatic activation to be maintained constant, have clearly illustrated the effect of this tonic abdominal contraction on inspiration.[8,9] When the patients

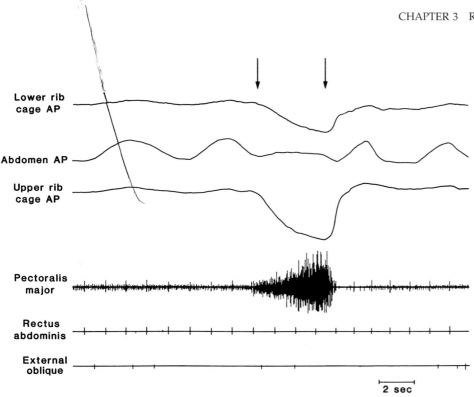

Lower rib cage AP

Abdomen AP

Upper rib cage AP

Pectoralis major

Rectus abdominis

External oblique

2 sec

FIGURE 3-10 Pattern of chest wall motion and respiratory muscle use during voluntary expiration from functional residual capacity in a C6 quadriplegic subject. The changes in anteroposterior (AP) diameter of the abdomen, the lower rib cage, and the upper rib cage are shown (increase upward). Arrows mark the onset and the end of the expiratory effort. Expiration elicits a large amount of electromyographic activity in the pectoralis major (clavicular portion) and causes a marked decrease in the AP diameter of the upper rib cage. The abdominal muscles show no activity and the AP diameter of the abdomen paradoxically increases under the influence of abdominal pressure (From De Troyer et al, [57] with permission.)

were supine, the unassisted paced diaphragm was able to generate an adequate tidal volume. However, when the patients were tilted head-up or moved to the seated posture, the weight of the abdominal viscera and the absence of abdominal muscle activity caused the stomach wall to protrude. The tidal volume produced by pacing in this posture was markedly reduced relative to the supine posture, but the reduction was significantly diminished when a pneumatic cuff was inflated around the abdomen to mimic tonic abdominal muscle contraction. Thus, by contracting throughout the breathing cycle in the standing posture, the abdominal muscles make the diaphragm longer at the onset of inspiration and prevent it from shortening excessively during inspiration; in accordance with the length-tension characteristics of the muscle, its ability to generate pressure is therefore increased.

Respiratory Muscle Function in Diseases

QUADRIPLEGIA

As pointed out earlier, the particular distribution of muscle paralysis in patients with traumatic transection of the lower cervical cord causes distinct abnormalities in the pattern of chest wall motion during breathing (Fig. 3-9). Because diaphragmatic function is preserved in these patients, the expansion of the abdomen during inspiration is associated with an expansion of the lower rib cage. However, whereas in healthy subjects the entire rib cage expands synchronously and uniformly, the lower rib cage in quadriplegic patients expands predominantly over its lateral walls, where the area of apposed diaphragm is greater (greater appositional force).[11] In addition, the paralysis of the rib cage inspiratory muscles, in particular the scalenes and the parasternal intercostals, is such that many quadriplegic patients at rest have

an inspiratory decrease (paradoxical motion) of the anteroposterior diameter of the upper rib cage.[10,11]

Quadriplegic patients also have complete paralysis of all the well-recognized muscles of expiration (abdominal muscles, internal intercostals, triangularis sterni). As a result, the expiratory reserve volume (ERV) is markedly reduced, and RV is usually greater than normal. The peak pleural pressures developed during cough are also less than normal, and indeed, in such patients, the efficiency of cough and the clearance of bronchial secretions are severely impaired. Several studies, however, have demonstrated that most quadriplegic patients have residual expiratory muscle function due to the action of the clavicular portion of the pectoralis major.[57,58] In patients with transection at the C6 segment or below, this muscle bundle invariably contracts during voluntary expiration (Fig. 3-10) and during cough, and its insertions on the humerus and the medial half of the clavicle make it displace the manubrium sterni and the upper ribs in a caudal direction when it contracts on both sides of the chest.[57] In so doing, it produces collapse of the upper rib cage and partial emptying of the lung. In a number of patients, the clavicular portion of the pectoralis major may even induce dynamic compression of the intrathoracic airways,[59] thus indicating that cough in this setting is not necessarily a passive phenomenon as conventionally thought.

DIAPHRAGMATIC PARALYSIS

Paralysis or severe weakness of both hemidiaphragms is seen usually in the context of generalized respiratory muscle weakness, but in occasional patients the diaphragm is specifically or disproportionately affected. Selective paralysis of the diaphragm results in a compensatory increase in the activation of the inspiratory rib cage muscles so that the inspiratory expansion of the rib cage compartment of the

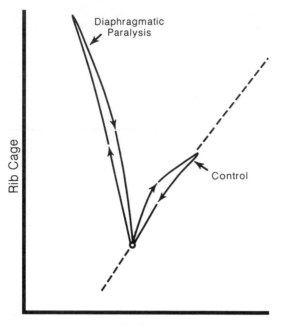

FIGURE 3-11 Pattern of chest wall motion during resting breathing in a supine anesthetized dog before (control) and after bilateral section of the phrenic nerves in the neck (diaphragmatic paralysis). The changes in abdominal cross section are on the abscissa (increase rightward), and the changes in rib cage cross section are on the ordinate (increase upward). The broken line represents the relaxation curve of the thoracoabdominal system, and the solid loops represent tidal volume cycles; arrows indicate the direction of the loops; and the open circle corresponds to end expiration. During breathing in the control condition, the chest wall moves on its relaxed configuration. After induction of diaphragmatic paralysis, however, the rib cage expands markedly during inspiration, but the abdomen moves paradoxically inward. (Adapted from De Troyer and Kelly,[17] with permission.)

chest wall is accentuated.[17,60] In addition, whereas in healthy subjects the simultaneous contraction of the diaphragm and the rib cage inspiratory muscles causes a rise in abdominal pressure associated with a fall in pleural pressure, in the presence of diaphragmatic paralysis the fall in pleural pressure is transmitted through the flaccid diaphragm such that abdominal pressure falls as well. As a result, the abdomen moves paradoxically inward, opposing the inflation of the lung[17] (Fig. 3-11).

Some patients also compensate for diaphragmatic paralysis by contracting the abdominal muscles during expiration, thus displacing the abdomen inward and the diaphragm cranially into the thorax. Relaxation of the abdominal muscles at the onset of inspiration therefore may result in outward abdominal motion and passive descent of the diaphragm.[61,62] Such a contraction of the abdominal muscles during expiration seems to be particularly frequent in the erect patient, and when present, it may remove the inspiratory inward motion of the abdomen that is the cardinal sign of diaphragmatic paralysis on clinical examination. However, this does not occur in the supine posture, where the abdominal muscles usually remain relaxed during the whole respiratory cycle.

CHRONIC OBSTRUCTIVE PULMONARY DISEASE (COPD)

Measurements of thoracoabdominal motion during breathing have shown that patients with COPD and hyperinflation have relatively greater expansion of the rib cage and smaller expansion of the abdomen than healthy subjects.[63,64] The normal inspiratory positive swing of abdominal pressure is also attenuated,[63–65] whereas the fall in pleural pressure is greater than normal due to the increased airflow resistance and the reduced dynamic pulmonary compliance. In patients with severe disease, abdominal pressure may even become negative during inspiration, and the abdomen may move paradoxically inward, as if the diaphragm were paralyzed.[63,64,66] This altered pattern has led to the widespread belief that these patients have more use of the rib cage inspiratory muscles and less use of the diaphragm than healthy subjects, possibly due to diaphragmatic fatigue.[64,67]

In agreement with this idea, the scalenes and parasternal intercostals feel tense on palpation in many patients with severe COPD. Recent electromyographic studies using concentric needle electrodes also have shown that although most of these patients do not contract the sternocleidomastoids or the trapezii when breathing at rest,[68] they have increased firing frequencies in the parasternal intercostal and scalene motor units compared with normal subjects.[69] The patients also had a greater number of active motor units in these two muscles. On the other hand, diaphragmatic motor units also demonstrated substantial increases in firing frequency during resting breathing, thus indicating that COPD is associated with an increase in neural drive not only to the rib cage inspiratory muscles but also to the diaphragm.[70] This suggests that the altered thoracoabdominal motion seen during inspiration in these patients results from mechanical factors alone.

The diaphragm in such patients is characteristically flat and low compared with normal subjects, and the zone of apposition is reduced in size. Therefore, irrespective of the degree of neural activation, the ability of the diaphragmatic dome to descend is impaired, and hence the rise in abdominal pressure and the outward displacement of the abdominal wall must be reduced. In some patients with severe hyperinflation, the zone of apposition has virtually disappeared, and the normal curvature of the diaphragm is even reversed, with its concavity facing upward rather than downward. The muscle fibers at their insertions on the ribs then run transversely inward rather than cranially. In this situation, contraction of the diaphragm cannot result in any descent of the dome. Instead, the vigorous contraction of the rib cage inspiratory muscles, resulting in a greater than normal elevation of the ribs, will tend to pull the diaphragm cranially and to displace the ventral abdominal wall inward. Contraction of this flat diaphragm, however, produces an inspiratory decrease in the transverse diameter of the lower rib cage (Hoover's sign).[71]

Patients with severe COPD also have a greater than normal neural drive to the abdominal muscles. Indeed, in contrast to normal subjects, many resting patients with severe COPD have phasic expiratory contraction of the abdominal muscles, in particular the transversus abdominis.[72] This causes a decrease in abdominal dimensions associated with an increase in abdominal pressure,[73] and in occasional patients it produces a paradoxical increase in the anteroposterior diameter of the lower rib cage.[71] Although this expiratory muscle contraction might be considered as a compensation for the relatively ineffective diaphragm, its usefulness is uncertain. As pointed out previously (see "Respiratory Function of the Abdominal Muscles" above), expiratory contraction of the abdominal muscles is a natural component of the response of the normal respiratory system to increased stimulation. In the absence of expiratory flow limitation, this expiratory muscle contraction is appropriate because it allows the work of breathing to be shared between the inspiratory and expiratory muscles. In patients with severe COPD and airflow limitation, however, this "automatic" response to increased ventilatory stimulation might be present during resting breathing without producing significant deflation of the respiratory system.[72]

Conclusions

Although the diaphragm is the main respiratory muscle in humans, it is not the only important contracting muscle. It expands the abdomen and the lower rib cage, but the expansion of the cranial half of the rib cage is accomplished by other inspiratory muscles, in particular the scalenes and the parasternal intercostals. Additional muscles, such as the transversus abdominis and the triangularis sterni, are also frequently involved in the act of breathing, particularly when the ventilatory requirements are increased. These muscles are usually considered to be expiratory because they displace the respiratory system below its resting volume. By relaxing at end-expiration, however, they also cause an increase in lung volume, thereby reducing the load on the inspiratory muscles. Moving the chest wall during breathing is thus a complex, integrated process that involves many muscles, and the control mechanisms that promote coordinated use of these different muscles are critically important to maintaining alveolar ventilation within acceptable limits. These mechanisms already play an important role in healthy subjects, but they become absolutely essential to life in conditions where the diaphragm is less effective or paralyzed.

References

1. Konno K, Mead J: Measurement of the separate volume changes of rib cage and abdomen during breathing. *J Appl Physiol* 22:407, 1967.
2. Jordanoglou J: Vector analysis of rib movement. *Respir Physiol* 10:109, 1970.
3. Wilson TA, Rehder K, Krayer S, et al: Geometry and respiratory displacement of human ribs. *J Appl Physiol* 62:1872, 1987.
4. De Troyer A, Decramer M: Mechanical coupling between the ribs and sternum in the dog. *Respir Physiol* 59:27, 1985.
5. De Troyer A, Estenne M, Vincken W: Rib cage motion and muscle use in high tetraplegics. *Am Rev Respir Dis* 133:1115, 1986.
6. Mead J: Functional significance of the area of apposition of diaphragm to rib cage. *Am Rev Respir Dis* 119:31, 1979.
7. D'Angelo E, Sant'Ambrogio G: Direct action of contracting diaphragm on the rib cage in rabbits and dogs. *J Appl Physiol* 36:715, 1974.
8. Danon J, Druz WS, Goldberg NB, Sharp JT: Function of the isolated paced diaphragm and the cervical accessory muscles in C1 quadriplegics. *Am Rev Respir Dis* 119:909, 1979.
9. Strohl KP, Mead J, Banzett RB, et al: Effect of posture on upper and lower rib cage motion and tidal volume during diaphragm pacing. *Am Rev Respir Dis* 130:320, 1984.
10. Mortola JP, Sant'Ambrogio G: Motion of the rib cage and the abdomen in tetraplegic patients. *Clin Sci Mol Med* 54:25, 1978.
11. Estenne M, De Troyer A: Relationship between respiratory muscle electromyogram and rib cage motion in tetraplegia. *Am Rev Respir Dis* 132:53, 1985.
12. De Troyer A, Sampson M, Sigrist S, Macklem PT: Action of costal and crural parts of the diaphragm on the rib cage in dog. *J Appl Physiol* 53:30, 1982.
13. Loring SH, Mead J: Action of the diaphragm on the rib cage inferred from a force-balance analysis. *J Appl Physiol* 53:756, 1982.
14. Urmey WF, De Troyer A, Kelly SB, Loring SH: Pleural pressure increases during inspiration in the zone of apposition of diaphragm to rib cage. *J Appl Physiol* 65:2207, 1988.
15. Duchenne GB: *Physiologie des mouvements*. Paris, Baillière, 1867.
16. Hamberger GE: *De Respirationis Mechanismo et usu genuino*. Jena, Germany, 1749.
17. De Troyer A, Kelly S: Chest wall mechanics in dogs with acute diaphragm paralysis. *J Appl Physiol* 53:373, 1982.
18. Decramer M, De Troyer A: Respiratory changes in parasternal intercostal length. *J Appl Physiol* 57:1254, 1984.
19. De Troyer A, Legrand A, Wilson TA: Rostrocaudal gradient of mechanical advantage in the parasternal intercostal muscles of the dog. *J Physiol (Lond)* 495:239, 1996.
20. De Troyer A, Farkas GA: Inspiratory function of the levator costae and external intercostal muscles in the dog. *J Appl Physiol* 67:2614, 1989.
21. De Troyer A, Kelly S, Zin WA: Mechanical action of the intercostal muscles on the ribs. *Science* 220:87, 1983.
22. Ninane V, Gorini M, Estenne M: Action of intercostal muscles on the lung in dogs. *J Appl Physiol* 70:2388, 1991.
23. Decramer M, Kelly S, De Troyer A: Respiratory and postural changes in intercostal muscle length in supine dogs. *J Appl Physiol* 60:1686, 1986.
24. Saumarez RC: An analysis of action of intercostal muscles in human upper rib cage. *J Appl Physiol* 60:690, 1986.
25. Wilson TA, De Troyer A: Respiratory effect of the intercostal muscles in the dog. *J Appl Physiol* 75:2636, 1993.
26. De Troyer A, Farkas GA: Mechanics of the parasternal intercostals in prone dogs: Statics and dynamics. *J Appl Physiol* 74:2757, 1993.
27. Greer JJ, Martin TP: Distribution of muscle fiber types and EMG activity in cat intercostal muscles. *J Appl Physiol* 69:1208, 1990.
28. De Troyer A, Farkas GA: Contribution of the rib cage inspiratory muscles to breathing in baboons. *Respir Physiol* 97:135, 1994.
29. Bainton CR, Kirkwood PA, Sears TA: On the transmission of the stimulating effects of carbon dioxide to the muscles of respiration. *J Physiol (Lond.)* 280:249, 1978.
30. Sears TA: Efferent discharges in alpha and fusimotor fibres of intercostal nerves of the cat. *J Physiol (Lond)* 174:295, 1964.
31. Hilaire GG, Nicholls JG, Sears TA: Central and proprioceptive influences on the activity of the levator costae motoneurones in the cat. *J Physiol (Lond)* 342:527, 1983.
32. De Troyer A, Ninane V: Respiratory function of intercostal muscles in supine dog: An electromyographic study. *J Appl Physiol* 60:1692, 1986.
33. Loring SH, Woodbridge JA: Intercostal muscle action inferred from finite-element analysis. *J Appl Physiol* 70:2712, 1991.
34. Da Silva KMC, Sayers BMA, Sears TA, Stagg DT: The changes in configuration of the rib cage and abdomen during breathing in the anesthetized cat. *J Physiol (Lond)* 266:499, 1977.
35. De Troyer A: Inspiratory elevation of the ribs in the dog: Primary role of the parasternals. *J Appl Physiol* 70:1447, 1991.
36. De Troyer A, Yuehua C: Intercostal muscle compensation for parasternal paralysis in the dog: Central and proprioceptive mechanisms. *J Physiol (Lond)* 479:149, 1994.
37. Taylor A: The contribution of the intercostal muscles to the effort of respiration in man. *J Physiol (Lond)* 151:390, 1960.

38. Delhez L: *Contribution électromyographique à l'étude de la mécanique et du contrôle nerveux des mouvements respiratoires de l'homme.* Liège, Belgium, Vaillant-Carmanne, 1974.

39. Whitelaw WA, Feroah T: Patterns of intercostal muscle activity in humans. *J Appl Physiol* 67:2087, 1989.

40. Duron B, Jung-Caillol MC, Marlot D: Myelinated nerve fiber supply and muscle spindles in the respiratory muscles of cat: Quantitative study. *Anat Embryol* 152:171, 1978.

41. De Troyer A: Differential control of the inspiratory intercostal muscles during airway occlusion in the dog. *J Physiol (Lond)* 439:73, 1991.

42. Whitelaw WA, Ford GT, Rimmer KP, De Troyer A: Intercostal muscles are used during rotation of the thorax in humans. *J Appl Physiol* 72:1940, 1992.

43. De Troyer A, Ninane V: Triangularis sterni: A primary muscle of breathing in the dog. *J Appl Physiol* 60:14, 1986.

44. Hwang JC, Zhou D, St John WM: Characterization of expiratory intercostal activity to triangularis sterni in cats. *J Appl Physiol* 67:1518, 1989.

45. De Troyer A, Ninane V, Gimartin JJ, et al: Triangularis sterni muscle use in supine humans. *J Appl Physiol* 62:919, 1987.

46. Raper AJ, Thompson WT Jr, Shapiro W, Patterson JL Jr: Scalene and sternomastoid muscle function. *J Appl Physiol* 21:497, 1966.

47. De Troyer A, Estenne M: Coordination between rib cage muscles and diaphragm during quiet breathing in humans. *J Appl Physiol* 57:899, 1984.

48. De Troyer A, Cappello M, Brichant JF: Do the canine scalene and sternomastoid muscles play a role in breathing? *J Appl Physiol* 76:242, 1994.

49. De Troyer A, Sampson M, Sigrist S, Kelly S: How the abdominal muscles act on the rib cage. *J Appl Physiol* 54:465, 1983.

50. D'Angelo E, Prandi E, Bellemare F: Mechanics of the abdominal muscles in rabbits and dogs. *Respir Physiol* 97:275, 1994.

51. Mier A, Brophy C, Estenne M, et al: Action of abdominal muscles on rib cage in humans. *J Appl Physiol* 58:1438, 1985.

52. Farkas GA, Estenne M, De Troyer A: Expiratory muscle contribution to tidal volume in head-up dogs. *J Appl Physiol* 67:1438, 1989.

53. Farkas GA, Schroeder MA: Mechanical role of expiratory muscles during breathing in prone anesthetized dogs. *J Appl Physiol* 69:2137, 1990.

54. De Troyer A, Estenne M, Ninane V, et al: Transversus abdominis muscle function in humans. *J Appl Physiol* 68:1010, 1990.

55. Abe T, Kusuhara N, Yoshimura N, et al: Differential respiratory activity of four abdominal muscles in humans. *J Appl Physiol* 80:1379, 1996.

56. Floyd WF, Silver PHS: Electromyographic study of patterns of activity of the anterior abdominal wall muscles in man. *J Anat* 84:132, 1950.

57. De Troyer A, Estenne M, Heilporn A: Mechanism of active expiration in tetraplegic patients. *N Engl J Med* 314:740, 1986.

58. Estenne M, De Troyer A: Cough in tetraplegic subjects: an active process. *Ann Intern Med* 112:22, 1990.

59. Estenne M, Van Muylem A, Gorini M, et al: Evidence of dynamic airway compression during cough in tetraplegic subjects. *Am Rev Respir Dis* 150:1081, 1994.

60. De Troyer A: The electro-mechanical response of canine inspiratory intercostal muscles to increased resistance: The cranial rib-cage. *J Physiol (Lond)* 451:445, 1992.

61. Newsom Davis J, Goldman M, Loh L, Casson M: Diaphragm function and alveolar hypoventilation. *Q J Med* 45:87, 1976.

62. Kreitzer SM, Feldman NT, Saunders NA, Ingram RH: Bilateral diaphragmatic paralysis with hypercapnic respiratory failure: A physiologic assessment. *Am J Med* 65:89, 1978.

63. Sharp JT, Goldberg NB, Druz WS, et al: Thoracoabdominal motion in chronic obstructive pulmonary disease. *Am Rev Respir Dis* 115:47, 1977.

64. Martinez FJ, Couser JI, Celli BR: Factors influencing ventilatory muscle recruitment in patients with chronic airflow obstruction. *Am Rev Respir Dis* 142:276, 1990.

65. Levine S, Gillen M, Weiser P, et al: Inspiratory pressure generation: Comparison of subjects with COPD and age-matched normals. *J Appl Physiol* 65:888, 1988.

66. Ashutosh K, Gilbert R, Auchincloss JH Jr, Peppi D: Asynchronous breathing movements in patients with chronic obstructive pulmonary disease. *Chest* 67:553, 1975.

67. Cohen CA, Zagelbaum G, Gross D, et al: Clinical manifestations of inspiratory muscle fatigue. *Am J Med* 73:308, 1982.

68. De Troyer A, Peche R, Yernault JC, Estenne M: Neck muscle activity in patients with severe chronic obstructive pulmonary disease. *Am J Respir Crit Care Med* 150:41, 1994.

69. Gandevia SC, Leeper JB, McKenzie DK, De Troyer A: Discharge frequencies of parasternal intercostal and scalene motor units during breathing in normal and COPD subjects. *Am J Respir Crit Care Med* 153:622, 1996.

70. De Troyer A, Leeper JB, McKenzie DK, Gandevia SC: Neural drive to the diaphragm in patients with severe COPD. *Am J Respir Crit Care Med* 155:1335, 1997.

71. Gilmartin JJ, Gibson GJ: Mechanisms of paradoxical rib cage motion in patients with chronic obstructive pulmonary disease. *Am Rev Respir Dis* 134:684, 1986.

72. Ninane V, Rypens F, Yernault JC, De Troyer A: Abdominal muscle use during breathing in patients with chronic airflow obstruction. *Am Rev Respir Dis* 146:16, 1992.

73. Ninane V, Yernault JC, De Troyer A: "Intrinsic PEEP" in patients with severe chronic obstructive pulmonary disease: Role of expiratory muscles. *Am Rev Respir Dis* 148:1037, 1993.

RESPIRATORY MUSCLES—STRUCTURAL CONSIDERATIONS

VINOD SAHGAL

SEVGI TETIK

Part I _____

The respiratory muscles are morphologically and functionally the skeletal muscles with the primary task of displacing the chest wall rhythmically to pump air in and out of the lungs. Understanding the actions of the respiratory muscles requires a clear understanding of their structure, function, and biochemical composition as well as the mechanical properties of the chest wall.[1]

Gross Anatomy of the Respiratory Muscles

The respiratory muscular system is divided into the rib cage and the abdominal muscles, separated by the diaphragm (Fig. 4-1).

DIAPHRAGM

The diaphragm is a dome-shaped, movable musculotendinous partition between the thoracic and abdominal cavities,[2] and it is the principal muscle of respiration.

The diaphragm is composed of two portions: a peripheral muscular part and a central aponeurotic part, the central tendon[1] (Fig. 4-1).

MUSCULAR PART OF THE DIAPHRAGM

The diaphragm is anatomically unique among skeletal muscles in that its muscle fibers radiate from a central tendinous structure (the central tendon) to insert peripherally into solid structures.[1] Because of the distinct attachments (origins), the muscular part is divided into three parts (sternal, costal, and lumbar)[3] (Fig. 4-1).

STERNAL PART OF THE DIAPHRAGM

This portion consists of two small muscular slips that are attached to the posterior aspect of the xiphoid process of sternum. These slips converge radially to the central tendon.

COSTAL PART OF THE DIAPHRAGM

This portion consists of wide muscular slips that arise from the internal surfaces of the inferior six ribs and their costal cartilage on each side. These slips interdigitate with the slips of the transversus abdominis muscles. The costal parts from the right and left hemidiaphragms (domes) are visible on radiographs of the chest.[3]

LUMBAR PART OF THE DIAPHRAGM

This portion arises from the lumbar vertebrae by two musculotendinous crura, which are attached on each side of the

aorta to the anterolateral surfaces of the superior two (left) or three (right) lumbar vertebrae and the intervening intervertebral discs. The crura of the diaphragm blend with the anterior longitudinal ligament of the vertebral column. These are united opposite the disc between T12 and L1 vertebrae by a tendinous band or narrow arch, called the *median arcuate ligament.* It passes over the anterior surface of the aorta and provides attachment for some fibers of the right crus of the diaphragm. The diaphragm on each side is attached to the medial and lateral arcuate ligaments.

CENTRAL PART OF THE DIAPHRAGM

The muscular fibers of the diaphragm converge radially to a strong, sheetlike tendon or aponeurosis called the *central tendon,* which is fused with the inferior surface of the fibrous pericardium. The central tendon has no bony attachments and is divided into three segments, which resemble a clover leaf, giving it a C-shape appearance.[3]

Although the older literature repeatedly has suggested the possibility of an intercostal motor innervation of some portions of the diaphragm, it now is clearly established that the only motor supply to the diaphragm is through the phrenic nerves (C3-5). After bilateral sectioning of these nerves, the whole muscle becomes electrically silent and eventually undergoes denervation atrophy.[1]

RIB CAGE

The rib cage is a complex structure consisting of a series of skeletal arches. Developmentally, these reflect the segmental organization of the trunk and are constituted by the thoracic vertebrae, the bony ribs, the costal cartilages, and the sternum. All these skeletal supports are connected by articulations and ligaments that dictate the respiratory movements of the rib cage.[1]

MUSCLES OF THE RIB CAGE

INTERCOSTAL MUSCLES

Typically, the space between the ribs, called intercostal spaces, contain three layers of muscle (Fig. 4-1). The superficial layer is the external intercostal muscle, the middle layer is the internal intercostal muscle, and the deepest layer is discontinuous. This comprises three individual muscles: anteriorly the transverse thoracic (sternocostalis), laterally the innermost intercostalis, and posteriorly the subcostalis. They are innervated by 12 pairs of thoracic nerves[2] (Fig. 4-1).

EXTERNAL INTERCOSTAL MUSCLES

The principal inspiratory muscles of the rib cage are the external intercostalis. Each of the 11 pairs of muscles occupies the intercostal spaces from the tubercles of the ribs posteriorly to the costochondral junctions anteriorly. Anteriorly the muscles fibers are replaced by the external intercostal membranes. The muscles run inferoanteriorly from the rib above to the rib below. Each muscle is attached superiorly to the inferior border of the rib above and inferiorly to the superior border of the rib below. The external intercostal muscles are continuous inferiorly with the external oblique muscles of the anterolateral abdominal wall[3] (Fig. 4-1).

INTERNAL INTERCOSTAL MUSCLES

The 11 pairs of muscles run deeply to and at right angles to the external intercostal muscles. Their fibers run inferopos-

INSPIRATORY MUSCLES   **EXPIRATORY MUSCLES**

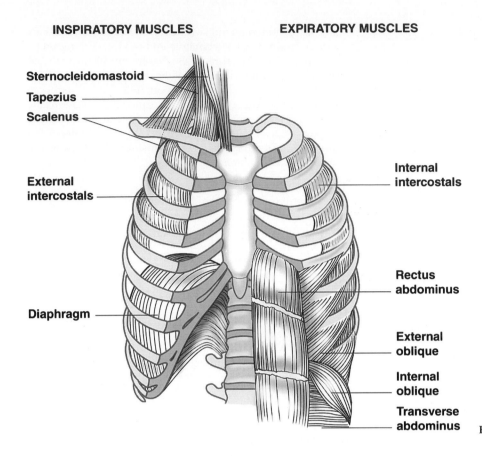

FIGURE 4-1 Muscles of respiration.

teriorly from the floors of the costal grooves to the superior borders of the ribs inferior to them. The internal intercostal muscles attach to the shafts of the ribs and their costal cartilages as far anteriorly as the sternum and as far posteriorly as the angles of the ribs. Between the ribs posteriorly, the internal intercostal muscles are replaced by the internal intercostal membranes. The inferior intercostal muscles are continuous with the internal oblique muscles of the anterolateral abdominal wall[3] (Fig. 4-1).

INNERMOST INTERCOSTAL MUSCLES
These muscles are the deep portion of the internal intercostal muscles. They are separated from the internal intercostal muscles by the intercostal nerves and vessels and pass between the internal surfaces of adjacent ribs.[3]

SUBCOSTAL MUSCLES
These muscle are thin slips that extend from the internal surface of the angle of the rib to the internal surface of the rib inferior to it, crossing one or two intercostal spaces. They run in the same direction as the internal intercostal muscles and lie internal to them.[3]

TRANSVERSUS THORACIC MUSCLES
These thin muscles consist of four or five slips that are attached posteriorly to the xiphoid process, the inferior part of the body of the sternum, and the adjacent costal cartilages. They pass superolaterally and are attached to the second to sixth costal cartilages. The transversus thoracic muscles are continuous inferiorly with the transversus abdominis muscle.

SCALENES
These muscles originate from the transverse processes of the lower five cervical vertebrae and are innervated by these spinal segments (Fig. 4-1). From their origins, the muscles slope caudally and insert on the upper surface of the first rib (scalene anterior and medial) and the second rib (scalene posterior).[1]

ACCESSORY MUSCLES OF INSPIRATION
There are many muscles that run between the head and rib cage, between the spine and the shoulder girdle, or between the shoulder girdle and rib cage and can operate to elevate the ribs. These include the pectoralis major and minor, the trapezii, the serratii, and the sternocleidomastoideus, as well as some laryngeal muscles. These muscles generally are included under the term *accessory muscles* of inspiration because they are inactive during quiet breathing. The sternocleidomastoid descends from the mastoid process to the ventral surface of the manubrium sterni and the medial third of the clavicle[1] (Fig. 4-1).

Innervation is from the cranial nerve XI and branches of the second and third cervical nerves.

ABDOMINAL MUSCLES
The abdominal muscles that have significant respiratory activity are those that constitute the ventrolateral wall of the abdomen. These are the rectus abdominis ventrally and the external and internal oblique and transversus abdominis laterally. These muscles are supplied by branches of the lower six thoracic nerves (T7-12) and first lumbar nerve[1] (Fig. 4-2).

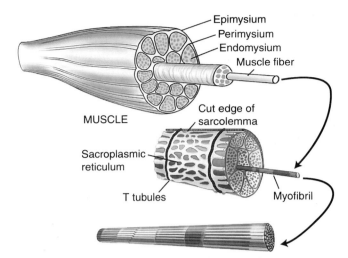

FIGURE 4-2 Structure of skeletal muscle. (Note the epimysium covering the entire muscle, perimysium covering the muscle bundle, and endomysium separating muscle fibers.)

Light Microscopic Anatomy and Histochemistry

ORGANIZATION OF SKELETAL MUSCLE FIBERS

The masses of fibers that make up the different types of muscle are not grouped in random fashion but are arranged in regular bundles surrounded by the *epimysium,* an external sheath of dense connective tissue surrounding the entire muscle. From the epimysium thin septa of connective tissue extend inward, surrounding the bundles of fibers with a muscle. The connective tissue around each bundle of muscle fibers is called the *perimysium.* Each muscle fiber is itself surrounded by a delicate layer of connective tissue, the *endomysium,* composed mainly of a basal lamina and reticular fibers (Fig. 4-2).

Skeletal muscle consists of muscle fibers. These are bundles of very long (up to 30 cm) cylindrical multinucleated cells with a diameter of 10 to 100 μm.[4]

As observed with the light microscope, longitudinally sectioned muscle cells or fibers show cross-striations of alternating light and dark bands. The darker bands are called A bands (anisotropic, i.e., birefringent in polarized light); the lighter bands are called I bands (isotropic, i.e., does not alter polarized light).[4]

HISTOCHEMICAL CHARACTERISTICS OF HUMAN RESPIRATORY MUSCLES

DIAPHRAGM

In general, muscle fibers are composed of two contractile protein filaments, myosin (thick filament) and actin (thin filament). Fibers containing myosin with high ATPase activity are classified as fast fibers, and those containing myosin with lower ATPase activity are slower fibers[5] (Fig. 4-3).

Fibers containing high concentrations of mitochondria and oxidative enzymes [the reduced form of nicotinamide-adenine dinucleotide (NADH), succinic dehydrogenase] have a high capacity for oxidative phosphorylation and are thus classified as oxidative fibers[5] (Fig. 4-3). These fibers also

have numerous capillaries and high myoglobin content. The large amounts of myoglobin give the muscle a dark red color; thus, oxidative fibers are also referred to as *red muscle.* In contrast, glycolytic fibers have few mitochondria but possess a high concentration of glycolytic enzymes with a large store of glycogen. These fibers, which have few blood vessels and contain little myoglobin, are glycolytic fibers and are referred to as *white muscle.*[5]

On the basis of these histochemical characteristics, the three types of diaphragmatic skeletal muscle fibers are referred to as type I, slow oxidative fibers; type IIA, fast oxidative fibers; and type IIB, fast glycolytic fibers (Table 4-1)[6] (Fig. 4-3).

The average fiber size of the coastal diaphragm determined using the cross-sectional area is 2200 μm^2 in normal subjects.[7,8] Type I fibers are slightly smaller than both type IIA and type IIB fibers. Thus, the size of diaphragmatic muscle fibers is relatively small compared with that of limb skeletal muscles.[9]

The relative occurrence of different fiber types and fiber sizes in the diaphragm has been described in animals[10,11] and humans,[12,13] including the histochemical differences between the crural and the costal parts of the diaphragm.[14]

From postmortem studies (where diaphragm muscle samples were obtained from previously healthy individuals who had suffered a sudden accidental death), the mean relative occurrence of type I fibers was approximately 50 percent.[7] The remaining proportion was evenly divided into type IIA (25 percent) and type IIB fibers (25 percent). Thus fiber type distribution of the diaphragm resembles the pattern exhibited in the limb muscles of untrained subjects.

INTERCOSTAL MUSCLES

The morphologic characteristics of the parasternal muscles, which are inspiratory, and the external intercostal muscles (EXT), which are also inspiratory, are quite different from the lateral internal intercostal muscles (INT), which are expiratory. It has been shown that fiber morphology and capillary supply of the intercostal muscles are a result of functional differences rather than their anatomic location.[7]

The relative occurrence of type I fibers is the same for all the intercostal muscles (62 percent), whereas the expiratory INT have more type IIA fibers (35 percent) than the parasternal INT and EXT (22 percent).[7,8] Accordingly, the expiratory INT have far fewer type IIB fibers (1 percent) than the inspiratory intercostal muscles (19 percent). Both the inspiratory and expiratory intercostal muscles have at least 10 percent more type I fibers than the diaphragm and most other skeletal muscles.[15]

The mean fiber cross-sectional area for the expiratory INT is large (4300 μm^2) compared with inspiratory INT and EXT (2900 μm^2). The inspiratory intercostal muscles show no significant difference in the cross-sectional area between sites and have a similar value to the diaphragm. The larger fiber area of expiratory INT is reflected by a greater area for both type I (3700 μm^2) and the type IIA fibers (5400 μm^2).[7] Thus the expiratory INT have large muscle fibers, and type IIA fibers are the largest. This result is in contrast to the inspiratory intercostal muscles, in which a similar area is seen among different fiber types.

The expiratory INT have a greater number of capillaries per fiber (2.3) than the inspiratory INT and EXT (1.6). Accord-

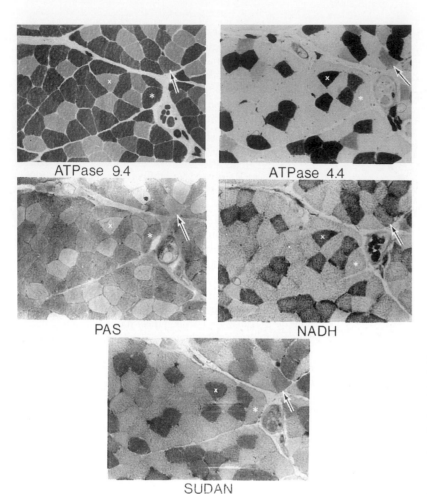

ATPase 9.4

ATPase 4.4

PAS

NADH

SUDAN

FIGURE 4-3 Histochemical profile of human skeletal muscle. ATPase pH 9.4: *, dark type 2B fibers; →, intermediate type 2A fibers; x, light type 1 fibers; Type 1 fibers, dark; type 2 fibers, light; type 2A fibers, intermediate color. PAS: Reactive type 2 fibers are dark; intermediate type 1 fibers are light; chain fibers are dark. NADH: Tetrazolium reductase close type 2 fibers are light; intermediate type 1 fibers are dark; SUDAN: Stain type 1 fibers are dark; type II fibers are light; intermediate color are reacting.

ingly, more capillaries are found around both type I and type IIA fibers (five to six) than in the inspiratory intercostal muscles.[7]

Enzyme Activities and Substrate Contents

MITOCHONDRIAL AND GLYCOLYTIC ENZYME ACTIVITIES

Mitochondrial enzyme activities, represented, for example, by citrate synthase (CS) and 3-hydroxyacyl-coenzyme A dehydrogenase (HAD), are within the range of values reported for skeletal muscles in the extremities of nonathletes.[15]

In patients with normal ventilatory function, HAD activity is slightly higher in the costal diaphragm than in both the EXT and expiratory INT. CS activity as well as glycolytic enzyme activities, represented as hexokinase (HK) and lactate dehydrogenase (LDH), are similar among these muscles.[16]

GLYCOGEN AND LACTATE

Like limb skeletal muscles, the average glycogen content of the diaphragm and intercostal muscles is 190 to 380 μmol

TABLE 4-1 The Characteristics of Diaphragmatic Muscle Fibers

Characteristics	Type I	Type IIA	Type IIB
Shortening velocity	Slow	Fast	Fast
ATPase activity	Low	High	High
Oxidative enzymes	High	High	Low
Mitochondrial content	High	High	Low
Capillary density	High	Intermediate	Low
Myoglobin content	High	High	Low
Primary source of ATP	Oxidative	Oxidative	Glycolytic
Glycogen content and enzymes	Low	Intermediate	High
Fiber diameter	Small	Intermediate	Large
Endurance	High	Intermediate	Low
Resistance to fatigue	High	Intermediate	Low
Force	Lowest	Intermediate	Highest
Recruitment order	First	Second	Third

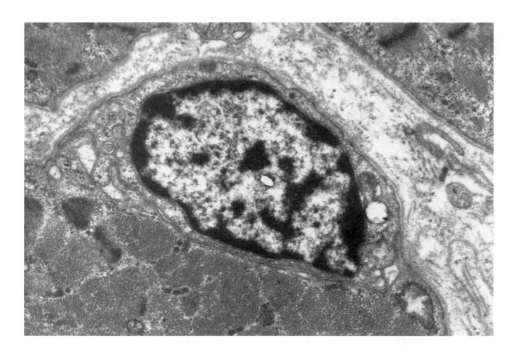

FIGURE 4-4 Oblique section of the diaphragm. (Note thick Z band, dark A band with gray M line, light I band, and sarcolemma, myonucleus, and mitochondria.)

per gram of dry weight, and lactate varies from 7 to 20 μmol per gram of dry weight.[9]

PHOSPHAGEN

Mean values of adenosine triphosphate (ATP) concentration in the diaphragm and intercostal muscles range between 10 and 20 μmol per gram of dry weight. The concentration of phosphocreatine ranges from 60 to 70 μmol per gram of dry weight. These values are similar to those reported for limb skeletal muscles.[15]

Ultrastructure

The ultrastructure of the respiratory muscles is like that of other skeletal muscles. With electron microscopy each I band can be observed to be bisected by a dark transverse line, the Z line (Fig. 4-3). The smallest repetitive subunit of the contractile apparatus, the sarcomere, extends from Z line to Z line and is about 2.5 μm long in resting muscle.

The sarcoplasm is filled with long, cylindrical, filamentous bundles called *myofibrils*. The myofibrils, which have diameter of 1 to 2 μm and are parallel to the long axis of the muscle fiber, consist of an end-to-end, chainlike arrangement of sarcomeres. Sarcomere pattern is due mainly to the presence of two types of filaments—thick and thin—that lie parallel to the long axis of the myofibrils in an asymmetric pattern.

The thick filaments are 1.6 μm long and 15 nm wide; they occupy the A band (Fig. 4-4), the central portion of the sarcomere. The thin filaments run between and parallel to the thick filaments and have one end attached to the Z line. Thin filaments are 1.0 μm long and 8 nm wide. Close observation of the A band shows the presence of a lighter zone in its center, the H band, that corresponds to a region consisting only of the rootlike portions of the myosin molecule. Bisecting the H band is the M line, a region where lateral connections are made between adjacent thick filaments (Fig. 4-4). The major protein of the M line is creatine kinase. Creatine

kinase catalyzes the transfer of a phosphate group from phosphocreatine to adenosine diphosphate (ADP), thus providing the supply to ATP necessary for muscle contraction.

Thin and thick filaments overlap for some distance within the A band. As a consequence, a cross section in the region of filament overlap shows each thick filament surrounded by six thin filaments in the form of a hexagon.

Striated muscle filaments contain several proteins; the four main proteins are actin, tropomyosin, troponin, and myosin. Thin filaments are composed of the first three proteins, whereas thick filaments consist primarily of myosin. Actin filaments, which anchor perpendicularly on the Z line, exhibit opposite polarity on each side of the line.[4]

SARCOPLASMIC RETICULUM AND TRANSVERSE TUBULE SYSTEM

The depolarization of the sarcoplasmic reticulum membrane, which results in the release of Ca^{2+} ions, is initiated at a specialized myoneuronal junction on the surface of the muscle cell. Surface-initiated depolarization signals would have to diffuse throughout the cell to effect the release of Ca^{2+} from internal sarcoplasmic reticulum cisterna. To provide for a uniform contraction, skeletal muscle possesses a system of transverse (T) tubules. These fingerlike investigations of sarcolemma form a complex anastomosing network of tubules that encircle the boundaries of each sarcomere in every myofibril.

Adjacent to opposite sides of each T tubule are expanded terminal cisterna of the sarcoplasmic reticulum (SR). This specialized complex, consisting of a T tubule with two lateral portions of SR, is known as the *triad*. At the triad, depolarization of the sarcolemma-derived T tubules is transmitted to the sarcoplasmic reticulum membrane.[4]

MYONEURAL JUNCTION (MOTOR END PLATE)

Myelinated motor nerves branch out within the perimysial connective tissue, where each nerve gives rise to several

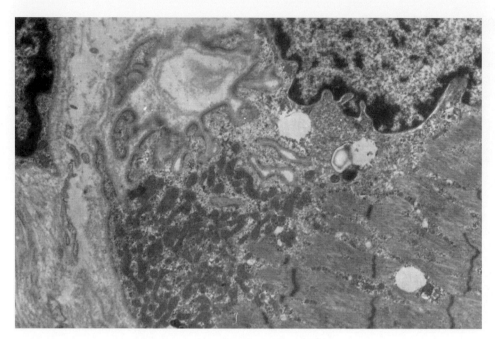

FIGURE 4-5 Ultrastructure of the myoneural junction from intercostal muscle. (Note the synaptic folds and clefts, subsarcolemmal collection of the mitochondria, and axon.)

terminal twigs. At the site of innervation, the nerve loses its myelin sheaths and forms a dilated termination that sits within a trough on the muscle cell surface. This structure is called the *motor end plate,* or *myoneural junction.* At this site, the axon is covered by a thin cytoplasmic layer of Schwann cells. Within the axon terminal are numerous mitochondria and synaptic vesicles, the latter containing the neurotransmitter acetylcholine. Between the axon and muscle is a space, the synaptic cleft, in which lies an amorphous basal lamina matrix. At the junction, the sarcolemma is thrown into numerous mitochondria, ribosomes, and glycogen granules[4] (Fig. 4-5).

MUSCLE SPINDLE AND GOLGI TENDON ORGAN

MUSCLE SPINDLE

All human striated muscles contain encapsulated proprioceptors known as muscle spindles. Each muscle spindle consists of up to about 10 muscle fibers enclosed in a connective tissue capsule. These structures consist of a connective tissue capsule surrounding a fluid-filled space that contains a few long, thick nuclear bag fibers and short, thinner nuclear chain fibers (collectively intrafusal fibers). Several sensory nerve fibers penetrate the muscle spindles, where they detect changes in the length of extrafusal muscle fibers and relay this information to the spinal cord[17] (Fig. 4-3).

GOLGI TENDON ORGAN

In tendons, near the insertion sites of muscle fibers, a connective tissue sheath encapsulates a number of large bundles of collagen fibers that are continuous with the collagen fibers that make up the myotendinous junction. Sensory nerves penetrate the connective tissue capsule. This structure, known as Golgi tendon organ, contributes to proprioception by detecting differences in tension in tendons.[18] This organ consists of a netlike collection of knobby nerve endings among the fascicles of a tendon. There are 3 to 25 nerve fibers per tendon organ. The fibers from the Golgi tendon organs

make up the Ib group of myelinated, rapidly conducting sensory nerve fibers.[17]

It is known that the chest wall spindles and tendon organs play a major role in the conscious perception of breathing,[19] although they are not the only neural structures involved in this sensation. The fact that intercostal muscles are rich in spindles, which act as a proprioceptive control mechanism, whereas the diaphragm is not, suggests the possibility that the diaphragm may be designed to perform the routine act of inspiration, but that the intercostal muscles are called into play with added loads on the system.[20]

Part II

Correlation of Structure with Physiologic Function (Strength, Endurance, Fatigue)

RESPIRATORY MUSCLES AS SKELETAL MUSCLES

Embryologically, morphologically, and by functional characteristics, the respiratory muscles are essentially striated skeletal muscles.[21] The respiratory muscles function both voluntarily (as in breath holding) as well as anatomically or involuntarily (as in sleeping). The nervous control of the voluntary and automatic breathing are separate. In addition to breathing, these muscles also serve multiple functions such as maintenance of posture, air movement for speech, and coughing.[22]

Compared with peripheral skeletal muscles, respiratory muscles fibers are characterized by increased fatigue resistance, increased maximal blood flow, greater oxidative capacity, and higher capillary density.[21,22] Respiratory muscles, unlike other skeletal muscles, contract against resistive (airways) and elastic (chest wall and lungs) loads, rather than inertial forces. Their resting position is uniquely determined by a balance of recoil forces of lung and chest wall.[23]

Finally, the muscles of respiration must function, like the heart, throughout life without periods of prolonged rest. To do this, they must metabolize primarily aerobically, but they must be able to function, when necessary, anaerobically.[24]

FIBER TYPES

The muscle fibers differ in terms of size and force development. Glycolytic fibers are larger in a diameter than oxidative fibers. The larger diameter of a muscle fiber, the greater force or tension it can develop. Consequently, type IIB fibers (strength-oriented) generate more force than type I fibers during contraction.[5]

The muscle fiber types differ in terms of motor unit recruitment order.[25] For a heterogenous muscle like the diaphragm, the earliest recruited motor units are the type 1, slow oxidative fibers with a rich capillary supply adapted to sustain aerobic work. At intermediate levels of force with moderate respiratory muscle loading, the type IIA motor units also will be active; at higher levels of force with significant muscle loading, the type IIB motor unit fibers (the largest and most fatigable units) are subsequently recruited. The size principle ensures recruitment of motor units in order of increasing fatigability (or decreasing endurance).[25]

All muscles contain varying amounts of each fiber type depending on its function. Fiber type composition may change over time in response to a variety of factors; such as aging, protein-calorie malnutrition, disuse, training, and chronic respiratory loading.[26] The latter two factors lead to cellular adaptation, with improved oxidative capacity, whereas the others result in fiber atrophy. Type I atrophy results in reduced endurance, where muscle strength decreases with atrophy of type II fibers.[27]

DIAPHRAGM

In general, the diaphragm is an endurance-oriented (low-tension, high-repetition activity), not strength-oriented (high-tension, low-repetition activity), muscle because the muscle mass is composed of type I slow oxidative fibers. In fact, it is capable of impressive feats of endurance. For example, an Olympic marathon runner in training can maintain high minute ventilation of approximately 50 L/min for several hours a day for many days in succession. Despite this endurance performance, the diaphragm can be fatigued in a matter of minutes by an increased resistance to flow or increased duration of muscle contraction.[5]

Regional differences in muscle fiber size indicate an adaptive response to differences in function. The costal parts of diaphragm function in inspiration not only to lower the central aponeurosis but also to expand the lower rib cage.[28] This finding may imply that the costal part carries relatively larger loads during contractions.

Determinants of Respiratory Muscles

STRENGTH

There are six major determinants of respiratory muscle strength in normal subjects. Age, sex, and general muscular development all reflect the state of the contractile machinery when the muscle is contracting under optimal conditions. The other factors reflect either the state of actin-myosin interaction (force-length, force-velocity relationships) or the state of muscle activation (force-frequency relationship).[29]

The force-length relationship indicates that when the muscle is stimulated at its optimal resting length, it produces its maximum contractile force.[29] When the muscle is either stretched beyond the optimal resting length or, alternatively, is foreshortened prior to contraction, supramaximal stimulation of the muscle produces submaximal force.[29]

Respiratory muscle length depends on the lung volume, and for the diaphragm, muscle's optimal length occurs slightly below functional residual capacity (FRC).[23] Chest wall configuration determines diaphragmatic length at any given lung volume.

The diaphragm is rarely if ever overstretched, but at lung volumes above normal FRC, the diaphragm and other inspiratory muscles are foreshortened and their contractile force is curtailed.[30] In contrast, expiratory muscle contraction force is reduced by low lung volumes.

At any muscle length, maximum contractile force is greatest when the muscle is prevented from shortening. If the muscle is allowed to shorten during its contraction, its contractile force declines hyperbolically as a function of the velocity with which the muscle shortens. This is termed the *force-velocity relationship*.[29] With increasing load on the muscles, velocity of shortening approaches zero (maximal isometric contraction). Maximal velocity of shortening occurs when no load is placed on the muscles. The shape of the curve depends on muscle fiber composition so that respiratory muscles demonstrate force-velocity behavior between that seen with fast and slow limb muscles.[6]

The third factor that modulates the contractile force of the respiratory muscles is the rate at which they are stimulated. The force-frequency response of the diaphragm and intercostals is similar to that of nonrespiratory skeletal muscles.[31] During everyday activities, phrenic nerve firing frequency is approximately 10 to 30 Hz[31] with increasing stimulation frequency, a force plateau is reached between 50 and 100 Hz.[32] Higher frequencies can be sustained for only a few seconds.[31]

When the diaphragm becomes fatigued following maximal contractile efforts, the force-frequency curve is depressed at all stimulation frequencies. The force-frequency relationship is an important mechanism for modulating the force of respiratory muscle contraction during both voluntary and involuntary efforts.[29]

ENDURANCE

Ventilatory endurance can be quantified by relating the level of ventilation to the time that ventilatory level can be sustained. It has been repeatedly established in normal subjects that the maximum voluntary ventilation (MVV) is sustainable for only 15 to 30 s, whereas 75 percent of the MVV can be sustained for about 4 min and 60 percent of the MVV can be sustained for 15 min.[29] Since the curve relating ventilation to endurance time appears asymptomatic at 60 percent of MVV, this level has been referred to as the maximum sustainable ventilation (MSV), or maximum sustainable ventilatory capacity (MSVC).[29] The fact that MSV is below MVV has been attributed to early fatigue of the type IIA fibers.[33]

Ventilatory endurance clearly depends on respiratory

muscle endurance. Since respiratory muscle strength (RMS) is an important determinant of the level of MVV, it would be expected that RMS would affect the level of MSV as well. In addition, the distribution of muscle fiber types and muscle blood flow are important determinants of endurance time for large but submaximal ventilatory efforts.[29]

Fixler and colleagues found in their exercise studies in dogs that the diaphragm receives the largest percentage of blood flow of all the muscles in the body, including the heart.[34] Furthermore, when shock is present, the diaphragm continues to receive the maximum amount of blood that can be perfused at a given blood pressure.[35] However, in the diaphragm as in other skeletal muscles, blood flow can be impeded by the high pressures generated inside the muscle when it contracts.[36] While under some circumstances this mechanism can limit diaphragmatic blood flow, its importance as a factor limiting endurance is not well established, provided that arterial blood pressure and cardiac output are normal.

However, in experimental cardiogenic shock the blood supply to the diaphragm can be made inadequate. As a result, diaphragm muscle lactate concentration increases, the diaphragm fatigues, and acute respiratory acidosis ensues.[37]

FATIGUE

Respiratory muscle fatigue is defined as a loss of the capacity to develop force and/or velocity in response to a load, which is reversible with rest.[38] In 1977, Roussos and Macklem showed that the diaphragm, like other skeletal muscles, was subject to fatigue.[39] Fatigue has been demonstrated in the sternomastoid and in expiratory muscles and occurs independently in each muscle group.[40]

The causes of fatigue include (1) inhibition of neural drive, (2) failure of transmission across neuromuscular junction, (3) excessive force and duration of contraction, (4) impaired muscle blood supply, (5) impaired excitation-contraction coupling, and (6) depletion of muscle energy stores.[29]

Fatigue can result from inadequate central nervous system drive, perhaps because of a reflex inhibition secondary to discomfort. Muscle fatigue can also result from alteration of motor nerve activity or by motor end-plate dysfunction, at least in isolated fatigued diaphragm strips.[41] However, the major cause of fatigue appears to lie within the muscle cell, involving the excitation-contraction coupling mechanism and muscle energy metabolism.[29]

Although the cellular and molecular mechanisms of respiratory muscle fatigue are not fully understood, it is clear that the development of fatigue is closely linked to the force and duration of muscle contraction.[41] In the case of diaphragm, the force of contraction can be expressed as the ratio of force per breath (Pdi) to the maximum force of diaphragmatic contraction during a static effort (Pdimax). The duration of diaphragmatic contraction can be expressed as the ratio of the duration of inspiration (T_I) to the total duration of the breath (Ttot). The product (Pdi/Pdimax) × (T_I/Ttot) is referred to as tension-time index of the diaphragm (TTI).[23]

The load on the respiratory muscles has been estimated by determining the TTI. In most circumstances T_I/Ttot changes little; thus Pdi/Pdimax is most crucial for determining the TTI.[23]

In experiments with inspiratory resistive loads in which T_I/Ttot was kept at approximately 0.5, diaphragmatic fatigue did not occur so long as Pdi per breath was less than 40 percent of Pdimax. Similar results were obtained for the inspiratory muscles as a whole, except that the critical level of inspiratory pressure (PI) per breath was about 60 percent of maximum inspiratory pressure (PImax).[42]

Fatigue is more likely to occur when maximal muscle pressures are decreased (weakness) or when the pressure needed on any given breath is increased, as when respiratory resistance is increased or compliance decreased. The fatigue threshold in normal individuals occurs when the Pdi/Pdimax is greater than or equal to 0.4 or when the TTI is greater than 0.15 to 0.2 or 0.3.[42] The higher the TTI, the shorter the endurance time before fatigue develops.[23] Presumably, when the demand of diaphragm exceeds 0.15 to 0.20, sufficient energy supplies are not available.[43] This threshold TTI is related to the limitation of blood perfusion and oxygen delivery to the muscles.[6]

Respiratory fatigue, characterized by a fall in the maximal pressure generated by a respiratory muscle, occurs anywhere along the path from the brain to sarcomere, and three types have been defined.[43] If phrenic nerve stimulation, superimposed on a maximal voluntary effort, results in an increase in maximal inspiratory pressure (Pmax), a central inhibitory component is suggested.[44] This central fatigue results from reflex inhibition caused by a chemical in muscles or by proprioceptive information, inhibitory effects on the brain stem or cortex, or the release of endogenous opioids.[45] In contrast, transmission fatigue, resulting from impulse blockade, is characterized by both decreased EMG amplitude and Pmax.[45] With contractile fatigue (high and low frequency), phrenic stimulation after a maximal voluntary effort produces normal EMG activation but no further increase in the reduced Pmax.[46]

Evidence suggests that high-frequency fatigue (HFF) results from impaired propagation of action potentials into the T-tubular system and a subsequent decrease in free intracellular Ca^{2+}.[47] Repeated stimulation at low frequencies (10 to 30 Hz, seen with everyday activity) or successive submaximal contractions lead to a slowly developing decrease in force production [low-frequency fatigue (LFF)].[37] Force is selectively reduced at low frequencies, whereas maximal force can still be generated by a high-frequency stimulus. Unlike the rapid recovery of HFF (minutes), LFF may last for 24 or more hours. Low-frequency fatigue appears to result from impaired excitation-contraction coupling due to reduced Ca^{2+} release from the sarcoplasmic reticulum, reduced myofibril Ca^{2+} sensitivity, and/or reduced maximum Ca^{2+}-activated tension.[47]

Part III

Respiratory Muscles in Disease

Respiratory muscle failure occurs either when thoracopulmonary diseases increase the work of breathing beyond the endurance capacity of the respiratory muscles or when the muscles become so weak that they cannot even sustain the work of normal quiet breathing. Often, there is mixed derangement of respiratory muscle function, for example, impaired contractile force combined with increased ventilatory work.[29]

Among the first to document abnormal function of respiratory muscles in a patient with pulmonary disease were Cournand and coworkers.[48] They described hypertonicity and spasticity of respiratory muscles and poor coordination between muscles of the rib cage and the diaphragm in a dyspneic patient with pulmonary fibrosis.

Christie noted abnormal patterns of breathing in patients with chronic obstructive pulmonary disease (COPD) and described a low, flattened diaphragm with greatly diminished movement.[49]

CHRONIC OBSTRUCTIVE PULMONARY DISEASE

COPD is a group of conditions characterized by airway obstruction. The term *chronic obstructive pulmonary disease* usually refers to a combination of primarily chronic bronchitis and emphysema but can include other conditions such as asthma, bronchiectasis, and cystic fibrosis.[50]

The function of the respiratory muscles is affected profoundly by the presence of COPD, because of the increase in the work of breathing and because COPD decreases the capacity of the muscles to cope with the increased ventilatory load. Several factors contribute to this imbalance.[51]

It is hypothesized that the respiratory muscles in individuals with COPD are more susceptible to respiratory muscle fatigue.[52] More recently, it is postulated that weakness rather than fatigue is present in the respiratory muscles of some groups of patients with COPD.[53] Regardless of whether weakness or fatigue is the cause, poor inspiratory muscle function is an important factor contributing to exertional dyspnea, exercise intolerance, and, as diseases progress, to hypercapnic ventilatory failure in patients with COPD.[52,53]

Patients with COPD must breathe at high lung volumes to maintain patency of their narrowed airways.[54] Under resting conditions, many patients with COPD have a slightly increased minute ventilation.[51]

The work of energy cost of breathing, however, is elevated markedly because of increased airway resistance and hyperinflation. The O_2 cost of breathing increases from about 2.5 in healthy subjects to 30 mL/min in patients with COPD.[55] In addition, ventilatory reserve is diminished markedly in these patients, such that resting ventilation constitutes about 40 percent of maximum ventilatory capacity compared with about 5 percent in healthy subjects.[56] Although expiratory airflow is severely limited, the increased work of breathing is performed primarily by the inspiratory muscles.[51]

The major abnormality of resting muscle function in patients with COPD is thought to be a mechanical disadvantage caused by this hyperinflation, which depresses the dome of the diaphragm, shortens its fibers, and forces it to work on an ineffective portion of its length-tension curve.[54]

Data from studies in normal dogs[57] and humans[30] indicate that the force-length relationship is the major or even the sole geometric factor which determines contractile force between normal residual volume (RV) and normal total lung capacity (TLC). As inflation of the lung exceeds predicted TLC, the diaphragm's radius of curvature (Rdi) increases. In other words, the diaphragm flattens. Under these circumstances, whatever tension (Tdi) is developed in the contracting muscle is poorly converted to transdiaphragmatic pressure (Pdi).[51]

The importance of the diaphragmatic curvature is best understood in terms of Laplace's law: Pdi = 2Tdi/Rdi. Tension developed in a tightly curved diaphragm (small Rdi), therefore, is converted more effectively into transdiaphragmatic pressure than is the tension developed in a flatter diaphragm (31/265). A completely flattened diaphragm, with an infinite radius of curvature, is incapable of generating any useful inspiratory pressure.[51] Indeed in this case, diaphragmatic contraction may pull in the lower rib cage, so it functions as an expiratory muscle.[51]

Hyperinflation has an adverse effect on the elastic recoil of the thoracic cage.[58] Resting lung volume, or FRC, normally is determined by the static equilibrium between inwardly directed elastic recoil of the lungs and outwardly directed elastic recoil of the thoracic cage. Thus, thoracic elastic recoil normally assists the action of the inspiratory muscles in inflating the lungs. When FRC is increased markedly, as in hyperinflation, thoracic elastic recoil becomes directed inward. This means that the inspiratory muscles must work not only against the elastic recoil of the lungs but also against that of the thoracic cage.[51]

Hyperinflation decreases the size of the zone of apposition.[59] As lung volume increases, this zone decreases, with the result that diaphragmatic contraction causes less effective rib cage expansion.[51] The axial direction of the diaphragmatic fibers is altered by hyperinflation. In this situation, diaphragmatic contraction has an expiratory action which can be detected clinically and is known as *Hoover's sign*.[60]

Hyperinflation may adversely affect muscle blood supply.[51] Recent animal experiments indicate that diaphragmatic blood flow decreases. TTI increases as it does with overinflation.[61]

RESPIRATORY MUSCLE STRENGTH AND ENDURANCE

Reduced respiratory muscle strength in COPD may be due to mechanical factors affecting the efficiency of the inspiratory muscles. Hyperinflation causes a shortening of inspiratory muscles so that the fibers are not at their optimal length for contraction. In addition, inspiratory muscle weakness in COPD could be related to malnutrition and respiratory muscle fiber atrophy; patients who have COPD may be inadequately nourished, and studies have shown a relationship between inspiratory muscle strength and nutrition in the absence of COPD.[62]

Undernutrition, with body weight less than 85 percent predicted, occurs in approximately 20 percent of patients with chronic obstructive pulmonary disease. It is accompanied by a reduction in diaphragm muscle mass and by a reduction in the thickness of the sternocleidomastoid muscle.[63] In this study, 65 percent of the variance in maximum expiratory pressure (Pemax) could be explained by body weight.[63] On the other hand, some patients who have airflow obstruction might develop respiratory muscle hypertrophy from the overload. Thus an increase in muscle fiber size could occur if there is a sufficient increase in resistive loading in association with obstructive pulmonary disease.[62]

Ventilatory endurance is usually quantified in terms of the fraction of maximum voluntary ventilation that can be sustained for prolonged periods of time. Patients with COPD have a decreased MVV, but are able to sustain fractions of MVV that are at least equal to those observed in healthy subjects: approximately 90 percent of MVV for 4 min and 59 to 76 percent for 15 min.[64]

MVV in healthy subjects is primarily related to respiratory muscle strength.[51] Aldrich and colleagues found that the degree of airway obstruction was the major determinant of MVV in patients with COPD, but MVV also was dependent to a small but significant extent on Pimax; the role of hyperinflation was not assessed.[65]

DIAPHRAGMATIC MUSCLE DIMENSIONS AND TYPE

It is conceivable that the diaphragm might become hypertrophied in response to the increased work of breathing in COPD or, alternatively, it may decrease in size because of malnutrition or sarcomere loss.[51]

In postmortem studies of COPD patients, measurements of the total size of the diaphragm have revealed conflicting results indicating both hypertrophy and atrophy. Muscle atrophy has been attributed to an impaired use of the diaphragm, as seen on radiography.[66] A small muscle mass of the diaphragm in COPD is related to the low body weight of the patients.[67] Consequently, the increased ventilatory work in COPD is not reflected by an increase in muscle fiber size of the diaphragm. On the contrary, a 16 percent reduction is the least diameter of diaphragmatic muscle fibers that has been found, and this reduction in fiber size is present in both type I (15 percent) and type II fibers (18 percent).[14]

It is known that atrophy of type II fibers in respiratory muscles is mostly a nonspecific finding in patients with COPD.[5,68] This type of atrophy is common in aging, with disuse, and with malnutrition,[69] three states which also characterize advanced COPD. Like the diaphragm, patients with COPD have a 15 percent reduction in the least diameter of type II fibers of the expiratory INT.[27,68] On the contrary, this reduction is not observed in the inspiratory EXT.

The small muscle fiber size of the diaphragm in COPD patients may indicate overuse atrophy as observed in limb skeletal muscle of extremely endurance-trained athletes.[70] However, at present, this is debated, since values are not available on either subgroups of type II fibers or capillary supply in the diaphragm of COPD patients. Furthermore, the effect of COPD on the diaphragm is probably more complicated than disuse or overuse atrophy, because COPD patients have generalized muscle weakness due to different factors.[71]

ENZYME ACTIVITIES AND SUBSTRATE CONTENTS

In biopsies obtained from patients with COPD, mitochondrial enzyme activities in both inspiratory and expiratory intercostal muscles are higher than in other skeletal muscles.[72] In COPD patients both hexokinase and lactic dehydrogenase activities (glycolytic enzyme activities) in the costal diaphragm are lower than in intercostal muscles, whereas citrate synthase and 3-hydroxyacyl-coenzyme A activities (mitochondrial enzyme activities) are similar. In both inspiratory EXT and expiratory INT, CS and HAD activity are higher in patients with moderate COPD than in patients with normal ventilatory function.[72] However, in patients with severe COPD, mitochondrial enzyme activity is the same for both the inspiratory EXT and expiratory INT. The ventilatory problems of patients with COPD appear to be reflected by

a high lactate concentration in the inspiratory intercostal muscles.[73]

ASTHMA

Asthma is a chronic obstructive airway disease characterized by airway blockage and hyperresponsiveness. The obstruction may be totally or partially reversible in response to therapy or with time.[74]

Airway resistance is increased to two to three times normal in asthmatic patients during a remission, and it is increased 5 to 15 times normal during an acute attack.[75] Hyperinflation in asthma is closely correlated with the increase in pulmonary resistance, and it occurs independently of expiratory airflow limitation.[74]

The capacity of the inspiratory muscles to deal with this load is impaired by the concomitant hyperinflation.[51]

Analysis of transthoracic pressure during bronchoconstriction indicates a substantial degree of negative work of inspiratory muscles in expiration, predominantly owing to inspiratory intercostal and accessory muscles.[74] Sternocleidomastoid and intercostal muscle retraction frequently are observed in patients during severe asthma attacks.[54] In addition, active recruitment of the abdominal muscles takes place during expiration.[74] During increased levels of ventilation in exercise or with increased chemical drive the respiratory muscles in asthma act in a coordinated fashion to optimize diaphragmatic function.

Respiratory muscle strength, however, may be increased in patients with asthma. Taking hyperinflation into account, it is estimated that Pimax was 125 percent of predicted in a group of asthmatic patients.[75] The sternomastoid muscles were about 25 percent thicker than normal in these patients, which seems to represent actual hypertrophy because it was seen when there was no evidence of muscle shortening.[75]

THORACIC RESTRICTIVE DISEASE

Obesity sufficient to elevate body weight by 50 percent or more increases the work of breathing, in part through mass loading of the chest wall and through secondary effects which reduce lung compliance. Patients with obesity-hyperventilation syndrome (OHS) may have pronounced lung and chest wall abnormalities but so do many equally obese eucapnic subjects.

It is known that eucapnic obese subjects have somewhat above normal inspiratory and expiratory muscle strength, whereas OHS patients have modest inspiratory and expiratory muscle weakness.[29] For approximately equivalent degrees of obesity, inspiratory muscle strength in OHS is about two-thirds that in simple obesity.[76] The role of inspiratory muscle weakness in the pathogenesis of carbon dioxide retention in OHS remains unquantified but undoubtedly contributes to the observed alterations in VC and MVV so characteristic of OHS group.[77]

A number of diseases affect movement of the thoracic cage; scoliosis, ankylosing spondylitis, pectus excavatum, fibrothorax, and thoracotomy.[51] These disorders compromise respiratory muscle function to varying degrees.[29] The role of respiratory muscle dysfunction in the pathogenesis of hypercapnic respiratory failure in these disorders has yet to be quantified.[29]

Kyphoscoliosis distorts the spine and rib cage, thus changing the position and length of the diaphragm and intercostal muscles. The work of breathing and its oxygen cost are markedly increased. Respiratory failure with carbon dioxide retention is related to the severity of kyphoscoliosis, as judged from the degree of spinal curvature.[29]

Patients with ankylosing spondylitis display a marked reduction in chest wall compliance,[78] associated with decreased rib cage movement and a greater than normal excursion of the diaphragm during breathing. In contrast to the other causes of thoracic deformity, FRC is elevated in more than half of these patients.[79] Patients with ankylosing spondylitis rarely, if ever, develop ventilatory failure, unless there is superimposed pulmonary disease.[51]

INTERSTITIAL LUNG DISEASE

Patients with interstitial lung disease (idiopathic pulmonary fibrosis, pneumoconiosis, sarcoidosis) have small stiff lungs, which may increase the length-tension advantage of the diaphragm because of the greater doming and stretching of its fibers. In one report, respiratory muscle strength in patients with interstitial lung disease was 72 percent of predicted. Their MVV was 56 percent of predicted and highly dependent on respiratory muscle strength.[65]

Investigators reported a significant decrease in P_{Imax} in patients with interstitial lung disease.[80] Taking this reduction in lung volume into account, De Troyer and Yernault[80] found a normal P_{Imax} at several lung volumes and an increase in the static recoil pressure at TLC in 12 patients with interstitial lung disease.

NEUROMUSCULAR DISEASE

A variety of neuromuscular disorders significantly compromise respiratory muscle function and lead to hypercapnic respiratory failure.[29]

STROKE

Respiratory function depends on the integrity of multiple structures of the central nervous system. The study of respiratory dysfunction after a cerebrovascular accident depends on the site and the extent of the lesion. In addition, changes in respiratory pattern may be related to the cause and the prognosis of stroke.[81]

Stroke is generally associated with a striking reduction in EMG activity of the diaphragm and parasternal intercostal muscles on the paralyzed side.[51] The decrease in diaphragmatic activity is less than that of the intercostal muscles. This involvement may contribute to the development of bronchopulmonary infections in these patients, but this remains to be determined.

SPINAL CORD INJURIES

High cervical (C1-2) spinal cord injuries disrupt the automatic respiratory pathway in the ventral cord as well as voluntary pathways in the lateral columns. Since the phrenic motor neuron pool is spared, ventilation can be maintained by pacing the phrenic nerve.[29] Patients develop hypertrophy of their sternomastoid and trapezius muscles, which are spared because they are innervated by the eleventh cranial nerve.[51] In addition, phasic inspiratory EMG activity has been observed in the platysma, mylohyoid, and sternohyoid mus-

cles. These patients can be conditioned to breathe for hours using only these muscles or by employing the technique of glossopharyngeal breathing.[82]

Midcervical (C3-5) cord injuries damage the phrenic motor neurons, and the resultant diaphragmatic paralysis is unresponsive to phrenic pacing.

Lower cervical (C6-8) and upper thoracic (T1-6) cord injuries paralyze intercostal and abdominal muscles, but leave the diaphragm and neck muscle intact. There is little influence on ventilatory endurance, because the diaphragm is functional.[83] All the well-recognized muscles of expiration are paralyzed, with the result that cough is defective and clearance of bronchial secretions impaired.[51]

AMYOTROPHIC LATERAL SCLEROSIS

Amyotrophic lateral sclerosis (ALS) is a progressive neurodegenerative disorder of the voluntary motor system that is characterized by loss and degeneration of motor neurons and their outflow tracts.[84]

Respiratory involvement occurs when the muscles subserving respiratory function become affected. Respiratory muscle weakness, particularly in the intercostal muscles and diaphragm, leads to hypoventilation and, ultimately, respiratory failure.[84]

Most commonly, hypoventilation develops in the setting of established limb and bulbar muscle involvement, at which time the diagnosis of ALS has already been established.[84] Patients have decreased respiratory muscle strength and rapid shallow breathing.[51] Occasionally, however, ALS can present with respiratory insufficiency as the main symptom. In these cases, the pathologic lesions preferentially involve the phrenic motor neurons located within the cervical spinal cord.[85]

Neuromuscular disorders such as ALS produce alveolar hypoventilation during the day, and this worsens with sleep.[84] The slope of the ventilatory response to hypercapnia is decreased, and, although it is correlated with the level of respiratory muscle strength and VC, these account for only 25 to 50 percent of the variance in CO_2 sensitivity.[51]

POLIOMYELITIS

In the first half of this century, poliomyelitis was the major neuromuscular disease affecting respiration, and some of these patients are still being treated for respiratory failure.[51]

MOTOR END-PLATE DISORDERS

Myasthenia gravis (MG) is an acquired disorder of the neuromuscular junction caused by antibodies directed against the acetylcholine receptor. MG frequently affects the respiratory system, causing respiratory muscle weakness as evidenced by a reduction in global respiratory muscle strength, diaphragmatic weakness, reduced VC, and a reduction in static compliance.[86] It may also affect the regulation of breathing, resulting in rapid shallow breathing and in a blunted ventilatory response to hypercapnia.[86] Respiratory muscle involvement is rare early in the course of MG (1 to 4 percent) but eventually becomes significant in 50 to 60 percent of patients.[87]

Ventilatory failure also has been noted in patients with the Lambert-Eaton myasthenic syndrome.[88]

PERIPHERAL NEUROPATHY

Guillain-Barré syndrome (GBS) is the most common peripheral neuropathy causing respiratory failure. Respiratory muscle weakness is the most serious complication and occurs in about one-third of patients.[89] Early detection of respiratory failure is essential because approximately 20 to 45 percent of afflicted patients require mechanical ventilation.[90]

MUSCULAR DYSTROPHY AND OTHER MYOPATHIES

Respiratory dysfunction occurs in a wide spectrum of myopathic disorders and is manifested by hypoventilation due to muscle weakness, increased risk of aspiration, and disturbances of breathing during sleep.[91] Respiratory failure is the major cause of death in 75 percent of patients with Duchenne's dystrophy.[92] Respiratory muscle weakness occurs early in the disease, but the diaphragm remains relatively spared, with the result that hypercapnia is uncommon except as a terminal event.[88] In contrast, diaphragmatic involvement occurs relatively early in patients with limb-girdle dystrophy, and these patients seem more likely to develop hypercapnia.[92]

Patients with myotonic dystrophy frequently develop respiratory insufficiency even when limb weakness is mild. This development is due to multiple factors, including weakness and myotonia of the respiratory musculature, pharyngoesophageal dysfunction, central hypoventilation, and excessive daytime somnolence.[91] Altered ventilatory response to hypoxia and hypercapnia has been well described in myotonic dystrophy and is generally attributed to respiratory weakness and fatigability with preservation of chemosensitivity.[91]

PART IV

Effects of Exercise Training on Respiratory Muscles

For life to be maintained, the respiratory muscles must possess sufficient strength to overcome resistive elastic forces of the lung and chest wall and sufficient endurance to produce phasic contractions continuously and indefinitely.[93]

It is possible to increase both the endurance and strength of respiratory muscles with specific training programs, in both normal subjects and patients with COPD.[94]

The response to specific training regimens appears to depend on the intensity of the training, the pattern of breathing employed, and the frequency and duration of the training program.[95] Moreover, the principle of specificity of skeletal muscle training indicates that optimal results on muscle performance are achieved when training mimics the function which needs to be enhanced.[95] Therefore, it should not be expected that all types of inspiratory muscle training will achieve similar effects on muscle function.[95]

Although there is sufficient evidence to conclude that the respiratory muscles respond to specific training programs in a manner similar to other skeletal muscles, there still is controversy regarding the true role of respiratory muscle training in the management of patients with neuromuscular and pulmonary disease.[96] It has been demonstrated repeatedly that improvement in pulmonary mechanics and gas exchange do not result from exercise training programs.[54]

The purpose of training the respiratory muscles is to improve their performance. On the other hand, in a variety of disease states, respiratory muscle performance may not be limiting and respiratory muscle training may not have a role in therapy.[96] Good examples of limitation caused by reduced respiratory muscle performance are a variety of neurologic, muscular, endocrine, and metabolic disease involving the respiratory muscles. In these disorders, severe inspiratory muscle weakness may lead to respiratory failure, or respiratory failure may occur when the weak inspiratory muscles are placed under added loads. Expiratory muscle weakness may be associated with a failure to clear secretions and the development of hypostatic pneumonia. Decreased respiratory muscle strength and endurance in such patients may contribute to exercise limitation, although it is more likely that associated weakness of limb muscles primarily is responsible for exercise limitation.[97]

Patients with COPD are typically limited in their exercise tolerance by the level of ventilation they can sustain.[8] Significant symptoms usually do not occur at rest until COPD is severe.[98] It seems likely that strategies that lower ventilatory requirement at a given level of exercise will increase exercise tolerance. It is demonstrated that in normal subjects, a program of exercise training is able to substantially reduce the ventilatory requirement for heavy exercise. The most likely mechanism for the reduction in ventilation is the concomitant reduction in lactic acidosis.[8] These changes act to increase the capacity for aerobic work and forestall the onset of lactic acidosis.[45] Such a training response might well be of benefit to the patient with COPD by removing some of the acid stimulus to breathing, thereby lowering the ventilatory requirement.[8]

RESPIRATORY MUSCLE TRAINING

Strength training of the respiratory muscles can be suggested for patients with respiratory muscle weakness.[96] This is reasonable when respiratory muscle fatigue is the cause of the weakness, but when the weakness is severe, then the respiratory muscles require rest, not training.[99]

Clinically, it may be difficult to distinguish between respiratory muscle weakness and fatigue. Respiratory muscle weakness is suggested by a chronic reduction in strength and chronic elevation of the Pa_{CO_2} or the acute development of paradoxical abdominal wall motion.[99]

Patients with COPD have excessive occasionally intolerable respiratory workloads due to increased airway resistance. In such cases, the continuous increase in respiratory work does not appear to induce hypertrophy of respiratory muscles.[93] Most studies have, in fact, shown decreases in respiratory muscle mass, strength, and endurance.[93] On the other hand, specific training programs utilizing intermittent resistive loading techniques have been shown to increase respiratory muscle strength and endurance in patients with and without COPD.[100]

RESPIRATORY MUSCLE STRENGTH TRAINING

In patients with COPD and normal subjects,[101] several authors have reported that respiratory muscle training decreases dyspnea and increases maximum inspiratory (MIP) and expiratory (MEP) pressures, which are indicators of respiratory muscle strength. It has been shown that the repetition of maximal forced inspiratory maneuvers produces an increase in vital capacity.[102] Variable increases in strength have been reported in patients in response to inspiratory resistive loading. The reason for the difference probably is related to the fact that, in some studies, the load applied to the inspiratory muscles was insufficient to increase strength. An alteration in breathing pattern during training may have caused a reduction in inspiratory load.[96]

RESPIRATORY MUSCLE ENDURANCE TRAINING

Endurance training of respiratory muscles can be achieved by both specific and nonspecific conditioning programs. The obvious nonspecific program is total body exercise. If exercise is of sufficient intensity and duration, minute ventilation may be increased to a degree sufficient to have an endurance training effect on the respiratory muscle of both normal and diseased humans.[103]

In COPD patients, the exercise minute ventilation is relatively low and thus is suboptimal for producing a training response. Specific respiratory muscle endurance training programs therefore should be used in such patients.[96] The most commonly used techniques for specific respiratory muscle endurance training programs are inspiratory resistive or threshold loading or isocapnic hyperventilation.[95]

However, there are many doubts about the use of such specific training for three very different reasons, depending on whether the respiratory muscles of the COPD patients are considered weak, chronically fatigued, or normal: (1) If they are weak, they may already be close to their fatiguing threshold. Any further increase in the work of breathing by inspiratory muscle training (IMT) may, therefore, not strengthen the inspiratory muscles but, on the contrary, be potentially hazardous. (2) If they are chronically fatigued, rest and not training should be the treatment to improve respiratory muscle function. (3) It probably makes no sense to train respiratory muscles if their function is well preserved.[104,105]

The development of animal models has been useful in the investigation of changes produced in respiratory muscle structure and function by resistive loading and training. One study looked for an increase in the number of mitochondria and quantity of aerobic enzymes in the respiratory muscles of the rat after chronic loading.[106] Akabas and coworkers showed that intermittent respiratory resistive loading in sheep improves diaphragm function (oxidative enzyme activity and in vivo diaphragm endurance), but they did not report the effect on diaphragm mass or maximal transdiaphragmatic pressure.[107] Recently, Tarasiuk and colleagues showed an increase in diaphragm mass of rats after 5 to 6 weeks of chronic resistive loading but only when the diaphragm mass was normalized for body weight. They also observed significant increases of in vitro contractility without any obvious change in endurance.[94]

Prezant and coworkers showed that the diaphragm of rats can adapt to long-term chronic respiratory resistance.[93] In contrast to Tarasiuk's study, they observed a decrease in diaphragm contractility and an increase in endurance. This finding might be explained as follows. The diaphragm adapts by shifting to those fibers that can most efficiently sustain prolonged isometric contractions (type I endurance fibers), but this is not without the expense of a decrease in contractility.[93]

The Effects of Mechanical Ventilation on Respiratory Muscles

The management of respiratory failure often includes the use of mechanical ventilation in a wide range of clinical settings to totally support or assist respiration. Although the goal of artificial ventilation is to achieve adequate oxygenation and ventilation, in recent years, ventilatory assist devices have been prescribed specifically in the management of acute and chronic respiratory muscle fatigue.[108]

Mechanical ventilators can be classified into two major categories, based on their effect on airway pressure: negative-pressure ventilators and positive-pressure ventilators. Positive-pressure ventilators may be subcategorized into conventional (low-frequency) ventilators and high-frequency ventilators which, either intermittently or continuously, apply positive pressure to the airway and provide partial support of ventilation.[109]

TOTAL VENTILATORY SUPPORT

Full ventilatory support is achieved by controlled mechanical ventilation (CMV), where the ventilator provides inflations at a preset volume and frequency. Respiratory muscle rest is attained if the patient is completely relaxed, which most often necessitates sedation and curarization. Respiration muscle depletion of glycogen, creatine phosphate, and adenosine triphosphate has been documented in patients with COPD and acute respiratory failure, which was corrected after a period of rest by mechanical ventilation.[95] Although this result was observed after several weeks of treatment, animal experiments suggest that metabolic repletion of muscles requires only several hours to a few days of rest. Longer rest may be required for recovery if respiratory muscle fibers have been damaged by work overload. On the other hand, complete rest of the respiratory muscles exposes them to the risk of atrophy. Skeletal muscle atrophy develops rapidly during complete rest, but the rate of respiratory muscle atrophy during full ventilatory support is not precisely known. A 46 percent fall in maximal transdiaphragmatic pressure and 37 percent fall in ventilatory endurance was reported in three baboons after 11 days of full ventilatory support.

PARTIAL VENTILATORY SUPPORT

Assisted or assist control mechanical ventilation (AMV) is a mode in which the ventilator provides assisted breaths of a preset volume in response to every patient-initiated inspiratory effort. Thus, the work of breathing performed by the patient (Wp) could be expected to be minimal. It has been demonstrated that during AMV, the Wp was approximately 60 percent of that during spontaneous breathing.[110] It is also found that the main determinants of Wp during AMV were the inspiratory drive and the inspiratory muscle strength. This observation implies that the inspiratory muscles are not easily inhibited during AMV.

During synchronized intermittent mechanical ventilation

(SIMV), the patient receives assisted breaths at a preset frequency and is also able to breathe spontaneously between assisted cycles.[96] Using electromyography, Imsand and colleagues[111] explored the neuromuscular output directed to the inspiratory muscles during SIMV. They found that the duration of EMG activity of the diaphragm and of the sternocleidomastoid muscle was unchanged with various levels of SIMV support, as well as between assisted and spontaneous breaths. Their results indicated that the degree of respiratory muscle rest achieved by SIMV is much less than anticipated. They also demonstrated that the inspiratory neural output is maintained constant for a given average load and is not regulated on a breath-by-breath basis in SIMV.

With inspiratory pressure support (IPS) ventilation, the patient quickly receives a positive airway pressure after having triggered the machine by an inspiratory effort. The pressure is maintained constant throughout inspiration until a preset fall in airflow occurs, usually 25 percent of peak inspiratory flow. The effect of IPS was described by Brochard and coworkers.[112] It is demonstrated that a higher degree of inspiratory muscle rest is achieved by IPS than by the other usual modes of inspiratory support.

NONINVASIVE VENTILATORY SUPPORT

Noninvasive mechanical ventilation can be provided either by intermittent negative pressure around the thorax or by intermittent nasal or facial positive pressure. Negative pressure ventilation (NPV), by means of an iron lung, a cuirass, or a poncho, is able to offer respiratory muscle rest. Shapiro and colleagues showed that NPV was difficult to apply and ineffective when used with the aim of resting the respiratory muscles in patients with stable COPD.[113,114] However, other groups showed that the degree of EMG inhibition achieved by negative pressure ventilation is variable among individuals, from very partial to nearly complete.[95]

Positive pressure ventilation through a nasal or facial mask may provide a marked inhibition of inspiratory muscles, even in patients with acute ventilatory failure. It is shown that the degree of inhibition of diaphragmatic EMG activity was significantly greater with positive pressure than with negative pressure ventilation.[115]

Electrical Activation of the Respiratory Muscles

ELECTRICAL ACTIVATION OF THE DIAPHRAGM

Electrical activation of the diaphragm is a relatively new and infrequently utilized technology that opens new potential avenues for treatment of respiratory failure, particularly in the areas of neuromuscular control.[108] The possibility of utilizing electrical stimulation of the phrenic nerve as a method of ventilation was recognized by Hufeland in 1783 and used by Boulogne and others as a technique for resuscitation. The concept of artificially stimulating the diaphragm to assist or totally support respiration in chronic respiratory disorders has been appealing conceptually but has been limited in application to a small patient group because of physiologic and clinical problems associated with the technique.[108] Van Lunteren and coworkers have suggested that the costal and

crural parts of the diaphragm functionally are distinct. It also has demonstrated apparent differences in the neural control of the two muscles. Clinical diaphragm pacing is designed to activate a maximum number of lower motor neuron fibers and thus results in electrical activation of nerve fibers supplying both costal and crural areas.[116]

INTERCOSTALS, SCALENES, AND OTHER MUSCLES OF INSPIRATION

Contraction of the parasternal intercostals, scalenes, and diaphragm acts to expand the rib cage and lung during inspiration. These other inspiratory muscles have been used experimentally to trigger the external electrical stimulus to the diaphragm in an attempt to produce a "closed loop" respiratory pacing system.[108] If inspiration is performed with the diaphragm remaining relaxed (as in phrenic nerve paralysis), the fall in pleural pressure required to inflate the lung is transmitted to the abdomen across the flaccid diaphragm. Under these circumstances, in contrast with diaphragmatic contraction, abdominal pressure falls and the abdominal wall is displaced inward instead of outward.[108]

Recent studies by DiMarco and coworkers have demonstrated the effect of spinal cord stimulation in developing respiratory pressure changes with the isolated intercostal muscles using phrenicotomized animal preparations.[116a] Effective pleural pressure changes for ventilation were produced, and this technique may have usefulness in inducing a "cough" in quadriplegics.

Danon and colleagues studied quadriplegic patients with high cervical cord lesions (C1).[117] These patients breathed only with their accessory muscles, with electrically paced diaphragms, or with a combination of the two. It is demonstrated that the diaphragm functioning alone did not drive the rib cage along its relaxation curve, but instead produced paradoxical inward movement of the upper rib cage. This apparently was because of the absence of accessory muscle activity that normally would support the rib cage.

Candidates for Diaphragmatic Pacing

QUADRIPLEGIA WITH RESPIRATORY PARALYSIS

Damage to the spinal cord above the origin of the phrenic nerve roots (C3-4-5) results in complete paralysis of the diaphragm as well as the intercostal muscles.[118] Prior to the development of the phrenic pacer, these patients were destined to be permanently dependent on a mechanical ventilator.[108]

These patients require full-time ventilatory support, which until recently could be achieved only by pacing each hemidiaphragm for 12 h. Continuous pacing of a phrenic nerve had resulted in a fatigue-like phenomenon. Glenn demonstrated that continuous pacing of the diaphragm was possible using a very low-frequency electrical stimulus (11 to 13 Hz).[119]

Disuse of the diaphragm in the first months following acute injury, when patients with high quadriplegia are on mechanical ventilation, probably results in muscle atrophy that must be reversed by a process of conditioning. Two weeks following implantation of the pacers, the optimal electrical parameters for achieving the required tidal volume are obtained and the pacing periods are lengthened gradually over a period of weeks.[108]

CENTRAL HYPOVENTILATION SYNDROMES

Central hypoventilation syndromes are characterized by an abnormally low ventilatory drive to the respiratory muscles that may be congenital or idiopathic or a result of anatomic damage to the respiratory center. These patients are able to maintain normal blood gases while awake but have significant hypoventilation and apnea most prominent during sleep. These patients are candidates for phrenic nerve pacing that often is required only at night to maintain normal oxygenation and adequate ventilation; unilateral pacing is attempted first. The decision to implant pacers in those patients who have ventilatory function is much more difficult than in quadriplegics.[108]

As in quadriplegic patients, diaphragm pacing, particularly during sleep, may induce episodes of upper airway closure that impair ventilation and oxygenation. Patients who have episodes of obstructive sleep apnea when not paced have an exaggeration of the problem during pacing.[120] It is likely that the augmented inspiratory action of the diaphragm collapses parts of the upper airway. Airway obstruction also occurs because the inspiratory action of the diaphragm is not coordinated in time with that of the upper airway muscles.[121] The patients in general appeared to benefit from pacing in terms of increasing P_{O_2} and lowering P_{CO_2}.[108]

DIAPHRAGMATIC PACING

Despite the remarkable advances made by Glenn with this technique, the application of phrenic pacing continues to be limited.[108] Despite experimental data suggesting that prolonged electrical stimulation of the canine phrenic nerve is of itself not injurious,[122] the potential risk of permanent damage to the nerve from the operative procedure or local injuries from effects of the electrode remain significant limiting factors.

Nochomovitz and coworkers reported, if properly placed, that intramuscular electrodes in one hemidiaphragm can produce the same degree of diaphragm contraction and subsequent tidal volume as that produced with whole nerve stimulation. The respiratory pressure–generated and –related surface movements are indistinguishable. This technique does not risk damage to the phrenic nerve, and previous studies have not documented damage to muscle function after prolonged use. This approach may have clinical application as an alternative technique for diaphragm pacing, with the advantage of not risking phrenic nerve damage, which would be particularly significant to nonquadriplegic patients, with a significant component of central hypoventilation to their respiratory failure.[123]

Dunn and coworkers reported the use of suture-type intramuscular electrodes for diaphragm and accessory respiratory muscle stimulation.[124] They concluded that intramuscular electrodes not only are capable of nerve stimulation but also can produce local inspiratory support from thoracic muscles. Thoracic support for diaphragm-driven respiration should provide a more effective system which over the long term is less prone to fatigue and failure.[124]

Effects of Pharmacotherapy on Respiratory Muscles

Recognition of respiratory muscle failure in respiratory diseases has an important therapeutic implication.[125,126]

In some instances, such as acute respiratory failure, the primary goal is to reduce afterload.[125–127] This can be accomplished by mechanical ventilation or by removing the underlying obstruction as in asthma or tracheal stenosis. In chronic respiratory system disorders, such as COPD and thoracic restrictive disorders, it may be difficult to reduce afterload or to correct the mechanical disadvantage to inspiratory muscles.

In recent years, attention has been focused on the possibility of enhancing respiratory muscle function with drugs.[125] Drugs that prove to have a positive inotropic effect on respiratory muscles include the xanthines and sympathomimetic amines.

XANTHINES

In respiratory medicine, the two compounds commonly used are caffeine (1,3,7-trimethylxanthine) and theophylline (1,3-dimethylxanthine), respectively. Both stimulate the central nervous system, act on the kidney to produce diuresis, stimulate cardiac and skeletal muscle, and relax smooth muscle, notably bronchial muscle. Theophylline and caffeine differ, however, in the intensity of their actions on various structures.[126]

There is no doubt that methylxanthines, including aminophylline and theophylline, enhance the contractility of skeletal muscle. Studies have clearly demonstrated this positive inotropic effect on single muscle fiber and muscle strip preparations. It is well known that the methylxanthines increase minute ventilation in anesthetized animals.[128]

Very few studies are available regarding the effects of caffeine on respiratory muscles in humans. It has been reported that diaphragmatic contractility increases 40 percent after administration of therapeutic doses of caffeine.[129] However, no data are available concerning the effect of caffeine on respiratory muscle function in patients with respiratory disease.[126]

The ventilatory response to methylxanthines has been attributed to several mechanisms. Eldridge and colleagues[130] showed that intravenously administered aminophylline and theophylline increased phrenic activity in paralyzed, vagotomized, and glomectomized cats to exclude any change in both chemical feedback and muscular function. The results obtained by Aubier and coworkers[131] in anesthetized dogs suggested that aminophylline also increases ventilation by improving diaphragm contractility, even if there is little change in respiratory drive.

In anesthetized dogs, aminophylline may promote expiratory muscle activity.[132] This effect was observed when there was no significant change in inspiratory muscle activation, but an increase in abdominal pressure suggests that expiratory muscle could contribute to the observed increase in minute ventilation.

In normal humans (1) breathing at rest increases ventilation, promoting larger tidal volume[133]; (2) this effect is due to great motor drive to inspiratory muscles; (3) aminophylline does not produce appreciable expiratory muscle activity or distortion in the pattern of chest wall motion.[128]

It has been reported that these drugs increase the ventilatory response to hypoxia and hypercapnia, a phenomenon that has been uniformly observed.[128]

The positive action of theophylline, however, seems to be small, and the use of those potentially toxic drugs is likely to be limited.[125]

SYMPATHOMIMETIC AMINES

Beta-adrenergic stimulation is involved in the normal training-induced increase in oxidative capacity in both locomotor and respiratory skeletal muscle.[134] Beta-adrenergic agonists have been shown to increase skeletal muscle contractility in vitro[135] and also may affect respiratory muscle contractility and prevent fatigue.[126] An abundance of beta receptors has been found in the diaphragm.[126]

The effect of isoproterenol on the fatigued diaphragm has been studied in dogs.[136] Fatigue was produced by electrophrenic stimulation. It was found that Pdi at therapeutic dosages (2 to 5 mg/min) was increased by 10 percent at low frequencies of stimulation but remained unchanged at high frequencies of stimulation. Similarly, Pdi increased by 5 to 10 percent with isoproterenol for a given diaphragmatic electromyogram during spontaneous inspiratory effort with the upper airway occluded. Isoproterenol also shortened the one-half relaxation time and increased the peak twitch tension of the diaphragm. The effect of the beta$_2$ sympathomimetic drug, terbutaline, on the contractile properties of the fresh and fatigued diaphragm of the dog in vivo has also been examined.[137] Terbutaline had no effect on Pdi at any frequency of stimulation in the fresh diaphragm, although heart rate increased by 30 percent. Because the diaphragm is composed of equal amounts of both slow and fast contracting fibers, it is possible that terbutaline elicited opposite effects within each population.

On the other hand, terbutaline exerted an important positive inotropic effect on the fatigued diaphragm at the same dosage.[137] Following administration of the drug, twitch tension and Pdi at low frequencies of stimulation increased by 25 percent, whereas Pdi at high frequencies increased by 15 percent. This effect likely resulted from the drug's direct action on the muscle fiber,[138] given that a similar increase in Pdi was obtained during stimulation directly or via the phrenic nerves. Furthermore, no change was observed in the electrical activity of the diaphragm during phrenic nerve stimulation before and after the administration of terbutaline.

Tulobuterol is reported to have greater specificity and potency in vitro than either salbutamol or terbutaline to the beta$_2$ adrenoreceptor.[139] Lanigan and coworkers reported that terbutaline and tulobuterol had no beneficial effects on either respiratory or limb muscle strength and endurance in humans.[140]

Clearly these studies indicated that at the present time the action of these drugs cannot be predicted accurately.[126] Despite recent concern about their safety, β_2 agonists are likely to remain an important drug for prevention and relief of bronchospasm. The long-acting β_2 agonists, salmeterol[141] and formoterol,[142] have been shown to be capable of improving control of airflow obstruction in asthma.[143]

CORTICOSTEROIDS

Corticosteroids in high doses and for prolonged periods are frequently used in the treatment of many pulmonary diseases.[144] Inhaled corticosteroids are recognized as having a central role in the treatment of asthma[145] and, even though other drugs may become available in the next 10 years, it is unlikely that inhaled steroids will be supplanted from this important role. The adverse effect of the drug on the respiratory muscles might have great potential relevance to patients already suffering from dyspnea due to their respiratory disorder.[144]

Patients who received high-dose steroids for several weeks developed inspiratory muscle weakness, which seemed to be reversible following withdrawal of the drug treatment.[144] One study found that muscle weakness was preventable by using specific inspiratory muscle training (SIMT) during corticosteroid treatment.[144]

References

1. De Troyer A, Estenne M: Functional anatomy of the respiratory muscles. *Clin Chest Med* 9:175–210, 1988.
2. Christensen JB, Telford IR: *Synopsis of Gross Anatomy.* Hagerstown, MD, Harper & Row, 1978; chap 3, pp 88–108.
3. Moore KL (ed): *Clinically Oriented Anatomy,* 3d ed. Philadelphia, Williams & Wilkins, 1992.
4. Junqueira LC, Carneiro J, Kelley RO: Muscle tissue, in Junqueira LC, Carneiro J, Kelley RO (eds): *Basic Histology,* 8th ed. Norwalk, CT, Appleton & Lange, 1995; pp 181–201.
5. Tuman KJ: Respiratory muscle loading and the work of breathing. *J Cardiothor Vasc Anesth* 9:192–204, 1995.
6. Braun NMT, Faulkner J, Hughes RL, et al: When should respiratory muscles be exercised? *Chest* 84:76–84, 1983.
7. Mizuno M, Secher NH: Histochemical characteristics of human expiratory and inspiratory intercostal muscles. *J Appl Physiol* 67:592–598, 1989.
8. Casaburi R, Patessio A, Ioli F, et al: Reductions in exercise lactic acidosis and ventilation as a result of exercise training in patients with obstructive lung disease. *Am Rev Respir Dis* 143:9–18, 1991.
9. Mizuno M: Human respiratory muscles: Fibre morphology and capillary supply. *Eur Respir J* 4:587–601, 1991.
10. Maxwell LC, McCarter RJM, Kuehl TJ, et al: Development of histochemical and functional properties of baboon respiratory muscles. *J Appl Physiol* 54:551–561, 1983.
11. Reid MB, Ericson GC, Feldman HA, et al: Fiber types and fiber diameters in canine respiratory muscles. *J Appl Physiol* 62:1705–1712, 1987.
12. Hanson J: Effects of repetitive stimulation on membrane potentials and twitch in human and rat intercostal muscle fibers. *Acta Physiol Scand* 92:238–248, 1974.
13. Keens TG, Bryan AC, Levison H, et al: Development pattern of muscle fiber types in human ventilatory muscles. *J Appl Physiol* 44:909–913, 1978.
14. Sanchez J, Medrano G, Debesse B, et al: Muscle fiber types in costal and crural diaphragm in normal men and in patients with moderate chronic respiratory disease. *Bull Eur Physiopathol Respir* 21:351–356, 1985.
15. Saltin B, Gollnick PD: Skeletal muscle adaptability. Significance for metabolism and performance, in Peachey LD, Adrian RH (eds): *Handbook of Physiology,* sec 10. Bethesda, MD, American Physiological Society, 1983; pp 555–631.
16. Sanchez J, Bastien C, Medrano G, et al: Metabolic enzymatic activities in the diaphragm of normal men and patients with

moderate chronic obstructive pulmonary disease. *Bull Eur Physiopathol Respir* 20:535–540, 1984.

17. Slonim NB, Hamilton LH: Neural regulation of pulmonary ventilation, in Carson D (ed): *Respiratory Physiology.* St Louis, MD, Mosby, 1987; chap 14, pp 179–186.

18. Junqueira LC, Carneiro J, Kelley RO (eds): Basic histology, sec 24, *The Sense Organs,* 8th ed. Norwalk, CT, Appleton & Lange, 1995; p 447.

19. Bakers JHCM, Tenney SM: The perception of some sensations associated with breathing. *Respir Physiol* 10:85, 1970.

20. Derenne JPH, Macklem PT, Roussos CH: The respiratory muscles: Mechanics, control, and pathophysiology. *Am Rev Respir Dis* 118:373–390, 1978.

21. Edwards RHT, Faulkner JA: Structure and function of the respiratory muscles, in Roussos C, Macklem PT (eds): *The Thorax,* part A. New York, Marcel Dekker, 1986; p 297–326.

22. Sharp JT: Respiratory muscle function in respiratory care, in O'Donohue WJ (ed): *Current Advances in Respiratory Care.* Park Ridge, IL, American College of Chest Physicians, 1984; p 21.

23. Epstein SK: An overview of respiratory muscle function. *Clin Chest Med* 15(4):619–639, 1994.

24. Rochester DF, Brisco AM: Metabolism of the working diaphragm. *Am Rev Respir Dis* 119:101, 1979.

25. McKenzie DK, Gandevia SC: Skeletal muscle properties: Diaphragm and chest wall, in Crystal RG, West JB (eds): *The Lung: Scientific Foundations.* New York, Raven, 1991; pp 649–659.

26. Druz WS, Danon J, Fishman HC, et al: Approaches to assessing respiratory muscle function in respiratory disease. *Am Rev Respir Dis* 119(2 Pt 2):145–149, 1979.

27. Campbell JA, Hughes RL, Sahgal V, et al: Alterations in intercostal muscle morphology and biochemistry in patients with obstructive lung disease. *Am Rev Respir Dis* 122:679–686, 1980.

28. De Troyer A, Sampson MG, Sigrist S, et al: Action of costal and crural pats of the diaphragm on the rib cage in dog. *J Appl Physiol* 53:30–39, 1982.

29. Rochester DF, Arora NS: Respiratory muscle failure. *Med Clin North Am* 67:573–597, 1983.

30. Braun NMT, Arora NS, Rochester DF: Force-length relation of the normal human diaphragm. *J Appl Physiol* 53:405, 1982.

31. Moxham J, Morris AJR, Spiro SG, et al: Contractile properties and fatigue of the diaphragm in man. *Thorax* 36(3):164–168, 1981.

32. Edwards RHT: The diaphragm as a muscle: Mechanisms underlying fatigue. *Am Rev Respir Dis* 119:81–84, 1979.

33. Faulkner JA, Maxwell LC, Rutt GL, et al: The diaphragm as a muscle: Contractile properties. *Am Rev Respir Dis* 119:89, 1979.

34. Fixler DE, Atkins JM, Mitchell JM, et al: Blood flow to respiratory cardiac and limb muscles in dogs during graded exercises. *Am J Physiol* 213:1515, 1976.

35. Grimby G, Goldman MD, Mead J: Respiratory muscle action inferred from rib cage and abdominal v-p partitioning. *J Appl Physiol* 41:739, 1976.

36. Bellemare F, Wight D, Lavigne CM, et al: Limitation of diaphragmatic blood flow in dogs. *Fed Proc* 441:1255, 1982.

37. Aubier M, Trippenbach T, Roussos C: Respiratory muscle fatigue during cardiogenic shock. *J Appl Physiol* 51:499, 1981.

38. NHLBI Workshop summary: Respiratory muscle fatigue. *Am Rev Respir Dis* 142:474–480, 1990.

39. Roussos C, Macklem PT: Diaphragmatic fatigue in man. *J Appl Physiol* 43:189–197, 1977.

40. Wilson SH, Cooke NT, Moxham J, et al: Sternomastoid muscle function and fatigue in normal subjects and in patients with chronic obstructive pulmonary disease. *Am Rev Respir Dis* 129:460–464, 1984.

41. Kelson SG, Nochomovitz ML: Fatigue of the mammalian diaphragm in vitro. *J Appl Physiol* 53:440, 1982.

42. Roussos C, Fixley M, Gross D, et al: Fatigue of inspiratory muscles and their synergic behavior. *J Appl Physiol* 46:897–904, 1979.

43. Grassino A, Macklem PT: Respiratory muscle fatigue and ventilatory failure. *Ann Rev Med* 35:625–647, 1984.

44. Bellemare F, Bigland-Ritchie B: Central components of diaphragmatic fatigue assessed by phrenic nerve stimulation. *J Appl Physiol* 62:1307–1316, 1987.

45. Aldrich TK: Central and transmission fatigue. *Semin Resp Med* 12:322–330, 1991.

46. Moxham J, Edwards RHT, Aubier M, et al: Changes in EMG power spectrum (high-to-low ratio) with force fatigue in humans. *J Appl Physiol* 53:1094–1099, 1982.

47. Westerblad H, Lee JA, Lannergren J, et al: Cellular mechanisms of fatigue in skeletal muscle. *Am J Physiol* 261(C):195–209, 1991.

48. Cournand A, Brock HJ, Rappaport J, et al: Disturbance of action of respiratory muscles as a contributing cause of dyspnea. *Arch Intern Med* 57:1008, 1986.

49. Christie RV: Emphysema of the lungs. *Br Med J* 1:105, 1944.

50. Fishman AP: The spectrum of chronic obstructive disease of the airways, in Fishman AP (ed): *Pulmonary Diseases and Disorders.* New York, McGraw-Hill, 1988; chap 70.

51. Tobin MJ: Respiratory muscles in diseases. *Clin Chest Med* 9:263–286, 1988.

52. Roussos C: Ventilatory failure and respiratory muscles, in Roussos C, Macklem PT (eds): *The Thorax.* New York, Marcel Dekker, 1985; p 29.

53. Rochester DF: Respiratory muscle weakness, pattern of breathing, and CO_2 retention in chronic obstructive pulmonary disease. *Am Rev Respir Dis* 143:901–903, 1991.

54. Luce JM, Culver BH: Respiratory muscle function in health and disease. *Chest* 81:82–90, 1982.

55. Levison H, Cherniack RM: Ventilatory cost of exercise in chronic obstructive pulmonary disease. *J Appl Physiol* 25:21–27, 1968.

56. Pardy RL, Hussain SNA, Macklem PT: The ventilatory pump in exercise. *Clin Chest Med* 5:35–49, 1984.

57. Kim MJ, Druz WS, Danon J, et al: Mechanics of canine diaphragm. *J Appl Physiol* 41:369, 1976.

58. Sharp JT: The respiratory muscles in emphysema. *Clin Chest Med* 4:421–432, 1983.

59. Belman MJ, Sieck GC, Mazar A: Aminophylline and its influence on ventilatory endurance in humans. *Am Rev Respir Dis* 131: 226–229, 1985.

60. Hoover CF: The diagnostic significance of inspiratory movements of costal margins. *Am J Med Sci* 159:633–646, 1920.

61. Bark H, Supinski GS, Lamanna JC, et al: Relationship of changes in diaphragmatic muscle blood flow to muscle contractile activity. *J Appl Physiol* 62:291–299, 1987.

62. Hards JM, Reid WD, Pardy RL, et al: Respiratory muscle fiber morphometry. *Chest* 97:1037–1044, 1990.

63. Arora NS, Rochester DF: Effect of chronic obstructive pulmonary disease on sternocleidomastoid muscle. *Am Rev Respir Dis* 125:252, 1982.

64. Belman MJ, Mittman C: Ventilatory muscle training improves exercise capacity in chronic obstructive pulmonary disease patients. *Am Rev Respir Dis* 121:273–280, 1980.

65. Aldrich TK, Arora NS, Rochester DF: The influence of airway obstruction and respiratory muscle strength on maximal voluntary ventilation in lung disease. *Am Rev Respir Dis* 126:195–199, 1982.

66. Barach AL: Restoration of diaphragmatic function and breathing exercises in pulmonary emphysema. *NY State J Med* 56:3319–3332, 1956.

67. Arora NS, Rochester DF: COPD and human diaphragm muscle dimension. *Chest* 91:719–724, 1987.

68. Hughes RL, Katz H, Sahgal V, et al: Fiber size and energy

metabolites in five seperate muscles from patients with chronic obstructive lung disease. *Respiration* 44:321–328, 1983.

69. Engel WK: The essentiality of histo- and cytochemical studies of skeletal muscles in the investigation of neuromuscular disease. *Neurology* 12:788–794, 1972.

70. Jansson E, Kaijser L: Muscle adaptation to extreme endurance training in man. *Acta Physiol Scand* 100:315–324, 1977.

71. Decramer M: Effects of hyperinflation on the respiratory muscles. *Eur Respir J* 2:299–302, 1989.

72. Sanchez L, Brunet A, Medrano G, et al: Metabolic enzymatic activities in the intercostal and serratus and in the latissimus dorsi of middle-aged normal men and patients with moderate obstructive pulmonary disease. *Eur Respir J* 1:376–383, 1988.

73. Gertz I, Hedenstierna G, Hellers G, et al: Muscle metabolism in patients with chronic obstructive lung disease and acute respiratory failure. *Clin Sci Mol Med* 52:395–403, 1977.

74. Martin J, Powell E, Shore S, et al: The role of respiratory muscles in the hyperinflation of bronchial asthma. *Am Rev Respir Dis* 121:441–447, 1980.

75. Rochester DF, Arora NS: The respiratory muscle in asthma, in Lavietes MH, Reichman L (eds): *Symposium on Bronchial Asthma*. New York, Purdue Frederick, 1982; pp 27–38.

76. Arora NS, Rochester DF: Respiratory muscle function in obesity and obesity hypoventilation syndrome. *Clin Res* 27:394, 1979.

77. Rochester DF, Arora NS: Respiratory failure from obesity, in Mancini M, Lewis E, Cuntaldo F (eds): *Medical Complications of Obesity*. New York, Academic, 1980; p 180.

78. Sharp JT, Sweeney SK, Henry JP: Lung and thoracic compliance in ankylosing spondylitis. *J Lab Clin Med* 63:254–263, 1964.

79. Bergofsky EH: Thoracic deformities, in Roussos C, Macklem PT (eds): *The Thorax*. New York, Marcel Dekker, 1985; pp 941–978.

80. DeTroyer A, Yernault JC: Inspiratory muscle force in normal subjects and patients with interstitial lung disease. *Thorax* 35:92–100, 1980.

81. Vingerhoets F, Bogousslavsky J: Respiratory dysfunction in stroke. *Clin Chest Med* 15(4):729–737, 1994.

82. Mazza FG, Dimarco AF, Altose MD, et al: The flow-volume loop during glossopharyngeal breathing. *Chest* 85:638–640, 1984.

83. Wicks AB, Menter RR: Long-term outlook in quadriplegic patients with initial ventilatory dependency. *Chest* 90:406–410, 1986.

84. Kaplan LM, Hollander D: Respiratory dysfunction in amyotrophic lateral sclerosis. *Clin Chest Med* 15(4):675–681, 1994.

85. Meyrignac C, Poirier J, Degos JD: Amyotrophic lateral sclerosis presenting with respiratory insufficiency as the primary complaint. *Eur Neurol* 24:115–120, 1985.

86. Zulueta JJ, Fanburg BL: Respiratory dysfunction in myasthenia gravis. *Clin Chest Med* 15:683–691, 1994.

87. Kaminski MJ, Young RR: Neuromuscular and neurological disorders affecting respiration, in Roussos C, Macklem PT (eds): *The Thorax*. New York, Marcel Dekker, 1985; pp 1023–1087.

88. Smith PE, Calverley MB, Edwards RH, et al: Practical problems in the respiratory care of patients with muscular dystrophy. *N Engl J Med* 316:1197–1205, 1987.

89. Teitelbaum JS, Borel CO: Respiratory dysfunction in Guillain-Barre syndrome. *Clin Chest Med* 15:705–714, 1994.

90. Gracey DR, McMichan JC, Divertie MB, et al: Respiratory failure in Guillain-Barre syndrome. *Mayo Clin Proc* 57:742–746, 1982.

91. Lynn DJ, Woda RP, Mendell JR: Respiratory dysfunction in muscular dystrophy and other myopathies. *Clin Chest Med* 15:661–673, 1994.

92. De Troyer A, Pride NB: The respiratory system in neuromuscular disorders, in Roussos C, Macklem PT (eds): *The Thorax*. New York, Marcel Dekker, 1985; pp 1089–1121.

93. Prezant DJ, Aldrich TK, Richner B, et al: Effects of long-term continuous respiratory resistive loading on rat diaphragm function and structure. *J Appl Physiol* 74:1212–1219, 1993.

94. Tarasiuk A, Scharf SM, Miller MJ: Effect of chronic resistive loading on respiratory muscles in rats. *J Appl Physiol* 70:216–222, 1991.

95. Tolep K, Kelson SG: Effect of aging on respiratory skeletal muscles. *Clin Chest Med* 14:363–378, 1993.

96. Pardy RL, Reid WD, Belman MJ: Respiratory muscle training. *Clin Chest Med* 9:287–296, 1988.

97. Nochomovitz ML, Peterson DK, Stellato TA: Electrical activation of the diaphragm. *Clin Chest Med* 9:349–358, 1988.

98. Gallagher CG: Exercise limitation and clinical exercise testing in chronic obstructive pulmonary disease. *Clin Chest Med* 15:305–325, 1994.

99. Rochester DF, Arora NS: Respiratory muscle failure. *Med Clin North Am* 67:573–597, 1983.

100. Aldrich TK, Karpel JP, Uhrlass RM, et al: Weaning from mechanical ventilation: Adjunctive use of inspiratory muscle resistive training. *Crit Care Med* 17:143–147, 1989.

101. Harver A, Mahler DA, Daubenspeck A: Targeted inspiratory muscle training improves respiratory muscle function and reduces dyspnea in patients with chronic obstructive pulmonary disease. *Ann Intern Med* 111:117–124, 1989.

102. Leith DE, Bradley M: Ventilatory muscle strength and endurance training. *J Appl Physiol* 41:508–516, 1976.

103. Keens TG, Krastins IRB, Wanamaker EM, et al: Ventilatory muscle endurance training in normal subjects and patients with cystic fibrosis. *Am Rev Respir Dis* 116:853–860, 1977.

104. Wanke T, Formanek D, Lahrmann H, et al: Effects of combined inspiratory muscle and cycle ergometer training on exercise performance in patients with COPD. *Eur Respir J* 7:2205–2211, 1994.

105. Pardy RL, Rivington RN, Despas PJ, et al: The effects of inspiratory muscle training on exercise performance in chronic airflow limitation. *Am Rev Respir Dis* 123:426–433, 1981.

106. Askew EW, Dohn GL, Huston RL, et al: Response of rat tissue lipases to physical training and exercise. *Proc Soc Exp Biol Med* 141:123–129, 1972.

107. Akabas SR, Bazzy AR, DiMaura S, et al: Metabolic and functional adaptation of the diaphragm to training with resistive loads. *J Appl Physiol* 66:529–535, 1989.

108. Nickerson BG, Keens TG: Measuring ventilatory muscle endurance in humans as sustainable inspiratory pressure. *J Appl Physiol* 52:768–772, 1982.

109. Popovich J: The physiology of mechanical ventilation and the mechanical zoo: IPPB, PEEP, CPAP. *Med Clin North Am* 67:621–631, 1983.

110. Marini JJ, Rodriguez RM, Lamb V: The inspiratory workload of patient-initiated mechanical ventilation. *Am Rev Respir Dis* 134:902–909, 1986.

111. Imsand C, Feihl F, Perret C, et al: Regulation of inspiratory neuromuscular output during synchronized intermittent mechanical ventilation. *Anesthesiology* 80:13–22, 1994.

112. Brochard L, Harf A, Lorino H, et al: Inspiratory pressure support prevents diaphragmatic fatigue during weaning from mechanical ventilation. *Am Rev Respir Dis* 139:513–521, 1989.

113. Shapiro SH, Ernst P, Gray-Donald K, et al: Effect of negative pressure ventilation in severe chronic obstructive pulmonary disease. *Lancet* 340:1425–1429, 1992.

114. Fitting JW: Respiratory muscles during ventilatory support. *Eur Respir J* 7:2223–2225, 1994.

115. Belman MJ, Soo Hoo GW, Kuei JH, et al: Efficacy of positive vs negative pressure ventilation in unloading the respiratory muscles. *Chest* 98:850–856, 1990.

116. Van Lunteren E, Haxhiu MA, Cherniack NS, et al: Effects of posture and hypercapnia on chest wall muscle activity. *Fed Proc* 42:1012, 1983.

116a. DiMarco AF, Romaniule JR, Kowalski KE, Supinski GS: Efficacy of combined inspiratory intercostal and expiratory muscle pacing to maintain artificial ventilation. *Am J Respir Crit Care Med* 156(1):122–126, 1997.

117. Danon J, Druz WS, Goldberg NB, et al: Function of the isolated paced diaphragm and cervical accessory muscles in the C1 quadriplegic. *Am Rev Respir Dis* 119:909–919, 1979.

118. Colin MA, Howland AJ, Gilbert R, et al: Pulmonary function, ventilatory control and respiratory complications in quadriplegic subjects. *Am Rev Respir Dis* 100:526, 1969.

119. Glenn WW: Twenty years of experience in phrenic nerve stimulation to pace the diaphragm. *PACE* 9:780–784, 1986.

120. Glenn WW, Gee JBL, Cold DR, et al: Combined central alveolar hypoventilation and upper airway obstruction. *Am J Med* 64:50–60, 1978.

121. Gottfried SB, Strohl KP, DiMarco AF, et al: Upper airway resistance during phrenic stimulation in anesthetized dogs. *Am Rev Respir Dis* 125:219, 1983.

122. Kim JH, Manuelidis EA, Glenn WW, et al: Light and electron microscopic studies of phrenic nerves after long-term electrical stimulation. *J Neurosurg* 58:84–91, 1983.

123. Nochomovitz ML, Dimarco AF, Mortimer JT, et al: Diaphragm activation with intramuscular stimulation in dogs. *Am Rev Respir Dis* 127:325–329, 1983.

124. Dunn RB, Walter JS, Walsh J: Diaphragm and accessory respiratory muscle stimulation using intramuscular electrodes. *Arch Phys Med Rehabil* 76:266–271, 1995.

125. Moxham J: Aminophylline and respiratory muscles: An alternative view. *Clin Chest Med* 9(2):325–336, 1988.

126. Aubier M: Pharmacotherapy of respiratory muscles. *Clin Chest Med* 9(2):311–324, 1988.

127. Juan G, Calverly P, Talamo C, et al: Effect of carbon dioxide on diaphragmatic function in human beings. *N Engl J Med* 310:874–879, 1984.

128. Gorini M, Duranti R, Misuri G, et al: Aminophylline and respiratory muscle interaction in normal humans. *Am J Respir Crit Care Med* 149:1227–1234, 1994.

129. Supinski GS, Deal EC Jr, Kelson SG: Comparison of the effects of aminophylline and caffeine on diaphragmatic contractility in man. *Am Rev Respir Dis* 130:429–433, 1984.

130. Eldridge FL, Millhorn DE, Waldrop TG, et al: Mechanism of respiratory effects of methylxanthines. *Respir Physiol* 53:239–261, 1983.

131. Aubier M, Murciano D, Viires N, et al: Increased ventilation caused by improved diaphragmatic efficiency during aminophylline infussion. *Am Rev Respir Dis* 127:148–154, 1983.

132. DeCramer M, Descheppes K, Jiang TX, et al: Effects of aminophylline on respiratory muscle interaction. *Am Rev Respir Dis* 144:797–802, 1991.

133. Rall TW: Central nervous stimulants: The methylxanthines, in Gilman AG, Goodman LD, Rall TW, Murad F (eds): *The Pharmacological Basis of Therapeutics*, 7th ed. New York, Macmillan, 1985; pp 589–603.

134. Powers SK, Wade M, Criswell D, et al: Role of beta-adrenergic mechanisms in exercise training-induced metabolic changes in respiratory and locomotor muscle. *Int J Sports Med* 16:13–18, 1995.

135. Goffart M, Ritchie JM: The effect of adrenaline on the contractility of mammalian skeletal muscle. *J Physiol* 116:357–371, 1952.

136. Howell S, Roussos C: Isoproterenol and aminophylline improve contractility of fatigued canine diaphragm. *Am Rev Respir Dis* 129:118–124, 1984.

137. Aubier M, Viires N, Murciano D, et al: Effects and mechanisms of action of terbutaline and diaphragmatic contractility and fatigue. *J Appl Physiol* 56:922–929, 1984.

138. Fell R, Lizzo F, Cervoni P, et al: Effect of contractile activity on rat skeletal muscle beta-adrenoreceptor properties. *Proc Soc Exp Biol Med* 180:527–532, 1985.

139. Raaijmakers J, Terpstra G: Tulobuterol, a new beta 2-sympatheticomimetic drug: An in vitro comparison with terbutaline and salbutamol. *Bull Eur Physiopathol Respir* 22:100S, 1986.

140. Lanigan C, Howes TQ, Borzone G, et al: The effects of beta 2-agonists and caffeine on respiratory and limb muscle performance. *Eur Respir J* 6:1192–1196, 1993.

141. Ball DI, Brittain RT: Salmeterol, a novel, long-acting β2 adrenoreceptor agonist characterization of pharmacological activity in vitro and in vivo. *Br J Pharmacol* 104:665–671, 1991.

142. Anderson GP: Pharmacology of formoterol: An innovative bronchodilator. *Agents Actions* 34:97–115, 1991.

143. Dahl R, Earshaw JS, Palmer JBD: Salmeterol: A four week study of long-acting beta-adrenoreceptor agonist for the treatment of reversible airways disease. *Eur Respir Dis J* 4:1178–1184, 1991.

144. Weiner P, Azgad Y, Weiner M: Inspiratory muscle training during treatment with corticosteroids in humans. *Chest* 107:1041–1044, 1995.

145. British Thoracic Society Guidelines for the management of asthma in adults with chronic persistent asthma. *BMJ* 301:651–653, 1990.

Chapter 5

MECHANISMS OF RESPIRATORY RHYTHM GENERATION AND THEIR DISTURBANCE

DIETHELM W. RICHTER

KLAUS BALLANYI

PETER M. LALLEY

In all mammalian species, gas exchange between the external environment and the organism is controlled by a neuronal respiratory network within the lower brain stem. A network of ventral respiratory neurons produces rhythmic activity and, through activation of spinal motoneurons, finally leads to periodic contractions of diaphragmatic, thoracic, and abdominal muscles. The respiratory rhythm oscillates in three neural phases: inspiration, postinspiration, and expiration.

The bilateral pre-Bötzinger complex is the center of the respiratory network and contains six subtypes of neurons, which are identified by their activity profile as pre-, early-, through-, late-, and postinspiratory and expiratory neurons. The neural mechanisms of rhythm and pattern generation involve synaptic interactions between neurons and cooperative adjustments of intrinsic membrane properties. All these processes are influenced by neuromodulators and can be manipulated by pharmacologic agents.

Here we describe our present view about the basic mechanisms of rhythm generation and methods of their modulation. Such knowledge may open new approaches to the treatment of respiratory disturbances such as rapid shallow breathing, involuntary breath holding/apneusis, or central apnea.

The primary function of respiration is the exchange of gases between the external environment and the organism. In mammals, this occurs through coordinated rhythmic actions of the respiratory and cardiovascular control systems. The respiratory system controls rhythmic ventilation of the lung; the cardiovascular system handles the transportation of O_2 in the bloodstream from the lung to various organs and of CO_2 from organ tissues to the lungs. All these processes are adjusted by a coupled cardiorespiratory control mechanism.

Ventilation of the lungs depends on the rhythmic movements of respiratory muscles innervated by spinal motoneurons that are activated by oscillatory bulbospinal outputs of the respiratory network within the lower brain stem. This oscillatory activity is to some extent independent of peripheral feedback. This chapter deals with the mechanisms underlying respiratory rhythm generation and pattern formation of respiratory activities. It also describes some neural processes leading to disturbance of rhythmic respiratory activity and indicates new ways to treat them.

Respiratory Movements and Neural Phases of the Respiratory Rhythm

Inspiratory and expiratory neural activities control the movements of the thorax, the diaphragm, and the abdominal wall.[1] This produces periodic swings in thoracic volume that determine the flow of the air into and out of the lungs and thus the volume and duration of inhalation and exhalation. The dimensions of the upper airways, such as the pharynx, the larynx, and the bronchial tree, are controlled by cranial motoneurons. These motoneurons are synaptically coupled with the medullary respiratory network[2-6] and adjust airflow resistance.[7] This regulation is also used for vocalization.[8,9]

Inhalation and exhalation are controlled by three neural phases[10]: inspiration (I phase), postinspiration (PI phase, which is synonymous with *passive expiration*), and expiration (E phase, which corresponds to *active expiration*) (Fig. 5-1; see below). These are actively controlled by three classes of medullary neurons (see Fig. 5-1). The different neural activities can be easily discerned in the motor outflow to the diaphragm spinal segments (C4–6), to the external intercostals (T4–10) or the internal intercostal spinal (T4–10) segments, to abdominal muscles, and also to laryngeal muscles such as the thyroarytenoid muscle (see Fig. 5-1) (for review, see Feldman[11]). The lungs are filled with air during the I phase by expansion of the intrathoracic volume resulting from a steadily augmenting contraction of the diaphragm and inspiratory intercostal muscles. Such augmenting inspiratory muscle contraction originates from recruitment and a ramplike increase in discharge of motoneurons. Laryngeal abductor muscles are also activated during inspiration and dilate the larynx[8,12] (see Fig. 5-1). The energy for exhalation is accumulated during inspiration and is stored in the recoil forces of lung tissue. It is released during postinspiration when lung volume is slowly reduced by relaxation of the diaphragm due to a declining postinspiratory "afterdischarge" of phrenic motoneurons.[13,14] Additionally, early expiratory airflow is retarded by contraction of laryngeal adductor muscles (e.g., the thyroarytenoid muscle), which increases upper airway resistance.[7,12] This regulatory postinspiratory activity pattern is visible during postinspiration in the declining discharge of recurrent laryngeal nerves, which, among others, innervate laryngeal adductor muscles (see Fig. 5-1). During the final part of exhalation, expiratory airflow can be reinforced by an active contraction of expiratory intercostal and abdominal muscles. Phrenic and inspiratory intercostal nerves are completely silent during this phase of the respiratory cycle (see Fig. 5-1).

Respiratory Center within the Brain Stem

The rhythmic nervous outflow from spinal motoneurons to the respiratory muscles is controlled by a bilaterally organized ventral respiratory group (VRG) of neurons within the lower brain stem.[11,15-17] The VRG extends rostrocaudally in close proximity to the nucleus ambiguus and forms a "distributed" network. There exists a *vital point* on both sides of the brain stem that is essential for respiratory rhythm generation. Rhythmic respiratory output disappears when

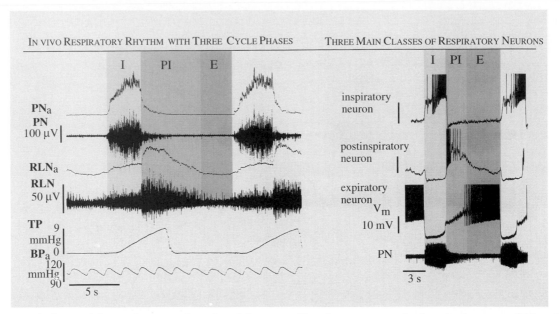

FIGURE 5-1 Neural phases of the respiratory cycle and medullary neurons. The left side of the figure illustrates the three phases of the respiratory cycle: inspiratory (I), postinspiratory (PI), and expiratory (E) phases, as recorded from motor nerves innervating the diaphragm and laryngeal muscles. Recordings illustrate phrenic nerve (PN) and recurrent laryngeal nerve activities (RLN) and their respective average discharge (PN$_a$, RLN$_a$). The shaded areas define the onset and duration of each phase.

Also shown are records of tracheal pressure (TP) and arterial blood pressure (BP). On the right side are recordings of membrane potential (V$_m$) from the three main classes of medullary respiratory neurons that control the three neural respiratory phases together with a neurogram of phrenic nerve activity (PN) to reveal the time relationship of V$_m$ fluctuations to the phases of the respiratory cycle. See text for a more detailed description.

neuronal activity within this specific point is blocked by local injection of tetrodotoxin or conotoxins.[18,19] It contains a kernel network of various subtypes of respiratory neurons that are thought to be necessary for respiratory rhythm generation.[20–22] The kernel network can be isolated in in vitro slice preparations and continues to generate rhythmic respiratory-like activity.[18,23,24] Histologically, this point is not identifiable as a "nucleus" but rather forms a loose complex of respiratory neurons within the ventral region just caudal to the retrofacial nucleus, referred to as the *pre-Bötzinger complex*[20,23,25,26] (Fig. 5-2). The name *pre-Bötzinger* identifies a location that is caudal to the Bötzinger region.[27–29] However, since the name *Bötzinger* is a fantasy name without any specific morphologic meaning (see comments in Feldman[11]), one could equally well label the pre-Bötzinger complex region the *respiratory center*.

Slightly more rostral to this respiratory center there is the classical area of "central chemosensitivity."[30,31] There is also partial overlap with the region of rostroventrolateral medulla, where sympathetic vasomotor tone seems to be generated.[32,33] Such close proximity of regions raises the question as to whether "cardiorespiratory" functions may be controlled by a common "cardiorespiratory center" representing a kernel of the more extensive respiratory and cardiovascular control networks in the brain stem.[34,35]

Medullary Respiratory Neurons

Medullary respiratory neurons do not have a *resting membrane potential* because they receive ongoing inhibitory or excitatory and inhibitory "synaptic drive" inputs that sum-

mate to produce long-lasting fluctuations of membrane potential[36–39] (Fig. 5-3). It might be important in this regard to note that, already at birth, inhibitory postsynaptic potentials (IPSPs) hyperpolarize neurons in vivo in the cat[40] and even in developmentally immature rodents.[41,42] The resting membrane potential of respiratory neurons can only be estimated when synaptic interaction is blocked pharmacologically or when animals are hyperventilated, which causes the disappearance of most of the synaptic drives and central apnea[43] (see Fig. 5-3).

Rhythmic synaptic bombardment produces metabolic and biophysical changes in the neurons that affect neuronal excitability. Inhibitory transmitters such as gamma-aminobutyric acid (GABA) and glycine activate inhibitory postsynaptic currents (IPSCs) carried by Cl$^-$ that is combined with a HCO$_3^-$ efflux that leads to significant intracellular acidification and produces a low cytosolic pH in respiratory neurons[39,44–48] (see Fig. 5-3). Excitatory postsynaptic cation inward currents (EPSCs) and membrane depolarization lead to excitation of neurons and activate Ca^{2+} influx.[39,49,50] Elevated cytosolic [Ca^{2+}] (see Fig. 5-3) then initiates Ca^{2+}-dependent K$^+$ currents.[51-54] These processes lead to a more than threefold increase in somatic membrane conductance[43] that effectively depresses the voltage-dependent "intrinsic properties" of neurons during most of the respiratory cycle (see below).

Respiratory neurons are subdivided into six subtypes that are identified by the timing and pattern of their ongoing membrane potential oscillations eliciting patterned bursts of action potential discharge during membrane depolarization.[10,20,55–58] The neurons are classified as preinspiratory (pre-I), early-inspiratory (early-I), through-inspiratory

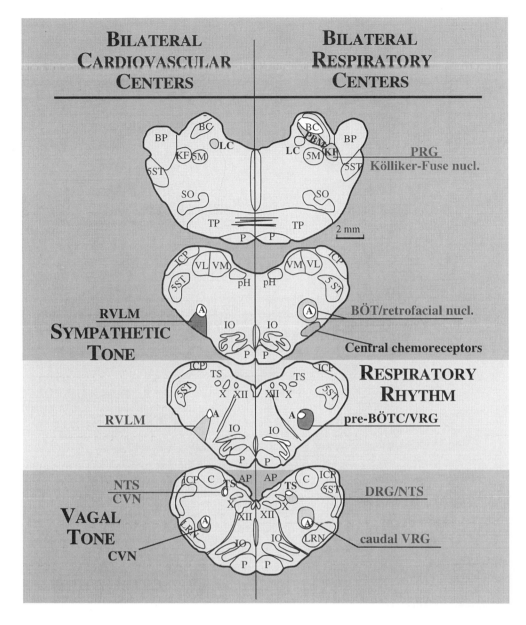

FIGURE 5-2 Location of the respiratory and cardiovascular centers within the brain stem. Schematic illustration of bilaterally organized regions in the brain stem that are essential for the production of normal respiratory rhythmicity and cardiovascular tone. Coronal sections are from the pons and the medulla oblongata. The relevant respiratory regions, identified on the right side, are (1) the pontine respiratory group (PRG), consisting of the medial parabrachial region (PBM) and Kölliker-Fuse nucleus (KF), (2) the Bötzinger (BÖT) region in the retrofacial nucleus of the medulla, (3) the central chemoreceptive region in ventrolateral medulla, (4) the dorsal respiratory group (DRG), including the nucleus of the solitary tract (NTS), (5) The pre-Bötzinger (pre-BÖT) complex within the ventral respiratory group (VRG), (6) the nucleus ambiguus (A), and (7) the region of the nucleus retroambigualis, medial to A in the VRG. Cardiovascular regions, identified on the left, are (1) the rostral ventrolateral medulla (RVLM), where presympathetic neurons are localized that generate the vasomotor tone, (2) the medial region of the NTS, and (3) the nucleus ambiguus, where cardiac vagal neurons are located.

(through-I), late-inspiratory (late-I), postinspiratory (PI), and expiratory (E) neurons (Fig. 5-4).

Early-I and PI neurons have certain activity patterns that point to specific cellular properties and network interconnections: Early-I neurons exhibit a rapid membrane depolarization and onset of discharge occurring up to 100 to 200 ms prior to the onset of the inspiratory discharge in the phrenic nerves. This "preinspiratory" onset of discharge indicates that these neurons might be involved in triggering inspiratory activity in the medullary network. Thereafter, discharge frequency declines, and the neurons stop firing during the second half of inspiration.[57] This decline of activity cannot be explained by synaptic inhibition alone.[59] A functionally more important mechanism seems to be an activity-related intracellular accumulation of Ca^{2+} and a consequent activation of Ca^{2+}-dependent mechanisms (such as Ca^{2+}-dependent K^+ conductances). Normally, early-I neurons are maximally inhibited during the PI phase and remain suppressed during most of the E phase (see Fig. 5-4). The membrane potential

oscillations of pre-I neurons are not very different from those seen in early-I neurons, despite a slowly increasing discharge during the late period of expiration.[20,22] Therefore, we believe that pre-I neurons represent a subgroup of early-I neurons receiving either a stronger tonic activation or a weaker declining pattern of synaptic inhibition during the E phase, allowing them to begin discharging earlier, during the "preinspiratory" (i.e., expiratory) period.

Similarly to early-I neurons, PI neurons also show a rapid membrane depolarization and low-threshold action potential discharge slightly before termination of inspiratory phrenic nerve activity. The frequency of action potential discharge also declines, and the neurons normally cease firing before the end of the expiratory interval[10,60,61] (see Fig. 5-4). The initial burst and the following adaptation of discharge are not heavily influenced by postsynaptic activities. Thus also this subtype of neurons seems to be transiently controlled by cellular properties responsible for rapid activation[62,63] and then for subsequent adaptation.[54] PI neurons are synaptically

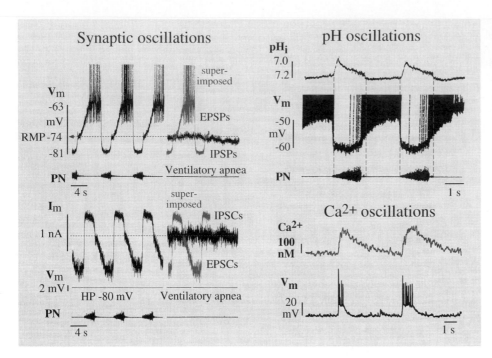

FIGURE 5-3 Synaptically mediated oscillations of membrane potential, membrane currents, intracellular pH, and Ca^{2+} in medullary respiratory neurons. (*Left*) Traces are membrane potential (V_m) and membrane currents (I_m) recorded from an expiratory neuron, and phrenic nerve activity (PN). During eupnea, V_m and I_m exhibit respiration-related oscillations, in synchrony with PN. Mechanical hyperventilation eliminates chemoreceptor-mediated excitatory synaptic drive, resulting in central apnea, as signaled by the absence of PN and elimination of oscillations of I_m resulting in a stable "resting membrane potential" of the E neuron. (*Right*) Respiratory oscillations of intracellular pH and intracellular Ca^{2+} measured in an expiratory (*upper*) and inspiratory (*lower*) neuron. Cytosolic pH becomes transiently more acidic during the period of synaptic inhibition, while intracellular Ca^{2+} concentration increases during every respiratory burst discharge.

inhibited during the E phase but often show a second membrane depolarization together with a second burst of spike discharge before the end of the E phase.[38,64] PI neurons are maximally suppressed during early inspiration.[10]

Through-I neurons start to depolarize with the beginning of inspiration, and some of them continue to depolarize almost linearly. Such linearly augmenting depolarization cannot result from recurrent excitatory loop connections alone[65–67] but likely arises from its integration with early-I inhibitory synaptic inputs.[10,16] Medullary through-I neurons are inhibited during the PI phase and remain suppressed during the E phase. Late-I neurons do not discharge action potentials before the second half of inspiration. This results from pronounced early-I inhibition, which shunts all excitatory drives arriving early in inspiration.[44] However, when released from early-I inhibition, late-I neurons rapidly discharge a short burst of action potentials. Afterwards they are inhibited again during the PI and E phases (see Fig. 5-4).

E neurons start to depolarize at the end of inspiration and often show a transient depolarization before onset of the PI phase. Thereafter, the neurons are synaptically inhibited again. The membrane potential starts to depolarize gradually as PI inhibition fades during quiet breathing and approaches a plateau potential turning to a steady discharge of action potentials. The augmenting pattern of action potential discharge of E neurons thus appears to result from a declining pattern of synaptic inhibition. E neurons are maximally suppressed during early inspiration and receive synaptic inhibition during late expiration.[29,45,68,69] During rapid shallow breathing or panting,[70] E neurons are inhibited throughout the cycle and remain silent[34] (see Fig. 5-3), indicating that the respiratory rhythm does not require expiratory neurons and oscillation and thus really oscillates in only two phases, i.e., inspiration and postinspiration.

Neurotransmitters

There is substantial information about the neurotransmitters used by the neurons of the respiratory network.[15,71] Synaptic activation seems to be mediated mainly through glutamate acting via non-NMDA (i.e., AMPA) receptors[72–74] as well as via NMDA receptors.[21,74–77] Most of the inhibitory synaptic events in respiratory neurons are mediated by $GABA_A$ receptor-activated Cl^- channels.[78–80] In addition, $GABA_B$ receptor-activated K^+ channels contribute to synaptic inhibition.[62,81–83] Synaptic inhibition of inspiratory neurons during early-I and PI phases is strychnine-sensitive.[78,79,84] This provides strong evidence that glycinergic inhibition also controls primary rhythm generation in vivo.

Neuromodulation and Intracellular Second Messengers

The excitability of respiratory neurons is continuously adjusted by neuromodulators such as catecholamines,[85–88] serotonin,[43,89–92] dopamine,[93,94] adenosine,[49,95–99] acetylcholine,[100,101] substance P,[92,102] somatostatin,[103] cholecystokinin,[104] and opioids.[105–109] Nitric oxide also seems to be important.[88,110] Most of the neuromodulators alter inotropic channel conductances by activation of G proteins, the subunits of which directly modulate membrane channels or act indirectly through intracellular second messengers. Cyclic 3',5'-adenosine monophosphate (cAMP), cAMP-dependent protein kinase A (cAMP-PKA), diacyl glycerol (DAG), protein kinase C (PKC), phosphatidylinositol-triphosphate (IP_3), and Ca^{2+} modulate receptors as well as voltage- and ligand-controlled channel activities.[111–115]

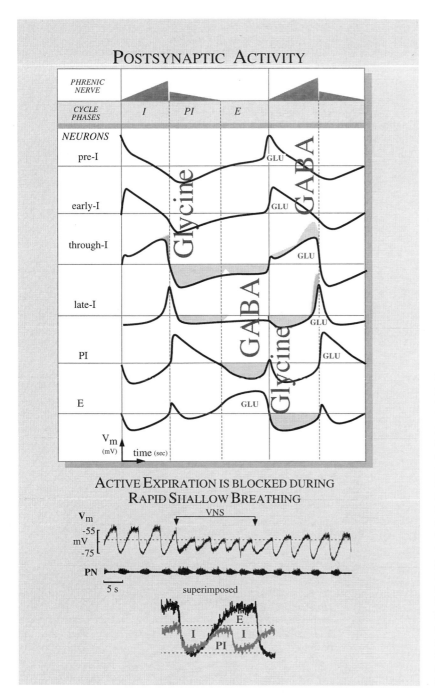

POSTSYNAPTIC ACTIVITY

ACTIVE EXPIRATION IS BLOCKED DURING RAPID SHALLOW BREATHING

FIGURE 5-4 Oscillations of membrane potential in medullary respiratory neurons. The scheme in the upper panel illustrates oscillations of membrane potential V_m, synchronized with phrenic nerve activity, that are typical for each subtype of medullary respiratory neuron. Shaded areas denote the pattern of synaptic inhibition (mediated primarily by GABA and glycine). Phases of synaptic depolarization are mediated principally by the neurotransmitter glutamate (GLU). Conversion of a three-phasic rhythm to two-phasic rhythm occurs during rapid shallow breathing, as shown in the lower panel. Stimulation of pulmonary afferents in the vagus nerve converts the normal three-phasic patterns of phrenic nerve (PN) activity and membrane potential (V_m) in a medullary expiratory (E) neuron into two-phasic patterns. The two-phasic pattern during vagus nerve stimulation (VNS) is evident from (*a*) absence of an expiratory phase–related silent period in PN activity and (*b*) arrest of V_m depolarization at the termination of the postinspiratory phase, followed immediately by inspiratory phase hyperpolarization of V_m.

Increased levels of cytosolic Ca^{2+} affect the duration of burst discharges by determining the degree of adaptation that contributes to phase-terminating activity. The underlying mechanism involves an increase in K^+ conductances. When intracellular $[Ca^{2+}]$ is experimentally reduced by injecting Ca^{2+} buffers, membrane resistance is increased and adaptation is reduced, leading to prolonged discharges.[52-54]

As studied at the single-cell level in intact adult mammals, activation of the cAMP-PKA system increases respiratory neuronal excitability by downregulating persistently activated K^+ channels[116,117] and IPSCs, as well as upregulating EPSCs.[83,118] "Systemic" activation of the cAMP-PKA pathway

in neonatal in vitro preparations, besides depolarizing VRG neurons,[105] also leads to increased respiratory frequency.[119] A good example of second messenger–mediated neuromodulation is the effects of serotonin (5HT) acting on $5HT_{1A}$ and $5HT_{2A}$ receptors. Activation of postsynaptic $5HT_{1A}$ receptors evokes downregulation of cAMP-PKA and hence leads to activation of persistent K^+ conductances and enforcement of IPSCs.[43,83,118] As discussed below, this was found to be important for the treatment of respiratory disturbances resulting from pathologically depressed inhibitory function or enhanced excitability of respiratory neurons leading to apneusis.[73,74,120-122] $5HT_{1A}$ receptor agonists or perhaps other neuromodulators that downregulate PKA may turn out to be effective in treating disorders in which apneustic breathing occurs.[123,124]

Activation of PKC, e.g., through $5HT_{2A}$ receptors, preferentially enhances EPSCs, whereas selective inhibition of PKC results in decline of IPSCs and EPSCs.[90,117,125] The excitatory effect of PKC is attributed to (1) decreased current flow through K^+ channels and (2) upregulation of postsynaptic EPSCs, including NMDA and AMPA types of glutamatergic currents. The PKC effects on neuronal inhibition are complex, since enhancement of GABA- and glycine-regulated channels is counteracted by depression of K^+ conductances.[125]

Network Structure and Modeling

The comparison between the patterns of action potential discharge of a particular subtype of VRG neurons and the patterns of postsynaptic activity elicited in other subtypes of neurons has allowed important inferences to be made about the basic connectivity within the respiratory network.[17] Many of these presumed connections are consistent with results obtained by cross-correlating the discharges of different neurons[65–67,126–132] and averaging unitary synaptic potentials in one neuron using the spike discharge of another neuron as a trigger.[22,29,58,68,133–135] Computer simulations based on such connectivity patterns reveal that the connectivity model can produce "normal" respiratory activity and also can explain disturbances to the rhythm, such as rapid shallow breathing, inspiratory apneusis, postinspiratory arrest, and apnea.[64,136,137]

Proposals for the Mechanism of Respiratory Rhythm Generation

What the principal mechanism of respiratory rhythm generation is remains a matter of controversy. Discussions of mechanisms concentrate on two theories. The *pacemaker theory* postulates that a biphasic respiratory rhythm, in both in vitro and in vivo conditions, arises from respiratory pacemaker cells within a hybrid network.[23,138–142] The *network theory* assumes that the three-phasic respiratory rhythm originates in vivo from a more complex network function that involves synaptic interactions between neurons that set narrow time windows for cellular bursting and for organizing synaptic off-switching of phase activities rather than via a pacemaker.[17,64,136,137,143]

PACEMAKER THEORY

The assumption that pacemaker cells generate the respiratory rhythm is based on the following findings in in vitro experiments: First, the in vitro isolated brain stem spinal cord of neonatal rats[138,144] and slices of the medulla from neonatal and mature rats[18,23,24,145] contain the pre-Bötzinger complex, and these slices continue to generate rhythmic activity that occurs in synchrony with the respiratory discharge of phrenic and/or hypoglossal motoneurons. Second, this in vitro rhythm persists when inhibitory synaptic transmission ($GABA_{A,B}$ and glycine) is blocked in "wild type" rats and mice[18,140,141,144,146,147] and in the mutant *oscillator* mouse that does not express the adult form of the glycine receptor.[148] Third, respiratory neurons continue to generate a rhythmic burst discharge when synaptic transmission and activation of output motoneurons are blocked by lowering extracellular calcium ion concentrations.[140,144]

Although all types of VRG neurons have been observed to generate such spontaneous in vitro bursting,[142] Onimaru and colleagues[146,147] have proposed as the primary pacemaker a respiratory neuron type that they called *pre-I neurons* ("Onimaru type"). The group of Feldman and Smith[149,150] postulated that another type of pre-I neurons ("Smith type") are the essential pacemaker cell. So far, however, clear intrinsic bursting behavior has been studied only in inspiratory and nonrespiratory VRG neurons in situations when synaptic interaction was not blocked.[23,147] Such neurons reveal endogenous bursting and, essentially so, a change in burst frequency when their membrane potential reaches the voltage range of -55 to -45 mV.[23] While the neurons are described as having inhibitory synaptic interactions, these connections do not seem to be essential for rhythm production, although they modify the rhythm, as shown theoretically in computer simulations.[150]

NETWORK THEORY

The network theory emphasizes that besides cellular bursting features of respiratory neurons, there are other factors deemed necessary for rhythm generation under in vivo conditions. These factors can be summarized as follows: First, a rhythmic bombardment with excitatory and inhibitory synaptic inputs underlies all the membrane potential changes within the crucial voltage range of -70 to -40 mV.[10] Second, synaptically controlled (especially inhibitory) processes are present that reduce neuronal input resistance of respiratory neurons by 50 to 80 percent[43] and override any spontaneous nonsynaptic conductance changes during prolonged periods of the respiratory cycle.[151–153] Inward currents that might operate through endogenously activated cation conductances effectively would be counteracted by persistent K^+ and inhibitory synaptic currents, thus blocking any tendency to pacemaker-like membrane depolarization during most periods of the respiratory cycle. This became obvious from in vitro[39,50,51] and in vivo[19,153] experiments performed to analyze voltage-dependent Na^+ and Ca^{2+} currents. Prior to blockade of persistent K^+ and synaptically controlled conductances, all sorts of inward cation currents effectively were counterbalanced by prominent outward currents between a voltage range of -100 and $+10$ mV.[49,51]

The network theory assumes that mutual inhibition of reciprocally connected (e.g., early-I and PI) neurons plays the key role in rhythm generation because it (1) opens a narrow time window of transiently increased neuronal input resistance restricted to the time when dominance of synaptic inhibition fades, which is the condition for "cellular bursting," (2) shapes the activity patterns of various types of respiratory neurons, (3) irreversibly "off-switches" phasic burst activities, and finally (4) sets the condition for rapidly inactivating membrane conductances.[143,153,154] The assumption that periods of inhibitory synaptic hyperpolarization are essential for on-switching and off-switching rhythmic burst activity is consistent with the observation that the in vivo cat blockade of $GABA_A$ receptor-mediated synaptic inhibition within the pre-Bötzinger complex on both sides induces apneustic respiratory discharges. Respiratory activity oscillates at greatly reduced frequencies, and additional blockade of glycinergic inhibition leads to further disturbance or even complete blockade.[19] It also agrees with the observation that the respiratory rhythm is arrested under in vivo conditions when synaptic inhibition is reduced and blocked during hypoxia.[155] Similar responses have been observed previously when synaptic inhibition was blocked in the perfused brain stem of adult rats[156] or when inhibitory synaptic interaction was blocked in the longitudinal brain stem slice preparation of mature mouse that includes a more complex respiratory network on one side.[145] These findings lead us to postulate that the mechanisms of respiratory rhythm generation are different when studied in vitro and in vivo. Such differences have to be considered when respiratory disturbances in humans are evaluated. The conclusion is that malfunction of synaptic inhibition results in severely disturbed breathing patterns in vivo (see Wilken et al.[124]).

Bursting Properties

The respiratory rhythm seems to be effectively controlled by a neuronal network that is activated by peripheral and central chemoreceptors[30,59,157–159] and by extrinsic sources such as the reticular formation.[160–162] The activating synaptic input need not be rhythmically modulated and could in fact be tonic. Tonic activity can be converted within the network into a rhythmic output by synaptic interaction that sets and modifies specific membrane properties of respiratory neurons[17,143] (Fig. 5-5).

Modulation of intrinsic properties of neurons by synaptic interaction means the following: Whenever the discharge declines in one subtype of neuron, postsynaptic inhibition diminishes in an antagonistically interconnected neuron type. The membrane potential escapes the hyperpolarizing "functional voltage clamp" of IPSCs and depolarizes slowly while input resistance increases, making the neuron susceptible to intrinsic voltage-dependent conductance changes. At a certain voltage range, below the threshold for Na$^+$-spike discharge, this disinhibition leads to activation of the low-voltage-activated Ca^{2+} current (Ca$_T$)[49,50,153] and probably a persisting Na$^+$ current (Na$_P$).[50,152] This results in rebound membrane depolarization that activates the intermediate-voltage-activated Ca^{2+} current (Ca$_P$)[39,49,50] and the fast-inactivating Na$^+$ current (Na$_{HH}$),[163] triggering a spike discharge. The action potentials bring the membrane potential into the voltage range where the high-voltage-activated Ca^{2+} currents (Ca$_{L,N}$)[39,49,50] are activated. Most of these conductances promote extensive Ca^{2+} influx, leading to an activity-dependent accumulation of intracellular, Ca^{2+}.[51] The accumulated Ca^{2+} activates calcium-dependent K$^+$ (K$_{Ca}$)[52–54] and possibly Cl$^-$ (Cl$_{Ca}$) currents.[164] These currents lead to repolarization of the membrane potential, independent of synaptic inhibition and adaptation of the spike discharge. Adaptation of discharge means that the inhibitory synaptic suppression of antagonistic populations of neurons vanishes so that these neurons activate their Ca$_T$ and Na$_P$ conductances. Antagonistic neurons are then phasically inhibited and hyperpolarize long enough to allow Ca$_T$ and Na$_{HH}$ conductances to deinactivate and intracellular Ca^{2+} to be transported into intracellular stores or out of the cells. In essence, synaptic inhibition plays an essential role in respiratory rhythm gener-

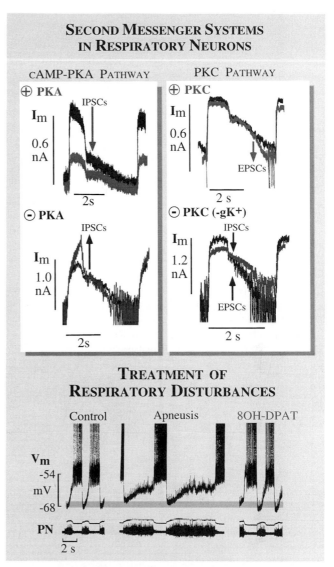

FIGURE 5-5 Burst generation in neurons of the respiratory network. The scheme illustrates how synaptic interactions between brain stem respiratory neurons modulate intrinsic membrane currents, resulting in generation and amplification of bursts of action potential discharges. Inspiratory neurons receive periodic and/or tonic synaptic drive from external sources. Excitatory synaptic drive (+) mediated by glutamate (GLU) depolarizes neurons and at certain voltages activates intrinsic membrane calcium (Ca) and sodium (Na) currents that boost the depolarizing voltage changes, thus leading to generation of bursts of action potentials. Duration and intensity of bursts are amplified (+) by recurrent excitatory synaptic transmission within the network. Bursts are terminated by calcium-activated potassium and chloride currents (K$_{Ca}$, Cl$_{Ca}$) and by inhibitory synaptic input that is mediated by glycine (GLY) and GABA released from antagonistically interconnected neurons.

ation under in vivo conditions by (1) producing long-lasting periods of stable membrane hyperpolarization, with increased neuronal conductances that suppress potential pacemaking fluctuations of membrane potential, (2) resetting inactivating voltage-dependent conductances, and (3) providing long-lasting intervals in the range of seconds for adequate control of ionic homeostasis.[17]

Another voltage-dependent K$^+$ current, such as I$_A$, is expressed in respiratory neurons[165,166] but seems not to play a significant role under normal conditions of quiet breathing.[151] The potential pacemaking, nonspecific Na$^+$/K$^+$ current (I$_H$) that is activated by membrane hyperpolarization and, besides Ca$_T$, is essential for rhythmic bursting in thalamic relay neurons[167] is so far not found in medullary respiratory neurons.

Activity Patterning

Pattern formation of the network involves integrative mechanisms. The linearly rising inspiratory ramp activity results from neural integration of recurrent excitation within a population of through-I neurons[65,67] and early-I inhibition.[10,44,168] The activity pattern of late-I neurons results from integration of excitatory and inhibitory inspiratory activities.[10]

Besides patterning of inspiratory and expiratory activities,[44,45,60,168] early-I and PI neurons also directly or indirectly control the timing of the inspiratory off-switching mechanism.[60,61,169-171] Early-I inhibition is responsible for the delayed discharge of late-I neurons, which are assumed to produce an initially graded and reversible inspiratory off-switch, while inspiration is irreversibly brought to an end by PI inhibition when the primary oscillator has moved to its antagonistic phase. Both inspiratory-terminating mechanisms are activated by pulmonary afferents that measure lung expansion.[11,169]

Summarizing the various processes of in vivo rhythm generation, we propose that the following cellular processes are sequentially activated during a normal respiratory cycle:

1. *Respiratory drive.* The network is activated from external sources. One possible source could be the reticular activating system.
2. *Inspiratory on-switch.* Release from synaptic inhibition triggers pre-I neurons and rebound excitation of early-I or through-I neurons.
3. *Inspiratory bursting.* Disinhibition and rebound depolarization provokes cellular bursting (see Fig. 5-5).
4. *Inspiratory pattern generation.* Recurrent excitation within the population of through-I neurons augments inspiratory burst strength (see Fig. 5-5) and, by integration of excitatory and inhibitory inputs, produces linearly rising membrane depolarization and augmenting excitation of inspiratory neurons. This activity pattern is fed to the inspiratory bulbospinal output and thence to phrenic motoneurons.
5. *Reversible off-switch of inspiration.* Adaptation of early-I neurons and disinhibition of late-I neurons leads to late-I inhibition of through-I neurons that effectively shunts recurrent excitatory inputs.[172] Apneustic breathing patterns occur when this sort of inhibition is disturbed (see below).
6. *Phase switching of the oscillator and irreversible inhibition of inspiration.* Decreasing inspiratory synaptic inhibition of PI neurons leads to rebound excitation of PI neurons. Rapid onset of their discharge irreversibly terminates inspiration by effective synaptic inhibition. The respiratory network comes to transient arrest during this PI phase because PI inhibition of E neurons suppresses onset of expiration, as well as the external tonic drive via reticular neurons.[10] PI neurons are further activated, and the PI phase is often prolonged by excitatory inputs from the pontine region,[173-175] from laryngeal afferents,[60,73,176,177] and probably from the cortical and subcortical regions during vocalization.[8,12,178]
7. *Phase switching in the oscillator and on-switching of expiration.* Adaptation of PI neurons leads to disinhibition of E neurons, which become active and slow the rhythm. Activated E neurons inhibit early-I and PI neurons but also through-I and late-I neurons. Activation of E neurons is, however, blocked during rapid shallow breathing (see Fig. 5-4).
8. *Phase switching in the oscillator and off-switching of expiration.* The late-E discharge of pre-I and PI neurons terminates the burst of E neurons and enables phase switching to inspiration.

Disturbances of Respiratory Rhythm

RAPID SHALLOW BREATHING

Stimulation of pulmonary C fibers induces rapid shallow breathing,[70] during which the E phase is absent. The rhythm oscillates only between the antagonistic inspiratory and postinspiratory phases[34] (see Fig. 5-4). This biphasic rhythm demonstrates that medullary expiratory activity is not necessary for central rhythm generation (see above); i.e., expiratory activity does not represent the primary antagonistic phase to inspiration. When activated, however, expiratory activity is effective in slowing the rhythm. A biphasic oscillation of breathing also occurs during panting in some animals. Such rapid respiratory oscillations that are used for thermoregulation produce only dead-space ventilation that does not affect acid-base balance or gas exchange.

INSPIRATORY APNEUSIS

The respiratory rhythm can be trapped in inspiration when inhibitory synaptic inputs to and within the network are reduced or blocked because the postinspiratory off-switching is impaired. Arrest of rhythmic breathing during apneusis causes hypoxia and hypercapnia because the lungs are no longer ventilated.[123,124] Weakening or blockade of inhibitory synaptic processes might occur as a result of lesioning of the brain stem–pons regions,[121,124,179] mild acute or chronic hypoxia, ischemia within the respiratory network,[155,180-182] or blockade of inhibitory interneurons due to overdose with barbiturates[123] or blockade of their activation through NMDA receptor antagonists.[73,75]

POSTINSPIRATORY APNEA

Stabilization of the PI phase can result in a "functional apnea" that also leads to systemic hypoxia and could possibly cause sudden death.[183] Such disturbance can occur easily when afferents from laryngeal receptors or bronchial irritant receptors[60,61,176,177,184] are activated or when pontine[173-175] or cortical regions[185] are strongly excited.

HYPOXIC RESPONSE

The response to severe systemic hypoxia or brain stem ischemia is biphasic, an initial augmentation turning into a secondary depression of respiratory activity and slowing of respiratory rate that finally terminates in respiratory arrest.[186-188] The biphasic response to hypoxia is also found in vitro in brain

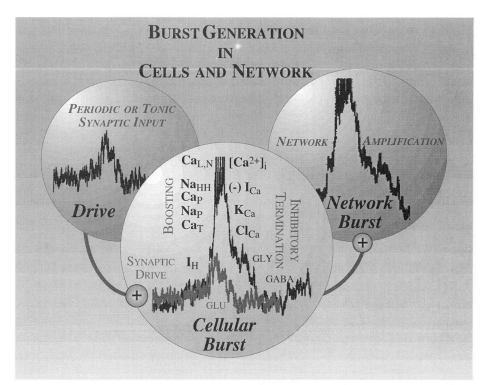

FIGURE 5-6 Second messenger–mediated modulation of respiratory neurons. (*Upper panels*) The functional importance of the cyclic-3′,5′-adenosine monophosphate–dependent protein kinase A (cAMP-PKA) and protein kinase C (PKC) second messenger pathways in modulating excitatory and inhibitory synaptic inputs to medullary respiratory neurons is illustrated. Pairs of superimposed traces are synaptic currents recorded from medullary expiratory neurons. For each pair, the darker trace is a control response recorded before alteration of PKA or PKC activity. Increasing (+) cAMP-PKA activity (*upper left*) markedly suppresses inhibitory postsynaptic currents ($\downarrow$IPSCs) and increases excitatory drive currents. When cAMP-PKA activity is suppressed (−, *lower left*), IPSCs are significantly enhanced ($\uparrow$). Increased PKC activity (*upper right*) leads to increased excitability by augmenting EPSCs and depressing IPSCs. Suppression (−) of PKC activity results in depression of EPSCs and IPSCs (*lower right*) after persistent K^+ currents were suppressed by TEA. (*Lower panel*) Treatment of an apneustic respiratory disorder by downregulating cAMP-PKA in the respiratory network with 8-OHDPAT, a $5HT_{1A}$ receptor agonist. Traces show membrane potential (V_m) of an expiratory (E) neuron, phrenic nerve activity (PN), and its moving average (*middle trace*). Horizontal reference bar denotes changes in maximum level of synaptic inhibition during the inspiratory phase. Control respiratory cycles are shown to the left. Middle panel shows apneustic disturbances produced by intravenous injection of the glutamate (NMDA) receptor blocker MK-801 (0.3 mg/kg). Apneusis is signaled by prolonged PN discharges and delayed discharges of the E neuron. Right panel shows reestablishment of a normal respiratory rhythm after increasing cAMP-PKA activity in the respiratory network by injecting 8-OHDPAT (10 μg/kg IV).

stem preparations,[189–191] which points to a central mechanism that is enforced by hypoxic depression of arterial chemoreceptive drive of the respiratory network.[59,158]

There are considerable developmental changes in the sensitivity of the respiratory network to hypoxia.[192–195] Neonatal rats survive anoxia for up to 1 h, whereas in mature animals respiratory efforts stop after only a few minutes.[196–199] Different from the adult in isolated brain stem preparations of neonatal rodents, long-lasting anoxic periods result in depression of respiratory frequency without occurrence of apneustic or apneic activity patterns.[191] There are also no major changes in extracellular [K^+] or [Ca^{2+}], indicating that there is effective utilization of anaerobic metabolism that enables rodents, which are born more immaturely than humans,[200] to maintain respiratory network functions shortly after birth.[201–205] Under in vitro conditions, respiratory neurons of the neonatal rat are only slightly depolarized by increased spontaneous EPSP activity during the early period of anoxia, but inspiration-related inhibition of E neurons is blocked (Fig. 5-6). Later, during hypoxia, the majority of neonatal respiratory neurons hyperpolarizes due to increased K^+ conductances. The amplitudes of inspiratory synaptic drive potentials are greatly reduced at the same time, leading to arrest of rhythmic discharges in more than 50 percent of cells (see Fig. 5-6). This reduction of network activity may help protect the network against activity-related damage.[206]

The respiratory network of adult cats and rabbits depends more critically on aerobic metabolism. Extracellular [K^+] rises maximally to 10 to 15 mM[207–209] during anoxic periods of more than 5 min. These changes do not originate from an irreversible damage of respiratory neurons; they rather represent activation of several K^+ conductances, such as ATP-dependent and adenosine-activated K^+ conductances[49,210] that stabilize the membrane potential of neurons at fairly negative values of −40 to −50 mV. Additional pre- and/or postsynaptic mechanisms may stabilize the membrane potential of neurons during hypoxia, such as acidosis effects on synaptic transmission,[211–213] endogenous opioids,[102,108,109,214,215] monoamines,[43,87,89,211,217] nitric oxide,[88] and/or other neuroactive substances. These mechanisms render the mature respiratory

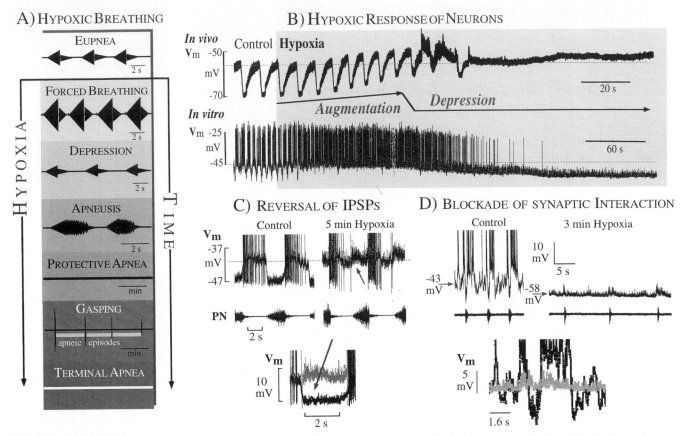

FIGURE 5-7 Disturbances of respiratory rhythm during hypoxia.
(*A*) Schematic representation of progressive changes in phrenic nerve activity during hypoxia, beginning with forced breathing at the onset of hypoxia (*upper trace*) and terminating in apnea during prolonged hypoxia (*lower trace*). (*B*) Progression of membrane potential changes during hypoxia in medullary respiratory neurons in the adult cat in vivo (*upper*) and in neonatal in vitro rat (*lower*). The membrane potential (V_m) of the expiratory neuron recorded in vivo is below threshold for action potential discharge before hypoxia (control). Dashed line denotes maximum level of depolarization under control conditions. In the in vitro record of the inspiratory neuron, action potential threshold under control conditions is represented by the dashed line. Hypoxia produces initial augmentation of EPSPs and action potential discharges, followed by membrane hyperpolarization and EPSP depression in the neonatal in vitro preparation. In the adult in vivo cat, hypoxia leads to an initial augmentation of re-

spiratory activity, followed by blockade of IPSPs that leads to augmentation of EPSPs. During prolonged hypoxia, the membrane potential is stabilized at a level below −50 mV. (*C*) Hypoxic reversal of IPSPs in in vivo cat. V_m records are taken from a postinspiratory (PI) neuron. After 5 min of hypoxia, IPSPs during the inpiratory phase were reversed to depolarizing IPSPs (*ascending arrow*) that occasionally generated action potentials. Superimposed traces further illustrate depolarization of inspiratory phased IPSP waves in the PI neuron. Dark trace and descending arrow denote control recording. (*D*) Hypoxic blockade of synaptic interactions in in vitro neonatal rat. After 3 min of exposure to hypoxia, V_m in a PI neuron was hyperpolarized, EPSPs and IPSPs were severely depressed, and action potential discharges were arrested. Changes are further illustrated in superimposed traces that show V_m under control (*dark trace*) and hypoxic conditions.

network quite tolerant to oxygen depletion, and normal breathing patterns can be reestablished even after periods of more than 15 min of hypoxia.[218–220]

HYPOXIC APNEUSIS
An important consequence of even moderate hypoxic membrane depolarization in adult respiratory neurons, however, is the tendency of the intact network to produce apneustic breathing patterns.[155,220,221] The reason for this is the reduction of synaptic inhibition and the reversal of normally hyperpolarizing IPSPs to depolarizing potentials (Fig. 5-7). The latter change seems to be reinforced when acidosis is treated with HCO_3^- infusion.[155] Reduced efficacy of late-I inhibition of inspiratory neurons results in failure of the inspiratory off-

switching and prolonged (apneustic) inspiratory bursts in phrenic nerves.

PROTECTIVE HYPOXIC APNEA
Synaptic inhibition decreases further as hypoxia progresses (see Fig. 5-7). The adult respiratory network seems to be very sensitive to hypoxic blockade of synaptic inhibition, since central respiratory activity finally comes to arrest. There is complete arrest of spontaneous spike discharge in nearly all subtypes of neurons; however, a few expiratory neurons discharge tonically at low frequencies.[155,222,223] It is of vital importance to know that this blockade of spontaneous action potential discharge does not occur because of irreversible cell damage or uncontrolled release of transmitters, as assumed

before.[224] The microdialysate from VRG regions shows that extracellular GABA and glutamate levels are elevated only during the initial hypoxic period of augmented synaptic interaction but are reduced below normal levels during the period of central apnea.[19,225] All respiratory neurons remain excitable during this period of hypoxic apnea, which therefore can be considered to be "protective" (see Fig. 5-7). This protective apnea is reversible in cats in vivo for periods of up to 30 min. The mature brain stem has a higher tolerance to hypoxia than the cardiovascular system, which can collapse during this period.[155,220]

TERMINAL HYPOXIC APNEA

Hypoxic respiratory arrest progresses to *irreversible apnea*, which is interrupted by gasping efforts that occur with declining strength and frequency.[224,226–229] This signals the beginning of serious damage to the respiratory network. Gasps are probably organized by medullary structures in the lateral tegmental field of the medulla,[227,230] which is located outside the primary respiratory network.[19,231] It is therefore possible that other brain stem regions also may be disturbed in this situation. A declining pattern of hypoxic gasping may signal the ultimate period when reestablishment of oxygen supply might rescue brain stem functions.[219,232–235]

Acknowledgments

We would like to thank Anne Bischoff for superb technical assistance in the preparation of this review and for important contributions to previous manuscripts.

References

1. Monteau R, Hilaire G: Spinal respiratory motoneurons. *Prog Neurobiol* 37:83–144, 1991.
2. Eyzaguirre C, Taylor JR: Respiratory discharge of some vagal motoneurons. *J Neurophysiol* 26:61–78, 1963.
3. Hwang J-C, Bartlett D Jr, St John WM: Characterization of respiratory-modulated activities of hypoglossal motoneurons. *J Appl Physiol Respir Environ Exerc Physiol* 55:793–798, 1983.
4. Grélot L, Barillot JC, Bianchi AL: Pharyngeal motoneurones: Respiratory-related activity and responses to laryngeal afferents in the decerebrate cat. *Exp Brain Res* 78:336–344, 1989.
5. Grélot L, Barillot JC, Bianchi AL: Activity of respiratory-related oropharyngeal and laryngeal motoneurones during fictive vomiting in the decerebrate cat. *Brain Res* 513:101–105, 1990.
6. Bianchi AL, Denavit-Saubié M, Champagnat J: Neurobiology of the central control of breathing in mammals: Neuronal circuitry, membrane properties and neurotransmitters involved. *Physiol Rev* 75:1–45, 1995.
7. Harding R: Function of the larynx in the fetus and newborn. *Ann Rev Physiol* 46:645–659, 1984.
8. Bartlett D: Respiratory functions of the larynx. *Physiol Rev* 69:33–57, 1989.
9. Wetzel DM, Kelly DB, Campbell BA: Central control of ultrasonic vocalizations in neonatal rats: I. Brain stem motor nuclei. *J Comp Physiol Psychol* 94:596–605, 1980.
10. Richter DW: Generation and maintenance of the respiratory rhythm. *J Exp Biol* 100:93–107, 1982.
11. Feldman JL: Neurophysiology of breathing in mammals, in Bloom FE (ed): *Handbook of Physiology*, sec I: *The Nervous System*. Bethesda, American Physiological Society, 1986, pp 463–524.
12. Bartlett D, Remmers JE, Gauthier H: Laryngeal regulation of respiratory airflow. *Respir Physiol* 18:194–204, 1973.
13. Gesell R, White F: Recruitment of muscular activity and the central neurone after-discharge of hyperpnea. *Am J Physiol* 122:48–56, 1938.
14. Shee CD, Loysongsang Y, Milic-Emili J: Decay of inspiratory muscle pressure during expiration in conscious humans. *J Appl Physiol* 58:1859–1865, 1985.
15. Richter, DW: in Elsner N, Richter DW (eds): *Rhythmogenesis in Neurons and Networks*. Stuttgart, Thieme Verlag, 1992, p 57.
16. Richter DW: Neural regulation of respiration: Rhythmogenesis and afferent control, in Greger R, Windhorst U (eds): *Comprehensive Human Physiology: From Cellular Mechanisms to Integration*, vol 2. Berlin, Springer-Verlag, 1996, pp 2079–2095.
17. Richter DW, Ballanyi K, Ramirez JM: Respiratory rhythm generation, in Miller AD, Bianchi AL, Bishop BP (eds): *Neural Control of the Respiratory Muscles*. Boca Raton, FL, CRC Press, 1996, pp 119–130.
18. Ramirez JM, Quellmalz UJA, Richter DW: Postnatal changes in the mammalian respiratory network as revealed by the transverse brainstem slice of mice. *J Physiol (Lond)* 491:799–812, 1996.
19. Pierrefiche O, Ramirez JM, Richter DW: Respiratory rhythm is blocked by injection of TTX or conotoxins into pre-BÖT complex in the cat in vivo. In preparation, 1997.
20. Smith JC, Greer JJ, Liu G, Feldman JL: Neural mechanisms generating respiratory pattern in mammalian brain stem-spinal cord in vitro: I. Spatiotemporal patterns of motor and medullary neuron activity. *J Neurophysiol* 64(4):1149–1169, 1990.
21. Connelly CA, Dobbins EG, Feldman JL: Pre-Bötzinger complex in cats: Respiratory neuronal discharge patterns. *Brain Res* 590:337–340, 1992.
22. Schwarzacher SW, Smith JC, Richter DW: Pre-Bötzinger complex in the cat. *J Neurophysiol* 73:1452–1459, 1995.
23. Smith JC, Ellenberg H, Ballanyi K, et al: Pre-Bötzinger complex: A brainstem region that may generate respiratory rhythm in mammals. *Science* 254:726–729, 1991.
24. Paton JFR, Ramirez J-M, Richter DW: Functionally intact in vitro preparation generating respiratory activity in neonatal and mature mammals. *Pflugers Arch* 428:250–260, 1994.
25. Ellenberger HH, Feldman JL: Brainstem connections of the rostral ventral respiratory group of the rat. *Brain Res* 513:35–42, 1990.
26. Ellenberger HH, Feldman JL: Subnuclear organization of the lateral tegmental field of the rat: I. Nucleus ambiguus and ventral respiratory group. *J Comp Neurol* 294:202–211, 1990.
27. Lipski J, Merrill EG: Electrophysiological demonstration of the projection from expiratory neurones in rostral medulla to contralateral dorsal respiratory group. *Brain Res* 197:521–524, 1980.
28. Merrill EG: Where are the real respiratory neurons? *Fed Proc* 40:2389–2394, 1981.
29. Ezure K, Manabe M: Decrementing expiratory neurons in the Bötzinger complex: II. Direct inhibitory synaptic linkage with ventral respiratory group neurons. *Exp Brain Res* 72:159–166, 1988.
30. Loeschcke HH: Central chemosensitivity and the reaction theory. *J Physiol (Lond)* 332:1–24, 1982.
31. Schlaefke ME: Central chemosensitivity: A respiratory drive. *Rev Physiol Biochem Pharmacol* 90:171–244, 1981.
32. Sun MK, Young BS, Hackett JT, Guyenet PG: Reticulospinal pacemaker neurons of the rat rostral ventrolateral medulla with putative sympathoexcitatory function: An intracellular study in vitro. *Brain Res* 442:229–239, 1988.
33. Guyenet PG: Role of the ventral medulla oblongata in blood pressure regulation, in Loewy AD, Spyer KM (eds): *Central Regulation of Autonomic Function*. Oxford, England, Oxford University Press, 1990, pp 145–167.
34. Richter DW, Spyer KM: Cardio-respiratory control, in Loewy AD, Spyer KM (eds): *Central Regulation of Autonomic Function*. Oxford, England, Oxford University Press, 1990, pp 189–207.
35. Richter DW, Spyer KM, Gilbey MP, et al: On the existence of

a common cardiorespiratory network, in Koepchen H-P, Huopaniemi T (eds): *Cardiorespiratory and Motor Coordination*. München, Springer-Verlag, 1991, pp 118–130.

36. Salmoiraghi GC, von Baumgarten R: Intracellular potentials from respiratory neurones in brain-stem of cat and mechanism of rhythmic respiration. *J Neurophysiol* 24:203–218, 1961.

37. Mitchell RA, Herbert DA: Synchronized high-frequency synaptic potentials in medullary respiratory neurons. *Brain Res* 75:350–355, 1974.

38. Richter DW, Heyde F, Gabriel M: Intracellular recordings from different types of medullary respiratory neurons of the cat. *J Neurophysiol* 38:1162–1171, 1975.

39. Onimaru H, Ballanyi K, Richter DW: Calcium-dependent responses in neurons of the isolated respiratory network of newborn rats. *J Physiol (Lond)* 491(3):677–695, 1996.

40. Lawson EE, Schwarzacher SW, Richter DW: Postnatal development of the medullary respiratory network in cat, in Elsner N, Richter DW (eds): *Rhythmogenesis in Neurons and Networks*. Stuttgart, Thieme, 1992, p 69.

41. Smith JC, Ballanyi K, Richter DW: Whole-cell patch-clamp recordings from respiratory neurons in neonatal rat brainstem in vitro. *Neurosci Lett* 134:153–156, 1992.

42. Onimaru H, Homma I: Whole cell recordings from respiratory neurons in the medulla of brainstem-spinal cord preparations isolated from newborn rats. *Pflugers Arch* 420:399–406, 1992.

43. Lalley PM, Bischoff AM, Richter DW: 5HT-1A receptor-mediated modulation of medullary expiratory neurones in the cat. *J Physiol (Lond)* 476:117–130, 1994.

44. Richter DW, Camerer H, Meesmann M, Röhrig N: Studies on the synaptic interconnection between bulbar respiratory neurones of cats. *Pflugers Arch* 380:245–257, 1979.

45. Ballantyne D, Richter DW: The non-uniform character of inhibitory synaptic activity in expiratory bulbospinal neurones of the cat. *J Physiol (Lond)* 370:433–456, 1986.

46. Bormann J, Hamill OP, Sakmann B: Mechanism of anion permeation through channels gated by glycine and γ-aminobutyric acid in mouse cultured spinal neurones. *J Physiol (Lond)* 385:243–286, 1987.

47. Lückermann M, Trapp S, Ballanyi K: GABA- and glycine-mediated fall in intracellular pH in rat medullary neurons in situ. *J Neurophysiol* 77:00–00, 1997.

48. Ballanyi K, Mückenhof K, Bellingham MC, et al: Activity-related pH changes in respiratory neurones and glial cells of cats. *Neuroreport* 6:33–36, 1994.

49. Pierrefiche O, Haji A, Richter DW: In vivo analysis of voltage-dependent Ca^{2+} currents contributing to respiratory bursting. *Soc Neurosci Abstr* 22:1746, 1996.

50. Elsen FP, Tellgkamp P, Ramirez JM, Richter DW: Calcium currents in neurons of the isolated respiratory system of mice. *Soc Neurosci Abstr* 22:1595, 1996.

51. Frermann D, Richter DW, Keller BU: Simultaneous patch clamp and intracellular calcium measurements in a rhythmically active neuronal network. *Jahrestag Dtsch Ges Biophys Leipzig* 99, 1996.

52. Mifflin SW, Ballantyne D, Backman SB, Richter DW: Evidence for a calcium activated potassium conductance in medullary respiratory neurones, in Bianchi AL, Denavit-Saubiè M (eds): *Neurogenesis of Central Respiratory Rhythm*. Lancaster, PA, MTP Press, 1985, pp 179–182.

53. Richter DW, Champagnat J, Jacquin T, Benacka R: Calcium and calcium-dependent potassium currents in medullary respiratory neurones. *J Physiol (Lond)* 470:23–33, 1993.

54. Pierrefiche O, Champagnat J, Richter DW: Calcium-dependent conductances control neurones involved in termination of inspiration in cats. *Neurosci Lett* 184:101–104, 1995.

55. Nesland R, Plum F: Subtypes of medullary respiratory neurons. *Exp Neurol* 12:337–348, 1965.

56. Cohen MI: Discharge patterns of brain-stem respiratory neurons during Hering-Breuer reflex evoked by lung inflation. *J Neurophysiol* 32:356–374, 1969.

57. Merrill EG: Finding a respiratory function for the medullary respiratory neurons, in Bellairs R, Gray EG (eds): *Essays on the Nervous System*. Oxford, England, Clarendon Press, 1974, pp 451–486.

58. Ezure K: Synaptic connections between medullary respiratory neurons and considerations on the genesis of respiratory rhythm. *Prog Neurobiol* 35:429–450, 1990.

59. Lawson EE, Richter DW, Ballantyne D, Lalley PM: Peripheral chemoreceptor inputs to medullary inspiratory and postinspiratory neurons of cats. *Pflugers Arch* 414:523–533, 1989.

60. Remmers JE, Richter DW, Ballantyne D: Reflex prolongation of stage I of expiration. *Pflugers Arch* 407:190–198, 1986.

61. Richter DW, Ballantyne D, Remmers JE: The differential organization of medullary postinspiratory activities. *Pflugers Arch* 410:420–427, 1987.

62. Haji A, Takeda R: Variations in membrane potential trajectory of post-inspiratory neurons in the ventrolateral medulla of the cat. *Neurosci Lett* 149:233–236, 1993.

63. Takeda R, Haji A: Mechanisms underlying post-inspiratory depolarization in post-inspiratory neurons of the cat. *Neurosci Lett* 150:1–4, 1993.

64. Oglivie MD, Gottschalk A, Anders K, et al: A network model of respiratory rhythmogenesis. *Am J Physiol* 263:R962–R975, 1992.

65. Feldman JL, Sommer D, Cohen MI: Short time scale correlations between discharges of medullary respiratory neurons. *J Neurophysiol* 43:1284–1295, 1980.

66. Feldman JL, Speck DF: Interactions among inspiratory neurons in dorsal and ventral respiratory groups in cat medulla. *J Neurophysiol* 49:472–490, 1983.

67. Madden KP, Remmers JE: Short time scale correlations between spike activity of neighboring respiratory neurons of nucleus tractus solitarius. *J Neurophysiol* 48:749–760, 1982.

68. Anders K, Ballantyne D, Bischoff AM, et al: Inhibition of caudal medullary expiratory neurones by retrofacial inspiratory neurones in the cat. *J Physiol (Lond)* 437:1–25, 1991.

69. Klages S, Bellingham MC, Richter DW: Late expiratory inhibition of stage 2 expiratory neurons in the cat: A correlate of expiratory termination. *J Neurophysiol* 70:1307–1315, 1993.

70. Coleridge HM, Coleridge JCG, Roberts AM: Rapid shallow breathing evoked by selective stimulation of airway C-fibres in dogs. *J Physiol (Lond)* 340:415–433, 1983.

71. Bonham AC: Neurotransmitters in the CNS control of breathing. *Respir Physiol* 101:219–230, 1995.

72. Greer JJ, Smith JC, Feldman JL: Role of excitatory amino acids in the generation and transmission of respiratory drive in neonatal rat. *J Physiol (Lond)* 437:727–749, 1991.

73. Feldman JL, Windhorst U, Anders K, Richter DW: Synaptic interaction between medullary respiratory neurones during apneusis induced by NMDA-receptor blockade in cat. *J Physiol (Lond)* 450:303–323, 1992.

74. Pierrefiche O, Foutz AS, Champagnat J, Denavit-Saubié M: NMDA and non-NMDA receptors may play distinct roles in timing mechanisms and transmission in the feline respiratory network. *J Physiol (Lond)* 474(3):509–523, 1994.

75. Pierrefiche O, Foutz AS, Champagnat J, Denavit-Saubié M: The bulbar network of respiratory neurons during apneusis induced by a blockade of NMDA receptors. *Exp Brain Res* 89:623–639, 1992.

76. Foutz AS, Pierrefiche O, Denavit-Saubié M: Combined blockade of NMDA and non-NMDA receptors produces respiratory arrest in the adult cat. *Neuroreport* 5:481–484, 1994.

77. Kashiwagi M, Onimaru H, Homma I: Effects of NMDA on respiratory neurons in newborn rat medulla in vitro. *Brain Res Bull* 32:65–69, 1993.

78. Champagnat J, Denavit-Saubié M, Moyanova S, Ronduin G:

Involvement of amino acids in periodic inhibitions of bulbar respiratory neurones. *Brain Res* 327:351–365, 1982.

79. Schmid K, Foutz AS, Denavit-Saubie M: Inhibition mediated by glycine and $GABA_A$ receptors shape the discharge pattern of bulbar respiratory neurons. *Brain Res* 710:150–160, 1996.
80. Haji A, Takeda R, Remmers JE: Evidence that glycine and GABA mediate postsynaptic inhibition of bulbar respiratory neurons in the cat. *J Appl Physiol* 73:2333–2342, 1992.
81. Lalley PM: Effects of baclofen and gamma-aminobutyric acid on different types of medullary respiratory neurons. *Brain Res* 376:392–395, 1986.
82. Pierrefiche O, Foutz AS: Effects of $GABA_B$ receptor agonists and antagonists on the bulbar respiratory network in the cat. *Brain Res* 605:77–84, 1993.
83. Lalley PM, Pierrefiche O, Bischoff AM, Richter DW: cAMP-dependent protein kinase modulates expiratory neurons in vivo. *J Neurophysiol* 77:1119–1131, 1997.
84. Pierrefiche O, Schmid K, Foutz AS, Denavit-Saubié M: Endogenous activation of NMDA and non-NMDA glutamate receptors on respiratory neurones in cat medulla. *Neuropharmacology* 30:429–440, 1991.
85. Champagnat J, Denavit-Saubié M, Henry JL, Leviel V: Catecholaminergic depressant effects on bulbar respiratory mechanisms. *Brain Res* 160:57–68, 1979.
86. Hilaire G, Monteau R, Errchidi S: Possible modulation of the medullary respiratory rhythm generator by the noradrenergic A_5 area: An in vitro study in the newborn rat. *Brain Res* 485:325–332, 1989.
87. Errchidi S, Monteau R, Hilaire G: Noradrenergic modulation of the medullary respiratory rhythm generator in the newborn rat: An in vitro study. *J Physiol (Lond)* 443:477–498, 1991.
88. Ohta A, Takagi H, Matsui T, et al: Localization of nitric oxide synthase–immunoreactive neurons in the solitary nucleus and ventrolateral medulla oblongata of the rat: Their relation to catecholaminergic neurons. *Neurosci Lett* 158:33–35, 1993.
89. Arita H, Ochiishi M: Opposing effects of 5-hydroxytryptamine on two types of medullary inspiratory neurons with distinct firing patterns. *J Neurophysiol* 66:285–292, 1991.
90. Lalley PM, Bischoff AM, Schwarzacher SW, Richter DW: 5HT-2 receptor controlled modulation of medullary respiratory neurones. *J Physiol (Lond)* 497(3):653–661, 1995.
91. Morin D, Monteau R, Hilaire G: Serotonin and cervical respiratory motoneurones: Intracellular study in the newborn rat brainstem-spinal cord preparation. *Exp Brain Res* 84:229–232, 1991.
92. Rampin O, Pierrefiche O, Denavit-Saubié M: Effects of serotonin and substance P on bulbar respiratory neurons in vivo. *Brain Res* 622:185–193, 1993.
93. Srinivasan M, Yamamoto Y, Persson H, Lagercrantz H: Birth-related activation of preprotachykinin-A mRNA in the respiratory neural structures of the rabbit. *Pediatr Res* 29:369–371, 1991.
94. Berkenbosch A, De Goede J, Olievier CN, Ward DS: Effect of exogenous dopamine on the hypercapnic ventilatory response in cats during normoxia. *Pflugers Arch* 407:504–509, 1986.
95. Hedner T, Hedner J, Jonason J, Wessberg P: Effects of theophylline on adenosine-induced respiratory depression in the preterm rabbit. *Eur J Respir Dis* 65:153–156, 1984.
96. Lagercrantz H, Yamamoto B, Fredholm N, et al: Adenosine analogs depress ventilation in rabbit neonates: Theophylline stimulation of respiration via adenosine receptors? *Pediatr Res* 18:387–390, 1984.
97. Darnall RA: Aminophylline reduces hypoxic ventilatory depression: Possible role of adenosine. *Pediatr Res* 19:706–710, 1985.
98. Norsted T, Jonzon A, Sedin G: Respiratory response to adenosine in newborn lambs is modified by hypoxemia and by heat stress. *Biol Neonate* 58:296–304, 1990.
99. Runold M, Lagercrantz H, Prabhakar NR, Fredholm BB: Role of adenosine in hypoxic ventilatory depression. *J Appl Physiol* 67:541–546, 1988.
100. Böhmer G, Dinse HRO, Fallert M, Sommer TJ: Microelectrophoretic application of agonists of putative neurotransmitters onto various types of bulbar respiratory neurons. *Arch Ital Biol* 117:13–22, 1979.
101. Takeda R, Haji A: Synaptic response of bulbar respiratory neurons to hypercapnic stimulation in peripherally chemodenervated cats. *Brain Res* 561:307–331, 1991.
102. Morin-Surun MP, Jordan D, Champagnat J, et al: Excitatory effects of iontophoretically applied substance P on neurons in the nucleus tractus solitarius of the cats: Lack of interaction with opiates and opioids. *Brain Res* 307:388–392, 1984.
103. Jacquin T, Champagnat J, Madamba S, et al: Somatostatin depresses excitability in neurons of the solitary tract complex through hyperpolarization and augmentation of I_M, a non-inactivating voltage-dependent outward current blocked by muscarinic agonists. *Proc Natl Acad Sci USA* 85:948–952, 1988.
104. Branchereau P, Champagnat J, Roques BP, Denavit-Saubié M: CCK modulates inhibitory synaptic transmission in the solitary complex through CCK_B sites. *Neuroreport* 3:909–912, 1992.
105. Ballanyi K, Lalley PM, Hoch B, Richter DW: cAMP-dependent reversal of opioid- and prostaglandin-mediated depression of the isolated respiratory network in newborn rats. *J Physiol (Lond)* 504:127–134, 1997.
106. Chernick V, Craig RJ: Naloxone reverses neonatal depression caused by fetal asphyxia. *Science* 216:1252–1253, 1982.
107. De Boeck C, Van Reempts P, Rigatto H, Chernick V: Naloxone reduces decrease in ventilation induced by hypoxia in newborn infants. *J Appl Physiol* 56:1507–1511, 1984.
108. Morin-Surun MP, Boudinot E, Fournie-Zaluski MC, et al: Control of breathing by endogenous opioid peptides: Possible involvement in sudden infant death syndrome. *Neurochem Int* 20:103–107, 1992.
109. Moss IR, Friedman E: Beta-endorphin: Effects on respiratory regulation. *Life Sci* 23:1271–1276, 1978.
110. Ling L, Karius DR, Fiscus RR, Speck DF: Endogenous nitric oxide required for an integrative respiratory function in the cat brain. *J Neurophysiol* 68(5):1910–1912, 1992.
111. Blackstone C, Murphy TH, Moss SJ, et al: Cyclic AMP and synaptic activity-dependent phosphorylation of AMPA-preferring glutamate receptors. *J Neurosci* 14:7585–7593, 1994.
112. Krishek BJ, Xie X, Blackstone C, et al: Regulation of $GABA_A$ receptor function by protein kinase C phosphorylation. *Neuron* 12:1081–1095, 1994.
113. Marek GJ, Aghajanian GK: Protein kinase C inhibitors enhance the 5-HT2A receptor-mediated excitatory effects of serotonin on interneurons in rat piriform cortex. *Synapse* 21(2):123–130, 1995.
114. Tanaka C, Nishizuka Y: The protein kinase C family for neuronal signaling. *Ann Rev Physiol* 17:551–567, 1994.
115. Wickman K, Clapman DE: Ion channel regulation by G proteins. *Physiol Rev* 75:865–885, 1995.
116. Champagnat J, Richter DW: Second messengers-induced modulation of the excitability of respiratory neurones. *Neuroreport* 4:861–863, 1993.
117. Champagnat J, Richter DW: The roles of K^+ conductance in expiratory pattern generation in anaesthetized cats. *J Physiol (Lond)* 4791:127–128, 1994.
118. Richter DW, Lalley PM, Pierrefiche O, et al: Intracellular signal pathways controlling respiratory neurons. *Respir Physiol* 110:113–123, 1997.
119. Arata A, Onimaru H, Homma I: Effects of cAMP on respiratory rhythm generation in brainstem-spinal cord preparation from newborn rat. *Brain Res* 605:193–199, 1993.
120. Sears TA: The respiratory motoneurone and apneusis. *Fed Proc* 36:2412–2420, 1977.
121. Berger AJ, Herbert DA, Mitchell RA: Properties of apneusis produced by reversible cold block of rostral pons. *Respir Physiol* 33:323–337, 1978.
122. Monteau R, Errchidi S, Gauthier P, et al: Pneumotaxic centre

and apneustic breathing: Interspecies differences between rat and cat. *Neurosci Lett* 99:311–316, 1989.

123. Lalley PM, Bischoff AM, Richter DW: Serotonin 1A-receptor activation suppresses respiratory apneusis in the cat. *Neurosci Lett* 172:59–62, 1994.

124. Wilken B, Lalley PM, Bischoff AM, et al: Treatment of apneustic respiratory disturbance with serotonin receptor agonists. *J Pediatr* 130:89–94, 1997.

125. Haji A, Pierrefiche O, Lalley PM, Richter DW: Protein kinase C pathways modulate respiratory pattern generation in the cat. *J Physiol (Lond)* 494:297–306, 1996.

126. Cohen MI, Piercey MF, Gootman PM, Wolotsky P: Synaptic connections between medullary inspiratory neurons and phrenic motoneurons as revealed by cross-correlation. *Brain Res* 81:319–324, 1974.

127. Graham K, Duffin J: Cross-correlation of medullary dorsomedial neurones in the cat. *Exp Neurol* 75:627–643, 1981.

128. Graham K, Duffin J: Cross-correlation of medullary expiratory neurons in the cat. *Exp Neurol* 73:451–464, 1981.

129. Hilaire G, Monteau R, Bianchi AL: A cross-correlation study of interactions among respiratory neurons of dorsal, ventral and retrofacial groups in cat medulla. *Brain Res* 302:19–31, 1984.

130. Lindsey BG, Segers LS, Morris KF, et al: Distributed actions and dynamic associations in respiratory-related neuronal assemblies of the ventrolateral medulla and brain stem midline: Evidence from spike train analysis. *J Neurophysiol* 72:1830–1851, 1994.

131. Segers LS, Shannon R, Lindsey BG: Interactions between rostral pontine and ventral medullary respiratory neurones. *J Neurophysiol* 54:318–334, 1985.

132. Segers LS, Shannon R, Saporta S, Lindsey B: Functional associations among simultaneously monitored lateral medullary respiratory neurons in the cat: I. Evidence for excitatory and inhibitory actions of inspiratory neurons. *J Neurophysiol* 57:1078–1100, 1987.

133. Geitz KA, Richter DW, Gottshalk A: The influence of chemical and mechanical feedback on ventilatory pattern in a model of the central respiratory pattern generator. *Adv Exp Med Biol* 393:23–28, 1995.

134. Fedorko L, Duffin J, England S: Inhibition of inspiratory neurons of the nucleus retroambigualis by expiratory neurons of the Bötzinger complex in the cat. *Expl Neurol* 106:74–77, 1989.

135. Onimaru H, Homma I, Iwatsuki K: Excitation of inspiratory neurons by preinspiratory neurons in rat medulla in vitro. *Brain Res Bull* 29:879–882, 1992.

136. Botros SM, Bruce EN: Neural network implementation of the three-phase model of respiratory rhythm generation. *Biol Cybernet* 63:143–153, 1990.

137. Gottschalk A, Ogilvie MD, Richter DW, Pack Al: Computational aspects of the respiratory pattern generator. *Neural Comp* 6:56–68, 1994.

138. Onimaru H, Arata A, Homma I: Localization of respiratory rhythm-generating neurons in the medulla of brainstem-spinal cord preparations from newborn rats. *Neurosci Lett* 78:151–155, 1987.

139. Onimaru H, Arata A, Homma I: Primary respiratory rhythm generator in the medulla of brainstem–spinal cord preparation from newborn rat. *Brain Res* 445:314–324, 1988.

140. Onimaru H, Arata A, Homma I: Firing properties of respiratory rhythm generating neurons in the absence of synaptic transmission in rat medulla in vitro. *Exp Brain Res* 76:530–536, 1989.

141. Feldman JL, Smith JC, Ellenberger HH, et al: Neurogenesis of respiratory rhythm and pattern: Emerging concepts. *Am J Physiol* 259:R879–R886, 1990.

142. Johnson SM, Smith JC, Funk GD, Feldman JL: Pacemaker behavior of respiratory neurons in medullary slices from neonatal rat. *J Neurophysiol* 72(6):2598–2608, 1994.

143. Ramirez JM, Richter DW: The neuronal mechanisms of respiratory rhythm generation (1996/97). *Curr Opin Neurobiol* 6:817–825, 1996.

144. Feldman JL, Smith JC: Cellular mechanisms underlying modulation of breathing pattern in mammals. *Ann NY Acad Sci* 563:114–130, 1989.

145. Paton JFR, Ramirez J-M, Richter DW: Mechanisms of respiratory rhythm generation change profoundly during early life in mice and rats. *Neurosci Lett* 170:167–170, 1994.

146. Onimaru H, Arata A, Homma I: Inhibitory synaptic inputs to the respiratory rhythm generator in the medulla isolated from newborn rats. *Pflugers Arch* 417:425–432, 1990.

147. Onimaru H, Arata A, Homma I: Intrinsic burst generation of preinspiratory neurons in the medulla of brainstem–spinal cord preparations isolated from newborn rats. *Exp Brain Res* 106:57–68, 1995.

148. Smith JC, Koshiya N, Simon ES: Generation of respiratory oscillations after disruption of inhibitory neurotransmission during postnatal development: In vitro and in vivo studies with mutant and normal mice. *Neurosci Abstr* 22:1595, 1996.

149. Feldman JL, Smith JC, Liu G: Respiratory pattern generation in mammals: In vitro en bloc analyses. *Curr Opin Neurobiol* 1:590–594, 1991.

150. Smith JC, Funk GD, Johnson SM, Feldman JL: Cellular and synaptic mechanisms generating respiratory rhythm: Insights from in vitro and computational studies, in Trouth CO, Mils R, Kiwull-Schone H, Schlaefke M (eds): *Ventral Brainstem Mechanisms and Control of Respiration and Blood Pressure.* New York, Marcel Dekker, 1995, pp 463–496.

151. Richter DW, Champagnat J, Mifflin SW: Membrane properties involved in respiratory rhythm generation, in von Euler C, Lagercrantz H (eds): *Neurobiology of the Control of Breathing.* New York, Raven Press, 1986 pp 141–147.

152. Richter DW, Ballantyne D, Mifflin S: Interaction between postsynaptic activation and membrane properties in medullary respiratory neurones, in Bianchi AL, Denavit-Saubié M (eds): *Neurogenesis of Central Respiratory Rhythm.* Lancaster, PA, MTP Press, 1985, pp 172–178.

153. Richter DW, Pierrefiche O, Lalley PM, Polder HR: Voltage-clamp analysis of neurons within deep layers of the brain. *J Neurosci Methods* 67:121–131, 1996c.

154. Richter DW, Ballanyi K, Schwarzacher S: Mechanisms of respiratory rhythm generation. *Curr Opin Neurobiol* 2:788–793, 1992.

155. Richter DW, Bischoff A, Anders K, et al: Response of the medullary respiratory network of the cat to hypoxia. *J Physiol (Lond)* 443:231–256, 1991.

156. Hayashi F, Lipski J: The role of inhibitory amino acids in control of respiratory motor output in an arterially perfused rat. *Respir Physiol* 89:47–63, 1992.

157. Hanson MA, Kumar P, Williams BA: The effect of chronic hypoxia upon the development of respiratory chemoreflexes in the newborn kitten. *J Physiol (Lond)* 411:563–574, 1989.

158. Kholwadwala D, Donnelly DF: Maturation of carotid chemoreceptor sensitivity to hypoxia. *J Physiol (Lond)* 453:461–473, 1992.

159. Lee LY, Millhorn HT: Central ventilatory responses to O_2 and CO_2 at three levels of carotid chemoreceptor stimulation. *Respir Physiol* 25:319–333, 1975.

160. Magoun HW: Caudal and cephalic influences of the brain stem reticular formation. *Physiol Rev* 30:459–474, 1950.

161. Hugelin A, Bonvallet M, Dell P: Activation reticulaire et corticale d'origine chemoreceptive au cours de l'hypoxie. *Electroencephalogr Clin Neurophysiol* 11:325–340, 1959.

162. Hugelin A, Cohen MI: The reticular activating system and respiratory regulation in the cat. *Ann NY Acad Sci* 109:586–603, 1963.

163. Hodgkin AL, Huxley AF: Currents carried by sodium and potassium ions through the membrane of the giant axon of Loligo. *J Physiol (Lond)* 116:449–472, 1952.

164. Su CK, Feldman JL: Identification of Ca^{2+}-dependent Cl^--con-

ductance in neonatal rat phrenic motoneurons. *Soc Neurosci Abstr* 22:1026, 1996.

165. Champagnat J, Jaquin T, Richter DW: Voltage-dependent currents in neurones of the nuclei of the solitary tract of rat brainstem slices. *Pflugers Arch* 406:372–379, 1986.

166. Mifflin SW, Richter DW: Effects of QX-314 on medullary respiratory neurones. *Brain* 420:22–31, 1987.

167. McCormick DA, Pape HC: Properties of a hyperpolarization-activated cation current and its role in rhythmic oscillation in thalamic relay neurones. *J Physiol (Lond)* 431:291–318, 1990.

168. Ballantyne D, Richter DW: Post-synaptic inhibition of bulbar inspiratory neurones in the cat. *J Physiol (Lond)* 348:67–87, 1984.

169. von Euler C: On the central pattern generator for the basic breathing rhythmicity. *J Appl Physiol* 55:1647–1659, 1983.

170. Gauthier H, Remmers JE, Bartlett D Jr: Control of the duration of expiration. *Respir Physiol* 18:205–221, 1973.

171. Younes MK, Remmers JE, Baker J: Characteristics of inspiratory inhibition by phasic volume feedback in cats. *J Appl Physiol Respir Environ Exer Physiol* 45:80–86, 1978.

172. von Euler C: Brain stem mechanisms for generation and control of breathing pattern, in Fishman AP, Cherniack NS, Widdicombe JG, Geiger SR (eds): *Handbook of Physiology*, sec III: *The Respiratory System*. Bethesda, American Physiological Society, 1986, pp 1–67.

173. Feldman JL, Cohen MI, Wolotsky P: Powerful inhibition of pontine respiratory neurones by pulmonary afferent activity. *Brain Res* 104:341–346, 1976.

174. Bianchi AL, St John WM: Medullary axonal projections of respiratory neurons of pontile pneumotaxic center. *Respir Physiol* 48:357–373, 1982.

175. Dick TE, Bellingham MC, Richter DW: Pontine respiratory neurons in anaesthetized cats. *Brain Res* 636:259–269, 1994.

176. Remmers JE, Bartlett D Jr: Reflex control of expiratory airflow and duration. *J Appl Physiol* 42:80–87, 1977.

177. Lawson EE, Richter DW, Czyzyk-Krzeska MF, et al: Respiratory neuronal activity during apnea and other breathing patterns induced by laryngeal stimulation. *J Appl Physiol* 70:2742–2749, 1991.

178. Bassal M, Bianchi AL: Effects de la stimulation des structures nerveuses centrales sur les activités respiratoires efférentes chez le chat: I. Réponses à la stimulation corticale. *J Physiol (Paris)* 77:741–757, 1981.

179. Lumsden T: Observations on the respiratory centres in the cat. *J Physiol (Lond)* 57:153–160, 1923.

180. Bellingham MC, Schmidt C, Richter DW: The inspiratory offswitch is disturbed during hypoxia. *Pflugers Arch* 418:R16, 1991.

181. Griggs GA, Findley LJ, Suratt PM, et al: Prolonged relaxation rate of inspiratory muscles in patients with sleep apnea. *Am Rev Respir Dis* 140:706–710, 1989.

182. Ballanyi K, Völker A, Richter DW: Anoxia induced functional inactivation of neonatal respiratory neurones in vitro. *Neuroreport* 6:165–168, 1994.

183. Downing SE, Lee JC: Laryngeal chemosensitivity: A possible mechanism of sudden infant death. *Pediatrics* 55:640–649, 1975.

184. Sant'Ambrogio G: Information arising from the tracheobronchial tree of mammals. *Physiol Rev* 62:531–569, 1982.

185. Waragai M, Niwa N, Iwabuchi S: Acute disseminated encephalomyelitis presented with apnea in the acute stage. *Rinsho Shinkeigaku* 34:347–350, 1994.

186. West JB: The 1988 Stevenson Memorial Lecture: Physiological responses to severe hypoxia in man. *Can J Physiol Pharmacol* 67:173–178, 1989.

187. Lawson EE, Long WW: Central origin of biphasic breathing pattern during hypoxia in newborns. *J Appl Physiol* 55:483–488, 1983.

188. Cherniack NS, Edelman NH, Lahiri S: Hypoxia and hypercapnia as respiratory stimulants and depressants. *Respir Physiol* 11:113–126, 1971.

189. Ballanyi K, Kuwana S, Völker A, et al: Developmental changes in the hypoxia tolerance. *Neurosci Lett* 148:141–144, 1992.

190. Morawietz G, Ballanyi K, Kuwana S, Richter DW: Hypoxic and ischemic responses of the in vitro respiratory network of adult rats. *Pflugers Arch* 422:R129, 1993.

191. Völker A, Ballanyi K, Richter DW: Anoxic disturbance of the isolated respiratory network of neonatal rats. *Exp Brain Res* 103:9–19, 1995.

192. Bureau MA, Begin R: Postnatal maturation of the respiratory response to O_2 in awake newborn lambs. *J Appl Physiol* 52:428–433, 1982.

193. Bonora M, Marlo D, Gauthier H, Duron B: Effects of hypoxia on ventilation during postnatal development in conscious kittens. *J Appl Physiol* 56:1464–1471, 1984.

194. Haddad GG, Mellins RB: Hypoxia and respiratory control in early life. *Ann Rev Physiol* 46:629–643, 1984.

195. Henderson-Smart DJ, Read DJC: Ventilatory responses to hypoxemia during sleep in the newborn. *J Dev Physiol* 1:195–208, 1980.

196. Fazekas JF, Alexander FAD, Himwich HE: Tolerance of the newborn to anoxia. *J Physiol (Lond)* 134:282–287, 1941.

197. Adolph EF: Regulations during survival without oxygen in infant mammals. *Respir Physiol* 7:356–368, 1969.

198. Stafford A, Weatherall JAC: The survival of young rats in nitrogen. *J Physiol (Lond)* 153:457–472, 1960.

199. Duffy TE, Kohle SJ, Vannucci RC: Carbohydrate and energy metabolism in perinatal rat brain: Relation to survival in anoxia. *J Neurochem* 24:271–276, 1975.

200. Alling HC: Biochemical maturation of the brain and the concept of vulnerable periods, in Ryberg U et al (eds): *Alcohol and the Developing Brain*. New York, Raven Press, 1985, pp 5–10.

201. Hansen AJ: Effect of anoxia on ion distribution in the brain. *Physiol Rev* 65:101–148, 1985.

202. Haddad GG, Donnelly DF: O_2 deprivation induces a major depolarisation in brainstem neurons in the adult but not in the neonatal rat. *J Physiol (Lond)* 429:411–428, 1990.

203. Haddad GG, Jiang C: O_2 deprivation in the central nervous system: On mechanisms of neuronal response, differential sensitivity and injury. *Proc Neurobiol* 40:277–318, 1993.

204. Trippenbach T, Richter DW, Acker H: Hypoxia and ion activities within the brain stem of newborn rabbits. *J Appl Physiol* 68:2494–2503, 1990.

205. Himwich HE, Bernstein AO, Herrlich H, et al: Mechanism for the maintenance of life in the newborn during anoxia. *Am J Physiol* 135:387–391, 1942.

206. Ballanyi K, Völker A, Richter DW: Functional relevance of anaerobic metabolism in the isolated respiratory network of newborn rats. *Pflugers Arch* 432:741–748, 1996.

207. Richter DW, Camerer H, Sonnhof U: Changes in extracellular potassium during the spontaneous activity of medullary respiratory neurones. *Pflugers Arch* 376:139–149, 1978.

208. Richter DW, Acker H: Respiratory neuron behavior during medullary hypoxia, in Lahiri S, (ed): *Chemoreceptors and Reflexes in Breathing: Cellular and Molecular Aspects*. Oxford, England, Oxford University Press, 1989, pp 267–274.

209. Melton JE, Chae LO, Neubauer JA, Edelman NH: Extracellular potassium homeostasis in the cat medulla during progressive brain hypoxia. *J Appl Physiol* 70:1477–1482, 1991.

210. Schmidt C, Bellingham MC, Richter DW: Adenosinergic modulation of respiratory neurones and hypoxic responses in the anaesthetized cat. *J Physiol (Lond)* 483(3):769–781, 1995.

211. Kiley JP, Eldridge FL, Millhorn DE: The roles of medullary extracellular and cerebrospinal fluid pH in control of respiration. *Respir Physiol* 59:117–130, 1985.

212. Taira T, Smirnov S, Voipio J, Kaila K: Intrinsic proton modula-

tion of excitatory transmission in rat hippocampal slices. *Neuroreport* 4:93–96, 1993.

213. Pasternack M, Smirnov S, Kaila K: Dual modulation of GABA$_A$ receptors by external H$^+$ ions in acutely isolated rat hippocampal neurones. *Soc Neurosci Abstr* 21(Suppl):1–3, 1995.

214. Grunstein MM, Hazinski TA, Schlueter HA: Respiratory control during hypoxia in newborn rabbits: Implied action of endorphines. *J Appl Physiol* 51:122–130, 1981.

215. Jansen AH, Loffe S, Chernick V: Influence of naloxone on fetal breathing and the respiratory response to hypercapnia. *Respir Physiol* 78:187–196, 1989.

216. Lalley PM, Benacka R, Bischoff AM, Richter DW: Nucleus raphe obscurus evokes 5HT-1A receptor-mediated inhibition of respiratory neurons. *Brain Res* 747:156–159, 1997.

217. Voss MD, De Castro D, Lipski J, et al: Serotonin immunoreactive boutons form close appositions with respiratory neurons of the dorsal respiratory group in the cat. *J Comp Neurol* 295:208–218, 1990.

218. Carley DW, Shannon DC: Relative stability of human respiration during progressive hypoxia. *J Appl Physiol* 65:1389–1399, 1988.

219. Pluta R, Romaniuk JR: Recovery of breathing pattern after 15 min of cerebral ischemia in rabbits. *J Appl Physiol* 69:1676–1681, 1990.

220. Richter DW, Ballanyi K: Response of the medullary respiratory network to hypoxia: A comparative analysis of neonatal and adult mammals, in Haddad GG, Lister G (eds): *Tissue Oxygen Deprivation: Developmental, Molecular and Integrated Function.* Hong Kong, Marcel Dekker, 1996, pp 751–777.

221. LaFramboise WA, Woodrum DE: Elevated diaphragm electromyogram during neonatal hypoxic ventilatory depression. *J Appl Physiol* 59:1040–1045, 1985.

222. Sears TA, Berger AJ, Phillipson EA: Reciprocal tonic activation of inspiratory and expiratory motoneurones by chemical drives. *Nature (Lond)* 299:728–730, 1982.

223. Bainton CR, Kirkwood PA: The effect of carbon dioxide on the tonic and the rhythmic discharges of expiratory bulbospinal neurones. *J Physiol (Lond)* 296:291–314, 1979.

224. Neubauer JA, Melton JE, Edelman NH: Modulation of respiration during brain hypoxia. *J Appl Physiol* 68:441–449, 1990.

225. Schmidt-Garcon P, Nagel H, Richter DW: Role of adenosine in the hypoxic response of central respiratory activity, in Elsner N, Heisenberg M (eds.): *Gene-Brain-Behaviour.* Stuttgart, Thieme Verlag, 1992.

226. Guntheroth WG, Kawabori I: Hypoxic apnea and gasping. *J Clin Invest* 56:1371–1377, 1975.

227. St John WM: Neurogenesis, control and functional significance of gasping. *J Appl Physiol* 68:1305–1315, 1990.

228. Zhou D, Wasicko MJ, Hu J-M, St. John WM: Differing activities of medullary respiratory neurons in eupnea and gasping. *J Appl Physiol* 70:1265–1270, 1991.

229. Wang W, Fung ML, Darnall RA, St John WM: Characterizations and comparisons of eupnoea and gasping in neonatal rats. *J Physiol (Lond)* 490:277–292, 1996.

230. Fung ML, Wang V, St John WM: Medullary loci critical for expression of gasping in adult rats. *J Physiol (Lond)* 480:597–611, 1994.

231. Ramirez JM, Tellgkamp P, Elsen FP, Richter DW: Gasp-like activity in the transverse rhythmic slice preparation of mice. *Soc Neurosci Abstr* 22:1373, 1996.

232. Tomori Z, Benacka R, Donic V, Tkacova R: Reversal of apnoea by aspiration reflex in anaesthetized cats. *Eur Respir J* 4:1117–1125, 1991.

233. Yang L, Weil MH, Noc M, et al: Spontaneous gasping increases the ability to resuscitate during experimental cardiopulmonary resuscitation. *Crit Care Med* 22:879–883, 1994.

234. Sanocka UM, Donnelly DF, Haddad GG: Autoresuscitation: A survival mechanism in piglets. *J Appl Physiol* 73:749–753, 1992.

235. Gershan WM, Jacobi MS, Thach BT: Mechanisms underlying induced autoresuscitation failure in BALB/c and SWR mice. *J Appl Physiol* 72:677–685, 1992.

Chapter 6

CONTROL OF BREATHING

MIECZYSLAW POKORSKI

The principal role of the brain stem in the generation and control of spontaneous respiratory activity was settled in the first half of this century. The discovery of the arterial sensors of chemical environment followed shortly afterwards and led to a multitude of studies. Despite, and perhaps due to, all the progress at the time, the early investigators could not predict the difficulties ahead on the way to unraveling the details of the mechanisms whereby respiration is generated and controlled. Over the years, a number of new techniques have been used, including the anatomic, histologic, immunohistochemical, and neurochemical approaches, to study the structure and function of the respiratory system.

This chapter reviews the mechanisms that allow the muscles of breathing to flexibly meet the demands imposed on them. Both central and peripheral control of respiration may be subdivided into two main but interrelated domains: neural and chemical. These two components consist of a number of tonic and phasic inputs that merge in the central nervous system. Respiration is initiated spontaneously in the medulla as a cycle of inspiration and expiration that is driven by discharges of the groups of neurons. The respiratory areas of the medulla are reasonably well worked out. These regions are subject to regulation by other important sites in the brain, lungs, and airways from sensors in the blood and from muscle receptors. These inputs sustain pulmonary ventilation at a level adequate for metabolic function but also allow breathing during prioritized functions such as vocalization or swallowing. Attention will be paid to chemical transmitters, since it is clear that they are heavily involved in the modulation of respiratory activity.

Central Control

MEDULLARY RESPIRATORY AREAS

Maintenance of an optimal level of O_2 and CO_2 tension in the arterial blood (Pa_{O_2} and Pa_{CO_2}) depends on the cyclic activity of the respiratory muscles by neural mechanisms. The respiratory rhythm is continuous and switches automatically from inspiratory to expiratory discharges. The control of the rhythm is basically automatic, but the rhythm also may be modulated behaviorally or voluntarily. These features make the respiratory rhythm distinctly different from the majority of other rhythms generated in the central nervous system (CNS), which usually are not subject to volitional control. This rhythm bears some resemblance to the automatic rhythm generated in the sinus node of the heart, i.e., a rhythm that may be generated without extrinsic inputs and reflexes. It is therefore not surprising that the theories of rhythm generation have included the existence of a respiratory pacemaker. Along this line of thinking, the bulbospinal fibers running down to the phrenic nerve and respiratory muscle motoneurons might be considered the conduction pathways of this system.

The popularity of the pacemaker theory has swayed back and forth over the years, and the pacemaker has been assigned to various localizations within the circumscribed areas of the brain stem. The most recent one places conditional pacemaker cells in the pre-Bötzinger complex, a small area caudal to the retrofacial nucleus. In a slice preparation from the medulla of the neonatal rat, these neurons exhibit oscillatory membrane potentials in synchrony with motor output of the hypoglossal nerve during a depolarizing input.[1] Another group of pacemaker-like neurons, which fire even in the absence of synaptic inputs, has been delineated in the ventral medulla of the neonatal rat in an vitro brain stem–spinal cord preparation.[2,3] In a similar type of preparation, periodic thoracic movements can be observed in synchrony with the phrenic nerve discharge.[4] Transection at the medullary–cervical spinal cord junction does not abolish the movements. Moreover, the spinal rhythm characteristics are similar to those of medullary rhythm. Therefore, areas other than in the brain stem are capable of generating a respiratory-like rhythm. The pacemaker theory may be an oversimplification, as is also the concept of a reciprocal inhibition between functionally opposing groups of medullary neurons[5] giving the appearance of an oscillator or a metronome-like mechanism. The strict inspiratory and expiratory sequence of firing of respiratory neurons likely depends on a complex interplay between intrinsic neuronal membrane properties and postsynaptic potential changes, underlain by chemical transmission and ionic conductances, and containing a sizable degree of redundancy. (Respiratory rhythm generation mechanisms are discussed in detail in Chap. 5 of this book.)

MEDULLARY RESPIRATORY NETWORKS

Respiratory neurons in the medulla are organized into two bilateral, symmetric networks. Each network is represented by two aggregates of both bulbospinal and cranial neurons named the *dorsal respiratory group* (DRG) and the *ventral respiratory group* (VRG).[6,7] The DRG is located in the region of the nucleus of the tractus solitarius and extends about 2.5 mm rostrally from the obex (Fig. 6-1*B*). There are mainly two types of inspiratory neurons and a fraction of expiratory neurons there. The inspiratory neurons have been distinguished by their response to lung inflation. R_α neurons are inhibited by lung inflation. They send collaterals to the phrenic motoneurons on the contralateral side and to the inspiratory neurons of the VRG on the same side. R_β neurons are stimulated by lung inflation. Besides their role in driving phrenic nerve activity and, therefore, the diaphragm, the DRG neurons appear to be the initial processing site of sensory information. They receive inputs from vagal and arterial chemoreceptor afferents and integrate them with the central pattern generator (CPG), which shapes the respiratory motor output (Fig. 6-3).

The VRG constitutes an elongated column of respiratory neurons in the ventrolateral medulla extending nearly from the bulbopontine to the bulbospinal border (Fig. 6-1*B*). This group includes the nucleus ambiguus (NA), paraambigualis (NPA), and retroambigualis (NRA) and the caudal portion of the nucleus retrofacial (NRF) encompassing the Bötzinger

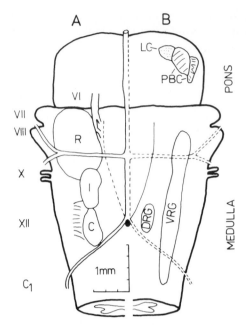

FIGURE 6-1 A topographic outline of positional relationships of the brain stem respiratory regions as viewed from the ventral (A) and dorsal (B) sides. (A) The three classical chemosensitive areas on the ventral surface of the medulla: rostral, intermediate, and caudal (R, I, and C). The vertebral arteries conjoining into the basilar artery are diagrammed. The Roman numerals on the left correspond to the roots of the cranial nerves of interest. The black point in the midline at the bifurcation of the vertebral arteries is a projection of the obex. (B) For comparison, an outline of the fourth ventricle and locations of the two neuronal aggregates in the medulla: dorsal (DRG) and ventral (VRG) respiratory groups. The pontine areas, locus ceruleus (LC) and parabrachial complex (PBC), are outlined in the rostral pons.

complex (BC). The neuronal content of the NA is mixed: inspiratory and expiratory. These neurons send their axons to laryngeal motoneurons and also to visceral and autonomic motoneurons for thoracic and abdominal viscera. The NPA contains mostly inspiratory-related neurons whose axons project to the contralateral phrenic and external (inspiratory) intercostal muscle motoneurons. These neurons receive projections from the DRG, but not the other way around. The NRA contains mostly the expiratory-related neurons. Their axons descend to the contralateral side of the spinal cord and make monosynaptic excitatory contacts with motoneurons that innervate the internal (expiratory) intercostal muscles. These neurons receive ipsilaterally an inhibitory input during the inspiratory phase from the inspiratory-related neurons of the NPA and an excitatory one from the expiratory-related neurons of the BC. The BC neurons project to the contralateral DRG, inhibiting the inspiratory-related neurons there during the expiratory phase. Recently, a respiratory neuronal circuit has been described in the upper cervical cord.[4] These spinal, inspiratory-related neurons receive excitatory inputs from the inspiratory neurons of the contralateral DRG and VRG and inhibitory inputs from the raphe region.[8] They project to the ipsilateral phrenic and respiratory muscle motoneurons.[9]

Studies using a technique of antidromic stimulation of the ventrolateral spinal cord or retrograde neuronal labeling have refined our knowledge of the medullary cells' projections. The detailed morphologic and functional characteristics of each group of respiratory neurons, their interactions, and membrane properties are beyond the scope of this chapter. These details and references may be obtained from recent reviews.[6,7]

Either half of the medulla is sufficient for generating rhythmic respiratory activity, but there are species differences concerning the synchrony of action. Whereas a midsagittal section of the medulla in the rabbit results in a near-normal firing of both phrenic nerves, it desynchronizes these nerves in the monkey and elevates the CO_2 threshold for rhythmic excitation in the cat; that is, hypercarbia is required to sustain the firing in the latter case.[10,11] Transverse intramedullary connections are thus not so much germane to rhythm generation as they are to matching the action of the two bilateral respiratory networks. Although a majority of axons of the medullary respiratory neurons decussate in the obex area,[12,13] those which descend ipsilaterally apparently provide a sufficient synaptic excitatory input to the phrenic motoneurons.

SUPRAMEDULLARY CONTROL OF RESPIRATION

Structures rostral to the medulla affect respiration. Elimination of these structures does not abolish rhythmogenesis but modifies it.

PONS

Respiratory-related neurons of the upper pons are involved in a pneumotaxic mechanism which is responsible for the termination of inspiration and switching over to expiration. These neurons facilitate the inspiratory off-switch mechanism, the function played alongside the volume-related vagal feedback[14] (see "Lung and Airways" under "Peripheral Control"). The corollary is that removal of this mechanism prolongs the phrenic discharge and leads to the apneustic pattern of respiration. This has been shown by a variety of techniques, ranging from focal tissue destructions[15] or cooling[16] to midpontine transections,[17] all of which lead to apneustic respiration in vagotomized and anesthetized animals. The converse, stimulation of the pneumotaxic mechanism, activates the inspiratory off-switch, terminating prematurely the phrenic discharge.[18] In 1923, Lumsden[19] defined apneustic respiration as sustained inspiratory discharges interrupted by short expirations. It is worthwhile to note that in some of the later studies on the pneumotaxic mechanism, the prolongation of both inspiratory (T_I) and expiratory (T_E) times was often observed after lesions in the upper pons.[16,20] The T_E prolongation does not fulfill the criteria of apneustic respiration and represents a mere slowing of respiration, which is a qualitatively different state.

It seems unquestionable that there is a functional pneumotaxic mechanism, but the localization of the underlying neuronal structures is less certain. Currently, most investigators consider this site to be the medial parabrachial and Kölliker-Fuse nuclear complex in the upper pons[21,22] (Fig. 6-1B). However, the exact location has variously been identified throughout this century in the locus ceruleus,[23] the rostral tegmentum,[24] and more recently in the nucleus raphe magnus[25] or the motor trigeminal nucleus.[26] Only a small fraction or about 10 percent of phase-spanning respiratory neurons and even fewer inspiratory- or expiratory-related neurons in the parabrachial complex project down to the medullary respiratory groups.[27] This existence of other controlling pathways has been envisioned, and the search has continued for other sites at which the pneumotaxic mechanism may be used.

Electrical stimulation of the raphe magnus terminates inspiration in a manner similar to that of the parabrachial complex. Monosynaptic projections from the parabrachial complex to the raphe region have been found.[25] These findings raise the possibility that the inspiratory off-switch effect originating in the rostral pons might be relayed in the raphe magnus on the way to the motoneurons in the spinal cord. The possibility of a raphe-spinal functional connection is strengthened by the finding of projections descending from the raphe region to the upper cervical inspiratory neurons.[8]

Using more refined techniques of chemical lesioning and electrical stimulation, Fung and St. John[28,29] showed that the loci involved with the pneumotaxic mechanism extended beyond the pontine parabrachial complex rostrally to the region of the nucleus of the lateral lemniscus and caudally and ventrally to the regions of the superior vestibular and spinal trigeminal nuclei. This report and those earlier by Bassal and Bianchi[30,31] showed that stimulations of even remotely more rostral areas with respect to the pons may induce respiratory phase switching. This finding raises the possibility that the pneumotaxic effects observed during the manipulations in the rostral pons may be nonspecific, resulting from effects on fibers originating elsewhere but passing through the pontine areas in question. Recently, attention once again has been brought back to the rostral pons by studies that show that the off-switching and on-switching functions of inspiration can each be influenced by distinct pontine areas. Neurons in the lateral tegmentum at the pontomesencephalon border regulate the length of T_I, whereas neurons in the parabrachial complex regulate the T_E.[29]

The pontine respiratory neurons are relatively separate from the medullary ones. Less than 50 percent of medullary respiratory neurons project directly upward to pontine counterparts, which, in turn, project down indirectly through relay structures, like the raphe magnus. The pontine neurons underlie the operation of a time-dependent volume threshold. This function is highly sensitive to lung stretch, which decreases the off-switch threshold and facilitates termination of inspiration (see ''Lungs and Airways'' under ''Peripheral Control''). However, even in the absence of vagal afferents, these neurons are capable of matching the respiratory phases.[22] This independent action of pontine neurons is suppressed in the presence of volume-related feedback, but the exact mechanism of the off-switching of inspiration remains unsettled.

Besides pneumotaxic and vagal mechanisms, there appears to be several other sources of inspiratory inhibition whose suppression may lead to apneustic respiration. These include the inputs from the reticular formation,[32] the ventrolateral spinal cord,[33] and the cerebellum.[34]

The pons also participates in the integration of central and peripheral chemoreceptor inputs. This integration is differential. Ablation of the rostral pons suppresses the frequency response to hypercapnia but not hypoxia. In contrast, interruption of the caudal pons suppresses the volume and elevates the frequency response to both stimuli.[35]

Thus the pontine neurons modulate the respiratory rate and depth, slow the rhythm, and tune respiration to both suprapontine and peripheral inputs.

SUPRAPONTINE BRAIN

Respiratory influences have been described that are exerted by the cerebral cortex, the diencephalon and mesencephalon, the reticular formation stretching through the midbrain and forebrain, and the cerebellum. Participation of the cortex is widely recognized in behavioral and volitional control of respiration that can interrupt temporarily (automatic involuntary rhythmic breathing). The contentious issue is whether the voluntary influence is due to direct control of respiratory spinal motoneurons by the cortex or via the neurons in medulla. Electrical stimulation of the cortex is known to stimulate respiratory bulbospinal neurons.[36] Behaviorally conditioned cats stop inspiration by inactivating medullary inspiratory cells.[37] Studies like these argue strongly for an indirect control of spinal motoneurons.

On the other side, there are data showing that electrical[38] or magnetic[39] stimulation of the motor cortex produces short-latency excitation of the human diaphragm, which is compatible with a direct motor projection to the motoneurons. A number of cortical areas have been implicated in contralateral phrenic nerve excitation, including the pericruciate, sensorimotor, and cingulate cortex and the visual areas.[40–42] The stimulation experiments have been substantiated by the anatomic identification of corticospinal projections, e.g., from the pericruciate cortex to the phrenic motoneurons.[43] However, similar projections also have been identified to brain stem areas, which does not help resolve the issue of the separateness of the behavioral and automatic respiratory functions. Interestingly, sensory projections from the phrenic motoneurons to the cortex do not overlap with the motor sites.[44] Thus an intercortical link must relay the phrenic sensory-to-motor flow of information. The connections found are not evidence for their use in behavioral control of breathing. Such use seems likely but is difficult to prove in conscious subjects. It is plausible that one function predominates over the other in various physiologic or experimental conditions. The voluntary function may predominate in rapid eye movement sleep, whereas the automatic function may predominate in deep wave or anesthetic-like sleep.

The state of vigilance has a controlling influence over respiration, which may be attributed to the function of higher brain structures. Apneustic respiration cannot be induced in the awake cat, even after bilateral vagotomy and a pneumotaxic lesion.[45] It is crucially dependent on anesthesia or mesencephalic decerebration, the common denominator of both procedures being the interruption of signal descending from the higher structures to the pontine respiratory controller. Similarly, posthyperventilation apnea cannot be readily induced in the awake as opposed to the anesthetized human subject[46] due to counteracting excitatory influences that are capable of maintaining respiration in the face of hypocapnia.

Besides anesthetics, sleep affects respiration. Sleep, in general, decreases pulmonary ventilation by action on both the frequency and volume components of breathing[47] and on the respiratory responses to hypoxia and hypercapnia.[48,49] The higher nervous system also supervises the drive descending to pharyngeal muscles, which ensures that the pharynx remains open during sleep. During sleep, this control is damp-

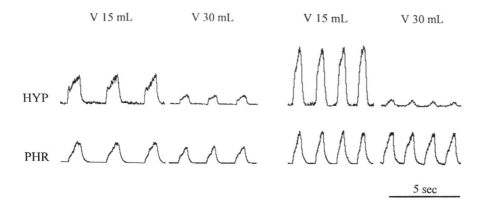

NORMOXIA   HYPOXIA

FIGURE 6-2 Hypoglossal (HYP) and phrenic (PHR) nerve responses to the doubling of tidal volume in normoxia (21% O_2 in N_2 inspired) and hypoxia (12% O_2 in N_2 inspired). Integrated neural activities are presented. Note disproportions between the hypoglossal and phrenic changes, which are increased by hypoxia. (U Jernajczyk and M Pokorski, unpublished observations.)

ened, and therefore, motor output to pharyngeal muscles is compromised. When this happens against the background of pharyngeal narrowing caused by anatomic abnormalities, occlusive episodes and sleep disruption typical of sleep apnea ensue. The patency of the pharynx depends on the balance of intrapharyngeal suction pressure developed by contracting inspiratory muscles and outward pull generated by pharyngeal muscles. It is plausible that deactivation of the higher nervous system in sleep endangers a preferential suppression of upper airway muscles as compared with inspiratory muscles, increasing the propensity for pharyngeal collapse. Disproportional changes in the motor activities running to these two groups of muscles have been found in experimental work. In the rabbit, periods of deep and accelerated respiration, which is a feature of the sleep apnea syndrome, strongly decrease the hypoglossal nerve activity with little change in the phrenic nerve activity.[49a] These disproportional changes are exaggerated by hypoxia, another characteristic feature of the syndrome (Fig. 6-2).

The diencephalon and mesencephalon exert their respiratory effects through the reticular activating system. The hypothalamus, which is part of the diencephalon, seems to be an especially active region with regard to respiratory control. Electrical stimulation of the region produces the arousal[50] or defense-like[51] reactions that are typically associated with increased respiration. Focal heating creates an excitatory input to the bulbar neurons and markedly increases respiration.[52] Of note is that respiratory activation by temperature diminishes the ability of the system to respond to other stimuli.[53] Respiratory responsiveness may become saturated, or the hypothalamic drive excites concomitantly interneurons that inhibit other inputs to the medullary respiratory network.

The facilitation of respiration by midbrain mechanisms is subject to inhibitory control by the cortex. In the normoxic cat, decortication alone increases baseline room air respiration and, particularly, the response to hypoxia.[54] The blunted hypoxic response in the chronically hypoxic cat is also relieved by decortication.[55]

In the face of stimuli that require a prompt and complex response to maintain metabolic homeostasis, such as, for example, exercise, the hypothalamus generates signals that become the commanding driving force for the respiratory

system.[56] This central command appears to be the essential feedforward force that is able to override other control mechanisms of the negative feedback type and which couples the respiratory, cardiovascular, and locomotive responses.

The cerebellum exerts an inhibitory effect on respiration, which has been found during both normal and apneustic respiration in the cat.[34] The anterior lobe of the cerebellum, which is also the area of respiratory muscle coordination, is the source of this inhibitory influence. The cerebellum receives connections from the reticular nuclei of the brain stem and from the spinal cord through the spinocerebellar tract. The sensory information from the chest wall joint mechanoreceptors,[57] which play a role in the perception of posture, may be relayed in the cerebellum on the way to the areas controlling respiration in the brain stem. The cerebellar projections involved with respiratory modulation have not yet been investigated in detail.

NEUROTRANSMITTERS

Research has begun to characterize the transmitters used for chemical communication in the central respiratory pathways. Classical transmitters such as indolamines, serotonin catecholamines, or peptides have been localized in brain stem respiratory structures.[58] It is unlikely that these transmitters are the determinants of the rapid, millisecond synaptic transmissions that should operate between neurons generating the respiratory rhythm because of their relatively slow and prolonged action. These classical transmitters couple to signaling G proteins and, via a multistep intracellular cascade of events, produce a cellular response. They may have a major part in modulation of the respiratory neural system, changing cellular and synaptic operation sometimes fundamentally but over a slower time scale. This function of neural modulation and molding may explain the diverse results of the studies employing these transmitters and their agonists and antagonists on respiration. Nevertheless, some generalizations may be drawn.

Serotonergic transmission is mostly inhibitory for respiratory motor output, the effects being exerted on both presynaptic and postsynaptic components of the brain stem respiratory network.[58] Catecholamines appear to have an antagonistic action to that of serotonin on the central respiratory network. Dopamine and norepinephrine act in concert to increase neuronal activity and the effector responses.[58] They are especially capable of influencing the respiratory timing mechanism. The action of central dopamine would thus oppose the action of dopamine peripherally in arterial chemoreceptors (see "Arterial Chemoreceptors" under "Peripheral Control"). Analysis of the effects of catecholamines is hampered by their actions on many receptor types and numerous interactions with other transmitter systems.

Thyrotropin-releasing hormone and substance P may be examples of peptide transmitters influencing respiration.[58] Their interactions with the respiratory drive result in stimulatory responses. These peptides have an important effect also on respiratory timing. Thyrotropin-releasing hormone especially is able to increase minute ventilation by causing pronounced tachypnea. These peptides coexist with serotonin in brain stem respiratory nuclei, which may help maintain a proper excitatory-inhibitory modulatory balance.

The processing of information and communication on only the respiratory neurons in the central nervous system are based on brief changes in ionic conductances and the resulting generation of excitatory and inhibitory postsynaptic potentials. This fast synaptic transmission uses either excitatory amino acids (primarily glutamate) or inhibitory amino acids [primarily γ-aminobutyric acid (GABA)].

Respiratory neurons are equipped with excitatory amino acid receptors. Activation of both glutamate N-methyl-D-aspartate (NMDA) and non-NMDA receptors has been incriminated in both respiratory rhythmicity generation and its modulation.[1,59-64] These receptors are inotropic receptors that are ligand-gated ion channels permeable to selective cations.

Excitatory amino acids appear necessary for respiratory rhythm generation in both in vitro and in vivo preparations. There are differences concerning the receptor type involved. In the in vitro rat brain stem–spinal cord preparation, respiratory rhythm generation depends on the activity of medullary non-NMDA receptors.[59] Selective activation of these receptors increases and blockade decreases respiratory firing rate; the NMDA receptors appear not to be involved.[59] Injection of a non-NMDA antagonist into the pre-Bötzinger area, which is an area involved with respiratory rhythmogenesis, abolishes respiratory motor activity.[1]

In the in vivo preparation, the function of either NMDA or non-NMDA receptors suffices for basic rhythm generation. Blockade of either receptor in the cat or rat pre-Bötzinger area causes little changes in respiratory pattern, whereas simultaneous blockade of the two receptor types results in respiratory arrest.[60,61] The difference between the in vivo and in vitro preparations may stem from sensory inputs emanating in vivo from both the rostral brain and the periphery that use excitatory amino acid transmission. Examples of such inputs, which cannot be present in the isolated brain stem preparation, are the carotid body–mediated excitation of the expiratory bulbospinal neurons of the caudal VRG, which depends on NMDA receptors,[62] and the pulmonary stretch receptor–mediated Hering-Breuer inflation reflex, which depends on non-NMDA receptor activation.[63] The cooperation of the two types of glutamate receptors may be germane to rhythmicity modulation.

Excitatory amino acid involvement in phase switching goes beyond that of the reflex effects on expiratory neurons

mediated by the carotid body and on inspiration termination mediated by the vagal volume-related feedback. Blockade of NMDA receptors in animals whose vagal nerves are severed results in inspiratory prolongation, which culminates in apneusis, similar to that induced by ablation of the pontine parabrachial region[64] (see "Supramedullary Control of Respiration" under "Central Control"). The similarity of apneusis strongly suggests that the pontine control of inspiratory duration is mediated by NMDA receptors. Excitatory amino acid transmission also has been established in the descending drive to spinal phrenic and intercostal motoneurons.[59]

There is cogent evidence that GABA is the major inhibitory neurotransmitter at various levels of the respiratory system. GABA-containing neurons have been found in the parabrachial area[65] and the raphe nucleus[66] that are involved in the inspiratory off-switch mechanism, in the Bötzinger area of the retrofacial nucleus[67] that participates in the respiratory rhythm generation, in the medullary respiratory groups,[68,69] and in the phrenic motor nucleus in the spinal cord.[70] GABA acts mainly through $GABA_A$ and $GABA_B$ receptors, and both receptor types are present on respiratory neurons. $GABA_A$ receptors are inotropic recognition sites that upon coupling with an agonist cause an increase in Cl^- permeability, hyperpolarization, and neuronal inhibition. $GABA_B$ receptors are metabotropic and act through G proteins that initiate an intracellular second messenger cascade.

Activation of $GABA_A$ receptors results in an overall respiratory depression in vivo[58] and in in vitro brain stem–spinal cord preparations.[71] These receptors have been implicated in periodic postsynaptic inhibition of both inspiratory and expiratory bulbar neurons.[69] The GABAergic system thus may influence respiratory rhythm and drive by affecting reciprocal neuronal inhibition. The $GABA_A$ also has been associated with the mechanism of central hypoxic depression.[72] It is probable that the GABAergic system exerts a tonic inhibitory influence on the respiratory neural network because GABA antagonism alone increases respiration.[71,73]

Activation of $GABA_B$ receptors has much less clear respiratory effects. The $GABA_B$ agonist baclofen is used most commonly as a pharmacologic tool. The effects on both bulbar respiratory neurons and respiratory motor output are variable, depending on the dose, the route of application, the species, etc. An interesting feature of baclofen is that it may cause apneustic respiration[74] that is similar to that caused by an NMDA antagonist.[64] The possibility arises that $GABA_B$ may mediate the inhibition of glutamate release, which would attenuate the inspiratory off-switch mechanism through NMDA receptors. Interference with transmitter release and turnover may yet be the most important function of $GABA_B$ in respiratory control.

HYPOXIC VENTILATORY DEPRESSION

The ventilatory effect of hypoxia consists of two opposing components: stimulation through the peripheral chemoreceptors (see "Arterial Chemoreceptors" under "Peripheral Control") and inhibition due to the central depressant effect. With the peripheral chemoreceptors intact, the net effect is stimulation. However, the central depressant effect gains in magnitude with the duration of hypoxic exposure. This is the reason why after the initial hypoxic stimulation, the rise in ventilation is attenuated, and after a while, ventilation may fall even below the baseline level. The central depression underlies the biphasic ventilatory response to steady-state hypoxia and attenuation of the rate of rise of ventilatory stimulation in progressive hypoxia in humans or animals. The depressant response to hypoxia dominates in the neonatal state, in which the carotid chemoreceptors are not yet fully operational. In chemodenervated animals, hypoxia has a progressively inhibitory effect on ventilation, eventually leading to cessation of respiration. The determinants of the central hypoxic depression seem multiple and are under debate. They involve the elaboration of inhibitory neurotransmitters in the CNS such as GABA[72] or endogenous opioids,[75] the latter acting at the central chemoreceptor, and a decrease in excitatory biogenic amines.[76] An increase in cerebral blood flow due to a hypoxic vasodilatation may cause an alkaline shift at the medullary chemoreceptors, which adds to ventilatory inhibition.[77]

MEDULLARY CHEMORECEPTORS

The respiratory neural network is able to respond to changes in the chemical composition of its environment. Respiratory motor output and its executive arm—pulmonary ventilation—are adjusted in such a way as to bring this environment back to its homeostatic level. This chemical control of respiration is brought about by a negative feedback system. The chemosensor is presumed to reside in the superficial layer (~200 μm) of the ventral medullary surface (VMS). The classical concept has it that there are three circumscribed chemosensitive areas there: the rostral, caudal, and intermediate areas (see Fig. 6-1A). The rostral and caudal areas detect changes in chemical stimuli, and their inputs converge on the intermediate area, from which the information is relayed to deeper medullary structures.[78–80] Consistent with this organization of the medullary areas, ablation of the intermediate area by focal cooling or coagulation greatly diminishes the ventilatory response to CO$_2$ and virtually eliminates it after concomitant denervation of peripheral chemoreceptors.[79,80] Despite this seemingly straightforward organization, the nature of the chemosensor remains elusive. There are, indeed, neuronal elements in the two chemosensitive areas that react in an opposite manner on acidosis and alkalosis.[81] However, these neurons are intermingled with others that are insensitive or react to nonspecific stimuli. Moreover, the chemoreactive cells also may be found beyond the outlines of the chemosensitive areas, albeit their responses are less regular and reproducible and the direction of the response has no relationship to the kind of stimulus.[79]

The stimulus is the [H$^+$] in the extracellular fluid (ECF) surrounding the chemoreceptor cells.[80] Acidity may be changed in a metabolic or respiratory manner. In the latter case, hydration of CO$_2$, catalyzed by carbonic anhydrase, leads to the rapid formation of H$^+$, according to the equation

$$CO_2 + H_2O \rightleftharpoons H_2CO_3 \rightleftharpoons HCO_3^- + H^+$$

In the steady-state condition, the ECF composition is thought to be in equilibrium with that of the adjacent ventral medullary interstices, which, in turn, equilibrate with the cerebrospinal fluid (CSF). The [H$^+$] at the chemoreceptor can thus be affected by way of the CSF. In both animals and humans, a unit decrease of pH in the CSF causes at least a doubling

of pulmonary ventilation.[80] Decreased pH also facilitates synaptic transmission and increases excitatory postsynaptic potentials, which may fill a role as a biologic amplifier of other inputs.

In general, CSF [H$^+$] changes are not a straight reflection of those in blood. As opposed to blood, CSF has very limited protein and noncarbon buffers. Changes in the brain [H$^+$] that follow those in the arterial [H$^+$] are minimized by rapid adjusting mechanisms linked, on the one side, to the arterial chemoreceptors and, on the other, to cerebral blood flow regulation. For example, a rise in arterial P_{CO_2} triggers a rapid increase in pulmonary ventilation mediated by the arterial chemoreceptors, whose response time is faster than that of the medullary chemoreceptors.[82] Additionally, increased central P_{CO_2} dilates cerebral blood vessels. An increased blood flow counteracts the rise in P_{CO_2} in the brain.

The blood-brain barrier (BBB) is another constraint for transmission of arterial blood acid-base disturbances into the brain ECF. The BBB is relatively impermeable to polar solutes such as H$^+$ or HCO$_3^-$.[83] The BBB is a heterogeneous structure that comprises such functionally different components as the cerebral capillary and choroid plexus interfaces that form plasma ultrafiltrate and CSF, respectively. Both active and passive ionic transport systems have been invoked to explain the regulation of the [H$^+$] in ECF.[83] It has been demonstrated that there is a potential difference across the BBB[84] that amounts to about +6.5 mV. This difference changes as a function of arterial [H$^+$]; a positive shift has been demonstrated in most species. The electrical force should influence movement and thus concentration of solutes on both sides of the barrier.

The time course of the ventilatory response to a step change in arterial P_{CO_2} has a fast and two slower components.[82] The former is believed to be the action of arterial chemoreceptors, and the other two stem from the differential kinetics of CO$_2$ equilibration between the relatively spacious compartments of tissue and fluids that affect central chemoreceptors.[82]

The morphologic substrate of the central chemosensors have not been identified. Thus chemoreceptor properties and responses cannot be studied directly. The level of H$^+$ in the extracellular fluid may not be as important as intracellular pH or the pH gradient along some submicroscopic elements of the system. The uniqueness of the [H$^+$] as a stimulus has been questioned too. Independent of [H$^+$] changes, some component of the response may be caused by molecular CO$_2$, as originally postulated by Nielsen.[85] This holds true also for the arterial chemoreceptors as well, which at constant [H$^+$] respond to CO$_2$ with an extra stimulatory effect.[86,87] These uncertainties have led some investigators to postulate that central chemosensitivity is in actuality a more or less specific feature of respiratory neurons themselves and is scattered throughout the medulla.

The physiologic effects of the central chemosensors may be mediated by defined structures such as the retrotrapezoid nucleus and the nucleus paragigantocellularis lateralis (NPGL). These neuronal clusters are located near the rostral ventral surface but beyond the outline of the major respiratory neuronal groups. Both nuclei send projections to the ventral and dorsal respiratory groups[88] and are clearly engaged in respiratory alterations, the source of which is at the ventral medullary surface. The role of the NPGL may even extend to rhythm generation. Its focal cooling results in apnea, i.e., cessation of inspiratory activator.[89] Besides the control of respiration, both the ventral medulla and the structures below it are involved in cardiovascular functions. Of these, relay in the baroreceptor reflex and possibly cerebral blood flow regulation are significant. The rostral ventrolateral medulla is the vasomotor area from which neurons send direct projections to the sympathetic preganglionic neurons, which control cardiac and vasomotor tone, in the intermediolateral cell columns of the spinal cord.[90]

Central chemosensitive pathways use neuroactive substances. A cholinergic link has been proposed. Topical application of acetylcholine (ACh) or its agonists to the VMS increases ventilation in a manner similar to that of [H$^+$] and in the spots that coincide with those for [H$^+$].[80] Moreover, in VMS slice preparations, neurons that respond to H$^+$ are also stimulated by ACh.[80] Other neuroactive substances may be involved too. Topical application of an opiate to the intermediate area depresses respiration, the effect being reversed by naloxone, an opiate antagonist.[91] Microinjections of glutamate into the rostral chemosensitive area also have clear ventilatory effects.[92]

Spinal Control

SPINAL RESPIRATORY NEURONS AND MOTONEURONS

Respiratory neurons have been demonstrated in the intermediate gray matter of the C1–C3 spinal segments.[4,9] These neurons are inspiratory-associated in the cat. Their axons project ipsilaterally as far down as to the lumbar segments, collateralizing along the way at the cervical phrenic and thoracic intercostal motoneurons.[93,94] These neurons are controlled by the medullary respiratory network. They receive excitatory inputs from the sensorimotor cortex, the nucleus tractus solitarius, and the inspiratory neurons of the nucleus paraambigualis and inhibitory ones from the raphe region.[8,66] The raphe magnus–induced depressant effects on medullary and upper cervical respiratory neurons are apparently mediated by GABA$_A$ receptors. The presumed function of the upper cervical respiratory neurons is to integrate and coordinate the descending supraspinal inputs on the way to the respiratory muscle motoneurons.

The phrenic motor nucleus consists of cells extending through several segments of the ventral aspect of the cervical ventral horn. There are interspecies and intraspecies differences in diaphragmatic innervation by segmental phrenic roots. In humans, the innervating roots come from C3, C4, and C5. The intercostal muscle motoneurons consist of a longitudinal cluster of cells extending throughout the thoracic spinal cord. These cells, belonging to α and γ motoneurons, drive the inspiratory external and parasternal intercostal muscles and the expiratory internal intercostal, abdominal, and triangularis sterni muscles.

SPINAL PATHWAYS

Both descending and ascending spinal pathways affect breathing. Lesions in the inferior reticular nucleus cause degeneration in the anterior column and in the anterior part of the lateral column of the spinal cord.[95] Conversely, hemi-cordotomies of the cervical spinal cord cause ascending degeneration to the inferior reticular nucleus. A major projection of afferent fibers to the medullary and pontine reticular formation has been confirmed in other studies employing anterolateral cordotomies.[96,97]

Most studies have been concerned with the descending respiratory pathways.[98,99] These pathways are organized in a discrete and systematic way. There is a physical separation of the pathways subserving the voluntary and involuntary respiratory drives. The former run in the corticospinal and corticorubrospinal tracts of the dorsolateral funiculus and the latter in the reticulospinal tracts of the ventrolateral funiculus of the spinal cord.[100] Accordingly, interruption of the dorsolateral funiculus abolishes the cortically evoked response but leaves rhythmic respiratory activity intact. Conversely, interruption of the anterolateral funiculus abolishes the rhythmic activity but leaves the cortical modulation of respiration intact. These findings in experimental animals are consistent with those in humans. Subjects with cervical anterolateral cordotomy exhibit suppressed rhythmic ventilatory drive, but their ability to voluntarily change respiration remains grossly unaffected.[101,102] Thus testing the subject's response to voluntary breathing acts may help discern the anatomic localization of a spinal cord lesion.

The separation of the voluntary and involuntary respiratory responses requires qualification, since they may, to some extent, be interactive. A number of fibers of the corticospinal tract branch off in the course of their descent through the pons and medulla to form a corticobulbar bundle that innervates, among other things, the motor nuclei of the trigeminal and hypoglossal nerves, the nuclei known to be engaged in the automatic respiratory control. Descending fibers also collateralize throughout the length of the spinal cord to segmental interneurons.

The spatial separation of descending fibers advances even further in the ventrolateral funiculus of the cervical cord. The expiratory descending fibers constitute a fairly distinct bundle lying medially to the inspiratory ones. Indeed, it is possible to lesion the spinal cord in such a way that the inspiratory action of the diaphragm is abolished but the expiratory activity of the abdominal muscles is preserved.[103]

Respiratory muscle motoneurons also receive inputs from supraspinal sources that are unrelated to the respiratory function. Neuronal structures integrating such involuntary reflexes as the hiccup, cough, or micturition lie in the vicinity of the brain stem respiratory networks. The descending pathways transmitting these reflexes run alongside those for the rhythmic respiratory drive in the ventral columns. These reflexes are integrated into a respiratory muscle response at the segmental level.

SEGMENTAL REFLEXES

Sensors in the respiratory muscles can alter the activity of the spinal respiratory motoneurons through segmental reflexes. These receptors belong to a class of mechanoreceptors and consist of muscle spindle endings and tendon organs that are generally considered as proprioceptors. The spindle endings are of two types: primary endings innervated by group Ia fibers and secondary endings innervated by group II fibers. The spindle is placed in the muscle in parallel to the extrafusal fibers and functionally behaves like a slowly adapting stretch receptor. The primary spindles excite monosynaptically α motoneurons, whereas the secondary ones use a polysynaptic method. The tendon organ, another of the slow adapting type of stretch receptors, is innervated by group Ib fibers and placed in series with muscle fibers. Tendons via an organ afferent have an inhibitory effect on α motoneurons. Muscle spindle endings sense changes in length, the primary spindles underlie the dynamic and the secondary spindles the static component of the response to stretch, whereas tendon organs respond to force exerted by the muscle.

The diaphragm is relatively poorly equipped with receptors. Estimates of the sensory component of phrenic nerve fibers vary from 10 to 25 percent.[104] The phrenic nerve contains about 500 sensory fibers in the cat or rat.[105,106] The majority of them carry information from tendon organs, and just a fraction can be traced to spindles. Fibers arising from tendon organs constitute the basis of a phrenic-to-phrenic reflex, which functions to limit phrenic activity and thereby diaphragmatic contraction.[107]

In contrast, about 45 percent of fibers in intercostal nerves are sensory. Muscle spindles and fusimotor activation play a dominant role in the segmental control of the intercostal muscles.[108,109] Two spinal reflexes are of greatest interest: the intercostal to intercostal and the intercostal to phrenic. Usually both inspiratory and expiratory proprioceptors are activated; therefore, the motor response is the net effect of the sensory information flowing from the two kinds of muscles and the two types of receptors affected. Muscle spindle afferents from external and internal intercostal muscles activate corresponding α motoneurons in the same or neighboring segments.[109] Stretching of an intercostal space causes external intercostal motor activity to increase in the same space and to decrease in a distant space.[108] The increase in external intercostal activity in the same space is largely ascribable to the excitatory effect of external intercostal primary muscle spindle endings and possibly of internal intercostal muscle spindles through interconnections[109] on external intercostal α motoneurons. The excitatory effect outweighs the inhibitory effect of the external and internal intercostal muscle tendon organs via an interneuron on the same motoneurons. The inhibitory effect of tendon organs prevails in distance spaces. Thus segmental control wanes with distance from the motoneurons concerned.

Proprioceptive activation due to intercostal muscle stretching[110] or lower intercostal nerve stimulation[111] in partially or wholly spinalized cats leads to phrenic activation with a relatively long latency of a polysynaptic manner. The likely role of such an intercostal-to-phrenic reflex is to coordinate the action of the intercostals and the diaphragm. Interestingly, these intercostal-to-phrenic reflexes are under an inhibitory supraspinal influence, since the phrenic activation is greater after spinal cord transection.[112]

The exact segmental arrangement of abdominal expiratory muscle spindle endings and tendon organs or their interaction with chest muscles is unknown. Their afferents run in the caudal thoracic nerves, so the mechanisms known for the chest muscles may be applicable to the expiratory abdominal muscles.

The segmental proprioceptive control of respiratory muscles may have a part in adjusting the contractile work of various muscle groups to meet the challenge of external (e.g., changes in posture) and internal (e.g., pathology within the inspiratory tract) strains imposed on the system.

Peripheral Control

One major function of the central respiratory network is to optimize the volume and frequency components of pulmonary ventilation. To do so, the system should receive inputs regarding the effectiveness of respiratory action, i.e., whether and how lung volume is actually changing. These inputs may be categorized into extravagal and vagal feedback loops. The extravagal reflexes emanate mainly from respiratory muscle afferents. The vagal reflexes originate mainly in the lower airway receptors and will be described subsequently.

RESPIRATORY MUSCLE AFFERENTS

Receptors in the respiratory muscles can influence respiration by supraspinal pathways.[108] The afferent fibers of the reflexes initiated in these receptors ascend in the dorsal columns and synapse on medullary and pontine respiratory neurons whose axons run down to spinal respiratory motoneurons. Respiratory modulation may be ascribed to these afferents, since sectioning of the thoracic dorsal roots markedly diminishes intercostal motoneuron activity[113] and abolishes proprioceptive reflexes.[114] Since midcollicular decerebration does not abolish these reflexes,[115] respiratory proprioceptive activity is processed within the brain stem. An understanding of the action on the central respiratory network of respiratory muscle afferents comes mostly from electrical or mechanical stimulation experiments.

There are two major problems concerning electrical stimulation. First, the separation among group Ia (primary muscle spindle endings), group Ib (tendon organs), and group II (secondary muscle spindle endings) afferents is based on differences in stimulus threshold and conduction velocities. Owing to the considerable overlap of these parameters, a clear separation is seldom feasible. Second, the internal intercostal nerves contain bundles of fibers that run, in the upper thorax, to the expiratory internal intercostal and inspiratory parasternal muscles and, in the lower thorax, to the expiratory internal intercostal and abdominal muscles. The internal intercostal nerves also contain an admixture of fibers innervating cutaneous tissue. These bundles are inseparable, and therefore, selective stimulation is unfeasible.

Taken as a whole, available evidence suggests that stimulation of afferent fibers in both external and internal intercostal nerves inhibits the activity of medullary VRG and DRG inspiratory neurons.[57,116-118] There may be a decrease in neuronal discharge rate or faster termination of inspiratory activity, which results in a reduction in phrenic and inspiratory intercostal motor output. The inhibitory effects have been ascribed to group I fibers,[57,117] but electrical stimulation could not distinguish whether these effects are mediated by group Ia or group Ib afferents. Cutaneous afferents innervating the skin over the respiratory muscles, having similar electrical properties to group Ib fibers[109] and running along the respiratory proprioceptors, might be stimulated concurrently. These afferents also have an inhibitory influence on medullary inspiratory and expiratory neuronal activities and may add to overall inspiratory motor inhibition.[117]

A greater selectivity of fiber excitation can be obtained with mechanical stimulation. Various modes of mechanical stimulation have been employed, such as intercostal muscle stretch, contraction, or vibration, ranging from a single space to larger areas of the chest wall. Selective excitation of tendon organs without increasing muscle spindle ending activity in a single intercostal space may be achieved by impeding the electrically induced contraction of the intercostal muscles in the space.[118] Excitation of muscle spindle endings, on the other hand, is achieved by choosing the optimal vibration amplitudes: 40 and 90 μm for the internal and external intercostal muscle spindle endings, respectively.[118] Higher vibration amplitudes progressively recruit tendon organs. Using such a selective experimental paradigm in the decerebrate and anesthetized cat, Bolser and colleagues[118] have found that both external and internal intercostal tendon organs, but not muscle spindle endings, have an inhibitory influence on both medullary inspiratory and phrenic nerve activities. The inhibition of the medullary inspiratory neurons is propagated to the pontine inspiratory neurons, causing their attenuation.[115] The inhibitory action of tendon organs is backed by a similar influence of mechanoreceptors of the costovertebral joints[57] and of lung mechanoreceptors whose afferents run in the thoracic sympathetic chain.[119]

Likewise, stimulation of both external and internal intercostal nerve afferents is inhibitory for the expiratory bulbospinal neurons of the VRG, whose axons project to intercostal and abdominal expiratory muscle motoneurons, the tendon organs being the determinants of the responses again.[120] Interestingly, despite the direct inhibitory effect on medullary expiratory neurons, their activity may be paradoxically prolonged because of concomitant withdrawal of the reciprocal inhibitory action of the inspiratory neurons on expiratory neurons.

Tendon organs have an opposing, excitatory effect on the expiratory laryngeal motoneurons[120] of the retroambigualis area. These motoneurons drive the laryngeal abductor muscles, such as the thyroarytenoid muscle that fulfills an expiratory resisting role, as opposed to an expiratory forcing role played by the intercostals. The opposing effect of tendon organs on the two pools of medullary expiratory motoneurons is thus accounted for by the different functions played by the two groups of muscles.

The inspiration inhibitory influence of intercostal proprioceptors is diminished by hypercapnia or hypoxia.[57] Such responses require a higher level of respiratory motor activation and are typically associated with the feeling of respiratory distress. Studies carried out in awake humans suggest that the higher the respiratory motor activity and consequently sensory input, the less is the feeling of respiratory distress. Respiratory sensations are increased when respiratory movement is constrained below that occurring freely at a given level of the CO_2 stimulus.[121] In general, respiratory distress is more when tidal volume is small than when it is large for the same level of the CO_2 stimulus.[122] This implicates the reflexes associated with the chest and lung movement in conveying information about the intensity of the respiratory stimulus. The information is intended for the cortex and therefore should be transmitted through suprapontine structures. In support of this hypothesis, it has been found in the cat that sensory signals from both chest wall muscles and carotid chemoreceptors affect the firing pattern of midbrain neurons, the effect of the signal from the latter being unaffected by high cervical transection.[123] The possibility thus arises that the suprapontine brain receives signals on the intensity of respiratory drive that, besides the chest wall muscles, emanate as a corollary discharge from medullary neurons.[124]

The diaphragm also contains tendon organs and a smaller fraction of spindle endings that can regulate diaphragmatic function over a supraspinal reflex.[125] Recent studies with afferent stimulation of the phrenic nerve in cats and dogs have unraveled excitatory, mono- or paucisynaptic projections going especially to the DRG inspiratory neurons[126] that have an excitory effect on respiration.[127] Increased inspiratory activity at the premotor medullary level may be opposed or even overridden by an inhibitory diaphragmatic reflex at the spinal level,[107,126] either of which can be mediated by the same diaphragmatic afferents.

The physiologic significance of the respiratory proprioceptive reflexes is unclear. Their role seems to be meager in both eupneic and stimulated breathing. The reflexes may assume greater importance in the condition of an increased respiratory muscle force when inhibition of the inspiratory drive is desirable, as in a Valsalva maneuver. They may have a role in adjusting the pattern of breathing to changes of the mechanical state of the chest-lung system, e.g., by detecting disproportional changes in the intrafusal and extrafusal fiber lengths when muscle shortening is impeded in the low-compliance state. The proprioceptors also may be important for cortical perception of the intensity of respiratory motor action that underlies the feeling of respiratory discomfort.

LUNGS AND AIRWAYS

RECEPTORS

Stretch Receptors
Stretch receptors are located about equally in the lower extrapulmonary and pulmonary airways. They are in series with airway smooth muscles[128] and respond to changes in intramural tension, being affected mostly by circumferential stretch of the airway wall. The receptors undergo adaptation to a sustained stimulus and may belong to a slowly or rapidly adapting type. The adaptation process depends also on the kinetics of volume, i.e., airway or lung distention, change.[129] For the same volume, a rapid distention causes a greater receptor activation than a slow one. The receptor threshold is within the range of the eupneic tidal volume. The receptors increase and decrease their discharge with each lung inflation and deflation, respectively, although some may fire throughout the respiratory cycle,[130] or their discharge may increase during deflation.[129] Another feature of airway stretch receptors is their sensitivity to CO_2.[131] They are stimulated by a decrease and inhibited by an increase in inspired P_{CO_2}. This responsiveness is separate from that to stretch and may be underlain by CO_2-induced pH changes. It remains unclear whether physiologic fluctuations in alveolar P_{CO_2} are strong enough to stimulate stretch receptors. Larger increases in inspired P_{CO_2} do increase the ventilatory rate by cutting expiratory time, which is an action consistent with an attenuation of the stretch receptor.[132] The relative role and importance of different types of receptors are clouded by the fact that they respond to many of the same stimuli.

J-Receptors
J-receptors, also referred to as *bronchopulmonary C-fiber receptors*, are juxtacapillary receptors of the lung parenchyma. The afferent pathway runs in slowly conducting nonmyelinated vagal fibers. The receptors respond to increased interstitial fluid volume outside the capillaries. Accordingly, they are

stimulated by conditions such as pulmonary embolism, lung edema, inhalation of irritant gases such as ammonia or volatile anesthetics, injection of chemicals such as capsaicin or phenyldiguanide into the pulmonary circulation, and a number of neuromodulators such as histamine, acetylcholine, and serotonin.[133] The reflex responses they induce consist of tachypnea, rapid and shallow breathing, and apnea. J-receptors do not seem germane to the control of normal respiration because they are silent in eupneic breathing. Their role comes to the fore in the diseased or congested lung, for example, in pneumonia, when they may develop a tonic discharge that modulates the pattern of respiration.[134]

Irritant Receptors

Irritant receptors are located in and around the walls of the trachea and large bronchi. They are rapidly adapting stretch receptors with afferents in myelinated vagal fibers. Generally, they respond to inhalation of irritant gases, chemicals, and the like. The reflex effects are cough, secretion of mucus, bronchoconstriction, and tachypnea. Those in the airway epithelium mostly give rise to cough, whereas those located deeper in the lungs produce tachypnea. The irritant receptors are also stimulated by atelectasis, pneumothorax, deep inflation and deflation,[135] and mediators such as histamine.[136] Their role is unclear, but apart from participating in defense reactions and inflammatory conditions of the airways, such as asthma, they may initiate the appearance of spontaneous augmented breaths.

REFLEXES

Classical Stretch Receptor–Mediated Reflexes

HERING-BREUER INFLATION REFLEX   In 1868, Hering and Breuer demonstrated that breathing can be interrupted by tracheal occlusion or increased intratracheal pressure at or close to the peak of inspiration, that is, by occluding expiration. This reflex originates in slowly adapting airway stretch receptors. The afferents are large myelinated vagal fibers. Inspiration in the occluded breath is terminated, and the next inspiration is delayed due to a prolonged expiratory pause. This is thus an expiration-promoting reflex. The next, delayed inspiration, which occurs even though the stimulus persists, is called *vagal escape*. The inflation reflex is readily evocable in animals but not humans, except during the neonatal state. The reflex is rather weak in unanesthetized animals and becomes more strongly expressed during anesthesia. The reflex is integrated in the brain stem, since neither midcollicular decerebration nor decortication abolishes it. The reflex's volume threshold in a conscious human is about 800 to 1000 mL, which is much higher than the normal tidal volume. The reflex may play a protective role, especially during breathing with large tidal volumes, but its real function is unclear.

PARADOXICAL REFLEX OF HEAD   In 1889, Head observed that if the inflation reflex is blocked by cooling the vagus nerve to 8°C, distention of the lungs causes an additional inspiratory effort, that is, further inflation rather than termination of inspiration. This reflex is then the reverse of the Hering-Breuer inflation reflex. The receptors are different and are the rapidly adapting mechanoreceptors in the lung parenchyma. The role of the reflex is unclear, but it might be engaged in "big breathing" phenomena such as gasping,

sighing, hyperinflation of exercise, and generation of the first breath in the newborn baby.

DEFLATION REFLEX   Airway occlusion during expiration or provoking lung deflation by applying negative pressure produces an inspiratory-promoting reflex that makes the next inspiration appear sooner and its volume smaller. The receptors for this reflex are in the lower airways. The reflex might be responsible for the hyperpnea of chest compression or pneumothorax. It also could have to do with the generation of spontaneous augmented breaths, "sighs," that appear occasionally in both normal and diseased breathing and help prevent atelectasis.

Inspiration Facilitation: A Positive Feedback Reflex

Besides the above-mentioned reflexes, stretch receptors exert a critical control over the timing and magnitude of each breath. Lung volume increments during inspiration cause facilitation of inspiratory activity in both phrenic and external intercostal motoneurons, the latter motoneurons displaying a much stronger facilitatory response.[137] The reflex originates in slowly adapting stretch receptors, is vagally mediated, and is observable in some species, such as the cat or dog, under light or no anesthesia.[137,138] The reflex has a low-volume threshold, that is, is elicited by small lung expansions, which are well below the eupneic tidal volume. This inspiration-facilitating reflex constitutes a positive feedback acting to reinforce the ascending inspiratory activity in each breath and precedes a negative feedback, inspiration-terminating reflex mediated by the same receptors. The latter reflex is initiated when the *inspiratory off-switch threshold* is reached. The bulbospinal pathways of the facilitatory reflex are unclear. The presence of the reflex in humans is not established, but it might provide the rationale for the increasing contribution of the chest muscles to breathing with increased tidal volumes.[139]

Inspiration Termination: A Negative Feedback Reflex

Stretch receptors are essential for the volume-related, vagally mediated effect on the bulbopontine mechanism regulating the frequency and depth of breathing. When lung distention reaches a certain threshold, inspiration is terminated. This is the inspiratory off-switch mechanism that switches the respiratory cycle over to expiration. The location of the off-switch mechanism in the brain stem respiratory network is not precisely determined, but its dependence on bulbopontine integrity and vagal input is. The inspiratory terminating effect of the pontine pneumotaxic mechanism has been discussed under "Central Control." The role of vagal input in terminating inspiration is just as important. We owe an understanding of the issue, to great extent, to the studies by Clark and von Euler.[140] Inspiration is terminated when a centrally generated, rising inspiratory activity combined with increasing afferent pulmonary stretch receptor activity reaches a critical threshold. If there were no vagal input, the central activity would be enough to switch inspiration off, but at a higher level, thus requiring a longer time of inspiration. The inspiratory off-switch manifests above a certain threshold, inhibiting further inspiration, but has little effect on the force or duration of ascending inspiratory activity below that threshold.

Inspiratory duration is thus set by one or both of two

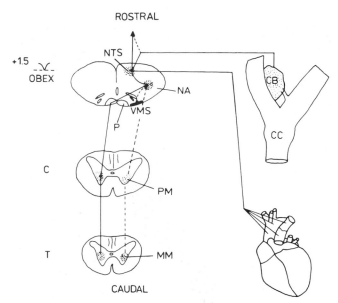

FIGURE 6-3 Somatotopic organization of the arterial chemoreceptors (*Right*) Schematic representation of the carotid and aortic bodies and their sensory innervation (CB, carotid body; CC, common carotid artery). (*Left*) Transverse section at three levels of the CNS showing the brain stem intermediates of the chemoreceptor input and the motor projections. Continuous lines designate proved and dashed lines unproved projections. The upper section is approximately 1.5 mm rostrally from the obex (NTS, nucleus tractus solitarius; NA, nucleus ambiguus; VMS, ventral medullary surface; P, pyramid; PM, phrenic motoneurons, MM, respiratory muscle motoneurons; C and T stand for cervical and thoracic segments, respectively).

different mechanisms: a bulbopontine mechanism and a vagal feedback mechanism linked to changes in lung volume. Concerning the vagal mechanism, the duration of TI shortens with increasing volume along a hyperbolic curve. The duration of TE depends on the duration of the preceding TI, but the timing within each breath is independent of the preceding breaths. These inspiratory characteristics and timing relationship underlie the control of depth and frequency of respiration in both conscious humans and anesthetized cats.[140] Moreover, it appears that afferent vagal input remains pretty fixed over a range of conditions, for example, temperature or respiratory loads,[141] but its effect depends on the precise setting of the bulbopontine mechanism by these conditions.

ARTERIAL CHEMORECEPTORS

Peripheral arterial chemoreceptors are specialized sensory cells that detect changes in the level of the "natural" chemical stimuli P_{O_2}, P_{CO_2}, and [H$^+$] in the arterial blood, the hypoxic stimulus being the most powerful one. Effect on respiration is the main response to arterial chemoreceptor stimulation, although their excitation also elicits cardiovascular and metabolic changes.

The arterial chemoreceptors reside in both carotid and aortic bodies (Fig. 6-3). The carotid bodies are paired organs located bilaterally at the bifurcations of the common carotid arteries. The aortic bodies are multiple organs; usually there are seven to nine of them scattered around the arch of the aorta and along the main trunk of the pulmonary artery. The

carotid body is innervated by the carotid sinus nerve, also called the *nerve of Hering,* which is a branch of the glossopharyngeal nerve carrying additionally sympathetic fibers from the superior cervical ganglion. The aortic body is innervated by the depressor nerve, which is a branch of the vagus nerve. Sensory information from the arterial chemoreceptors enters the nucleus tractus solitarius of the medulla (see Fig. 6-3), where it is relayed to the supramedullary structures and to the bulbospinal neurons of the ventral respiratory group. The latter neurons project to the contralateral, and possibly in part ipsilateral, phrenic and respiratory muscle motoneurons.

The ultrastructure of the carotid body parenchyma is shown in Fig. 6-4. The organ consists of two main types of cells. Type I, or glomus, cells are the chemoreceptor cells, and type II cells are supporting cells. Sinus nerve endings are in synaptic apposition to type I cells, which form clusters surrounded by a dense capillary network. The chemoreceptor cells are derived from the neural crest. A characteristic feature of type I cells is the presence of dense-core cytoplasmic vesicles containing transmitters, notably catecholamines.

Both carotid and aortic chemoreceptors discharge at a low frequency of less than two impulses per second per fiber under normal conditions. Functionally, the aortic bodies are of negligible significance in some species, including humans.[87,142,143] In further discussion, except for when there is a basic difference between the carotid and aortic chemoreceptors, referrals to the peripheral or arterial chemoreceptors will mean the carotid chemoreceptors. In 1930, Heymans and coworkers[144] reported their discovery of the chemoreflex ventilatory function of the carotid body. This discovery was a major breakthrough in the respiratory physiology of the time, for which Heymans received a Nobel prize in 1938. Hyperpnea produced by hypoxia is for all practical purposes mediated solely by the arterial chemoreceptors. The chemoreceptors are also of importance in driving ventilation during exposure to acidosis and exercise, but their role in resting ventilation is, at best, debatable.

CAROTID CHEMORECEPTOR AND VENTILATORY RESPONSES

Recording from a single- or paucifiber preparation of the distal, emerging from the carotid body, end of the cut sinus nerve has been used extensively as a method of studying chemoreceptor properties. The steady-state carotid chemoreceptor and ventilatory responses are compared in the anesthetized cat in Fig. 6-5. Carotid chemoreceptor afferent activity increases roughly hyperbolically with decreasing Pa_{O_2} at a constant Pa_{CO_2}. The ventilatory response follows closely that of chemoreceptors (see Fig. 6-5A). Both responses accelerate when Pa_{O_2} falls below 90 mmHg.

The same chemoreceptors that respond to Pa_{O_2} respond also to increasing Pa_{CO_2} at a constant Pa_{O_2} (see Fig. 6-5B). The CO_2 response is approximately linear over a wide range of Pa_{CO_2}, and so is the corresponding ventilatory response. The stimulatory effect of CO_2 on carotid chemoreceptor activity, and accordingly on ventilation, is also seen at a constant [H$^+$] and is greater at a higher Pa_{CO_2}.[145] This suggests that there is an effect of CO_2 that is independent of the associated change in [H$^+$]. The carotid chemoreceptor and ventilatory responses to increases in pH at constant Pa_{O_2} and Pa_{CO_2} show a linear

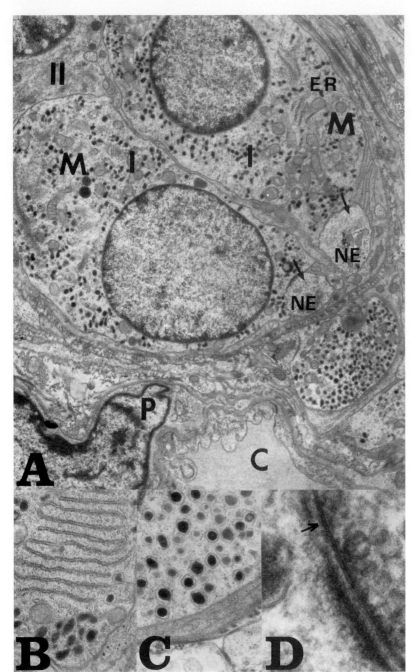

FIGURE 6-4 Electron micrographs of cat carotid body. (*A*) Cross section through the carotid body parenchyma (I, chemoreceptor cells; II, sustentacular cell; M, mitochondria; ER, endoplasmic reticulum; NE, nerve endings in apposition to the chemoreceptor cells; arrows show presynaptic projections; C, capillary vessel; P, pericyte associated with the capillary). Note the dense-core vesicles in the cytoplasm of the chemoreceptor cells (~×12,000). The most characteristic elements are shown magnified at the bottom. (*B*) Endoplasmic reticulum (~×35,000) (*C*) Dense-core vesicles (~×30,000). (*D*) Synaptic cleft; arrow shows the presynaptic projection (~×230,000). (M Walski and M Pokorski, unpublished observations.)

inhibitory pattern (see Fig. 6-5*C*). The ventilatory response to CO_2-H^+ is mediated through both peripheral and central chemoreceptors, the contribution of the peripheral chemoreceptors being smaller.[145]

A combination of stimuli, in particular that of hypoxia and hypercapnia, has a multiplicative effect on the response of both carotid chemoreceptor afferents and ventilation.[145,146] The slope of the chemoreceptor CO_2 response curve increases as Pa_{O_2} decreases, giving the appearance of a "fan" of curves.[146]

The combination of Pa_{O_2} and Pa_{CO_2} values at which the chemoreceptor discharge is nearly silent is defined as the *threshold stimulus*.[146] In the anesthetized cat, most chemoreceptors may be silenced at a Pa_{O_2} of about 30 mmHg by lowering the Pa_{CO_2} to about 10 mmHg.[147] The Pa_{CO_2} threshold

decreases with increasing intensity of hypoxia. Hypoxia alone is not enough to sustain the chemoreceptor discharge. The ventilatory stimulus threshold follows a similar pattern of Pa_{O_2}-Pa_{CO_2} interaction[147] but is higher, which means that a lower Pa_{O_2} and a higher Pa_{CO_2} are required to start respiration once apnea is produced than to start the discharge of chemoreceptors once they are silenced. In the carotid body–denervated animal, the Pa_{CO_2} threshold increases in hypoxia, which indicates that there is a depressant effect of hypoxia on the central chemoreceptors. The Pa_{O_2}-Pa_{CO_2} threshold may have practical implications in the rehabilitation of patients with severe hypoxia, for example, due to chronic obstructive pulmonary disease. When severe hypoxia is combined with a decrease in Pa_{CO_2} due to hyperventilation, this may give rise to a hypocapnic apnea. The lower the Pa_{CO_2} level, the

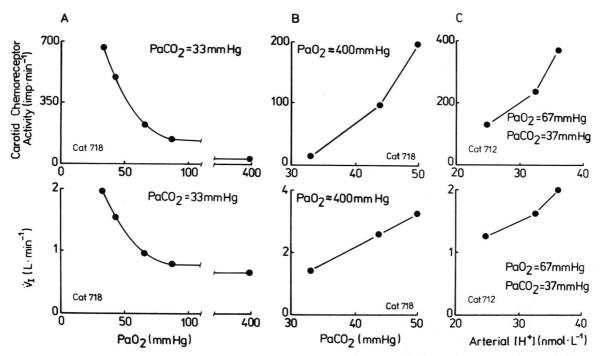

FIGURE 6-5 Carotid chemoreceptor and ventilatory responses to hypoxia (*A*), hypercapnia (*B*), and hydrogen ion (*C*) in the anesthetized cat. See details in the text. (*A* and *B* from M Pokorski and S Lahiri, unpublished observations; *C* adapted, with permission, from Pokorski and Lahiri.[145])

longer is the duration of apnea. The hypoxic rise in the central chemoreceptor Pa_{CO_2} threshold further impairs the resumption of breathing.

The contribution of the carotid chemoreceptors to respiratory control is highlighted by studies on humans who underwent bilateral removal of carotid bodies as a treatment for severe asthma. Honda[143] studied the ventilatory responses in a group of such patients about 20 years after their carotid bodies had been removed surgically. The ventilatory response to sustained or single-breath hypoxia was essentially gone, except for a residual component that might have been dependent on the action, possibly greater than normal, of the aortic bodies. The hypercapnic response was preserved but attenuated. On the basis of the magnitude of the responses, it was concluded that in humans, 90 percent of the hypoxic and 30 percent of the hypercapnic responses originate in the carotid chemoreceptors, the remaining part being provided by the aortic chemoreceptors and by the CO_2-H^+-sensitive central chemoreceptors in the case of hypercapnia.

The relative contribution to ventilation of peripheral chemoreceptors, as assessed from the linear relationship between carotid chemosensory activity and ventilation at graded levels of Pa_{O_2} in the cat,[145] is small in normocapnic hyperoxia, amounting to 10 percent. This contribution increases severalfold with the increased hypoxic or hypercapnic stimulus but fails short of the above-mentioned percentage figures for humans.

Hypoxia, which stimulates ventilation solely through peripheral chemoreceptor activity, has less of an effect on ventilation for the same increase in the chemosensory activity than hypercapnia.[145] Hypercapnia is thus a more powerful ventilatory stimulant, and its effect is dominated by the central chemoreceptors.[148]

A comparison of the normal pattern of breathing with those obtained at the peak of progressive hypoxic and hypercapnic responses in healthy humans is shown in Fig. 6-6. Hypercapnia causes a stronger increase in *central inspiratory activity,* which is manifest by an increase in the rate of rise of inspiration. The high flow with which subjects inspire leads to much higher tidal volumes with only a little short-

FIGURE 6-6 Spirograms constructed from mean values of tidal volume and inspiratory and expiratory times for 17 healthy subjects during normoxic (NVR; Sa_{O_2} = 98%, $P_{ET_{CO_2}}$ = 37 mmHg), hypoxic (HVR; Sa_{O_2} = 80%, $P_{ET_{CO_2}}$ = 37 mmHg), and hypercapnic (HCVR; Sa_{O_2} = 100%, $P_{ET_{CO_2}}$ = 55 mmHg) ventilatory responses. Hypercapnia causes a stronger increase in the slope of the ascending part of the spirogram corresponding to inspiratory drive and flow. (Used with permission, from Pokorski et al.[148])

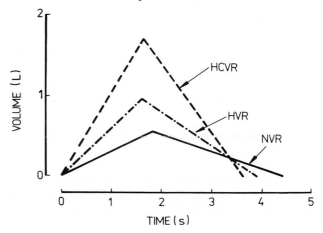

ened T_I. In conscious subjects, the T_I shortening is no match for the greater decrease in T_E in the face of both O_2 and CO_2 stimuli.[148] Here, too, hypercapnia has a stronger effect, which leads to a higher ventilatory rate and an overall stimulation of minute ventilation.

CAROTID VERSUS AORTIC CHEMORECEPTORS

It is commonly presumed that the physiology of aortic and carotid chemoreceptors is the same. There are, however, differences between the two pools of chemoreceptors. Quantitative differences concern the responses to natural stimuli. The excitatory response of aortic chemoreceptors to hypercapnia and many other stimuli is only a fraction of that of carotid chemoreceptors.[87,142] The sluggish response of the aortic chemoreceptors may be a reason, at least in part, for their small ventilatory effects.

Aortic chemoreceptor discharge is sensitive to small changes in systemic arterial blood pressure, even within the physiologic range, which may then cause a significant excitatory response.[149] This is in opposition to the carotid chemoreceptor discharge, which is pretty resistant to blood pressure changes and does not increase until the blood pressure falls to below 60 mmHg. The latency of the aortic chemoreceptor responses to inhaled chemical stimuli is much longer than that of the carotid ones.[143] This difference may have to do with an abundant blood flow in the carotid body as opposed to the rather restricted perfusion of the aortic body. The difference in perfusion kinetics also may underlie the excitatory response of the aortic chemoreceptor discharge to a decrease in the O_2 content,[143] which is not displayed by the carotid body.

TRANSDUCTION OF THE STIMULUS

Various hypotheses have been put forward to explain how chemoreceptor cells transduce the arriving hypoxic stimulus into a nerve discharge. The older theories linked chemoreception to energy metabolism, based on the observation that inhibitors of mitochondrial electron transfer and uncouplers of oxidative phosphorylation all lead to chemoreceptor stimulation. A decrease in cellular energy metabolism and hence in the capability to carry out the ATP-dependent processes was thought to be at the core of chemoreceptor events. However, hypoxia and other stimuli at the strength that fully excites the chemoreceptor activity do not necessarily lead to decreased ATP content.[150]

Another theory is based on the premise that low P_{O_2} causes type I cells to release a chemical that activates the sensory fibers. A potpourri of substances is enumerated in Table 6–1 that have been suggested as mediators of carotid body stimulation.

Electrophysiologic and pharmacologic studies have shown that neuroactive substances and their analogs are capable of altering the chemosensory discharge and its responses to stimuli. Further studies, therefore, have concentrated on the synthesis, release, turnover, and site of action of putative neurotransmitters in the carotid body, yielding supportive evidence on the involvement of these substance in the chemoreception process.

Acetylcholine has been proposed as the main neurotransmitter in the carotid body. The evidence supporting this proposal consists chiefly of the presence of acetylcholine in the chemoreceptor cell, its release on stimulation, and the

TABLE 6-1 Putative Neuroactive Substances in the Carotid Body

I. Neuropeptides
   Tachykinins, notably substance P
   Opiate peptides, notably enkephalins
   Neuropeptide Y
   Cholecystokinin
   Neurotensin
   Bombesin
   Galanin
   Vasoactive intestinal peptide
   Calcitonin gene–related peptide
   Atrial natriuretic peptide
II. Biogenic amines
   Dopamine
   Norepinephrine
   5-Hydroxytryptamine
III. Gaseous neurotransmitters
   Nitric oxide
   Carbon monoxide
IV. Other neurotransmitters and neuromodulators
   Acetylcholine
   Adenosine
   GABA
   Prostacyclines

stimulatory effects on chemoreceptor afferents of cholinergic agonists.[151] Recently, both nicotinic and muscarinic receptors have been identified in the chemoreceptor cell, the former mediating an excitatory and the latter an inhibitory action on chemoreceptors.[152] However, the cholinergic blockers, even when they inhibit chemoreceptor responses to acetylcholine, do not block the chemoreceptor or ventilatory responses to hypoxia or other stimuli.[152]

Enkephalin-like peptides are involved in chemoreceptor responses. A close upstream injection of met-enkephalin in the common carotid artery inhibits carotid body activity in the cat, and this effect is blocked by the specific opiate antagonist naloxone.[153] Naloxone alone stimulates the responses of both carotid chemoreceptors and ventilation to hypoxia.[153] Opioid peptides coexist with catecholamines in the secretory vesicles in the chemoreceptor cell.[154] Opioid content decreases along with dopamine during acute hypoxic exposure in the rabbit, which suggests that the two are coreleased and that a specific ratio of these neuromodulators may be required for an optimal chemoreceptor response to hypoxia.[152]

The rate of dopamine production in the carotid body is one of the most studied and yet most perplexing and contentious issues in contemporary carotid body research. Dopamine fulfills all the criteria of an ideal neurotransmitter in the carotid body, but its function remains controversial. Tyrosine hydroxylase, a rate-limiting enzyme in dopamine synthesis, is present, and dopamine is abundant in the chemoreceptor cell. D_2 receptors are present on both presynaptic and postsynaptic sites and are fully activated. Hypoxia and other stimuli elicit an exocytotic Ca^{2+}-dependent release of dopamine that is in proportion not only to the intensity of the stimulus but also to the chemoreceptor firing rate.[152]

However, dopamine does not regularly excite chemoreceptors. The effects of dopamine on both the chemoreceptor discharge and ventilation are variable, depending on the species, the dose, the experimental conditions, and the experimenter. Overall, the most frequently reported effect of systemically administered dopamine is inhibition of carotid body activity. Dopamine may be excitatory in some species, such as the rabbit,[155] or at high doses regardless of the species used.[152] A recent concept that attempts to reconcile the dopamine discrepancy has it that a low exogenous dose of dopamine would act preferentially on the high-affinity presynaptic D_2 receptors to inhibit dopamine release and thus the chemoreceptor discharge. At higher doses, the presynaptic inhibition would be overcome by an excitatory effect exerted at the postsynaptic site of lower affinity. This site would then be the place where the endogenously released dopamine would act to stimulate the chemoreceptor discharge.[152]

Chemoreceptor cells are excitable and have K^+, Ca^{2+}, and Na^+ voltage-gated channels. The existence of such channels has been well established in recent years using the patch-clamp technique on isolated chemoreceptor cells from different animal species.[152] Studies of the channel physiology have led to new concepts of O_2 transduction. According to this scheme, the initial event in the chemotransduction is inhibition of the outward K^+ currents of type I cells by hypoxia, leading to chemoreceptor cell depolarization. The depolarization, in turn, would activate the voltage-gated L-type Ca^{2+} channels and initiate a massive influx of extracellular Ca^{2+} into the cell. The increasing cytosolic Ca^{2+} would release dopamine and/or other neurotransmitters from the chemoreceptor cell.[152] It is of interest that the release of dopamine depends on external Ca^{2+} and is inhibited by Ca^{2+} channel blockers.[156] K^+ channel sensitivity to hypoxia may not be the whole story.

A maximum inhibition of the O_2-dependent K^+ current was found at a Pa_{O_2} of about 85 mmHg,[156] which, at best, corresponds to mild hypoxia and in no way correlates with the level of hypoxia needed to cause maximum carotid sinus nerve discharge increase or dopamine release. The increase in cytosolic Ca^{2+} may originate, at least in part, from internal Ca^{2+} stores.[157] A recent study has shown that inhibition of K^+ channels of type I cells does not inhibit the excitatory response of the carotid sinus nerve discharge to hypoxia.[158] Finally, transduction of the acidic stimulus does not seem to involve cell depolarization and Ca^{2+} influx through voltage-gated Ca^{2+} channels but rather a Ca^{2+} exchange by way of antiporters.[156] Another idea is that O_2-sensor may be a hemoglobin-like molecule.[159] Cytochrome a_3 is a prime candidate, since CO-induced changes of carotid chemosensory activity are reversed by illumination of the carotid body with the light wavelength typical of the CO compound of this cytochrome.[160] Another possibility is a heme-linked NADPH oxidase[161] that decreases the production of H_2O_2 in response to hypoxia and, by changing the redox state of glutathione, alters membrane ionic conductances.

The role of second messengers as initiators of cellular responses in the carotid body remains largely unexplored. The few available data implicate both adenosine-3′,5′-cyclic monophosphate and lipid-derived second messengers. Cyclic AMP is present in the cat and rabbit carotid body. Hypoxia increases its content, the effect being abolished by inhibition of the adenylyl cyclase.[162] Other carotid chemoreceptor stimuli, however, have inconsistent effects on the cyclic AMP content.[163] The modulatory effect on chemoreceptor activity of cyclic AMP also may be due to its ability to inhibit O_2-sensitive K^+ currents and to increase the exocytotic release of catecholamines from the chemoreceptor cell.[152]

Phosphoinositides also appear to shape carotid body responses. Phosphoinositide breakdown is increased by hypoxia in the carotid body.[164]

Endogenous CO also may function as a chemical messenger in the carotid body. A CO-generating enzyme, hemoxygenase, has been found in type I cells. CO has an inhibitory effect on chemosensory discharge due to modulation of voltage-gated Ca^{2+} channels.[165]

References

1. Smith JC, Ellenberger HH, Ballanyi K, et al: Pre-Bötzinger complex: A brainstem region that may generate respiratory rhythm in mammals. *Science* 254:726, 1991.
2. Onimaru H, Arata A, Homma I: Primary respiratory rhythm generator in the medulla of brainstem-spinal cord preparation from the newborn rat. *Brain Res* 445:314, 1988.
3. Onimaru H, Arata A, Homma I: Firing properties of respiratory rhythm generating neurons in the absence of synaptic transmission in rat medulla in vitro. *Exp Brain Res* 76:530, 1989.
4. Aoki M, Mizuguchi A: Spinal generation of respiratory rhythm: A study in an in vitro brainstem-spinal cord preparation of newborn rat. *Adv Biosci* 79:51, 1991.
5. Salmoiraghi GC, von Baumgarten R: Intracellular potentials from respiratory neurons in brainstem of cat and mechanism of rhythmic respiration. *J Neurophysiol* 24:203, 1961.
6. Long S, Duffin J: The neuronal determinants of respiratory rhythm. *Prog Neurobiol* 27:100, 1986.
7. Bianchi AL, Denavit-Saubie M, Champagnat J: Central control of breathing in mammals: Neuronal circuitry, membrane properties, and neurotransmitters. *Physiol Rev* 75:1, 1995.
8. Aoki M, Fujito Y, Kurosawa Y, et al: Descending inputs to the upper cervical inspiratory neurons from the medullary respiratory neurons and the raphe nuclei in the cat, in Sieck C, Gandevia SC, Cameron WE (eds): *Respiratory Muscles and Their Neuromotor Control*. New York, Alan R Liss, 1987, pp 73–82.
9. Aoki M, Kasaba T, Kurosawa Y, et al: The projection of cervical respiratory neurons to the phrenic nucleus in the cat. *Neurosci Lett Suppl* 17:S49, 1984.
10. Gromysz H, Karczewski WA: Phrenic motoneurone activity in split-brainstem cats and monkeys. *Respir Physiol* 50:51, 1982.
11. Gromysz H, Karczewski WA: The split-respiratory centre in the cat: Responses to hypercapnia. *Respir Physiol* 57:225, 1984.
12. Bianchi AL: Localisation et étude des neurones respiratoires bulbaires. *J Physiol (Paris)* 36:5, 1971.
13. Merrill EG: Finding a respiratory function for the medullary respiratory neurons, in Bellairs R, Gray EG (eds): *Essays on the Nervous System*. New York, Oxford University Press, 1974, pp 451–486.
14. von Euler C, Marttila I, Remmers JF, et al: Effects of lesions in the parabrachial nucleus on the mechanisms for central and reflex termination of inspiration in cat. *Acta Physiol Scand* 96:324, 1976.
15. St John WM, Glasser RL, King RA: Apneustic breathing after vagotomy in cats with chronic pneumotaxic center lesions. *Respir Physiol* 12:239, 1971.
16. Berger AJ, Herbert DA, Mitchell RA: Properties of apneusis produced by reversible cold block of the rostral pons. *Respir Physiol* 33:323, 1978.
17. Glasser RL, Tippett JW: Dissociation of facilitatory mechanisms in the midpontile decerebrate cat. *Nature* 205:810, 1965.
18. St John WM: Pneumotaxic mechanisms influence phrenic, hypoglossal, and trigeminal activities. *Exp Neurol* 97:301, 1987.
19. Lumsden T: Observations on the respiratory centres in the cat. *J Physiol (Lond)* 57:153, 1923.
20. St John WM: Differential alteration by hypercapnia and hypoxia

of the apneustic respiratory pattern in decerebrate cats. *J Physiol (Lond)* 287:467, 1979.

21. Bertrand F, Hugelin A: Respiratory synchronizing function of nucleus parabrachialis medialis: Pneumotaxic mechanisms. *J Neurophysiol* 34:189, 1971.

22. Feldman JL, Gautier H: Interaction of pulmonary afferents and pneumotaxic center in control of respiratory pattern in cats. *J Neurophysiol* 39:31, 1976.

23. Johnson FH, Russel GH: The locus ceruleus as a pneumotaxic center. *Anat Rec* 112:348, 1952.

24. Tang PC: Localization of the pneumotaxic center in the cat. *Am J Physiol* 172:645, 1953.

25. Gang S, Mizuguchi A, Aoki M: Axonal projections from the pontine pneumotaxic region to the nucleus raphe magnus in cats. *Respir Physiol* 85:329, 1991.

26. Pokorski M, Gromysz H: Trigeminal motor nucleus and pontile respiratory regulation. *Adv Exp Med Biol* 393:59, 1995.

27. Bianchi AL, St John WM: Pontile axonal projections of medullary respiratory neurons. *Respir Physiol* 45:142, 1981.

28. Fung M-L, St John WM: Electrical stimulation of pneumotaxic center: Activation of fibers and neurons. *Respir Physiol* 96:71, 1994.

29. Fung M-L, St John WM: Separation of multiple functions in ventilatory control of pneumotaxic mechanism. *Respir Physiol* 96:83, 1994.

30. Bassal M, Bianchi AI: Effects de la stimulation des structures nerveuses centrales sur les activities respiratoires efferentes chez le chat: I. Reponses a la stimulation corticale. *J Physiol (Paris)* 77:741, 1981.

31. Bassal M, Bianchi AI: Effets de la stimulation des structures nerveuses centrales sur les activites respiratoires efferentes chez le chat: I. Reponses a la stimulation sous-corticale. *J Physiol (Paris)* 77:759, 1981.

32. Hugelin A: Regional effects of nembutal anesthesia on brainstem respiratory neurons, in Fitzgerald RS, Gautier H, Lahiri S (eds): *The Regulation of Respiration during Sleep and Anesthesia.* New York, Plenum Press, 1978, pp 5–15.

33. Krieger AJ, Christensen HD, Sapru HN, et al: Changes in ventilatory patterns after ablation of various respiratory feedback mechanisms. *J Appl Physiol* 33:431, 1972.

34. Glasser RL, Tippett JW, Davidian VA: Cerebellar activity, apneustic breathing, and the neural control of respiration. *Nature* 209:810, 1966.

35. St John WM: Integration of peripheral and central chemoreceptor stimuli by pontine and medullary respiratory centers. *Fed Proc* 36:2421, 1977.

36. Planche D, Bianche AL: Modification de l'activite des neurons respiratoires bulbaires provoquee par stimulation corticale. *J Physiol (Paris)* 64:69, 1972.

37. Orem J, Trotter RH: Behavioral control of breathing. *News Physiol Sci* 9:228, 1994.

38. Gandevia SC, Rothwell JC: Activation of the human diaphragm from the motor cortex. *J Physiol (Lond)* 384:109, 1987.

39. Murphy K, Mier A, Adams L, et al: Putative cerebral cortical involvement in the ventilatory response to inhaled CO_2 in conscious man. *J Physiol (Lond)* 420:1, 1990.

40. Lipski J, Bektas A, Porter R: Short latency inputs to phrenic motoneurons from the sensorimotor cortex in the cat. *Exp Brain Res* 61:280, 1986.

41. Kremer WF: Autonomic and somatic reactions induced by stimulation of the cingular gyrus in dogs. *J Neurophysiol* 10:371, 1974.

42. Kaada BR: A study of responses from the limbic, subcallosal, orbito-insular, piriform and temporal cortex, hippocampus-fornix and amygdala. *Acta Physiol Scand* 24(suppl 83):1, 1951.

43. Rickard-Bell GC, Bystrzycka EK, Nail BS: Cells of origin of corticospinal projections to phrenic and thoracic respiratory motoneurones in the cat as shown by retrograde transport of HRP. *Brain Res Bull* 14:39, 1985.

44. Warner JJ, Coffey JP, Thompson FJ, et al: Afferent-efferent organization and cytoarchitecture of phrenic sensorimotor cortex in the cat. *Neurosci Abstr* 14:462, 1988.

45. St John WM, Glasser RL, King RA: Rhythmic respiration in awake vagotomized cats with chronic pneumotaxic area lesions. *Respir Physiol* 15:233, 1972.

46. Fink BR: Influence of cerebral activity in wakefulness on regulation of breathing. *J Appl Physiol* 16:15, 1961.

47. Bulow K: Respirations and wakefulness in man. *Acta Physiol Scand* 59:1, 1963.

48. Honda Y, Natsui T: Effects of sleep on ventilatory response to CO_2 in severe hypoxia. *Respir Physiol* 3:220, 1967.

49. Robin ED, Whaley RD, Crump CH, et al: Alveolar gas tensions, pulmonary ventilation and blood pH during physiologic sleep in normal subjects. *J Clin Invest* 37:981, 1958.

49a. Pokorski M, Jernajczyk U: Disproportional changes of the hypoglossal and phrenic nerve activities induced by large respiration in the rabbit. *Eur J Respir Dis* 10(suppl 25): 355, 1997.

50. Cohen MI, Hugelin A: Suprapontine reticular control of intrinsic respiratory mechanisms. *Arch Ital Biol* 103:317, 1965.

51. Evans MH, Pepler PA: Respiratory effects mapped by focal stimulation in the rostral brain stem of the anaesthetized rabbit. *Brain Res* 75:41, 1974.

52. Pleschka K, Wang SC: The activity of respiratory neurons before and during panting in the cat. *Pflugers Arch* 353:303, 1975.

53. Budzinska K: Effects of hyperthermia and stimulation of the hypothalamus on the activity of the phrenic nerve in hypo-, normo- and hypercapnic rabbits. *Acta Neurobiol Exp* 35:227, 1975.

54. Tenney SM, Ou LC: Ventilatory response of decorticate and decerebrate cats to hypoxia and CO_2. *Respir Physiol* 29:81, 1977.

55. Tenney SM, Ou LC: Hypoxic ventilatory response of cats at high altitude: An interpretation of "blunting". *Respir Physiol* 30:185, 1977.

56. Eldridge FL, Millhorn DE: Hypothalamic central command and exercise hyperpnea, in von Euler C, Lagercrantz H (eds): *Neurobiology of the Control of Breathing.* New York, Raven Press, 1986, pp 35–43.

57. Shannon R: Respiratory pattern changes during costovertebral joint movement. *J Appl Physiol Respir Environ Exer Physiol* 48:862, 1980.

58. Mueller RA, Lundberg DBA, Breese GR, et al: The neuropharmacology of respiratory control. *Pharmacol Rev* 34:255, 1982.

59. Greer JJ, Smith JC, Feldman JL: Role of excitatory amino acids in the generation and transmission of respiratory drive in neonatal rat. *J Physiol (Lond)* 437:727, 1991.

60. Abrahams TP, Hornby PJ, Walton DP, et al: An excitatory amino acid(s) in the ventrolateral medulla is (are) required for breathing to occur in the anesthetized cat. *J Pharmacol Exp Ther* 259:1388, 1991.

61. Connelly CA, Feldman JL: Synergistic roles for NMDA and non-NMDA receptors in brainstem respiratory control in adult rats. *Soc Neurosci Abstr* 18:488, 1992.

62. Dogas Z, Stuth EAE, Hopp A, et al: NMDA receptor-mediated transmission of carotid body chemoreceptor input to expiratory bulbospinal neurones in dogs. *J Physiol (Lond)* 487:639, 1995.

63. Karius DR, Ling L, Speck DF: Blockade of N-methyl-D-aspartate (NMDA) receptors has no effect on certain inspiratory reflexes. *Am J Physiol* 261:L443, 1991.

64. Pierrefiche O, Foutz AS, Champagnat J, et al: The bulbar network of respiratory neurons during apneusis induced by a blockade of NMDA receptors. *Exp Brain Res* 89:623, 1992.

65. Mugnaini E, Oertel WH: An atlas of the distribution of GABA-ergic neurons and terminals in the rat CNS as revealed by GAD immunohistochemistry, in Bjorklund A, Hokfelt T (eds): *Handbook of Chemical Neuroanatomy,* vol 4, part 1. Amsterdam, Elsevier, 1985, pp 436–608.

66. Aoki M, Nakazono Y: Raphe magnus-induced inhibition of medullary and spinal respiratory activities in the cat, in Honda Y, et al (eds): *Control of Breathing and Its Modeling Perspective.* New York, Plenum Press, 1992, pp 15–23.

67. Nagai T, Maeda T, Imai H, et al: Distribution of GABA-T-intensive neurons in the rat hindbrain. *J Comp Neurol* 231:260, 1985.

68. Lipski J, Waldvogel HJ, Pilowski P, et al: GABA-immunoreactive boutons make synapses with inspiratory neurons of the dorsal respiratory group. *Brain Res* 529:309, 1990.

69. Haji A, Takeda R, Remmers JE: GABA-mediated inhibitory mechanisms in control of respiratory rhythm, in Takishima T, Cherniack NS (eds): *Control of Breathing and Dyspnea*. New York, Pergamon Press, 1991, pp 61–63.

70. Zhan WZ, Ellenberger HH, Feldman JL: Monoaminergic and GABAergic terminations in phrenic motor nucleus of rat identified by immunocytochemical labeling. *Neuroscience* 31:105, 1989.

71. Hayashi F, Lipski J: The role of inhibitory amino acids in the control of respiratory motor output in an arterially perfused rat. *Respir Physiol* 89:47, 1992.

72. Melton JE, Neubauer JA, Edelman NH: GABA antagonism reverses hypoxic respiratory depression in the cat. *J Appl Physiol* 69:1296, 1990.

73. Hedner J, Hedner T, Wessberg P, et al: An analysis of the mechanisms by which γ-aminobutyric acid depresses ventilation in the cat. *J Appl Physiol Respir Environ Exerc Physiol* 56:849, 1984.

74. Pierrefiche O, Foutz AS, Denavit-Saubie M: Effects of $GABA_B$ receptor agonists and antagonists on the bulbar respiratory network in cat. *Brain Res* 605:77, 1993.

75. Neubauer JA, Posner MA, Santiago TV, et al: Naloxone reduces ventilatory depression of brain hypoxia. *J Appl Physiol* 63:699, 1987.

76. McNamara MC, Gingras-Leatherman JL, Lawson EE: Effect of hypoxia on brainstem concentration of biogenic amines in postnatal rabbits. *Dev Brain Res* 25:253, 1986.

77. Neubauer JA, Santiago TV, Posner MA, et al: Ventral medullary pH and ventilatory responses to hyperperfusion and hypoxia. *J Appl Physiol Respir Environ Exerc Physiol* 58:1659, 1985.

78. Mitchell RA, Loeschcke HH, Severinghaus JW, et al: Regions of respiratory chemosensitivity on the surface of the medulla. *Ann NY Acad Sci* 109:661, 1963.

79. Schlaefke ME: Central chemosensitivity: A respiratory drive. *Rev Physiol Biochem Pharmacol* 90:171, 1981.

80. Loeschcke HH: Central chemosensitivity and the reaction theory. *J Physiol (Lond)* 332:1, 1982.

81. Pokorski M: Neurophysiological studies on central chemosensor in medullary ventrolateral areas. *Am J Physiol* 230:1288, 1976.

82. Gelfand R, Lambertsen CJ, Kemp RA: Dynamic respiratory response to abrupt change of inspired CO_2 at normal and high P_{O_2}. *J Appl Physiol* 35:903, 1973.

83. Bledsoe SW, Hornbein TF: Central chemoreceptors and the regulation of their chemical environment, in Hornbein TF (ed): *Regulation of Breathing*, part I. New York, Marcel Dekker, 1981, pp 347–428.

84. Held D, Fencl V, Pappenheimer JR: Electrical potential of cerebrospinal fluid. *J Neurophysiol* 27:942, 1964.

85. Nielsen M: Studies on the regulation of breathing in man with special reference to the nature of the chemical stimulus. *Scand Arch Physiol Suppl* 10:83, 1936.

86. Pokorski M, Lahiri S: Inhibition of aortic chemoreceptor responses by metabolic alkalosis in the cat. *J Appl Physiol Respir Environ Exerc Physiol* 53:75, 1982.

87. Pokorski M, Lahiri S: Aortic and carotid chemoreceptor responses to metabolic acidosis in the cat. *Am J Physiol Reg Integr Comp Physiol* 244:R652, 1983.

88. Smith JC, Morrison DE, Ellenberger HH, et al: Brainstem projections to the major respiratory neuron populations in the medulla of the cat. *J Comp Neurol* 281:69, 1989.

89. Budzinska K, von Euler C, Kao FF, et al: Effects of graded focal cold block in rostral areas of the medulla. *Acta Physiol Scand* 124:329, 1985.

90. Agarwal SK, Calaresu FR: Monosynaptic connection from caudal to rostral ventrolateral medulla in the baroreceptor reflex pathway. *Brain Res* 555:70, 1991.

91. Pokorski M, Grieb P, Wideman J: Opiate system influences central respiratory chemosensors. *Brain Res* 211:221, 1981.

92. McAllen RM: Location of neurons with cardiovascular and respiratory function at the ventral surface of the cat's medulla. *Neuroscience* 18:43, 1986.

93. Miller AD, Ezure K, Suzuki I: Control of abdominal muscles by brain stem respiratory neurons in the cat. *J Neurophysiol* 54:155, 1985.

94. Lipski J, Duffin J: An electrophysiological investigation of propriospinal inspiratory neurons in the upper cervical cord of the cat. *Exp Brain Res* 61:625, 1986.

95. Pitts RF: The respiratory center and its descending pathways. *J Comp Neurol* 72:605, 1940.

96. Mehler WE, Feferman ME, Nauta WJH: Ascending axon degeneration following anterolateral cordotomy. *Brain* 83:718, 1960.

97. Rossi GT, Brodal A: Terminal distribution of spinoreticular fibers in the cat. *Arch Neurol Psychiatry* 78:439, 1957.

98. Hukuhara T, Nakayma S, Okada H: Action potentials in the normal respiratory centers and its centrifugal pathways in the medulla oblongata and spinal cord. *Japn J Physiol* 4:145, 1954.

99. Nathan PW: The descending respiratory pathways in man. *J Neurol Neurosurg Psychiatry* 26:487, 1963.

100. Aminoff MJ, Sears TA: Spinal integration of segmental, cortical and breathing inputs to thoracic respiratory motoneurons. *J Physiol (Lond)* 215:557, 1971.

101. Belmusto L, Brown E, Owens G: Clinical observation on respiratory and vasomotor disturbance as related to cervical cordotomies. *J Neurosurg* 20:225, 1963.

102. Rosomoff HL, Krieger AJ, Kuperman AS: Effects of percutaneous cervical cordotomy on pulmonary function. *J Neurosurg* 31:620, 1969.

103. Newsom Davis J, Plum F: Separation of descending spinal pathways to respiratory motoneurons. *Exp Neurol* 34:78, 1972.

104. Hinsey JC, Hare K, Phillips RA: Sensory components of the phrenic nerve of the cat. *Proc Soc Exp Biol Med* 41:411, 1939.

105. Longford LA, Schmidt RF: An electron microscopic analysis of the left phrenic nerve in the rat. *Anat Rec* 205:207, 1983.

106. Larnicol N, Rose D, Duron B: Identification of phrenic afferents to the external cuneate nucleus: A fluorescent double-labeling study in the cat. *Neurosci Lett* 62:163, 1985.

107. Gill PK, Kuno M: Excitatory and inhibitory actions on phrenic motoneurones. *J Physiol (Lond)* 168:274, 1963.

108. Remmers JE: Inhibition of inspiratory activity by intercostal muscle afferents. *Respir Physiol* 10:358, 1970.

109. Sears TA: Some properties and reflex connexions of respiratory motoneurones of the cat's thoracic spinal cord. *J Physiol (Lond)* 175:386, 1964.

110. Decima EE, von Euler C, Thoden U: Intercostal-to-phrenic reflexes in the spinal cat. *Acta Physiol Scand* 75:568, 1969.

111. Garcia Ramos J, Lopez Mendoza E: On the integration of respiratory movements: II. The integration at spinal level. *Acta Physiol Latinamer* 9:257, 1959.

112. Downman CBB: Skeletal muscle reflexes of splanchnic and intercostal nerve origin in acute spinal and decerebrate cats. *J Neurophysiol* 18:217, 1955.

113. Andersen P, Sears TA: Medullary activation of intercostal fusimotor and alpha motoneurons. *J Physiol (Lond)* 209:739, 1970.

114. Remmers JE, Tsiaras WG: Effect of lateral cervical cord lesions on the respiratory rhythm of anaesthetized decerebrate cats after vagotomy. *J Physiol (Lond)* 233:63, 1973.

115. Shannon R, Lindsey BG: Intercostal and abdominal muscle afferent influence on pneumotaxic center respiratory neurons. *Respir Physiol* 52:85, 1983.

116. Remmers JE, Martilla I: Action of intercostal muscle afferents on the respiratory rhythm of anesthetized cats. *Respir Physiol* 24:31, 1975.

117. Shannon R, Freeman DL: Nucleus retroambigualis respiratory neurons: Responses to intercostal and abdominal muscle afferents. *Respir Physiol* 45:357, 1981.

118. Bolser DC, Lindsey BG, Shannon R: Medullary inspiratory activity: Influence of intercostal tendon organs and muscle spindle endings. *J Appl Physiol* 62:1046, 1987.

119. Kostreva DR, Hopp FA, Zuperku EJ, et al: Respiratory inhibition with sympathetic afferent stimulation in the canine and primate. *J Appl Physiol Respir Environ Exerc Physiol* 44:718, 1978.

120. Shannon R, Bolser DC, Lindsey BG: Medullary expiratory activity: Influence of intercostal tendon organs and muscle spindle endings. *J Appl Physiol* 62:1057, 1987.

121. Schwartzstein RM, Simon PM, Weiss JW et al: Breathlessness induced by dissociation between ventilation and chemical drive. *Am Rev Respir Dis* 139:1231, 1989.

122. Opie LH, Smith AC, Spalding JMK: Conscious appreciation of the effects produced by independent changes of ventilation volume and of end-tidal P_{CO_2} in paralyzed patients. *J Physiol (Lond)* 149:494, 1959.

123. Chen Z, Eldridge FL, Wagner PG: Respiratory-associated thalamic activity is related to level of respiratory drive. *Respir Physiol* 90:99, 1992.

124. Eldridge FL, Chen Z: Respiratory-associated rhythmic firing of midbrain neurons is modulated by vagal input. *Respir Physiol* 90:31, 1992.

125. Sant'Ambrogio G, Wilson MF, Frazier DT: Somatic afferent activity in reflex regulation of diaphragmatic function in the cat. *J Appl Physiol* 17:829, 1962.

126. Speck DF, Revelette WR: Excitation of dorsal and ventral respiratory group neurons by phrenic nerve afferents. *J Appl Physiol* 62:946, 1987.

127. Road JD, West NH, Van Vliet BN: Ventilatory effects of stimulation of phrenic afferents. *J Appl Physiol* 63:1063, 1987.

128. Mortola JP, Sant'Ambrogio G: Mechanics of the trachea and behavior of its slowly adapting stretch receptors. *J Physiol (Lond)* 286:577, 1979.

129. Bartlett D Jr, Sant'Ambrogio G, Wise JCM: Transduction properties of tracheal stretch receptors. *J Physiol (Lond)* 258:421, 1976.

130. Guz F, Trenchard DW: Pulmonary stretch receptor activity in man: A comparison with dog and cat. *J Physiol (Lond)* 213:329, 1971.

131. Coleridge HM, Coleridge JCG, Banzett RB: Effect of CO_2 on afferent vagal endings in the canine lung. *Respir Physiol* 24:135, 1978.

132. Bartoli A, Cross BA, Guz A, et al: The effect of carbon dioxide in the airways and alveoli on ventilation: A vagal reflex studied in the dog. *J Physiol (Lond)* 240:91, 1974.

133. Paintal AS: Vagal sensory receptors and their reflex effects. *Physiol Rev* 53:159, 1973.

134. Trenchard D, Guz A: Role of pulmonary vagal afferent nerve fibers in the development of rapid shallow breathing in lung inflammation. *Clin Sci* 42:251, 1972.

135. Sellick H, Widdicombe JG: Vagal deflation and inflation reflexes mediated by lung irritant receptors. *Q J Exp Physiol* 55:153, 1970.

136. Koller EA: Afferent vagal impulses in anaphylactic bronchial asthma. *Acta Neurobiol Exp* 33:51, 1973.

137. DiMarco AF, von Euler C, Romaniuk JR, et al: Positive feedback facilitation of external intercostal and phrenic inspiratory activity by pulmonary stretch receptors. *Acta Physiol Scand* 113:375, 1981.

138. Cross BA, Jones PW, Guz A: The role of vagal afferent information during inspiration in determining phrenic motoneurone output. *Respir Physiol* 39:149, 1980.

139. Sharp J, Goldberg T, Druz NB, et al: Relative contributions of rib cage and abdomen to breathing in normal subjects. *J Appl Physiol* 39:608, 1975.

140. Clark FJ, von Euler C: On the regulation of depth and rate of breathing. *J Physiol (Lond)* 222:267, 1972.

141. Grunstein MM, Younes M, Milic-Emili J: Control of tidal volume and respiratory frequency in anesthetized cats. *J Appl Physiol* 35:463, 1973.

142. Pokorski M, Mokashi E, Mulligan T, et al: Responses of aortic chemoreceptors before and after pneumothorax in the cat. *J Appl Physiol Respir Environ Exerc Physiol* 51:665, 1981.

143. Honda Y: Role of carotid chemoreceptors in control of breathing at rest and in exercise: Studies on human subjects with bilateral carotid body resection. *Jpn J Physiol* 35:535, 1985.

144. Heymans C, Bouckhaert JJ, Dautrebande L: Sinus carotidien et reflexes respiratoires: II. Influences respiratoires reflexes de l'acidose de l'alkalose, de l'anhydride carbonique, de l'ion hydrogene et de l'anoxeme. Sinus carotidiens et l'changes respiratoires dans les poumons et au dela des poumons. *Arch Int Pharmacodyn* 39:400, 1930.

145. Pokorski M, Lahiri S: Relative peripheral and central chemosensory responses to metabolic alkalosis. *Am J Physiol Reg Integr Comp Physiol* 245:R873, 1983.

146. Lahiri S, Delaney RG: Stimulus interaction in the responses of carotid chemoreceptor single afferent fibers. *Respir Physiol* 24:249, 1975.

147. Lahiri S, Mokashi A, Delaney RG, et al: Arterial PO_2 and PCO_2 stimulus threshold for carotid chemoreceptors and breathing. *Respir Physiol* 34:359, 1978.

148. Pokorski M, Morikawa T, Honda Y: Breathing pattern in tetraplegics during exposure to hypoxia and hypercapnia. *Mater Med Pol* 27:97, 1995.

149. Lahiri S, Nishino T, Mokashi A, et al: Relative responses of aortic body and carotid body chemoreceptor to hypotension. *J Appl Physiol Respir Environ Exerc Physiol* 48:781, 1980.

150. Verna A, Talib N, Roumy M, et al: Effects of metabolic inhibitors and hypoxia on the ATP, ADP and AMP content of the rabbit carotid body in vitro: The metabolic hypothesis in question. *Neurosci Lett* 116:156, 1990.

151. Nishi K, Eyzaguirre C: The action of some cholinergic blockers on carotid body chemoreceptors in vivo. *Brain Res* 33:37, 1971.

152. Gonzalez C, Almaraz L, Obeso A, et al: Carotid body chemoreceptors: From natural stimuli to sensory discharges. *Physiol Rev* 74:829, 1994.

153. Pokorski M, Lahiri S: Effects of naloxone on carotid body chemoreception and ventilation in the cat. *J Appl Physiol Respir Environ Exerc Physiol* 51:1533, 1981.

154. Hansen JT, Brokaw J, Christie D, et al: Localization of enkephalin-like immunoreactivity in the cat carotid and aortic body chemoreceptors. *Anat Rec* 203:405, 1982.

155. Monti-Bloch L, Eyzaguirre C: A comparative pharmacological study of carotid body chemoreceptors. *Neurosci Abstr* 3:458, 1977.

156. Gonzalez C, Almaraz L, Obeso A, et al: Oxygen and acid chemoreception in the carotid body chemoreceptors. *Trends Neurosci* 15:146, 1992.

157. Biscoe TJ, Duchen MR, Eisner DA, et al: Measurements of intracellular Ca^{2+} in dissociated type I cells of the rabbit carotid body. *J Physiol (Lond)* 416:421, 1989.

158. Cheng PM, Donnelly DF: Relationship between changes of glomus cell current and neural response of rat carotid body. *J Neurophysiol* 74:2077, 1995.

159. Lahiri S: Chemical modification of carotid body chemoreception by sulfhydryls. *Science* 212:1065, 1981.

160. Wilson DF, Mokashi A, Chugh D, et al: The primary oxygen sensor of the cat carotid body is cytochrome a_3 of mitochondrial respiratory chain. *FEBS Lett* 351:370, 1994.

161. Cross AR, Henderson L, Jones OTG, et al: Involvement of an NAD(P)H oxidase as a P_{O_2} sensor protein in the rat carotid body. *Biochem J* 272:743, 1990.

162. Delpiano MA, Acker H: Hypoxia increases the cyclic AMP content of the cat carotid body in vitro. *J Neurochem* 57:291, 1991.

163. Perez-Garcia MT, Almaraz L, Gonzalez C: Effects of different types of stimulation on cyclic AMP content in the rabbit carotid body: Functional significance. *J Neurochem* 55:1287, 1990.

164. Pokorski M, Strosznajder R: P_{O_2}-dependence of phospholipase C in the cat carotid body. *Adv Exp Med Biol* 337:191, 1993.

165. Prabhakar NR, Dinerman JL, Agani FH: Carbon monoxide: A role in carotid body chemoreception. *Proc Natl Acad Sci USA* 92:1994, 1995.

Chapter 7
BREATHING IN EXERCISE

CRAIG A. HARMS
THOMAS J. WETTER
JEROME A. DEMPSEY

Muscular exercise makes unique and multifaceted demands on the respiratory system. The increase in CO_2 production by the locomotor muscles and therefore in CO_2 flow to the lung with increasing work rate means that there is little room for error in the magnitude and proportionality of the ventilatory response. This gas-exchange requirement becomes an especially demanding problem in strenuous exercise because the buffering of metabolic acids produced by the locomotor muscles greatly augments both the CO_2 load presented to the lung and the circulating hydrogen ion concentration, both of which must be compensated. In addition to this substantial requirement for gas exchange, feedback and feedforward mechanisms must be available and highly sensitive to protect against incurring excessively high levels of mechanical work and energy expenditures on the part of the chest wall muscles to meet ventilatory requirements. Finally, ventilation has structural characteristics that limit lung expansion, increases in airflow rates, and the strength and endurance of the respiratory muscles. This chapter focuses on the regulation of ventilation, breathing pattern, and respiratory muscle function during exercise in health, with specific attention paid to neurochemical regulation, mechanical efficiency, cardiorespiratory interactions, and the effects of the structural characteristics of the lung and chest wall.

Alveolar Gases: First Line of Defense of Gas Transport

The critical, bottom-line role for exercise hyperpnea is that the increased alveolar ventilation must match the heightening of tissue O_2 consumption and CO_2 production by the exercising muscles, which in turn rise in direct proportion to the increasing power output. These relationships are governed by the following equations*, which dictate the regulation of alveolar P_{O_2} and P_{CO_2}:

$$P_{A_{O_2}} = \text{Inspired } P_{O_2} - \frac{O_2 \text{ Consumption/min } (\dot{V}_{O_2})}{\text{Alveolar Ventilation/min } (\dot{V}_A)} \cdot K$$

* Calculation of alveolar gases may be made from these equations if $\dot{V}_{O_2}$ is expressed in milliliters per minute, while $\dot{V}_A$ is expressed in liters per minute. The constant K then becomes 0.863. For example, if inspired P_{O_2} is 150 mmHg, $\dot{V}_{O_2}$ is 240 mL/min STPD, and $\dot{V}_A$ is 4.0 L/min BTPS, alveolar P_{O_2} is 98 mmHg. The same applies to CO_2 exchange between alveoli and atmosphere, only this is simplified because CO_2 is virtually absent in inspired air.

$$P_{A_{CO_2}} = \frac{CO_2 \text{ production/min } (\dot{V}_{CO_2})}{\text{Alveolar Ventilation/min } (\dot{V}_A)} \cdot K$$

In mild and strenuous exercise, $\dot{V}_{CO_2}$ and $\dot{V}_{O_2}$ are about five to ten times greater than resting levels, and $\dot{V}_A$ needs to increase proportionately, i.e., to about 25 and 50 L/min, in order to ensure that alveolar gases are maintained near resting levels. If increases in alveolar ventilation during exercise were disproportionately smaller than the increases in $\dot{V}_{CO_2}$, CO_2 would quickly accumulate in the body, leading to the acidification of the arterial blood and tissues, including exercising skeletal muscle. Fortunately, increasing $\dot{V}_A$ closely tracks increases in $\dot{V}_{CO_2}$ throughout exercise. Furthermore, $\dot{V}_A$ increases at a slightly greater rate than does $\dot{V}_{O_2}$ (and cardiac output) during exercise, so the overall ventilation : perfusion ratio ($\dot{V}_A/\dot{Q}$) is increased (Fig. 7-1). This allows alveolar P_{O_2} to increase steadily during exercise and protects arterial P_{O_2} in the face of a gradually rising alveolar-to-arterial P_{O_2} difference ($D_{A-a_{O_2}}$) with increasing exercise (Fig. 7-2).

The widening of the $D_{A-a_{O_2}}$ during exercise is caused by a slight increase in the intraregional maldistribution of $\dot{V}_A/\dot{Q}$ during exercise and a fixed 1 to 2 percent anatomic shunt—both of which have an increasing influence on widening $D_{Aa_{O_2}}$ as $D_{a-\bar{v}_{O_2}}$ increases and mixed venous O_2 ($C_{\bar{v}_{O_2}}$) falls with increasing exercise. There is also the potential for a significant contribution from a diffusion disequilibrium between alveolar gas and pulmonary capillary blood to the widening of the $D_{A-a_{O_2}}$ during exercise, even at normal levels of $V_{max_{O_2}}$.[1] In very strenuous and maximal exercise, alveolar hyperventilation commonly occurs, and $P_{a_{CO_2}}$ falls. The degree of hyperventilation varies substantially among normal subjects, with $P_{a_{CO_2}}$ ranging from the high twenties to only 2 or 3 mmHg less than resting levels. This hyperventilatory response serves two important compensatory responses, namely, to lessen the magnitude of metabolic acidosis induced by muscle lactate production in strenuous exercise and to prevent serious arterial hypoxemia as $D_{A-a_{O_2}}$ widens to an average of 20 to 30 mmHg at maximal exercise.

Breathing Patterns, Lung Volumes, and Mechanics

Contributions from both increasing frequency and tidal volume (V_T) are used to accomplish the increasing $\dot{V}_A$ with increasing work rate. From light- to moderate-intensity exercise, increases in V_T dominate, and these are accomplished by encroaching on both inspiratory and expiratory reserve volumes, since end-expiratory lung volume falls during exercise on average between 300 and 700 mL less than (relaxation) functional residual capacity (FRC) (see Fig. 7-4). Once 50 to 60 percent of vital capacity (VC) is reached, further increases in ventilation are accomplished only by increasing frequency.[2]

This response has several advantages to both gas exchange and inspiratory muscle function: (1) V_D/V_T falls with increasing V_T so that more than 80 percent of each tidal volume is useful alveolar ventilation, (2) V_T is limited, with increases occurring only along the linear portion of

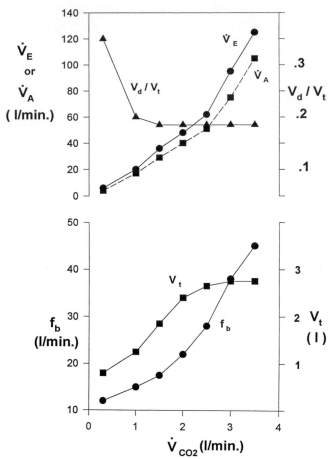

FIGURE 7-1 Ventilation and breathing pattern during steady-state exercise to maximum in healthy young adult males ($Vmax_{O_2}$ = 40 to 50 mL/kg per minute) (data from the authors' laboratory).

the Ppl/V relationship (this decreases the work of breathing because it avoids volume increases to levels where there is increased lung stiffness), (3) the reduced end-expiratory lung volume (EELV) (below FRC) is accomplished by active expiratory muscle effort, and therefore, on relaxation at end-expiration, the lung and chest wall tend to recoil back to FRC, thereby assisting inspiratory effort, and (4) the reduced lung volume means that the diaphragm and other inspiratory muscles are lengthened and therefore operate at a more optimal position for generating force during the subsequent inspiration.

Airway resistance during exercise remains near resting levels during both inspiration and expiration despite fivefold increases in flow rates. Several factors maintain and even enhance airway diameter: (1) the diameter of the extrathoracic upper airway increases because of strong rhythmic and tonic activation of upper airway skeletal muscles that abduct (e.g., at the laryngeal glottal aperture) and "stiffen" the upper airway so that it can resist the negative intrathoracic pressure generated during forceful inspiration,[3] (2) at levels of ventilation approximating five to six times resting levels, there is a shift from predominately nasal to oral ventilation,[2] and (3) significant bronchodilation of intrathoracic airways occurs during exercise, thereby increasing the maximum flow-volume envelope.

Neurochemical Regulation of Exercise Hyperpnea and Hyperventilation

The age-old problem of what factors regulate levels of exercise hyperpnea still lacks a definitive answer (Fig. 7-3). Nevertheless, two very specific locomotor-linked neural stimuli to hyperpnea have emerged from animal models that have simulated locomotion. First, *descending feedforward neural drives* originating in locomotor areas of the higher central nervous system (CNS) are capable of producing parallel activation of medullary respiratory neurons and motor pathways to limb locomotor muscles. This "central command" type of stimulus requires no feedback from the periphery.[4] Second, an *ascending sensory input* carried via type III-IV afferent fibers from contracting skeletal muscle also may contribute to increasing hyperpnea in proportion to the mechanical and chemical feedback stimuli generated by the locomotor muscle force output.[5] Very little is as yet understood about precisely how and where these neural influences are incorporated into the respiratory pattern generator and how they are integrated with other ongoing metabolic and chemoreceptor inputs to control the final ventilatory output that so precisely matches increasing metabolic requirements. Analogous

FIGURE 7-2 Alveolar and arterial blood gases and acid-base status during progressive steady-state exercise to maximum in healthy young adult males ($Vmax_{O_2}$ = 40 to 50 mL/kg per minute) (data compiled from the authors' laboratory).

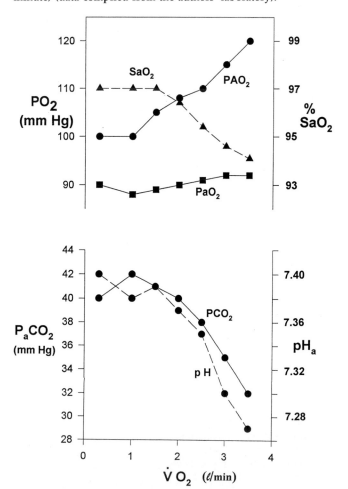

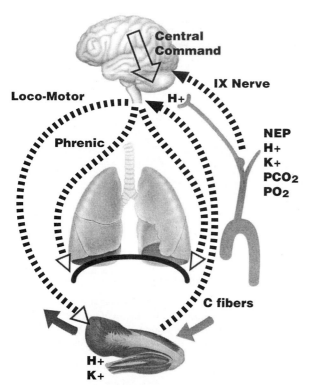

FIGURE 7-3 Schema including major primary and feedback neural pathways proposed for exercise hyperpnea. Central command *descending* from supermedullary locomotor areas (feedforward) and feedback *ascending* via type III-IV afferents from chemoreceptors in contracting skeletal muscle are proposed as the primary feedforward stimuli to exercise hyperpnea. Peripheral chemoreceptors may play a modulatory role because circulating humoral stimuli increase during high exercise intensities. Medullary (H+] chemoreceptors are also shown, but their role is unknown. Not shown are sensory vagal feedback pathways sensitive to lung stretch and motor pathways via cranial nerves that innervate the "respiratory" muscles of the upper airway (please see text).

feedforward and feedback mechanisms are also purported to be responsible for the linear increases in cardiac output in relation to V_{O_2} during exercise. Amazingly, the contribution to exercise hyperpnea from an increasing metabolic CO_2 production or "CO_2 flow" to the lung remains unresolved, even though based on purely correlative evidence and the intuitive need for metabolic feedback regulation, V_{CO_2} must somehow play a key role in determining the degree of hyperpnea.[6]

The *hyperventilation of heavy exercise* coincides with the appearance of three strong humoral stimuli in the arterial blood, metabolic H^+, K^+ (which actually increases linearly throughout exercise), and norepinephrine. Since all these stimuli have been shown to excite carotid chemoreceptors, they must contribute to some extent to the extra ventilation of strenuous exercise, perhaps by means of a strong interaction with the neural locomotor stimuli (see above). Nonetheless, at rest, the gain of the response to each of these humoral stimuli is not substantial, and an increasing lactacidosis has been shown not to be required for the hyperventilatory response.[7] Furthermore, animal studies involving bilateral denervation of the carotid body showed that the hyperventilatory re-

sponse to heavy exercise was actually *greater* following denervation[8]; perhaps the accompanying arterial hypocapnia provides a very strong disfacilitory effect on the carotid chemoreceptor's response to coexisting stimuli.[9] An alternative hypothesis for this hyperventilatory response is that increases in the central command are mainly responsible (just as they may be in moderate exercise). More and more motor units in the locomotor skeletal muscle must be recruited when muscle fatigue intensifies during strenuous exercise, and this increased recruitment also should mean greater feedforward stimulation of medullary respiratory neurons.[7]

Mechanoreceptor Feedback Control of Exercise Hyperpnea

Observations of the response to exercise suggest that the mechanical efficiency of each breath is regulated. These observations include the fact that V_T is limited below maximal possible levels, the extrathoracic airways are maximumly dilated, and expiratory muscle activation drives EELV below FRC, thereby optimizing and sparing inspiratory muscle function, and so on. In exercising dogs, use of reversible vagal blockade has indeed shown a strong effect of pulmonary stretch receptor (PSR) feedback on breathing pattern and on the recruitment of expiratory muscle activity.[10] Humans exhibit a Herring-Breuer inhibitory reflex from lung stretch receptors that becomes significant above 1.0 to 1.5 L of lung inflation,[11] and T_I is prolonged significantly when normal tidal inflation is prevented via airway occlusion.[12] This inhibitory reflex appears to be much more powerful in the newborn than in the adult human. In humans, the physiologic role of PSR can be examined in lung transplant patients, who lack a Herring-Breuer reflex after transplantation.[11] Post-lung transplant patients also do *not* prolong their inspiratory time during airway occlusion initiated at normal end-expiration. During exercise, there is some evidence that V_T increases to a slightly greater percentage of VC and that T_I is slightly prolonged in the lung transplant patient.[13] Given the wide range of normal breathing patterns during exercise, the response of the lung-denervated patient is not strikingly different from that of the intact person. In the adult human, PSRs may be important for the within-breath regulation of cardiovascular function because the normally occurring respiratory sinus arrhythmia is absent in patients after lung transplantation.[14] In addition, within-breath modulation of muscle sympathetic nerve activity at high tidal volumes is greatly blunted.[15] What cannot be ruled out is that at least a portion of our ventilatory response to exercise—both ventilatory volume and breathing pattern—may be "preprogrammed" by the higher CNS regions based on experience gained during repetitive motor acts.

Mechanical feedback from the chest wall respiratory muscles and lung stretch receptors during exercise is the source of dyspneic sensations. We do not know all of the neural pathways over which sensory inputs from the chest wall and lungs travel to the medulla and in turn are transmitted to the midbrain. When the inputs become substantial, they are manifested as an awareness of hyperpnea that eventually leads to unpleasant and often painful sensations of dyspnea. Fortunately, in health, the work of the respiratory muscles during even moderately strenuous exercise is maintained at

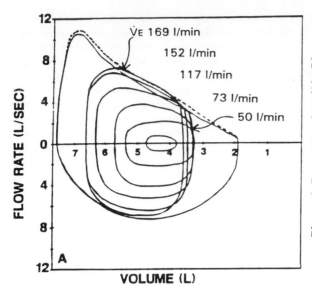

FIGURE 7-4 Flow-volume and pleural pressure-volume relationships during execise in young adult males. The largest envelope is the mean maximal volitional effort for all subjects. Note that all subjects show a reduced EELV during mild to moderate exercise, untrained subjects (Vmax$_{O_2}$ = 35 to 50 mL/kg per minute) with a mean VE of 117 L/min at maximal exercise show no significant flow limitation, and highly trained subjects (Vmax$_{O_2}$ = 60 to 83 mL/kg per minute) with a mean VE of 150 to 190 L/min but a normal maximal-flow-volume envelope showed significant expiratory flow limitation during strenuous and maximal exercise.

a relatively low level (see above) compared with the maximal capacity for force development. Accordingly, we are rarely aware of our increased ventilation during almost all types rhythmic exercise of moderate intensity, and it is only in very exceptional circumstances that the healthy, normally fit young adult experiences true dyspneic sensations. Such instances may include the termination of exhaustive exercise or strenuous exercise carried out in hypoxic or hot environments or with small muscle groups, i.e., arm work. Vagal feedback from the lung may play some role in dyspnea, as shown by (1) observations that the dyspnea of breath holding can be relieved by movement of the lung and chest wall in normal, intact subjects but to a much lesser extent in the lung transplant patient[16] and (2) the report in a case study that unilateral vagal denervation in a patient with chronic pulmonary hypertension and edema markedly relieved the patient's tachypnea and dyspnea, especially during exercise.[17]

Mechanical Reserves: Airways and Respiratory Muscles

The maximum (volitional) flow-volume envelope defines the limits of the airways and respiratory muscles to produce flow and volume during exercise. In health, the airways are clearly overbuilt for the ventilatory challenge demanded by even maximal exercise, since ventilations up to 120 to 130 L/min fit well within the normal maximum flow-volume loop (Fig. 7-4). Furthermore, the force output required of the inspiratory muscles to produce the required flow rates and tidal volumes is usually only 40 to 60 percent of the maximal dynamic force output available at the muscle length (i.e., lung volumes) and velocity of shortening (flow rates) achieved at maximal exercise. The capacity of the respiratory muscles

for maximal force generation is preserved by the increasing length (i.e., reduced EELV) and the absence of respiratory muscle fatigue, at least in short-term maximum exercise (also see below). The work of the respiratory muscles required to overcome elastic recoil and airway resistance increases linearly in ventilation and at the normal Vmax$_{O_2}$ of 40 to 50 mL/kg per minute and VE of 100 to 120 L/min requires an energy expenditure of about 8 to 10 percent of the Vmax$_{O_2}$. The diaphragm increases its V$_{O_2}$ during exercise in a manner similar to limb skeletal muscles by increasing both blood flow and O$_2$ extraction (see below).

Cardiovascular Consequences of Exercise Hyperpnea

The ventilatory response to exercise commands substantial changes in intrathoracic pressure and in the work output and metabolic rate of the respiratory muscles. In turn, these effects may exert significant influences on the cardiovascular response to exercise, both total cardiac output and its distribution.

RESPIRATORY MUSCLE BLOOD FLOW DURING EXERCISE

Metabolic demands are usually the most important determinant of respiratory muscle blood flow under normal conditions. Many reports have investigated the relationship between diaphragmatic metabolic demands and blood flow,[18,19] but there is much less work on respiratory muscle blood flow during exercise. Respiratory muscle blood flow has not been quantified in humans during exercise; however, studies measuring blood flow in exercising dogs,[18] pigs,[19] and rats[20] show substantial increases in blood flow to the diaphragm and inspiratory and expiratory muscles that often approximate the blood flow to locomotor muscles during moderate to maximal exercise. Increased blood flow to the respiratory muscles during exercise is directly related to muscle activity.[21]

It is still unknown, however, whether diaphragmatic blood flow reaches maximal values during physical exercise. Hsai and colleagues[22] have reported that in dogs exercising at maximal workloads, blood flow to the diaphragm remained lower than predicted maximal values. However, Manohar's studies in the exercising pony showed that at $Vmax_{O_2}$ (~120 to 130 mL/kg per minute and Pa_{CO_2} of 25 to 30 mmHg), diaphragm V_{O_2} (estimated via the Fick principle) increased from 0.4 mL/min per 100 g at rest to 45 mL/min per 100 g because of a 20- to 30-fold increase in blood flow and more than 80 percent O_2 extraction by the diaphragm.[23-25] Intercostal muscle blood flow also increased many times greater than rest, but their peak blood flow was less than half that of the diaphragm. Attempts to further lower diaphragm vascular resistance and to increase blood flow at maximal exercise either by infusion of adenosine or by raising ventilatory work (via airway resistive loading) suggest that the diaphragm may have been maximally vasodilated. The myocardium, on the other hand, showed a significant vasodilator reserve at peak exercise. In addition, the highest values for diaphragm blood flow were equal to or even slightly more than blood flow per 100 g to the primary locomotor muscles of the limbs (e.g., gluteus medius and biceps femoris) at peak exercise.

The diaphragm therefore may be an exception to the generalization that some degree of sympathetically mediated vasoconstriction occurs during moderate and strenuous exercise in active limb muscles.[26] Apparently, this ongoing vasoconstriction in limb muscles is necessary for maintaining perfusion pressure. The maximal available capillary blood volume in the diaphragm perhaps is sufficiently large to maintain enough long red cell transit times to ensure maximal O_2 offloading and extraction. The study of the pony[25] also provides extensive data on arterial to phrenic venous metabolite differences that demonstrate the extraordinary aerobic capacity of the diaphragm and its suitability for meeting and sustaining high metabolic requirements during prolonged strenuous exercise. In over 30 min of high-intensity exercise, the pony showed progressive hyperventilation with very high breathing frequencies and yet maintained blood flow and high O_2 extraction rates of the diaphragm throughout. Arterial blood lactate and NH_3 concentrations rose throughout exercise, but there was no net production of either metabolite by the diaphragm so that arterial-to-phrenic venous concentration differences were absent.[25] Similar findings were observed in studies of the diaphragm of awake sheep who were subjected to high resistive loads for prolonged periods.[27] These data are consistent with the notion that the working diaphragm, much like cardiac muscle, may take up and use lactate as a substrate during prolonged exercise. This is also suggested by the high levels of tissue diaphragmatic lactate found in the absence of substantial glycogen depletion in the rat diaphragm following exhaustive exercise.[28]

EFFECTS OF RESPIRATORY MUSCLE WORK ON LIMB LOCOMOTOR BLOOD FLOW

During strenuous exercise in highly fit humans, when the level of ventilatory requirement is such that severe expiratory flow limitation is realized, the oxygen cost of breathing may approach 15 percent of total V_{O_2}.[29] Theoretically, the metabolic cost of breathing required by the primary respiratory and stabilizing muscles of the chest wall, plus their demand for perfusion to meet this oxygen cost, could limit the blood flow available for locomotor muscles and thereby limit their work output. This would likely depend in part on the relative strength of local and autonomic controlled reflexes in the different muscle vascular beds[30] and also on the magnitude of the increased respiratory muscle work. The fact that high and progressively increasing levels of ventilation occur throughout prolonged exercise would indicate that total respiratory muscle power output remains unaffected and meets the requirements of CO_2 elimination. Accordingly, it seems reasonable to postulate that the respiratory muscles would receive a preferential share of blood flow at the expense of limb locomotor muscles under conditions where total cardiac output is at or near maximal. This postulate would require that vasoconstriction occur in working limb muscles during strenuous exercise (see above) and that there is a redistribution of blood flow to the chest wall.

Most of the work investigating this idea of competition between different vascular beds has used the technique of adding arm work to leg exercise during submaximal exercise. Secher and colleagues[31] determined that adding arm work when the legs are already exercising submaximally resulted in reduced blood flow to the legs. They surmised that increased blood flow was made available to the working arms at the expense of blood flow to the legs. However, several recent reports have failed to corroborate these findings.[32-34] In these investigations, adding arm work was shown to increase leg vascular resistance[35] and to increase NE spillover across the working muscle.[32-34] However, with added arm work, Richter and colleagues[33] reported that systemic pressure also rose sufficiently to preserve flow to the working limb. Thus the consensus from these studies is that added working muscle mass does not decrease blood flow to the exercising lower limbs. However, these four studies were all conducted only at submaximal exercise intensities. Perhaps clear, consistent demonstration of blood flow redistribution and local vasoconstriction might only occur when muscle mass is added to situations closer to maximal work intensities.

We have recently investigated whether changes in work of breathing and respiratory muscle loading and unloading (via proportional assist ventilation) affect leg blood flow, V_{O_2}, and vascular resistance during maximal exercise.[35] Our findings suggest that increases in the amount of working respiratory muscle mass at maximal exercise significantly reduced leg blood flow and V_{O_2} and increased leg vascular resistance, whereas decreases in working respiratory muscle mass increased leg blood flow and V_{O_2} and decreased vascular resistance (Fig. 7-5). This implies that respiratory muscles may compete more effectively than limb muscles for total cardiac output during maximal exercise. This possibility is also suggested by the increase in diaphragm blood flow and decrease in limb locomotor muscle blood flow during submaximal exercise in rats when the work of breathing was presumably increased via experimental congestive heart failure.[36] This substantial redistribution effect between locomotor and respiratory muscles may reflect two important properties of respiratory muscles. First, the diaphragm and

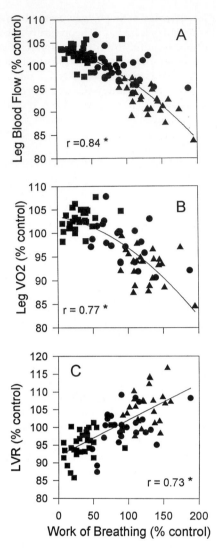

FIGURE 7-5 Relative effects of changing work of breathing on leg blood flow (*A*), leg V_{O_2} (*B*), and leg vascular resistance (LVR) (*C*) at $Vmax_{O_2}$ (*n* = 7) (*circles*, control; *squares*, inspiratory muscle unload; *triangles*, inspiratory muscle load). *$P < .05$. (See Harms et al.[35])

accessory respiratory muscles are of high oxidative capacity; accordingly, their resistance vessels may be especially responsive to local vasodilator influences, as shown by the vasculature of limb muscle in highly trained individuals.[37,38] Second, increased work by the respiratory muscles has been shown to promote reflex sympathoexcitation and vasoconstriction of systemic vascular beds,[39] similar to the reflex pressor responses attributed to type III and IV afferents from contracting limb muscles.[5,40]

What is the mechanism responsible for blood flow redistribution at maximal exercise between respiratory muscles and locomotor muscles when the work of breathing is altered? Changes in NE spillover have been shown to be related to changes in leg vascular resistance.[32,34,35] This suggests an increased muscle sympathetic nerve activity (MSNA) and vasoconstriction with respiratory muscle loading and reduced MSNA and vasodilation with respiratory muscle unloading. The vasodilatory effect in response to respiratory

muscle unloading is consistent with the concept that a significant level of sympathetically mediated vasoconstriction is normally present in active limb skeletal muscle at maximal exercise.[41] These findings further imply that a significant portion of this vasoconstrictor sympathetic outflow during maximum exercise may emanate from tonically active respiratory muscle chemoreflexes, a sensitive feedback mechanism known to originate from type III and IV afferents in contracting limb muscles[41] and in the diaphragm.[39] On stimulation of their thin-fiber phrenic afferent pathways in the diaphragm, sympathoexcitation and vasoconstriction in both respiratory and resting limb skeletal muscle can be induced.[39]

The effects of partial respiratory muscle *unloading* on increasing leg muscle blood flow speaks directly to the question of the physiologic relevance of the work of breathing normally achieved during maximal exercise to oxygen transport to locomotor muscles. It is not unexpected that the respiratory muscle work normally achieved in maximal exercise would require a significant share of maximal cardiac output. Again, we found that reducing the work of breathing at maximum exercise by about 50 percent increased leg blood flow and leg muscle V_{O_2} (see Fig. 7-5). Along with this *increase* in V_{O_2} of the legs, however, respiratory muscle unloading also *reduced* total-body V_{O_2} (also see below).

MECHANICAL AND METABOLIC EFFECTS OF HYPERPNEA ON CARDIAC OUTPUT

It is generally accepted that venous return increases during inspiration and decreases during expiration. Inspiration is associated with more negative intrathoracic pressure. As the diaphragm descends, intraabdominal pressure increases, and this increases the pressure gradient between the right side of the heart and the abdomen, causing the inferior vena cava to discharge blood centrally and enhancing venous return. Expiration, on the other hand, has the opposite effect on these pressures, although venous return is somewhat maintained due to the release of blood outflow from the level that was mechanically limited during inspiration.[42] The effects of ventilation on preload are in contrast to those on afterload. During inspiration, as right atrial and ventricular volumes are increased, left ventricular stroke volume is decreased. This is thought to be an effect of the limited space within the pericardium, as evidenced by diminished stroke volume changes in patients with pericardiectomy.[42] In addition, mechanical effects on the heart (e.g., an increase in transmural pressure) due to an increase in lung volume during inspiration may decrease cardiac output via decreased stroke volume. In a one-way system (e.g., venous valves), the net effect of the changes in intrathoracic pressure is to act as a pump (respiratory pump) that is thought to aid venous return, especially during exercise, when oscillations in pressure differences are increased.

It has been proposed that high negative intrathoracic pressures might collapse the veins during inspiration and limit venous return.[43] However, it appears that collapse of vessels is time dependent and flow is decreased only if inspirations are prolonged and deep.[44] Wexler and associates[45] directly measured vena caval flow during mild supine exercise with a velocity transducer inserted into the inferior vena cava of conscious humans. Pulsatile changes in blood flow were noted and corresponded with respiration (e.g., increased with inspiration, decreased with expiration). Differences existed, however, depending on type of breathing. Primarily diaphragmatic inspirations or Muller maneuvers resulted in decreases in blood flow, which were thought to result from collapse of the vessel just below the diaphragm.

Because respiration increases both preload and afterload, the net effect over an entire cardiac cycle could be either an increase or decrease in cardiac output. Giesbrecht and colleagues[46] tested whether these oscillations in pleural pressure affect cardiac output at rest and during light exercise (50 W). By changing the amplitude of these respiratory fluctuations with elastic loading (increases pressure amplitude) or unloading (decreases amplitude), they found no effect on breath-by-breath measures of V_{O_2} in the first three breaths following the changes in loading. This argues against a large effect of changes in intrathoracic pressure in altering cardiac output at least during mild exercise.

Other forces that occur with breathing also may influence cardiac output. As the diaphragm descends during inspiration and intrathoracic pressure falls, abdominal pressure is raised. This, in turn, could serve to limit venous return by decreasing the pressure gradient from the lower body. In addition, direct compression of the blood vessels in the abdominal compartment may occur during contraction of the diaphragm. This idea was tested by Williput and colleagues,[47] who examined the effects of the respiratory pattern of breathing on femoral venous blood flow. They found that in supine resting humans, femoral blood flow was decreased when inspiration was accomplished primarily by contraction of the diaphragm. These results, however, cannot be generalized beyond the supine condition because the increased gravitational forces while standing may increase intraluminal pressure and serve to keep the vessel open.

While it is clear that the mechanical forces that accompany hyperpnea can have effects on cardiac output, it is also true that the O_2 requirement of respiratory muscles could influence cardiac output, especially when the work of breathing is increased as in exercise. Coast and associates[48] examined the time course of cardiac output changes during loaded breathing while at rest. Cardiac output increased significantly during loaded breathing, clearly showing the cardiovascular effects of an increased work of breathing. However, mechanical effects did not appear to be the major factor causing the increased cardiac output because the rise in cardiac output was delayed until 20 s after the load was imposed, consistent with a metabolic effect. Further strengthening the lack of important mechanical effects, a significant increase in heart rate (but not stroke volume) was found to account for the change in cardiac output. This metabolic effect of increased respiratory muscle work on cardiac output at rest is consistent with the reduced V_{O_2} observed during maximal exercise when respiratory muscles were unloaded (see above).[35]

It is well established then that mechanical factors associated with respiration can transiently influence venous return and affect afterload on the left ventricle. However, the effects on cardiac output over an entire cardiac cycle and over even longer periods of time are not as well established. During exercise when muscle activity is increased, the effects of the muscle pump on modulating the respiratory-induced pulsatile nature of venous return remains to be determined.

All Is Not Perfect: Demand Greater than Respiratory System Capacity during Exercise

Under the normal "textbook" circumstances described to date for the standard "reference" young, healthy, normally fit adult male, it is clear that structural and functional capacity of the respiratory system, including the lung and chest wall and the supporting neural control system, exceeds the demands placed on them for flow rate, volume, and O_2 and CO_2 exchange by even maximal short-term exercise. Accordingly, while much evidence supports the view that maximal systemic O_2 transport (i.e., the product of arterial O_2 content and blood flow) is the critical determinant of $Vmax_{O_2}$, it is clearly the constraint on maximum systemic blood flow and not the completeness (or physiologic cost) of oxygenating arterial blood that is crucial. On the other hand, there are several special circumstances in which the respiratory system limits the response to strenuous exercise even in healthy people.

ENDURANCE EXERCISE–INDUCED DIAPHRAGM FATIGUE

The diaphragm appears to be ideally built for the increased ventilatory requirements of muscular exercise. Mechanically, it expands the rib cage in a highly efficient manner by both lowering its floor and laterally expanding the lower ribs indirectly by using the compressible abdominal contents as a fulcrum. Structurally, the diaphragm's mixed fiber composition, high capillary density, and high aerobic enzymatic capacity means that this primary respiratory muscle is highly fatigue resistant. Accordingly, the human (at rest) can sustain up to six to eight times the resting diaphragmatic force output for 10 to 15 min without inducing significant fatigue of the diaphragm and without evidence of volitional "task failure" of the diaphragm.[49] Furthermore, sustained force outputs of the diaphragm that were 1.5 to 2 times those normally experienced in exhaustive exercise were required to cause diaphragm fatigue when the subject was in the resting state and increased ventilation voluntarily. This evidence would support the idea of the high resistance to fatigue of the respiratory muscles. However, very strenuous exercise to exhaustion caused the diaphragm to fatigue (Fig. 7-6), as judged by a 20 to 40 percent reduction of trans-diaphragmatic pressure (Pdi) in response to the supramaximal bilateral phrenic nerve stimulation (1 to 20 Hz), and the diaphragm did not recover after 1 h or more of rest following the exercise. To elicit diaphragmatic fatigue required that the exercise be sustained for longer than 10 min and that the intensity be very high. Thus, at 80 to 85 percent of $Vmax_{O_2}$ about one-half of subjects showed diaphragm fatigue, whereas at 90 to 95 percent of $Vmax_{O_2}$ almost all subjects showed exercise-induced diaphragm fatigue. Young, healthy subjects of all fitness levels ($Vmax_{O_2}$ of 40 to 80 ml/kg per minute) showed equal amounts of diaphragm fatigue when carrying out strenuous endurance exercise to exhaustion.[49–51]

Although the magnitude of the sustained increase in diaphragm force output is a significant determinant of diaphragm fatigue, the whole-body exercise itself appears to be a critical prerequisite that greatly lowers the threshold of force output by the diaphragm required for its fatigue (see

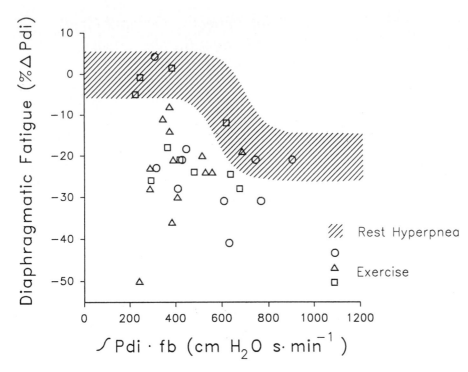

FIGURE 7-6 Force output of the diaphragm versus diaphragm fatigue, the latter determined by bilateral phrenic nerve stimulation. Percentage change in Pdi reflects the change in stimulated Pdi (sum of 1-, 10-, and 20-Hz stimulations) from control to after hyperpnea. The shaded area shows the fatigue incurred by hyperpnea of different magnitudes in the subject at rest. Note that the threshold force output of the diaphragm for fatigue averaged about 500 $cmH_2O \cdot s \cdot min^{-1}$ (or approximately four times resting levels) in the resting subject. The superimposed points for individual subjects show that following whole body exercise to exhaustion, significant diaphragm fatigue occurred at much lower sustained force outputs of the diaphragm; i.e., the fatigue threshold for the diaphragm was substantially reduced during the endurance exercise (see Johnson et al.[51]).

Fig. 7-6). Why is this fatigue threshold lowered during exercise? Perhaps the acid milieu created by strenuous endurance exercise of the locomotor muscles might precipitate fatigue. In support of this, it is known that exercising rats accumulate large quantities of lactic acid in the diaphragm during exercise,[38] and metabolic acidosis per se will precipitate diaphragm fatigue.[52] This does not mean that the amount of diaphragm force output incurred during exercise is not important in fatigue; to the contrary, the greater the force of muscle contraction, the greater is the uptake of lactate,[53] and rested muscles (e.g., of the hand) do not show fatigue when the legs exercise at high intensities to exhaustion.[49] An alternative explanation for the decreased diaphragm fatigue threshold during exercise might be that the diaphragm must compete with working limb muscles for the limited amount of available cardiac output during exercise, whereas during sustained hyperpnea trials at rest, availability of blood flow to the diaphragm is far greater (also see above).

What are the consequences of exercise-induced diaphragm fatigue? Certainly, alveolar ventilation appears to be adequate, since, with few exceptions, arterial P_{CO_2} falls and arterial P_{O_2} rises throughout heavy endurance exercise. The only clear evidence of an effect of exercise-induced diaphragm fatigue is that force output from the diaphragm tends to plateau (or occasionally even falls slightly) beyond the initial few minutes of strenuous exercise, even though ventilation and total inspiratory muscle force output continue to rise throughout exercise.[49–51] Thus the diaphragm contributes less and less to total inspiratory muscle work as exercise continues. Theoretically, this increasing use of "accessory" respiratory muscles as exercise continues might be a mechanically inefficient means of producing ventilation because of chest wall distortion, which might in turn translate into a higher cost of breathing and command a higher blood flow to the chest wall muscles.

HIGHLY TRAINED YOUNG ADULT MALES

The extraordinarily high $Vmax_{O_2}$ (and $Vmax_{CO_2}$) in the highly fit demands high levels of alveolar ventilation; however, with very few exceptions, the airway diameter and lung volumes in athletes are similar to those of their less fit contemporaries with much lower $Vmax_{O_2}$ values. Accordingly, significant expiratory flow limitation beginning, for example, at 15 to 20 percent of tidal volume begins to occur even in strenuous submaximal exercise and becomes progressively more severe with increasing exercise to maximum. Several highly trained athletes at $Vmax_{O_2}$ filled the entire "available" flow-volume loop and their V_E was truly maximized so that further imposed increases in chemoreceptor stimuli (achieved by breathing carbon dioxide) at maximum exercise did not increase V_E further (Fig. 7-4). Under these circumstances, ventilatory demand does indeed exceed or at least match the capacity of the airways for increasing flow rate. Limitation of expiratory flow rate, even when only 20 percent of V_T is flow-limited during submaximal exercise, becomes a significant constraint on the exercise hyperpnea. This is shown by the increased ventilation achieved when the maximum flow-volume envelope was increased by breathing a low-density helium-oxygen gas mixture. The onset of expiratory flow limitation in these fit subjects also caused EELV to increase back toward resting FRC with subsequent shortening of inspiratory muscles during exercise and a reduction in the force-generating capacity of these inspiratory muscles (Fig. 7-4). Accordingly, respiratory muscle force output at peak exercise in the highly trained often exceeded 90 percent of (their reduced) capacity.[55]

The consequence of these ventilatory limitations in highly trained subjects was commonly, but not always, a lessened hyperventilation (but again, never frank CO_2 retention) during strenuous and maximal exercise. When combined with the lack of equilibrium between alveolar gases and capillary blood in these highly trained subjects, this constrained ventilatory response contributed to the significant arterial hypoxemia experienced by many of these subjects during strenuous exercise.[55] Furthermore, the magnitude of respiratory muscle work achieved during inspiration and expiration reached very high levels in these subjects, resulting in an oxygen cost of ventilation that averaged 13 to 16 percent of $Vtot_{O_2}$ at maximal exercise.[29]

GENDER EFFECTS

Postpubertal females have narrower-diameter airways (and reduced maximum flow-volume envelopes), smaller lung volumes, a reduced number of alveoli, and smaller surface areas for diffusion than do males.[56,57] This occurs in part because women are generally of smaller stature and trunk size than are males, but these differences in lung volumes, flow rates, and diffusion surface persist even when stature and body size are taken into account. Accordingly, during exercise, young adult women experience significant expiratory flow limitation with substantial increases in EELV at minute ventilations of 90 to 100 L/min, i.e., well below the V_E required for flow limitation in their male contemporaries.[58] Accordingly, mechanical constraints on exercise hyperpnea are more common in females, and the work and oxygen cost of exercise hyperpnea are probably higher at a given V_E. Furthermore, in a high percentage of fit females at above-average $Vmax_{O_2}$, $DA\text{-}a_{O_2}$ widened substantially during strenuous but submaximal work loads, which in combination with a reduced (mechanically constrained) hyperventilatory response caused significant exercise-induced arterial hypoxemia.

AGING EFFECTS

Healthy aging, especially noticeable at and beyond the sixth decade, causes reductions in lung elastic recoil, vital capacity, diffusion surface area, and chest wall compliance. Accordingly, in highly fit elderly individuals, significant expiratory flow limitation with an accompanying increase in the EELV and increased ventilatory work begins during submaximal exercise at V_E values in the 70 to 80 L/min range.[59] Exercise-induced arterial hypoxemia also occurs in the highly fit elderly persons at $Vmax_{O_2}$ values in the 40 to 60 mL/kg per minute range (1.5 to 2.5 times age-predicted normal $Vmax_{O_2}$ values), but the prevalence of hypoxemia is less than in younger highly fit males at much higher $Vmax_{O_2}$ values.[60] Apparently then in most fit, healthy subjects the age-related decline in $Vmax_{O_2}$ and in pulmonary O_2 transport capacity are similar. Given the gender effects on lung structure and function in young adults, aging females might be even more susceptible to pulmonary limitations in exercise performance.

ENVIRONMENTAL HYPOXIA AND HEAT

In the hypoxia of high altitudes, the sojourner from sea level hyperventilates even at "mild" exercise intensities. This response is critical to minimizing the arterial hypoxemia of high altitudes, especially during exercise. However, there are also many consequences of this hyperventilatory response, since flow limitation and high levels of ventilatory work occur throughout moderate exercise because of the hyperventilation. Furthermore, exercise-induced diaphragmatic

fatigue occurs after shorter exercise durations and longer recovery times are required to relieve this diaphragm fatigue following the exercise.[61] Even more troublesome is the awareness of hyperventilation, tachypnea, and dyspnea during exercise in hypoxia. Uncoupling of locomotion from respiration, i.e., respiratory frequency from foot-plant frequency, creates especially unpleasant sensations in breathing during exercise in hypoxia, apparently because the combination of carotid chemoreceptor stimulation and locomotor-linked stimuli to breathe are multiplicative in their effect on respiratory motor output and breathing frequency.

Long-term heavy exercise causes a time-dependent "drift" in breathing frequency and in the degree of hyperventilation. When endurance exercise is carried out under hot, humid environmental conditions, tachypnea and hyperventilation intensify, and rarely, breathing frequencies may exceed 80 to 90 breaths per minute.[62] Consequently, even though locomotor muscle fatigue sets in and exercise performance and V_{CO_2} fall over time, a tachypneic hyperventilation persists, increasing dead space ventilation and at times leading to a rise in arterial P_{CO_2}. These examples illustrate that in rare circumstances the demand for alveolar ventilation during exercise exceeds respiratory system capacity.

References

1. Torre-Bueno JR, Wagner PD, Saltzman HA, et al: Diffusion limitation in normal humans during exercise at sea level and simulated altitude. *J Appl Physiol* 58:989–995, 1985.
2. Dempsey JA, Adams L, Ainsworth D, et al: Airway lung and respiratory muscle function during exercise, in Rowell L, Shepard J (eds): *Handbook of Physiology* sec. XII: *Exercise*. New York, Oxford University Press, 1996, pp 448–515.
3. England SJ, Bartlett D Jr, Knuth SL: Changes in respiratory movements of the human vocal cords during hyperpnea. *J Appl Physiol* 52:780–785, 1982.
4. Eldridge FL, Milhorn DE, Kily JP, Waldrop TG: Stimulation by central command of locomotion, respiration and circulation during exercise. *Respir Physiol* 59:313–337, 1985.
5. Kaufman MP, Forster HV: Reflexes controlling circulatory, ventilatory and airway responses to exercise, in Rowell L, Shepard J (eds): *Handbook of Physiology*, sec. XII: *Exercise*. New York, Oxford University Press, 1996, pp 381–442.
6. Phillipson EA, Bpwes G, Towssend ER, et al: Carotid chemoreceptors in ventilatory responses to venous CO_2 load. *J Appl Physiol* 51:1398–1403, 1981.
7. Duffin J: Neural drives to breathing during exercise. *Can J Appl Physiol* 19:289–304, 1994.
8. Pan LG, Forster HV, Bisgard GE, et al: Independence of exercise hyperpnea and acidosis during high intensity exercise in ponies. *J Appl Physiol* 60:1016–1024, 1986.
9. Smith CA, Saupe KW, Henderson KS, Dempsey JA: Ventilatory effects of specific carotid body hypocapnia in dogs during wakefulness and sleep. *J Appl Physiol* 79(3):689–699, 1995.
10. Ainsworth DM, Smith CA, Johnson BD, et al: Vagal modulation of respiratory muscle activity in awake dogs during exercise and hypercapnia. *J Appl Physiol* 72(4):1362–1367, 1992.
11. Iber CP, Simon PM, Skatrud JB, et al: The Breuer-Hering reflex in humans. *Am J Respir Crit Care Med* 152:217–224, 1995.
12. Polacheck J, Strong R, Arens J, et al: Phasic vagal influence on inspiratory motor output in anesthetized human subjects. *J Appl Physiol* 49:609–619, 1980.
13. Sciurba FC, Owens GR, Sanders MH, et al: Evidence of an altered pattern of breathing during exercise in recipients of heart-lung transplants. *N Engl J Med* 319:1186–1192, 1988.

14. Taha B, Simon PM, Dempsey JA, et al: Respiratory sinus arrhythmia in humans: An obligatory role for vagal feedback from the lungs. *J Appl Physiol* 78(2):638–645, 1995.

15. Seals DR, Suwarno NO, Joyner MJ, et al: Respiratory modulation of muscle sympathetic nerve activity in intact and lung denervated humans. *Circ Res* 72:440–454, 1993.

16. Flume PA, Eldridge FL, Edwards LJ, Mattison LE: Relief of the ''air hunger'' of breath holding: A role for pulmonary stretch receptors. *Respir Physiol* 103:221–232, 1996.

17. Davies SF, McQuaid KR, Iber C, et al: Extreme dyspnea from unilateral pulmonary venous obstruction. *ARRD* 136:184–188, 1982.

18. Fixler DE, Atkins JM, Mitchell JH, Horwitz LD: Blood flow to respiratory, cardiac, and limb muscles in dogs during graded exercise. *Am J Physiol* 231:1515, 1976.

19. Sanders M, White F, Bloor C: Cardiovascular responses of dogs and pigs exposed to similar physiological stress. *Comp Biochem Physiol |A|* 58:365, 1977.

20. Musch TI, Friedman DB, Pitetti KH, et al: Regional distribution of blood flow of dogs during graded exercise. *J Appl Physiol* 63:2269, 1987.

21. Hussain SNA: Invited review: Regulation of ventilatory muscle blood flow. *J Appl Physiol* 81:1455, 1996.

22. Hsia CC, Ramanathan WM, Pean JL, Johnson RL Jr: Respiratory muscle blood flow in exercising dogs after pneumonectomy. *J Appl Physiol* 73:240, 1992.

23. Manohar M: Vasodilator reserve in respiratory muscles during maximal exertion in ponies. *J Appl Physiol* 60:1571, 1986.

24. Manohar M: Costal versus crural diaphragmatic blood flow during submaximal and near-maximal exercise in ponies. *J Appl Physiol* 65:1514, 1988.

25. Manohar M, Hassan AS: The diaphragm does not produce ammonia or lactate during high intensity short-term exercise. *Am J Physiol* 28(Heart Circ. Physiol. 28):H1185, 1990.

26. Rowell LB: *Human Cardiovascular Control.* New York: Oxford University Press, 1993, p 331.

27. Bazzy AR, Pang LM, Akabas SR, Haddad GG: O₂ metabolism of the sheep diaphragm during flow resistive loaded breathing. *J Appl Physiol* 66:2305, 1989.

28. Fregosi R, Dempsey JA: The effects of exercise in normoxia and acute hypoxia on respiratory muscle metabolites. *J Appl Physiol* 60:1274, 1986.

29. Aaron EA, Seow KC, Johnson BD, Dempsey JA: Oxygen cost of exercise hyperpnea: Implications for performance. *J Appl Physiol* 72:1818, 1992.

30. Rowell L, O'Leary DS, Kellog DL: Integration of cardiovascular control systems in dynamic exercises, in Rowell L, Shepard J (eds): *Handbook of Physiology* New York: Oxford University Press, 1996, p 770.

31. Secher NH, Clausen JP, Klausen K, et al: Central and regional circulatory effects of adding arm exercise to leg exercise. *Acta Physiol Scand* 100:288, 1977.

32. Richardson RS, Kennedy B, Knight DR, Wagner PD: High muscle blood flows are not attenuated by recruitment of additional muscle mass. *Am J Physiol* 269(*Heart Circ Physiol* 38)J1545, 1995.

33. Richter EA, Kiens B, Hargreaves M, Kaejer M: Effect of arm cranking on leg blood flow and noradrenaline spillover during leg exercise in man. *Acta Physiol Scand* 144:9, 1992.

34. Savard GK, Richter EA, Strange S, et al: Norepinephrine spillover from skeletal muscle during exercise: Role of muscle mass. *Am J Physiol* 257(*Heart Circ Physiol* 26):H1812, 1989.

35. Harms CA, Babcock MA, McClaran SR, et al: Respiratory muscle work compromises leg blood flow during maximal exercise. *J Appl Physiol* 82(5):1573, 1997.

36. Musch TI: Elevated diaphragmatic blood flow during submaximal exercise in rats with chronic heart failure. *Am J Physiol* 265(*Heart Circ Physiol* 34):H1721, 1993.

37. Laughlin MH, Klabunde RE, Delp MD, Armstrong RB: Effects of dipyridamole on muscle blood flow in exercising miniature swine. *Am J Physiol* 257(*Heart Circ Physiol* 26):H1507, 1989.

38. Laughlin MH, McAllister RM: Exercise training-induced coronary vascular adaptation. *J Appl Physiol* 73:2209, 1992.

39. Hussain S, Chatillon A, Comtois A, et al: Chemical activation of thin fiber phrenic afferents: 2. Cardiovascular responses. *J Appl Physiol* 70:77, 1991.

40. Pickar JG, Hill JM, Kaufman MP: Dynamic exercise stimulates group III muscle afferents. *J Neurophysiol* 71:753, 1994.

41. Rowell LB, O'Leary DS: Reflex control of the circulation during exercise: Chemoreflexes and mechanoreflexes. *J Appl Physiol* 69:407, 1990.

42. Rowell LB: *Human Cardiovascular Control* New York, Oxford University Press, 1993.

43. Guyton AC, Jones CE, Coleman TG: *Circulatory Physiology: Cardiac Output and Its Regulation,* 2d ed. Philadelphia, WB Saunders, 1973.

44. Brecher GA: *Venous Return* New York, Grune and Stratton, 1956.

45. Wexler L, Bergel DH, Gabe IT, et al: Velocity of blood flow in normal human venae cavae. *Circ Res* 23:349–359, 1968.

46. Giesbrecht GG, Ali F, Younes M: Short-term effect of tidal pleural pressure swings on pulmonary blood flow during rest and exercise. *J Appl Physiol* 71:465, 1991.

47. Williput R, Rondeux C, De Troyer A: Breathing affects venous return from legs in humans. *J Appl Physiol* 57:971, 1984.

48. Coast JR, Jensen RA, Cassidy SS, et al: Cardiac output and O₂ consumption during inspiratory threshold loaded breathing. *J Appl Physiol* 64:1624, 1988.

49. Babcock MA, Pegelow DF, McClaran SR, et al: Contribution of diaphragmatic power output to exercise-induced diaphragm fatigue. *J Appl Physiol* 78(5):1710–1719, 1995.

50. Babcock MA, Pegelow DF, Johnson BD, Dempsey JA: Aerobic fitness effects on exercise-induced low-frequency diaphragm fatigue. *J Appl Physiol* 8(5):2156–2164, 1996.

51. Johnson BD, Babcock MA, Suman OE, Dempsey JA: Exercise-induced diaphragmatic fatigue in healthy humans. *J Physiol (Lond)* 460:385–405, 1993.

52. Fitzgerald RS, Hauer MX, Bierkamper GG, Raff H: Responses of in vitro rat diaphragm to changes in acid base environment. *J Appl Physiol* 57:1202–1210, 1984.

53. Gladden B, Crawford R, Webster M: Effect of lactate concentration and metabolic rate on net lactate uptake. *Am J Physiol* 35:R1095–1101, 1994.

54. Johnson BD, Saupe KW, Dempsey JA: Mechanical constraints on exercise hyperpnea in endurance athletes. *J Appl Physiol* 73:874–886, 1992.

55. Dempsey JA, Hanson PG, Henderson K: Exercise-induced arterial hypoxemia in healthy humans at sea level. *J Physiol (Lond)* 355:161–175, 1984.

56. Schwartz J, Katz SA, Fegley RW, Tockman MS: Analysis of spirometic data from a national sample of healthy 6–24 year olds (NHANES II). *Am Rev Respir Dis* 121:339–342, 1980.

57. Thurlbeck WM: Postnatal human lung growth. *Thorax* 37:564–571, 1982.

58. Harms CA, McClaran SR, Nichele GA, Pegelow DF, Nelson WB, Dempsey JA: Exercise-induced arterial hypoxemia in healthy young women. *J Physiol* 507.2:619–628, 1998.

59. Johnson BD, Reddan WG, Seow KC, Dempsey JA: Mechanical constraints on exercise hyperpnea in an aging population. *Am Rev Respir Dis* 143:968–977, 1991.

60. Johnson BD, Badr MS, Dempsey JA: Impact of the aging pulmonary system on the response to exercise. *Clin Chest Med* 15(2):229–246, 1994.

61. Babcock MA, Johnson BD, Pegelow DF, et al: Hypoxic effects on exercise-induced diaphragmatic fatigue in normal healthy humans. *J Appl Physiol* 78(1):82–92, 1995.

62. Hanson P, Claremont A, Dempsey JA, Reddan WA: Determinants and consequences of ventilatory responses to competitive endurance running. *J Appl Physiol* 52:615–623, 1982.

PART II
PATHOPHYSIOLOGY

Chapter 8
PATHOPHYSIOLOGY OF ASTHMA

KENJI MINOGUCHI
MITSURU ADACHI

Bronchial asthma is characterized by persistent airway inflammation that is associated with increased airway responsiveness, airflow limitation, and respiratory symptoms. Although many different cells are involved in the pathogenesis of atopic asthma, CD4+ T cells play an important role in promoting airway inflammation by producing cytokines, such as interleukin (IL-4, IL-5, and IL-13). Mast cells are other important cells that initiate and maintain allergic inflammation; mast cells release histamine, leukotrienes, and prostaglandins after aggregation of its high affinity IgE receptors by allergen. This in turn is followed by release of cytokines including IL-4, IL-5, and tumor necrosis factor α (TNF-α). In nonatopic asthma, the precise mechanisms that induce allergic inflammation remain unknown, but analysis of bronchial tissue specimens by immunocytochemistry and in situ hybridization demonstrates that CD4+ T cells are also activated and produce IL-5. These allergic reactions result in the recruitment of eosinophils into the airway from the microvasculature through interaction with specific adhesion molecules, lead to airway epithelium damage, and enhance airway reactivity. Epithelial cells are thought to protect the airways from pathogens, but these cells also act as effector cells by secreting cytokines and chemokines. Remodeling of the airways might be caused by persistent activation of the repair process by transforming growth factor (TGF)-β and platelet derived growth factor (PDGF).

Introduction

In 1962 the Committee on Diagnostic Standards of the American Thoracic Society defined asthma as a disease characterized by an increased responsiveness of the trachea and bronchi to a wide variety of stimuli and manifested by widespread narrowing of the airway that changes in severity either spontaneously or as a result of therapy.

However, recent studies have revealed that asthma is a chronic inflammatory disorder of the airway that leads to airway hyperreactivity, airflow limitation, and respiratory symptoms as wheezing, coughing, and dyspnea.[1] The tissue specimens obtained from patients with asthma show an active process with mast cells, T cells, eosinophils, and neutrophils infiltrating the airway. Sequestration of epithelium, mucus plugs, and swelling of the airway are also characteristic features of asthma. Similar findings are observed even in asymptomatic patients.

In 1995, the Global Initiative for Asthma (GINA) proposed the following definition[2]:

1. Asthma—whatever the severity—is a chronic inflammatory disorder of the airway.
2. Airway inflammation is associated with airway hyperresponsiveness, airflow limitation, and respiratory symptoms.
3. Airway inflammation produces four forms of airflow limitation: acute bronchoconstriction, swelling of the airway wall, chronic mucus plug formation, and airway wall remodeling.
4. Atopy, the predisposition for developing an IgE-mediated response to common environmental allergens, is the strongest identifiable predisposing factor for developing asthma.
5. Considering asthma an inflammatory disorder has implications for the diagnosis, prevention, and management of the disorder.

Pathology of Asthma

Examination of specimens obtained postmortem demonstrate thickening of the airway wall from the trachea to the terminal bronchioles. The airways are occluded by mucus plugs, consisting of shed epithelial and inflammatory cells. Eosinophils and lymphocytes are found infiltrating the walls of the airway. Blood vessels are dilated.[3–6] Because of persistent airway inflammation, airway epithelium is lost and subepithelial fibrosis occurs with the deposition of collagen types III and V, as well as fibronectin.[7] Airway smooth muscle hypertrophy and hyperplasia of the mucous glands and goblet cells can be observed. The pathologic changes can be divided into reversible and irreversible changes. Airway remodeling leading to irreversible hypertrophy of the smooth muscle and subepithelial fibrosis is caused by chronic inflammation.

Recent evidences support the idea that activated eosinophils produce TGF-β and PDGF which contribute to the permanent change in the airway.[8,9] These irreversible changes are greater in severe asthma. Pathologic findings from postmortem specimens are described in Fig. 8-1.

Symptoms of Asthma

Wheezing, dyspnea, cough, and sputum are the major symptoms of asthma which arise from expiratory airflow limitations. Chronic asthmatic inflammation causes increased airway hyperresponsiveness, which is the characteristic of asthma. Furthermore, triggers such as an upper respiratory infection, inhalation of cold air, and specific allergens lead to the airway narrowing (Fig. 8-2). The many factors involved in airflow limitation including swelling of the airway, remodeling of the airway, chronic mucus plug formation, and airway smooth muscle contraction (Fig. 8-2).[1,2]

Airway Inflammation

A number of studies support the concept that asthma is a chronic inflammatory disorder.[10,11] Specimens obtained by

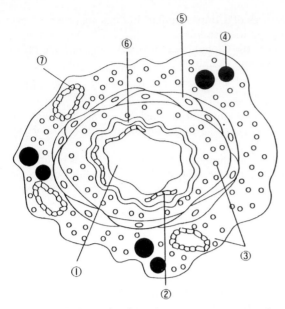

FIGURE 8-1 Pathology of asthma from post-mortem specimens. 1, mucus plug; 2, epithelial sequestration; 3, infiltration of inflammatory cells and edema; 4, congestion; 5, hypertrophy of airway smooth muscle; 6, thickening of basement membrane (subepithelial fibrosis); 7, hyperplasia of mucous gland and goblet cells.

bronchoscopy have provided additional information showing that there is distinct airway inflammation even in mild and subclinical asthma.[12-14] As in autopsy, the inflammatory processes include epithelial sloughing, edema, leukocyte infiltration, and mucus secretion.

Specimens from bronchoalveolar lavage and biopsy show that mast cells, T cells, eosinophils, epithelial cells, and macrophages are key inflammatory cells independent of whether asthma is atopic or nonatopic.[15] In atopic asthma CD4[+] T cells and mast cells play a central role in initiating and perpetuating airway inflammation. Possible mechanisms of airway inflammation in atopic asthma are summarized in Fig. 8-3.

Inflammatory Cells

MAST CELLS

The number of mast cells is increased in the bronchial epithelium, submucosa, and lung parenchyma in asthma. Mast cells release chemical mediators by allergen-IgE-mediated activation in atopic asthma.[16,17] Bronchoprovocation with sensitized allergen or instillation of allergen in segmental airways causes an immediate rise of histamine and tryptase released from stores in the mast cells.[18,19] In addition, mast cells generate and release, when activated, sulfidepeptide leukotrienes (LTs), LTC4, D4, E4, and thromboxane (TX)A$_2$.[20-22] Although these chemical mediators mainly contribute to bronchoconstriction, some of them also alter vascular permeability. The role of mast cells in chronic airway inflammation is not fully elucidated. However, some mediators work as chemotactic factors for eosinophils and neutrophils. Furthermore, recent reports suggest that mast cells generate cytokines, including IL-3, IL-4, IL-5, and granulo-

cyte macrophage–colony stimulating factor (GM-CSF).[16,23,24] In nonatopic asthma the exact mechanisms are not clear, but an increase in the number of mast cells and their activity in the airway have been reported.

T CELLS

CD4+ T cells can be divided into three subsets according to their profile of cytokine production, T helper (Th)0, Th1, and Th2 cells.[25-29] Th1 cells produce predominantly IFN-γ and are important in cell-mediated immunity. Th2 cells produce IL-4, IL-5, and IL-13 and are important in humoral immunity and allergy (Fig. 8-4). Th1 and Th2 cells are derived from common precursor cells which secrete only IL-2. These precursor cells differentiate into Th0 cells depending on environmental stimuli and then further differentiate into polarized Th1 or Th2 cells. Differentiation of precursor cells into distinct phenotypes of Th cells is influenced by the antigen type, antigen dose, types of antigen presenting cells, cytokines, and co-stimulatory molecules.[30-32] In atopic asthma there is an increase in the expression of messenger RNA of Th2 type cytokines such as IL-4 and IL-5 in CD4+ T cells. These findings suggest that Th2 cells are persistently activated and release Th2-type cytokines in the airway.[33-36] IL-4 and IL-13 help promote immunoglobulin (Ig)E synthesis. IL-5 activates eosinophils. In nonatopic asthma, an increase in the production of IL-5 but not IL-4 has been reported.[37] However, in another study, both IL-4 and IL-5 in the bronchial biopsy specimens were found from subjects with atopic as well as nonatopic asthma.[38] Further studies of the phenotype and function of T cells in nonatopic asthma are needed.

EOSINOPHILS

The presence of eosinophils in the airway is a characteristic feature of asthma, and indeed asthma has been termed *chronic*

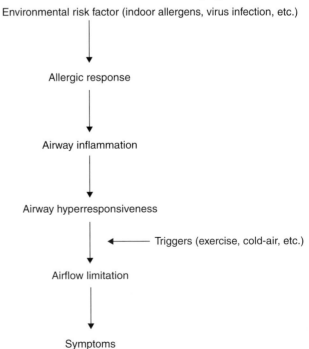

FIGURE 8-2 Mechanisms underlying asthma.

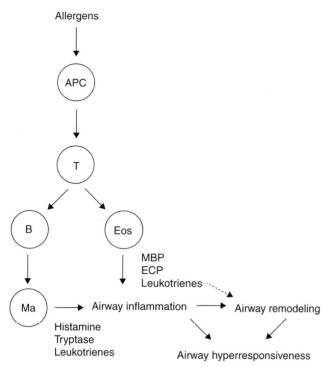

FIGURE 8-3 Mechanisms of airway inflammation in atopic asthma. APC, antigen-presenting cells; T, CD4+ T helper cells; B, B cells; Ma, mast cells; Eos, eosinophils.

eosinophilic bronchitis.[39,40] There is a close relationship between the number of eosinophils in peripheral blood, bronchoalveolar lavage, or biopsy specimen and the severity of asthma and the degree of airway hyperresponsiveness. Increases in eosinophil granule proteins, including eosinophil cationic protein (ECP), major basic protein (MBP), and eosinophil peroxidase (EPO) are also detected in specimens and may contribute to the airway epithelial damage.[41] Chemokines, such as RANTES, macrophage inflammatory protein (MIP)-1, and eotaxin, are involved in the recruitment of eosinophils into the airway.[42–45] Furthermore, eosinophils in active asthma are hypodense, and these cells may arise from the activation by cytokines like IL-3, IL-5, and GM-CSF or chemical mediators including LTC4 and platelet activating factor (PAF). Eosinophils themselves also produce these cytokines and chemical mediators. Recent studies revealed that these cytokines suppress the programmed cell death of eosinophils by apoptosis.[46]

NEUTROPHILS

Several animal studies indicate that neutophils are important in airway inflammation induced by ozone exposure and viral infection, but the role of neutrophils in human asthma is less certain. There seems to be an association between broncho-constriction and recruitment and activation of neutrophils in the airway in nocturnal asthma.[47] Analysis of bronchoalveolar lavage fluid revealed increased numbers of neurophils in sensitized subjects with asthma after allergen and diisocyanate challenges.[48–50] Neutrophils seem to be important for the exacerbation of asthma since they are present in large numbers in postmortem bronchial specimens, but in these cases airway infection, another cause of neutrophilia was not completely excluded.[51]

EPITHELIAL CELLS

Epithelial cell damage is associated with airway hyperresponsiveness.[52] A number of different insults such as virus infections, ozone exposure, and allergen exposure result in the epithelial disruption.[53,54] The release of MBP and oxygen derivatives from inflammatory cells leads to disruption of epithelial cells from airways. These cells then clump and form the so-called Creola body. Recent findings suggest that epithelial cells act not only as a barrier to external stimuli but also participate in the allergic inflammation by producing eicosanoids, neutral-endopeptidase degrading neuropeptides, as well as cytokines such as IL-6, IL-8, TNF-α, GM-CSF, TGF-β, and RANTES.[55–58] Eotaxin, one of the newly discovered chemokines, is also released and attracts eosinophils. An increase in eotaxin in bronchoalveolar lavage fluid and airway epithelium has been reported in asthma.[59]

MACROPHAGES

The marked increase in the number of macrophages in biopsy specimens and bronchoalveolar lavage fluid after allergen challenge suggests that these cells may play some important role in asthma.[60–62] When macrophages are activated, they release a variety of chemical mediators, including LTC4, prostaglandin (PG)F$_{2\alpha}$, TXB2, and PAF.[63] Furthermore these cells also produce IL-1, IL-8, IL-10, GM-CSF, and TNF-α.[64]

Another important role of macrophages is acting as antigen-presenting cells to T cells. In the airways, dendritic cells act more effectively as antigen-presenting cells than alveolar macrophages. Presence of certain cytokines such as IL-12 and IL-4 at the time of antigen presentation also affects phenotypic differentiation of naive T cells into Th1 or Th2 cells.

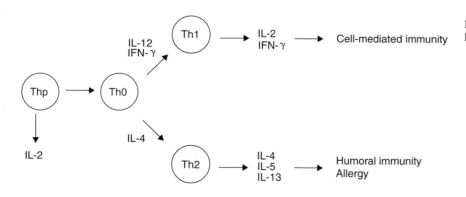

FIGURE 8-4 Differentiation of CD4+ T helper cells and their function.

Airway Remodeling

Chronic inflammation is associated with a healing process which results in repair and replacement of tissues.[65] Sometimes this leads to reconstitution of fibrosis. Chronic inflammation is characterized by proliferation of fibroblasts, angiogenesis, increase in connective tissue, and tissue destruction.[66–69] Inflammatory cells present in the chronic state produce TNF-α, IL-1, IL-6, IL-8, GM-CSF, TGF-β, PDGF, epidermal growth factor (EGF), fibronectin, and MIP-1. TGF-β and PDGF, which are mainly produced by eosinophils, seem to be closely associated with airway remodeling, especially in asthma.[8,9]

Pseudothickening of basement membrane caused by subepithelial fibrosis and hypertrophy of smooth muscle eventually occurs. Until recently this thickening of basement membrane was thought to be one of the characteristic features of asthma, but ultrastructural study and immunohistochemistry show that basement membrane thickness in asthmatic patients is actually normal. Immunohistochemistry indicates the deposition of immunoglobulins and collagen type III and IV and fibronectin in the subepithelial lesion.[7] A significant decrease in the pseudothickening of basement membrane has been reported by asthma treatment, although fibrotic changes are not affected.[70] Furthermore, tenascin, a component of the basement membrane, was also significantly reduced after treatment with inhaled glucocorticoids.[71]

Hypertrophy and hyperplasia of airway smooth muscle are part of remodeling. Studies in patients who died from an asthma exacerbation showed an increase in smooth muscle. Autopsy specimens revealed that muscles occupied up to 20 percent of the bronchial wall thickness.[72–75]

Chemical Mediators

Mediators released from inflammatory cells are responsible for the abnormal physiology of asthma.[76] A large number of potential candidate mediators seem to be important. Among these are lipid mediators produced from arachidonic acid like the cysteinyl LTs, TXA_2, and PAF. Arachidonic acid is released by the action of phospholipase A_2 in the cell membrane. It is subsequently metabolized by the enzyme cyclooxygenase to produce prostaglandins, or by 5-lipoxygenase to produce leukotrienes. Through another pathway platelet-activating factor is also produced from arachidonic acid.

Cysteinyl Leukotriene

Cysteinyl leukotrienes are potent bronchoconstrictive mediators both in vivo and in vitro and are important in asthma. Inhalation of LTD4 results in the bronchoconstriction and leads to an increase in airway responsiveness.[77,78] Eosinophil recruitment was observed after inhalation of LTE4 in asthmatic subjects.[79] LTs have other reactions including stimulation of afferent neurons, increasing microvascular permeability, stimulation of mucus secretion, stimulation of ion transport across epithelial cells, and promotion of smooth muscle proliferation (by LTD4). An increase in LTE4 in urine was reported in subjects with nocturnal asthma, suggesting that

LTs were released during the night.[80] Clinical studies using the LT receptor antagonist or the 5-lipoxygenase inhibitor have demonstrated the importance of LT in asthma. Treatment with these drugs inhibits both the early and late allergic reactions after inhaling allergen, exercise-induced asthma, aspirin-induced asthma, and cold-air–induced bronchoconstriction.[81,82] In addition, improvement of asthma symptoms, increased peak expiratory flow (PEF), and decreased usage of rescue medications and inhaled corticosteroids were reported.

Thromboxane and PAF

To investigate the role of TX and PAF, inhibitors for these mediators have been examined in asthma. Studies with a TXA_2 receptor antagonist or synthetase inhibitor resulted in slight but significant inhibition of allergen-induced early asthmatic response but failed to suppress late asthmatic response and allergen-induced airway hyperresponsiveness.[83] PAF receptor antagonists have also been examined in the study of allergen-induced asthma, but no inhibitory effect of this type of drug was reported.[84,85] These results suggest that TXA_2 and PAF do not play major roles in asthma.

Airway Hyperresponsiveness

The increased responsiveness of the airway to a wide variety of physical or chemical stimuli is a consistent feature of asthma. The factors that influence airway hyperresponsiveness are closely related to those that produce clinical symptoms. Airway hyperresponsiveness correlates closely with the severity of the asthma, and hence measurement of airway responsiveness is important in estimating the clinical severity of the asthma.[86] There are many studies which indicate a close relationship between genetic factors and airway hyperresponsiveness. Townley and coworkers studied the incidence of bronchial hyperresponsiveness and found that it occurred in the families in which the proband had asthma.[87] These studies suggest that familial and possible genetic factors influence the development of asthma. Postma and colleagues analyzed the genetic susceptibility to asthma and found that airway hyperresponsiveness was coinherited with a major gene for atopy.[88] On the other hand Ohe and coworkers reported that abnormality of β-adrenoceptor was associated with airway responsiveness.[89] Because airway tone is controlled by the balance of bronchoconstrictory and bronchodilatory factors, the dysfunction of β-adrenoceptor directly influences the airway responsiveness. Candidate genes for airway hyperresponsiveness may be discovered soon.

Another factor that determines airway hyperresponsiveness is airway inflammation.[90,91] In asthma, inflammatory cells release chemical mediators, such as PGs, LTs, and PAF.[92] These mediators themselves have potent bronchoconstrictory effect, but even lower when present in threshold, amounts increase responsiveness to other spasmogens. Damage of airway epithelium also affects the airway responsiveness by stimulating the c-fiber endings by an axon reflex that leads to the release of neuropeptides.[93] Airway remodeling is another important mechanism which can increase airway responsiveness.

Clinically, bronchial responsiveness is measured by the

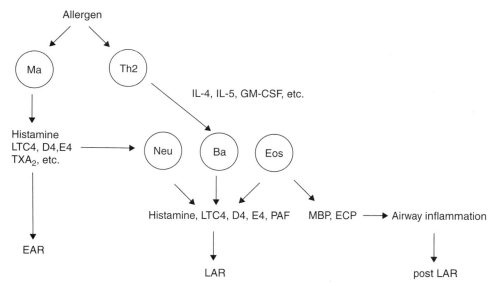

FIGURE 8-5 Allergen-induced EAR and LAR in atopic asthma.

inhalation of increasing concentrations of nonspecific spasmogens such as metacholine or histamine until FEV_1 is decreased by 20 percent of the baseline value. Results are expressed as the provocative concentration causing a 20 percent decrease in FEV_1 (PC_{20}).

Early Asthmatic Response (EAR) and Late Asthmatic Response (LAR)

Cross-linking of IgE on mast cells induces aggregation of high-affinity IgE receptor (FcϵRI) followed by the release of chemical mediators from those cells.[76] Early asthmatic response (EAR) occurs within a minute and continues to 1 to 2 h after allergen inhalation challenge. This acute phase bronchoconstriction usually disappears spontaneously. The chemical mediators released during EAR act to narrow airways, increase vascular permeability, and act as chemoattractants for inflammatory cells. Major mediators of bronchoconstriction are histamine, LTC4, D4, E4, PGD2, TXA$_2$, and PAF. Several cytokines such as TNF-α and IL-5 are also released that lead to the recruitment of eosinophils into the airway and induce late asthmatic response (LAR) that occurs 3 to 5 h after allergen inhalation in 50 to 60 percent of patients.[94] Allergen-specific T cells, especially Th2-type cells are activated and release IL-4, IL-5, and IL-13. IL-4 increases the expression of VCAM-1 on the endothelium which binds VLA-4 on eosinophils.[95,96] IL-5 and LTC4 attract eosinophils into the airway and then activate them to release mediators.[97,98] Eosinophil activation leads to the exacerbation of allergic inflammation, which continues after LAR for several days and is accompanied by an increase in the airway hyperresponsiveness (Fig. 8-5). Steroids are the most potent drug for the treatment of LAR, because they reduce the inflammatory reaction.

Factors that Influence the Acute Exacerbation of Asthma

It has been well known that respiratory infections, especially virus infection, are associated with the development and acute exacerbation of asthma.[99] Many have revealed that virus infections can lead to sensitization to aeroallergens, β-adrenergic blockade, increase in cytokine production by epithelial cells, stimulation of sensory nerves, and loss of epithelium-derived relaxing factors and enkephalinase degrading enzymes. These complex reactions exacerbate airway inflammation and enhance airway responsiveness. For example, experimental rhinovirus infection leads to asthmatic exacerbations.[100] Infection of epithelial cells with influenza virus in vitro results in the release of cytokines including IL-6, IL-8, GM-CSF, and RANTES into the culture supernatant and may explain airway eosinophilia after virus infection in vivo.[101]

Exercise, cold air inhalation, and alcohol drinking sometimes induce asthma. Physical factors which determine exercise-induced asthma (EIA) are the type, intensity, and duration of exercise. Furthermore, appearance of EIA depends on the temperature and humidity of inhaled air and the state of airway responsiveness. In addition, histamine, PGs, and LTs released from mast cells are involved in the induction of EIA.[102]

References

1. International Asthma Management Project (NHLBI, NIH): International consensus report on diagnosis and treatment of asthma. *Clin Exp Allergy* 22:S1, 1992.
2. NHLBI/WHO Workshop report: Global initiatives for asthma: Global strategy for asthma management and prevention. NIH Publication 95:3659, 1995.
3. Dunnill MS, Massarella GR, Anderson JA: A comparison of the quantitive anatomy on the bronchi in normal subjects, in status asthmaticus, in chronic bronchitis and emphysema. *Thorax* 24:176, 1969.
4. Arm JP, Lee TH: The pathobiology of bronchial asthma. *Adv Immunol* 51:323, 1992.
5. Dunnill MS: The pathology of asthma, with special reference to changes in the bronchial mucosa. *J Clin Pathol* 13:27, 1960.
6. Djukanovic R, Roche WR, Wilson JW, et al: Mucosal inflammation in asthma. *Am Rev Respir Dis* 142:434, 1990.
7. Roche WR, Beasley R, Williams JH, et al: Subepithelial fibrosis in the bronchi of asthmatics. *Lancet* 1:520, 1989.

8. Vignola AM, Chanez P, Chlappara G, et al: Transforming growth factors' expression in mucosal biopsies in asthma and chronic bronchitis. *Am J Respir Crit Care Med* 156:591, 1997.

9. Ohno T, Nilta Y, Yamaguchi K, et al: Eosinophils as a potential source of platelet-derived growth factor-B chain (PDGF-B) in nasal polyposis and bronchial asthma. *Am J Respir Cell Mol Biol* 13:639, 1996.

10. Poston RN, Chanez P, Lacoste JY, et al: Immunohistochemical characterization of the cellular infiltration in asthmatic bronchi. *Am Rev Respir Dis* 145:918, 1992.

11. Wardlaw AJ, Dunnette S, Gleich GJ, et al: Eosinophils and mast cells in bronchoalveolar lavage in subjects with mild asthma. *Am Rev Respir Dis* 137:62, 1988.

12. Beasley R, Roche WR, Roberts JA, et al: Cellular events in the bronchi in mild asthma and after bronchial provocation. *Am Rev Respir Dis* 139:806, 1989.

13. Laitinen LA, Laitinen A, Haatela T: Airway mucosal inflammation even in patients with newly diagnosed asthma. *Am Rev Respir Dis* 147:697, 1993.

14. Vignola AM, Chanez P, Campbell AM, et al: Airway inflammation in mild intermittent and in persistent asthma. *Am J Respir Crit Care Med* 157:403, 1998.

15. Busse WW, Calhoun WL, Sedgwick JD, et al: Mechanisms of airway inflammation in asthma. *Am Rev Respir Dis* 147:S20–S24, 1993.

16. Church MK, Levi-Schaffer F: The human mast cell. *J Allergy Clin Immunol* 99:155, 1997.

17. Marshall JS, Blenenstock J: The role of mast cells in inflammatory reactions of the airways, skin, and intestine. *Curr Opin Immunol* 6:853, 1994.

18. Agius R, Godfrey RC, Holgate ST: Mast cell and histamine content of human bronchoalveolar lavage fluid. *Thorax* 40:760, 1985.

19. Liu MC, Bleecker ER, Lichtenstein LM, et al: Evidence for elevated levels of histamine, prostaglandin D2, and other bronchoconstricting prostaglandins in the airways of subjects with mild asthma. *Am Rev Respir Dis* 142:126, 1990.

20. Lam S, Chan H, LeRiche JC, et al: Release of leukotrienes in patients with bronchial asthma. *J Allergy Clin Immunol* 81:711, 1988.

21. Hint KC, Leung KBP, Hudspith BN, et al: Bronchoalveolar mast cells in extrinsic asthma: A mechanism for the initiation of antigen specific bronchoconstriction. *Br Med J* 291:923, 1985.

22. Kirby JG, Hargreeve FE, Gleich GJ, et al: Bronchoalveolar lavage profiles of asthmatics and non asthmatic subjects. *Am Rev Respir Dis* 136:379, 1987.

23. Bradding P, Feather IH, Wilson S, et al: Immunolocalization of cytokines in the nasal mucosa of normal and perennial rhinitic subjects. The mast cell as a source of IL-4, IL-5, IL-6 in human allergic mucosal inflammation. *J Immunol* 151:3853, 1993.

24. Pawanker R, Okuda M, Yssel H, et al: Nasal mast cells in perennial allergic rhinitis exhibit increased expression of the FCεRI, CD40, IL-4, and IL-13, and can induce IgE synthesis in B cells. *J Clin Invest* 99:1492, 1997.

25. Mosmann TR, Coffman RL: TH1 and TH2 cells: Different patterns of lymphokine secretion lead to different functional properties. *Ann Rev Immunol* 7:145, 1989.

26. Wierenga EA, Snoek M, de Groot C, et al: Evidence for compartmentalization of functional subjects of CD4+ T-lymphocytes in atopic patients. *J Immunol* 144:4651, 1990.

27. Romagnani S: Lymphokine production by human T cells in disease states. *Annu Rev Immunol* 12:227, 1994.

28. Umetsu DT, DeKruyff RH: Th1 and Th2 CD4+ cells in human allergic diseases. *J Allergy Clin Immunol* 100:1, 1997.

29. Mosmann TR, Sad S: The expanding universe of T-cell subsets: Th1, Th2 and more. *Immunol Today* 17:138, 1996.

30. Hosken NA, Shibuya K, Heath AW, et al: The effect of antigen dose on CD4+ T helper cell phenotype development in a T cell receptor-alpha beta-transgenic model. *J Exp Med* 182:1579, 1995.

31. Gajewski TF, Pinnas M, Wong T, et al: Murine Th1 and Th2 clones proliferate optimally in response to distinct antigen-presentating cell populations. *J Immunol* 146:1750, 1991.

32. Thompson CB: Distinct role of the costimulatory ligands B7-1 and B7-2 in T helper cell differentiation? *Cell* 81:979, 1995.

33. Robinson DS, Hamid Q, Ying S, et al: Predominant TH2-like bronchoalveolar T-lymphocyte population in atopic asthma. *N Engl J Med* 3 26:298, 1992.

34. Ricci M, Rossi O, Bertoni M, et al: The importance of TH2-like cells in the pathogenesis of airway allergic inflammation. *Clin Exp Allergy* 23:360, 1993.

35. Corrigan CJ, Hartnell A, Kay AB: T lymphocyte activation in acute severe asthma. *Lancet* 1:1129, 1988.

36. Kay AB, Ying S, Vayney V, et al: Messenger RNA expression of the cytokine gene cluster, interleukin (IL)-3, IL-4, IL-5, and granulocyte/macrophage colony stimulating factor, in allergen-induced late-phase cutaneous reactions in atopic patients. *J Exp Med* 173:775, 1991.

37. Walker C, Bode E, Boer L, et al: Allergic and nonallergic asthmatics have distinct pattern of T cell activation and cytokine production in peripheral and bronchoalveolar lavages. *Am Rev Respir Dis* 146:109, 1992.

38. Humbert M, Durham SR, Ying S, et al: IL-4 and IL-5 mRNA and protein in bronchial biopsies from patients with atopic and nonatopic asthma: Evidence against intrinsic asthma being a distinct immunopathologic entity. *Am J Crit Care Med* 154:1497, 1996.

39. Weller PF: Human eosinophils. *J Allergy Clin Immunol* 100:283, 1997.

40. Bousquet J, Chanez P, Lacoste JY: Eosinophilic inflammation in asthma. *N Engl J Med* 323:1033, 1990.

41. Gleich GJ, Flavahan NA, Fujisawa T, et al: The eosinophil as a mediator of damage to respiratory epithelium: A model for bronchial hyperreactivity. *J Allergy Clin Immunol* 81:776, 1988.

42. Baggiolini M, Dahinden CA: CC chemokines in allergic inflamation. *Immunol Today* 15:127, 1994.

43. Rot A, Krieger M, Brunner T, et al: RANTES and macrophage inflammatory protein 1 alpha induce the migration and activation of normal human eosinophil granulocytes. *J Exp Med* 176:1489, 1992.

44. Jose PJ, Adcock IM, Griffiths-Johnson DA, et al: Cloning of an eosinophil chemoattractant cytokine and increased mRNA expression in allergen-challenged guinea-pig lungs. *Biochem Biophys Res Commun* 205:788, 1994.

45. Moqbel R, Hamid Q, Ying S, et al: Expression of mRNA and immunoreactivity for the granulocyte/macrophage colony-stimulating factor in activated human eosinophils. *J Exp Med* 174:749, 1991.

46. Woolley KL, Gibson PG, Carty K, et al: Eosinophil apoptosis and resolution of airway inflammation in asthma. *Am J Respir Crit Care Med* 154:237, 1996.

47. Kraft M, Torvik JA, Trudeau JB, et al: Theophylline: Potential anti-inflammatory effects in nocturnal asthma. *J Allergy Clin Immunol* 97:1242, 1996.

48. Fabbri LM, Boschetto P, Zocca E, et al: Bronchoalveolar neutrophilia during late asthmatic reactions induced by toluene diisocyanate. *Am Rev Respir Dis* 136:36, 1987.

49. Kraft M, Pak BS, Borish M, et al: Theophylline's effect on neutrophil function and the late asthmatic response. *J Allergy Clin Immunol* 98:251, 1996.

50. Diaz PC, Gonzalez MC, Galleguilos FR, et al: Leukocytes and mediators in bronchoalveolar lavage during allergen-induced late-phase asthmatic reactions. *Am Rev Respir Dis* 139:1383, 1989.

51. Fahy JV, Kim KW, Liu J, et al: Predominant neutrophilic inflammation in sputum from subjects with asthma exacerbation. *J Allergy Clin Immunol* 95:843, 1995.

52. Laitinen LA, Heino M, Laitinen A, et al: Damage of the airway epithelium and bronchial reactivity in patients with asthma. *Am Rev Respir Dis* 131:599, 1985.

53. Laitinen LA, Heino M, Laitinen A, et al: Damage of the airway epithelium and bronchial respiratory tract in patients with asthma. *Am Rev Respir Dis* 131:599, 1985.

54. Lozewicz S, Wells C, Gomez E, et al: Morphological integrity of the bronchial epithelium in mild asthma. *Thorax* 45:12, 1990.

55. Hunter JA, Finkbeiner WE, Nadel JA, et al: Predominant generation of 15-lipoxygenase metabolites of arachidonic acid by epithelial cells from human trachea. *Proc Natl Acad Sci USA* 82: 4633, 1985.

56. Cromwell O, Hamid Q, Corrigan CJ, et al: Expression and generation of interleukin-8, IL-6, and granulocyte-macrophage colony-stimulating factor by bronchial epithelial cells and enhanced by IL-1 beta and tumor necrosis factor. *Immunology* 77:330, 1992.

57. Alam R, York J, Boyars M, et al: The involvement of chemokines in bronchial asthma. The detection of mRNA for MCP-1, MCP-3, RANTES and MIP-1 in the lavage fluid. *Am J Respir Crit Care Med* 149:A951, 1994.

58. Spriggs DR, Imamura K, Rodriguez C, et al: Tumor necrosis factor expression in human epithelial tumor cell lines. *J Clin Invest* 81:455, 1988.

59. Rothenberg ME, Luster AD, Lilly CM, et al: Constitutive and allergen-induced expression of eotaxin mRNA in the guinea pig lung. *J Exp Med* 181:1211, 1995.

60. Godard P, Chaintreuil J, Damon M, et al: Functional assessment of alveolar macrophages: Comparison of cells from asthmatics and normal subjects. *J Allergy Clin Immunol* 70:88, 1982.

61. Unanue ER, Allen PM: The basis for the immunoregulatory role of macrophages and other accessory cells. *Science* 236:551, 1987.

62. Viksman MY, Liu MC, Bickel CA, et al: Phenotypic analysis of alveolar macrophages and monocytes in allergic airway inflammation. 1. Evidence for the activation of alveolar macrophages, but not peripheral blood monocytes, in subjects with allergic rhinitis and asthma. *Am J Respir Crit Care Med* 155: 858, 1997.

63. Rankin JA, Hitchcock M, Merrill W, et al: IgE-dependent release of leukotriene C4 from alveolar macrophages. *Nature* 297:329, 1982.

64. Gant VA, Cluzel M, Shakoor Z, et al: Alveolar macrophage accessory cell function in bronchial asthma. *Am Rev Respir Dis* 146:900, 1992.

65. Rennard SI: Repair mechanisms in asthma. *J Allergy Clin Immunol* 98:S278, 1996.

66. Rennard SI: Extracellular matrix. *Am J Respir Crit Care Med* 153:S14, 1996.

67. Roche WR: Fibloblast and asthma. *Clin Exp Allergy* 21:545, 1991.

68. Brewster CEP, Howarth PH, Djukanovic R, et al: Myofibroblasts and epithelial fibrosis in bronchial asthms. *Am J Resp Cell Mol Biol* 3:507, 1990.

69. Gauldie J, Jordana M, Cox G, et al: Fibloblast and other structural cells in airway inflammation. *Am Rev Respir Dis* 145:S14, 1992.

70. Oliviell D, Chetta A, Donno MD, et al: Effect of short-term treatment with low-dose inhaled fluticasone propionate on airway inflammation and remodeling in mild asthma: A placebo-controlled study. *Am J Respir Crit Care Med* 155:1864, 1997.

71. Laitinen A, Altraja A, Kampe M, et al: Tenascin is increased in airway basement membrane of asthmatics and decreased by an inhaled steroid. *Am J Respir Crit Care Med* 156:951, 1997.

72. Heard BE, Hossain S: Hyperplasia of bronchial muscle in asthma. *J Pathol* 110:319, 1973.

73. Takizawa T, Thurlbeck WM: Muscle and mucus gland size in the major bronchi of patients with chronic bronchitis, asthma and asthmatic bronchitis. *Am Rev Respir Dis* 104:331, 1971.

74. James AL, Pare PD, Hogg JC: The mechanisms of airway narrowing. *Am Rev Respir Dis* 139:242, 1989.

75. Wiggs BR, Moreno R, Hogg JC, et al: A model of the mechanics of airway narrowing. *J Appl Physiol* 69:849, 1990.

76. Bames PJ, Chung KF, Page CP: Inflammatory mediators and asthma. *Pharmacol Rev* 40:49, 1988.

77. Kaye MG, Smith LJ: Effect of inhaled leukotriene D4 and platelet activating factor on airway reactivity in normal subjects. *Am Rev Respir Dis* 141:993, 1990.

78. Diamant Z, Hiltermann JT, van Rensen EL, et al: The effect of inhaled leukotriene D4 and methacholine on sputum cell differentials in asthma. *Am J Respir Crit Care Med* 155:1247, 1997.

79. Arm JP, Spur BW, Lee TH: The effect of inhaled leukotriene E4 on the airway responsiveness to histamine in subjects with asthma and normal subjects. *J Allergy Clin Immunol* 82:654, 1988.

80. Bellia V, Bonanno A, Cibella F, et al: Urinary leukotriene E4 in the assessment of nocturnal asthma. *J Allergy Clin Immunol* 97:735, 1996.

81. Taylor IK, O'Shaughnessy KM, Fuller RW, et al: Effect of cysteinyl-leukotriene receptor antagonist ICI 204,219 on allergen-induced bronchoconstriction and airway hyperreactivity in atopic subjects. *Lancet* 337:690, 1991.

82. Manning PJ, Watson RM, Margolskee DJ, et al: Inhibition of exercise-induced bronchoconstriction by MK-571, a potent leukotriene D4-receptor antagonist. *N Engl Med* 323:1736, 1990.

83. Beasley RCW, Fetherstone RL, Church MK, et al: Effect of a thromboxane receptor antagonist on PGD2- and allergen-induced bronchoconstriction. *J Appl Physiol* 66:1685, 1989.

84. Freitag A, Watson RW, Matsos G, et al: The effect of a platelet activating factor antagonist, WEB2086, on allergen-induced asthmatic responses. *Thorax* 48:594, 1993.

85. Kultert LM, Hui KP, Uthayakumar S, et al: Effect of a platelet activating factor (PAF) antagonist, UK 74,505 on allergen-induced early and late responses. *Am Rev Respir Dis* 147:82, 1993.

86. Josephs LK, Gregg I, Mullee MA, et al: Non-specific bronchial reactivity and its relationship to the clinical expression of asthma. *Am Rev Respir Dis* 140:350, 1989.

87. Townley RG, Bewtra A, Wilson AF, et al: Segregation analysis of bronchial response to methacholine inhalation challenge in families with and without asthma. *J Allergy Clin Immunol* 77: 101, 1986.

88. Postma DS, Bleecker ER, Amelung PJ, et al: Genetic susceptibity to asthma: Bronchial hyperresponsiveness coinherited with a major gene for atopy. *N Engl J Med* 333:894, 1995.

89. Ohe M, Munakata M, Hizawa N, et al: β2-adrenergic receptor gene restriction fragment length polymorphism and bronchial asthma. *Thorax* 50:353, 1995.

90. Chung KF: Role of inflammation in the hyperresponsiveness. *Thorax* 41:657, 1986.

91. O'Byrne PM, Hargreeve FE, Kirby JG: Airway inflammation and hyperresponsiveness. *Am Rev Respir Dis* 136:S35, 1987.

92. Kelly CA, Ward C, Stenton SC, et al: Numbers and activity of cells obtained at bronchoalveolar lavage in asthma, and their relationship to airway responsiveness. *Thorax* 43:684, 1988.

93. Bames PJ: Asthma as an axon reflex. *Lancet* 1:242, 1986.

94. Pelikan Z, Pelikan-Filipek M: The late asthmatic response to allergen challenge—Part 1. *Ann Allergy* 56:414, 1986.

95. Bochner BS, Luscinskas FW, Gimbrone MA, et al: Adhesion of human basophils, eosinophils, and neutrophils to IL-1 activated human vascular endothelial cell: Contributions of endothelial cells adhesion molecules. *J Exp Med* 173:1553, 1991.

96. Bentley AM, Durham Sr, Robinson DS, et al: Expression of endothelial and leukocyte adhesion molecules intracellular adhesion molecule-1, E-selectin, and vascular cell adhesion molecule-1 in the bronchial mucosa in steady state and allergen-induced asthma. *J Allergy Clin Immunol* 92:857, 1993.

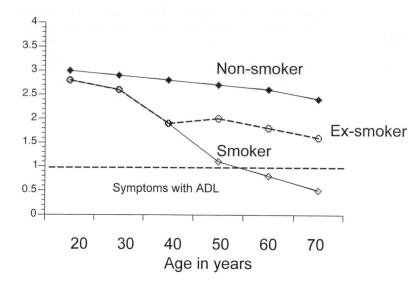

FIGURE 9-1 Changes in forced expiratory volume in 1 s (FEV₁) over time. Notice the gradual decline in normal subjects. In contrast susceptible smokers manifest a steeper decline and reach levels that are clinically significant at a relatively young age. Smoking cessation is associated with some recovery of lung function and an interruption in the decline of FEV₁.

chronic bronchitis and occasionally with bronchiectasis. Patients may also have increased frequency of nonspecific airway hyperactivity. The onset of disease is accelerated by smoking. Dyspnea begins at a median age of 40 years in smokers and 50 years in nonsmokers who develop disease. Not all patients with AAT levels below threshold will go on to emphysema, especially if they are not exposed to cigarettes or pollution. Patients should be screened for AAT deficiency if they present with premature onset of COPD (before age 50), predominance of basilar emphysema (by radiographs), presence of nonremitting asthma in a young person, and cirrhosis without apparent risk factors.

Natural History of COPD

The decline in lung function with age is shown in Fig. 9-1. Normal nonsmokers lose between 25 to 35 mL yearly. The rate of decline is steeper for smokers than for nonsmokers.[9] The heavier the smoking, the steeper the decline, likewise the lower the initial FEV₁, the faster will FEV₁ drop. Patients with COPD will manifest decreases in FEV₁ of around 90 mL a year. This decline can be reversed after smoking cessation. The Lung Health Study showed the important observation that patients who stopped smoking had a mean post-bronchodilator FEV₁ increase of 57 mL at the first annual visit compared with a mean FEV₁ decline of 38 mL for those who continued to smoke.[10] This indicates that not only will the decline decrease, but lung function may actually improve after smoking cessation. It is clear that the natural rate of decline accelerates dramatically in susceptible smokers. The rate of decline returns toward normal soon after smoking cessation in most patients. As is seen in Fig. 9-1, the development of symptoms with minimal activities will occur much earlier in current than in former smokers.

Clinical Features

HISTORY

The typical patient with COPD has usually been smoking more than 20 pack-years before symptoms develop. Patients commonly present with productive cough or an acute chest illness in their fifth decade. Dyspnea usually does not occur until the sixth or seventh decade, but it may become the dominant feature. When severe, dyspnea may be crippling and lead to severe deconditioning as ever less intense exercise precipitates worsening of the symptom. This vicious cycle is one of the most important problems in patients with advanced COPD.

Sputum initially occurs only in the morning and is usually mucoid. Over time, and especially during exacerbations, it may become purulent. Acute chest illnesses characterized by increased cough, purulent sputum, wheezing, dyspnea, and occasionally fever may occur intermittently. The history of wheezing and dyspnea may lead to the erroneous diagnosis of asthma.

As the disease progresses, the intervals between exacerbations shorten. Late in the course, the patient may develop hypoxemia, which if severe enough may result in clinical cyanosis; later the disease is accentuated by erythrocytosis. The occurrence of morning headache suggests hypercapnia. Weight loss occurs in some patients. Cor pulmonale with right heart failure and edema may develop in patients with hypoxemia and hypercapnia. Most episodes of hemoptysis are due to mucosal erosion and not to carcinoma. However, since bronchogenic carcinoma occurs with increased frequency in smokers with COPD, an episode of hemoptysis raises the possibility that a carcinoma has developed and it should prompt an evaluation to rule out this possibility.

PHYSICAL EXAMINATION

At the beginning, physical examination of the chest may show wheezes only on forced expiration. As obstruction progresses, hyperinflation becomes evident and the anteroposterior diameter of the chest increases. The diaphragm is depressed and limited in its motion. Breath sounds are decreased at this stage, and heart sounds often become distant. Coarse crackles are often heard at the lung bases. An excessively prolonged forced expiratory time (more than 4 s with the stethoscope over the trachea) may be seen in patients with a significant degree of airflow limitation.

The patient with end-stage COPD may adopt positions which relieve dyspnea, such as leaning forward, with arms outstretched and weight supported on the palms. The accessory respiratory muscles of the neck and shoulder girdle are in full use. Expiration often takes place through pursed lips. Paradoxical indrawing of the lower interspaces is a classic finding, first described by William Stokes in 1837. Cyanosis may be present. An enlarged tender liver indicates heart failure. Neck vein distention, especially during expiration, may be observed in the absence of heart failure because of increased intrathoracic pressure. Asterixis may be seen with severe hypercapnia.

Laboratory Findings

CHEST RADIOGRAPHY

Since emphysema is defined in anatomic terms, posteroanterior and lateral chest roentgenogram provides evidence of its presence.[11] Overdistention is indicated by a low, flat diaphragm; an increased retrosternal airspace; and a long, narrow heart shadow. Rapid tapering of the vascular shadows accompanied by hypertransparency of the lungs is a sign of emphysema; bullae, presenting as radiolucent areas larger than 1 cm in diameter and surrounded by arcuate hairline shadows, are proof of its presence. However, bullae reflect only locally severe disease and are not necessarily indicative of widespread emphysema. Studies correlating lung structure and the chest radiograph show that emphysema is consistently diagnosed when the disease is severe, is not diagnosed when the disease is mild, and is diagnosed in about half the instances when moderate.

Right ventricular hypertrophy does not result in cardiomegaly in COPD. Comparison with previous chest radiographs may show the enlargement. The hilar vascular shadows are prominent, and the heart shadow encroaches on the retrosternal space as the right ventricle enlarges anteriorly. Lung cancer and heart disease are associated with the same risk factor as COPD, namely, smoking. Therefore, a chest roentgenogram is indicated not only to find evidence of emphysema but equally important to rule out the presence of any of the diseases that may present with similar symptoms.

COMPUTERIZED TOMOGRAPHY

Computerized tomography (CT), especially high-resolution CT scan (collimation of 1 to 2 mm), has much greater sensitivity and specificity than standard chest radiography.[12] It may identify the specific anatomic type of emphysema. However, since this rarely alters therapy, CT has no place in the routine care of patients with COPD. It is the main imaging tool for evaluating the benefit of pulmonary resection for giant bullous disease and for diagnosing bronchiectasis. It also is gaining ground as a good tool to evaluate potential candidates for lung volume reduction surgery.

Pathophysiologic Effects of COPD

Functionally, COPD is characterized by decrease in airflow which is more prominent on maximal efforts. The airflow limitation is not uniform in nature. This causes uneven distribution of ventilation and blood perfusion,[13-15] which in turn

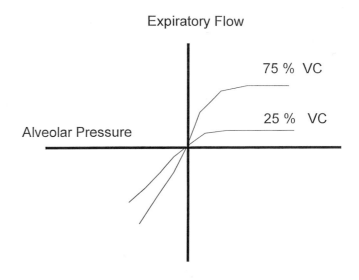

FIGURE 9-2 Inspiratory flow is proportional to inspiratory pressure. In contrast, expiratory flow at any given lung volume (expressed in this graph as percent of the vital capacity) does not increase with increasing expiratory pressure.

results in arterial hypoxemia (decreased Pa_{O_2}). If overall ventilation is decreased, as occurs in the most severe cases, Pa_{CO_2} will increase. In those patients with an important component of emphysema or bullous disease, total lung volume increases, resulting in hyperinflation. Each of these interrelated elements is important in the adaptive changes seen in these patients. Their presence helps explain the clinical manifestations of the disease. The relationship between structure and function in COPD is not well understood. Whether due to loss of attachments or tethering forces and/or due to inflammation and mucous secretions, patients with COPD have decreased airflow.

To move air in and out, the bellows must force air through the conducting airways. The resistance to flow is given by the interaction of air molecules with each other and with the internal surface of the airways. Therefore, airflow resistance depends on the physical property of the gas and the length and diameter of the airways. For a constant diameter, flow is proportional to the applied pressure. This relationship holds true on normals for inspiratory flow measured at fixed lung volume as shown in Fig. 9-2. In contrast, expiratory flow is linearly related to the applied pressure only during the early portion of the maneuver. Beyond a certain point, flow does not increase despite further increase in driving pressure. This flow limitation is due to the dynamic compression of airways as force is applied around them during forced expirations. This can be readily understood in the commonly determined flow-volume expression of the vital capacity. The left panel of Fig. 9-3 shows the flow-volume loop of a normal individual. It is clear that as effort increases, expiratory flow increases up to a certain point (outer envelope), beyond which further efforts result in no further increase in flow. During tidal breathing (inner tracing) only a small fraction of the maximal flow is used, and therefore flow is not limited under these circumstances. In contrast the flow-volume loop of patients with COPD is markedly different as shown in

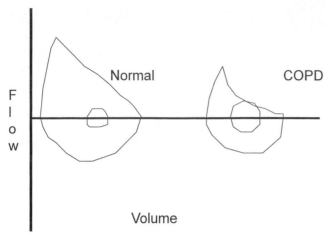

FIGURE 9-3 Flow-volume loops of a normal person (*left panel*), and that of a patient with COPD (*right panel*). Notice that patients with severe COPD may reach airflow limitation even during tidal breathing.

the right panel of Fig. 9-3. The expiratory portion of the curve is caved out. This shape is due to the lower flow at each lung volume, since the decreased diameter of the intrathoracic airways is reduced even more during forced exhalation. The airflow limitation can be so severe that it can be reached even during tidal breathing, as represented in this diagram. A patient so afflicted cannot increase flow with increased ventilatory demand. As is seen later, increased demands can be met only by increased respiratory rate, which in turn is detrimental to the expiratory time, a crucial problem in patients with COPD.

The precise reason for the development of airflow obstruction in COPD is not entirely clear, but it may very likely be multifactorial. In pure emphysema, destruction of the tissue around the airways decreases the forces that act to keep the airways open.[16] In those patients with a component of airway inflammation, the problem is compounded by intrinsic narrowing of the airways.[8,17,18] As shown above, the obstruction is physiologically more evident during exhalation. Therefore, COPD has been thought to be a problem of "expiration." This is not entirely correct because inspiration is also affected. Inspiratory resistance is increased, and more importantly, the inability to expel the inhaled air coupled with parenchymal destruction leads to static and dynamic hyperinflation.[19,20]

HYPERINFLATION

As the parenchymal destruction of emphysema progresses, the distal air spaces enlarge. The loss of the lung elastic recoil resulting from this destruction increases resting lung volume. In a pervasive way the loss of elastic recoil and airway attachments narrows even more the already constricted airways. The decrease in airway diameter increases resistance to airflow and worsens the obstruction. Decreased lung elastic recoil, therefore, is a major contributor of airway narrowing in emphysema.[19,21,22] Since in most patients the distribution of emphysema is not uniform, portions of lung with low elastic recoil may coexist with portions with more normal elastic recoil. It follows that ventilation to each of those portions will not be uniform. This helps explain some of the differences in gas exchange. It also explains why reduction

of the uneven distribution of recoil pressures by procedures that resect more afflicted lung areas (bullectomy) results in better ventilation of the remainder of the lung and improved gas exchange.

When breathing frequency increases, hyperinflation worsens.[19,23] The reason is that expiratory time shortens, even if patients simultaneously shorten their inspiratory time. The resulting "dynamic" hyperinflation is very detrimental to lung mechanics and helps explain many of the clinical findings associated with higher ventilatory demand, such as is seen during exercise.

ALTERATION IN GAS EXCHANGE

Based on the uneven distribution of airway obstruction and emphysema, it becomes easier to understand the changes in blood gases. The lungs of a patient with COPD can be modeled as composed of two portions: one more emphysematous and obstructed and another more normal one. The pressure-volume curve of the emphysematous lung is displaced up and to the left compared with that of the normal lung (Fig. 9-4). At low lung volume the more emphysematous portion of the lung undergoes greater volume changes than the normal lung. In contrast, at higher lung volume, the emphysematous lung is overinflated and accepts less volume change than the normal lung. Therefore, the distribution of ventilation depends on the relative differences of the pressure-volume relationship and the difference in pressure acting on each region. The emphysematous and bullous areas of the lung are underventilated compared with the normal lung. Because perfusion is even more compromised than ventilation in these areas, they have a high ventilation/perfusion ratio and behave as dead space. Indeed, this wasted ventilation portion (V_D/V_T) corresponds with approximately 0.3 to 0.4 of a tidal breath in a normal person, whereas it has been measured to

FIGURE 9-4 Pressure-volume relationship in portions of "normal" and "emphysematous" lung. At low lung volume (*A*), small changes in pressure cause a larger volume change in the emphysematous lung. In contrast, at higher lung volume (*B*), similar changes in pressure result in minimal changes in volume in the emphysematous lung. This portion will behave as if it were "restricted," and larger pressure changes are needed to produce airflow.

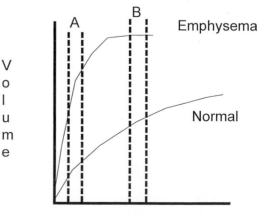

be higher in patients with severe emphysema.[24] At the same time, narrower bronchi in other areas may not allow appropriate ventilation to reach relatively well perfused areas of the lung. This low ventilation/perfusion ratio contributes to venous admixture and hypoxemia.[15,25]

Because of the increased work of breathing, the patient with emphysema must attempt to increase ventilation to deliver the oxygen demanded by the working respiratory muscles. Alveolar ventilation must also be sufficient to eliminate the produced CO_2. If this does not occur, Pa_{CO_2} will increase. Indeed, the arterial blood-gas changes over time in patients with COPD parallel this sequence. Initially Pa_{O_2} progressively decreases but is compensated by increased ventilation. When the ventilation is insufficient, the Pa_{CO_2} rises sometimes to levels that further compromise oxygenation.[4] Therefore, severe hypoxemia and the presence of hypercarbia are ominous changes that confer a poor prognosis to patients who manifest it.[26]

Control of Ventilation in COPD

As mentioned above, for gas exchange to occur it is necessary to move air in and out of the lung. This is done by the respiratory pump, which is composed of the respiratory centers; the nerves that carry the signals from those centers; the respiratory muscles, which are the pressure generating structures; and the rib cage and abdomen. These components are linked and ordinarily function in a well orchestrated manner, whereby ventilation goes unnoticed and utilizes very little energy.[27,28]

The central controller, or respiratory center, is located in the upper medulla and integrates input from the periphery, specific chemoreceptors, and other parts of the nervous system.[29] The output of this generator is modulated not only by mechanical, cortical, and sensory input but also by the state of oxygenation (Pa_{O_2}), CO_2 concentration, and acidemia (pH). Once generated, the output is distributed by the conducting nerves to the respiratory muscles, which shorten, deform the rib cage and abdomen, and generate intrathoracic pressures. These pressure changes displace volume, and air moves in and out depending on the direction of the pressure changes. The relation between "drive" and inspiratory pressure or volume is referred to as *coupling*. Coupling is usually smooth and occurs with minimal effort. This is the reason breathing is perceived as effortless. Whenever the act of breathing requires effort and this "effort" is perceived as "work," the symptom is labeled dyspnea. The interaction between the central drive (controller output) and the final output (ventilation) is complex and involves many components.[30,31] This complexity renders it very difficult to ascribe dyspnea to any individual portion of the system and is also the reason dyspnea is the most frequent symptom reported by patients with important airflow obstruction.

Ventilatory control can be assessed at different levels. The simplest is the minute ventilation (VE), which reflects the final effectiveness of the ventilatory drive. Further insight can be obtained by measuring the two contributors to VE, the tidal volume (VT) represented by the volume of air inhaled in a breath and the respiratory frequency, or breathing rate. Analysis of these variables in COPD reveals that as the disease progresses, VE increases.[31] This is expected, since the need to keep oxygen uptake and CO_2 removal constant is challenged by the changes in lung mechanics leading to increased impedance and by worsening ventilation/perfusion coupling. The increase in VE is achieved first by an increase in VT, but as the resistive work due to airflow obstruction worsens, tidal volume decreases (right panel in Fig. 9-5). At this point respiratory rate increases[32] (left panel in Fig. 9-6), a feature that is detrimental because it leads to shortened expiratory time with all its consequences.

The VE can also be expressed in terms of the mean inspiratory flow rate. This is obtained by relating the VT to the inspiratory time (VT/TI) and the fractional duration of inspiration (TI/Ttot). VT/TI reflects drive, and TI/Ttot reflects timing. Both are affected by the need to increase VE in COPD.

A relatively noninvasive way to measure central drive is the mouth occlusion pressure measured 0.1 s after the onset of inspiration ($P_{0.1}$).[33] With increased drive the increase in $P_{0.1}$ is higher than that of VT/TI.[34] This is due to airflow impedance that decreases mean inspiratory flow measured at the mouth compared with $P_{0.1}$, which is measured in conditions of no airflow. $P_{0.1}$ has been shown to increase as the degree of obstruction worsens (Fig. 9-6). It is clear that the central drive increases as the degree of airflow obstruction progresses, reaching its maximum in patients in respiratory failure.[35-37]

The drive is effectively "coupled" to increased VT in the early stages of obstruction, but VT actually drops, as the work to move air becomes very high. The only alternative left is to increase respiratory rate. This also occurs, but as determined by the flow limitation characteristics of these patients, this adaptive phenomenon may result in further hyperinflation. As described earlier, hyperinflation displaces diseased portions of lung higher in their pressure/volume relationship. This effectively turns many portions of the lung to behave as "restrictive" tissue. At this point, respiration is least demanding (in terms of work or pressure changes) when a fast and shallower ventilatory pattern is achieved. This indeed is the observed pattern in patients with the most severe COPD,[32,37] as shown in Figs. 9-4 and 9-5. This situation has important negative consequences on the respiratory muscles and mechanics of rib cage and abdomen that are discussed later.

Respiratory Muscles

Breathing depends on the coordinated action of different groups of muscles. The respiratory muscles can be divided into those that help inflate the lungs (inspiratory) and those that have an expiratory action. In addition, there are upper airway muscles (tongue and muscles of the palate, of the pharynx, and of the vocal cords), the function of which is to contract at the beginning of inspiration and hold the upper airways open through the inhalatory phase. Although very important in function, they play a limited role in pure COPD and are not discussed further.

The diaphragm and the other inspiratory muscles are innervated by a wide array of motoneurons that range from cranial nerve XI (C-11) to lumbar roots L2–3. The respiratory cycle is regulated by a complex series of centrally organized neurons. This complex arrangement maintains rhythmic breathing that usually goes unnoticed, but can be voluntarily

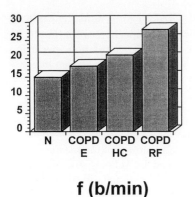

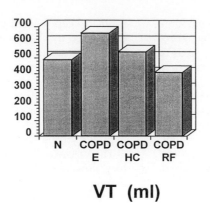

f (b/min)   VT (ml)

FIGURE 9-5 As COPD progresses and work of breathing increases, respiratory frequency increases (*left panel*) whether the panel is eucapnic (E), hypercapnic (H) or in respiratory failure (RF). In contrast, tidal volume (VT) initially increases, but as the disease progresses and the overall impedance worsens, VT decreases, reaching its lowest value during respiratory failure.

overridden by cortical connections. This unique feature of the respiratory system can be used to modulate and change the breathing pattern when under conditions of physiologic demand the system has responded in a primitive way. Indeed, some of the techniques that are thought to benefit patients with symptomatic severe COPD, such as pursed lips breathing and breathing retraining, are aimed at using the cortex to influence the breathing pattern.

The most important inspiratory muscle is the diaphragm.[35] It is well suited to perform its work because of its anatomic arrangement and histochemical composition. Its long fibers extend from the noncontractile central tendon and are directed down and outward to insert circumferentially in the lower ribs and upper lumbar spine. This concave shape allows the muscle its lifting action as the fibers contract. The diaphragm can shorten up to 40 percent between full expiration and end inspiration.[38] During quiet breathing, it accounts for most of the force needed to displace the rib cage. Other inspiratory muscles, the scalene and parasternal intercostal, are also agonists during quiet breathing and contribute to inspiratory effort. There are yet other muscles (truly accessory in nature) that are not active during quiet breathing in normal subjects, but may contribute to ventilation in situations of increased demand. Muscles such as the sternomas-

toid, pectoralis minor, latissimus dorsi, and trapezius are some of these truly "accessory" muscles.[27,28]

The abdominal muscles are expiratory in action, since their contractions will decrease lung volume.[39] Inasmuch as they provide tone to the abdominal wall, they help the diaphragm, since they contribute to the generation of the gastric pressure needed for diaphragmatic contraction to be effective. Under this analysis, the abdominal muscles may help inspiration by forcefully contracting during an obstructive expiration and help push the diaphragm up, that is to say helping lengthen it so that it may then contract from a better position in its length-tension relationship during the following inspiration.

It has been postulated that the automatic and voluntary neuroventilatory pathways are different and that the respiratory and tonic functions of these muscles are driven from different central nervous areas and integrated at the spinal level. To perform nonventilatory work, patients in whom some of these muscles are participating in respiration must maintain a high degree of coordination. Either because of the load or because of competing central integration, muscle function may become dyscoordinated and result in dysfunction. This has been shown to occur in patients with COPD who perform unsupported arm exercise. This type of exercise leads to early fatigue of the muscles involved in arm positioning and to dyssynchrony between rib cage and diaphragm-abdomen. Dyssynchrony could also be caused by competing outputs of the various driving centers that control rhythmic respiratory and tonic activities of the accessory ventilatory muscles and the diaphragm. This dyssynchrony may be perceived as dyspnea. Its occurrence has been observed in normal subjects made to breath against resistive loads and in patients with COPD during voluntary hyperventilation.[40,41] Likewise, it has been observed in patients immediately after disconnection from ventilators but before evidence of contractile fatigue. This suggests that the dyssynchrony is a consequence of the load and not an indication of fatigue itself. Whatever the reason, an uncoordinated breathing pattern is ineffective and is associated with respiratory muscle dysfunction.[31,40] Unfortunately, very little is known about the exact nature of this phenomenon and even less about possible therapeutic interventions. Perhaps new breathing retraining techniques using biofeedback and other tools that may modify breathing strategies may help patients who manifest this breathing pattern.

Patients with COPD stop exercising because of dys-

FIGURE 9-6 Value of mouth occlusion pressure (a measure of central drive) in centimeters of water at 0.1 s of an occluded tidal breath. The $P_{0.1}$ increases as a function of the severity of COPD. It is lower in normal (N) subjects than in eucapnic (E) and hypercapnic (H) patients and highest in patients with respiratory failure (RF).

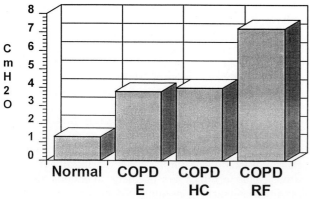

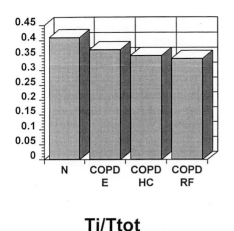

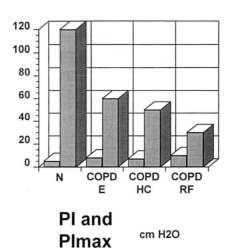

Ti/Ttot

PI and PImax cm H2O

FIGURE 9-7 As COPD worsens, the ratio of inspiratory time (TI) over the total duration of the breathing cycle (Ttot) shortens minimally. In contrast, the maximal inspiratory pressure (PImax) decreases as the disease progresses. In contrast the load to breath (PI) increases in eucapnic (E) and hypercapnic (H) patients and during respiratory failure (RF).

pnea.[24,42,43] Recent evidence indicates that dyspnea relates better to respiratory muscle function with hyperinflation rather than to airflow obstruction.[19,42,43] It has been shown that dyspnea increases as the ratio between the pressure needed to ventilate and the maximal pressure that the muscles can generate (Pbreath/PImax) increases. Dyspnea also worsens in proportion to the duration of the inspiratory contraction (TI/Ttot) and respiratory frequency. These are also the factors that are associated with electromyographic evidence of respiratory muscle fatigue.[44] Although respiratory muscle fatigue has been documented in patients with COPD suffering from acute decompensation,[45] its presence in stable patients remains in doubt. It is fair to state that the respiratory muscles of patients with severe COPD are functioning at a level closer to the fatigue threshold (Fig. 9-7) but are not fatigued. It is also believed that restoration of the respiratory muscles to a better contractile state should improve the dyspnea of these patients. This difficult goal may now be achievable with surgery aimed at reducing the increased lung volume of selected patients. Using computerized tomography, ventilation-perfusion lung scans, and plethysmographically determined lung volumes, it is possible to select hyperin-

flated areas that can then be targeted for resection. Although the results are preliminary, they seem encouraging and a national randomized study now in progress will help answer this question.[46-52] The other possible way to restore normal mechanics is using lung transplants, but the lack of sufficient donors and the frequent occurrence of important posttransplant complications make this a last resort form of therapy. The means to best select candidates for these procedures remain to be fully determined.

Integrative Approach

The overall action of the respiratory system can be represented by the model shown in Fig. 9-8. Central to the model is the problem of airway narrowing and hyperinflation. To reverse the model to a normal state, it is necessary to resolve those two problems. Efforts to prevent the disease from developing (smoking cessation) must be associated with methods aimed at reversing airflow obstruction. Indeed, pharmacotherapy including bronchodilators, antibiotics, and corticosteroids are given to improve airflow. If this is effec-

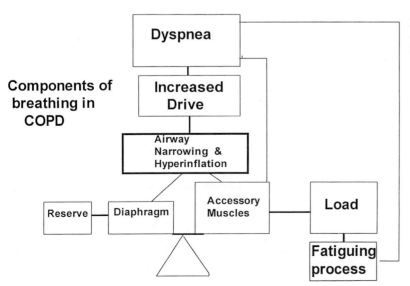

FIGURE 9-8 Model that represents the different components of breathing in patients with COPD. See text for details.

tive, hyperinflation will consequently decrease. One alternative option is to resect the portions of the lungs which are severely diseased. This has been effective in those cases of large bullae.[48,53] Whether partial resection of lesser evident (but still unevenly distributed) emphysematous areas is effective remains to be determined. From a strict pathophysiologic point of view, lung resection in patients with COPD whose main problem is inflammatory airways disease is not justifiable. On the other hand, improving the reserve of the system, using rehabilitation and exercise, has proved effective for the majority of symptomatic patients with COPD. Significant improvement has been documented for exercise endurance, for perception of breathlessness at rest and with exercise, and in quality of life.[54]

In summary, a thorough understanding of the pathophysiology of COPD can help plan treatment in a logical way. A rational approach is outlined for each of the possible pathways in the different chapters in this book.

References

1. Mitchell RS, Stanford RE, Johnson JM, et al: The morphologic features of bronchi, bronchioles and alveoli in chronic airway obstruction. *Am Rev Respir Dis* 114:137–145, 1976.
2. Thurlbeck WM: Pathophysiology of chronic obstructive pulmonary disease. *Clin Chest Med* 11:389-403, 1990.
3. Higgins MW, Thom T: Incidence, prevalence, and mortality: Intra- and intercountry differences, in Hensley MJ, Saunders NA (eds): *Clinical Epidemiology of Chronic Obstructive Pulmonary Disease.* New York, Marcel Dekker, 1990.
4. Feinlieb M, Rosenberg HM, Collins JG, et al: Trends in COPD morbidity in the United States. *Am Rev Respir Dis* 140:S9–S18, 1989.
5. Redline S, Weiss ST: Genetic and perinatal risk factors for the development of chronic obstructive pulmonary disease, in Hensley MJ, Saunders NA (eds): *Clinical Epidemiology of Chronic Obstructive Pulmonary Disease.* New York, Marcel Dekker, 1989; pp 139–168.
6. Buist SA: Smoking and other risk factors, in Murray JF, Nadel JA (eds): *Textbook of Respiratory Medicine,* 2d ed. Philadelphia, Saunders; 1994; pp 1259–1287.
7. Snider GL: Pulmonary disease in alpha-1 antitrypsin deficiency. *Ann Intern Med* 111:957–959, 1989.
8. Postma DS, Sluiter HJ: Prognosis of chronic obstructive pulmonary disease: The Dutch experience. *Am Rev Resp Dis* 140:S100–S105, 1989.
9. Fletcher C, Peto R: The natural history of chronic airflow obstruction. *Br Med J* 1:1645–1648, 1977.
10. Anthonisen NR, Connett JE, Kiley JP, et al, for the Lung Health Study Group 1994: The effects of smoking intervention and the use of an inhaled anticholinergic bronchodilator on the rate of decline of FEV_1: The Lung Health Study. *JAMA* 272:1497–1505, 1994.
11. Sanders C: The radiographic diagnosis of emphysema. *Radiol Clin North Am* 29:1019–1030, 1991.
12. Klein JS, Gamsu G, Webb WR, et al: High resolution CT diagnosis of emphysema in symptomatic patients with normal chest radiographs and isolated low diffusing capacity. *Radiology* 182:817–821, 1992.
13. Berend N, Woolcock AJ, Marlin GE: Correlation between the function and the structure of the lung in smokers. *Am Rev Respir Dis* 119:695–702, 1979.
14. Buist AS, Van Fleet DL, Ross BB: A comparison of conventional spirometric tests and the tests of closing volume in one emphysema screening center. *Am Rev Respir Dis* 107:735–740, 1973.
15. Rodriguez-Roisin R, Roca J: Pulmonary gas exchange, in Calverley PM, Pride N (eds): *Chronic Obstructive Pulmonary Disease.* London, Chapman and Hall, 1995; pp 161–184.
16. Nagai A, Yamawaki I, Takizawa T, Thurlbeck WM: Alveolar attachments in emphysema of human lungs. *Am Rev Respir Dis* 144:888–891, 1991.
17. Bosken C, Hards J, Gatter K, Hogg J: Characterization of the inflammatory reaction in the peripheral airways of cigarette smokers using immunocytochemistry. *Am Rev Respir Dis* 145:911–917, 1992.
18. Saetta M, Kim WD, Izquierdo J, et al: Extent of centrilobular and panacinar emphysema in smoker's lungs: Pathological and mechanical implications. *Eur Respir J* 7:664–671, 1994.
19. O'Donnell D, Webb K: Exertional breathlessness in patients with chronic airflow limitation. *Am Rev Respir Dis* 148:1351–1357, 1993.
20. Bates DV: *Respiratory Function in Disease,* 3d ed. Philadelphia, Saunders, 1989; pp 172–187.
21. Greaves IA, Colebatch HJ: Elastic behavior and structure of normal and emphysematous lung postmortem. *Am Rev Respir Dis* 68:566–587, 1980.
22. Hogg JC, Macklem PT, Thurlbeck WA: Site and nature of airways obstruction in chronic obstructive lung disease. *N Engl J Med* 278:1355–1359, 1968.
23. O'Donnell SE, Sanil R, Anthonisen NR, Younis M: Effect of dynamic airway compression on breathing pattern and respiratory sensation in severe chronic obstructive pulmonary disease. *Am Rev Respir Dis* 135:912–918, 1987.
24. Javahari S, Blum J, Kazemi H: Pattern of breathing and carbon dioxide retention in chronic obstructive lung disease. *Am J Med* 71:228–234, 1981.
25. Parot S, Miara B, Milic-Emili J, Gauthier H: Hypoxemia, hypercapnia and breathing patterns in patients with chronic obstructive pulmonary disease. *Am Rev Respir Dis* 126:882–886, 1982.
26. Anthonisen NR: Prognosis in chronic obstructive pulmonary disease: Results from multicenter clinical trials. *Am Rev Respir Dis* 133:95–99, 1989.
27. Celli BR: Respiratory muscle function. *Clin Chest Med* 7:567–584, 1986.
28. Roussos CH, Macklem PT: The respiratory muscles. *N Engl J Med* 307:786–797, 1982.
29. von Euler C: On the central pattern generator for the basic breathing rhythmicity. *J Appl Physiol* 55:1647–1659, 1983.
30. Derenne JP, Macklem PT, Roussos CH: The respiratory muscles: Mechanics, control and pathophysiology. *Am Rev Respir Dis* 119:119–133, 1978.
31. Sears TA: Central rhythm and pattern generation. *Chest* 97:47–45, 1990.
32. Martinez FJ, Couser JI, Celli BR: Factors influencing ventilatory muscle recruitment in patients with chronic airflow obstruction. *Am Rev Respir Dis* 142:276–282, 1990.
33. Murciano D, Broczkowski J, Lecocguic M, et al: Tracheal occlusion pressure. A simple index to monitor respiratory muscle fatigue during acute respiratory failure in patients with chronic obstructive pulmonary disease. *Ann Intern Med* 108:800–805, 1988.
34. Milic-Emili J, Grassino AE, Whitelaw WA: Measurement and testing of respiratory drive, in Horbein TF (ed): *Regulation of Breathing. Lung Biology in Health and Disease.* New York, Marcel Dekker, 1981; pp 675–743.
35. Rochester DF: The diaphragm contractile properties and fatigue. *J Clin Invest* 75:1397–1402, 1985.
36. Sassoon CS, Te TT, Mahutte CR, Light R: Airway occlusion pressure. An important indicator for successful weaning in patients with chronic obstructive pulmonary disease. *Am Rev Respir Dis* 135:107–113, 1987.
37. Loveridge B, Est P, Anthonisen NR, Krugger MH: Breathing

patterns in patients with chronic obstructive pulmonary disease. *Am Rev Respir Dis* 130:730–733, 1984.

38. Braun NM, Arora NS, Rochester DF: The force-length relationship of the normal human diaphragm. *J Appl Physiol* 53:405–412, 1982.

39. DeTroyer A, Estenne M: Functional anatomy of the respiratory muscles. *Clin Chest Med* 9:175–193, 1988.

40. Sharp JT: The respiratory muscles in emphysema. *Clin Chest Med* 4:421–432, 1983.

41. Tobin MJ, Perez W, Guenther SM, et al: Does rib-cage abdominal paradox signify respiratory muscle fatigue? *J Appl Physiol* 63:857–860, 1987.

42. Killian K, Jones N: Respiratory muscle and dyspnea. *Clin Chest Med* 9:237–248, 1988.

43. LeBlanc P, Bowie DM, Summers E, et al: Breathlessness and exercise in patients with cardiorespiratory disease. *Am Rev Respir Dis* 133:21–25, 1986.

44. Bellemare F, Grassino A: Force reserve of the diaphragm in patients with chronic obstructive pulmonary disease. *Am Rev Respir Dis* 143:905–912, 1991.

45. Cohen C, Zagelbaum G, Gross D, et al: Clinical manifestations of inspiratory muscle fatigue. *Am J Med* 73:308–316, 1982.

46. Brantigan OC, Mueller E, Kress MB: A surgical approach to pulmonary emphysema. *Am Rev Respir Dis* 80:194–202, 1959.

47. Cooper JD, Trulock ER, Triantafillou AN, et al: Bilateral pneumonectomy (volume reduction) for chronic obstructive pulmonary disease. *J Thor Cardiovasc Surg* 109:106–119, 1995.

48. Knudson RJ, Gaensler E: Surgery for emphysema. *Ann Thor Surg* 1:332–362, 1965.

49. Sciurba F, Rogers R, Keenan R, et al: Improvement in pulmonary function and elastic recoil after lung-reduction surgery. *N Engl J Med* 334:1095–1099, 1996.

50. Gelb A, Zamel N, McKenna R, Brenner M: Mechanism of short term improvement in lung function after emphysema reduction. *Am J Respir Crit Care Med* 154:945–951, 1996.

51. O'Donnell D, Webb K, Bertley J, et al: Mechanism of relief of exertional breathlessness following unilateral bullectomy and lung volume reduction surgery in emphysema. *Chest* 110:18–27, 1996.

52. Martinez F, Montes de Oca M, Whyte R, et al: Lung volume reduction improves dyspnea, dynamic hyperinflation and respiratory muscle function. *Am J Respir Crit Care Med* 155:2018–2023, 1997.

53. Fitzgerald MX, Keelan PJ, Cugell DW, Gaensler EA: Long-term results of surgery for bullous emphysema. *J Thor Cardiovasc Surg* 68:556–587, 1974.

54. Celli BR: Is pulmonary rehabilitation an effective treatment for chronic obstructive pulmonary disease? *Am J Respir Crit Care Med* 155:781–783, 1997.

Chapter 10

PATHOPHYSIOLOGY OF INTERSTITIAL LUNG DISEASE

RALPH J. PANOS

TALMADGE E. KING, JR.

The interstitial lung diseases (ILDs) encompass a broad spectrum of pulmonary disorders with overlapping clinical, radiographic, physiologic, and histopathologic features. Approximately 15 percent of patients seen by pulmonologists in the United States have ILD, and these disorders account for between 5000 and 6000 deaths per year.[1,2] In addition, a rising rate of mortality from pulmonary fibrosis has been identified in several countries.[3-5] The prevalence of ILD is slightly higher among males, 80.9 per 100,000, compared with females, 67.2 per 100,000.[6] Pulmonary fibrosis and idiopathic pulmonary fibrosis are the most common diagnoses and account for approximately 45 percent of all ILD cases.[6] Occupational and environmental exposures, connective tissue disease, and sarcoid are the next most prevalent forms of ILD.

At least 150 types of ILD have been described, and the number of different disorders continues to increase as new histopathologic patterns are characterized and additional causes of parenchymal lung disease recognized. Based on these methods of identification, most classification schemes for ILD reflect either the pattern of lung parenchymal derangement or its cause (Table 10-1). Although many ILDs have characteristic histopathologic patterns, others are doubly redundant; one agent or associated disease may produce multiple, different histopathologic patterns, and a particular histopathologic pattern may be seen in different forms of ILD. In addition, the pathogenesis of these disorders has not been completely elucidated. Over the past several decades, important insights have been made into the types of cells, cytokines, and other biologic factors involved in parenchymal fibrosis. However, a complete understanding of their interactions and the complex mechanisms initiating and propagating the inflammatory and fibrotic processes that characterize these disorders remain elusive. Thus, until ILDs can be classified based on their pathogenic mechanisms,[7] these disorders must be categorized based on either their histopathologic pattern or the inciting agent or disease.

This chapter presents an overview of ILD from the perspective of the clinician evaluating a patient who presents with a diffuse parenchymal process. The clinical, physiologic, radiographic, and histopathologic manifestations of ILD are reviewed and unique characteristics of individual disease processes presented. Lastly, therapy and management of these disorders are discussed.

Clinical History

The initial evaluation should include a complete history and physical examination. Patients with ILD commonly come to clinical attention because of the onset of progressive breathlessness with exertion (dyspnea) and/or a persistent nonproductive cough. Other important symptoms and signs include hemoptysis, wheezing, and chest pain.

The history is the most valuable clue in the determination of the cause of ILD (Table 10-2). A diagnosis was established based on the history in nearly one-third of 381 patients with diffuse lung disease.[8] Occupational and environmental exposures, previous or concurrent diseases, drugs (prescribed, over the counter, and illicit), therapeutic treatments, and family history of similar or other inherited diseases may suggest causes for interstitial disorders.

GENDER

Lymphangioleiomyomatosis occurs exclusively in premenopausal women. Also, ILD in the connective tissue diseases is more common in women; the exception is ILD in rheumatoid arthritis, which is more common in men.

AGE

The patient's age may be helpful, given that the majority of patients with sarcoidosis and connective tissue disease present between the ages of 20 and 40 years. Conversely, most patients with idiopathic pulmonary fibrosis are older than 60 years.[9]

SYMPTOMS AND SIGNS

Progressive breathlessness with exertion is the usual presenting complaint in most patients with ILD. In many cases, the shortness of breath progresses insidiously and patients often gradually reduce their activity level to compensate for their worsening respiratory impairment. These patients may, in fact, not complain of breathlessness because they have adapted their activities of daily living by reducing or eliminating strenuous tasks to alleviate the sensation of shortness of breath. The duration and tempo at which dyspnea progresses may suggest different etiologies for a diffuse parenchymal process. A short, rapid onset of symptoms and radiographic findings (weeks) may occur in eosinophilic pneumonia,[10] hypersensitivity pneumonitis,[11] acute interstitial pneumonia (Hamman-Rich syndrome),[12] alveolar hemorrhage syndromes,[13] and ILD associated with collagen vascular diseases, especially systemic lupus erythematosis[14] and bronchiolitis obliterans organizing pneumonia.[15] Because these processes may be accompanied by systemic symptoms including fever, they are often difficult to distinguish from atypical pulmonary infections. In most ILDs, breathlessness is usually chronic and slowly progresses over months to years, especially idiopathic pulmonary fibrosis (IPF, also called cryptogenic fibrosing alveolitis).

Systemic symptoms of weight loss, diminished energy, and fatigue occur frequently. Another common symptom is a dry, nonproductive cough, which occurs frequently in IPF and forms of ILD that affect the airways including sarcoid,[16] respiratory bronchiolitis,[17] bronchiolitis with organizing pneumonia,[18] eosinophilic granuloma,[19] and hypersensitivity pneumonitis.[20]

Chest pain occurs infrequently in most ILDs, although chest discomfort and vague substernal pain can be a trouble-

TABLE 10-1 Classification of Interstitial Lung Diseases

Occupational and environmental exposures
  Inorganic dusts
    Silica
    Asbestos
    Beryllium
    Tin
    Coal and mineral particles
    Hard metals (cobalt)
  Organic (hypersensitivity pneumonitis)
    Bacteria
    Fungi
    Animal proteins
  Toxic gases
    Chlorine
    Sulfur dioxide
    Nitrogen dioxide
Drug or medication induced
  Chemotherapeutic agents
  Cardiovascular medications
  Radiation exposure
  Oxygen
Collagen vascular diseases
  Scleroderma
  Polymyositis-dermatomyositis
  Systemic lupus erythematosis
  Rheumatoid arthritis
Neoplasms
  Bronchoalveolar cell carcinoma
  Lymphangitic carcinomatosis
  Lymphoma
Metabolic disorders
  Gaucher's disease
  Neimann-Pick disease
  Hermansky-Pudlak syndrome
Unknown etiologies
  Idiopathic pulmonary fibrosis
    Familial
    Sporadic
  Sarcoid
    Familial
    Sporadic
  Lymphangioleiomyomatosis
  Tuberous sclerosis
  Eosinophilic granuloma
  Nonspecific (nonclassifiable) interstitial pneumonia
  Bronchiolitis obliterans organizing pneumonia
  Respiratory bronchiolitis–interstitial lung disease

sarcoid. Ocular symptoms including anterior uveitis suggest sarcoid or ILD associated with collagen vascular disease.

OCCUPATIONAL HISTORY

The occupational history should elicit not only job titles but also descriptions of the actual work performed and all potentially hazardous materials encountered, dust exposures, use or misuse of protective respiratory devices, and similar symptoms in coworkers.

ENVIRONMENTAL EXPOSURES

Environmental factors include recreational activities and hobbies, travel, and pets in the home or regularly frequented areas.

MEDICATION AND TREATMENT HISTORY

Drug-induced pulmonary fibrosis may be caused by many different medications, including chemotherapeutic agents, cardiovascular drugs, and antibiotics. Previous radiation treatments with ports encompassing the chest may lead to the diagnosis of radiation-induced pulmonary fibrosis[26] or bronchiolitis obliterans organizing pneumonia (BOOP).[27]

FAMILY HISTORY

Various inherited disorders of metabolism are associated with diffuse parenchymal processes, including Neimann-Pick disease,[28] Hermansky-Pudlak disease,[29] and Gaucher's

TABLE 10-2 Historical Clues to the Cause of an Interstitial Pulmonary Process

Medications
  Chemotherapeutic agents
  Antibiotics
  Antiinflammatory agents
  Cardiovascular agents
Risks for hypersensitivity pneumonitis
  Pets, especially birds
  Hot tubs or swimming pools
  Evaporative coolers (swamp coolers)
  Mold or mildew at home or in the workplace
Occupational exposures
  Silica
    Hard rock mining
    Foundry work
    Sandblasting
    Glassmaking
    China and ceramics industries
  Asbestos
    Shipyards
    Plumbing, boilermaker
    Railroads
    Welding
    Construction trades
  Talc
  Hard metals (cobalt, tungsten, carbide, beryllium)
    Metal foundry
    Tool and parts makers
    Lathe workers
    Aluminum pot room workers
  Symptoms or history of collagen vascular diseases
  Radiation therapy

some complaint in patients with sarcoidosis, and uncommonly in eosinophilic granuloma (from rib involvement). Pleurisy may accompany ILD associated with collagen vascular diseases, especially systemic lupus erythematosis or be caused by drug reactions. The rapid onset of pleuritic chest pain may be precipitated by a pneumothorax in patients with IPF,[21] eosinophilic granuloma,[19] lymphangioleiomyomatosis,[22,23] or tuberous sclerosis.[24,25]

Musculoskeletal complaints may accompany ILD associated with collagen vascular disease, including rheumatoid arthritis, systemic lupus erythematosis, or dermatomyositis-polymyositis. Cutaneous findings such as malar rash, skin thickening, and maculopapular rashes occur in patients with ILD due to systemic lupus erythematosis, scleroderma, and disease.[30] There are also familial forms of sarcoid and IPF, sarcoidosis, tuberous sclerosis, and neurofibromatosis.

SMOKING HISTORY

Smoking history may also aid in the determination of the etiology of a diffuse parenchymal process. Eosinophilic granuloma, desquamative interstitial pneumonia, and respiratory bronchiolitis–associated ILD occur almost exclusively in smokers, and a history of smoking is associated with the development of IPF.[31] Conversely, the incidence of hypersensitivity pneumonitis[32] and sarcoidosis appears to be reduced in active smokers. The clinical course of patients with IPF[33] and Goodpasture's syndrome may be influenced by active smoking.

Physical Examination

The respiratory rate of patients with ILD is often elevated. This tachypnea is due to an alteration in the breathing pattern to compensate for decreased lung compliance and increased work of breathing. Patients usually take rapid, shallow breaths, and this pattern is accentuated during exertion.[34] Auscultation of the chest frequently reveals bilateral dry, end-inspiratory rales (Velcro crackles) that are more prominent in the lung bases. Wheezing occurs infrequently in the ILD but may accompany parenchymal processes with airways involvement such as eosinophilic granuloma, respiratory bronchiolitis-associated ILD, and sarcoid. Clubbing is a common finding in IPF. As pulmonary fibrosis progresses and causes physiologic deterioration and hypoxemia, signs of cor pulmonale and right heart strain such as an increased P2 and elevated jugular venous pressure may develop.

Other physical examination findings may provide diagnostic clues to the cause of a diffuse parenchymal process. Ophthalmologic signs of uveitis may lead to the diagnosis of sarcoidosis or collagen vascular disease, whereas keratoconjunctivitis sicca suggests lymphocytic interstitial pneumonitis associated with Sjögren's syndrome. Dermatologic findings of erythema nodosum occur in sarcoidosis and collagen vascular diseases, facial rashes in systemic lupus erythematosis, or dermatomyositis, and maculopapular rashes may accompany drug-induced lung disease, collagen vascular disorders, as well as metabolic diseases. Skin nodules or calcifications may be found in patients with rheumatoid arthritis or scleroderma. Arthritis occurs in collagen vascular diseases and sarcoid. Although these patterns of physical examination findings may suggest a cause for ILD, they are not usually diagnostic and require corroborative studies.

Effect of ILD on Lung Function

The inflammatory processes which stimulate the accumulation of cells, edema, and extracellular components as well as the subsequent architectural derangements in the lung parenchyma cause alterations in lung mechanics. Although the reductions in lung volumes are believed to be caused predominantly by fibrosis rather than inflammation,[35] the site of the structural abnormality may determine the nature of the change. In disorders such as lymphangioleiomyomatosis, tuberous sclerosis, eosinophilic granuloma, and sarcoid, the airways may become obstructed, causing air trap-

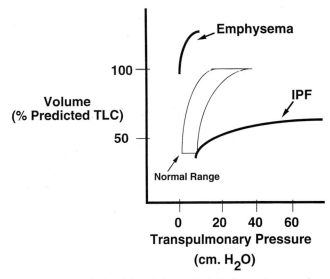

FIGURE 10-1 Relationship of the static deflation volume and pressure in idiopathic pulmonary fibrosis (PIF) compared with emphysema. The percent predicted TLC is plotted against the static transpulmonary pressure (centimeters of water) for a patient with ILD. In general, the compliance, maximum static transpulmonary pressure, and the coefficient of retraction (the maximum transpulmonary pressure to TLC) tend to correlate with the extent of parenchymal lung involvement observed on lung biopsy.

ping and increased lung volumes. In addition, mixed processes in which emphysema accompanies ILD may result in normal lung volumes. Although pulmonary function testing in patients with ILD may be normal during early disease, the physiologic hallmark of ILD is restriction. The pressure-volume curve is flattened owing to diminished lung compliance, and its position is shifted down and to the right (Fig. 10-1). All lung volume compartments including total lung capacity, thoracic gas volume, and residual volume are decreased. Spirometric indices of airflow, forced vital capacity (FVC), and forced expiratory volume in 1s (FEV_1), are usually diminished due to the reduction in lung volumes. The ratio of FEV_1 to FVC may be normal or increased owing to augmented flow rates (Fig. 10-2).

Gas exchange is frequently disturbed in ILD. The diffusing capacity for carbon monoxide (DL_{CO}) is decreased, and its reduction may precede alterations in lung volumes.[36] During the early stages of ILD, the resting arterial oxygen tension (Pa_{O_2}) may be normal, but with exercise the Pa_{O_2} decreases and the alveolar-arterial oxygen gradient $P(A-a)_{O_2}$ increases.[37] As the parenchymal derangement progresses, resting hypoxemia and widening of the $P(A-a)_{O_2}$ occur. Although mismatching of ventilation and perfusion is the major cause of these gas-exchange abnormalities at rest,[37] impaired oxygen diffusion may be a contributing factor during exertion.[37] The ventilation-perfusion imbalance occurs both at the alveolar level where poorly ventilated units are perfused and at the organ level owing to a redistribution of pulmonary blood flow to the upper lung zones.[38] Other alterations in the arterial blood gas may include respiratory alkalosis. Hypercarbia is rare in ILD.

Patients with ILD have a characteristic ventilatory response to exercise. They increase their minute ventilation by

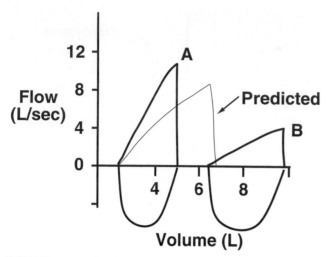

FIGURE 10-2 Maximal expiratory flow volume (MEFV curve). *A.* **Shown are the MEFV curves at presentation in idiopathic pulmonary fibrosis. At any given lung volume, the flow rates are higher than expected because of elevated driving pressure due to an increased elastic recoil.** *B.* **Shows the MEFV curve for a patient with chronic obstructive lung disease. The FEV_1 and FVC values are low relative to the predicted values, and the lung volumes are increased.**

raising their respiratory rate rather than their tidal volume. This breathing pattern is an effort to conserve energy and reduce the work of breathing. Because the lungs are stiff and noncompliant, less energy is utilized in rapid, shallow breaths than in slow, deep respirations. This panting breathing pattern results in an increase in the dead space to tidal volume ratio, V_D/V_T, because of the reduction in V_T. Normally during exercise V_D/V_T decreases due to the increase in V_T and increased cardiac output with augmented perfusion to the upper lung zones; however, in patients with ILD, V_D/V_T either remains constant or increases further with exercise. Measurements of gas exchange at rest and with exercise have been shown to be the most useful physiologic gauges of disease severity and clinical course in ILD.[39]

Alterations in cardiopulmonary hemodynamics frequently accompany diffuse parenchymal fibrosis. Pulmonary hypertension develops due to hypoxemic vasoconstriction and obliteration of the vascular bed by parenchymal fibrosis.[40,41] The severity of pulmonary hypertension correlates with the diminution in vital capacity and level of hypoxemia.[42,43] With disease progression, cor pulmonale and right heart failure develop.

The incidence of apneas is reduced, and elevations in the breathing frequency persist during sleep indicating an increased respiratory drive and a failure of sleep to inhibit the neural reflexes which stimulate and maintain the rapid breathing pattern in patients with ILD.[44,45] Sleep is fragmented with alterations in the distribution of sleep stages. Patients with ILD spend more sleep time in stage 1 and less time in rapid eye movement (REM) sleep than do normal individuals.[45] Patients with resting Sa_{O_2} less than 90 percent have greater sleep disturbances than those who are normoxemic. Sa_{O_2} falls during REM sleep, and these desaturations may be more severe than the decreases in Sa_{O_2} that occur during maximal exercise.[44]

Chest Imaging

CHEST RADIOGRAPH

The chest roentgenogram may be normal in up to 10 percent of individuals with ILD.[46] More commonly, the chest radiograph is abnormal with parenchymal abnormalities. There are several radiographic patterns in ILD: ground glass opacification, reticular or nodular opacities, and honeycombing or end-stage lung disease. *Ground glass opacification* is a nonspecific term for a hazy increase in lung opacity which does not obscure the underlying vessels. *Air-space consolidation* is an alveolar filling process which appears as a diffuse haziness overlying the pulmonary parenchyma and may contain air bronchograms. This pattern appears to correlate with cellular and proteinaceous exudate within the intraalveolar space and may represent early, inflammatory disease. A *reticular pattern* is characterized by lacy, gossamer lines; the *nodular pattern* consists of diffusely distributed small densities. *Honeycombing* or end-stage lung disease consists of thick walled cysts up to 1 cm in diameter within a coarse reticular opacity. This pattern correlates with severe parenchymal fibrosis. Other less common findings in ILD include dense alveolar opacities in bronchiolitis obliterans organizing pneumonia and chronic eosinophilic pneumonia.

Most interstitial opacities occur predominantly in the lower lung zones and progress to involve the upper lung zones. However, the upper lobes may be preferentially involved in several ILDs including sarcoid, silicosis, eosinophilic granuloma, ankylosing spondylitis, and berylliosis. Concomitant with the progression of interstitial opacities, lung volumes often decrease. The trachea may deviate to the right due to the marked reduction in lung volume. As pulmonary hypertension develops, the right ventricle dilates.

FIGURE 10-3 Pulmonary lymphangioleiomyomatosis. The HRCT scan shows multiple thin-walled cystic airspaces of varying sizes.

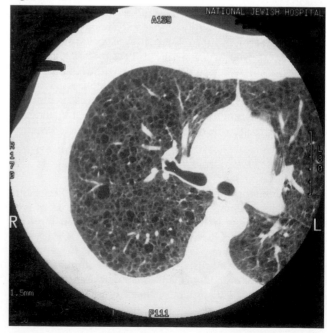

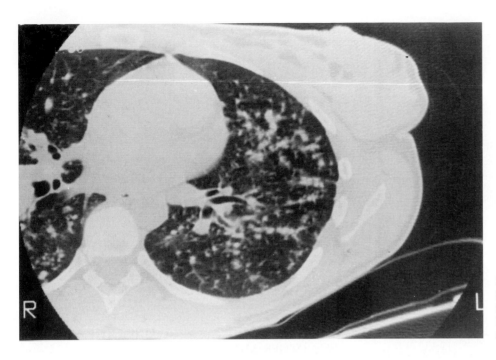

FIGURE 10-4 Sarcoidosis (Stage III). HRCT shows the beaded or irregular thickening of the bronchovascular bundles; nodules along bronchi, vessels, and subpleural regions.

In lymphangioleiomyomatosis, tuberous sclerosis, eosinophilic granuloma, and sarcoid, lung volumes may be preserved or even increased.

Pleural effusions occur infrequently in most of the ILD but may accompany parenchymal lung disease associated with collagen vascular disorders. Pleural plaques and effusions occur in asbestos-related lung disease. Chylous pleural effusions may be present in lymphangioleiomyomatosis. Eosinophilic granuloma, tuberous sclerosis, and lymphangioleiomyomatosis are associated with pneumothorax. Hilar adenopathy occurs commonly in sarcoid, berylliosis, and bronchogenic or metastatic neoplasms.

CHEST CT

High-resolution thin section computed tomography (HRCT) has rapidly become the best imaging modality in the evaluation of ILD. Reduced scan times and collimation widths along with other technical refinements eliminate the superimposition of images that occurs in the routine chest radiograph and provide enhanced spatial resolution and morphologic detail in the images of the lung parenchyma.[47–50] HRCT scans can delineate the components of the secondary pulmonary lobule, an anatomic unit bounded by pulmonary veins and lymphatics within interlobular septae and encompassing the alveolar sacs supplied by three to five terminal bronchioles with their adjacent pulmonary arteries. Current technology does not permit the imaging of the alveolar wall.

The HRCT findings of diffuse parenchymal disease can be classified into several patterns: linear, cystic, nodular, and ground glass. Thickened interlobular septae are seen as linear opacities which extend to the pleura peripherally and appear as polygons centrally. Located within these structures are dotlike or branching shapes which are the bronchioles, arteries, and supporting tissue composing the intralobular septae. Interlobular septal thickening is seen commonly in many forms of ILD but is rarely the predominant pattern (sarcoidosis and asbestosis). *Cysts* are areas of decreased attenuation

which are distinguished from the lesions of emphysema by well defined walls (Fig. 10-3). The cystic spaces of honeycombing are usually subpleural and can range from several millimeters to several centimeters in diameter. They are characterized by thick, clearly definable, fibrous walls. Associated findings consistent with extensive fibrosis include traction bronchiectasis and bronchiolectasis. *Nodules* as small as 1 to 2 mm in diameter can be recognized by HRCT and appear as heterogenous opacifications with different shapes and borders (Fig. 10-4). "Well-defined" nodules usually represent interstitial lesions while "ill-defined" nodules are usually airspace in origin. *Ground glass attenuation* is characterized by a hazy opacification which does not always obscure the linear markings of the interlobular septae (Fig. 10-5). Because not all lobules are simultaneously and equally involved in the ILD, areas of increased, hazy attenuation may be interspersed with normal lobules. Ground glass opacities usually suggest an active and potentially reversible process. *Airspace consolidation* results in increased lung opacity with obscuration of the underlying vessels (Fig. 10-6). Based on these patterns and their distribution, many types of ILD are sufficiently well characterized to establish a radiographic diagnosis (Table 10–3).

Because it is more sensitive than routine chest radiographs, HRCT is useful in the evaluation of suspected ILD in individuals with normal chest roentgenograms. This technique can also be used to determine the extent and severity of parenchymal involvement, provide the optimal location for biopsy, monitor disease progression, and assess the response to therapy.

GALLIUM SCINTIGRAPHY

Gallium 67 (^{67}Ga) citrate is a radiopharmaceutical which is injected intravenously and its thoracic uptake assessed 2 to 3 days later by chest scintigraphy. Normal lung tissue does not accumulate ^{67}Ga, but it is believed to localize to areas of inflammation, especially within activated macrophages.[51]

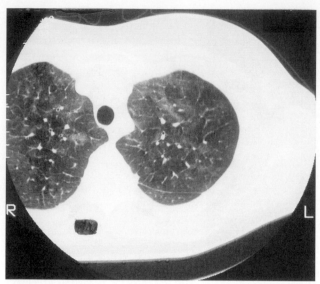

FIGURE 10-5 Respiratory bronchiolitis-associated interstitial lung disease. HRCT shows extensive ground-glass opacities in the upper lung zones. These opacities resolved with smoking cessation.

The mechanisms regulating its accumulation within the lung are not completely known, however. [67]Ga scanning has been used to assess pulmonary inflammation in numerous forms of ILD including sarcoid, the pneumoconioses, IPF, collagen vascular-related lung disease, and drug-induced pulmonary fibrosis.[51] Numerous methods have been used to quantitate gallium scans and to correlate the ^{67}Ga index with various physiologic, radiographic, histopathologic, and bronchoalveolar lavage findings.[51–54] However, because of the differences in quantitation techniques, interobserver variations in

FIGURE 10-6 Wegener's granulomatosis. This CT scan shows diffuse alveolar hemorrhage in the right lung. There is airspace consolidation with air bronchograms.

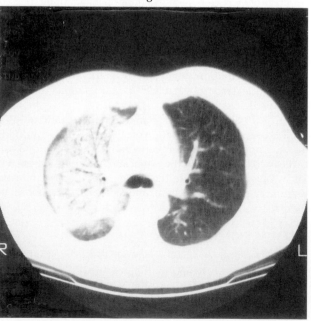

interpretation, and utilization of bronchoalveolar lavage to sample directly the number and types of inflammatory cells within the intraalveolar space, gallium scanning is now used infrequently in the evaluation of ILD.

Laboratory Studies

ROUTINE LABORATORY STUDIES

Although routine blood studies and urine analysis may suggest potential causes of ILD, they are usually not specific and require additional laboratory tests. Eosinophilia may occur in eosinophilic pneumonia, drug reaction, sarcoid, or vasculitis. Anemia may accompany connective tissue disorders, sarcoid, or alveolar hemorrhage syndromes. Connective tissue disorders, vasculitis, alveolar hemorrhage syndromes, and drug reactions may cause an active urinary sediment. The serum angiotensin converting enzyme level is elevated in numerous parenchymal lung diseases and is not specific for a particular disorder.

ANTINEUTROPHIL CYTOPLASMIC ANTIBODIES AND OTHER AUTOANTIBODIES

Antineutrophil cytoplasmic antibodies (ANCAs) are autoantibodies directed against cytoplasmic components of neutrophils and monocytes. Most ANCAs are IgG isotypes. Two predominant patterns are observed when neutrophils are stained with serum containing ANCA: cANCA, diffuse cytoplasmic staining which spares the nucleus, and pANCA,

TABLE 10-3 High-Resolution Thin Section Computed Tomography (HRCT) Patterns in Interstitial Lung Disease

Linear or reticular
    Idiopathic pulmonary fibrosis
    Asbestosis
    Lymphangitic carcinomatosis
    ILD associated with connective tissue disease
Cysts
    Lymphangiomyomatosis
    Eosinophilic granuloma
    End-stage honeycomb lung
Nodules
    Sarcoid
    Silicosis
    Eosinophilic granuloma
    Hypersensitivity pneumonitis
    Silicosis, coal worker's pneumoconiosis
    Lung metastases
Ground glass pattern
    Desquamative interstitial pneumonitis (DIP)
    Hypersensitivity pneumonitis
    Respiratory bronchiolitis associated ILD
    BOOP
    Drug toxicity
Airspace consolidation
    BOOP
    Eosinophilic pneumonia (chronic or acute)
    Pulmonary alveolar proteinosis
    Alveolar hemorrhage
    Lymphoma
    Aspiration
    Alveolar carcinoma

staining around the periphery of the nucleus. The pANCA pattern is a preservation artifact due to the movement of cytoplasmic antigens to the perinuclear region during fixation in alcohol.[55] PR3, a multifunctional protein within azurophilic granules, is the predominant antigen for cANCA. The major antigen for pANCA is myeloperoxidase (MPO) but lactoferrin, elastase, lysozyme, cathepsin, and bactericidal permeability increasing protein may also be targets.[56]

The cANCA staining pattern occurs in up to 90 percent of individuals with active Wegener's granulomatosis (upper respiratory, lung, and kidney involvement) but is present occasionally in other forms of vasculitis.[57] In "limited" Wegener's granulomatosis (i.e., without active glomerulonephritis), or in inactive disease, the sensitivity of the cANCA may be as low as 65 to 70 percent.[58] In addition, reports of false negatives and the presence of positive cANCA in conditions other than Wegener's results are increasing. Positive cANCA results have been demonstrated in other vasculitic processes: in about 50 percent of patients with necrotizing (pauci-immune) glomerulonephritis in combination with systemic small-vessel vasculitis but without granulomatous inflammation of the respiratory tract, for example, microscopic polyarteritis; in 40 percent of patients with polyangiitis overlap syndrome; in 30 percent of patients with idiopathic crescentic glomerulonephritis; in 10 percent of patients with Churg-Strauss syndrome; in 10 percent of patients with classic polyarteritis nodosa[59]; and in alveolar hemorrhage syndromes with or without glomerulonephritis. In addition, positive cANCA results occur in patients with infections (tuberculosis, HIV, endocarditis), nasal septal perforation, drug-induced Wegener-like disease, monoclonal gammopathy, neoplastic disease, and peripheral neuropathy.[58]

False-negative cANCA tests are extremely rare such that in the presence of suspected vasculitis a negative cANCA test is likely a true negative result.[60] However, in some instances repeated testing will yield a positive result that might be missed if only performed once. Also, one or more negative cANCA tests does not completely rule out a diagnosis of Wegener's granulomatosis, especially in the setting of limited disease where up to one-third of the cases may be missed if cANCA is used as the only diagnostic criterion.[61]

The level of the cANCA titer has been used to follow the disease course of patients with Wegener's granulomatosis. Increases in cANCA titers precede or parallel relapses and support increases in or reinstitution of immunosuppressive therapy.[62–64] However, the specific level of the cANCA titer does not correlate well with the disease activity.[65] Many patients with inactive Wegener's granulomatosis will continue to have high cANCA titers for years following successful treatment.

pANCA due to antibodies against MPO occurs in up to 90 percent of individuals with microscopic polyangiitis and pauci-immune rapidly progressive glomerulonephritis which may be associated with alveolar hemorrhage.[66,67] The pANCA staining pattern may also occur in individuals with rheumatoid arthritis and systemic lupus erythematosis.[68]

Autoantibodies directed against other intracellular components may also be detected in many of the connective tissue diseases.[69] In addition to assisting in the diagnosis of these disorders, autoantibody titers may correlate with the presence of ILD. In patients with systemic sclerosis, the presence of antibodies to histones or DNA topoisomerase I (Scl-70) correlates with more severe systemic disease including interstitial fibrosis.[69] The prevalence of ILD in patients with scleroderma and autoantibodies to the RNA polymerases is reduced.[70,71] The presence of autoantibodies to tRNA synthetases characterizes a group of patients with polymyositis with arthralgia and pulmonary fibrosis, decreased responsiveness to treatment, and higher mortality.[72] The Jo-1 autoantibody defines a subgroup of patients with polymyositis and interstitial lung disease.[73,74] In contrast, the incidence of interstitial lung disease is reduced or absent in adult patients with polymyositis and antibodies to signal recognition particle[75,76] and with dermatomyositis and antibodies to Mi-2.[77]

Precipitating antibodies may be present in hypersensitivity pneumonitis. However, the presence of reactive antibodies to a specific antigen merely reflects exposure to a particular agent and does not necessarily demonstrate a causative role in pulmonary disease.[78] Furthermore, the presence of serum precipitins can fluctuate with time despite continued exposure to an offending substance.[79] Finally, unless meticulous care is taken with antigen preparation and testing, the absence of precipitating antibodies to a specific substance does not exclude it as an inciting factor.

Bronchoalveolar Lavage

Bronchoalveolar lavage (BAL) is a technique to sample the cellular and biochemical components of the bronchoalveolar lining fluid. Under local anesthesia, a fiberoptic bronchoscope is wedged in a distal airway and saline is instilled and recovered. The procedure is usually very well tolerated and there are few side effects.[80] The total instilled volume ranges from 100 to 300 mL and is generally divided into 50- to 100-mL aliquots. The initial bolus is believed to sample preferentially the bronchial lining fluid, and the remainder of the lavage is representative of the intraalveolar space.[81] In normal volunteers, the majority of cells are macrophages, <15 percent lymphocytes, <3 percent neutrophils, and <0.5 percent eosinophils.[82]

BAL has been used for the diagnosis, staging, and monitoring of disease activity, response to therapy, predicting prognosis, and identifying various cytokines and mediators which may be involved in the pathogenesis of ILD. In general, the BAL fluid is classified by elevations in the proportion of various cell types, either neutrophil, lymphocyte, or eosinophil (Table 10-4). Individuals with increases in the percentage of BAL lymphocytes may be further categorized by the ratio of CD4 to CD8 cells (helper to suppressor cells). Decreased CD4/CD8 ratios occur in hypersensitivity pneumonitis, silicosis, and drug-induced lung disease, whereas elevated ratios are present in sarcoid, berylliosis, and asbestosis. Mononuclear cells in the BAL fluid of patients with berylliosis proliferate when incubated with beryllium.[83] Substantial increases in the percentage of eosinophils to >40 to 50 percent occur almost exclusively in eosinophilic pneumonia.[84–86] In IPF, the cellular composition of the BAL fluid may predict the response to corticosteroid therapy. Patients with a lymphocytosis tend to respond better than those with eosinophilia.[87,88] In contrast, there does not appear to be a correlation between the proportion of lymphocytes and responsiveness to corticosteroids in sarcoid.[89–91]

TABLE 10-4 Bronchoalveolar Lavage in ILD

Increased cell type
  Lymphocytes
    Sarcoidosis
    Hypersensitivity pneumonitis
    Berylliosis
    Lymphocytic interstitial pneumonitis
    Pulmonary lymphoma
    Drug-induced lung disease
    Collagen vascular disease
    Asbestosis
    Idiopathic pulmonary fibrosis
  Eosinophils
    Eosinophilic pneumonia
    Drug-induced lung disease
    Collagen vascular disease
    Idiopathic pulmonary fibrosis
    Churg-Strauss syndrome
  Neutrophils
    Idiopathic pulmonary fibrosis
    Collagen vascular disease
    Asbestosis
    Pneumoconioses
    Eosinophilic granuloma
    Respiratory bronchiolitis-ILD
  Langerhans' cells
    Eosinophilic pneumonia
  Malignant cells
    Metastatic carcinoma
    Alveolar cell carcinoma
    Lymphoma
  Other constituents
    Protein
      Pulmonary alveolar proteinosis
    Asbestos bodies
      Asbestos exposure

In addition to alterations in the proportions or absolute numbers of the usual cells within BAL fluid, the finding of other cell types may be diagnostic for various pulmonary disorders. Eosinophilic granuloma may be diagnosed by the presence of numerous Langerhans' cells, which are recognized by characteristic pentalaminar inclusions within the cytoplasm or immunocytochemically by OKT6 antibodies.[92] Cytopathologic confirmation of bronchogenic or metastatic neoplasms is established by the presence of neoplastic cells.

Bronchoalveolar lavage is also used to sample the noncellular constituents of the intraalveolar space. The presence of opaque fluid which is positive on periodic acid-Schiff staining, does not react with Alcian blue, and contains few alveolar macrophages can establish the diagnosis of alveolar proteinosis.[93] Although other biochemical markers including cytokines and mediators are measured in BAL fluid from patients with ILD, the clinical usefulness of these parameters is not well established. Nevertheless, their identification and quantitation has significantly aided research studies which have implicated these factors in the cellular and biochemical processes that culminate in parenchymal fibrosis.

Lung Biopsy

Although a diagnosis can be established in approximately one-third of ILD cases based on the history and additional physiologic, radiographic, and bronchoalveolar lavage studies may assist in the evaluation of many of the remaining cases, histopathologic examination of lung tissue is often required. Lung specimens can be obtained by transbronchial biopsies through the fiberoptic bronchoscope or by surgical procedures, either open thoracotomy or video-assisted thoracoscopic surgery (VATS).

Transbronchial biopsies demonstrating noncaseating granulomas aid in the diagnosis of sarcoid or hypersensitivity pneumonitis in the correct clinical setting. The diagnosis of lymphangitic carcinomatosis or eosinophilic granuloma may also be established by this procedure. Because of the small size of transbronchial biopsies and the heterogenous presentation and distribution of many of the ILDs, histopathologic evaluation of these specimens is frequently indeterminate and a larger, surgical biopsy is required.[94]

VATS has largely supplanted open thoracotomy as the preferred surgical approach to obtain lung tissue for the diagnosis of a diffuse parenchymal process.[95-98] The diagnostic yield is comparable for the two procedures, 92 to 100 percent for VATS and 92 percent for open biopsies.[97,98] The duration of chest tube drainage and hospital stay as well as morbidity are less with VATS.[95,97] Because the lung undergoing biopsy must be deflated to allow the surgeon access to the thorax and room to manipulate surgical instruments during VATS, the patient must have sufficient pulmonary reserve to undergo single lung ventilation for the duration of the operative procedure. It is important that the surgeon obtain an adequate sample (at least 2 cm or greater diameter) usually from several sites.[99] Specifically, the surgeon should avoid obtaining only subpleural tissue (especially if pleuritis is present) and avoid the dependent segments of the right middle lobe and lingula. This approach decreases the sampling error that often occurs when a single, small piece is obtained. (Frequently only nonspecific scar tissue is found.) More importantly, it allows the pathologist to better define the pattern of the lesions present (key to making the diagnosis) and the extent and severity of the inflammation and fibrosis (key to suggesting stage of disease).

Histopathology

NORMAL ANATOMY OF THE ALVEOLAR WALL

The alveoli emerge from the alveolar ducts as saclike structures which are 150 to 200 μm in diameter. The interalveolar walls are composed of alveolar epithelial, interstitial, and endothelial cells along with their associated extracellular matrix components. More than 90 percent of the alveolar surface is lined by alveolar type I cells, which are flat, squamous epithelial cells that contain few intracytoplasmic organelles. These cells may be as thin as 0.2 μm. This membranous shape and reduced metabolic capacity are believed to permit maximal gas exchange but cause these cells to be extremely vulnerable to injurious agents. The other alveolar epithelial cell is the type II cell, which has a cuboidal shape with apical microvilli and is thought to be metabolically more robust with abundant intracytoplasmic organelles. Type II cells produce surfactant, the complex mixture of lipids and proteins which maintains alveolar patency at the end of exhalation. These cells produce numerous components of the extracellular matrix, cytokines, and complement components, as well as transporting ions across the alveolar surface. In addition, type II cells appear to be the stem cells for the alveolar epithelium. They proliferate in response to alveolar damage, differentiate into type I cells, and restore the integrity of the epithelium during alveolar repair after lung injury.

The alveolar capillaries are lined by nonfenestrated endothelial cells which are united by tight junctions. Like type I alveolar epithelial cells, they are highly susceptible to injury; however, the endothelial cells retain the capacity to proliferate and appear to have increased synthetic capabilities. These cells produce vasoactive peptides and amines, eicosanoids, and components of the clotting cascade. They secrete basement membrane components which fuse with the alveolar type I cell basal lamina along parts of the alveolar wall reducing the distance between red blood cells and the intraalveolar space to as little as 0.5 μm. In the remainder of the alveolar wall, the interstitial space composed of cells and extracellular matrix components occupies the area between the alveolar epithelium and the capillary endothelial cells. The interstitial cells include fibroblasts, myofibroblasts, migratory inflammatory cells such as lymphocytes and macrophages, and dendritic cells. These cells are metabolically active and produce various cytokines, eicosanoids, and enzymes. The major extracellular components of the interstitial space are collagen, mainly type I and III, and elastin.

ALVEOLAR FILLING PROCESSES

The intraalveolar space may be filled with fluid, cells, blood, or protein. In *desquamative interstitial pneumonitis* (DIP), the alveoli are homogenously filled with macrophages and the epithelium is lined with hypertrophic, hyperplastic alveolar type II cells. The descriptive term *desquamative* is a misnomer because the intraalveolar cells are not shed epithelial cells but mainly macrophages.[100] This inflammatory infiltrate reaches into the interstitium, and the fibrosis associated with DIP is usually uniform in appearance. Eosinophils and macrophages are the predominant alveolar inflammatory cells in eosinophilic pneumonia. These cells extend into the interstitium and, in some areas, there may be foci of necrosis and proteinaceous debris termed *eosinophilic microabscesses*. In lymphocytic interstitial pneumonitis, the lymphoid infiltrate involves both the interstitium and the alveolar space. In some cases, lymphoid follicles are dispersed throughout the lung parenchyma. In alveolar proteinosis, the alveolar space is filled with dense eosinophilic proteinaceous material and there is a paucity of inflammatory cells. Red blood cells may fill the alveoli in the pulmonary hemorrhage syndromes and in the vasculitides, including Wegener's granulomatosis and capillaritis.

INFLAMMATION AND DESTRUCTION OF THE ALVEOLAR WALL

Many of the ILDs can be categorized based on the pattern of histopathologic derangement that occurs within the alveolar wall. *Usual interstitial pneumonitis* (UIP) is a quite distinct pattern characterized by predominantly subpleural and marked irregular replacement of the alveolar septal walls by mature collagen. The degree of inflammation is diminished compared with DIP and involves the interstitium more than the alveolar space (Fig. 10-7). The alveolar walls are thickened with increased numbers of fibroblasts

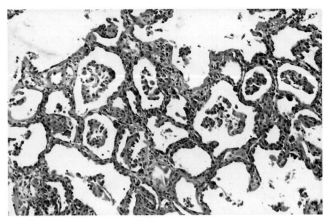

FIGURE 10-7 Usual interstitial pneumonia. Photomicrograph of an area of biopsy that reveals intraalveolar chronic inflammatory cells (mainly macrophages, DIP-like reaction) with inflammation and thickening of the alveolar walls (H&E stain).

and noncellular material. Widening of the interstitium occurs not only by deposition of collagen and other extracellular matrix components but also by alveolar collapse, apposition of alveolar walls, and obliteration of the intraalveolar space.[101,102] Fibroblastic foci are also present within the alveolar spaces.[103] In IPF, the lung is heterogenously involved with areas of inflammation interspersed with more fibrotic regions and occasionally normal lung parenchyma. Eventually the fibrotic process progresses to destroy the lung architecture totally and the interstitium is replaced with dense, acellular material arranged around small cysts which resemble honeycombs. The cysts are lined by metaplastic epithelial cells, and few inflammatory cells are present within the cysts or the interstitium (Fig. 10-8). End-stage lung is a nonspecific histopathologic pattern that occurs in the final stages of many ILDs (Table 10-5).

Granulomatous processes may alter the interstitium in sarcoidosis and hypersensitivity pneumonitis, as well as mycobacterial and fungal infectious processes. In sarcoidosis, these

FIGURE 10-8 Usual interstitial pneumonia (honeycombing). Photomicrograph of an area of biopsy that reveals end-stage honeycomb lung. The fibrotic process has destroyed the normal lung architecture replacing it with dense, acellular fibrous material arranged around small cysts (H&E stain).

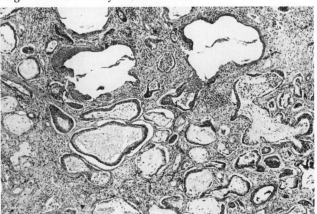

TABLE 10-5 Causes of End-Stage or Honeycomb Lung

Idiopathic pulmonary fibrosis (IPF)
ILD due to drugs
ILD associated with collagen vascular diseases
Sarcoid
Berylliosis
Hypersensitivity pneumonitis
Radiation-induced ILD
Eosinophilic granuloma
Lymphocytic interstitial pneumonitis

granulomas are tightly formed, well circumscribed, and have minimal surrounding inflammation (Fig. 10-9). They are not necrotizing and occur along pulmonary lymphatics, vessels, bronchi, and the pleura. In contrast, the granulomas of hypersensitivity pneumonia are less tightly formed and have a more random distribution within the interstitium and alveolar septae. In addition, there is greater inflammation within the interstitium, which may also involve the bronchioles. Fibrosis is usually present only in severe, chronic hypersensitivity pneumonitis.

The histopathologic manifestations of parenchymal lung involvement in lymphangioleiomyomatosis (LAM) and tuberous sclerosis are characterized by the proliferation of smooth muscle-like cells along the lymphatics and extending into the parenchymal interstitium. The morphology of these cells varies from elongated spindle-shaped to plump and round. They stain positively for HMB-45 and, upon electron microscopic examination, contain dense intracytoplasmic inclusions. The lung parenchyma is replaced with cysts of varying size up to 2 cm in diameter. The pathogenesis of these cysts is unclear but may be due to airway obstruction by the proliferating smooth muscle cells. Similar involvement of the lymphatics and thoracic duct may explain the increased incidence of chylous pleural effusions in LAM. In addition, renal smooth muscle cell tumors (angiomyolipomas) occur in nearly 40 percent of women with LAM.[104,105]

BRONCHIOLOCENTRIC ILD

In several forms of ILD including bronchiolitis obliterans organizing pneumonia, respiratory bronchiolitis-interstitial lung disease (RB-ILD), and eosinophilic granuloma, the site of structural derangement centers around the bronchiole from which it extends to involve adjacent lung parenchyma. Fibrosis arises within the airways in BOOP or cryptogenic organizing pneumonia. Few inflammatory cells and fibroblasts within myxomatous plugs of loose connective tissue (Masson's bodies) fill the distal bronchioles and reach into the peribronchiolar alveoli (Fig. 10-10). Although plasma cells and lymphocytes may infiltrate the interstitium, there is relatively little parenchymal fibrosis. Similarly in RB-ILD, the lung parenchyma is usually well preserved. Increased numbers of macrophages containing pigmented inclusions are present within the lumen and walls of the respiratory bronchioles, and the inflammatory process may extend into the surrounding alveoli. The dense intraalveolar macrophage congestion resembles DIP. Eosinophilic granuloma is characterized by the intramural accumulation of Langerhans' cells within bronchioles and alveolar ducts which are often accompanied by inflammatory cells, especially eosinophils. Langerhans' cells are defined by the ultrastructural presence of racket-shaped pentalaminar organelles or Birbeck granules and often stain positively for the S-100 protein. The inflammatory reaction extends outward into the lung parenchyma along the alveolar septae leading to the formation of a stellate nodule with a fibrotic, peribronchiolar center. As the disease progresses, small cysts or cavities develop which can be identified on gross examination of the lung. The processes regulating the formation of these cysts are not known.

ILD ASSOCIATED WITH COLLAGEN VASCULAR DISEASE, DRUGS, AND RADIATION THERAPY

The histopathologic manifestation of ILD associated with the collagen vascular diseases varies with both the underlying

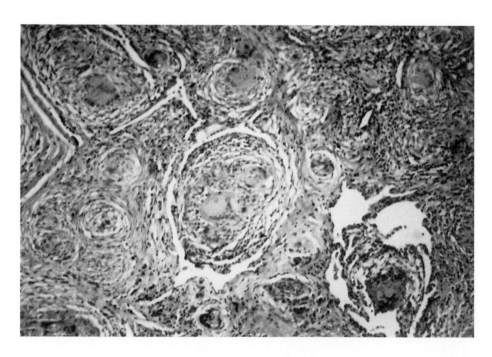

FIGURE 10-9 Sarcoidosis. Photomicrograph shows granulomatous inflammation. The granulomas has coalesced to form nodules several centimeters in size and identifiable on chest radiograph. Mutiple multinucleated giant cells are present.

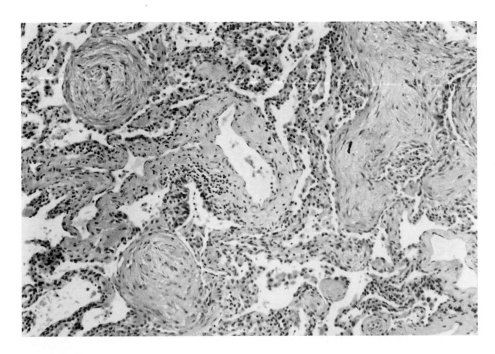

FIGURE 10-10 Cryptogenic Organizing Pneumonia. Photomicrograph of histopathologic specimen shows bronchiolitis obliterans with organizing pneumonia. Myxomatous plugs of loose connective tissue (Masson's bodies) fill the distal bronchioles and reach into the peribronchiolar alveoli.

disorder and the individual patient. Many patterns of parenchymal derangement have been described with each of the collagen vascular diseases, and a lung biopsy may exhibit either a single or several different forms of lung destruction (Table 10-6). Similarly, in drug-induced ILD, the histopathologic patterns are not pathognomonic for a particular agent,

TABLE 10-6 Parenchymal Manifestations of Collagen Vascular Diseases

Rheumatoid arthritis
   Desquamative interstitial pneumonitis (DIP)
   Nonspecific interstitial pneumonitis
   Bronchiolitis obliterans (BO)
   Bronchiolitis obliterans organizing pneumonia (BOOP)
   Eosinophilic pneumonia
   Vasculitis
Systemic lupus erythematosis
   Desquamative interstitial pneumonitis
   Nonspecific interstitial pneumonitis
   Lymphocytic interstitial pneumonitis
   Vasculitis
   Alveolar hemorrhage
   Bronchiolitis obliterans organizing pneumonia
Scleroderma
   Usual interstitial pneumonitis
   Pulmonary hypertension
   Bronchiolitis obliterans organizing pneumonia
Sjogren's syndrome
   Lymphocytic interstitial pneumonitis
   Nonspecific interstitial pneumonitis
   Amyloidosis
   Lymphoma and pseudolymphoma
   Bronchiolitis obliterans organizing pneumonia
   Vasculitis
Polymyositis-dermatomyositis
   Bronchiolitis obliterans organizing pneumonia
   Nonspecific interstitial pneumonitis
   Diffuse alveolar damage

and a particular drug may cause different forms of lung damage.

The risk of radiation-induced lung injury is enhanced by the mass of lung tissue irradiated, previous radiation treatments, total dose and fractionation of delivered radiation, and previous or concurrent sensitizing chemotherapeutic agents including bleomycin, cyclophosphamide, and doxorubicin. Both acute and chronic forms of lung damage occur after irradiation. Acute radiation pneumonitis develops 6 weeks to 6 months after the completion of treatment and is characterized by diffuse alveolar damage. Capillary endothelial cells are bloated and necrotic, and vessels may be occluded by detached cells and thrombi. The alveoli are filled with proteinaceous exudate and lined by hypertrophic alveolar type II cells with large, irregular nuclei containing prominent nucleoli. Epithelial cell damage may extend into the airways. Although there is not usually an extensive inflammatory reaction, these lesions are responsive to corticosteroids. The demonstration of T-helper cell predominant alveolitis by BAL has suggested that acute radiation pneumonitis may be a variant of hypersensitivity pneumonitis.[106] In chronic radiation lung injury, the lung parenchyma is replaced by extensive interstitial fibrosis, and pulmonary arterioles are obstructed by vascular sclerosis.

THERAPY AND MANAGEMENT

Treatment of ILD is based on the current idea of the pathogenic processes that mediate pulmonary fibrosis. Initially, these disorders are characterized by the accumulation of inflammatory and immune effector cells within the pulmonary parenchyma. If this alveolar and interstitial inflammatory reaction continues, alveolar wall, vascular, and airway damage ensues when reparative processes are inadequate or impaired, fibrosis develops. Eventually the lung parenchyma is irreversibly replaced with honeycombed cysts that are incapable of gas exchange, and ventilatory reserve is diminished to the point that symptoms of respiratory insufficiency

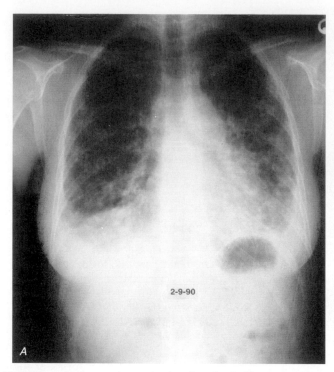

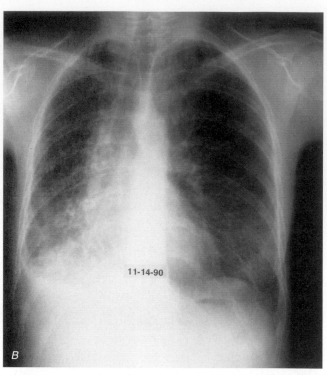

FIGURE 10-11 Progressive systemic sclerosis. *A.* Chest roent-genogram shows diffuse, reticular, and hazy opacities worse in the lower lung zones. *B.* Same patient as in *A.* Chest roentgeno-gram 5 months after left single-lung transplant shows normal left lung with small right lung and shift of the mediastinum to the right. The patient is alive 6 years after the transplant.

become apparent. No treatment other than lung transplantation is known to stop this process or to reverse parenchymal fibrosis.

Treatment of the ILD should begin with the identifying inciting agents such as inhaled antigens in hypersensitivity pneumonitis and occupational exposures, or medications known to cause parenchymal lung disease. The putative agent can be removed, and the clinical, radiographic, and physiologic course followed. If the patient improves, no further interventions are required other than avoiding further contact with the causative agent.

If the patient does not improve or no inciting factor is identified, therapeutic interventions are directed against the parenchymal inflammation to halt or delay the fibrotic process. The principal anti-inflammatory medications used in the treatment of the ILD are corticosteroids and cytotoxic drugs. In general, the more inflammatory disorders such as BOOP tend to be the most responsive to treatment, and the more fibrotic disorders, for example, honeycomb lung, are the least responsive.

Few prospective, randomized, double-blind, placebo-controlled trials have been performed to evaluate the efficacy of corticosteroids in the treatment of the most common forms of ILD, IPF,[107] and sarcoidosis.[108] The available studies indicate that approximately 20 to 30 percent of patients with IPF respond to steroids.[109,110] Based on the current evidence, treatment of pulmonary sarcoidosis with corticosteroids is justified for relief of symptoms and to control disabling systemic involvement.[108,111]

Corticosteroids are thought to have multiple anti-inflammatory actions including modification of neutrophil function as well as humoral processes. Although the optimal response to treatment is an improvement in lung function, steroids may prevent or reduce the rate of deterioration. Because the clinical course of ILD varies with the type of disease, its severity, and the individual patient, there is no single measurement which completely reflects disease activity and progression. Therefore, an approach which ranks and combines a number of parameters into a single CRP (clinical, radiographic, and physiologic) score, has been suggested to assess and follow the course of patients with IPF[88] and sarcoidosis.[112] The utility of these scales in the management of other forms of ILD awaits further assessment.

Cyclophosphamide, an alkylating agent that is activated by the P-450 system in the liver, has been used in the treatment of ILD. The active metabolites cross-link macromolecules interfering with their replication and function. Lymphocytes are particularly sensitive to this agent, and cyclophosphamide reduces both lymphocyte numbers and function. The usual dose is 1 to 2 mg/kg daily, and up to 6 months of treatment may be required to determine if there is a positive response to therapy. Between 20 and 60 percent of patients improve with cyclophosphamide.[87,113,114] Reduction in the white blood cell count, anemia, and thrombocytopenia are the major hematologic side effects. Hemorrhagic cystitis and secondary malignancies are other potential complications. Another alkylating agent, chlorambucil, has been shown to be effective in treating many collagen vascular disorders and may be useful in the treatment of sarcoid that is not responsive to corticosteroids.[115,116]

Azathioprine has been reported to be beneficial in the treatment of IPF.[117] This purine analog is metabolized to 6-mercaptopurine in the liver and acts by inhibiting DNA synthesis. In addition to its cytotoxic effects, azathioprine

TABLE 10-7 Criteria for Lung Transplantation

End-stage fibrosis, life expectancy <12–18 months
Age <65
No other systemic disease, end organ failure, infection
Normal body habitus
Prednisone <10–20 mg/d
Adequate cardiac function
Good general fitness and nutritional status
Psychosocial and family support systems
No recent alcohol, drug, tobacco abuse
Understanding of the transplant process and ability to comply
   with medical and rehabilitation programs

may diminish the humoral immune response. Hematologic, gastrointestinal, and pulmonary side effects as well as increased risk of secondary malignancies and teratogenic effects have been reported with azathioprine.

Cyclosporine is a cyclic endecapeptide which suppresses T-cell–mediated alloimmune and autoimmune responses, in part, by reducing interleukin 2 and γ-interferon production. It has been used as a steroid sparing agent in the treatment of ILD associated with dermatomyositis-polymyositis,[118] rheumatoid arthritis,[119] and systemic sclerosis.[120] In patients with IPF awaiting lung transplantation, cyclosporine may aid in the reduction of corticosteroid therapy.[121] However, cyclosporine has not been shown to be definitively beneficial in the treatment of IPF[122,123] or sarcoidosis.[124,125] The major complication of treatment with cyclosporine is renal toxicity.

Colchicine diminishes neutrophil function and inhibits the production of fibroblast growth factors by macrophages.[126] Based on these in vitro anti-inflammatory actions, it has been proposed as an agent in the treatment of IPF.[127] In a retrospective study of 23 patients, 22 percent improved, 39 percent stabilized, and 39 percent deteriorated over an average 23 months of therapy.[127] Many of these patients also received varying doses of prednisone. The usual dose of colchicine is 0.6 mg up to two times daily depending on gastrointestinal tolerance. Prospective trials examining the effectiveness of this agent in IPF are ongoing.

In addition to anti-inflammatory medications, other interventions may be used in the treatment of ILD. Supplemental oxygen is indicated for arterial oxygen levels below 55 mmHg at rest, with exercise, or during sleep. Oxygen flow rates should be titrated to ensure the prevention of desaturation and are frequently higher than for obstructive lung disease. The alleviation of hypoxemia may reduce right heart strain by decreasing hypoxic vasoconstriction and also improve mental acuity and exercise tolerance. Pulmonary rehabilitation and physical and occupational therapy may teach patients energy saving techniques and modifications of their activities of daily living that will allow them greater independence and relief from their respiratory insufficiency. Psychological and family counseling may aid in the acceptance of a chronic, debilitating disorder and, lastly, hospice care may lessen the discomfort of respiratory insufficiency during the terminal stages of ILD.

Lung replacement by transplantation is the only currently known treatment that "reverses" parenchymal fibrosis (Fig. 10-11). Criteria for lung transplantation are presented in Table 10-7. Single-lung transplantation is the preferred surgical procedure as long as right heart failure is the only cardiac

abnormality.[128] Although the 1-year survival after transplantation has improved to more than 60 percent, between one-third and two-thirds of patients die while awaiting surgery.[129,130] The development of bronchiolitis obliterans appears to be the limiting factor to prolonged survival after the initial postoperative period. Lastly, even with successful transplantation, several underlying systemic processes including sarcoid and lymphangioleiomyomatosis have recurred in the donor lung.[131–133] The long-term effect of these disorders on the transplanted lung is not yet known.

Common Forms of ILD

IDIOPATHIC PULMONARY FIBROSIS

IPF (cryptogenic fibrosing alveolitis) is one of the more commonly occurring interstitial lung diseases of unknown etiology. The pathogenesis of IPF is unknown, although genetic, viral, and immunologic aberrations are hypothesized. Clinical manifestations include dyspnea on exertion, nonproductive cough, and "Velcro"-type inspiratory crackles with or without digital clubbing noted on physical examination. The chest roentgenogram typically reveals diffuse interstitial opacities and honeycombing. HRCT findings in IPF include (1) ground glass opacification with patchy, predominantly peripheral, airspace infiltrates or a "hazy" increase in lung density (an increase in CT lung density that does not obscure the underlying lung parenchyma); (2) a lower lung zone predominant reticular pattern, consisting largely of thickened interlobular septae and intralobular lines; and (3) combined ground glass and reticular patterns. Honeycombing, traction bronchiectasis, and subpleural fibrosis also may be present (Fig. 10-12).

Pulmonary function tests often reveal restrictive impairment (decreased static lung volumes) (see Figs. 10-1 and 10-2), reduced diffusing capacity for carbon monoxide, and arterial hypoxemia exaggerated or elicited by exercise.

The confirmation of the diagnosis of IPF generally requires tissue obtained by VATS or open-lung biopsy. Pathologically, IPF is characterized by the UIP pattern, that is variable degrees of cellular infiltration of alveolar walls, fibroblast proliferation, collagen deposition, and cystic spaces in areas of advanced disease (the so-called honeycomb lung).

The clinical course is variable with a mean survival of 4 to 6 years after the time of diagnosis. Response to treatment of the disease is variable, but patients with a more cellular biopsy are more likely to improve with corticosteroid and/or cytotoxic therapy. For IPF, prednisone is usually started at 1.0 to 1.5 mg/kg as a single daily dose. This level is maintained for 3 months, then tapered to 0.5 to 1.0 mg/kg for 3 more months. Maintenance therapy at 0.25 mg/kg is continued for the following 6 months. At each reduction in dosage, the clinical, radiographic, and physiologic response is assessed. Cytotoxic drugs, particularly cyclophosphamide and azathioprine, have been the most commonly employed second line drugs in the management of patients with IPF.[134] Several newer agents are being tried in an effort to identify better treatments for IPF.[135,136]

SARCOIDOSIS

Sarcoidosis is a multisystem disease of unknown etiology and pathogenesis. The exact prevalence (10 to 20 per 100,000

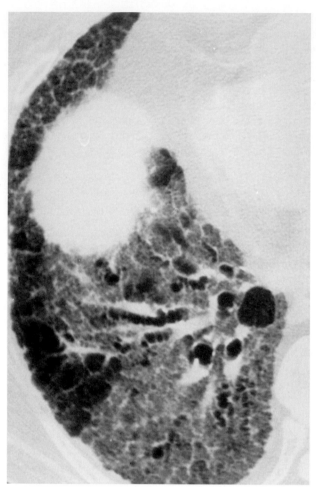

FIGURE 10-12 Idiopathic pulmonary fibrosis. HRCT shows extensive ground-glass opacities in the lower lung zone associated with marked traction bronchiectasis and bronchiolectasis. Biopsy revealed severe end-stage fibrosis. Parenchymal opacification on HRCT is usually associated with active alveolitis (From Leung et al.), however, parenchymal opacification in the presence of traction bronchiectasis or bronchiolectasis, anatomic distortion, and discernible cysts most likely represents fibrosis (From Leung AN, Miller RR, Muller NL: Parenchymal opacification in chronic infiltrative lung disease: CT-pathologic correlation. *Radiology* 188:209, 1993, and Nishimura K, Kitaichi M, Izumi T, et al: Usual interstitial pneumonia: Histologic correlation with high-resolution CT. Radiology 182: 337, 1992.

population) and annual incidence varies. Sarcoid is eight times more common in African Americans. The immunogenetic background of affected individuals may play a role in the clinical heterogeneity of sarcoidosis.[137]

The onset is usually between age 10 and 40 years (70 to 90 percent of cases). In 40 to 60 percent of patients the disease is discovered by routine chest x-ray before the development of symptoms. Dyspnea with or without exertion, nonproductive cough, and nonspecific chest pain are the most common complaints. Laboratory evaluation may reveal elevated liver function tests, hypercalcemia, and hypergammaglobulinemia. Serum angiotensin converting enzyme (ACE) levels, formerly thought to reflect the activity of the disease, are not consistently helpful. Pulmonary function tests may reveal normal function, a restrictive pattern, or an obstructive de-

fect, the latter inferring endobronchial sarcoid involvement. The $D_{L_{CO}}$ is commonly reduced, however, usually to a lesser degree than in other interstitial lung disorders.

The "classic" chest roentgenogram in sarcoidosis reveals bilateral hilar adenopathy, but this may be absent or occur in combination with parenchymal opacities, depending on the stage of disease (Fig. 10-13). Parenchymal opacities may be interstitial, alveolar, or both. Nodular lesions also occur. An upper-zone-predominant distribution of disease is typical.

The diagnosis of sarcoidosis is made histologically, by demonstrating noncaseating granulomas in a perivascular pattern. They may occur in any organ, although the lung, peripheral lymph nodes, skin, eyes, and liver are most commonly affected. The frequent involvement of the lung makes this organ the most accessible tissue for biopsy. Even if interstitial opacities are not present radiographically, the diagnosis may be made by transbronchial biopsy in more than 90 percent of cases.

Treatment of the disease with corticosteroids is indicated for patients with symptoms and for those who have significant vital organ involvement such (e.g., uveitis or central nervous system or heart involvement). Since a substantial number of patients experience spontaneous remission (especially younger ones with bilateral hilar adenopathy and a recent history of erythema nodosum), stable patients should be monitored for up to 6 months before instituting treatment.[112] Sarcoidosis is generally very responsive to corticosteroids. The effect of treatment on the long-term outcome of patients with sarcoidosis is unknown.[112]

DRUG-INDUCED ILD

Many drugs are known to have the potential to induce diffuse interstitial infiltrates with associated symptoms of dyspnea

FIGURE 10-13 Sarcoidosis. The chest radiograph shows bilateral hilar adenopathy (stage I).

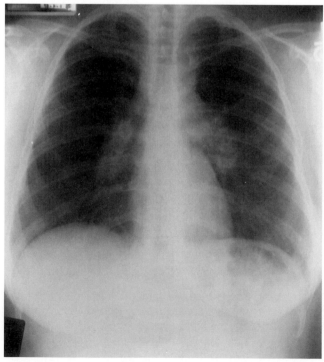

and nonproductive cough. In most cases, the pathogenesis of this aberrant pulmonary response to a given drug is unknown, although a combination of direct toxic effects of the drug (or its metabolite) and indirect inflammatory and immunologic events is likely. This topic is too extensive to discuss thoroughly, but several generalizations can be made: (1) the extent and severity of disease is usually dose-related; (2) many classes of drugs may cause disease; (3) the onset of illness may be insidious over weeks to months, or may be abrupt and fulminant; (4) treatment always includes discontinuation of any possible offending drug and supportive care; and (5) since the addition of corticosteroids is often ineffective, this is a decision that must be based on the available data for a given drug.

A syndrome of drug-induced lupus, manifested in the lung principally as pleural disease, can be seen (particularly with procainamide and rarely quinidine). Current evidence suggests a genetic predisposition to drug-induced lupus because patients who are "slow acetylators" of the aromatic amine group on procainamide are at greater risk for developing drug-induced lupus.[138] Like systemic lupus erythematosis (SLE), clinical manifestations of drug-induced lupus are protean, including fever, arthralgia, rashes, myositis, vasculitis, serositis, and Raynaud's phenomenon.[139] The pulmonary lesions associated with drug-induced lupus include pleuritis manifested by pleural effusions and pleurisy and diffuse parenchymal lung disease.[140] There are several features that distinguish drug-induced lupus from SLE. In drug-induced lupus renal and central nervous system involvement are extremely rare, serum complement level is usually normal, antibody to double-stranded DNA is negative, and there is no predilection for females.[141]

SILICOSIS

Miners, sandblasters, glass manufacturers, quarry workers, stone dressers, foundry workers, and boiler scalers can have silicosis. Radiographically, silicosis appears as bilateral multinodular rounded densities predominantly in the upper lung zones. The radiographic changes usually appear before the clinical and functional abnormalities. Progression from simple to progressive massive fibrosis occurs in a minority of patients.

Patients with silicosis are highly susceptible to infection by *Mycobacterium tuberculosis* and other atypical mycobacteria. Also, scleroderma and rheumatoid arthritis are unusually common in silicotics. Laboratory findings in simple silicosis may include an increased sedimentation rate, immunoglobulins, immune complexes, antinuclear antibodies, and anti-immunoglobulin antibodies (rheumatoid factors). There is no known effective treatment at present for silicosis.

ASBESTOSIS

Asbestos exposure is widespread because it has been used extensively as an insulation material, fire retardant, and noise reduction agent in many public facilities. More than 90 percent of the asbestos used is chrysolite, or white asbestos. Workers employed in the shipyard, automotive, insulation, cement, textile, and asbestos mining industries are at greatest risk. There is a long latent period between exposure and the development of lung diseases. In general, individuals who develop asbestos-induced disease will have markedly in-

creased numbers of asbestos fibers in their lung compared with the general population. Smoking appears to facilitate the damaging effects of asbestos inhalation.

It is important to distinguish evidence of asbestos exposure from asbestosis. Asbestosis is characterized by a history of exposure to asbestos and the presence of interstitial pulmonary fibrosis manifested by dyspnea, cough, and bibasilar inspiratory crackles with or without digital clubbing on examination. Bilateral pleural thickening along the lower or midthoracic walls, calcified pleural plaques occurring on the parietal pleura and diaphragm, and hazy opacities composed of irregular or linear small opacities especially in the lower lung zones are the most common roentgenographic changes.

Pulmonary function studies may reveal a restrictive pattern, and the $D_{L_{CO}}$ is often reduced. Asbestos-induced fibrosis of the visceral pleura can produce restrictive functional abnormalities. The clinical course of asbestosis is usually one of slow but progressive deterioration, and death is often a result of either respiratory compromise or cancer. Thirty to forty percent of patients with asbestosis will develop lung cancer. Pleural and peritoneal mesotheliomas and bronchogenic carcinoma are established complications of asbestos exposure. Pseudotumors, or rounded atelectasis (infoldings of lung caused by scarring of the overlying pleura) can be mistaken radiographically for tumors. The synergistic effect of cigarette smoking and asbestos exposure on the development of lung cancer is well established.

HYPERSENSITIVITY PNEUMONITIDES (EXTRINSIC ALLERGIC ALVEOLITIS)

This group of diseases is associated largely with repeated inhalation of finely dispersed organic dusts. This produces diffuse patchy interstitial and/or alveolar infiltrates in the lung following the formation of antigen-antibody complexes (Arthus reaction). Farmer's lung (exposure to moldy hay containing fungal spores) is the prototype. In urban areas, bird fancier's lung (due to exposure to bird proteins) and air conditioner or humidifier lung disease (due to fungal overgrowth and aerosolization) are more common.

Patients with hypersensitivity pneumonitis can present with either an acute or chronic illness. An abrupt onset (4 to 6 h later) of fever, chills, malaise, nausea, cough, chest tightness, and dyspnea without wheezing usually follows heavy exposure. Diffuse fine rales throughout the chest, mild hypoxemia, and a restrictive ventilatory defect accompanies these symptomatic episodes. A fleeting, micronodular, interstitial pattern in the lower and mid-lower zone may be identified on chest roentgenogram. Removal from exposure usually results in complete resolution within hours or days. Pathologically, this stage is characterized by noncaseating interstitial granulomatous pneumonitis.

An insidious or chronic form results if repeated acute episodes or continued antigen exposure occurs. A patient with chronic hypersensitivity pneumonitis may not have had any acute episodes. Disabling and frequently irreversible respiratory findings, i.e., pulmonary fibrosis, are characteristic. Mixed obstructive and restrictive physiology is often present on pulmonary function testing, as well as reduced diffusing capacity, and hypoxemia. The chest roentgenogram shows progressive fibrotic changes and loss of volume, particularly in the upper lobes. Diagnosis of the chronic form of hypersensitivity pneumonitis usually requires open or VATS lung biopsy. Besides the granulomatous pneumonitis, biopsy specimens at this stage reveal bronchiolitis obliterans with distal destruction of alveoli (honeycombing) in association with densely fibrotic zones.

The diagnosis of hypersensitivity pneumonitis is important since it is a reversible disease when diagnosed early. Measurement of serum precipitins to a general panel of possible antigens usually is not very helpful. Bronchoalveolar lavage with the measurement of antibodies, IgG, and IgM, and examination of immunoreactive cells for specific immune responses may eventually become a useful diagnostic procedure. A lavage lymphocytosis (usually >40 percent) suggests the diagnosis.

CONNECTIVE TISSUE DISORDERS

ILD associated with connective tissue disorders (CTD) usually occurs after the CTD has been recognized. Occasionally the ILD may precede the development of the characteristic systemic signs and symptoms of the particular CTD, especially rheumatoid arthritis or polymyositis. The most common form of radiographic change is a chronic interstitial pattern similar to that found in patients with IPF. In these diseases there is also a high incidence of lung disease caused by disease-associated complications of esophageal dysfunction (predisposing to aspiration and secondary infections), respiratory muscle weakness (atelectasis and secondary infections), therapeutic complications (opportunistic infections), and associated malignancies.

RHEUMATOID ARTHRITIS
Although rheumatoid arthritis (RA) itself is more common in women, the pulmonary disease associated with RA is more common in men. Manifestations of RA in the lung include pleurisy with or without effusion, interstitial lung disease (up to 20 percent of cases), necrobiotic nodules (nonpneumoconiotic intrapulmonary rheumatoid nodules) with or without cavities, Caplan's syndrome (rheumatoid pneumoconiosis), pulmonary hypertension secondary to rheumatoid pulmonary vasculitis, bronchiolitis obliterans, bronchiolitis obliterans organizing pneumonia, and upper airway obstruction due to arytenoid arthritis.

PROGRESSIVE SYSTEMIC SCLEROSIS
Progressive systemic sclerosis (PSS), or scleroderma, is a systemic disease characterized by dermatologic changes (skin thickening, ulcerations), visceral microvascular abnormalities, and esophageal dysfunction. The incidence of interstitial lung disease associated with PSS ranges from 14 to 90 percent in clinical studies and from 60 to 100 percent in autopsy studies. Pulmonary function tests usually have revealed a restrictive pattern with reduced lung compliance and impaired diffusing capacity, often before any clinical or radiographic evidence of lung disease appears. Pulmonary vascular disease alone or in association with pulmonary fibrosis, pleuritis, recurrent aspiration pneumonitis, and bronchiolar carcinoma also occur. The interstitial lung disease and pulmonary hypertension associated with scleroderma are strikingly resistant to current modes of therapy.

SYSTEMIC LUPUS ERYTHEMATOSUS
SLE is a systemic disorder of unknown etiology characterized by immunologically mediated tissue damage. Multiple organ systems may be involved including renal, central nervous, musculoskeletal, mucocutaneous, and other systems. Pleuritis with or without effusion is the most common pulmonary manifestation of SLE. Other lung manifestations include atelectasis, diaphragmatic dysfunction with loss of lung volume, pulmonary vascular disease, pulmonary hemorrhage, uremic pulmonary edema, infectious pneumonia, bronchiolitis obliterans, and ILD.

SJÖGREN'S SYNDROME
Sjögren's syndrome (SS) manifested by keratoconjunctivitis sicca, xerostomia, and recurrent swelling of the parotid gland may be associated with ILD. Lymphocytic interstitial pneumonitis (LIP), lymphoma, pseudolymphoma, bronchiolitis, and bronchiolitis obliterans are associated with SS. Open or VATS lung biopsy is frequently required to discern a precise pulmonary diagnosis in SS. In the absence of controlled trials, corticosteroids have been used in the management of SS-associated ILD with some degree of clinical success.

POLYMYOSITIS AND DERMATOMYOSITIS
ILD occurs in approximately 10 percent of patients with polymyositis and dermatomyositis (PM and DM), and the clinical features are similar to IPF. Less commonly, a rapidly progressive Hamman-Rich syndrome (diffuse alveolar damage) may occur with respiratory failure. Diffuse reticular or reticular-nodular opacities with or without an alveolar component occur radiographically, with a predilection for the lung bases. The response rate to corticosteroid therapy in patients with ILD has been reported to be higher than ILD associated with other CTD.

EOSINOPHILIC PNEUMONIA

CHRONIC EOSINOPHILIC PNEUMONIA
Chronic eosinophilic pneumonia (CEP) is often a fulminant illness characterized by fever, night sweats, weight loss, and progressive breathlessness and asthma (which accompanies or precedes the illness in 50 percent of cases). The chest radiographic findings of bilateral peripheral- or pleural-based opacities described as the *photographic negative* of pulmonary edema are virtually pathognomonic (Fig. 10-14). Peripheral blood eosinophilia, very high sedimentation rate, iron deficiency anemia, and thrombocytosis are frequent laboratory abnormalities. BAL eosinophilia (>40 percent) suggests the diagnosis.[142] BAL eosinophils show signs of activation with the release of eosinophil proteins.[143] Serial BAL may be helpful in following the course of the disease.[142] BAL eosinophilia (>40 percent) suggest the diagnosis. Histopathologic findings are characterized by interstitial and alveolar eosinophils and histiocytes including multinucleated giant cells. Necrosis of the alveolar exudate results in formation of eosinophilic abscesses. Fibrosis is minimal, and bronchiolitis obliterans with organizing pneumonia is a frequent associated finding. CEP has an excellent response to corticosteroids, but long-term treatment (months to years) may be required.

ACUTE IDIOPATHIC EOSINOPHILIC PNEUMONIA
Acute idiopathic eosinophilic pneumonia is a cause of acute respiratory failure.[10,144,145] The etiology is unknown, but an inhaled antigen is suspected. The diagnosis is based on the presence of an acute febrile illness associated with hypoxemic

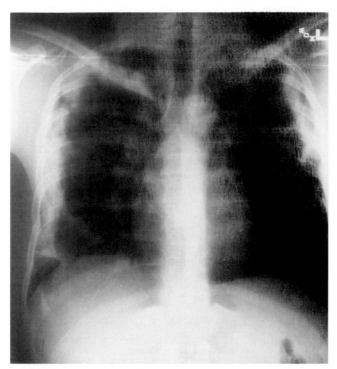

FIGURE 10-14 Chronic eosinophilic pneumonia. Chest roentgenogram shows dense bilateral peripheral alveolar opacities described as the *photographic negative* of pulmonary edema.

respiratory failure, diffuse pulmonary opacities, and BAL eosinophilia (>25 percent) without infection, asthma or atopic disease. There is often a dramatic response to corticosteroids without relapse after withdrawal.

CRYPTOGENIC ORGANIZING PNEUMONIA

Cryptogenic organizing pneumonia (COP, or idiopathic BOOP) is a distinct clinical entity of unknown incidence and prevalence (found in six to seven per 100,000 admissions[146]). The disease onset occurs usually in the fifth and sixth decade (mean age 58 years old) and affects men and women equally. Almost three-fourths of the patients have their symptoms for less than 2 months and few have symptoms for >6 months prior to diagnosis.[147]

A persistent and usually nonproductive cough is the most common presenting symptom (72 percent). Frequently, patients experience dyspnea with exertion (66 percent) and usually describe their onset as a flulike illness with fever (51 percent), malaise (48 percent), fatigue, and cough. Weight loss of usually more than 10 lb is a common complaint (57 percent). The clinical presentation frequently mimics that of community-acquired pneumonia. Physical examination may be normal[18] but most often reveals inspiratory rales (74 percent). Clubbing is rare (<5 percent).[148]

Routine laboratory studies are nonspecific.[149–151] A leukocytosis is seen in approximately half the patients. The initial erythrocyte sedimentation rate (ESR) is elevated (frequently reaching or exceeding 100 mm), and a positive C-reactive protein is observed in 70 to 80 percent of patients.[148,152] Autoantibodies are usually negative or only slightly positive.[152]

The roentgenographic manifestations of COP are quite distinctive—bilateral, diffuse alveolar opacities in the presence of normal lung volume (Fig. 10-15). This pattern was present in 79 percent of reported subjects where the radiographic appearance was detailed.[147] A peripheral distribution of the opacities, very similar to that thought to be "virtually pathognomic" for chronic eosinophilic pneumonia, is also seen in COP.[149,153,154] Rarely, the alveolar opacities may be unilateral. In addition, recurrent and migratory pulmonary opacities are common.[155] Irregular linear or nodular interstitial opacities or honeycombing are rarely seen at presentation. Computed tomography scans of the lung reveal patchy airspace consolidation, ground-glass opacities, small nodular opacities, and bronchial wall thickening and dilatation.[156,157] These patchy opacities occur more frequently in the periphery of the lung and are often in the lower lung zone. The CT scan may reveal much more extensive disease than is expected by review of the plain chest x-ray.

Pulmonary function is usually impaired with a restrictive defect being most common. Gas exchange abnormalities are extremely common. The diffusing capacity ($D_{L_{CO}}$) is reduced in the majority of patients (72 percent). Resting alveolar-arterial ($P_A-a_{O_2}$) gradient of >20 mmHg and/or exercise arterial hypoxemia are common (83 percent).

The histopathologic lesions characteristic of COP include an excessive proliferation of granulation tissue within small airways (proliferative bronchiolitis) and alveolar ducts associated with chronic inflammation in the surrounding alveoli. This organizing pneumonia is the most important process underlying the clinical and radiographic manifestations of COP.

The clinical and pathologic features of COP may be present in other disorders, such as bacterial pneumonia, hypersensitivity pneumonitis, chronic eosinophilic pneumonia, infec-

FIGURE 10-15 Cryptogenic organizing pneumonia. This posteroanterior roentgenogram shows bilateral patchy alveolar opacities. There was complete resolution following corticosteroid therapy; however, the disease recurred when the drug was stopped.

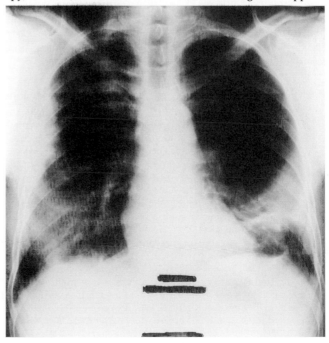

tion, drug reaction, or connective tissue disorder. Thus, the diagnosis of COP depends on both the clinical setting and finding the characteristic pathologic features of the disease (the prominent finding of the BOOP pattern in the absence of any other features suggestive of another process).[152] An open or thoracoscopic lung biopsy is recommended to confirm the diagnosis.

Corticosteroid therapy is the most common treatment. It results in clinical recovery, usually with complete clinical and physiologic improvement and normalization of the chest film, in two-thirds of the patients. Approximately one-third of patients demonstrate persistent disease.

Conclusion

The interstitial lung diseases are a diverse group of more than 150 different pulmonary disorders with overlapping clinical, radiographic, physiologic, and histopathologic characteristics. The clinical history is the most valuable factor in the assessment of patients with parenchymal lung disease. Velcro crackles are commonly present on auscultation of the chest, and restriction is the most frequent finding in pulmonary function testing. Widening of the alveolar-arterial oxygen gradient is a sensitive indicator of physiologic impairment which may detect early disease. High-resolution thin section computed tomography is the most valuable and informative chest imaging technique. Bronchoalveolar lavage allows the sampling and characterization of the types of cells and mediators within the alveolar space but is not necessarily representative of the processes within the interstitium. Lastly, histopathologic review of lung tissue remains the gold standard in the diagnosis and assessment of interstitial lung disease. In those cases in which an inciting agent can be identified, cessation of exposure is the principal therapeutic intervention. For the remaining patients in whom the cause of their ILD remains unknown, treatment with corticosteroids or cytotoxic medications is directed at interdicting the inflammatory processes which are believed to precede the development of fibrosis. Lung replacement by transplantation is the only known method of reverting dysfunctional fibrotic lung parenchyma. Thus, the interstitial lung diseases are challenges in diagnosis, evaluation, management, and treatment.

References

1. Division of Lung Diseases National Heart Lung Blood Institute: Report of task force on epidemiology of respiratory disease. Washington DC, US Department of Health and Human Services, NIH Publication no. 81-2019, 1980.
2. Coultas DB: Epidemiology of idiopathic pulmonary fibrosis. *Sem Respir Med* 14:181, 1993.
3. Johnston I, Britton J, Kinnear W, Logan R: Rising mortality from cryptogenic fibrosing alveolitis. *Br Med J* 301:1017, 1990.
4. Hubbard R, Johnston IDA, Coultas D, Britton J: Mortality rates from cryptogenic fibrosing alveolitis is seven countries. *Thorax* 51:711, 1996.
5. Mannino DM, Etzel RA, Parrish RG: Pulmonary fibrosis deaths in the United States, 1979–1991. An analysis of multiple-cause mortality data. *Am J Respir Crit Care Med* 153:1548, 1996.
6. Coultas DB, Zumwalt RE, Black WC, Sobonya RE: The epidemiology of interstitial lung disease. *Am J Respir Crit Care Med* 150:967, 1994.
7. Hogg JC: Chronic interstitial lung disease of unknown cause: A new classification based on pathogenesis. *AJR* 156:225, 1991.
8. Gaensler EA: Diagnostic techniques in diffuse or miliary lung diseases: Experience with 381 patients. *Adv Cardiopulmonary Dis* 3:81, 1966.
9. Wade JF III, King TE Jr: Infiltrative and interstitial lung disease in the elderly. *Clin Chest Med* 14:501, 1993.
10. Badesch DB, King TE, Jr., Schwarz MI: Acute eosinophilic pneumonia: A hypersensitivity phenomenon? *Am Rev Respir Dis* 139:249, 1989.
11. Fink JN: Hypersensitivity pneumonitis. *Clin Chest Med* 13:303, 1992.
12. Olson J, Colby TV, Elliott CG: Hamman-Rich syndrome revisited. *Mayo Clin Proc* 65:1538, 1990.
13. Leatherman JW: Immune alveolar hemorrhage. *Chest* 91:891, 1987.
14. Corley DE, Winterbauer RH: Collagen-vascular disease. *Sem Respir Infect* 10:78, 1995.
15. King TE Jr, Mortenson RL: Cryptogenic organizing pneumonia. The North American experience. *Chest* 102:8S, 1992.
16. Sharma OP, Johnson R: Airway obstruction in sarcoidosis: A study of 123 non-smoking black American patients with sarcoidosis. *Chest* 94:343, 1988.
17. Myers JL, Veal CF, Shin MS, Katzenstein ALA: Respiratory bronchiolitis causing interstitial lung disease: A clinicopathologic study of six cases. *Am Rev Respir Dis* 135:880, 1987.
18. Epler GR, Colby TV, McLoud TC, et al: Bronchiolitis obliterans organizing pneumonia. *N Engl J Med* 312:152, 1985.
19. Hance AJ, Cadranel J, Soler P, Basset F: Pulmonary and extrapulmonary Langerhans' cell granulomatosis (Histiocytosis X). *Sem Respir Med* 9:349, 1988.
20. Coleman A, Colby TV: Histologic diagnosis of extrinsic allergic alveolitis. *Am J Surg Path* 12:514, 1988.
21. Picado C, Gomez de Almeida R, Xaubet A, et al: Spontaneous pneumothorax in cryptogenic fibrosing alveolitis. *Respiration* 48:77, 1985.
22. Taylor JR, Ryu J, Colby TV, Raffin TA: Lymphangioleiomyomatosis. Clinical course in 32 patients. *N Engl J Med* 323:1254, 1990.
23. Kitaichi M, Nishimura K, Itoh H, Izumi T: Pulmonary lymphangioleiomyomatosis: A report of 46 patients including a clinicopathologic study of prognostic factors. *Am J Respir Crit Care Med* 151:527, 1995.
24. Dwyer JM, Hickie JB, Garvan J: Pulmonary tuberous sclerosis. Report of three patients and a review of the literature. *Quart J Med* 40:115, 1971.
25. Stefansson K: Tuberous sclerosis. *Mayo Clin Proc* 66:868, 1991.
26. Davis SD, Yankelevitz DF, Henschke CI: Radiation effects on the lung: Clinical features, pathology and imaging findings. *AJR* 159:1157, 1992.
27. Bayle JY, Nesme P, Bejui-Thivolet F, et al: Migratory cryptogenic organizing pneumonitis "primed" by radiation therapy. *Eur Respir J* 8:322, 1995.
28. Terry RD, Sperry WM, Brodoff B: Adult lipoidosis resembling Neimann-Pick disease. *Am J Pathol* 30:263, 1954.
29. Garay SM, Gardella JE, Fazzini EP, Goldring RM: Hermansky-Pudlak syndrome. Pulmonary manifestations of a ceroid storage disorder. *Am J Med* 66:737, 1979.
30. Schneider EL, Epstein CJ, Kaback MJ, Brandes D: Severe pulmonary involvement in adult Gaucher's disease. Report of three cases and review of the literature. *Am J Med* 63:475, 1977.
31. Baumgartner KB, Samet JM, Stidley CA, et al, and the Collaborating Centers: Cigarette smoking: A risk factor for idiopathic pulmonary fibrosis. *Am J Respir Crit Care Med*, 155:242, 1997.
32. Kusaka H, Homma Y, Ogasawara H, et al: Five-year follow-up of *Micropolyspora faeni* antibody in smoking and nonsmoking farmers. *Am Rev Respir Dis* 140:695, 1989.
33. Schwartz DA, Helmers RA, Galvin JR, et al: Determinants of

survival in idiopathic pulmonary fibrosis. *Am J Respir Crit Care Med* 149:450, 1994.

34. Kornbluth RS, Turino GM: Respiratory control in diffuse interstitial lung disease and diseases of the pulmonary vasculature. *Clin Chest Med* 1:91, 1980.

35. Keogh BA, Crystal RG: Clinical significance of pulmonary function tests: Pulmonary function testing in interstitial pulmonary disease. What does it tell us? *Chest* 78:856, 1980.

36. Englert M, Yernault JC, deCoster A, Clumeek N: Diffusing properties and elastic properties in interstitial diseases of the lung. *Prog Respir Res* 8:177, 1975.

37. Jernudd-Wilhelmsson Y, Hoernblad Y, Hedenstierna G: Ventilation-perfusion relationships in interstitial lung disease. *Eur J Respir Dis* 68:39, 1986.

38. McCarthy D, Cherinack RM: Regional ventilation-perfusion and hypoxia in cryptogenic fibrosing alveolitis. *Am Rev Respir Dis* 107:200, 1973.

39. Fulmer JD, Roberts WC, Von Gal ER: Morphologic-physiologic correlates of the severity of fibrosis and degree of cellularity in idiopathic pulmonary fibrosis. *J Clin Invest* 63:665, 1979.

40. Michel RP, Hakim TS, Freeman CR: Distribution of pulmonary vascular resistance in experimental fibrosis. *J Appl Physiol* 65:1180, 1988.

41. Sturani C, Papiris S, Galavotti V, Gunella G: Pulmonary vascular responsiveness at rest and during exercise in idiopathic pulmonary fibrosis; Effects of oxygen and nifedipine. *Respiration* 50:117, 1986.

42. Shivkumar K, Ravi K, Henry JW, et al: Right ventricular dilatation, right ventricular wall thickening, and Doppler evidence of pulmonary hypertension in patients with a pure restrictive ventilatory impairment. *Chest* 106:1649, 1994.

43. Hawrylkiewicz I, Izdebska-Makosa Z, Grebska E, Zielinski J: Pulmonary haemodynamics at rest and on exercise in patients with idiopathic pulmonary fibrosis. *Bull Eur Physiopathol Respir* 18:403, 1982.

44. Bye PTP, Issa F, Berthon-Jones M, Sullivan CE: Studies of oxygenation during sleep in patients with interstitial lung disease. *Am Rev Respir Dis* 129:37, 1984.

45. Perez-Padilla R, West P, Lertzman M, Kryger MH: Breathing during sleep in patients with interstitial lung disease. *Am Rev Respir Dis* 132:224, 1985.

46. Epler GR, McLoud TC, Gaensler EA, et al: Normal chest roentgenograms in chronic diffuse infiltrative lung disease. *N Engl J Med* 298:934, 1978.

47. Muller NL, Miller RR: Computed tomography of chronic diffuse infiltrative lung disease, Part 1. *Am Rev Respir Dis* 142:1206, 1990.

48. Muller NL, Miller RR: Computed tomography of chronic diffuse infiltrative lung disease, Part 2. *Am Rev Respir Dis* 142:1440, 1990.

49. Padley S, Gleeson F, Flower CD: Review article: Current indications for high resolution computed tomography scanning of the lungs. *Brit J Radiol* 68:105, 1995.

50. Corcoran HL, Renner WR, Milstein MJ: Review of high-resolution CT of the lung. *Radiographics* 12:917, 1992.

51. Line B: Scintigraphic studies of inflammation in diffuse lung disease. *Radiol Clin North Am* 29:1095, 1991.

52. Bisson G, Lamoureux G, Begin R: Quantitative gallium 67 lung scan to assess the inflammatory activity in the pneumoconioses. *Sem Nucl Med* 27:72, 1987.

53. Crystal RG, Gadek JE, Ferrans VJ, et al: Interstitial lung disease: Current concepts of pathogenesis, staging, and therapy. *Am J Med* 70:542, 1981.

54. Crystal RG, Bitterman PB, Rennard SI, et al: Interstitial lung diseases of unknown cause. Disorders characterized by chronic inflammation of the lower respiratory tract. *N Engl J Med* 310:154, 1984.

55. Gross WL, Schmitt WH, Csernok E. ANCA and associated diseases: Immunodiagnostic and pathogenetic aspects. *Clin Exp Immunol* 91:1, 1993.

56. Schnabel A, Hauschild S, Gross WL: Anti-neutrophil cytoplasmic antibodies in generalized autoimmune diseases. *Int Arch Allergy Immunol* 109:201, 1996.

57. Moder K: Use and interpretation of rheumatologic tests: A guide for clinicians. *Mayo Clin Proc* 71:391, 1996.

58. Rao JK, Weinberger M, Oddone EZ, et al: The role of antineutrophil cytoplasmic antibody (c-ANCA) testing in the diagnosis of Wegener's granulomatosis. A literature review and meta-analysis. *Ann Intern Med* 123:925, 1995.

59. Kallenberg CGM, Mulder AHL, Cohen Tervaert JW: Antineutrophil cytoplasmic antibodies: A still-growing class of autoantibodies in inflammatory disorders. *Am J Med* 93:675, 1992.

60. Rao JK, Allen NB, Feussner JR, Weinberger M: A prospective study of antineutrophil cytoplasmic antibody (c-ANCA) and clinical criteria in diagnosing Wegener's granulomatosis. *Lancet* 346:926, 1995.

61. King TE, Jr. A lung biopsy is necessary in the management of ANCA-positive patients with chest roentgenographic abnormalities. *Sarcoidosis* 13:238, 1996.

62. Cohen Tervaert JW, Huitema MG, Hene RJ, et al: Prevention of relapses in Wegener's granulomatosis by treatment based on antineutrophil cytoplasmic antibody titre. *Lancet* 336:709, 1990.

63. Kerr GS, Fleisher TA, Hallahan CW, et al: Limited prognostic value of changes in antineutrophil cytoplasmic antibody titer in patients with Wegener's granulomatosis. *Arthritis Rheum* 36:365, 1993.

64. Kallenberg CGM, Brouwer E, Weening JJ, Cohen Tervaert JW: Anti-neutrophil cytoplasmic antibodies: Current diagnostic and pathophysiological potential. *Kidney Int* 46:1, 1994.

65. Specks U, Wheatley BA, McDonald TJ, et al: Anticytoplasmic autoantibodies in the diagnosis and follow-up of Wegener's granulomatosis. *Mayo Clin Proc* 64:28, 1989.

66. Falk RJ, Jennette JC: Anti-neutrophil cytoplasmic autoantibodies with specificity for myeloperoxidase in patients with systemic vasculitis and idiopathic necrotizing and crescentic glomerulonephritis. *N Engl J Med* 318:1651, 1988.

67. Cohen Tervaert JW, Goldschmeding R, Elema JD, et al: Autoantibodies against myeloid lysosomal enzymes in crescentic glomerulonephritis. *Kidney Int* 37:799, 1990.

68. Gross W, Csernok E: Immunodiagnostic and pathophysiologic aspects of antineutrophil cytoplasmic antibodies in vasculitis. *Curr Opinion Rheumatol* 7:11, 1995.

69. Von Muehlen CA, Tan EM: Autoantibodies in the diagnosis of systemic rheumatic diseases. *Semin Arth Rheum* 24:323, 1995.

70. Kuwana M, Kaburaki J, Mimori T, et al: Autoantibody reactive with three classes of RNA polymerases in sera from patients with systemic sclerosis. *J Clin Invest* 91:1399, 1993.

71. Okano Y, Steen VD, Medsger TA Jr: Autoantibody reactive with RNA polymerase III in systemic sclerosis. *Ann Intern Med* 119:1005, 1993.

72. Love LA, Leff RL, Fraser DD, et al: A new approach to the classification of idiopathic inflammatory myopathy: Myositis-specific autoantibodies define useful homogeneous patient groups. *Medicine* 70:360, 1991.

73. Arnett FC, Hirsch TJ, Bias WB, et al: The Jo-1 antibody system in myositis: Relationship to clinical features and HLA. *J Rheumatol* 8:925, 1981.

74. Yoshida S, Akizuki M, Mimori T, et al: The precipitating antibody to an acidic nuclear protein antigen, the Jo-1, in connective tissue diseases. A marker for a subset of polymyositis with interstitial pulmonary fibrosis. *Arthritis Rheum* 26:604, 1983.

75. Targoff IN, Johnson AE, Miller FW: Antibody to signal recognition particle in polymyositis. *Arthritis Rheum* 33:1361, 1990.

76. Hirakata M, Mimori T, Akizuki M, et al: Autoantibodies to small nuclear and cytoplasmic ribonucleoproteins in Japanese patients with inflammatory muscle disease. *Arthritis Rheum* 35:449, 1992.

77. Targoff IN, Nilasena DS, Trieu EP, et al: Clinical features and

immunologic testing of patients with anti-Mi-2 antibodies (abstract). *Arthritis Rheum* 33:S72, 1990.

78. Burrell R, Rylander R: A critical review of the role of precipitins in hypersensitivity pneumonitis. *Eur J Respir Dis* 62:332, 1981.

79. Gariepy L, Cormier Y, Laviolette M, Tardif A: Predictive value of bronchoalveolar lavage cells and serum preciitins in asymptomatic dairy farmers. *Am Rev Respir Dis* 140:1386, 1989.

80. American Thoracic Statement: Clinical role of bronchoalveolar lavage in adults with pulmonary disease. *Am Rev Respir Dis* 142:481, 1990.

81. Crystal RG, Reynolds HY, Kalica AR: Bronchoalveolar lavage. The report of an international conference. *Chest* 90:122, 1986.

82. BAL Cooperative Group: Bronchoalveolar lavage constituents in healthy individuals, idiopathic pulmonary fibrosis, and selected comparison groups. *Am Rev Respir Dis* 141:S169, 1990.

83. Newman LS, Kreiss K, King TE Jr. et al: Pathologic and immunologic alterations in early stages of beryllium disease: Re-examination of disease definition and natural history. *Am Rev Respir Dis* 139:1479, 1989.

84. Lieske TR, Sunderranjan EV, Passamonte P: Bronchoalveolar lavage and technetium-99m glucopeptate imaging in chronic eosinophilic pneumonia. *Chest* 85:282, 1984.

85. Pesci A, Bertorelli G, Manganelli P, et al: Bronchoalveolar lavage in chronic eosinophilic pneumonia. Analysis of six cases in comparison with other interstitial lung diseases. *Respiration* 54 (Suppl):16, 1988.

86. Jederlinic PJ, Sicilian L, Gaensler EA: Chronic eosinophilic pneumonia. A report of 19 cases and a review of the literature. *Medicine* 67:154, 1988.

87. Haslam PL, Turton CWG, Lukoszek A, et al: Bronchoalveolar lavage fluid cell counts in cryptogenic fibrosing alveolitis and their relation to therapy. *Thorax* 35:328, 1980.

88. Watters LC, Schwarz MI, Cherniack RM, et al: Idiopathic pulmonary fibrosis: Pretreatment bronchoalveolar lavage cellular constituents and their relationships with lung histopathology and clinical response to therapy. *Am Rev Respir Dis* 135:696, 1987.

89. Baughman RP, Fernandez M, Bosken CH, et al: Comparison of gallium-67 scanning, bronchoalveolar lavage, and serum angiotensin-converting enzyme levels in pulmonary sarcoidosis: Predicting response to therapy. *Am Rev Respir Dis* 129:676, 1984.

90. Lawrence EC, Teague RB, Gottlieb MS, et al: Serial changes in markers of disease activity with corticosteroid treatment in sarcoidosis. *Am J Med* 74:747, 1983.

91. Turner-Warwick M, McAllister W, Lawrence R, et al: Corticosteroid treatment in pulmonary sarcoidosis: Do serial lavage lymphocyte counts, serum angiotensin converting enzyme measurements, and gallium-67 scans help management? *Thorax* 41: 903, 1986.

92. Chollet S, Soler P, Dournovo P, et al: Diagnosis of pulmonary histiocytosis X by immunodetection of Langerhans cells in bronchoalveolar lavage fluid. *Am J Pathol* 115:225, 1984.

93. Martin RJ, Coalson JJ, Rogers RM, et al: Pulmonary alveolar proteinosis: The diagnosis by segmental lavage. *Am Rev Respir Dis* 121:819, 1980.

94. Wall CP, Gaensler EA, Carrington CB, Hayes JA: Comparison of transbronchial and open biopsies in chronic infiltrative lung diseases. *Am Rev Respir Dis* 123:280, 1981.

95. Bensard DD, McIntyre RC Jr, Waring BJ, Simon JS: Comparison of video thoracoscopic lung biopsy to open lung biopsy in the diagnosis of interstitial lung disease. *Chest* 103:765, 1993.

96. Krasna MJ, White CS, Aisner SC, et al: The role of thoracoscope in the diagnosis of interstitial lung disease. *Ann Thorac Surg* 59: 348, 1995.

97. Ferson PF, Landreneau RJ, Dowling RD, et al: Comparison of open versus thoracoscopic lung biopsy for diffuse infiltrative pulmonary disease. *J Thorac Cardiovasc Surgery* 106:194, 1993.

98. Ferguson MK: Thoracoscopy for diagnosis of diffuse lung disease. *Ann Thorac Surg* 56:694, 1993.

99. Flint A, Martinez FJ, Young ML, et al: Influence of sample number and biopsy site on the histologic diagnosis of diffuse lung disease. *Ann Thorac Surg* 60:1605, 1995.

100. Tubbs RR, Benjamin SP, Reich NE, et al: Desquamative interstitial pneumonitis: Cellular phase of fibrosing alveolitis. *Chest* 72:159, 1977.

101. Burkhardt A: Alveolitis and collapse in the pathogenesis of pulmonary fibrosis. *Am Rev Respir Dis* 140:513, 1989.

102. Crouch E: Pathobiology of pulmonary fibrosis. *Am J Physiol Lung Cell Molec Biol* 259:L159, 1990.

103. Kuhn C III, Boldt J, King TE Jr, et al: An immunohistochemical study of architectural remodeling and connective tissue synthesis in pulmonary fibrosis. *Am Rev Respir Dis* 140:1693, 1989.

104. Kerr LA, Blute ML, Ryu JH, et al: Renal angiomyolipoma in association with pulmonary lymphangioleiomyoma: Forme fruste of tuberous sclerosis? *Urology* 41:440, 1993.

105. Bernstein SM, Newell JD, Adamczyk D, et al: How common are renal angiomyolipomas in patients with pulmonary lymphangioleiomyomatosis? *Am J Respir Crit Care Med* 152:2138, 1995.

106. Gibson PG, Bryant DH, Morgan GW, et al: Radiation-induced lung injury: A hypersensitivity pneumonitis? *Ann Intern Med* 109:288, 1988.

107. Mapel DW, Samet JM, Coultas DB: Corticosteroids and the treatment of idiopathic pulmonary fibrosis. *Chest* 110:1058, 1996.

108. du Bois RM: Corticosteroids in sarcoidosis: Friend or foe? *Eur Respir J* 7:1203, 1994.

109. Turner-Warwick M: Bronchoalveolar lavage fluid cell counts in cryptogenic fibrosing alveolitis and their relation to therapy. *Thorax* 35:328, 1980.

110. Wright PH, Heard BE, Steel SJ, Turner-Warwick M: Cryptogenic fibrosing alveolitis: Assessment by graded trephine lung biopsy histology compared with clinical, radiographic, and physiological features. *Br J Dis Chest* 75:61, 1981.

111. Sharma OP: Pulmonary sarcoidosis. *Am Rev Respir Dis* 147: 1598, 1993.

112. Gibson GJ, Prescott RJ, Muers MF, et al: Sarcoidosis Subcommittee of the Research Committee of the British Thoracic Society: British Thoracic Society Sarcoidosis study: Effects of long term corticosteroid treatment. *Thorax* 51:238, 1996.

113. Rudd RM, Haslam PL, Turner-Warwick M: Cryptogenic fibrosing alveolitis relationships of pulmonary physiology and bronchoalveolar lavage to treatment and prognosis. *Am Rev Respir Dis* 124:1, 1981.

114. Johnson MA, Kwan S, Snell NJC, et al: Randomized controlled trial comparing prednisolone alone with cyclophosphamide and low dose prednisolone in combination in cryptogenic fibrosing alveolitis. *Thorax* 44:280, 1989.

115. Kataria Y: Chlorambucil in sarcoidosis. *Chest* 78:36, 1980.

116. Israel HL, McComb BL: Chlorambucil treatment of sarcoidosis. *Sarcoidosis* 8:35, 1991.

117. Raghu G, Depaso WJ, Cain K, et al: Azathioprine combined with prednisone in the treatment of idiopathic pulmonary fibrosis: A prospective, double-blind randomized, placebo-controlled clinical trial. *Am Rev Respir Dis* 144:291, 1991.

118. Gruhn WB, Diaz-Buxo JA: Cyclosporine treatment of steroid resistant interstitial pneumonitis associated with dermatomyositis/polymyositis. *J Rheumatol* 14:1045, 1987.

119. Puttick MP, Klinkhoff AV, Chalmers A, Ostrow DN: Treatment of progressive rheumatoid interstitial lung disease with cyclosporine. *J Rheumatol* 22:2163, 1995.

120. Akesson A, Scheja A, Lundin A, Wollheim FA: Improved pulmonary function in systemic sclerosis after treatment with cyclophosphamide. *Arthritis Rheum* 37:729, 1995.

121. Venuta F, Rendina EA, Ciriaco P, et al: Efficacy of cyclosporine to reduce steroids in patients with idiopathic pulmonary fibrosis before lung transplantation. *J Heart Lung Transplant* 12:909, 1993.

122. Alton EW, Johnson M, Turner-Warwick M: Advanced crypto-

genic fibrosing alveolitis: Preliminary report on treatment with cyclosporin A. *Respir Med* 83:277, 1989.

123. Moolman JA, Bardin PG, Rossouw DJ, Joubert JR: Cyclosporin as a treatment for interstitial lung disease of unknown aetiology. *Thorax* 46:592, 1991.

124. Rebuck AS, Sanders BR, MacFadden DK, et al: Cyclosporin in pulmonary sarcoidosis. *Lancet* ii:1486, 1978.

125. Rebuck AS, Stiller CR, Braude AC, et al: Cyclosporin for pulmonary sarcoidosis. *Lancet* ii:1174, 1984.

126. Rennard SI, Bitterman PB, Ozaki T, et al: Colchicine suppresses the release of fibroblast growth factors from alveolar macrophages in vitro. The basis of a possible therapeutic approach to the fibrotic disorders. *Am Rev Respir Dis* 137:181, 1988.

127. Peters SG, McDougall JC, Douglas WW, et al: Colchicine in the treatment of pulmonary fibrosis. *Chest* 103:101, 1993.

128. McNeil K, Higenbottam T: The long-term outcome of lung transplantation in interstitial lung disease. *Clin Pulm Med* 3:137, 1996.

129. Breen TJ, Bennett LE, Daily OP, Hosenpud JD: The effect of diagnosis on survival before and after lung transplantation. *J Heart Lung Transplant* 14(Suppl):S49, 1995.

130. Hayden AM, Robert RC, Kriett JM, et al: Primary diagnosis predicts prognosis of lung transplant candidates. *Transplantation* 55:1048, 1993.

131. O'Brien JD, Lium JH, Parosa JF, et al: Lymphangiomyomatosis recurrence in the allograft after single-lung transplantation. *Am J Respir Crit Care Med* 151:2033, 1995.

132. Nine JS, Yousem SA, Paradis IL, et al: Lymphangioleiomyomatosis: Recurrence after lung transplantation. *J Heart Lung Transplant* 13:714, 1994.

133. Johnson B, Duncan S, Ohori N, et al: Recurrence of sarcoidosis in pulmonary allograft recipients. *Am Rev Respir Dis* 148:1373, 1993.

134. Dayton CS, Schwartz DA, Helmers RA, et al: Outcome of subjects with idiopathic pulmonary fibrosis who fail corticosteroid therapy. Implications for further studies. *Chest* 103:69, 1993.

135. Hunninghake GW, Kalica AR: Approaches to the treatment of pulmonary fibrosis. *Am J Respir Crit Care Med* 151:915, 1995.

136. Sullivan EJ, King TE Jr: Idiopathic pulmonary fibrosis, in Leff AR (ed): *Pulmonary and Critical Care Pharmacology and Therapeutics.* New York, McGraw-Hill, 1996, pp 1061, 1996.

137. Hueto-Perez-de-Heredia JJ, Dominguez-del-Valle FJ, Garcia E, et al: Chronic eosinophilic pneumonia as a presenting feature of Churg-Strauss syndrome. *Eur Respir J* 7:1006, 1994.

138. Uetrecht JP, Woosley RL: Acetylator phenotype and lupus erythematosus. *Clin Pharmacokinet* 6:118, 1981.

139. Katzenstein ALA, Myers JL, Mazur MT: Acute interstitial pneumonia. A clinicopathologic, ultrastructural, and cell kinetic study. *Am J Surg Pathol* 10:256, 1986.

140. Zitnik RJ: Drug-induced lung disease: Antiarrhythmic agents. *J Respir Dis* 17:254, 1996.

141. Hahn BH: Systemic lupus erythematosus, in Wilson, JD, Braunwald E, Isselbacher KJ, et al (eds): *Harrison's Principles of Internal Medicine,* 12th ed. New York, McGraw-Hill, 1991; p 1436.

142. Danel C, Israel-Biet D, Costabel U, et al: The clinical role of BAL in rare pulmonary diseases. *Eur Respir Rev* 2:83, 1991.

143. Janin A, Torpier G, Courtin P, et al: Segregation of eosinophil proteins in alveolar macrophage compartments in chronic eosinophilic pneumonia. *Thorax* 48:57, 1993.

144. Allen JN, Pacht ER, Gadek JE, Davis WB: Acute eosinophilic pneumonia as a reversible cause of noninfectious respiratory failure. *N Engl J Med* 321:569, 1989.

145. Buchheit J, Eid N, Rodgers G Jr, et al: Acute eosinophilic pneumonia with respiratory failure: A new syndrome? *Am Rev Respir Dis* 145:716, 1992.

146. Alasaly K, Muller N, Ostrow D, et al: Cryptogenic organizing pneumonia. A report of 25 cases and a review of the literature. *Medicine* 74:201, 1995.

147. King TE Jr: Bronchiolitis obliterans, in Schwarz MI, King TE Jr (eds): *Interstitial Lung Disease,* 2d ed. Philadelphia, Mosby-Year Book, 1993; pp 463, 1993.

148. Izumi T: The global view of idiopathic bronchiolitis obliterans organizing pneumonia, in Epler GR (ed): *Diseases of the Bronchioles.* New York, Raven, 1994; p 307.

149. Davison AG, Heard BE, McAllister WAC, Turner-Warwick MEH: Cryptogenic organizing pneumonitis. *Quart J Med* 52:382, 1983.

150. Yamamoto M, Ina Y, Kitaichi M: Bronchiolitis obliterans organizing pneumonia (BOOP): Profile in Japan, in Harasawa M, Fukuchi Y, Morinari H (eds): *Interstitial Pneumonia of Unknown Etiology.* Tokyo, University of Tokyo Press, 1989; p 61.

151. Cordier JF, Loire R, Brune J: Idiopathic bronchiolitis obliterans organizing pneumonia. Definition of characteristic clinical profiles in a series of 16 patients. *Chest* 96:999, 1989.

152. Cordier JF: Cryptogenic organizing pneumonitis. *Clin Chest Med* 14:677, 1993.

153. Muller NL, Guerry-Force ML, Staples CA, et al: Differential diagnosis of bronchiolitis obliterans with organizing pneumonia and usual interstitial pneumonia clinical, functional, and radiologic findings. *Radiology* 162:151, 1987.

154. Bartter T, Irwin RS, Nash G, et al: Idiopathic bronchiolitis obliterans organizing pneumonia with peripheral infiltrates on chest roentgenogram. *Arch Intern Med* 149:273, 1989.

155. Izumi T, Kitaichi M, Nishimura K, Nagai S: Bronchiolitis obliterans organizing pneumonia. Clinical features and differential diagnosis. *Chest* 102:715, 1992.

156. Nishimura K, Itoh H: Is CT useful in differentiating between BOOP and idiopathic UIP?, in Harasawa M, Fukuchi Y, Morinari H (eds): *Interstitial Pneumonia of Unknown Etiology.* Tokyo, University of Tokyo Press, 1989, p 317.

157. Muller NL, Staples CA, Miller RR: Bronchiolitis obliterans organizing pneumonia: CT features in 14 patients. *AJR* 154:983, 1990.

Chapter 11

DISORDERS OF THE CHEST WALL

JOHN M. SHNEERSON

Most of the disorders of the chest wall cause a restrictive ventilatory defect similar to that due to obesity, pleural disorders, and weakness of the respiratory muscles: Most of the individual skeletal abnormalities are uncommon, but together they form an important group that, unlike many lung diseases, can be treated effectively.

Pathophysiologic Effects

LUNG VOLUMES

The vital capacity (VC) is characteristically decreased in disorders of the chest wall.[1,2] The forced expiratory volume in 1 second (FEV$_1$) falls proportionately so that the forced expiratory ratio remains normal or may even increase. The total lung capacity (TLC) is reduced, usually with relatively little change in the residual volume (RV). The RV/TLC ratio increases. The reduction in total lung capacity is due to the reduced chest wall and lung compliance, together in some disorders with an additional component due to impaired inspiratory muscle strength. The functional residual capacity (FRC) usually falls to a similar extent to the total lung capacity so that the FRC/TLC ratio remains normal.

CHEST WALL AND LUNG COMPLIANCE

The chest wall compliance is reduced in almost all these conditions, except perhaps Marfan's and the Ehlers-Danlos syndromes, which are characterized by laxity of the soft tissues. The loss of compliance is more marked in older subjects, probably because of degenerative changes in the costovertebral and other joints. The compliance of the abdomen remains unchanged, but as the lung volume decreases, the lung compliance falls as well. This is thought to be due to closure of small airways with distal lung collapse. If the chest wall disorder arises early in life, it also may reduce lung compliance through a failure to develop the normal number of alveoli.

A consequence of the increased elastic work of breathing is that the respiratory pattern changes to one of rapid shallow breathing. This minimizes the work of respiration but increases the inspiratory muscle duty cycle and dead-space-to-tidal-volume ratio, which reduces alveolar ventilation.

RESPIRATORY MUSCLE FUNCTION

The small lung volume reduces the force that the expiratory muscles can generate because they contract at a shorter length than is optimal for them. Distortion of the rib cage, which is a feature of scoliosis and following a thoracoplasty, also puts both the inspiratory and expiratory muscles at a mechanical disadvantage through changing the configuration of the rib cage. The respiratory muscle strength and endurance are also reduced in primary neuromuscular diseases such as congenital myopathies that often cause chest wall deformities, particularly scoliosis.

RESPIRATORY DRIVE

The ventilatory response to chemical stimuli such as hypoxia and hypercapnia is usually reduced in diseases of the chest wall. This is probably not the result of an impairment of the respiratory drive itself but of an inability for this to be translated into a normal ventilatory response because of the impaired respiratory mechanics and reduced respiratory muscle function.[3] If, however, chronic hypercapnia develops, the increase in the cerebrospinal fluid (CSF) bicarbonate concentration reduces the ventilatory response to hypercapnia. Respiratory drive also may be reduced by chronic sleep deprivation due to respiratory-induced arousals from sleep.

BLOOD GAS ANALYSIS

The first abnormality of arterial blood gases is almost invariably a reduced P$_{O_2}$. This is due to mismatching of ventilation and perfusion, either as a result of basal airway closure or due to distortion of the rib cage. At a later stage, hypoventilation with an elevated P$_{CO_2}$ develops, initially usually during sleep. During sleep, the respiratory drive is reduced, and upper airway resistance increases. These changes are most marked during rapid eye movement sleep, in which chest wall muscle activity except for the diaphragm is also reduced. Daytime hypercapnia is a later manifestation (Table 11-1) but may be precipitated by an acute illness such as a chest infection.

RIGHT-SIDED HEART FAILURE AND PULMONARY HYPERTENSION

The pulmonary vascular resistance increases partly due to a reduction in the lung volume, with a corresponding loss of the pulmonary microcirculation, and partly due to the effect of hypoxia. This leads to pulmonary vasoconstriction, and if it is prolonged, structural changes in the pulmonary vessels appear. Polycythemia also may develop in response to hypoxia, and by increasing the blood viscosity, it contributes to pulmonary hypertension. Fluid retention related to responses of the renin-angiotensin system are also probably important but little understood at present. The degree of pulmonary hypertension and polycythemia appears to correlate with the mean oxygen saturation both during the day and at night, and it is therefore more severe if there is any coexisting lung disease that reduces the oxygen saturation.

LUNG DEVELOPMENT

The bronchi normally develop by 16 weeks' gestation, and bronchial development is therefore rarely influenced by chest wall disorders. The total number of alveoli, however, is only reached between the ages of 2 and 4 years. Their multiplication depends on the mechanical forces transmitted to the lungs by the respiratory muscles. Failure of the thoracic cavity to develop normally alters these mechanical forces and can result in a reduced number of alveoli. If the disease affects chest wall development at a later age, the normal dimensions of the alveoli may not be attained, with the result

TABLE 11-1 Ventilatory Failure in Thoracic Disorders

Never	Rare	Common	Usual
Pectus excavatum	Congenital rib abnormalities	Thoracoplasty	Asphyxiating thoracic dystrophy
Pectus carinatum	Ankylosing spondylitis	Scoliosis	
Straight back syndrome	Kyphosis		

that they either remain small or of variable size.[4] These considerations are particularly important in congenital and infantile idiopathic scoliosis, early onset kyphosis, and asphyxiating thoracic dystrophy, all of which affect the thoracic cage early in life.

PREGNANCY

The blood volume increases by up to 25 percent during pregnancy, and patients with preexisting pulmonary hypertension frequently develop right-sided heart failure, usually during the second half of pregnancy. The enlarging uterus elevates the diaphragm, probably through the increase in intraabdominal pressure, and this worsens the restrictive defect resulting from the chest wall disorder.[5] This may precipitate ventilatory failure during pregnancy. Termination of pregnancy may be required either for this reason or because of the appearance of right-sided heart failure.[6]

During labor, the pain of the contractions often increases ventilation and reduces the arterial P_{CO_2} unless analgesics are prescribed.[7] Cesarean section should be considered if the respiratory muscles are weak or the pelvic outlet is severely narrowed, but in other cases a trial of labor is usually indicated. Acute diaphragmatic fatigue has been demonstrated during labor,[8] but respiratory failure during spontaneous labor is unusual.

Disorders of the Sternum

Neoplastic and inflammatory conditions affecting the sternum usually have little effect on ventilation unless they are painful. An exception is a fractured sternum when it forms part of an anterior flail segment that can significantly impair alveolar ventilation. Paradoxical movement of the sternum also can be a problem with severe congenital defects such as agenesis or bifid sternum. Surgery in the neonatal period may be required to stabilize the anterior chest wall.[9]

There is also a wide range of protrusion and depression deformities of the sternum and adjacent structures. The two best defined are pectus excavatum and pectus carinatum.

PECTUS EXCAVATUM

Pectus excavatum is a depression deformity of the sternum that is often present at birth but may worsen during the adolescent growth spurt (Fig. 11-1). It is occasionally familial and may be associated with other skeletal abnormalities such as a thoracic kyphosis,[10] scoliosis,[11] or the straight back syndrome. Some patients with pectus excavatum also have Marfan's syndrome, Ehlers-Danlos syndrome, and hyperflexibility of the joints.[10]

The cause of pectus excavatum has been thought to be an overgrowth of the ribs pushing the sternum inward[12] or a congenitally short central tendon of the diaphragm,[13] but an increased inward pull on the sternum by the sternal diaphragmatic fibers or an abnormally compliant chest wall is more likely.[14] In neonates, transient paradoxical movement of the sternum during respiration may be apparent, particularly in the presence of upper airway obstruction or pneumonia, when the work of the inspiratory muscles, including the diaphragm, is increased. The sternal depression may become permanent, even if the cause, such as enlarged tonsils, resolves completely.[15]

In adults, it is unusual for pectus excavatum to cause any symptoms, although occasionally breathlessness on exertion or a feeling of precordial pressure may be noticed if this is severe.[16] The lung volumes, including TLC, FRC, RV, and VC, are normal or are only slightly reduced.[17] The FEV_1, forced vital capacity (FVC), and flow-volume loops are normal.[18] Any mild restrictive defect appears to be due directly to the small loss in volume of the thorax due to the sternal depression, since the chest wall mobility both at rest and after exercise is unimpaired.[19] Arterial blood gases are also normal, both at rest and during exercise.[20]

Pectus excavatum nevertheless can cause cardiac problems. The heart is displaced to the left of the sternum, and its rotation is responsible for the frequent finding of right-axis deviation and tall P waves in lead II on the electrocardiogram.[16] The function of the left ventricle is unimpaired, but

FIGURE 11-1 Pectus excavatum.

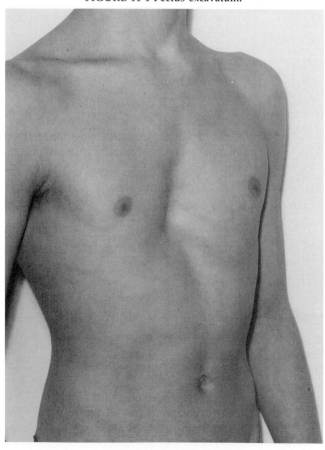

right ventricular filling is occasionally reduced because the heart is compressed between the depressed sternum and the spine.[16] The effect is similar to constrictive pericarditis. The pulmonary outflow tract also may be compressed, and particularly since it is close to the anterior chest wall this often results in a systolic murmur that is loudest during deep inspiration.[21] The restriction in right ventricular filling may be most marked during exercise, particularly in the sitting position, when the heart becomes more caudal. The fixed cardiac output may limited exercise,[22] and occasionally, supraventricular tachycardias or atrial fibrillation develop.[23,24]

The main indication for surgical correction of pectus excavatum is cosmetic, although the scar may be more noticeable than the original pectus excavatum.[25] Surgery has little effect on the restrictive defect or exercise ability[17,26,27] and may even worsen it,[28,29] except in the rare situation where right ventricular filling is impaired or atrial dysrhythmias are a problem.[30]

PECTUS CARINATUM

Pectus carinatum is a protrusion of the sternum, and this is often associated with narrowing of the chest transversely. Although the deformity may be present at birth, it usually becomes more pronounced during the adolescent growth spurt. This is probably due to excessive growth of the ribs or costal cartilages,[31] but excessive contraction of the lateral diaphragmatic fibers leading to narrowing of the chest and anterior protrusion of the sternum has been proposed.[32] Ventricular septal defects associated with pulmonary hypertension and a raised pulmonary vascular resistance can lead to protrusion of the upper sternum, whereas atrial septal defects usually cause a localized bulge over the hypertrophied right ventricle.[33]

Pectus carinatum is usually asymptomatic, but occasionally, chest pain may arise at the insertions of the intercostal muscles anteriorly or in the abnormally located costal cartilages and anterior ribs. The lung volumes are normal.[18] The inferior diaphragmatic surface is often larger than normal because of the shape of the thorax, but the significance of this is uncertain.[31] No data regarding the compliance of the chest wall are available.

Treatment is not usually required. Surgery does not improve respiratory function or exercise ability and is only indicated for cosmetic reasons.[34]

Disorders of the Ribs

Rib abnormalities are common but only occasionally interfere with respiration unless they cause pain. The most important conditions are as follows.

CONGENITAL ABNORMALITIES

The most common *congenital abnormalities* are bifid ribs, abnormal intercostal joints, and the presence of cervical ribs. It is unusual for them to cause any significant respiratory problems unless they are multiple or located in the region of the insertion of the diaphragm. Occasionally, the absence of several ribs leads to paradoxical chest wall movement.

GENERALIZED SKELETAL DISORDERS

Generalized bone disorders may affect the ribs, usually by making them more compliant, to a degree that ventilation is

reduced. Deformities of the rib cage such as symmetrical grooves along the line of the costochondral joints, Harrison's sulcus at the site of the insertion of the diaphragm, and enlargement of the costochondral joints are well recognized, but their physiologic significance has not been studied. Relapsing polychondritis may lead to inflammation of the costochondral joints, but this appears to be less important than the damage to the cartilage in the trachea and bronchi.[35]

ACHONDROPLASIA

Achondroplasia may lead to obstructive sleep apneas, probably due to abnormalities of vocal cord control associated with malformations of the base of the skull and spinal canal. Chest wall deformities such as kyphosis and pectus excavatum also occur, but the most common feature is a reduction in the vital capacity.[36] This, together with the TLC and RV, are reduced even when allowance is made for the short stature and short trunk height. The RV/TLC and FRC/TLC ratios are normal, and the reduction in lung volumes is probably due to the shortening of the ribs, which reduces the anteroposterior and possibly the lateral diameter of the rib cage. The lungs themselves appear to be normal.[37]

ASPHYXIATING THORACIC DYSTROPHY (JEUNE'S DISEASE)

Asphyxiating thoracic dystrophy is a cartilaginous disorder in which the most prominent changes are in the pelvis, phalanges, and other limb bones. The ribs, like other long bones, are shortened. The rib cage becomes narrower than normal and less compliant. Respiration depends on abdominal expansion.[38] The lungs fail to develop normally, and the number of alveoli is reduced.[38]

Respiratory failure usually develops in infancy or childhood,[39] but some patients die of renal failure before respiratory failure appears. Treatment by surgical reconstruction of the rib cage with splitting the sternum has been attempted but has been largely unsuccessful.[40]

FLAIL CHEST

A *flail chest* causes paradoxical movement of the chest wall during respiration and is usually due to multiple rib fractures. These may be associated with other complications such as pulmonary contusion, pneumothorax, hemothorax, or rupture of the aortic arch. In most patients, analgesia is sufficient to enable the patient to cough adequately and is all that is required, but if the paradoxical movement of the chest wall causes hypoventilation, positive-pressure ventilation may be required.[41]

THORACOPLASTY

Thoracoplasty was commonly carried out to treat pulmonary tuberculosis before chemotherapy was introduced. Most thoracoplasties were performed between 1930 and 1995. It has been estimated that between 1951 and 1960, about 30,000 operations were performed in the United Kingdom alone.[42] The principle of the procedure was that if that the tuberculous cavities could be closed, the disease could be arrested. Thoracoplasty was the most effective but also the most invasive of the surgical procedures carried out for tuberculosis and

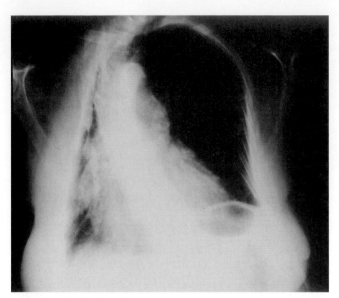

FIGURE 11-2 Chest radiograph of a thoracoplasty showing marked asymmetry of thorax due to extensive rib resection.

involved resection of varying lengths of several ribs (Fig. 11-2). As many as 11 ribs were resected, but less radical surgery was found to be equally effective and caused fewer respiratory problems and a less noticeable deformity. Following the introduction of effective antituberculous chemotherapy, the indication for thoracoplasty has become restricted to occasional patients with chronic infections, especially those involving the pleural space after pulmonary resection.

PATHOPHYSIOLOGY

Effects on Chest Wall and Lung Volumes
The total lung capacity is reduced to a greater extent by a thoracoplasty than the RV or FRC. The VC therefore falls. In most subjects, the FEV_1 is reduced disproportionately because of airflow obstruction. This may be due to coincidental smoking, but recent studies have shown that airflow obstruction may develop many years after the thoracoplasty and probably represents tuberculous endobronchitis due to persisting small airway inflammation.[43] In a few patients, large airway obstruction is due to posttuberculous stenoses or, occasionally, to damage to the airways from adjacent inflamed lymph nodes.

The severity of the restrictive defect varies according to the details of the surgical procedure, of which most important is the number of ribs resected. With 5-rib thoracoplasty, the reduction in FEV_1 and FVC is approximately 20 percent[44]; if 8 ribs were removed, then a 35 percent reduction is common[45]; and with a 9- to 11-rib resection, around 45 percent reduction develops.[45,46] The cause of the restrictive defect is complex. Resection of the ribs leads to an indrawing of the rib cage with loss of volume because the rib cage also becomes unstable, allowing it to move paradoxically. The surgery also requires dissection close to the pleura, and as a result, pleural thickening is common. Thoracoplasty leads to late degenerative changes in the thoracic cage that restrict the range of movement at the costovertebral joints. The chest wall compliance is also reduced by the appearance of a thoracic scoliosis that is almost invariable after a thoracoplasty.[47] The scoliosis

is convex to the side of the surgery, and its severity correlates with the number of ribs removed. It is also more marked if the head, neck, and tubercle of the ribs and the transverse processes of the vertebrae are removed[48,49] or if the anterior segments of the second to fourth ribs were resected.[50] The scoliosis often progresses for several years after the thoracoplasty, but about two-thirds of the final curvature is apparent within the first 6 months.[48]

Respiratory muscle function is impaired after a thoracoplasty. The maximum inspiratory pressure and transdiaphragmatic pressure are reduced. This may be due to direct damage to the intercostal and shoulder muscles by the surgery, but a more important mechanism is probably the distortion of the chest wall that puts the inspiratory muscles at a mechanical disadvantage. Diaphragm function is also impaired, particularly on the side of the thoracoplasty. Its excursion is reduced, as observed fluoroscopically,[51] but the exact cause of diaphragm dysfunction is not established.

Exercise Responses
The exercise capacity is reduced after a thoracoplasty and is usually limited by ventilatory rather than cardiovascular factors. Maximum exercise ventilation is related to FVC, maximum tidal volume, FEV_1, and maximum respiratory frequency. The latter two are partially determined by the degree of airflow obstruction, which may therefore be an important contributory factor in determining the exercise ability.[52] The maximum oxygen uptake does not correlate with the P_{O_2}, P_{CO_2}, angle of scoliosis, or number of ribs resected.[52]

Respiratory Failure
Hypoxia is almost invariable after a thoracoplasty. It is probably due both to the underlying lung disease and to regional ventilation and perfusion mismatching due to the rib cage deformity and pleural thickening. Both ventilation and perfusion are usually markedly reduced on the side of the thoracoplasty, and the P_{O_2} depends primarily on the function of the contralateral lung.

Hypoxia is more marked during sleep, particularly rapid eye movement sleep.[53] The respiratory drive is reduced, upper airway resistance increases, and during rapid eye movement sleep, the chest wall muscles other than the diaphragm are less active. Alveolar hypoventilation first develops during sleep. The degree of hypercapnia correlates with the fall in maximum inspiratory and maximum transdiaphragmatic pressures,[54] and it is more common if there is pleural thickening on the contralateral side, which presumably restricts the expansion of this lung.[55] Hypercapnic respiratory failure usually appears many years after a thoracoplasty and often develops quite rapidly over a period of weeks. It may be related to the combination of normal age-related reductions in respiratory drive, chest wall compliance, and respiratory muscle strength superimposed on the complications of the thoracoplasty. It may be precipitated by an intercurrent illness such as a chest infection.

Right-Sided Heart Failure
The pulmonary artery pressure rises as a result of an increase in the pulmonary vascular resistance.[56] Right-sided heart failure commonly develops,[57] usually around the stage that hypercapnia appears.

ASSESSMENT

The symptoms of nocturnal respiratory failure and arousals are often subtle, and a careful history is required to enquire into symptoms such as daytime tiredness, sudden awakening at night, early morning headaches, and ankle swelling rather than the conventional pulmonary symptoms such as cough and wheeze. If, however, a productive cough persists, a recurrence of the underlying tuberculosis should be suspected and investigated. On physical examination, the deformity of the rib cage with hypertrophy and use of the accessory respiratory muscles and paradoxical movement of the rib cage in the region of the thoracoplasty may be seen. Occasionally, the physical signs of hypercapnia and right ventricular hypertrophy or failure are present.

The electrocardiogram (ECG) is insensitive at detecting right ventricular hypertrophy, and echocardiography is often technically difficult. A transesophageal echocardiogram may be required. Measurement of lung volumes indicates the severity of the restrictive defect and of any airflow obstruction. Estimation of the maximum inspiratory and expiratory mouth pressures and transdiaphragmatic pressure can be used to assess respiratory muscle strength. Computed tomography (CT) will show the sequelae of the tuberculous infection and surgery most clearly, although a chest radiograph is employed more commonly. The presence of respiratory failure can be assessed by arterial blood gas analysis, although continuous recording of oxygen saturation or P_{O_2} and P_{CO_2} during sleep will demonstrate abnormalities at an earlier stage.

Disorders of the Spine

Spinal disorders may affect ventilation by compressing the spinal cord or peripheral nerves and by mechanical effects on the chest wall and lungs. Only the latter is discussed in this chapter.

ANKYLOSING SPONDYLITIS

The typical presentation of *ankylosing spondylitis* is with sacroiliac joint inflammation, but eventually, the intervertebral and costovertebral joints may become involved. Occasionally, the costochondral, chondrosternal, and sternomanubrial joints are also affected. After the active phase of the disorder, the joints often becomes ankylosed with calcification of the spinal ligaments. This results in a rigid rib cage with a pronounced kyphosis and little spinal mobility.[58]

PATHOPHYSIOLOGY

The changes in lung volumes in ankylosing spondylitis differ from those of all other chest wall disorders in that the FRC increases. This is a result of the rib cage becoming fixed at its own relaxation volume. This is greater than the normal FRC, which is also determined by the inward pull of the elastic recoil of the lungs. The TLC is slightly reduced, and the RV usually increases so that the VC falls.[59] The reduction in VC is related to the degree of vertebral ankylosis[60] and the reduction in chest wall compliance but does not correlate with the degree of kyphosis or the duration of the ankylosing spondylitis.[61]

The reduction in chest wall compliance, and in particular the expansion of the rib cage, leads to atrophy of the intercostal muscles.[62] Occasionally this can be severe enough to cause paradoxical movement of the rib cage during inspiration. Both maximal inspiratory and expiratory mouth pressures are reduced.[63] Respiration becomes increasingly dependent on diaphragmatic contraction. The excursion of the diaphragm is greater than normal.[62,64] This largely compensates for the rib cage immobility, and even during exercise, the ventilatory responses are virtually normal.[65]

The arterial blood gases are usually normal or virtually normal in ankylosing spondylitis. It might be anticipated that the lung expansion is mainly due to diaphragmatic contraction and that the bases would be disproportionately ventilated so that overall ventilation-perfusion matching might deteriorate. This, however, has not been confirmed.[66] Hypercapnia is very unusual in ankylosing spondylitis because of the ability of the diaphragm to compensate for the rib cage immobility, and if it does occur, other causes should be sought. These causes may be one of the recognized complications of ankylosing spondylitis such as the following.

Airflow Obstruction

This is most commonly the result of coincidental chronic obstructive pulmonary disease (COPD) related to smoking, but a few patients with ankylosing spondylitis develop cricoarytenoid arthritis. This may present with hoarseness of the voice, stridor, breathlessness, obstructive sleep apneas, or respiratory failure.[67] In the early stages, prednisolone may be effective, but once fibrosis has developed, a surgical approach such as a tracheostomy may be required.

Pleural Thickening and Effusion

Both pleural thickening[68] and pleural effusion[69] are associated with ankylosing spondylitis but are not related to its activity. The effusions may resolve with intrapleural prednisolone.[70]

Aspiration Pneumonia

This may be due to esophageal dysmotility related to ankylosing spondylitis.

Bullae

Fibrobullous lung disease is associated with ankylosing spondylitis. It may become infected with opportunist or pathogenic organisms such as *Aspergillus fumigatus* or saprophytic mycobacteria. Pulmonary tuberculosis was thought to be common in ankylosing spondylitis, but there is little evidence for this.

Abdominal Surgery

Diaphragmatic function is reflexly reduced by abdominal surgery, which therefore can precipitate respiratory failure. Thoracic surgery, however, has little effect on ventilation because of the small contribution that rib cage expansion plays to respiration.

ASSESSMENT

Sudden movement such as coughing and laughing may cause chest wall pain in the active phase of ankylosing spondylitis, but these symptoms usually subside as the joints become less mobile. Breathlessness is rarely a problem unless cricoarytenoid arthritis appears. The most prominent physical sign is the restriction of rib cage movement associated with prominent accessory muscle activity and abdominal expansion during inspiration due to diaphragmatic contraction.

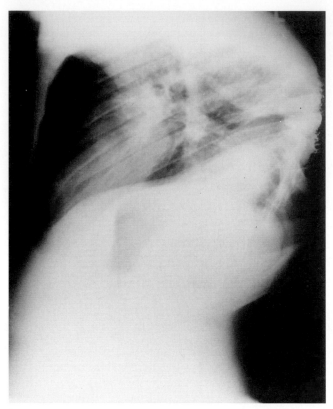

FIGURE 11-3 Lateral radiograph of thoracic spine showing sharp kyphosis following tuberculosis.

The chest radiograph may show pleural shadowing and apical fibrobullous disease, as well as calcification of the paraspinal ligaments (bamboo spine), especially on the lateral film. Arterial blood gases are usually normal, both at rest and during exercise, and the carbon monoxide transfer coefficient (K_{CO}) is usually normal or raised.

RIGID SPINE SYNDROME

The *rigid spine syndrome* is a rare disorder in which flexion of the cervical, thoracic, and lumbar spine is grossly reduced. The condition usually becomes apparent during childhood and is associated with a slowly progressive proximal muscle weakness that involves the respiratory muscles. A moderately severe scoliosis is common, but ventilatory failure is usually mainly determined by the degree of respiratory muscle weakness.[71,72] Death may be due to respiratory failure, right-sided heart failure, or pneumonia.

KYPHOSIS

The normal thoracic *kyphosis* is less than 40 degress, but even if this is increased, it is unusual for any significant respiratory deficit to appear. Even if there is a marked kyphosis due to vertebral collapse as a result of osteoporosis or malignancy, the effects on respiratory function are usually small.[73] The exception is when a very sharp kyphosis (gibbus) develops in childhood (Fig. 11-3). This is usually due to tuberculous osteomyelitis (Pott's disease). This infection often spreads across the intervertebral disk into at least two vertebrae, which collapse with considerable loss of height and angulation of the spine. The costovertebral joints usually becomes

ankylosed. This also limits expansion of the rib cage, and respiration becomes more dependent on the diaphragm. Although tuberculous osteomyelitis usually occurs at the thoracolumbar junction, respiratory problems usually are seen when the infection is higher in the thoracic spine.[74]

The characteristic effect of a kyphosis of this type is a restrictive defect in which the TLC is reduced more than the RV.[75] The restrictive defect appears to be most severe if the kyphosis develops in early childhood, probably because this prevents normal development of the lungs. Kyphosis appearing before the age of around 2 would be expected to be associated with a reduction in alveolar number, and a later-onset defect would be likely to reduce the growth of alveoli, but without reduction in their number.[76]

Ventilatory failure is almost always confined to patients in whom the kyphosis developed early in childhood, usually before the age of 4.[77] Right-sided heart failure with pulmonary hypertension[78] develops probably because of a combination of chronic hypoxia and a reduced size of the pulmonary vascular bed. Hypercapnia appears first during sleep, particularly rapid eye movement sleep, and later develops during wakefulness. Occasionally, respiratory failure is precipitated by an acute chest infection, asthma, or pregnancy. The enlarging uterus limits the excursion of the diaphragm and usually causes ventilatory failure during the second half of pregnancy.[79]

STRAIGHT BACK SYNDROME

The normal thoracic kyphosis is reduced or absent in *straight back syndrome*. This may lead to a mild restrictive defect,[80] but the cardiac complications are more prominent. They are similar to those which may develop with pectus excavatum and, as in this condition, are the result of compression of the heart between the spine and the sternum and the anterior rib cage. A systolic murmur may be audible,[81] and this is

FIGURE 11-4 Thoracic scoliosis with posterior rib hump following poliomyelitis.

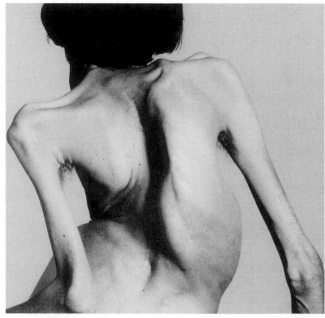

usually due to compression either of the right ventricular outflow tract or of the pulmonary artery. Mitral valve prolapse is also associated with this condition. Reduction in filling of the right ventricle may limit cardiac output, particularly during exercise.[82]

SCOLIOSIS

Scoliosis is a lateral curvature of the spine, but this is almost invariably linked with a rotation of the vertebral bodies as well. As a result, the spine forms an unstable lordosis rather than a kyphosis (Fig. 11-4). The term *kyphoscoliosis,* which is frequently used, is therefore inaccurate. It is common for a mild degree of scoliosis to be present, and although angles of curvature of 5 or 10 degrees have been used to define the abnormality, these are arbitrary figures. It is important to distinguish a postural scoliosis from a structural scoliosis. A postural scoliosis is temporary and disappears when the patient bends forward.

The cause of the scoliosis largely determines the age at which it develops and its natural history (Table 11-2). It usually appears during childhood or adolescence when there is an underlying neuromuscular disorder, and with poliomyelitis, it is usually apparent within about 2 years of the acute infection. In this condition as in many neuromuscular disorders (such as syringomyelia, Friedreich's ataxia, spinal muscular atrophy, Duchenne's muscular dystrophy, and some congenital myopathies), the scoliosis has a long C shape and may be severe. With congenital abnormalities such as hemivertebrae or segmentation defects, the scoliosis is usually noticed early in childhood. Neurofibromatosis and Marfan's syndrome usually lead to a severe and high thoracic scoliosis, whereas the scoliosis due to pleural or pulmonary disease, which is less common than previously now that chronic infections are less frequent, is usually less severe.

The most common form of scoliosis is the adolescent idiopathic type that develops during the pubertal growth spurt. About 80 percent of these scolioses are seen in girls, and the convexity of the deformity is on the right in 80 percent of patients. The scoliosis may continue to deteriorate slightly even after growth of the spine ceases. The infantile form of idiopathic scoliosis is less common, and while it usually resolves spontaneously, it can progress occasionally to a severe deformity.

TABLE 11-2 Causes of Scoliosis

Idiopathic	Infantile
	Adolescent
Osteogenic	Congenital
	Thoracoplasty
Neuromuscular	Syringomyelia
	Poliomyelitis
	Duchenne's dystrophy
Connective tissue disorders	Neurofibromatosis
	Marfan's syndrome
	Osteogenesis imperfecta
Pleuropulmonary	Empyema
	Pneumonectomy
	Unilateral lung fibrosis

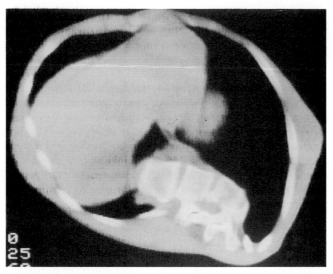

FIGURE 11-5 CT scan of chest in scoliosis showing marked asymmetry of the two hemithoraces.

PATHOPHYSIOLOGY

Lung Volumes and Compliance

The abnormal configuration of the spine and rib cage reduces the chest wall compliance[83] and the lung compliance.[84] This, together with the impaired function of the respiratory muscles, causes a restrictive defect. The exact severity of this may be difficult to determine because normal values for lung volumes are related to height, which is reduced by the spinal curvature. Several methods have been devised to correct for this, and the least unsatisfactory is division of the arm span by 1.03 to obtain an estimated value for the height.[85]

The TLC, FRC, and VC are all reduced in scoliosis, although the RV may increase slightly.[86] In idiopathic scoliosis these changes in lung volumes are proportional to the angle of scoliosis,[87] but this relationship is obscured in neuromuscular disorders because the loss of lung volume is also dependent on the degree of muscle weakness. The restrictive defect also may be worse if a lordosis is present as well as the scoliosis.[88] The VC is also smaller if the scoliosis is of early onset, presumably because of failure to develop the normal adult number of alveoli.[89] The VC usually falls when moving from the sitting to a supine position, indicating that diaphragm function is impaired.[90]

Respiratory Muscle Function

The hemithorax on the side of the concavity of the scoliosis is underinflated relative to the side of its convexity[91] (Fig. 11-5). The implication of this is that the inspiratory muscles are lengthened and would be expected to generate more force on the side of the concavity than on the convexity. The converse probably holds for the expiratory muscles. The deformity of the spine also shifts the axis of the neck of the ribs obliquely. The ribs continue to move parallel to this axis as in normal subjects. The rib cage therefore expands obliquely during inspiration. The abnormal configuration of the rib cage puts the respiratory muscles at a mechanical disadvantage, and the consequences of this and the other factors are that both the maximum inspiratory and expiratory pressures are reduced.[84] The maximum transdiaphragmatic pressure is often below normal, probably because of the inefficient configuration of the insertion of the diaphragm onto the distorted lower rib cage.

Exercise Capacity

The capacity for exercise may be severely reduced by scoliosis.[92] Oxygen consumption during everyday activities is increased by, for instance, the additional contraction of postural muscles to maintain balance and of the respiratory muscles to overcome the increased elastic work of breathing. Exercise capacity is further limited by a reduction in the maximum oxygen consumption,[93] although in younger subjects with mild deformities usually due to adolescent idiopathic scoliosis, physical unfitness rather than any direct effect of scoliosis is more commonly the limiting factor.[94] These subjects may show only minor abnormalities of ventilation during exercise.[95] In the presence of more severe deformities, the maximum exercise ventilation is reduced in proportion to the reduction in FEV_1.[93] Ventilation at any given oxygen uptake is greater than normal,[96] so the reduced maximal exercise ventilation is reached at a lower oxygen uptake than expected. The tidal volume increases initially to a maximum and then remains constant while the respiratory frequency rises. This maximum tidal volume is a higher percentage of the VC than in normal subjects, although in absolute terms it is usually less than normal.[93]

The blood gases usually remain unchanged during exercise and unless pulmonary hypertension is present cardiac output increases normally. The pulmonary artery pressure, however, may rise rapidly, particularly if the lung volume is reduced, as indicated by, for example, a reduction in VC. This suggests that exercise-induced pulmonary hypertension is primarily related to the anatomic limitation of the pulmonary vascular bed in the small lungs. Vascular distention and the recruitment of unperfused vessels that is a normal response appear not to be significant in the scoliotic.

Ventilatory Control

The ventilatory responses to both hypercapnia[83] and hypoxia[95] are reduced. This is probably not due to any central abnormality of respiratory control but to the inability of the respiratory muscles to increase ventilation normally in response to an increase in biochemical drive because of the reduction in the effectiveness of the respiratory muscles and the increased work of breathing. The ventilatory response correlates with the compliance of the lungs and chest wall, VC, and TLC.[83,97] It is likely that respiratory drive only falls if the CSF bicarbonate concentration increases as a result of chronic hypercapnia[86] or if other factors such as sleep deprivation due to respiratory-induced arousals from sleep are present.

Respiratory Failure

A slightly reduced arterial P_{O_2} is seen soon after the onset of scoliosis[98] and results from mismatching of ventilation and perfusion. This might be anticipated to differ considerably between the two lungs, but in practice it is only slightly abnormal at regional levels, as shown on isotope scans. Ventilation in general is reduced in the region of the convexity of the spine,[99] and the normal gradient of an increase in perfusion from the apex to the base of the lungs in the upright posture is lost.[100] This may be secondary

to hypoxic vasoconstriction at the bases caused by airway closure. The distribution of perfusion between the two lungs is usually equal.

Ventilatory failure usually develops gradually and is apparent initially during sleep. During rapid eye movement sleep, the reduction in respiratory drive together with an increased upper airway resistance due to loss of tone in the dilator muscles leads to underventilation. These effects are magnified during rapid eye movement sleep, when all the chest wall muscles except for the diaphragm are inactivated.[90,101] During rapid eye movement sleep, severe oxygen desaturations coupled with transient hypercapnia may be seen. Hypopneas and central sleep apneas are the most common features, but periods of rapid shallow breathing with an increased dead-space-to-tidal-volume ratio are common during both rapid eye movement and non-rapid eye movement sleep.

Hypercapnic respiratory failure during the day usually develops after it is apparent at night[90,101] and is to a certain extent predictable.[102,103] It is related to the following.

AGE OF ONSET OF SCOLIOSIS   If this appears before the age of about 4 years, the normal alveolar number may not be attained, and hypercapnic respiratory failure frequently appears. The later onset of adolescent idiopathic scoliosis is probably the main reason why ventilatory failure rarely occurs in this condition.

LEVEL OF SCOLIOSIS   In general, the higher the curve in the thoracic spine, the more marked are the respiratory and cardiovascular consequences. Thoracolumbar and lumbar scoliosis rarely cause significant respiratory effects.

SEVERITY OF SCOLIOSIS   The angle of scoliosis is closely linked to the reduction in lung volume in patients without an underlying neuromuscular disorder, in which the muscle weakness also contributes to the volume changes. When the angle of scoliosis is greater than around 100 degrees, hypercapnia frequently develops.

PRESENCE OF MUSCLE WEAKNESS   Respiratory failure is more common in neuromuscular disorders causing scoliosis than when muscle strength is normal.

LUNG VOLUMES   Respiratory failure usually occurs when the lung volumes are reduced to a degree such that the VC is less than 1.0 to 1.5 L.

Acute respiratory failure may be precipitated by an intercurrent illness such as a chest infection, even when these risk factors are absent.

Cardiovascular Complications

Right ventricular failure may occur transiently during episodes of acute respiratory failure, but chronic right ventricular failure is a late complication of severe scoliosis.[86] Autopsy series have shown that right ventricular hypertrophy may be present in around 75 percent of subjects.[104] Left ventricular hypertrophy also may be seen and is probably related to hypertension, chronic hypoxia, or other associated problems such as congenital renal or ureteric abnormalities.[104]

The cause of right ventricular hypertrophy is pulmonary hypertension due to an increased pulmonary vascular resistance. Pulmonary artery pressure while awake correlates with the degree of hypoxia,[105] which leads to vasoconstriction and, if prolonged, to smooth muscle hypertrophy as well.[106] Polycythaemia also may contribute to the increased pulmonary vascular resistance. During exercise, however, the pulmonary artery pressure relates more closely to the lung volumes (see above), indicating that the anatomic dimensions of the pulmonary vascular bed determine pulmonary vascular resistance.

Congenital heart disease is a recognized association of scoliosis. It occurs in about 3 percent of subjects with idiopathic scoliosis and 7 percent of those with congenital scoliosis.[107] Any type of congenital heart disease may be present, but Fallot's tetralogy, aortic coarctation, and mitral valve prolapse are seen most commonly. Specific cardiac abnormalities are a feature of certain disorders causing scoliosis, such as Friedreich's ataxia and Duchenne's muscular dystrophy.

ASSESSMENT

Breathlessness on exertion is a common feature of severe scoliosis, but it is when this deteriorates that hypoventilation should be suspected. Symptoms such as daytime somnolence due to sleep fragmentation, early morning headaches as a result of carbon dioxide retention, and frequent arousals from sleep at the end of central apneas may be present. Signs of right ventricular hypertrophy and right-sided heart failure may develop. The chest radiograph is usually unhelpful because the spine often obscures the cardiac outline and most of the lung fields. Serial assessments of lung volumes, maximum inspiratory and expiratory pressures, and transdiaphragmatic pressure may be useful. The ECG is insensitive at detecting right atrial or ventricular hypertrophy, and echocardiography is often technically difficult. Transesophageal echocardiograms may be required. Arterial blood gas analysis is essential if respiratory failure is suspected, and sleep studies provide further additional information.

EFFECTS OF BRACES AND SURGICAL TREATMENT

Any of the techniques for applying external support to the spine have the potential to restrict respiratory movements. Even lightweight braces can lower the VC, especially if the scoliosis is severe.[108] Resection of the posterior sections of the ribs comprising the rib hump (costectomy)[109] leads to little loss of respiratory function. The exercise ability is hardly influenced,[110] and lung volumes are only slightly reduced.[111]

Spinal fusion reduces the compliance of the respiratory system postoperatively, and considerable right-to-left shunting of blood through the lungs may occur.[112] The longer-term effects on respiratory mechanics of spinal fusion in patients without neuromuscular disorders are only slight. In adolescent idiopathic scoliosis, only minimal alterations in lung volumes, maximal inspiratory pressure,[113] ventilatory responses to hypercapnia,[114] and ventilation-perfusion matching have been recorded. The arterial blood gases hardly alter,[115] and there is little change in exercise ability.[116]

In contrast, the benefits of spinal fusion in scoliosis associated with neuromuscular disorders can be considerable. The rate of fall in VC in Duchenne's muscular dystrophy may slow significantly,[117] and in poliomyelitis, the VC can increase after surgery.[118]

References

1. Bergofsky EH: Respiratory failure in disorders of the thoracic cage. *Am Rev Respir Dis* 119:643–669, 1979.
2. Rochester DF, Lindley LJ: Neuromuscular and skeletal disease, in Murray JF (ed): *Pulmonary Complications of Systemic Disease.* New York, Marcel Dekker, 1992, pp 303–384.
3. Baydur A, Milic-Emili J: Respiratory mechanics in kyphoscoliosis. *Monaldi Arch Chest Dis* 48:69–71, 1993.
4. Davies G, Reid L: Effect of scoliosis on growth of alveoli and pulmonary arteries and on right ventricle. *Arch Dis Child* 46:623–632, 1971.
5. Shneerson JM: Pregnancy in neuro-muscular and skeletal disorders. *Monaldi Arch Chest Dis* 49:227–230, 1994.
6. Bender S: Pregnancy in a 31 in (77.5 cm) dwarf. *Br Med J* 2:1166, 1965.
7. Huang CT, Pelosi M, Langer A, Harrigan JT: Blood gas measurements in the kyphoscoliotic gravida and her fetus: Report of a case. *Am J Obstet Gynecol* 121:287–288, 1975.
8. Nava S, Zanotti E, Ambrosino N, et al: Evidence of acute diaphragmatic fatigue in a "natural" condition. *Am Rev Respir Dis* 146:1226–1230, 1992.
9. Martin LW, Helmsworth JA: The management of congenital deformities of the sternum. *JAMA* 179:82–84, 1962.
10. Gyllensward A, Irnell L, Michaelsson M, et al: Pectus excavatum: A clinical study with long term postoperative follow-up. *Acta Paediatr Scand Suppl* 255:1–14, 1973.
11. Lindskog GE, Felton WL 2d: Pectus excavatum: A report of eight cases with surgical correction. *Surg Gynecol Obstet* 95:615–622, 1952.
12. Naef AP: The surgical treatment of pectus excavatum: An experience with 90 operations. *Ann Thorac Surg* 21:53–66, 1976.
13. Lester CW: Funnel chest and allied deformities of the thoracic cage. *J Thorac Surg* 19:507–522, 1950.
14. Chin EF: Surgery of funnel chest and congenital sternal prominence. *Br J Surg* 44:360–376, 1957.
15. Fan I, Murphy S: Pectus excavatum from chronic upper airway obstruction. *Am J Dis Child* 135:550–552, 1981.
16. Fabricius J, Davidsen HG, Hansen AT: Cardiac function in funnel chest: Twenty-six patients investigated by cardiac catheterization. *Dan Med Bull* 4:251–257, 1957.
17. Orzalesi MM, Cook CD: Pulmonary function in children with pectus excavatum. *J Pediatr* 66:898–900, 1965.
18. Castile RG, Staats BA, Westbrook PR: Symptomatic pectus deformities of the chest. *Am Rev Respir Dis* 126:564–568, 1982.
19. Mead J, Sly P, le Souef P, et al: Rib cage mobility in pectus excavatum. *Am Rev Respir Dis* 132:1223–1228, 1985.
20. Weg JG, Krumholz A, Harkleroad LE: Pulmonary function in pectus excavatum. *Am Rev Respir Dis* 96:936–945, 1967.
21. Guller B, Hable K: Cardiac findings in pectus excavatum in children: Review and differential diagnosis. *Chest* 66:165–171, 1974.
22. Bevegard S: Postural circulatory changes at rest and during exercise in patients with funnel chest, with special reference to factors affecting the stroke volume. *Acta Med Scand* 171:693–713, 1962.
23. Majid PA, Zienkowicz BS, Roos JP: Pectus excavatum and cardiac dysfunction: A case report with pre-operative and postoperative haemodynamic studies. *Thorax* 34:74–78, 1979.
24. Ravitch MM: Pectus excavatum and heart failure. *Surgery* 30:178–194, 1951.
25. Jensen NK, Schmidt WR, Garamella JJ: Funnel chest: a new corrective operation. *J Thorac Cardiovasc Surg* 43:731–741, 1962.
26. Wynn SR, Driscoll DJ, Ostrom NK, et al: Exercise cardiorespiratory function in adolescents with pectus excavatum: Observations before and after operation. *J Thorac Cardiovasc Surg* 99:41–47, 1990.

27. Kaguraoka H, Ohnuki T, Itaoka T, et al: Degree of severity of pectus excavatum and pulmonary function in preoperative and postoperative periods. *J Thorac Cardiovasc Surg* 104:1483–1488, 1992.

28. Derveaux L, Ivanoff I, Rochette F, Demedts M: Mechanism of pulmonary function changes after surgical correction for funnel chest. *Eur Respir J* 1:823–825, 1988.

29. Haller JA Jr, Colombani PM, Humphries CT, et al: Chest wall constriction after too extensive and too early operations for pectus excavatum. *Ann Thorac Surg* 61:1618–1625, 1996.

30. Dorner RA, Keil PG, Schissel DJ: Pectus excavatum: Case report with pre- and post-operative angiocardiolgraphic studies. *J Thorac Surg* 20:444–453, 1950.

31. Lester CW: Pigeon breast (pectus carinatum) and other protrustion deformities of the chest of developmental origin. *Ann Surg* 137:482–489, 1953.

32. Brown AL: Cardio-respiratory studies in pre- and post-operative funnel chest (pectus excavatum). *Dis Chest* 20:378–391, 1951.

33. Davies H: Chest deformities in congenital heart disease. *Br J Dis Chest* 53:151–158, 1959.

34. Cahill JL, Lees GM, Robertson HT: A summary of preoperative and postoperative cardiorespiratory performance in patients undergoing pectus excavatum and carinatum repair. *J Pediatr Surg* 19:430–433, 1984.

35. Michet CJ Jr, McKenna CH, Luthra HS, O'Fallon WM: Relapsing polychondritis: Survival and predictive role of early disease manifestations. *Ann Intern Med* 104:74–78, 1986.

36. Stokes DC, Pyeritz RE, Wise RA, et al: Spirometry and chest wall dimensions in achondroplasia. *Chest* 93:364–369, 1988.

37. Stokes DC, Wohl MEB, Wise RA, et al: The lungs and airways in achondroplasia: Do little people have little lungs? *Chest* 98:145–152, 1990.

38. Finegold MJ, Katzew H, Genieser NB, Becker MH: Lung structure in thoracic dystrophy. *Am J Dis Child* 122:153–159, 1971.

39. Oberklaid F, Danks DM, Mayne V, Campbell P: Asphyxiating thoracic dysplasia: Clinical, radiological and pathological information on 10 patients. *Arch Dis Child* 52:758–765, 1977.

40. Barnes ND, Hull D, Milner AD, Waterston DJ: Chest reconstruction in thoracic dystrophy. *Arch Dis Child* 46:833–837, 1971.

41. Tzelepis GE, McCool FD, Hoppin FG Jr: Chest wall distortion in patients with flail chest. *Am Rev Respir Dis* 140:31–37, 1989.

42. Phillips MS, Kinnear WJM, Shneerson JM: Late sequelae of pulmonary tuberculosis treated by thoracoplasty. *Thorax* 42:445–451, 1987.

43. Phillips MS, Miller MR, Kinnear WJM, et al: Importance of airflow obstruction after thoracoplasty. *Thorax* 42:348–352, 1987.

44. Landis FB, Weisel W: Comparative study of pulmonary function loss with thoracoplasty versus small resection in surgery of tuberculosis. *J Thorac Surg* 27:336–348, 1954.

45. Little GM: Loss of ventilatory function after surgical procedures for tuberculosis. *Tubercle* 37:172–176, 1956.

46. Zeilhofer R, Sroka W: Spatunterschungen der Lungenfunktion nach Thoracoplastik. *Beitr Klin Tuberk* 122:48–70, 1960.

47. Lindahl T: Spirometric and bronchospirometric studies in five-rib thoracoplasties. *Thorax* 9:285–290, 1954.

48. Loynes RD: Scoliosis after thoracoplasty. *J Bone Joint Surg* 54B:484–498, 1972.

49. Iacob G: La scoliose de cause thoraco-pleuro-pulmonaaire. *Poumon Coeur* 23:439-451, 1967.

50. Powers SR Jr, Himmelstein A: Late changes in ventilatory function following thoracoplasty. *J Thorac Surg* 22:45–51, 1951.

51. Geensler EA, Strieder JW: Pulmonary function before and after extrapleural pneumothorax: A comparison with other forms of collapse and resection. *J Thorac Surg* 20:774–797, 1950.

52. Phillips MS, Kinnear WJM, Shaw D, Shneerson JM: Exercise responses in patients treated for pulmonary tuberculosis by thoracoplasty. *Thorax* 44:268, 1989.

53. Brander PE, Salmi T, Partinen M, Sovijarvi ARA: Nocturnal oxygen saturation and sleep quality in long-term survivors of thoracoplasty. *Respiration* 60:325–331, 1993.

54. Kinnear WJM, Phillips MS, Shneerson JM: Inspiratory muscle function after thoracoplasty. *Thorax* 41:244, 1986.

55. Moore NR, Phillips MS, Shneerson JM, et al: Appearances on computed tomography following thoracoplasty for pulmonary tuberculosis. *Br J Radiol* 61:573–578, 1988.

56. Huang CT, Lyons HA: Cardiorespiratory failure in patients with pneumonectomy for tuberculosis: Long-term effects of thoracoplasty. *J Thorac Cardiovasc Surg* 74:409-417, 1977.

57. Zimmerman HA: Hemodynamics: Studies on a group of patients who developed cor pulmonale following thoracoplasty. *J Thorac Surg* 22:94–98, 1951.

58. Hart FD, Maclagan NF: Ankylosing spondylitis: A review of 184 cases. *Ann Rheum Dis* 14:77–83, 1955.

59. Franssen MJAM, van Herwaarden CLA, van de Putte LBA, Gribnau FWJ: Lung function in patients with ankylosing spondilitis: A study of the influence of disease activity and treatment with nonsteroidal anti-inflammatory drugs. *J Rheumatol* 13:936–940, 1986.

60. Meister R, Merkel T: Beziehungen zwischen Wirbelsaulenfunktion und Atmung bei ankylosierender Spondylitis (M. Bechterew). *Prax Klin Pneumol* 37:691–694, 1983.

61. Sharp JT, Sweany SK, Henry JP, et al: Lung and thoracic compliances in ankylosing spondylitis. *J Lab Clin Med* 63:254–263, 1964.

62. Josenhans WT, Wang CS, Josenhans G, Woodbury JFL: Diaphragmatic contribution to ventilation in patients with ankylosing spondylitis. *Respiration* 28:331–346, 1971.

63. Travis DM, Cook CD, Julian DG, et al: The lungs in rheumatoid spondylitis: Gas exchange and lung mechanics in a form of restrictive pulmonary disease. *Am J Med* 29:623–632, 1960.

64. Hauge BN: Diaphragmatic movement and spirometric volume in patients with ankylosing spondylitis. *Scand J Respir Dis* 54:38–44, 1973.

65. Elliott CG, Hill TR, Adams TF, et al: Exercise performance of subjects with ankylosing spondylitis and limited chest expansion. *Bull Eur Physiopathol Respir* 21:363–368, 1985.

66. Parkin A, Robinson PJ, Hickling P: Regional lung ventilation in ankylosing spondylitis. *Br J Radiol* 55:833–836, 1982.

67. Libby DM, Schley S, Smith JP: Cricoarytenoid arthritis in ankylosing spondylitis. *Chest* 80:641–643, 1981.

68. Rosenow EC III, Strimlan CV, Muhm JR, Ferguson RH: Pleuropulmonary manifestations of ankylosing spondylitis. *Mayo Clin Proc* 52:641–649, 1977.

69. Kinnear WJM, Shneerson JM: Acute pleural effusions in inactive ankylosing spondylitis. *Thorax* 40:150–151, 1985.

70. Tanaka H, Itoh E, Shibusa T, et al: Pleural effusion in ankylosing spondylitis: Successful treatment with intra-pleural steroid administration. *Respir Med* 80:509-511, 1995.

71. Efthimiou J, McLelland J, Round J, et al: Diaphragm paralysis causing ventilatory failure in an adult with the rigid spine syndrome. *Am Rev Respir Dis* 136:1483–1485, 1987.

72. Ras GJ, van Staden M, Schultz C, et al: Respiratory manifestations of rigid spine syndrome. *Am J Respir Crit Care Med* 150:540–546, 1994.

73. Culham EG, Jimenez HAI, King CE: Thoracic kyphosis, rib mobility, and lung volumes in normal women and women with osteoporosis. *Spine* 19:1250–1255, 1994.

74. O'Brien JP: Kyphosis secondary to infectious disease. *Clin Orthop* 128:56–64, 1977.

75. Larmi TKI, Patiala J, Karvonen MJ: Studies of pulmonary function in kyphoscoliosis after tuberculous spondylitis. *Ann Med Intern Fenn* 44:57–69, 1955.

76. Berend N, Martin GE: Arrest of alveolar multiplication in kyphoscoliosis. *Pathology* 11:485–491, 1979.

77. Smith IE, Laroche CM, Jamieson SA, Shneerson JM: Kyphosis secondary to tuberculous osteomyelitis as a cause of ventilatory

failure: Clinical features, mechanisms and management. *Chest* 110:1105–1110, 1996.

78. Hanley T, Platts MM, Clifton M, Morris TL: Heart failure of the hunchback. *Q J Med* 27:155–171, 1958.

79. Kopenhager T: A review of 50 pregnant patients with kyphoscoliosis. *Br J Obstet Gynaecol* 84:585–587, 1977.

80. de Leon AC, Perloff JK, Twigg H, Majd M: The straight back syndrome: Clinical cardiovascular manifestations. *Circulation* 32:193–203, 1965.

81. Rawlings MS: Straight back syndrome: A new heart disease. *Dis Chest* 39:435–443, 1961.

82. Serratto M, Kezdi P: Absence of the physiologic dorsal kyphosis: Cardiac signs and hemodynamic manifestations. *Ann Intern Med* 58:938–945, 1963.

83. Kafer ER: Idiopathic scoliosis: Mechanical properties of the respiratory system and the ventilatory response to carbon dioxide. *J Clin Invest* 55:1153–1163, 1975.

84. Cooper DM, Rojas JV, Mellins RB, et al: Respiratory mechanics in adolescents with idiopathic scoliosis. *Am Rev Respir Dis* 130: 16–22, 1984.

85. Linderholm H, Lindgren U: Prediction of spirometric values in patients with scoliosis. *Acta Orthop Scand* 49:469-478, 1978.

86. Bergofsky EH, Turino GM, Fishman AP: Cardiorespiratory failure in kyphoscoliosis. *Medicine* 38:263–317, 1959.

87. Pehrsson K, Bake B, Larsson S, Nachemson A: Lung function in adult idiopathic scoliosis: A 20-year follow-up. *Thorax* 46:474–478, 1991.

88. Winter RB, Lovell WW, Georgia D, Moe JH: Excessive thoracic lordosis and loss of pulmonary function in patients with idiopathic scoliosis. *J Bone Joint Surg* 57A:972–977, 1975.

89. Muirhead A, Conner AN: The assessment of lung function in children with scoliosis. *J Bone Joint Surg* 67B:699–702, 1985.

90. Midgren B, Peterson K, Hansson L, et al: Nocturnal hypoxaemia in severe scoliosis. *Br J Dis Chest* 82:226–236, 1988.

91. Jones RS, Kennedy JD, Hasham F, et al: Mechanical inefficiency of the thoracic cage in scoliosis. *Thorax* 36:456–461, 1981.

92. Kesten S, Garfinkel FK, Wright T, Rebuck AS: Impaired exercise ability in adults with moderate scoliosis. *Chest* 99:663–666, 1991.

93. Shneerson JM: The cardiorespiratory response to exercise in thoracic scoliosis. *Thorax* 33:457–463, 1978.

94. Bjure J, Grimby G, Nachemson A, Lindh M: The effect of physical training in girls with idiopathic scoliosis. *Acta Orthop Scand* 40:325–333, 1969.

95. Smyth RJ, Chapman KR, Wright TA, et al: Ventilatory patterns during hypoxia, hypercapnia, and exercise in adolescents with mild scoliosis. *Pediatrics* 77:690–697, 1986.

96. Shneerson JM: Cardiac and respiratory responses to exercise in adolescent idiopathic scoliosis. *Thorax* 35:347–350, 1980.

97. Kafer ER: Idiopathic scoliosis: Gas exchange and the age dependence of arterial blood gases. *J Clin Invest* 58:825–833, 1976.

98. Buhlmann A, Gierhake W: Die Lungenfunktion bei der jugendlichen Kyphoskoliose. *Schweiz Med Wochenschr* 90:1153–1155, 1960.

99. Secker-Walker RH, Ho JE, Gill IS: Observations on regional ventilation and perfusion in kyphoscoliosis. *Respiration* 38:194–203, 1979.

100. Dollery CT, Gillam PMS, Hugh-Jones P, Zorab PA: Regional lung function in kyphoscoliosis. *Thorax* 20:175–181, 1965.

101. Sawicka EH, Branthwaite MA: Respiration during sleep in kyphoscoliosis. *Thorax* 42:801–808, 1987.

102. Anonymous: Respiratory function in scoliosis. *Lancet* 1:84–85, 1985.

103. Branthwaite MA: Cardiorespiratory consequences of unfused idiopathic scoliosis. *Br J Dis Chest* 80:360–369, 1986.

104. Bachmann M: Die Veranderungen der inneren Organe bei hochgradigen Skoliosen und Kyphoskoliosen. *Bibl Med Abteilung* 4:DI, 1899.

105. Shneerson JM, Venco A, Prime FJ: A study of pulmonary artery pressure, electrocardiography and mechanocardiography in thoracic scoliosis. *Thorax* 32:700–705, 1977.

106. Hasleton PS, Heath D, Brewer DB: Hypertensive pulmonary vascular disease in states of chronic hypoxia. *J Pathol Bacteriol* 95:431–440, 1968.

107. Shneerson JM, Sutton GC, Zorab PA: Causes of death, right ventricular hypertrophy, and congenital heart disease in scoliosis. *Clin Orthop* 135:52–57, 1978.

108. Noble-Jamieson CM, Heckmatt JZ, Dubowitz V, Silverman N: Effects of posture and spinal bracing on respiratory function in neuromuscular disease. *Arch Dis Child* 61:178–181, 1986.

109. Barrett DS, MacLean JGB, Bettany J, et al: Costoplasty in adolescent idiopathic scoliosis: Objective results in 55 patients. *J Bone Joint Surg* 75B:881–885, 1993.

110. Haber P, Kummer F: Der Einfluss der Rippen buckelresektion als Zweitoperation auf die Lungenfunktion und die aerobe Leistengs fahigkeit bei Skoliosepatienten nach dorsaler Spondylodese. *Acta Med Aust* 9:171–173, 1982.

111. Manning CW, Prime FJ, Zorab PA: Partial costectmy as a cosmetic operation in scoliosis. *J Bone Joint Surg* 55B:521–527, 1973.

112. Lin HY, Nash CL, Herndon CH, Andersen NB: The effect of corrective surgery on pulmonary function in scoliosis. *J Bone Joint Surg* 57A:1173–1179, 1974.

113. Cooper DM, Rojas JV, Mellins RB, et al: Respiratory mechanics in adolescents with idiopathic scoliosis. *Am Rev Respir Dis* 130: 16–22, 1984.

114. Levine DB: Pulmonary function in scoliosis. *Orthop Clin North Am* 10:761–768, 1979.

115. Kumano K, Tsuyama N: Pulmonary function before and after surgical correction of scoliosis. *J Bone Joint Surg* 64A:242–248, 1982.

116. Shannon DC, Riseborough EJ, Kazemi H: Ventilation perfusion relationships following correction of kyphoscoliosis. *JAMA* 217:579-584, 1971.

117. Rideau Y, Glorion B, Delaubier A, et al: The treatment of scoliosis in Duchenne muscular dystrophy. *Muscle Nerve* 7:281–286, 1984.

118. Lindh M, Bjure J: Lung volumes in scoliosis before and after correction by the Harrington instrumentation method. *Acta Orthop Scand* 46:934–948, 1975.

Chapter 12

DISORDERS OF THE RESPIRATORY MUSCLES

FRANCO LAGHI

MARTIN J. TOBIN

Several disease states affect the respiratory muscles both directly, as in the case of myopathies, and indirectly, as in the case of hyperinflation in obstructive lung disease. This chapter discusses some of the more common conditions. The interested reader is referred elsewhere for a detailed discussion of respiratory muscle involvement in additional disease entities.[1,2]

Chronic Obstructive Pulmonary Disease

Chronic obstructive pulmonary disease (COPD) has become the fourth leading cause of death in the adult population of the United States.[3] The most disabling symptom in patients with COPD, dyspnea, results primarily from a decreased capacity of the respiratory muscles to meet the increase in respiratory mechanical load.[4,5] This imbalance probably also leads to the development of acute respiratory failure in these patients.[6] Several factors contribute to the imbalance between load and capacity.

VENTILATORY AND ENERGY DEMANDS

Under resting conditions, many patients with COPD have an increased minute ventilation, approximately 9 L/min, compared with 6 L/min in healthy subjects.[7-9] Almost all patients with COPD have an increased work and energy cost of breathing due to hyperinflation[10,11] and, to a lesser extent, due to increased airway resistance[12-14] (Fig. 12-1).

HYPERINFLATION

A major pathophysiologic consequence of COPD is static hyperinflation due to a loss of pulmonary elastic recoil[12] and dynamic hyperinflation as airflow become limited secondary to a loss of tethering forces on the airways.[12] This may slow expiration sufficiently that some of the air inspired remains in the lungs and the inspiratory muscles have to overcome a threshold load that can be detected as a positive end-expiratory pressure intrinsic PEEP (PEEPi).

Hyperinflation has a number of other adverse effects on inspiratory muscle function (Fig. 12-2). Hyperinflation causes the inspiratory muscles to operate at an unfavorable position on the length-tension curve. As lung volume increases, the inspiratory muscles shorten, and their ability to generate negative inspiratory pressure decreases.[16-19] On changing from functional residual capacity (FRC) to total lung capacity (TLC) in patients with COPD and healthy control subjects, it has been estimated that the diaphragm shortens by 40 percent of its in situ resting length; the shortening of other muscles has been estimated to be about 20 percent or less of their in situ resting length.[21] Although

the rib cage muscles shorten relatively little as lung volume increases from FRC to TLC, their capacity to generate negative pleural pressure decreases substantially due to a shift in the orientation of the ribs from the usual oblique position to a more horizontal position.[22,23] This results in increased impedance to rib cage expansion[24] and greater mechanical disadvantage for the rib cage muscles than is the case for the diaphragm.[23]

Hyperinflation decreases the size of the zone of apposition,[25-27] the portion of the inner rib cage that lies in contact with the costal fibers of the diaphragm. Normally, an increase in abdominal pressure resulting from diaphragmatic contraction is transmitted directly to the lower rib cage through the zone of apposition, expanding the lower rib cage and aiding inspiration. As lung volume increases, the zone of opposition decreases, so diaphragmatic contraction is less effective in expanding the rib cage. When lung volumes approach TLC, the zone of apposition may disappear as the diaphragmatic fibers become directed medially or inward. In this situation, diaphragmatic contraction has an expiratory action[28]—detected clinically as an indrawing of the lateral rib cage on inspiration, such as Hoover's sign.[29]

Although hyperinflation affects the geometry of the respiratory muscles, particularly the curvature of the diaphragm, this may not be as important as diaphragmatic fiber length in determining the contractile force of the diaphragm over the range of normal vital capacity (VC).[25,30] In fact, employing a three-dimensional reconstruction of in vivo human diaphragmatic shape at different lung volumes, Gauthier and colleagues[25] showed that the radius of curvature in the coronal plane changed very little over the range of VC.

Hyperinflation has an adverse effect on the elastic recoil of the thoracic cage[31] (see Fig. 12-2). Resting lung volume, or FRC, is normally determined by the static equilibrium between inwardly directed elastic recoil of the lungs and outwardly directed elastic recoil of the thoracic cage. Thus thoracic elastic recoil normally assists the action of the inspiratory muscles in inflating the lungs. When FRC is markedly increased, as in hyperinflation, thoracic elastic recoil becomes directed inward. This means that the inspiratory muscles must work not only against the elastic recoil of the lungs but also against that of the thoracic cage.

RESPIRATORY MUSCLE STRENGTH AND ENDURANCE

In some patients with COPD, the observed reduction in maximal inspiratory pressure (Pimax) can be explained completely by hyperinflation-induced muscle shortening.[32] In other patients with COPD, however, the Pimax value is actually supranormal for the absolute increase in FRC.[33] This suggests that the inspiratory muscles of some patients with COPD adapt to hyperinflation,[34] possibly by loss of sarcomeres, as reported in the hamster model of emphysema.[35] This interpretation has been challenged, however, by autopsy data indicating that diaphragmatic length is similar in patients with and without COPD.[36] Moreover, following lung transplantation, patients with COPD exhibit more rapid recovery of transdiaphragmatic sniff pressure than can be explained by length adaptation of the muscle.[37] Furthermore, after correction for lung volume, diaphragmatic dimensions[27] and transdiaphragmatic pressure (Pdi) during stimulation

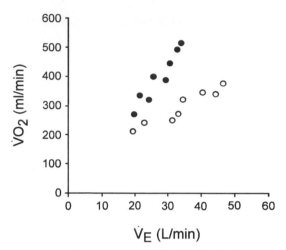

FIGURE 12-1 Total oxyen consumption (V_{O_2}) and minute ventilation (V_E) in a patient with COPD (*solid circles*) and in a healthy subject (*open circles*). As V_E increased, the rate of increase in V_{O_2} was greater in the patient than in the healthy subject, indicating an increased mechanical load and decreased efficiency of the respiratory muscles in patients with COPD than in healthy subjects. (Reproduced, with permission, from Shindoh et al: *Chest* 105: 790–797, 1994.)

of the phrenic nerves[19] are the same in patients with COPD and healthy control subjects. Hystologic data on sarcomere length in severe COPD are not yet available.

In some patients with COPD, it is possible to demonstrate not only a reduction in PImax but also a reduction in maximal expiratory pressure (PEmax).[32] Since the expiratory muscles should not be at a mechanical disadvantage in COPD, Rochester and Braun[32] proposed that some patients with COPD have generalized muscle weakness. This hypothesis is supported by the high correlation between PImax and PEmax ($r = 0.73$) that these investigators reported in a study of 32 patients with COPD.[32] Hypoxemia,[38,39] hypercapnia,[40] reductions in respiratory muscle adenosine triphosphate (ATP), phosphocreatine, glycogen,[41,42] and phosphorus,[43] fiber damage,[41,44] and malnutrition[45–47] may contribute to muscle weakness in patients with COPD. Other possible factors include cor pulmonale causing decreased blood supply to the muscles and steroid-induced myopathy.[48]

The ratios of contraction time to total respiratory cycle time (T_I/T_{tot}) and mean Pdi per breath to maximum static Pdi (Pdi/Pdimax) are critical determinants of respiratory muscle fatigue.[49,50] For the diaphragm, the product of these ratios is termed the *diaphragmatic tension-time index* (TTdi), and once a critical value of 0.15 has been reached, diaphragmatic fatigue can occur in certain situations.[49,50] In healthy subjects breathing at rest, TTdi is 0.02, i.e., an 8-fold reserve before the development of fatigue. In a study of stable patients with COPD,[51] TTdi was 0.05 (range 0.01–0.12) during resting breathing, indicating a low degree of functional reserve (33 percent of the critical TTdi value).

CLINICAL EVIDENCE OF RESPIRATORY MUSCLE DYSFUNCTION

Abnormalities in rib cage–abdominal motion are common in patients with COPD,[52] and they appear to indicate a poor prognosis.[53] The best recognized distortion is inspiratory paradoxical inward movement of the lateral rib cage, known as *Hoover's sign*.[29] The paradoxical movement occurs at the time of peak negative pleural pressure and peak Pdi and has been attributed to direct traction by the flattened diaphragm on the lateral rib margins.[54] Recently, Jubran and Tobin[55] have shown that acute hyperinflation produced minimal alterations in rib cage–abdominal motion in healthy subjects, suggesting that the primary cause of abnormal chest wall motion in patients with COPD is likely to be increased airway resistance.[56]

For a given fall in pleural pressure during resting breathing, patients with COPD exhibit a smaller increase in abdominal pressure[57,58] and lesser abdominal expansion than healthy subjects.[9] This finding suggests that the rib cage muscles make a greater contribution to tidal breathing in patients with COPD than in healthy subjects. The greater rib cage muscle contribution to tidal breathing is likely due to recruitment of the scalene and inspiratory intercostal muscles,[59] and contrary to the widely held belief, most patients with stable severe COPD and hyperinflation do not contract their sternomastoid or trapezii when breathing at rest.[59,60] Neither is the prominence of the sternomastoid muscles due to muscle hypertrophy[61] but instead results from sculpturing of the soft tissue because of decrease in overlying skin-fold thickness.[62]

Recently, Ninane and colleagues[63] investigated the pattern of abdominal muscle contraction in 40 stable patients with severe COPD. During resting breathing, the rectus abdominis

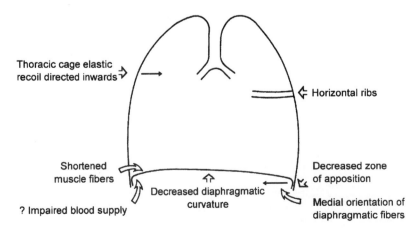

FIGURE 12-2 The detrimental effects of hyperinflation on respiratory muscle function (see text for discussion). (Reproduced, with permission, from Tobin MJ: *Clin Chest Med* 9:263–286, 1988.)

Thoracic cage elastic recoil directed inwards

Horizontal ribs

Shortened muscle fibers

Decreased zone of apposition

? Impaired blood supply

Decreased diaphragmatic curvature

Medial orientation of diaphragmatic fibers

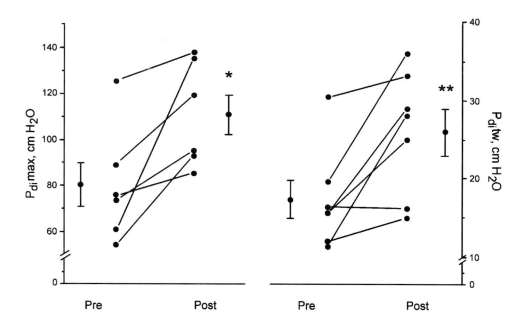

FIGURE 12-3 Voluntary maximal transdiaphragmatic pressure (Pdimax) (*right*) and transdiaphragmatic twitch pressure (Pditw) response to phrenic nerve stimulation (*left*) before and 3 months after lung volume-reduction surgery in seven patients with severe emphysema. Pdimax increased from 80.3 ± 9.5 (SE) before to 110.8 ± 9.3 cmH$_2$O after surgery (*p* = .03). Pditw increased from 17.2 ± 2.4 to 25.9 ± 3.0 cmH$_0$) (*p* = .02). Significant difference between pre- and postoperative values: **p* < .05; ***p* < .025. (Pdimax data are based on six patients because one was unable to perform a Mueller maneuver.) (Reproduced, with permission, from Laghi et al: *Am J Respir Crit Care Med* 155:A511, 1997.)

and external oblique muscles were virtually silent in all patients, invariable phasic activity of the transversus abdominis was noted in 17 patients, and intermittent activity of the latter muscle was noted in an additional 11 patients. Expiratory contraction of the transversus abdominis was related to the severity of airflow obstruction.[63] In a subsequent study, Ninane and colleagues[64] investigated the contribution of expiratory muscle activity to PEEPi and reported a significant correlation between the level of PEEPi and the expiratory increase in gastric pressure (*r* = 0.87). The investigators concluded that the PEEPi in their patients largely resulted from transmission through the relaxed diaphragm of an increase in abdominal pressure due to abdominal muscle contraction.

Contrary to earlier reports, some patients with COPD have been shown to have an increased respiratory drive,[8,65] although the increased output in hypercapnic patients is insufficient to achieve a normal Pa$_{CO_2}$. The level of hypercapnia has been correlated with lower inspiratory muscle strength and higher inspiratory muscle loads.[66] Other factors that may contribute to the development of hypercapnia in patients with COPD include inherited alterations of the respiratory drive,[67] ventilation-perfusion mismatch,[68] hypoxemia, and the metabolic milieu.[32]

In patients with COPD, Pitcher and Cunningham[11] recently investigated the effect of increasing tidal volume on the O$_2$ cost of breathing. While keeping minute ventilation constant, hypercapnic patients experienced a significant increase in the O$_2$ cost of breathing in response to increasing tidal volume, whereas eucapnic patients and healthy control individuals did not. The increase in O$_2$ cost of breathing was positively correlated with baseline Pa$_{CO_2}$ and the degree of diaphragmatic flattening. In other words, diaphragmatic flattening secondary to hyperinflation may produce mechanical inefficiency (increased chest wall elastic load; see above) that limits the effective operating range of the respiratory muscles during tidal breathing.

During exercise, healthy subjects decrease end-expiratory lung volume as a result of increased expiratory activation of the abdominal and expiratory rib cage muscles.[69] In contrast,

patients with COPD usually experience an exercise-induced increase in end-expiratory lung volume[5,70,71] that is proportional to the severity of airway obstruction.[70] As a result of marked shortening, the force-generating capacity of the inspiratory muscles is decreased compared with resting conditions (see above). Belman and associates[72] recently demonstrated that albuterol can partially prevent exercise-induced hyperinflation in patients with COPD. Although resting FRC was not significantly affected by albuterol, the degree of dynamic hyperinflation and breathlessness during progressive exercise was decreased by it.[72]

Lung-reduction surgery has been revived as a means of decreasing breathlessness and improving exercise tolerance in patients with severe COPD.[73] Laghi and colleagues[60] have recently reported improved diaphragmatic strength (Fig. 12-3) and a trend toward improved dynamic compliance following lung-reduction surgery. These changes resulted in an improved neuromechanical coupling of the diaphragm (Fig. 12-4), which in turn could be one of the mechanisms responsible for decreased dyspnea and increased exercise tolerance following surgery. Of interest, the improvement in diaphragmatic strength was out of proportion to improvement in lung hyperinflation.[60] Other mechanisms that may contribute to the physiologic and clinical improvements following lung-reduction surgery include improvements in lung[74-76] and chest wall[77] elastic recoil, improvements in the pattern of breathing,[9,79] and enhanced right ventricular function.[75,78]

Asthma

Patients with asthma experience airway obstruction and hyperinflation, but only intermittently, unlike the situation in COPD. The capacity of the inspiratory muscles to deal with the obstruction is impaired by the concomitant hyperinflation. However, in some asthmatic patients, respiratory muscle strength (corrected for hyperinflation)[80,81] and respiratory muscle endurance are increased.[82,83] On the other hand, asth-

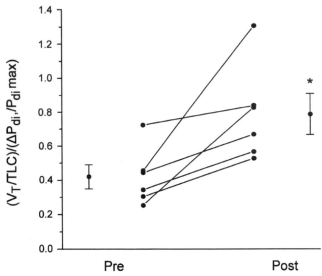

FIGURE 12-4 Diaphragmatic neuromechanical coupling, quantified as the quotient of tidal volume (normalized to total lung capacity) to tidal change in transdiaphragmatic pressure (normalized to maximal transdiaphragmatic pressure), that is, $(V_T/TLC)/(Pdi/Pdimax)$, before and 3 months after lung volume-reduction surgery in six patients with severe emphysema. Diaphragmatic neuromechanical coupling improved from 0.42 ± 0.05 (SE) to 0.78 ± 0.12 after lung volume-reduction surgery ($p = .025$). Significant difference between pre- and postoperative values: $*p < .05$). (Reproduced, with permission, from Laghi et al: *Am J Respir Crit Care Med* 155:A511, 1997.)

matic patients who require chronic systemic steroids have a decreased inspiratory muscle strength and endurance.[84]

The considerable airway narrowing increases the energy cost of breathing, which, combined with impaired function of the respiratory muscles, predisposes to respiratory muscle fatigue. Compensatory alterations that might decrease the likelihood of fatigue include a decrease in the duty cycle (T_I/T_{tot}), an increase in respiratory muscle strength, enhanced endurance of the respiratory muscles, and a decrease in maximal voluntary activation of the respiratory muscles. The duty cycle has been found to be decreased in patients with mild[8] and severe asthma.[85] A decrease in duty cycle tends to offset the negative effect of increased Pdi on the tension-time index (see above). McKenzie and Gandevia[83] have reported that the endurance of the respiratory muscles is enhanced in patients with frequent exacerbations of asthma, perhaps because repeated episodes of airflow obstruction may induce a "training response." This notion is supported by the recent observation that the thickness of the diaphragm at FRC, measured by high-resolution ultrasound, was greater in asthmatic patients than in healthy control subjects: 2.2 ± 0.4 (SD) versus 1.7 ± 0.3 mm ($p < .02$).[86] Finally, a reduced voluntary drive to breathe has been demonstrated by Allen and associates[87] in some asthmatic patients, and the investigators speculated that this reduced drive may predispose to ventilatory failure. This is in agreement with a study by Kikuchi and colleagues,[88] who reported reduced chemosensitivity to hypoxia and blunted perception of dyspnea in patients with a history of near-fatal asthma as compared with either healthy subjects or patients with asthma who were not susceptible to near-fatal attacks (Fig. 12-5).

Acute Respiratory Failure

Acute respiratory failure producing respiratory acidosis may result from a number of factors, including hypoventilation caused by decreased respiratory center output or respiratory muscle fatigue, impaired pulmonary gas exchange, and excessive ventilatory requirements (Fig. 12-6). The development of respiratory muscle fatigue has long been suspected in patients experiencing acute ventilatory failure, but unequivocal evidence of contractile fatigue has not been demonstrated. In one of the first studies to use weaning failure as a model of acute ventilatory failure, Cohen and colleagues[89] observed a shift in the power spectrum of the diaphragmatic electromyogram (EMG) and respiratory paradox, which they considered to signify fatigue. It is now recognized, however, that the EMG power spectrum is influenced by several factors and does not necessarily signify impaired muscle contractility,[90] and also that paradoxical motion of the rib cage and abdomen is neither sensitive nor specific for muscle fatigue but instead reflects an increased respiratory load.[56]

In five patients who failed a weaning trial, Goldstone and colleagues[91] observed a 44 percent decrease in the maximal relaxation rate measured from the decay portion of the Pdi signal. When mechanical ventilation was reinstituted, the maximum relaxation rate recovered within 10 min (Fig. 12-7). In contrast, four patients who were weaned successfully showed no change in relaxation rate. Slowing of the maximum relaxation rate has been interpreted as evidence of respiratory muscle fatigue.[90] However, like changes in the EMG power spectrum, the maximum relaxation rate changes very early in a fatiguing process and is not necessarily associated with a decrease in contractile force. As such, it is more closely related to an increased load on the respiratory system

FIGURE 12-5 Mean (±SE) perception of dyspnea (Borg score) during breathing at six levels of resistance in 11 patients with asthma who had suffered near-fatal attacks, 11 patients with asthma without near-fatal attacks, and 12 healthy subjects. Compared with the healthy subjects, the patients who had experienced near-fatal asthmatic attacks had a blunted perception of dyspnea following application of greater levels of resistance. (Reproduced, with permission, from Kikuchi et al: *N Engl J Med* 330:1329–1334, 1994.)

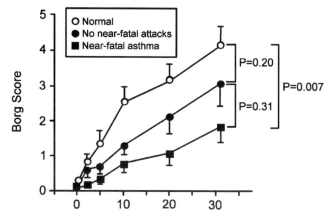

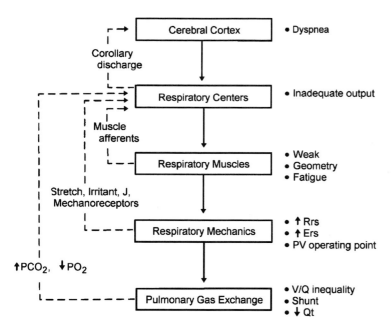

FIGURE 12-6 Model of the respiratory neuromuscular control system. Potential mechanisms of acute ventilatory failure are listed on the right side, and afferent stimuli arising at each site are shown on the left side. Abbreviations: Rrs, respiratory system resistance; Ers, respiratory system elastance; PV, pressure-volume; V/Q, ventilation-perfusion ratio; Q_T, cardiac output; P_{CO_2}, carbon dioxide tension; P_{O_2}, oxygen tension. (Reproduced, with permission, from Tobin MJ, Jubran A: *Schweiz Med Wochenschr* 124:2139–2145, 1994.)

rather than a direct reflection of neuromechanical uncoupling.

The major determinants of inspiratory muscle fatigue are inspiratory muscle strength, mean inspiratory pressure, and the duration of inspiratory effort; these can be combined together as the *tension-time index* (TTI) (see above).[49] In a recent study of 17 patients with COPD who developed acute respiratory distress during a trial of weaning from mechanical ventilation, TTI was 0.06 ± 0.01 (SE) at the onset of the trial, which was not different from the value observed in 14 patients who tolerated the trial and were extubated.[6] Over the course of the trial, TTI did not change in the success group, whereas 5 of the patients in the failure group developed an increase in TTI above the threshold of 0.15 (Fig. 12-8), all but one of whom exhibited increases in Pa_{CO_2} of 20 to 30 mmHg. Figure 12-9 shows a decrease in Pdi following stimulation of the phrenic nerves in a patient with spinal cord injury who failed a weaning trial. These data suggest that some patients who develop acute respiratory failure during a weaning trial probably develop respiratory muscle fatigue.

Neuromuscular Diseases

Respiratory muscle weakness in patients with neuromuscular disease frequently goes undetected until the precipitation of ventilatory failure by aspiration pneumonia or the development of cor pulmonale. The delay in diagnosis arises in part because impaired skeletal muscle function prevents patients from exceeding their limited ventilatory capacity.[92,93] Interestingly, some patients with mild peripheral neuromuscular disease who do not have respiratory symptoms may have severe reductions in P_{Imax} and P_{Emax}.[93]

Patients with respiratory muscle weakness typically present with a "restrictive" pattern on pulmonary function testing: markedly decreased VC, reduced TLC and FRC, and relatively normal forced expiratory volume in 1 s to forced vital capacity ratio (FEV_1/FVC).[94] As long as the expiratory muscles are not weak, residual volume (RV) remains relatively normal.[94] One of the earliest indications of respiratory muscle weakness is a reduced maximal voluntary ventilation.[2] Diffusing capacity (when related to lung volume) and gas exchange are relatively normal, unlike the situation in patients with restrictive pattern caused by infiltrative lung disease.[94] Many patients show a greater than expected loss of VC because of an associated decrease in the compliance of both the lungs and chest wall.[94-96] Previously it was thought that diffuse microatelectasis accounted for the decrease in lung compliance in patients with neuromuscular diseases. This concept was challenged recently by Estenne and colleagues,[95] who used high-resolution computed tomography

FIGURE 12-7 Maximum relaxation rate (MRR) calculated from transdiaphragmatic pressure (Pdi) tracings obtained (*A*) during mechanical ventilation, (*B*) during a trial of spontaneous breathing, and (*C*) following a weaning trial. The MRR remained constant over time in those patients who were weaned successfully (*closed symbols*), whereas the MRR slowed by 44 percent during the spontaneous breathing trial in the weaning failure group (*open symbols*) and then recovered fully 10 min after the reinstitution of mechanical ventilation. (Reproduced, with permission, from Goldstone et al: *Thorax* 49:54–60, 1994.)

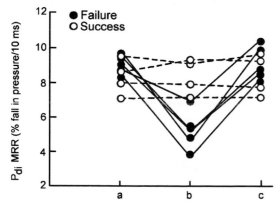

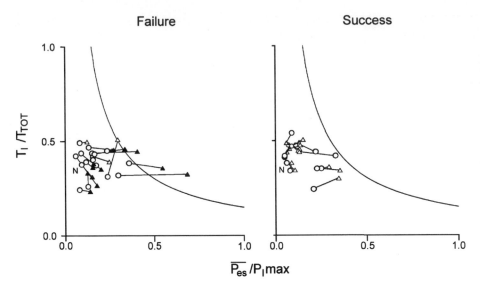

FIGURE 12-8 The relationship between mean esophageal pressure–maximum inspiratory pressure ratio (Pes/Pɪmax) and duty cycle (Tɪ/Ttot) in patients who failed and succeeded in a trial of spontaneous breathing. Circles and triangles represent values at the start and the end of the trial, respectively; closed symbols indicate patients who developed an increase in Pa_{CO_2} during the trial. Five of the 17 patients in the failure group developed a tension-time index of more than 0.15 (indicated by isopleth). *N* represents the value in a healthy subject. (Reproduced, with permission, from Jubran A, Tobin MJ: *Am J Respir Crit Care Med* 155:916–921, 1997.)

(CT) to evaluate the lung parenchyma of 8 patients with tetraplegia and 6 with generalized neuromuscular disorders. Despite a 30 percent reduction in lung compliance, 12 of the 14 patients had no evidence of atelectasis or any other parenchymal abnormality. Given that the elastic properties of a system are partly determined by the stresses to which the system is subjected, the decrease in lung compliance could be secondary to the persisting limited range of lung distention in patients with chronic respiratory muscle weakness.[94] Decreased chest wall compliance in these patients is likely due to stiffening of the rib cage tendons and rib cage ligaments and to ankylosis of the costosternal and thoracovertebral joints.[97]

The breathing pattern in patients with respiratory muscle weakness is characterized by rapid shallow breaths[98–102] and infrequent sighs.[103] The tachypnea may be caused by afferent signals arising in the weakened respiratory muscles and/or intrapulmonary receptors stimulated by decreased lung compliance. Arterial CO_2 tension may be reduced early in the disease,[94] but an elevated Pa_{CO_2} becomes likely when respiratory muscle strength falls to 39 percent of

the predicted normal value.[104] However, Gibson and associates[101] described several patients with neuromuscular disease who had a normal Pa_{CO_2} despite decreases in respiratory muscle strength to less than 20 percent of predicted. Conversely, some patients with only moderate respiratory muscle weakness displayed hypercapnia[101] (Fig. 12-10). In other words, reductions in muscle strength and VC do not consistently predict alveolar hypoventilation in this setting. Alterations in the pattern of breathing and gas exchange during sleep in patients with chronic neuromuscular disorders may induce resetting of the chemoreceptor sensitivity, which together with respiratory muscle weakness may produce daytime hypercapnia.[94,105] Long-term nocturnal ventilation improves Pa_{O_2} and Pa_{CO_2} during sleep and wakefulness in these patients[105] (Fig. 12-11). Such an improvement in Pa_{O_2} and Pa_{CO_2} may be due to a combination of improved respiratory muscle strength (Fig. 12-12) and normalization of chemoreceptor sensitivity.[105]

When considering respiratory involvement in neuromuscular disease, it is useful to recall the innervation of the different muscle groups (Fig. 12-13).

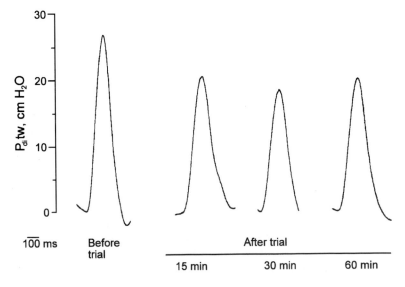

FIGURE 12-9 Recordings of transdiaphragmatic twitch pressure (Pditw) in a patient with C4 spinal cord injury 10 min before a trial of spontaneous breathing and at several intervals after the conclusion of the unsuccessful trial that lasted 31 min. The nadir in Pditw was reached 30 min after completion of the trial, and at 60 min Pditw was still less than that recorded 10 min before the trial of spontaneous breathing. This finding indicates the development of peripheral diaphragmatic fatigue.

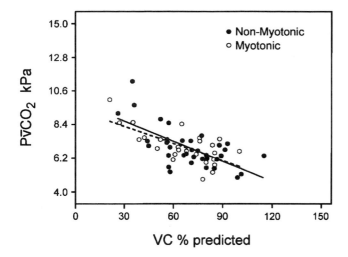

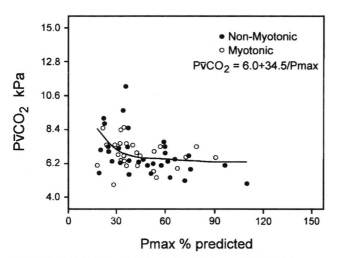

FIGURE 12-10 Relationship between vital capacity (VC) (*upper panel*) and respiratory muscle strength (*lower panel*) and mixed venous partial pressure of CO_2 ($P\bar{v}_{CO_2}$) in patients with respiratory muscle weakness. Respiratory muscle strength is the arithmetic sum of maximum static inspiratory and expiratory mouth pressures (Ptot = Pɪmax + Pᴇmax). The open circles represent patients with myotonic dystrophy, and the closed circles represent patients with a variety of nonmyotonic muscle diseases. As respiratory muscle weakness became more severe, $P\bar{v}_{CO_2}$ increased, although considerable variability was observed among patients. The regression lines were similar in the myotonic and nonmyotonic patients. [Reproduced, with permission, from Gibson et al: in Jones NL, Killian KJ, (eds): *Breathlessness*. The Campbell Symposium. Hamilton, Ontario, Boehringer-Ingelheim, 1992, pp 68–69.]

DISORDERS OF THE CENTRAL NERVOUS SYSTEM

Hemiplegia is generally associated with a striking reduction in EMG activity of the diaphragm and parasternal intercostal muscles on the paralyzed side.[106] Such involvement may contribute to the development of bronchopulmonary infections in these patients, although this remains to be proven. Using cranial magnetic stimulation, Similowski and colleagues[107] recently found asymmetrical conduction responses in pa-

tients with hemiplegia due to a capsular lesion—the diaphragmatic response on the paralyzed side was abolished or markedly delayed. Healthy control subjects and patients with a stroke not due to a capsular lesion displayed no such asymmetry.[107] These findings support the idea of "central diaphragmatic paralysis" in capsular strokes, and they also indicate the absence of bilateral cortical representation of each hemidiaphragm.

SPINAL CORD INJURY

The degree of impairment depends on the level of the lesion. *High cervical* cord lesions (C1 to C2) cause paralysis of the diaphragm, intercostal, scalene, and abdominal muscles.[108] Patients develop hypertrophy of their sternomastoid and trapezius muscles.[108] These patients can be conditioned to breathe for hours using only these muscles or by employing the technique of glossopharyngeal breathing.[109,110] In these patients, ventilation also can be sustained by a phrenic pacer.[108,111–114] Lesions of *middle cervical* cord (C3 to C5) destroy the phrenic motoneurons, causing diaphragmatic paralysis (see below) that is unresponsive to phrenic pacing.[111–114] Prognosis is better in patients with more caudal lesions; 40 percent of patients with a C3 lesion remain dependent on a ventilator compared with 14 and 11 percent of patients with C4 and C5 lesions, respectively.[115] Injuries of the *lower cervical* (C6 to C8) and *upper thoracic* (T1 to T6) cord denervate the intercostal and abdominal muscles but leave the diaphragm and neck muscles intact. Ventilatory endurance is not a problem, and few patients require prolonged mechanical ventilation because the diaphragm is functional.[115]

Although expiratory reserve volume is approximately zero within the first week of injury,[116] it increases to about 500 mL over time[117] as a result of expiratory contraction of the clavicular portion of the pectoralis major[117] (Fig. 12-14). This muscle receives its motor innervation from fibers originating in the C5 to C7 segments (see Fig. 12-12). In patients with C5–8 traumatic tetraplegia, contraction of the pectoralis muscle during cough usually can increase pleural pressure to an extent sufficient to cause dynamic compression of the intrathoracic airways, which is critical for the production of an effective cough.[118] Training of the pectoralis muscle might conceivably improve the effectiveness of cough in these patients.[118a]

MOTOR NEURON DISEASE

The most common cause of death in patients with amyotrophic lateral sclerosis is respiratory failure.[119] The decline in respiratory muscle strength tends to be linear over time, with a mean reduction in Pɪmax and Pᴇmax of 2.9 and 3.4 cmH_2O per month, respectively, although considerable interpatient variability exists.[120] The slope of the ventilatory response to hypercapnia is decreased,[99] but hypercapnia is uncommon until the terminal stages of the disease.[94] No treatment is effective except for the recent demonstration that an antiglutamate agent, riluzole, may slow the progression of the disease and improve survival in patients with disease of bulbar onset.[121]

PERIPHERAL NERVE DISORDERS

DIAPHRAGMATIC PARALYSIS

Unilateral diaphragmatic paralysis can result from malignancy, trauma, pneumonia, or herpes zoster or be idiopathic

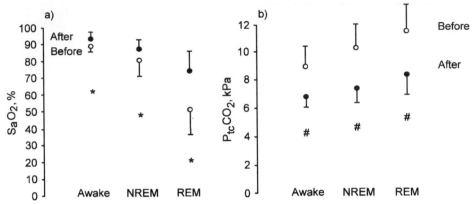

FIGURE 12-11 The minimum arterial oxygen saturation (Sa_{O_2}) and the maximum transcutaneous carbon dioxide tension (Ptc_{CO_2}) measured during spontaneous breathing before the institution of nocturnal nasal positive-pressure ventilation (*squares*) and during a night without nasal positive-pressure ventilation (*triangles*) in patients with chronic neuromuscular disorders. The use of nocturnal nasal positive-pressure ventilation resulted in significant increase in Sa_{O_2} (*$p < .002$) and decrease in Ptc_{CO_2} (#$p < .005$). NREM, non-rapid eye movement sleep; REM, rapid eye movement sleep. (Reproduced, with permission, Piper AJ, Sullivan CE: *Eur Respir J* 9:1515–1522, 1996.)

in origin.[122,123] It usually presents as an elevated hemidiaphragm that needs to be differentiated from a pleural or subpulmonic effusion. Lung volumes and inspiratory pressures are mild to moderately decreased[124,125] (Table 12-1). An additional fall in lung volume is observed on assuming the supine posture, associated with an 11 mmHg decrease in Pa_{O_2}.[124] Fluoroscopy is the method most commonly employed to make the diagnosis. Normally, the diaphragm descends during "sniffing," whereas the entire leaf of a paralyzed diaphragm should show at least 2 cm of paradoxical motion, provided the abdominal muscles are relaxed.[124] Unfortunately, paradoxical motion also may be observed in 6 percent of healthy subjects.[126] Demonstration of a delayed phrenic nerve conduction time is a more specific test.[127] High-resolution ultrasonographic quantification of diaphragmatic thickness at rest and following inhalation to TLC can help in the diagnosis of diaphragmatic paralysis.[128]

Bilateral diaphragmatic paralysis may be caused by diffuse neuropathies and myopathies or trauma or may be idiopathic.[122] Unlike unilateral diaphragmatic paralysis, patients with bilateral diaphragmatic paralysis demonstrate a marked reduction in FRC and RV[129] (see Table 12-1).[129] These findings are the result of decreased lung compliance secondary to atelectasis. On changing to the supine position, abdominal paradox develops and VC falls by approximately 50 percent.[130] Fluoroscopy can be a very misleading diagnostic method, and Newsom-Davis and colleagues[131] observed paradoxical diaphragmatic motion in only one of six patients. This occurs because some patients with paralyzed diaphragms contract their abdominal muscles during expiration, displacing the abdomen inward and the diaphragm into the rib cage. At the onset of inspiration, relaxation of the abdominal muscles causes outward recoil of the abdominal wall and diaphragmatic descent.[131]

GUILLAIN-BARRÉ SYNDROME

Guillain-Barré syndrome is the most common acute neurologic disease leading to paralysis or respiratory failure over a matter of days.[132] It accounts for more than half the patients with a primary neuromuscular disorder who are admitted

to intensive care units.[132] The course of the disorder is highly variable, and in an apparently healthy individual, the disease may progress rapidly over a period of hours to respiratory failure.[132] Accordingly, all patients with this syndrome should be hospitalized.[132] Early detection of ventilatory failure is essential because approximately 20 to 45 percent of afflicted patients require mechanical ventilation.[133–135]

The usefulness of either plasmapheresis or intravenous immune globulin in the treatment of Guillain-Barré syndrome has been demonstrated convincingly.[136,137] However, there is no convincing evidence that the combination of plasmapheresis and intravenous immune globulin is better than either therapy on its own.[137]

MOTOR END-PLATE DISORDERS

Myasthenia gravis is an acquired autoimmune disorder of neuromuscular transmission that can be worsened by several medications.[138] Respiratory muscle involvement is rare during the early course of this disease (1 to 4 percent) but eventually becomes significant in 50 to 60 percent of patients.[119,139,140] Patients with mild myasthenia have a normal pattern of breathing, whereas rapid shallow breathing is common in patients with moderate myasthenia.[102] Ventilatory failure may be precipitated by infections, surgery, or inappropriate use of cholinergic medications.[138] Conditions to be considered in the differential diagnosis include congenital myasthenic syndromes, Graves' disease, Lambert-Eaton myasthenic syndrome, botulism, progressive external ophthalmoplegia, and intracranial mass lesions.[138]

The major therapies employed for myasthenia gravis are anticholinesterase agents, thymectomy, long-term immunosuppressive treatment, and short-term immunotherapies.[138] Only anticholinesterase agents and short-term immunotherapies have an onset of action that is sufficiently rapid to assist with the discontinuation of mechanical ventilation in these patients.[138] If respiratory muscle strength shows little improvement with anticholinesterase agents, short-term immunotherapy, such as intravenous immuneglobulin or plasmapheresis, can be tried.[138]

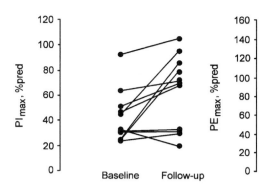
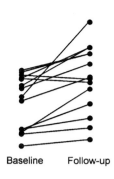

FIGURE 12-12 Individual changes in maximal inspiratory (PImax) and maximal expiratory (PEmax) mouth pressures (as percentage of predicted) before and after the institution of nocturnal nasal positive-pressure ventilation in patients with chronic neuromuscular disorders. The use of nasal positive-pressure ventilation resulted in significant improvements in PImax ($p < .003$) and PEmax ($p < .01$). (Reproduced, with permission, Piper AJ, Sullivan CE; *Eur Respir J* 9:1515–1522, 1996.)

MUSCLE DYSTROPHIES

DUCHENNE'S MUSCULAR DYSTROPHY

Respiratory failure is the major cause of death in 75 percent of patients with Duchenne's muscular dystrophy.[94] Respiratory muscle weakness occurs early in the disease, but the diaphragm remains relatively spared; consequently, hypercapnia is uncommon except as a terminal event.[92] Inspiratory muscle training can improve inspiratory and expiratory muscle function in the early stage of Duchenne's muscular dystrophy.[141] As is the case with other neuromuscular diseases, patients with Duchenne's muscular dystrophy develop a progressive decrease in lung volumes (see above). Raphael and colleagues[142] recently investigated whether nasal positive-pressure ventilation could prevent pulmonary deterioration in asymptomatic patients with an FVC of 20 to 50 percent of predicted, who were free of hypercapnia and hypoxemia. Unfortunately, noninvasive ventilation did not arrest the progressive decrease in lung function and instead was associated with increased mortality.[142]

MYOTONIC DYSTROPHY (STEINERT'S DISEASE)

Myotonic dystrophy, an autosomal dominant disease, is the most frequent adult form of muscular dystrophy.[143] Patients with myotonic dystrophy appear to suffer from disproportionate involvement of the respiratory muscles[143] and exhibit a high incidence of hypercapnia.[144] A combination of respiratory muscle weakness, increased respiratory elastance, and low central drive appears to be responsible for the chronic hypercapnia in these patients.[144] Many patients with myotonic dystrophy have a grossly chaotic pattern of breathing when awake.[101] It has been suggested that this abnormal

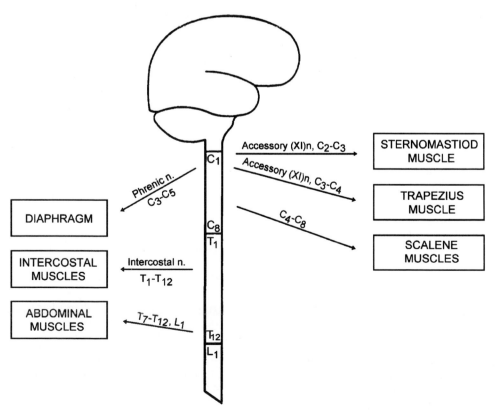

FIGURE 12-13 The motor innervation of the major respiratory muscle groups. (Reproduced, with permission, from Tobin MJ: *Clin Chest Med* 9:263–286, 1988.)

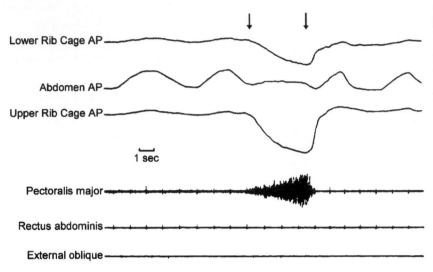

Lower Rib Cage AP

Abdomen AP

Upper Rib Cage AP

1 sec

Pectoralis major

Rectus abdominis

External oblique

FIGURE 12-14 Electromyogram of the abdominal (rectus abdominis and external oblique) and pectoralis major (clavicular portion) muscles during voluntary expiration in a patient with midcervical spinal cord injury. The changes in anteroposterior (AP) diameters of the abdomen and the rib cage are also shown (upward increase). Arrows mark the onset and the end of expiratory effort. Voluntary expiration caused a marked decrease in the anteroposterior diameter of the upper rib cage, a slight increase in the anteroposterior diameter of the abdomen, and a large amount of activity in the pectoralis major, while the abdominal muscles are silent. (Reproduced, with permission, from DeTroyer et al: *N Engl J Med* 314:740–744, 1986.)

pattern of breathing is the result of disordered afferent information from the muscle spindles.[101]

Deformity of the Thoracic Cage

A number of diseases affect movement of the thoracic cage: scoliosis, ankylosing spondylitis, pectus excavatum, fibrothorax, and thoracotomy.[145]

The severity of scoliosis is quantitated by Cobb's or Ferguson's method of measuring the angle between the upper and lower limbs of the spinal curve. While mild scoliosis (angle greater than 35 degrees) is common (incidence 1 in 1000), respiratory dysfunction becomes detectable only when the angle is greater than 70 degrees (incidence 1 in 10,000), and early cardiopulmonary failure is expected when the angle is greater than 120 degrees.[145] The risk of cardiopulmonary complications appears to be greater in patients whose scoliosis is apparent before 5 years of age compared with those developing it after age 11.[146] Moderate to severe scoliosis is associated with decreased lung volumes, chest wall compliance, ventilatory response to hypercapnia, and inspiratory

muscle strength.[147,148] Besides the angle of the scoliosis, other factors that contribute to pulmonary impairment include the number of vertebrae involved, cephalad location of the curve, and loss of the normal thoracic kyphosis.[149]

In patients with severe scoliosis, severe oxygen desaturation may occur at night, especially during rapid eye movement sleep.[150] Pulmonary hypertension and cor pulmonale are well-recognized complications but usually are observed only when the spinal angle is greater than 80 degrees.[145] Kinking or compression of the great vessels by the deformed chest wall does not play a role,[145] but the pulmonary hypertension has been shown to be related to the decreased lung volumes.[151] Hypoxic vasoconstriction is important, and lung deflation causing compression of the pulmonary vascular bed also may play a role.[145] While surgical correction of scoliosis in the adult population is of no benefit in improving respiratory function,[152] medical management, especially employing nighttime mechanical ventilation, can result in remarkable clinical improvement and increased longevity.[153-155]

Patients with ankylosing spondylitis display a marked reduction in chest wall compliance[156,157] associated with decreased rib cage movement and a greater than normal excursion of the diaphragm during breathing.[158] In contrast to the other causes of thoracic deformity, FRC is elevated in more than half these patients.[145] The elevated FRC is thought to occur because the stiffer rib cage causes the equilibrium point of the respiratory system (FRC) to move closer to the resting point of the rib cage, a volume that is about 1 L more than normal FRC.[156] Patients with ankylosing spondylitis rarely if ever develop ventilatory failure, unless there is superimposed pulmonary disease. Some patients with pectus excavatum have a mild restrictive ventilatory defect,[159] occasionally associated with respiratory symptoms that may require surgical correction.[160] A right ventricular filling defect has been reported in some patients with pectus excavatum.[161]

Conclusion

Respiratory muscle impairment occurs with numerous disease processes. Severe respiratory muscle weakness may be

TABLE 12-1 Comparison of Pulmonary and Respiratory Muscle Function in Unilateral and Bilateral Paralysis of the Diaphragm

Variable	Unilateral Diaphragm Paralysis	Bilateral Diaphragm Paralysis
Vital capacity	75%	45%
Total lung capacity	85%	55%
Functional residual capacity	100%	60%
Residual volume	100%	55%
Forced expiratory volume in 1 sec	70%	50%
PImax, cmH$_2$O	−70	−10 to −20
Pdimax, cmH$_2$O	70	0 to −10

NOTE: Values expressed as percentage of predicted normal values unless otherwise specified. PImax and Pdimax are maximal inspiratory and transdiaphragmatic pressures, respectively.

SOURCE: Reproduced, with permission, from Aldrich T, Rochester D: The lungs and neuromuscular diseases, in Murray JF, Nadel JA (eds): *Textbook of Respiratory Medicine*, 2d ed. Philadelphia, WB Saunders, 1994, p 2497.

recognized early in the disease process, as in the case of bilateral diaphragmatic paralysis, or it may go unrecognized until hypercapnic respiratory failure develops, as in the case of Duchenne's muscular dystrophy. Muscle weakness often leads to pulmonary aspiration and breathing disturbances during sleep. Dyspnea may not develop until respiratory impairment is so far advanced because activity sufficient to induce dyspnea is limited by associated weakness of the limb muscles. Accordingly, a high level of suspicion is necessary to recognize the presence of respiratory muscle impairment and allow the institution of specific therapies.

References

1. Roussos C (ed): *The Thorax*, part C. New York, Marcel Dekker, 1995.
2. Fanburg BL, Sicilian L (eds): Respiratory dysfunction in neuromuscular diseases. *Clin Chest Med* 15:607–810, 1994.
3. American Thoracic Society: Lung function testing: Selection of reference values and interpretative strategies. ATS statement. *Am Rev Respir Dis* 144:1202–1218, 1991.
4. O'Donnell DE, Webb KA: Exertional breathlessness in patients with chronic airflow limitation: The role of lung hyperinflation. *Am Rev Respir Dis* 148:1351–1357, 1993.
5. O'Donnell DE, Bertley JC, Chau LK, Webb KA: Qualitative aspects of exertional breathlessness in chronic airflow limitation: Pathophysiologic mechanisms. *Am J Respir Crit Care Med* 155: 109–115, 1997.
6. Jubran A, Tobin MJ: Pathophysiologic basis of acute respiratory distress in patients who fail a trial of weaning from mechanical ventilation. *Am J Respir Crit Care Med* 155:906–915, 1997.
7. Tobin MJ, Chadha TS, Jenouri G, et al: Breathing patterns: 1 Normal subjects. *Chest* 84:202–205, 1983.
8. Tobin MJ, Chadha TS, Jenouri G, et al: Breathing patterns: 2. Diseased subjects. *Chest* 84:286–294, 1983.
9. Block KE, Li Y, Zhang J, et al: Effect of surgical lung volume reduction on breathing patterns in severe pulmonary emphysema. *Am J Respir Crit Care Med* 156:553–560, 1997.
10. Donahoe M, Rogers RM, Wilson DO, Pennock BE: Oxygen consumption of the respiratory muscles in normal and in malnourished patients with chronic obstructive pulmonary disease. *Am Rev Respir Dis* 140:385–39, 1989.
11. Pitcher WD, Cunningham HS: Oxygen cost of increasing tidal volume and diaphragm flattening in obstructive pulmonary disease. *J Appl Physiol* 74:2750–2756, 1993.
12. Younes M: Mechanisms of ventilatory failure. *Curr Pulmonol* 14:243–291, 1993.
13. Shindoh C, Hida W, Kikuchi Y, et al: Oxygen consumption of respiratory muscles in patients with COPD. *Chest* 105:790–797, 1994.
14. Schols AMWJ, Fredix EWHM, Soeters PB, Westerterp KR: Resting energy expenditure in patients with chronic obstructive pulmonary disease. *Am J Clin Nutr* 54:983–987, 1991.
15. Baarends EM, Schols AMWJ, Pannemans DLE, et al: Total free living energy expenditure in patients with severe chronic obstructive pulmonary disease. *Am J Respir Crit Care Med* 155:549-554, 1997.
16. Rahn H, Otis AB, Chadwick LE, Fenn WO: The pressure-volume diagram of the thorax and lung. *Am J Physiol* 146:161–178, 1946.
17. Smith J, Bellemare F: Effect of lung volume on in vivo contraction characteristics of human diaphragm. *J Appl Physiol* 62:1893–1900, 1987.
18. Laghi F, Harrison MJ, Tobin MJ: Comparison of magnetic and electrical phrenic nerve stimulation in assessment of diaphragmatic contractility. *J Appl Physiol* 80:1731–1742, 1996.
19. Polkey MI, Kyroussis D, Hamnegard CH, et al: Diaphragm strength in chronic obstructive pulmonary disease. *Am J Respir Crit Care Med* 154:1310–1317, 1996.
20. Newman S, Road J, Bellemare F, et al: Respiratory muscle length measurements by sonomicrometry. *J Appl Physiol* 56:753–764, 1984.
21. Sharp JT, Beard GA, Sunga M, et al: The rib cage in normal and emphysematous subjects: A roentgenographic approach. *J Appl Physiol* 61:2050–2059, 1986.
22. Di Marco AF, Romaniuk JR, Supinski GS: Mechanical action of the interosseous intercostal muscles as a function of lung volume. *Am Rev Respir Dis* 142:1041–1046, 1990.
23. Brancatisano A, Engel LA, Loring SH: Lung volume and effectiveness of inspiratory muscles. *J Appl Physiol* 74:688–694, 1993.
24. De Troyer A, Kelly S, Macklem PT, Zin WA: Mechanics of intercostal space and actions of external and internal intercostal muscles. *J Clin Invest* 75:850–857, 1985.
25. Gauthier A, Verbanck S, Estenne M, et al: Three-dimensional reconstruction of the in vivo human diaphragm shape at different lung volumes. *J Appl Physiol* 76:495–506, 1994.
26. Pettiaux N, Cassart M, Paiva M, Estenne M: Three-dimensional reconstruction of human diaphragm with the use of spiral computer tomography. *J Appl Physiol* 82:998–1002, 1997.
27. Cassart M, Pettiaux N, Genois PA, et al: Effect of chronic hyperinflation of diaphragm length and surface area. *Am J Respir Crit Care Med* 156:504–508, 1997.
28. Minh VD, Dolan GF, Konopka RF, Moser KM: Effect of hyperinflation on inspiratory function of the diaphragm. *J Appl Physiol* 40:67–73, 1976.
29. Hoover CF: The diagnostic significance of inspiratory movements of the costal margins. *Am J Med Sci* 159:633–646, 1920.
30. Hubmayr RD, Litchy WJ, Gay PC, Nelson SB: Transdiaphragmatic twitch pressure. *Am Rev Respir Dis* 139:647–652, 1989.
31. Sharp JT: The respiratory muscles in emphysema. *Clin Chest Med* 4:421–432, 1983.
32. Rochester DF, Braun NMT: Determinants of maximal inspiratory pressure in chronic obstructive pulmonary disease. *Am Rev Respir Dis* 132:42–47, 1985.
33. Byrd RB, Hyatt RE: Maximal respiratory pressures in chronic obstructive lung disease. *Am Rev Respir Dis* 98:848–856, 1968.
34. Similowski T, Yan S, Gauthier AP, et al: Contractile properties of the human diaphragm during chronic hyperinflation. *N Engl J Med* 325:917–918, 1991.
35. Kelsen SG, Sexauer WP, Mardini IA, Criner GJ: The comparative effects of elastase-induced emphysema on costal and crural diaphragm and parasternal intercostal muscle contractility. *Am J Respir Crit Care Med* 149:168–173, 1994.
36. Arora NS, Rochester DF: COPD and human diaphragm muscle dimensions. *Chest* 91:719–724, 1987.
37. Wanke T, Merkle M, Formanek D, et al: Effect of lung transplantation on diaphragmatic function in patients with chronic obstructive pulmonary disease. *Thorax* 49:459-464, 1994.
38. Criner GJ, Celli BR: Ventilatory muscle recruitment in exercise with O₂ in obstructed patients with mild hypoxemia. *J Appl Physiol* 63:195–200, 1987.
39. Jardin J, Farkas G, Prefaut C, et al: The failing inspiratory muscles under normoxic and hypoxic conditions. *Am Rev Respir Dis* 124:274–279, 1981.
40. Juan G, Calverley P, Talamo C, et al: Effect of carbon dioxide on diaphragmatic function in human beings. *N Engl J Med* 310:874–879, 1984.
41. Campbell JA, Hughes RL, Sahgal V, et al: Alterations in intercostal muscle morphology and biochemistry in patients with obstructive lung disease. *Am Rev Respir Dis* 122:679–686, 1980.
42. Gertz I, Hedenstierna G, Hellers G, Wahren J: Muscle metabolism in patients with chronic obstructive lung disease and acute respiratory failure. *Clin Sci Mol Med* 52:395–403, 1977.
43. Fiaccadori E, Coffrini E, Fracchia C, et al: Hypophosphatemia

and phosphorus depletion in respiratory and peripheral muscles of patients with respiratory failure due to COPD. *Chest* 105: 1392–1398, 1994.

44. Hards JM, Reid WD, Pardy RL, Pare PD: Respiratory muscle morphometry: Correlation with lung function and nutrition. *Chest* 97:1037–1044, 1990.

45. Engelen MAM, Schols AMW, Baken WC, et al: Nutritional depletion in relation to respiratory and peripheral skeletal muscle function in an outpatient population with chronic obstructive pulmonary disease. *Eur Respir J* 7:1793–1797, 1994.

46. Laaban JP, Kouchakji B, Dore MF, et al: Nutritional status of patients with chronic obstructive pulmonary disease and acute respiratory failure. *Chest* 103:1362–1368, 1993.

47. Arora NS, Rochester DF: Effect of body weight and muscularity on human diaphragm muscle mass, thickness, and area. *J Appl Physiol* 52:64–70, 1982.

48. Decramer M, Lacquet LM, Fagard R, Rogiers P: Corticosteroids contribute to muscle weakness in chronic airflow obstruction. *Am J Respir Crit Care Med* 150:11–26, 1994.

49. Bellemare F, Grassino A: Effect of pressure and timing of contraction on human diaphragm fatigue. *J Appl Physiol* 53:1190–1195, 1982.

50. Bellemare F, Grassino A: Evaluation of human diaphragm fatigue. *J Appl Physiol* 53:1196–1206, 1982.

51. Bellemare F, Grassino A: Force reserve of the diaphragm in patients with chronic obstructive pulmonary disease. *J Appl Physiol* 55:8–15, 1983.

52. Celli BR, Rassulo J, Make BJ: Dyssynchronous breathing during arm but not leg exercise in patients with chronic airflow obstruction. *N Engl J Med* 314:1485–1490, 1986.

53. Gilbert R, Ashutosh K, Aucinloss JH, et al: Prospective study of controlled oxygen therapy: Poor prognosis of patients with asynchronous breathing. *Chest* 71:456–462, 1977.

54. Gilmartin JJ, Gibson GJ: Mechanisms of paradoxical rib cage motion in patients with chronic obstructive pulmonary disease. *Am Rev Respir Dis* 134:683–687, 1986.

55. Jubran A, Tobin MJ: The effect of hyperinflation on rib cage-abdominal motion. *Am Rev Respir Dis* 146:1378–1382, 1992.

56. Tobin MJ, Perez W, Guenther SM, et al: Does rib-cage abdominal paradox signify respiratory muscle fatigue? *J Appl Physiol* 63: 851–860, 1987.

57. Levine S, Gillen M, Weiser P, et al: Inspiratory pressure generation: Comparison of subjects with COPD and age-matched normals. *J Appl Physiol* 65:888–889, 1988.

58. Martinez FJ, Couser JI, Celli BR: Factors influencing ventilatory muscle recruitment in patients with chronic airflow obstruction. *Am Rev Respir Dis* 142:276–282, 1990.

59. De Troyer A, Peche R, Yernault J, Estenne M: Neck muscle activity in patients with severe chronic obstructive pulmonary disease. *Am J Respir Crit Care Med* 150:41–47, 1994.

60. Laghi F, Jubran A, Topeli A, et al: Effect of lung volume reduction surgery on neuromechanical coupling of the diaphragm. *Am J Respir Crit Care Med* 157:475–483, 1998.

61. Peche R, Estenne M, Gevenois PA, et al: Sternomastoid muscle size and strength in patients with severe chronic obstructive pulmonary disease. *Am J Respir Crit Care Med* 153:422–425, 1996.

62. Arora NS, Rochester DF: Effect of chronic obstructive pulmonary disease on sternocleidomastoid muscle. *Am Rev Respir Dis* 125:252, 1982 (abstr).

63. Ninane V, Rypens F, Yernault JC, De Troyer A: Abdominal muscle use during breathing in patients with chronic airflow obstruction. *Am Rev Respir Dis* 146:16–21, 1992.

64. Ninane V, Yernault JC, De Troyer A: Intrinsic PEEP in patients with chronic airflow obstruction. *Am Rev Respir Dis* 148:1037–1042, 1993.

65. Tobin MJ, Gardner WN: Monitoring of the control of breathing,

in Tobin MJ (ed): *Principles and Practice of Intensive Care Monitoring*. New York, McGraw-Hill, 1997, chap 26.

66. Begin P, Grassino A: Inspiratory muscle dysfunction and chronic hypercapnia in chronic obstructive pulmonary disease. *Am Rev Respir Dis* 143:905–912, 1991.

67. Scano G, Spinelli A, Duranti R, et al: Carbon dioxide responsiveness in COPD patients with and without chronic hypercapnia. *Eur Respir J* 8:78–85, 1995.

68. Rodriguez-Roisin R, Roca J: Pulmonary gas exchange, in Calverley P, Pride N (eds): *Chronic Obstructive Pulmonary Disease*. London, Chapman & Hall, 1995, pp 161–184.

69. Younes M: Determinants of thoracic excursions during exercise, in Whipp WJ, Wasserman K (eds): *Exercise: Pulmonary Physiology and Pathophysiology*. New York, Marcel Dekker 1991, pp 1–65.

70. Babb TG, Viggiano R, Hurley B, et al: The effect of mild–moderate airflow limitation on exercise capacity. *J Appl Physiol* 70:223–230, 1991.

71. Grimby G, Elgefors V, Oxhoj H: Ventilatory levels and chest wall mechanics during exercise in obstructive lung disease. *Scand J Respir Dis* 54:45–52, 1973.

72. Belman MJ, Botnick WC, Shin JW: Inhaled bronchodilators reduce dynamic hyperinflation during exercise in patients with chronic obstructive pulmonary disease. *Am J Respir Crit Care Med* 153:967–975, 1996.

73. Cooper JD, Trulock EP, Triantafillou AN, et al: Bilateral pneumonectomy (lung reduction) for chronic obstructive pulmonary disease. *J Thorac Cardiovasc Surg* 109:106–119, 1995.

74. Jubran A, Laghi F, Parthasarathy S, et al: Effect of lung reduction surgery on viscoelastic behavior of the lung. *Am J Respir Crit Care Med* 155:A520, 1997 (abstr).

75. Sciurba FC, Rogers RM, Keenan RJ, et al: Improvement in pulmonary function and elastic recoil after lung reduction surgery for diffuse emphysema. *N Engl J Med* 334:1095 1096, 1996.

76. Gelb AF, Zamel N, McKenna RJ, Brenner M: Mechanisms of short-term improvement in lung function after emphysema resection. *Am J Respir Crit Care Med* 154:945–951, 1996.

77. Hoppin FG: Theoretical basis for improvement following reduction pneumoplasty in emphysema. *Am J Respir Crit Care Med* 155:520–525, 1997.

78. Fein AM, Branman SS, Casiburi R, et al: Lung volume reduction surgery. ATS official statement. *Am J Respir Crit Care Med* 154: 1151–1152, 1996.

79. Benditt JO, Wood DE, McCool DF, et al: Change in breathing and ventilatory muscle recruitment patterns induced by lung volume reduction surgery. *Am J Respir Crit Care Med* 155:279–284, 1997.

80. Rochester DF, Arora NS: The respiratory muscles in asthma, in Lavietes MH, Reichman L (eds): *Symposium on Bronchial Asthma: Diagnostic Aspects and Management of Asthma*. New York, Purdue Frederick, 1982, pp 27–38.

81. Peress L, Sybrecht G, Macklem PT: The mechanisms of increase in total lung capacity during acute asthma. *Am J Med* 61:165–169, 1976.

82. Mak VH, Bugler JR, Spiro SG: Sternomastoid muscle fatigue and twitch maximum relaxation rate in patients with steroid dependent asthma. *Thorax* 48:979–984, 1993.

83. McKenzie DK, Gandevia SC: Strength and endurance of inspiratory, expiratory, and limb muscles in asthma. *Am Rev Respir Dis* 134:999–1004, 1986.

84. Perez T, Becquart L-A, Stach B, et al: Inspiratory muscle strength and endurance in steroid-dependent asthma. *Am J Respir Crit Care Med* 153:610–615, 1996.

85. Hillman DR, Prentice L, Finucane KE: The pattern of breathing in acute severe asthma. *Am Rev Respir Dis* 133:587–592, 1986.

86. De Bruin PF, Ueki J, Watson A, Pride NB: Size and strength of the respiratory and quadriceps muscles in patients with chronic asthma. *Eur Respir J* 10:59–64, 1997.

87. Allen GM, McKenzie DK, Gandevia SC, Bass S: Reduced voluntary drive to breathe in asthmatic subjects. *Respir Physiol* 93:29–43, 1993.

88. Kikuchi Y, Okabe S, Tamura G, et al: Chemosensitivity and perception of dyspnea in patients with a history of near-fatal asthma. *N Engl J Med* 330:1329–1334, 1994.

89. Cohen CA, Zagelbaum G, Gross D, et al: Clinical manifestations of inspiratory muscle fatigue. *Am J Med* 73:308–316, 1982.

90. Tobin MJ, Walsh J, Laghi F: Monitoring of respiratory neuromuscular function, in Tobin MJ (ed): *Principles and Practice of Mechanical Ventilation.* New York, McGraw-Hill, 1994, chap 43, pp 945–966.

91. Goldstone JC, Green M, Moxham J: Maximum relaxation rate of the diaphragm during weaning from mechanical ventilation. *Thorax* 49:54–60, 1994.

92. Smith PE, Calverly PM, Edwards RH, et al: Practical problems in the respiratory care of patients with muscular dystrophy. *N Engl J Med* 316:1197–1205, 1987.

93. Vicken W, Elleker MG, Cosio MG: Determinants of respiratory muscle weakness in stable chronic neuromuscular disorders. *Am J Med* 82:53–58, 1981.

94. De Troyer A, Estenne M: Respiratory system in neuromuscular disorders, in Roussos C (ed): *The Thorax,* part C. New York, Marcel Dekker, 1995, chap 74, pp 2177–2212.

95. Estenne M, Gevenois PA, Kinnear W, et al: Lung volume restriction in patients with chronic respiratory muscle weakness: The role of microatelectasis. *Thorax* 48:698–701, 1993.

96. Estenne M, Heilporn A, Delhez L, et al: Chest wall stiffness in patients with chronic respiratory muscle weakness. *Am Rev Respir Dis* 128:1002–1007, 1983.

97. Estenne M, De Troyer A: The effects of tetraplegia on chest wall statics. *Am Rev Respir Dis* 134:121–124, 1986.

98. Baydur A. Respiratory muscle strength and control of ventilation in patients with neuromuscular disease. *Chest* 99:330–338, 1991.

99. Loveridge BM, Dubo HI. Breathing pattern in chronic quadriplegia: *Arch Phys Med Rehabil* 71:495–499, 1990.

100. Spinelli A, Marconi G, Gorini M, et al: Control of breathing in patients with myasthenia gravis. *Am Rev Respir Dis* 145:1359–1366, 1992.

101. Gibson GJ, Gilmartin JJ, Veale D, et al: Respiratory muscle function in neuromuscular disease, in Jones NL, Killian KJ, (eds): *Breathlessness.* The Campbell Symposium. Hamilton, Ontario, Boehringer-Ingelheim, 1992, chap 10, pp 66–73.

102. Garcia RF, Prados C, Diez Tejedor E, et al: Breathing pattern and central ventilatory drive in mild and moderate generalized myasthenia gravis. *Thorax* 49:703–706, 1994.

103. McKinley AC, Auchincloss JH, Gilbert R, Nicholas JJ: Pulmonary function, ventilatory control, and respiratory complications in quadriplegic subjects. *Am Rev Respir Dis* 100:526–532, 1969.

104. Braun NMT, Arora NS, Rochester DF: Respiratory muscle and pulmonary function in polymyositis and other proximal myopathies. *Thorax* 38:616–623, 1983.

105. Piper AJ, Sullivan CE: Effects of long-term nocturnal nasal ventilation on spontaneous breathing during sleep in neuromuscular and chest disorders. *Eur Respir J* 9:1515–1522, 1996.

106. De Troyer A, De Beyl DZ, Thirion M: Function of the respiratory muscles in acute hemiplegia. *Am Rev Respir Dis* 123:631–632, 1981.

107. Similowski T, Catala M, Rancurel G, Derenne J-P: Impairment of central motor conduction to the diaphragm in stroke. *Am J Respir Crit Care Med* 154:436–441, 1996.

108. Danon J, Druz WS, Goldberg NB, Sharp JT: Function of the isolated paced diaphragm and the cervical accessory muscles in C1 quadriplegics. *Am Rev Respir Dis* 119:909–919, 1979.

109. Affeldt JE, Dail CW, Collier CR, Farr AF: Glossopharyngeal breathing: Ventilation studies. *J Appl Physiol* 8:111–113, 1955.

110. Mazza FG, DiMarco AF, Altose MD, Strohl KP: The flow-volume loop during glossopharyngeal breathing. *Chest* 85:638–640, 1984.

111. Moxham J, Sheerson JM: Diaphragmatic pacing. *Am Rev Respir Dis* 148:533–536, 1993.

112. Similowski T, Straus C, Attali V, et al: Assessment of the motor pathway to the diaphragm using cortical and cervical magnetic stimulation in the decision-making process of phrenic pacing. *Chest* 110:1551–1557, 1996.

113. Nochomovitz M, Hopkins M, Brodkey J, et al: Conditioning of the diaphragm with phrenic nerve stimulation after prolonged disuse. *Am Rev Respir Dis* 130:685–688, 1984.

114. Nava S, Rubini F, Zanotti E, Caldiroli D: The tension-time index of the diaphragm revisited in quadriplegic patients with diaphragm pacing. *Am J Respir Crit Care Med* 153:1322–1327, 1996.

115. Wicks AB, Menter RR: Long-term outlook in quadriplegic patients with initial ventilatory dependency. *Chest* 90:406–410, 1986.

116. Ledsome JR, Sharp JM: Pulmonary function in acute cervical cord injury. *Am Rev Respir Dis* 124:41–44, 1981.

117. De Troyer A, Estenne M, Heilporn A: Mechanism of active expiration in tetraplegic subjects. *N Engl J Med* 314:740–744, 1986.

118. Estenne M, van Muylem A, Gorini M, et al: Evidence of dynamic airway compression during cough in tetraplegic patients. *Am J Respir Crit Care Med* 150:1081–1085, 1994.

118a. Estenne M, Knoop C, Vanvaerembergh J, et al: The effect of pectoralis muscle training in tetraplegic subjects. *Am Rev Respir Dis* 139:1218–1222, 1989.

119. Lieberman SL, Young RR, Shefner JM: Neurological disorders affecting respiration, in Roussos C (ed): *The Thorax,* part C. New York, Marcel Dekker, 1995, chap 73, pp 2135–2175.

120. Shifman PL, Belsh JM: Pulmonary function at diagnosis of amyotrophic lateral sclerosis: Rate of deterioration. *Chest* 103:508–513, 1993.

121. Bensimon G, Lacomblez L, Meininger V: A controlled trial of riluzole in amyotrophic lateral sclerosis. ALS/Riluzole Study Group. *N Engl J Med* 330:585–591, 1994.

122. Wilcox PG, Pardy RL: Diaphragmatic weakness and paralysis. *Lung* 167:323–341, 1989.

123. Mulvey DA, Aquilina RJ, Elliott MW, et al: Diaphragmatic dysfunction in neuralgic amyotrophy: An electrophysiologic evaluation of 16 patients presenting with dyspnea. *Am Rev Respir Dis* 147:66–71, 1993.

124. Arborelius M, Lilia B, Senyk J: Regional and total lung function studies in patients with hemidiaphragmatic paralysis. *Respiration* 32:253–264, 1975.

125. Lisboa C, Pare PD, Pertuze J, et al: Inspiratory muscle function in unilateral diaphragmatic paralysis. *Am Rev Respir Dis* 134:488–492, 1986.

126. Alexander C: Diaphragm movements and the diagnosis of diaphragmatic paralysis. *Clin Radiol* 17:79–83, 1966.

127. Tobin MJ, Laghi F: Respiratory neuromuscular function, in Tobin MJ (ed): *Principles and Practice of Intensive Care Monitoring.* New York, McGraw-Hill, 1997, chap 28.

128. Gottesman E, McCool DF: Ultrasound evaluation of the paralyzed diaphragm. *Am J Respir Crit Care Med* 15:1570–1574, 1997.

129. McCredie M, Lovejoy FW, Kaltreider NL: Pulmonary function in diaphragmatic paralysis. *Thorax* 17:213–217, 1962.

130. Allen SM, Hunt B, Green M: Fall in vital capacity with posture. *Br J Dis Chest* 79:267–271, 1985.

131. Newsom-Davis J, Goldman M, Loh L, Casson M: Diaphragm function and alveolar hypoventilation. *Q J Med* 45:87–100, 1976.

132. Hanley DF, Cornblath DR: Peripheral nerve disease: Guillain-Barré syndrome, in Parrillo JE (ed): *Current Therapy in Critical Care Medicine,* 3d ed. St Louis, Mosby–Year Book, 1997, pp 313–317.

133. Gracey DR, McMichan JC, Divertie MB, Howard FM Jr: Respiratory failure in Guillain-Barré syndrome. *Mayo Clin Proc* 57:742–746, 1982.

134. Sunderrajan EV, Davenport J: The Guillain-Barré syndrome: Pulmonary neurologic correlations. *Medicine* 64:333–341, 1985.

135. Chevrolet J-C, Deleamont P: Repeated vital capacity measurements as predictive mechanical ventilation need and weaning success in Guillain-Barré syndrome. *Am Rev Respir Dis* 144:814–818, 1991.

136. Van der Meche FGA, Schmitz PIM, the Dutch Guillain-Barré Study Group: A randomized trial comparing intravenous immune globulin and plasma exchange in Guillain-Barré syndrome. *N Engl J Med* 326:1123–1129, 1992.

137. Plasma Exchange/Sandoglobulin Guillain-Barré Syndrome Trial Group: Randomized trial of plasma exchange, intravenous immunoglobulin, and combined treatments in Guillain-Barré syndrome. *Lancet* 349:225–230, 1997.

138. Drachman DB: Myasthenia gravis. *N Engl J Med* 330:1797–1810, 1994.

139. Mier A, Laroche C, Green M: Unsuspected myasthenia gravis presenting as respiratory failure. *Thorax* 45:422–423, 1990.

140. Zeolite JJ, Fanburg BL: Respiratory dysfunction in myasthenia gravis. *Clin Chest Med* 15:683–691, 1994.

141. Wanke T, Toifl K, Merkle M, et al: Inspiratory muscle training in patients with Duchenne's muscular dystrophy. *Chest* 105:475–482, 1994.

142. Raphael J-C, Chevret S, Chastang C, Bouvet F, for the French Multicenter Cooperative Group on Home Mechanical Ventilation Assistance in Duchenne de Boulogne Muscular Dystrophy: Randomized trial of preventive nasal ventilation in Duchenne's muscular dystrophy. *Lancet* 343:1600–1604, 1994.

143. Lynn JD, Woda RP, Mendell JR: Respiratory dysfunction in muscular dystrophy and other myopathies, in Fanburg BL, Sicilian L (eds): *Respiratory Dysfunction in Neuromuscular Diseases*. Philadelphia, WB Saunders, 1994, pp 661–674.

144. Begin P, Mathieu J, Almirall J, Grassino A: Relationship between chronic hypercapnia and inspiratory muscle weakness in myotonic dystrophy. *Am J Respir Crit Care Med* 156:133–139, 1997.

145. Bergofskv EH: Thoracic deformities, in Roussos C (ed): *The Thorax*, part C. New York, Marcel Dekker, 1995, chap 66, pp 1915–1949.

146. Branthwaite MA: Cardiorespiratory consequences of unfused idiopathic scoliosis. *Br J Dis Chest* 80:360–368, 1986.

147. Kafer ER: Idiopathic scoliosis: Mechanical problems of the respiratory system and the ventilatory response to carbon dioxide. *J Clin Invest* 55:1153–1163, 1975.

148. Lisboa C, Moreno R, Fava M, et al: Inspiratory muscle function in patients with severe kyphoscoliosis. *Am Rev Respir Dis* 132:48–52, 1985.

149. Kearon C, Viviani G, Kirkley A, Killian KJ: Factors determining pulmonary function in adolescent idiopathic thoracic scoliosis. *Am Rev Respir Dis* 148:288–294, 1993.

150. Mezon BL, West P, Israels J, Kryger M: Sleep breathing abnormalities in kyphoscoliosis. *Am Rev Respir Dis* 122:617–621, 1980.

151. Shneerson JM: Pulmonary artery pressure in thoracic scoliosis during and after exercise while breathing air and pure oxygen. *Thorax* 33:747–754, 1978.

152. Wong CA, Cole AA, Watson L, et al: Pulmonary function before and after anterior spinal surgery in adult idiopathic scoliosis. *Thorax* 51:534–536, 1996.

153. Fulkerson WJ, Wilkins JK, Esbenshade AM, et al: Life threatening hypoventilation in kyphoscoliosis: successful treatment with a molded body brace ventilator. *Am Rev Respir Dis* 129:185–187, 1984.

154. Zaccaria S, Zaccaria E, Zanaboni S, et al: Home mechanical ventilation in kyphoscoliosis. *Monaldi Arch Chest Dis* 48:161–164, 1993.

155. Woolf CR: Kyphoscoliosis and respiratory failure: A patient treated with assisted ventilation for 27 years. *Chest* 98:1297–1298, 1990.

156. Sharp JT, Sweeney SK, Henry JP: Lung and thoracic compliances in ankylosing spondylitis. *J Lab Clin Med* 63:254–263, 1964.

157. Van Noord JA, Cauberghs M, Van de Woestijne KP, Demedts M: Total respiratory resistance and reactance in ankylosing spondylitis and kyphoscoliosis. *Eur Respir J* 4:945–951, 1991.

158. Grimby C, Fugl-Meyer AR, Blomstrand A: Partitioning of the contributions of rib cage and abdomen to ventilation in ankylosing spondylitis. *Thorax* 29:179–184, 1974.

159. Mead J, Sly P, Le Souef P, et al: Rib cage mobility in pectus excavatum. *Am Rev Respir Dis* 132:1223–1228, 1985.

160. Goertzen M, Baltzer A, Schulitz KP: Late results following surgery for funnel chest. *Z. Orthop* 132:322–326, 1994.

161. Khan ZU, Gerson MC, Burwinkel PM: Right ventricular filling defect resulting from severe pectus excavatum. *Clin Nucl Med* 19:71, 1994.

Chapter 13

THE IMPACT OF ABNORMALITIES IN THE CONTROL OF BREATHING ON PULMONARY REHABILITATION

NEIL S. CHERNIACK

The adequacy of gas exchange depends on the ability of the respiratory control system to adjust ventilation in the face of disturbances in the environment, in metabolism, and in the performance of the lung and respiratory muscles. Briefly, this system consists of arterial and central chemoreceptors, mechanoreceptors in the airways as well as the lungs, and force and length sensors in the respiratory muscles that relay information to a network of neurons in the medulla.[1-8] Additional inputs of this network descend from higher brain centers and are transmitted centrally from the periphery via cardiovascular receptors and other receptors in the viscera. The medullary network, which includes neurons with pacemaker potential, generates a rhythmic output in which the depth of each breath and its frequency depend on an interplay of chemical and mechanical signals.[3] This oscillatory output drives the respiratory muscles of the thorax and abdomen and, in addition, modulates the activity of the skeletal muscle of the pharynx, larynx, and shoulder girdle as well as the discharge of the autonomic nerves to the airways and to the heart and blood vessels.[3,7]

In health, breathing is an automatic and largely reflex act. It occurs effortlessly and without awareness until exertion substantially increases metabolic demand for greater respiration.[6,9] However, the activity of the diaphragm (the main muscle of breathing) and the other respiratory muscles is also subject to voluntary control from the cortex. This voluntary control allows the breath to be held for a minute or so but, more important, allows the respiratory muscles to be used in speech, in expressing emotion, in eating, and in excretion. The respiratory muscles are also engaged in postural changes that alter their operating length and affect their mechanical advantage. The automatic control of the respiratory system is concerned with the coordination and proper sequencing of the contraction of the thoracic, abdominal, and upper airway muscles to maintain O_2 supplies despite changes in the environment, metabolic rate, and the force-generating ability of the muscles of breathing.

The sleep-wakefulness cycle has very considerable effects on breathing.[10-12] In general, respiratory responses to chemical and mechanical stimuli diminish or entirely disappear during sleep. In addition, in rapid eye movement sleep, the breathing rhythm becomes more irregular, and even in healthy people, brief periods of apnea can occur. In addition,

during sleep, the distribution of output to the respiratory muscles changes, with the diaphragm incurring a smaller reduction in motor outflow than the intercostals or the upper airway muscles. The horizontal position adopted during sleep increases the importance of coordinating thoracoabdominal and upper airway muscles movements so that the pharynx remains patent despite the negative intraluminal pressures produced during inspiration.

The adequacy of the O_2 supply is best measured by the level of arterial P_{CO_2} rather than P_{O_2}. While inadequate ventilation produces hypoxemia as well as hypercapnia, hypoxemia can occur even if ventilation is sufficient because of unevenness in the ratio of blood flow to ventilation within the lung. In the face of impaired gas exchange in the lung or suboptimal performance of the respiratory muscles, control system attempts to adjust ventilation can lead to breathlessness or dyspnea.[9] However, sometimes dyspnea arises directly from control system malfunction so that ventilation is driven excessively beyond the requirements of the body for oxygen.[6,9] Additionally, while the control system usually produces a quite regular rhythm with minimal fluctuations in arterial blood gas levels, control system abnormalities can cause the rhythm of breathing to become frankly irregular or periodic so that intermittent hypoxemia occurs.[13]

Disturbances in the Rhythm of Breathing

Usually the respiratory rhythm awake is quite regular. Breathing variations diminish during non-rapid eye movement (NREM) sleep, especially in stages 3 and 4, and are exaggerated in rapid eye movement (REM) sleep.[10]

APNEAS DURING SLEEP

Apneas can occur in normal individuals during sleep especially. In sleeping individuals, for example, a reduction in P_{CO_2} by even a few millimeters stops breathing. These apneas are usually less than a few seconds in duration and cause only small percentage changes in arterial O_2 saturation.[10,14] Less than 5 to 10 such brief apneas occur on average per hour of sleep. Apneas during sleep can be central; i.e., there is complete cessation of respiratory activity.[10,13] More often, however, they are obstructive so that even though the thoracoabdominal muscles contract, no air flows into the lungs because the upper airway is closed. Loss of muscle tone, poorly coordinated activity of the dilator muscles of the larynx and/or pharynx, or anatomically narrowed upper airway passages can lead to obstructive apnea.

In 4 or 5 percent of people above 65 years of age, apneas are more frequent and more prolonged because airway obstruction occurs.[10,13,14] In the more severe cases, serious hypoxemia during the apneic period gives rise to cardiac arrhythmias. The intermittent hypoxia may produce pulmonary arterial hypertension and right ventricular failure. Apneas are terminated in general by arousal. The poor quality of sleep that results may lead to daytime somnolence. Overall minute ventilation during sleep may decrease more than the reduction in metabolic rate so that arterial P_{CO_2} increases by even more than the 2- to 3-mmHg increase usually observed during sleep. This reduced ventilation can initiate CO_2 and bicarbonate retention that continues during wakefulness. Relief of sleep apnea by one of the several mechanical inter-

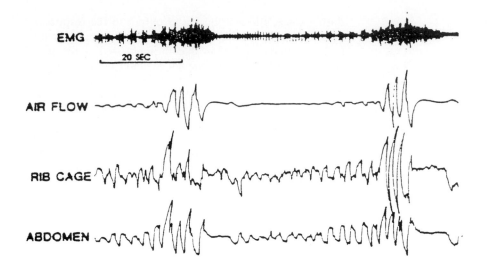

FIGURE 13-1 Tracing of electromyogram (EMG) measured from a chin surface electrode, airflow, and rib cage and abdominal movement in a patient with sleep apnea. Note that the airflow pattern resembles that seen in Cheyne-Stokes respiration. Associated with the waxing and waning of airflow are swings in the chin IMG (reflecting change in the activity of upper airway muscles). Note that chest wall movements peersist even in the absence of airflow so that the apnea is obstructive in type.

ventions that are readily available such as nasal continuous positive airways pressure (CPAP) reverses these changes in bicarbonate. While serious and potentially life-threatening consequences of apneas occur in only a fraction of those with obstructive apneas who have healthy lungs, lesser abnormalities in breathing during sleep may have serious effects on those with lung disease.[11,14]

PERIODIC BREATHING

Apneas, instead of occurring irregularly, may be associated with regular swings in the level of ventilation, with the apneas either central or obstructive occurring at the nadir of the ventilation swings (periodic breathing)[13,15] (Fig. 13-1). This kind of respiratory pattern is called *Cheyne-Stokes,* or *periodic, breathing*. It can occur in normal people during sleep, especially at altitude, but also occurs at sea level in patients with congestive heart failure or bilateral cerebral cortical disease.

Periodic breathing is believed to be an instability in respiratory control analogous to those which can appear in human-designed feedback control systems.[13,15] When these artificial control systems become unstable, output, rather than being maintained at some steady level, oscillates because of delays in information transfer around the feedback system or because controller gain is too high. Basically, it arises in these systems because the controller lacks adequate information about the state of the output.[15,16]

In the respiratory control system, information on the level of blood gas tensions in the lungs is relayed by the flow of blood to chemoreceptors from the alveoli. The time required for the blood to circulate between these points causes a delay that, when sufficiently long, causes the instability. This delay, which is normally quite short (less than 10 s), can become quite long in disorders such as congestive heart failure.

Hypoxia is one factor that increases the sensitivity of chemoreceptors to CO_2 (Fig. 13-2). Thus periodic breathing is more likely to occur against a background of reduced environmental P_{O_2} levels. The cortex normally has an inhibitory effect on ventilatory responsivity to CO_2. Strokes (often bilateral cortical infarcts), which destroy this inhibition, heighten CO_2 sensitivity and may lead to periodic breathing.[13,16] A

number of other factors such as increased thresholds for responses and the small size of the oxygen stores in the body that allow P_{O_2} to drop precipitously when breathing is arrested also contribute to periodic breathing. Sleep or hypoxia that lasts more than 30 min tends to eliminate the slow decay in ventilation that occurs when a respiratory stimulus is removed abruptly. This slow decay (also called *afterdischarge*) helps prevent periodic breathing.[17]

Other Breathing Rhythm Abnormalities

Severe injury to the respiratory neuronal network in the medulla can produce a grossly irregular *chaotic breathing*.[18] Sometimes tidal volume is uniform, but the frequency is not, producing *Biot's breathing* (Fig. 13-3). Slow deep inspirations lasting several seconds characterize *apneustic breathing*, which usually arises from damage to the pons. All the preceding changes in breathing indicate a quite poor prognosis.[19]

Metabolic acidosis as well as diseases or injury to the midbrain can produce greater than normal ventilation levels with an increase in tidal volume or frequency.[19] These disorders will be discussed in the next section.

HYPERVENTILATION

The respiratory control system is organized so that over a wide range of metabolic rates, ventilation can be adjusted to maintain arterial P_{CO_2} within normal limits (generally 35 to 45 mmHg). Hyperventilation occurs when arterial P_{CO_2} falls below this range in the steady state.

Minute ventilation can be considered to consist of two parts: alveolar ventilation, which equilibrates with blood in the lung, and dead space ventilation, which does not equilibrate because it fills the conducting airways or reaches areas of the lung that have no or inadequate blood flow. Generally, the smaller the tidal volume, the more is the dead space ventilation.[20]

Minute ventilation varies considerably in healthy individuals because of differences in body size and hence oxygen consumption and because of differences in dead space vol-

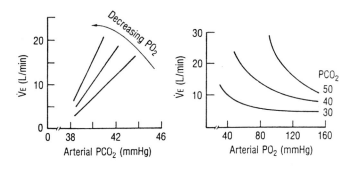

FIGURE 13-2 Left side: ventilatory response to CO_2; the slope of the response line increases with hypoxia. Right side: ventilatory response to hypoxia. Note how hypercapnia increases the curvature of the ventilatory response to hypoxia.

ume. Lung disease can enlarge the dead space substantially so that even when minute ventilation is greater, alveolar ventilation is unchanged. The diagnosis of hyperventilation can only be made by measuring arterial blood gas levels; measurements of minute ventilation do not suffice.

There are a number of different stimuli that can produce hyperventilation. These stimuli arise from three sources: the chemoreceptors, the mechanoreceptors, and areas of the brain above the pons.

Hypoxia and metabolic acidosis can reduce arterial P_{CO_2} substantially because of chemoreceptor stimulation.[21] If hypoxia or acidosis persists for long periods of time, renal excretion of barcarbonate can rise, restoring the elevated pH resulting from respiratory alkalosis toward normal levels.[22,23] Sojourn at altitude produces a persistent hyperventilation with hypocapnia that preserves the supply of O_2. The hyperventilation seen at altitude persists for several days after the return to sea level for reasons that are still not clear.[24-26] Persistent hyperventilation also occurs in pulmonary thrombosis and congestive heart failure, whereas transient hyperventilation is common during asthmatic attacks. In all these cases, hypoxemia contributes to the supernormal levels of alveolar ventilation, as well as heightened input from irritant receptors in the airways and J-receptors in the lung.[21]

FIGURE 13-3 Example of phrenic nerve tracings (moving average) in *A*, Cheyne-Stokes breathing; *B*, ataxic breathing; and *C*, Biot's breathing.

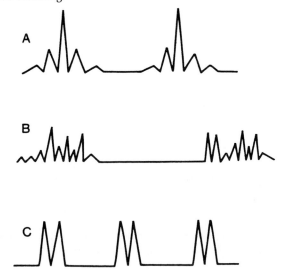

J-receptors have endings in the lung interstitium and can be excited by edema formation; they also stimulate breathing in left-sided heart failure.[21]

Fever acting on hypothalamic centers also can elevate alveolar ventilation disproportionately to metabolic need. During pregnancy, increased levels of progesterone can reduce arterial P_{CO_2}. Arterial P_{CO_2} fluctuates during the menstrual cycle in parallel to the changes in progesterone level.[21]

Transient hyperventilation can occur in attacks along with feelings of suffocation, breathlessness, depersonalization, and paresthesias in patients with panic disorder and agoraphobia.[27-30] Sometimes the attack produces chest pain mimicking coronary artery occlusion. Although the attacks can be relieved by rebreathing from a bag, and about half of those with panic disorder chronically hyperventilate, overventilation is now thought to be a consequence rather than the cause of the malady.[27] Panic attacks can be reproduced in those with the disorder by 5% CO_2 breathing for several minutes, 35% CO_2 in O_2 breathing for 30 s, or intravenous infusion of sodium lactate. This has led to the hypothesis that this disorder might be a result of chemoreceptor hyperactivity. Some but not all studies report increased ventilatory responsivity to CO_2 in panic disorder patients.

The anxiety that occasionally occurs in normal subjects with CO_2 inhalation occurs much more frequently in those with panic attacks. This behavioral effect of CO_2 seems to be fairly specific and does not appear in patients with other types of phobias, nor can it be reproduced by breathing through a resistance.[29]

Panic attacks can occur during sleep, and patients with the disorder tend to have more irregular breathing than normal subjects, particularly in NREM sleep stages 3 and 4 and during wakefulness.[30]

The acute episodes often can be treated successfully by selective serotonin reuptake inhibitors. Retraining in diaphragm breathing as well as behavioral therapy helps prevent the attacks from recurring.

HYPOVENTILATION

Hypoventilation, elevation of arterial P_{CO_2} (above 45 mmHg), in the vast majority of instances occurs in the presence of disease of the respiratory apparatus (the lungs, the airways, the thoracic cage, and the respiratory muscles).[21] Although hypercapnia is more frequent the more severe the disease, it has been recognized for a long time that in patients with equally severe lung or thoracic disease, only some will develop hypercapnia.[31,32] Therefore, it is believed that abnormal or subnormal respiratory control contributes to CO_2 retention in those who have it. Only rarely does hypercapnia occur when the thoracic bellows are normal.

HYPERCAPNIA IN THE PRESENCE OF LUNG DISEASE

Increased airway resistance and lung and chest wall elasticity can interfere with the movement of air into and out of the lung.[31,32] These mechanical changes act as a load for the respiratory muscles, inhibiting their shortening, and thus tend to reduce tidal volume.

The respiratory control system can compensate for loads in several ways.[33] Loads decrease the velocity of shortening of the respiratory muscle, and in all skeletal muscle, contractile force increases as velocity slows. Loads that act mainly during expiration (as in obstructive lung disease) tend to raise functional residual capacity, lengthening the expiratory muscles and thereby increasing the force they are able to produce, but they have the opposite effect on inspiratory muscles. Tonic contraction of expiratory muscles activated by muscle and lung stretch receptors tends to reduce lung volume toward normal and to lengthen the inspiratory muscles, helping to restore the force-producing ability. To a certain extent in humans, the decreased tidal volume caused by abnormalities in pulmonary mechanics slows breathing and in particular prolongs inspiratory time (by lung stretch receptor inhibition via the Hering-Breuer reflex), prolonging inspiratory muscle contraction. Any elevation in P_{CO_2} as a result of reduced alveolar ventilation increases drive to the muscles from the chemoreceptors. Muscle spindles that compare actual to chemoreceptor-demanded muscle shortening can act to augment motor output to the intercostal muscles if they do not shorten enough. Finally, awake unsedated humans increase the force of respiratory muscle contraction acutely as soon as a load is consciously detected.

In addition to loading the respiratory muscles, lung disease increases physiologic dead space so that tidal volume and minute ventilation must be above normal if eucapnia is to be maintained.[31] In some patients, minute ventilation is not increased, and hypercapnia results. It has been suggested that in these patients chemosensitivity to either CO_2 or low O_2 is blunted. Normal subjects vary tremendously in their respiratory responses to chemical stimuli. Patients with responses in the low-normal range may not be able to compensate completely for impaired lung thoracic function. Familial and/or hereditary factors have been shown to be important in determining chemosensitivity.[31,32] Chemoreceptor responses to CO_2 as well as to hypoxia have been reported to be less in relatives of patients who develop hypercapnia with lung disease than in relatives of patients who do not, lending support to the depressed chemosensitivity hypothesis.

Other patients with lung disease develop hypercapnia despite an augmented minute ventilation.[34] In these patients, some mechanism seems to restrict the increase in tidal volume so that it fails to rise enough to maintain alveolar ventilation. One study reported that hypercapnic patients had decreased inspiratory times that limited tidal volume. It was hypothesized that the reduced time of inspiration arose from hyperactive irritant receptors, since the hypercapnic patients frequently also had chronic bronchitis.

TABLE 13-1 Causes of Hypercapnia in Patients with or without Significant Respiratory Disease

Idiopathic
Sleep apnea syndrome
Metabolic alkalosis
Lateral spinal artery thrombosis
Platybasia
Severe diffuse cerebrovascular disease

The energy used by the respiratory muscles or the force they need to exert each breath also may be factors that restrict tidal volume.[35,36] One idea is that minute ventilation is determined by neurons that by some process algebraically sum the excitatory drive that arises from hypoxia and hypercapnia and a ventilatory inhibitory drive that arises from some sensor that can measure the work or energy cost of breathing. While no work sensor has been found, conscious humans can perceive and quantify the forces exerted by the respiratory muscles as well as the tidal volumes that are actually achieved.[37] It has been shown that the sensory effects of breathing are predominately the result of the effort expended during each breath. It is possible that tidal volumes are limited by patients with lung disease as a strategy to minimize the awareness of the difficult breathing.[38]

Hypercapnia also can be a consequence of neuromuscular diseases. There is a reasonable correlation between the maximal force that can be exerted by the inspiratory muscles and the occurrence of hypercapnia. Neuromuscular diseases such as paralysis of the diaphragm, in animals, enhances intercostal muscle activity even if changes in arterial blood gas tensions are prevented artificially. It is of interest that the increase in intercostal muscle activity seems to depend on vagal receptors. However, humans with spinal cord transection are less able than normal individuals to detect changes in resistance to airflow produced experimentally by the application of resistance devices to the mouth.[31–33]

Recent studies suggest that changes in the usual pattern and level of ventilation (whether they are increased or decreased) and the use of certain muscles such as the accessory muscles of the neck are dyspnogenic.[31,32]

Hypercapnia in Patients with a Normal Respiratory Apparatus

Table 13-1 lists some of the conditions in which hypercapnia occurs even in the absence of respiratory disease.[32,33] The most common of these conditions are sleep-disordered breathing, metabolic alkalosis, and the use of sedative drugs. Sleep apneas, in addition to producing rhythm disorders, can lead to an overall diminution in alveolar ventilation. Respiratory depression has been said to occur mainly when K^+ depletion is the cause of metabolic alkalosis. Elevated bicarbonate levels, even in the absence of alkalosis, may depress respiration, and sufficient chloride must be available for bicarbonate excretion.

Pain-killing medication (opiates) and hypnotics may depress responses to chemical stimuli and interfere with mechanisms to overcome respiratory loads. In the presence of respiratory disease, they may cause hypercapnia but rarely do so in the absence of such diseases.

A number of conditions such as birth at altitude and cyanotic congenital heart disease can cause blunting of hypoxic response without affecting the ventilatory response to CO_2. While these patients rarely present with hypercapnia because their central chemoreceptors are functioning adequately, they may tolerate hypoxia poorly.[39]

Anatomic deformities of the base of the skull and thrombosis of the lateral spinal arteries are other conditions that may reduce CO_2 sensitivity without proportionately affecting the response to hypoxia.

Nonetheless, the cause of most cases of depressed chemosensitivity in many patients with hypercapnia and normal lungs is unknown.

Implications of Abnormalities in the Control of Breathing for the Rehabilitation of Pulmonary Patients

The usually effortless supply of O_2 to the body by breathing is essential for normal daily activity and maintenance of the quality of life. Both dyspnea and hypoxia can severely limit functional capacity. Trauma or disease rarely causes defects isolated to the respiratory control system. Much more commonly, injuries or disease that interferes with respiratory function uncovers an inherent and perhaps hereditary attenuation of chemosensitivity.[31,32]

Respiratory diseases and their treatment can cause abnormalities in control. For example, the use of diuretics in right-sided heart failure can produce metabolic alkalosis, whereas some cough suppressants can depress breathing as well. The behavioral increase in drive that occurs with loading in normal awake individuals disappears in patients with chronic obstructive lung disease, perhaps because of endogenous release of opiates, though aging also may contribute to the absence of the anticipatory load-overcoming response.[33] Mechanical appliances such as splints and braces used in rehabilitating patients with nonpulmonary injuries can compromise movement of the respiratory muscles and respiratory function. Dyspnea may occur with any event that alters usual breathing patterns or the level of ventilation either up or down. Both the intermittent hypoxia of periodic breathing and the sustained hypoxia that results from chronic underventilation may cause pulmonary hypertension and right-sided heart failure.

A number of diagnostic tests have been devised to measure chemosensitivity and to quantify dyspnea. Table 13-2 lists methods of evaluating chemosensitivity. Relatively simple rebreathing methods with measurements of ventilation can be used to assess chemosensitivity in patients with no respiratory disease. These tests may be useful in identifying individuals with reduced chemosensitivity who have other illnesses that make them more susceptible to respiratory disease, for example, patients with stroke or paraplegics. In patients with lung disease, more complicated approaches must be used, including measurements of occlusion pressure or diaphragm electrical activity with surface or esophageal electrodes.

More practically, assessment of chemosensitivity can begin in patients with lung disease by taking a careful history to detect possible sleep-disordered breathing, measuring arterial blood gases and electrolytes to determine if hypoxia or

TABLE 13-2 Methods of Evaluating Chemosensitivity

Hypercapnia
   Steady-state ventilation response to CO_2
   Rebreathing ventilation response to CO_2
   Electromyographic response of diaphragm
   Occlusion-pressured response
   Breath-holding time
Hypoxia
   Steady state and rebreathing
   Ventilation response to low O_2
   Ventilation
   Response to single breaths of N_2
   Electromyogram of diaphragm
   Occlusion pressure

alkalosis are present, and determining lung volumes and flow rates by spirometry. In patients in whom respiratory muscle weakness may be a factor, measurements of maximal inspiratory and expiratory pressures are useful.

There is a significant inverse correlation between forced expiratory volume in 1 s ($FEV_{1.0}$) and P_{CO_2} and between maximal inspiratory force and P_{CO_2}. Patients who differ substantially from the usual relationship should be suspected of having abnormalities of respiratory control. Simple bedside tests that can be used to distinguish whether hypercapnia is the result of defective respiratory control or a defective respiratory apparatus include measurement of the breath-holding time of the patient compared with simultaneous breath hold by a healthy person and voluntary hyperventilation. The hypercapnic patients with the normal lungs can maintain a normal P_{CO_2} for several minutes by voluntary hyperventilation.

The effects of treatment of lung or muscle disease on dyspnea can be measured, as indicated in Table 13-3. These tests include evaluation of dyspnea during increased stimulation of breathing with a Borg or a visual analog scale as well as evaluation of the dyspnea brought about by normal daily activities. These measurements are particularly valuable in assessing the efficacy of rehabilitative interventions.

The limitation of lifestyle in patients with hypoxemia and dyspnea may contribute to mental distress. O_2 therapy will help relieve hypoxemia and sometimes dyspnea as well. Depression and anxiety are often features of the psychological stresses experienced by patients with breathing problems. Several studies have reported that the incidence of depression may be higher in patients with chronic obstructive lung disease than in other medical conditions. Rehabilitative programs either to produce general physical conditioning such as walking or specifically designed to improve respiratory muscle strength or endurance may reduce distress. Avoidance of routine activities because of anxiety concerning dyspnea can interfere with rehabilitative efforts. Dyspnea can

TABLE 13-3 Tests to Measure Dyspnea

Borg scale
Visual analog scale
Chronic respiratory questionnaire
Magnitude estimation and production
Dyspnea index (minute ventilation/maximum voluntary ventilation)

be accompanied by panic, leading to hyperventilation and so worsening the dyspnea. Depression and anxiety also may interfere with smoking cessation efforts or compliance with recommended use of bronchodilators. Behavioral modification, relaxation efforts, and desensitization to dyspnea all may help improve function when control system abnormalities worsen breathlessness or oxygenation in patients.

References

1. Loeschcke HH: Central chemosensitivity and the reaction theory. *J Physiol (Lond)* 332:1–24, 1982.

2. Raminez JM, Richter DW: The neuronal mechanisms of respiratory rhythm generation. *Curr Opin Neurobiol* 6(6): 817–825, 1996.

3. Blanche A, Denavit-Saubie M, Champagnat J: Neurobiology of the central control of breathing in mammals: Neuron circuitry, membrane properties and neurotransmitters involved. *Physiol Rev* 751:1–45, 1995.

4. Richter DW, Ballanyi K: Responses of the medullary respiratory network to hypoxia: A comparative analysis of neonatal and adult mammals, in Haddad GG, Lister G (eds): *Tissue Oxygen Deprivation: Developmental, Molecular, and Integrated Function.* New York, Marcel Dekker, 1996, pp 751–777.

5. Gonzalez C, Vicario I, Alvarez L, Rigual R: Oxygen sensing in the carotid body. *Biol Signals* 4:245–256, 1995.

6. Schwartzstein RM: Pathophysiology of dyspnea. *N Engl J Med* 333:1547–1553, 1995.

7. Taylor EW, Coote JH, Jordan D: Central control of cardiorespiratory interactions in aquatic, amphibious, and terrestrial vertebrates. *Physiol Rev* (in press).

8. Lahiri S: Chromophores in O_2 chemoreception: The carotid body model. *NIPS* 9:161–165, 1994.

9. Cherniack NS: Respiratory sensation as a respiratory controller, in Adams L, Guz A (eds): *Respiratory Sensation*, vol 90. New York, Marcel Dekker, 1996, pp 213–230.

10. Pack AI: Obstructive sleep apnea. *Adv Intern Med* 39:517–567, 1994.

11. Ballard RD, Clover CW, Suh BY: Influence of sleep on respiratory function in emphysema. *Am J Respir Crit Care Med* 151:945–951, 1995.

12. Sharp JT: Therapeutic considerations in respiratory muscle function. *Chest* 88:118–123, 1985.

13. Cherniack NS, Longobardo GS: Periodic breathing during sleep, in Saunders NA, Sullivan CE (eds): *Sleep and Breathing*, 2d ed. New York, Marcel Dekker, 1994, pp 157–190.

14. Strohl KP, Saunders NA, Sullivan CE: Sleep apnea syndrome, in Saunders NA, Sullivan CE (eds): *Sleep and Breathing*. New York, Marcel Dekker, 1984, pp 365–402.

15. Khoo MCK, Kronauer RE, Strohl KP, Slutsky AS: Factors inducing periodic breathing in humans: A general model. *J Appl Physiol* 53:644–659, 1982.

16. Cherniack NS: Sleep apnea and its causes. *J Clin Invest* 73:1501–1506, 1984.

17. Badr MS, Skatrod JB, Dempsey JA: Determinants of poststimulus potentiation in humans during NREM sleep. *J Appl Physiol* 73:1958–1971, 1992.

18. Powell AR, Buckley CE III, Cohen R, et al: Cheyne-Stokes respiration: A review of clinical manifestations and physiological mechanisms. *Arch Intern Med* 127:712–716, 1971.

19. Brown HW, Plum F: The neurological basis of Cheyne-Stokes respiration. *Am J Med* 30:899–891, 1961.

20. Severinghaus JW, Stuptel M: Alveolar dead space as an index of distribution of blood flow in pulmonary capillaries. *J Appl Physiol* 10:335–348, 1957.

21. Kelsen SA, Cherniack NS: Disorders of ventilatory control, in Simmons DH (ed): *Current Pulmonology,* vol 6, chap 2. New York, Wiley, 1985, pp 29–65.

22. Godfrey S, Edwards RHT, Copland GM, Gross PL: Chemosensitivity in normal subjects, athletes and patients with chronic airways obstruction. *J Appl Physiol* 30:193–199, 1971.

23. Arbus GA, Herbert LA, Levesque PR, et al: Characterization and clinical application of the "significance band" for acute respiratory alkalosis. *N Engl J Med* 280:117–123, 1969.

24. Milledge JS, Lahiri S: Respiratory control in lowlanders and Sherpa highlanders at altitude. *Respir Physiol* 2:310–322, 1967.

25. Ward MP, Milledge JS, West JB: *High Altitude Medicine and Physiology,* 2d ed. London, Chapman & Hall, 1995.

26. Bisgard GE, Forster HV: Ventilatory response to acute and chronic hypoxia, in Fregly MJ, Blatteis CM (eds): *Handbook of Physiology: Environmental Physiology.* New York, Oxford University Press, 1996, pp 1202–1240.

27. Liehowitz MR, Gorman JM, Fyer AJ, et al: Lactate provocation of panic attacks: II. Biochemical and physiological findings. *Arch Gen Psychiatry* 42:701–719, 1985.

28. Papp LA, Klein DF, Martinez J, et al: Diagnostic and substance specificity of CO_2 induced panic. *Am J Psychiatry* 150:250–257, 1993.

29. Perna G, Bertani A, Arancio C, et al: Laboratory response of patients with panic and obsessive-compulsive disorder to 35% CO_2 challenge. *Am J Psychiatry* 152:85–89, 1995.

30. Stein MD, Millar TW, Larsen DK, Kryger MH: Irregular breathing during sleep in patients with panic disorder. *Am J Psychiatry* 152:1168–1173, 1995.

31. Altose MD, Cherniack NS, Gothe B, et al: Nonchemical factors in the control of breathing in patients with pulmonary disorders, in von Euler C, Lager Krants H (eds): *Central Nervous Control Mechanisms in Breathing.* New York, Oxford University Press, 1979, pp 389–396.

32. Kelsen SG, Jammes Y, Cherniack NS: Control of motor activity to the respiratory muscles, in Roussos C, Macklem PT (eds): *The Thorax.* New York, Marcel Dekker, 1985, pp 493–529.

33. Cherniack NS, Milic-Emili J: Mechanical aspects of loaded breathing in the thorax, in Roussos C, Macklem PT (eds): *The Thorax.* New York, Marcel Dekker, 1985, pp 751–786.

34. Sorli J, Grassino A, Lorange G, Milic-Emili J: Control of breathing in patients with chronic obstructive pulmonary disease. *Clin Sci Mol Med* 54:295–304, 1978.

35. Otis AB: The work of breathing. *Physiol Rev* 34:449-458, 1958.

36. Poon CS: Ventilatory control in hypercapnia and exercise: Optimization hypothesis. *J Appl Physiol* 62:2447–2459, 1987.

37. Tack M, Altose MD, Cherniack NS: Effects of aging on sensation of respiratory force and displacement. *J Appl Physiol* 55:1433–1440, 1983.

38. Oku Y, Saidel GM, Altose MD, Cherniack NS: Perceptual contributions to optimization of breathing. *Ann Biomed Engr* 21:509–515, 1993.

39. Lahiri S, Delaney RG, Brody JS, et al: Relative role of environmental and genetic factors in respiratory adaptation to high altitude. *Nature* 261:133–135, 1976.

Chapter 14

DISORDERED BREATHING DURING SLEEP

ROBERT C. BASNER
ERGÜN ÖNAL

As pointed out in earlier chapters of this text, sleep represents a major and unavoidable stress to respiratory homeostasis in humans, the manifestations of which are often overlooked by the attending clinician and undertaught in our medical schools.[1,2] Sleep is not a homogeneous state in regard to breathing, and understanding the pathophysiologic events of the separate sleep states is important in delineating appropriate treatment for each patient with potential or documented disordered breathing during sleep.

At sleep-wake transitions and in light non-rapid eye movement (non-REM) sleep, periodicity of respiratory rate and volume may predominate, with loss of waking drive to breathe and dependence on metabolic control.[3] Propagation of this transitional state, as occurs with repetitive arousals (which themselves may be associated with increased upper airway resistance and obstruction), may manifest as a diathesis to central and obstructive sleep apnea.[4] Consolidated non-REM sleep is associated with more regular respiration, but minute ventilation decreases from light to deep non-REM sleep by up to 1.5 L/min, whereas Pa_{CO_2} increases on the order of 3 to 6 mmHg. Upper airway resistance also increases.[5] Thus, clinically important hypoventilation and upper airway obstruction may become manifest during non-REM sleep in predisposed patients. Finally, in rapid eye movement (REM) sleep, metabolic ventilatory responses are greatly decreased or absent, and respiration tends to be irregular in rate and volume. In REM sleep, active inhibition of postural muscles including upper airway and accessory ventilatory muscles occurs. Severe hypoxemia, hypoventilation, and upper airway obstruction may result. Thus it can be seen that many, if not most, patients with awake respiratory compromise, as well as many without such overt awake compromise, may require specific therapy for sleep-disordered breathing.

Consideration of patients for treatment of sleep-disordered breathing should begin with a thorough assessment of the patient's awake medical status; obesity, craniofacial or upper airway anatomic or physiologic defects (including chronic nasal congestion), medications, sleep habits, pulmonary function and gas exchange, and cardiac, renal, endocrine, and neurologic status should be delineated. Sleep studies to address the pathophysiologic concerns just noted are usually necessary; these ideally should be able to delineate the degree of sleep fragmentation, upper airway obstruction, alveolar hypoventilation, ventilation-perfusion mismatching, bronchospasm, and the combinations and overlap among these. Positional and sleep-stage components of the sleep-disordered breathing also should be delineated.

Treatment of Specific Disorders

SLEEP APNEA SYNDROMES

OBSTRUCTIVE SLEEP APNEA

Treatment Rationale

The rationale for treatment of *obstructive sleep apnea (OSA)* is to prevent or reverse life-threatening and debilitating sleepiness during usual awake hours and to prevent or reverse cardiovascular and respiratory morbidity and mortality. In the United States, epidemiologic data indicate that as many as 24 percent of adult men and 9 percent of adult women in the community manifest at least 5 obstructive respiratory events per hour of sleep.[6] In other countries, 26 percent of middle aged men and 8 percent of middle aged women in the community have been found to have 15 or more obstructive events per hour of sleep, whereas greater than 40 percent of geriatric (over 65 years of age) community-dwelling populations show similar obstructive event frequencies.[7] Vascular mortality in OSA appears to be increased when obstructive apneas and hypopneas occur with a frequency of as low as 10 to 20 per hour of sleep.[8–10] It is difficult to define a precise obstructive event or sleep fragmentation index for predicting symptomatic sleepiness or, indeed, for sleepiness that may involve work or traffic fatalities,[11,12] although it has been shown that increasingly severe OSA is more likely to be associated with motor vehicle accidents and fatalities.[2,12–14] However, quantification of sleepiness in the range associated with unintentional sleep intruding into awake time is available in the sleep laboratory in the form of the well-validated Multiple Sleep Latency Test.[15] Therefore, the clinician can and should be quite objective about who needs treatment and what the treatment goals must be.

Preliminary Treatment Considerations

Certain preliminary issues should be a part of the clinician's considerations in treating patients with diagnosed OSA. These are, among others, weight loss, avoidance of respiratory suppressants, assessment of anatomic and functional status of the upper airway, attention to sleep position, and avoidance of driving and other activities in which falling asleep suddenly might endanger the patient and others. Each of these will be reviewed briefly here.

Obesity is clearly linked pathophysiologically and epidemiologically to disordered breathing during sleep.[16] However, although there are accumulating data to argue that weight loss is both beneficial and feasible in many OSA patients, it is not clear how definitively weight loss will improve OSA acutely or over time.[16] In obese patients, it is reasonable to aim for a 10 to 15 percent decrease in weight to improve the sleep-disordered breathing,[17] but such weight loss alone may not be sufficient to treat more than mild OSA.

Ethanol, apart from its tendency to cause acute and chronic sleep disruption, may worsen sleep-disordered breathing in snorers as well as in patients with known OSA.[18,19] Other sedative-hypnotics, including benzodiazepines and barbiturates, as well as opioids, may have been prescribed for the OSA patient who complains of daytime sleepiness, anxiety, depression, or pain in association with poor sleep. Such medications, like ethanol, may worsen OSA.[20,21] We advise that the use of any sedative-hypnotic or opioid medication in patients diagnosed with, or suspected to have, OSA only be done with objective evidence of the patient's sleep and respiration while taking the medication.

"Shut your mouth and save your life" is the subtitle of a nineteenth century paper referring to the tendency to sleep-disordered breathing in people with nasal obstruction and mouth breathing during sleep.[22,23] Since then, it has been found that nasal breathing is important in the maintenance of upper airway muscle function[24] and normal sleep.[23,25] At the same time, it is difficult to show that relief of nasal obstruction, either functional, as with seasonal or chronic rhinitis, or anatomic, such as septal deviation, is curative in patients with OSA.[26] Other nasopharyngeal, oropharyngeal, and velopharyngeal defects, such as adenotonsillar hypertrophy, "redundant" tissue of the soft palate, elongated uvula, nasopharyngeal tumor, macroglossia, micro- and retrognathia, and vocal cord dysfunction, may be present, and these should be looked for in any patient suspected or known to have OSA.[27] In most adult patients, however, a specific abnormality amenable to surgical intervention will not be found,[27] nor can treatment of such abnormalities in adults always sufficiently reverse significant disordered breathing during sleep. We advocate otolaryngologic examination in OSA with the specific goal of allowing the patient to best tolerate nasal continuous positive airway pressure (CPAP). Nasal steroids, decongestants, antihistamines, or even surgery may be indicated for this. Otolaryngologic examination is also important to rule out lesions, as described above, that warrant treatment apart from their contribution to sleep-related apnea.

In some patients, obstructive events may be found to be more numerous in the supine as opposed to the lateral decubitus position, and treatments aimed at avoiding the supine position have been devised, such as placing a tennis ball in a sock and sewing this to the back of the night shirt.[28] However, it is our experience that few patients with clinically significant OSA are free of obstructive events and sleep fragmentation in the lateral decubitus or prone position versus the supine position, and we only occasionally rely on positional training alone in patients with significant OSA.

Finally, we consider it extremely important to explain to patients with diagnosed OSA that they are predisposed to falling asleep suddenly and inappropriately[2,11,12] and to advise that driving and other activities in which falling asleep suddenly would constitute a risk to the patient or others must be avoided until efficient therapy has been achieved. We routinely document this in the patient's medical record. In the United States, regulations regarding mandatory reporting of OSA and the liabilities regarding both reporting and nonreporting differ from state to state, and the clinician of record is advised to consult with legal counsel regarding these issues.[12]

Nasal Positive Airway Pressure

Except for a minority of situations in which a readily reversible anatomic or functional defect can be demonstrated and corrected, the primary and definitive therapy for OSA in adults is nasal positive airway pressure (PAP). The delivery of PAP involves the use of a tight-fitting mask, usually a nasal mask, secured by soft headgear and attached by flexible tubing to a portable electrically driven unit that can deliver pressurized air of up to 35 cmH_2O pressure, although 20 cmH_2O is generally the maximum pressure used in OSA. The pressure typically is set to be maintained throughout the respiratory cycle, thus creating continuous positive airway pressure, or CPAP. Positive airway pressure also can be delivered via mouthpiece or full-face mask, though these are generally less effective. From 1983 on, extensive data have accrued documenting the ability of CPAP to achieve immediate and long-standing improvement in cardiorespiratory and sleep parameters as well as daytime somnolence[29–32]; discontinuing CPAP use for one night may return patients to pretreatment levels of sleep disruption and daytime somnolence.[33] CPAP is the modality other than tracheostomy that has been shown to achieve decreased vascular mortality in OSA.[6] It is rather remarkable, then, that recent objective and subjective measures of long-term compliance with CPAP have shown surprisingly low rates.[33] In a study utilizing covert monitoring of 35 patients using CPAP for up to 30 months, only 46 percent used the CPAP properly at least 4 hours per day at least 70 percent of the days monitored; only 2 of the 35 patients used the modality properly at least 7 hours per day at least 70 percent of days monitored. Self-reports overestimated actual use.[33] Thus the treating clinician should not assume that patients who are initially successfully titrated on CPAP are receiving adequate therapy at home. The disappointing long-term compliance is not easily explained. The initial increase in sleep quality may be offset by increasing nasal dryness, congestion, burning, or facial discomfort, as well as social and personal inconvenience. The lack of uniform approaches and goals in titrating desirable levels of CPAP, even in accredited sleep laboratories,[34] also may be partly responsible, since CPAP levels may at times be prescribed in a more arbitrary fashion than previously thought. Similarly, maximally effective levels may vary from night to night in a given patient. Further, effective patient education and follow-up are likely to be lacking in many cases. Mask leak occurs frequently in the laboratory with position change and mouth opening; occult air leak from mask slippage or mouth opening at home may cause resumption of sleep-disordered breathing and loss of symptomatic relief, in return causing less investment in wearing the equipment nightly. Mask fit and comfort are clearly important issues in this regard, and these are issues that too often may not be closely addressed and followed. Similarly, improvement in daytime sleepiness and daytime function appears to be self-limited,[35] perhaps accounting for decreased use of therapy over time. On the other hand, perhaps effective treatment, by reversing sleepiness such that initial levels of prescribed CPAP are less well tolerated, may paradoxically contribute to decreased compliance. Warm air humidification of the CPAP circuit, particularly during the winter months, has been of decided benefit in increasing nasal comfort for many of our patients. Care should be taken to individualize the CPAP interface according to the fit and comfort of each patient. There are now many different sizes and styles of CPAP masks, including nasal "pillows" and minimasks that do not necessitate surrounding the entire nose. There are foam, air, silicone, and gel mask cushions to choose from as interfaces. We have found that a commercially available soft chin strap is effective in preventing severe air leak from the mouth when necessary. Finally, newer strategies of CPAP are being developed[36]; such units continuously self-adjust based on detection of inspiratory airflow limitation.

Although the ability to do this on a breath-to-breath basis has not been well established, such "smart CPAP" units have the theoretical advantages of more accurate overnight and night-to-night pressure delivery, thus possibly improving patient compliance as well as providing a more physiologically rational titration than is currently employed during routine laboratory titrations. The most important aspect of CPAP use is supervision by a knowledgeable clinician; this supervision should include patient teaching before the laboratory titration, accurate interpretation of diagnostic and titration data, and support and careful patient follow-up, with necessary adjustments with symptomatic and clinical changes. It should be remembered that failure to obtain relief from daytime sleepiness and related symptoms may indicate poor compliance but also, perhaps, reflect an inaccurate diagnosis or the presence of additional diagnoses.[37,38] Numerous CPAP machines are currently available that can monitor the minute-by-minute delivery of positive pressure; the clinician can obtain a printout not only of daily compliance, but of the actual amounts of effective pressures that were delivered. This should lead to more rational and effective treatment follow-up and planning.

Similar to CPAP described above, some systems can be adjusted to deliver an inspiratory pressure higher than the expiratory pressure, thus bilevel positive airway pressure (bilevel PAP), or Bi-PAP, as commonly referred to by many clinicians. This latter terminology is a trade name of a specific manufacturer of such units and should not be used to describe the generic concept of bilevel PAP. While some data have suggested that less positive pressure is necessary to overcome upper airway resistance in expiration as opposed to inspiration,[39] in practice, increasing inspiratory pressure during CPAP titration rarely allows for decreased amounts of expiratory pressure, and there are no data documenting that such bilevel pressure promotes improved patient compliance. Indeed, when studied, similar compliance rates with CPAP and bilevel PAP were found.[40] Thus the clinician should not expect bilevel PAP to solve problems of comfort and compliance experienced with CPAP. On the other hand, the ability of bilevel PAP to provide higher inspiratory pressure (up to 35 cmH$_2$O with some models) than expiratory pressure may be useful for those OSA patients in whom severe sleep-related hypoxemia persists despite regular breathing and adequate restoration of upper airway patency with maximal levels of CPAP (Fig. 14-1) (see also "Obesity Hypoventilation" below). There are also OSA patients in whom the "central" component of the respiratory events predominates, and in whom CPAP does not provide adequate cessation of apneas and arousals. Bilevel PAP, with or without a backup rate, may be useful in this setting, although documentation of the efficacy of such therapy remains anecdotal.

Other Medical Modalities

Oxygen alone is generally not recommended as definitive treatment of OSA. Such treatment does not necessarily treat the likely cardiovascular perturbations of obstructed breathing, nor the sleep fragmentation of OSA,[41–43] and may result in longer apnea length and worsened alveolar hypoventilation.[44] However, oxygen therapy often will eliminate severe oxygen desaturation during sleep in OSA and in some cases actually may reduce the frequency of obstructive events.[45]

When CPAP is not tolerated or effective, sleep-related hypoxemia is severe, and tracheostomy is not felt to be a desirable option, we sometimes will consider a laboratory titration of oxygen alone. Oxygen alone also may be helpful in OSA patients with pronounced respiratory periodicity and borderline awake oxygen saturation. In all these cases, it is desirable to measure CO$_2$ levels during O$_2$ administration to be certain that severe hypercarbia is not occuring. Finally, we and others[45] have found it useful to add supplemental O$_2$ to the CPAP circuit during a titration when a certain level of positive airway pressure shows itself to be maximally effective in terms of regularizing breathing and establishing good sleep consolidation, but significant hypoxemia, either in non-REM or REM sleep, remains.

Pharmacologic therapy unfortunately has not proven to be of significant benefit in the treatment of OSA. Tricyclic antidepressants, particularly the less sedating ones, have been used in OSA, the theoretical basis being suppression of REM sleep, the sleep stage commonly associated with worsened sleep-disordered breathing and hypoxemia. There are also data to show that such medication may be associated with increased upper airway nerve and muscle activity.[46,47] In practice, however, these medications do not appear to provide great or lasting benefit,[47–49] particularly in more severe OSA, and side effects such as urinary retention, impotence, postural hypotension, sedation, and cardiac arrhythmia may prevent therapeutic levels from being achieved. Respiratory stimulants such as medroxyprogesterone, theophylline, and acetazolamide have not been shown consistently to be of therapeutic benefit in OSA, although they may be used when OSA overlaps with other awake and sleep-related hypoventilation syndromes.[50]

Surgical Approaches to the Treatment of OSA

TRACHEOSTOMY   Tracheostomy is the oldest method of treating OSA[51]; it is also the method other than CPAP that has been shown to decrease mortality in this disorder.[52] Because of the numerous complications potentially associated with chronic tracheostomy and the availability of CPAP, it is no longer desirable to recommend tracheostomy routinely in OSA, although this modality continues to be indicated in patients with severe OSA who cannot or will not use CPAP effectively. Patients with OSA and craniofacial abnormalities that anatomically prevent successful CPAP therapy, for example, may need to be considered for tracheostomy.

PALATAL SURGERY   Numerous pharyngeal surgical procedures designed to widen the pharyngeal airspace have been used in an attempt to definitively treat OSA. Uvulopalatopharyngoplasty (UPPP) is the most commonly performed and well studied of these procedures. Even in those patients "preselected" as retropalatal obstructors by using cephalometry, fiberoptic endoscopy with Mueller maneuver, and segmental upper airway pressure measurements,[53–55] few with OSA in the range associated with significant morbidity and increased mortality prior to surgery are left without significant OSA after surgery.[56] Perioperative and early and late postoperative complications can be significant.[57] At this time, the cost and morbidity of this procedure do not appear to be readily justified in patients with more than mild OSA, nor does it appear justified to consider UPPP alone as definitive

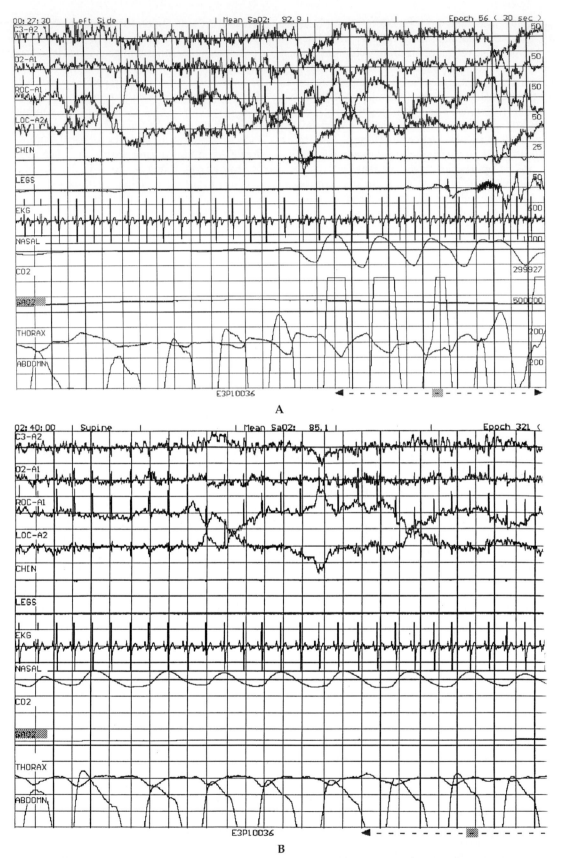

FIGURE 14-1 (*A*) Obstructive apnea in a 37-year-old man with obesity and hypersomnolence prior to treatment. C3-A2, O2-A1; central and occipital referential EEGs; ROC-A1, LOC-A2; right and left electrooculograms; NASAL, nasal/oral airflow; THORAX, thoracic respiratory effort; ABDOMN, abdominal respiratory effort. (*B*) Same patient during nasal continuous positive-airway pressure (CPAP) of 12 cmH₂O in REM sleep. Abbreviations are the same for (*A*). Respiration is regularized, without evidence of upper airway obstruction, and sleep quality is improved. However, REM-related hypoxemia, pictured here as 85 percent but falling as low as 65 percent at other times during REM continues.

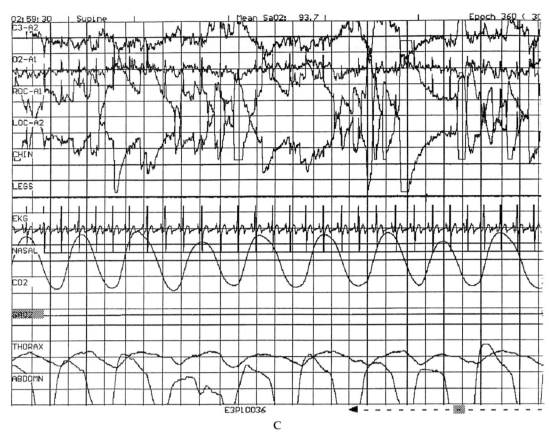

C

FIGURE 14-1 (*Continued*) (*C*) Same patient in REM sleep during nasal bilevel positive airway pressure (PAP) of 20 cmH$_2$O inspiratory pressure and 12 cmH$_2$O expiratory pressure. Abbreviations are the same as for (*A*). Sa$_{O_2}$ remains greater than 90 percent, with good sleep consolidation.

treatment for severe OSA. UPPP may make subsequent treatment with CPAP more difficult in some patients, possibly by creating increased air leak through the mouth, and compliance with CPAP, in turn, may suffer.[58] That UPPP may increase the subsequent efficacy of CPAP in some patients is also a reasonable possibility that remains to be investigated.

Much interesting work has been done to characterize the major site of upper airway obstruction and relate this to a specific surgical strategy. Utilizing UPPP for patients with retropalatal collapse, UPPP and inferior sagittal mandibular osteotomy and genioglossus advancement with hyoid myotomy and suspension for patients with combined retropalatal-retrolingual collapse, and inferior sagittal mandibular osteotomy and genioglossus advancement with hyoid myotomy and suspension alone for patients with retrolingual collapse as a first step, with the addition of maxillary, mandibular, and hyoid advancement to UPPP for others, some authors have reported high rates of meaningful responses in patients with even severe OSA. Responses were most impressive after the two-stage operations. Retropalatal obstructors, patients with lesser degrees of OSA, and less obese patients were more likely to have a good response.[59] Such an approach does not appear to be practical in most centers at the current time. Finally, in patients with OSA, medical complications can be expected peri- and postoperatively; cardiac arrhythmia was seen in 12 percent of patients in association with such surgeries in one series.[60]

Laser-assisted uvulopalatoplasty, a procedure developed for the treatment of snoring,[61] has gained rapid acceptance as an outpatient procedure for the treatment of OSA. Neither the efficacy nor the complications of this procedure have been established by adequate controlled studies, and this procedure is not currently recommended by the Standards of Practice Committee of the American Sleep Disorders Association,[62] nor by us, as treatment for OSA.

We cannot emphasize enough our feeling that implicit in the consideration of any of these surgeries for the treatment of OSA should be a sleep and/or respiratory expert's meaningful involvement in interpretation of polysomnographic data and assessment of the medical status of the patient regarding the ability to tolerate and benefit from such a procedure or procedures. The data are not sufficiently convincing at this point to encourage a patient with significant OSA to have any surgery done without the benefit of a thorough and meaningful attempt to use CPAP and achieve weight loss. Finally, careful follow-up, including polysomnography, should be agreed to by the patient and all treating clinicians prior to undertaking surgery for OSA. Follow-up should not rely solely on the patient and bed partner's report, which may underestimate postoperative sleep-disordered breathing and even the degree of snoring.[63]

Oral Appliances

The use of oral appliances in the treatment of OSA has been reviewed recently.[64] Oral appliances include a wide range of devices that widen the upper airway by changing mandible position or keeping the tongue from falling backward into the pharynx. Such devices may be thought of as possible noninvasive alternatives in the treatment of OSA patients who cannot or will not tolerate nasal CPAP. It also may be that such devices will prove to be useful as adjuncts to CPAP, but this is speculative at present. Overall, these devices appear to be better tolerated than nasal CPAP but not as effective in more compromised patients,[65] and in general, they demonstrate success rates similar to surgical therapies other than tracheostomy. As with surgical approaches, patients may have better success rates if screened; cephalometrics have appeared to be particularly useful in identifying patients with posterior airspace compromise who may more likely benefit from anterior mandibular positioning devices.[66]

Several investigators have had experimental success with stimulation of the genioglossus, an upper airway dilator muscle, in relieving upper airway obstruction during sleep.[67,68] While experimental results have been encouraging, routine clinical use of such therapy awaits further trials.[69]

OSA in the Elderly
Special note is made here concerning the treatment of OSA in elderly individuals. Morbidity, including cognitive impairment, and mortality of OSA have been difficult to define in elderly patients, despite the consistent reports of elevated apnea/hypopnea indices in this age group.[10,70] It should be noted that some data have in fact found increased mortality in elderly patients with OSA.[71] Diagnosis itself may be difficult; we have seen, for example, OSA diagnosed in elderly patients with predominant central apneas and frequent arousals with respiratory periodicity. It is our experience that CPAP therapy in this setting is, in general, poorly tolerated. Thus the diagnosis of OSA, the portent of such a diagnosis, and the efficacy of treatment of OSA in the elderly are particularly difficult to define at this time, and aggressive treatment strategies for OSA are not necessarily justified. The use of supplemental oxygen therapy alone in elderly patients with sleep-disordered breathing and a diagnosis of OSA requires further investigation but appears to have some rationale, particularly in those with prominent respiratory periodicity associated with transitions to sleep. If attempted, oxygen therapy should be monitored initially polysomnographically.

Summary
OSA is a relatively common and potentially life-threatening condition, particularly in patients with obstructive events of 10 per hour or more. Definitive therapy in such patients should be considered mandatory. Adjusting sleep position, weight loss, and attention to anatomic or physiologic upper airway defects are useful adjuncts in the treatment of OSA but rarely curative. Nasal positive airway pressure should be considered the therapy of first choice in all cases of significant OSA; surgery and oral appliances should be considered second-line therapies when and if nasal positive airway pressure is not effective. Patient education, careful prescription of CPAP, and attentive follow-up should be part of every CPAP experience. The clinician should be prepared for difficulties with compliance with CPAP and aware as well of concomitant respiratory and nonrespiratory illnesses and diagnoses that may be contributing to the overall syndrome of OSA and which may require adjustments to the positive airway pressure regimen or additional therapies.

UPPER AIRWAY RESISTANCE SYNDROME
The description of this entity grew out of the observation that in adults, just as in pediatric patients, repetitive or cyclic electroencephalographic (EEG) arousal without definable change in airflow or respiratory effort on standard polysomnography may occur, typically in the setting of known or suspected increased upper airway resistance due to anatomic or physiologic factors as well as complaints of daytime somnolence.[72] Such increased upper airway resistance may lead to arousals secondary to increased effort, chemostimulation, or mechanical stimulation without clear evidence of changed airflow or respiratory effort. Such a syndrome may occur even in the absence of prominent snoring. Accurate identification of such patients is difficult without sophisticated sleep studies. Although nasal CPAP has been described as treating this disorder successfully, there is no clear evidence that CPAP, even if successful in the laboratory, will be of long-term benefit.[72] Treatment of this disorder should include, as with OSA, consideration of treatment of anatomic and/or physiologic upper airway dysfunction, possible avoidance of the supine position, and weight loss, as well as consideration of problems with sleep deprivation or sleep schedule disorders that may be contributing to the patient's sleepiness.

CENTRAL SLEEP APNEA
The treatment of central sleep apnea, just as with obstructive sleep apnea, is as diverse and complicated as its etiologies. *Central sleep apnea* refers to a syndrome of repetitive pauses in respiration during sleep. One form of central sleep apnea occurs as an exaggeration of periodic breathing at sleep-wake transitioning and may be seen in patients with normo- and hypocapnia.[73] Such central sleep apnea is commonly seen in subjects at high altitude, as well as in elderly subjects. This syndrome also may be associated with frequent arousals due to pain and other chronic conditions and/or medications, which in turn predisposes to respiratory periodicity and central apnea at sleep transitions. Central sleep apnea in this setting may result in sleep fragmentation and complaints of disordered initiation and maintenance of sleep as well as excessive daytime somnolence; severe cardiorespiratory compromise during sleep is not typical. Treatment is often difficult. Supplemental oxygen, particularly where mild awake hypoxemia is present, has some rationale in that it may stabilize ventilation and improve sleep consolidation, but increased hypoventilation needs to be assessed during such therapy. Other strategies to better consolidate sleep, thus avoiding arousals and sleep-wake transitioning, may be tried. For example, sedatives have been used in this setting but, with their potential to cause worsening respiratory suppression and prolonged sedation, have limited usefulness.[74] Nasal CPAP in this setting may be tried but is not likely to be well tolerated chronically nor indeed to improve sleep quality in the long term. Respiratory stimulants have not been well studied for this condition but are unlikely to be well tolerated. In a small group of patients, the use of acetazolamide did result in improvement in sleep-disordered breathing and sleep quality.[75] Central sleep apnea also may overlap with OSA and may become particularly manifest during CPAP titration. In this situation, CPAP has been shown to have efficacy in treating both components of the sleep apnea,[76] but there are some patients who will not respond to CPAP in whom nocturnal positive-pressure ventila-

tion may be required, either with bilevel PAP in a ventilatory mode or with a ventilator set either for volume- or pressure-cycled ventilatory support.

Central sleep apnea, when associated with respiratory periodicity of the Cheyne-Stokes type, commonly occurs in the setting of congestive heart failure (CHF), renal insufficiency, and neurologic disorders, either congenital or acquired. A dramatic presentation of central sleep apnea is sometimes termed *Ondine's curse*—named for the legendary mermaid who afflicts her unfaithful lover with the need to consciously initiate each respiratory effort; this syndrome is typically a manifestation of cerebral or brain stem disease and may be thought of as a syndrome of central hypoventilation (see below). This condition generally will require assisted ventilation during sleep (Fig. 14-2). Such treatment may stabilize respiratory drive to the extent that awake respiration and gas exchange may stabilize or improve. However, it should be remembered that sleep and awake status may not be clinically or physiologically well delineated in such patients, who may thus be at risk of severe respiratory compromise at all times.

Treatment of Cheyne-Stokes respiration and central sleep apnea in the setting of CHF is well studied. The importance of such treatment, aside from the importance of treatment of the underlying disorder itself, derives from studies that have found increased mortality in CHF patients with Cheyne-Stokes breathing versus those without such breathing, the level of left ventricular dysfunction being similar.[77] Aside from using other modalities to control the underlying circulatory failure, the clinician should consider nasal CPAP as a possible therapy.[78] Its usefulness in this setting may derive from its ability to prevent upper airway collapse, which would otherwise tend to propagate arousals and periodicity.[79] Nasal CPAP may be effective in treating CSR in CHF even to the point of improvement in left ventricular function.[80,81] The treatment goal is to reduce the respiratory periodicity and onset of apnea. Oxygen administration alone in Cheyne-Stokes respiration with CHF may improve nocturnal hypoxemia as well as improve respiratory periodicity and sleep fragmentation.[82] CO_2 itself has been tried in this setting,[83] as have respiratory stimulants such as acetazolamide, theophylline, and progesterone; the efficacy of these treatments is not well established, particularly since side effects may outweigh or even override benefits.

HYPOVENTILATION SYNDROMES

PRIMARY AND CENTRAL ALVEOLAR HYPOVENTILATION

Primary alveolar hypoventilation refers to patients with awake hypoventilation without evidence of parenchymal lung disease, obesity, or chest wall or neuromuscular disorder. When a central nervous system (CNS) lesion is identifiable as the underlying cause of the hypoventilation, the term *central alveolar hypoventilation* is applied. The syndrome of central sleep apnea, as described above, may be considered a form of primary or central alveolar hypoventilation. Central alveolar hypoventilation syndromes are typically either congenital or sequelae of acquired CNS disease or damage. In both primary and central alveolar hypoventilation, sleep is typically associated with the most severe hypoventilation, since awake drive to breathe is lost and impaired metabolic control of respira-

tion remains as the main mediator of respiration.[3] Sleep evaluation, including polysomnography, should be considered in all patients diagnosed with primary or central alveolar hypoventilation. Ventilation during sleep may provide adequate amelioration of gas-exchange abnormality on a diurnal as well as nocturnal basis. Even when 24-h ventilation is necessary, the levels of required assisted ventilation may differ significantly when the patient is awake and asleep.

OBESITY HYPOVENTILATION

It has been recognized for many years that certain patients may have obesity, excessive daytime sleepiness, and awake gas-exchange abnormality, often with cor pulmonale. Formerly, such patients were likely to be referred to as *pickwickian*,[21,84] a term that has much literary but little clinical specificity. In current practice, the diagnosis of obstructive sleep apnea tends to be assumed in this situation. In reality, this clinical presentation is a difficult to define entity. When chronic alveolar hypoventilation is present in an obese patient without other specific respiratory or neuromuscular disorder, the term *obesity hypoventilation syndrome (OHS)* is commonly applied. Ventilatory responses tend to be blunted in such patients as compared with those with simple obesity,[85] thus potentially further contributing to sleep-related hypercarbia and hypoxemia associated with increasingly mismatched ventilation and perfusion and hypoventilation associated with abnormal respiratory mechanics. It is clear polysomnographically that such patients may have significant and even severe sleep hypoxemia and fragmentation yet show a spectrum ranging from little or no clinically significant increase in upper airway resistance during sleep to frequent decreases in airflow consistent with partial or total upper airway obstruction and arousal. Thus the sleep-related breathing disorder in such a patient appears to represent some overlap among obesity, obesity hypoventilation syndrome, and obstructive sleep apnea. Further, many such obese patients (male and female) will demonstrate typical features of OSA polysomnographically yet when titrated to maximally effective CPAP in non-REM sleep continue to display significant hypoxemia during REM sleep, even in the presence of regularized respiration (see Fig. 14-1A and B). It is not clear whether this represents hypoventilation or exaggerated ventilation-perfusion mismatch or both, but in such situations, bilevel PAP often can be applied successfully (see Fig. 14-1C). This therapy may allow upper airway patency throughout the respiratory cycle and thus regularized respiration and improved sleep architecture, as well as normoxemia, presumably on the basis of increased ventilation or increased recruitment of lung units. Many patients with OHS, with or without concomitant OSA, may be unable to tolerate such therapy on a long-term basis, and tracheostomy with ventilation needs to be considered in this situation. It is not known, in fact, whether positive-pressure ventilation, delivered either noninvasively or by tracheostomy, decreases long-term morbidity or mortality in this setting. Alternatives to increased pressure or volume to provide better Sa_{O_2} levels are to opt for lower levels of support with the addition of O_2 to the circuit. This is particularly rational when good sleep quality is achieved, respiration is regularized, but Sa_{O_2} remains unacceptably low, and increased ventilatory support results in increased arousals and fragmented sleep and perhaps worsened respiration as a result. The long-term effects

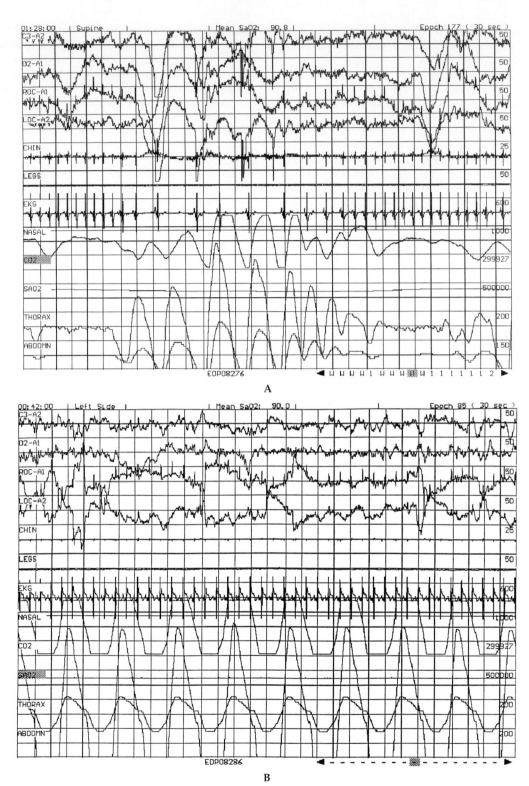

FIGURE 14-2 (*A*) A 45-year-old man with kyphoscoliosis, obesity, and type 2 Arnold-Chiari malformation, with hypersomnolence, recurrent syncope, and chronic awake hypoxemia (Pa_{O_2} = 56 mmHg) and hypercapnic (Pa_{CO_2} = 59 mmHg). Periodicity of respiratory effort, concurrent with periodic cycling between sleep and arousal, is displayed. This pattern continued throughout the night, with Sa_{O_2} falling to as low as 74 percent. Note the severe bradycardia during periods of increasing ventilation. C3-A2, O2-A1, central and occipital referential EEGs; ROC-A1, LOC-A2, right and left electrooculograms; NASAL, nasal/oral airflow; THORAX, thoracic respiratory effort; ABDOMN, abdominal respiratory effort. (*B*) Same patient during nasal bilevel positive airway pressure ventilation (inspiratory pressure = 20 H_2O, expiratory pressure = 8 cmH_2O, with a backup rate of 16 per minute) in REM sleep. Abbreviations are the same as for (*A*). Respiratory effort and ECG have become regular, sleep is well consolidated, and Sa_{O_2} is now 90 percent. Awake hypercapnia, hypersomnolence, and syncope were resolved at 1-month follow-up on this nocturnal regimen.

of using less ventilatory support but adding O_2, treatment with supplemental O_2 alone, or high ventilatory support without O_2 is unknown in this patient population, and it is difficult to extrapolate from data in chronic obstructive pulmonary disease (COPD) patients that show similar efficacy among such treatments.[86] With any of these measures, the issue of weight loss should be addressed continuously. We have seen hypoventilation reversed with loss of weight; conversely, patients who neither lose weight nor can be managed effectively with nocturnal ventilatory support appear to be at significant risk for chronic morbidity as well as sudden death.

As distinguished from OHS and sleep-disordered breathing as described above, some obese patients with awake hypoventilation and hypersomnolence associated with a prominent component of OSA may demonstrate reversal of sleep-disordered breathing and awake gas-exchange abnormality and sleepiness with CPAP or tracheostomy alone[87,88] and therefore do not require nocturnal ventilation. The choice of treatment modalities among the overlapping syndromes of severe sleep-disordered breathing described in the foregoing section is obviously as difficult as the distinction among the various diagnoses.

OTHER DISORDERS WITH SLEEP-RELATED HYPOVENTILATION

Alveolar hypoventilation may be a component of other disorders affecting both awake and sleep respiration; such disorders include neuromuscular disease and chronic obstructive pulmonary disease (COPD). The treatment of these other conditions of sleep-related hypoventilation is detailed in the following sections relating hypoventilation to specific accompanying respiratory disorders.

NEUROMUSCULAR DISORDERS

Disorders of the neuromuscular system generally have in common an awake respiratory pattern of rapid and shallow breathing with the use of accessory muscles of respiration. Such a pattern is likely to result in hypoventilation and exaggerated mismatching of ventilation and perfusion of lung units awake and thus significant hypoventilation and hypoxemia during sleep. Sleep fragmentation is also common in these disorders, undoubtedly mediated by the arousal-inducing chemical and mechanical stimuli of blood gas perturbations and increased work of breathing. Increased upper airway resistance or outright obstructive apnea also may occur.[89] Among the more common neuromuscular disorders associated with such sleep-disordered breathing are the muscular dystrophies, postpolio syndrome, multiple sclerosis, motor neuron disease, and traumatic spinal cord disorders. Cerebrovascular accident and other neurologic disorders, as outlined above under ''Central Sleep Apnea'' and ''Central Alveolar Hypoventilation,'' also may be considered in this category.

Except in cases of virtually normal awake gas exchange, it has been shown that patients with neuromuscular disease may have severe sleep-related oxygen desaturation, and as with other disorders of hypoxemia during sleep, awake parameters may not accurately predict which patients will show the most severe desaturations.[90] What may not be intuitive regarding this situation is that providing ventilatory support during sleep can improve 24-h respiratory functioning and quality of life; this latter may include reversal of awake gas-exchange abnormalities and/or daytime hypersomnolence.[91] As with OSA and other disorders discussed in this chapter in which hypoventilation and hypoxemia occur awake and/or asleep, the use of supplemental oxygen alone during sleep is often not sufficient therapy and may worsen hypoventilation and hypercarbia. Reversal of acute respiratory failure by both invasive and noninvasive ventilation has been well documented in virtually all clinical situations of hypercapnic respiratory failure, although the utility of nocturnal ventilation alone in such situations is not established.[92] Nocturnal ventilation, both invasive and noninvasive, does have established efficacy in treating chronic respiratory insufficiency and hypoventilation due to restrictive defect, including that of neuromuscular disease.[93–96] There are no firm data regarding the decision as to when to initiate nocturnal ventilation for chronic respiratory insufficiency, however. Current strategies generally include awake hypercarbia as one indication. Symptoms associated with sleep-related hypoventilation and/or sleep disruption (which would include morning headache and daytime fatigue or somnolence) or polysomnographic evidence of nocturnal hypoxemia, increased work of breathing, or sleep fragmentation also would be reasonable criteria. It is difficult to clearly demonstrate increased survival with nocturnal ventilation due in part to the heterogeneous nature of these disorders and their variable progression. Nevertheless, some data and the experience of numerous clinicians are encouraging in this regard.[97]

As referred to earlier, nocturnal ventilation can be accomplished via tracheostomy (i.e., invasive), via negative pressure applied to the thorax, or with positive pressure via a mask applied to the nose, mouth, or full face.[98,99] Tracheostomy complications are considerable, ranging from local pain and irritation, the need for frequent suctioning, infection, hemorrhage, and mucus plugging, to chronic pulmonary aspiration. The presence of a tracheostomy also makes assisted coughing difficult, important in such patients for preventing pulmonary complications. In all, tracheostomy ventilation may be poorly tolerated long term by many patients, although some patients actually may find such ventilation more comfortable. The clinician should not hesitate to recommend tracheostomy-assisted nocturnal ventilation when such ventilation is indicated and noninvasive ventilation is not successful.

While negative-pressure ventilation has been a successful noninvasive therapy for many years, this mode of ventilatory support during sleep may present difficulties for some patients with neuromuscular disorders. The cuirass may be difficult to fit in and sleep in comfortably, and any system of negative-pressure ventilation risks provoking upper airway obstruction during inspiration, particularly during REM sleep.[96] Likewise, the rocking bed is not conducive to good sleep quality, and its role in nocturnal ventilation is thereby limited. Diaphragm pacing has been used in congenital central hypoventilation syndromes and in spinal cord lesions; as with negative-pressure ventilation, the upper airway is prone to collapse during pacing, and tracheostomy is generally required. This method is also very expensive. Its use as a method of nocturnal ventilation is not well established.[100]

Nocturnal noninvasive ventilation via positive airway pressure applied to a face mask now has almost 10 years of documented successful application to patients with restrictive ventilatory defects and chronic respiratory failure. Such ventilation can be delivered via nasal, oral, or oronasal interface,[98] and this mode of ventilation is probably the therapy of first choice in patients with neuromuscular disorders who can tolerate it (Fig. 14-3). Upper airway muscle function must be intact in order to clear secretions and prevent relapse of soft tissue. With volume-cycled ventilation, we prefer to begin with assist control mode, using a backup rate of 2 to 4 breaths per minute higher than the average spontaneous respiratory rate during which Sa_{O_2} is consistently low. Adjustment of the inspiratory time is important. Leak from around the mask or through the mouth is common with nasal masks in particular, and some leak must be tolerated; thus effective volumes are typically considerably higher than those set for invasive ventilation. Pressure alarms generally are not useful in this setting and indeed may be sleep-disrupting to the patient. We usually ask that these alarms be set at zero for the low and 100 cmH_2O for the high pressure alarms. For bilevel positive airway pressure machines, we generally ventilate with expiratory positive airway pressures (EPAP) set as low as possible in order to abolish any upper airway collapse while improving functional residual capacity; usually, EPAP will be in the 6 to 10 cmH_2O range, and the IPAP will be 20 cmH_2O or possibly higher if necessary and the particular machine allows it. Backup rates are provided similar to assist control modes. It should be pointed out that these settings are arrived at throughout a night of titration, using quality of sleep consolidation, Sa_{O_2} levels, and often transcutaneous CO_2 levels as titration parameters. As with all disorders of hypoventilation, one cannot always aim to completely reverse hypoventilation and hypoxemia during sleep by increasing ventilatory rate, volume, or pressure, particularly if such increased support comes at the expense of worsened sleep. We generally do not place arterial catheters for blood gas measurements but usually will obtain awake arterial blood gases in the evening before and the morning after ventilation titrations.

As with CPAP, all positive-pressure ventilatory setups must be checked often to see that the interface is sufficient to avoid leak. Leak of air from the mouth is common during nasal ventilation, and numerous types of chin straps are available that may ameliorate this problem. The addition of a warm air humidifier to the PAP circuit may be very helpful in preventing nasal dryness and irritation, particularly in the winter months.

For all patients undergoing nocturnal positive-pressure ventilation and particularly during nocturnal ventilation via tracheostomy, the risk of hyperventilation and severe alkalosis is present, particularly if the patient is awake for a prolonged time. Conversely, levels of necessary ventilatory support actually may be less during sleep than awake in some patients who are not able to coordinate respiratory efforts with the ventilator awake, while such coordination is quite characteristic once consolidated sleep is attained.

For all clinical syndromes requiring nocturnal ventilatory support, the patient must be included as a decision maker, and the clinician must be flexible enough to consider changing modes of ventilation, as well as interfaces, as the need arises. Further, many of these disorders may involve progressive defects, either neurologic or thoracic, despite nocturnal ventilation, and the efficacy of a chosen therapy should be assessed carefully at appropriate intervals. Clinical goals should include decreased fatigue or reversal of outright sleepiness, improved nocturnal sleep, and improved or stable respiratory function as supported by awake arterial blood gas testing.

DISORDERS OF THE CHEST WALL

Much of what has been noted earlier for sleep-disordered breathing related to neuromuscular disorders may be applied to patients with restrictive ventilatory defects due to disorders of the chest wall. The prototype and most common of these conditions is kyphoscoliosis.[101] While alveolar hypoventilation is of particular concern, this condition is also associated with obstructive apneas during sleep,[102] again emphasizing the theoretical advantage of positive-pressure over negative-pressure ventilation. Nocturnal titration aims, as with the neuromuscular disorders, include regularization of respiration, blunting of hypoventilation, prevention of hypoxemia, and establishment of good sleep consolidation.

INTERSTITIAL LUNG DISEASE

The treatment of sleep-disordered breathing in patients with interstitial lung disease in many ways may be considered similar to that of patients with COPD, as discussed below.[103,104] Sleep-related hypoxemia may be severe and may not always correlate with awake Sa_{O_2} levels, particularly in REM sleep.[105] If loud snoring, other clinical evidence of OSA, or sequellae of hypoxemia out of proportion to awake Pa_{O_2} exists, polysomnography should be considered. Neither nocturnal O_2 supplementation for patients without indications for awake supplementation nor nocturnal ventilation has been well studied in terms of survival benefit in patients with interstitial lung disease. However, given the commonly seen morbidity and mortality related to cor pulmonale, and extrapolating from supplemental oxygen trials in COPD,[106,107] prevention of severe nocturnal hypoxemia as well as possible hypoventilation may well be interventions that generally have been overlooked in the treatment of such patients.[103,105] We have noted frequent idiopathic arousals leading to significant sleep fragmentation in patients with interstitial lung disease, particularly sarcoidosis, with and without the use of steroids. It is unclear that any specific intervention, other than protecting the sleep period from external interruption, would be of benefit in this situation once severe nocturnal hypoxemia is ruled out.

OBSTRUCTIVE DISORDERS OF THE LARGE AIRWAYS

ASTHMA

The major point concerning treatment of sleep-related bronchospasm is that the severity of the nocturnal disorder is correlated with awake lung function. Thus therapeutic intervention in nocturnal asthma most rationally focuses on control of daytime signs and symptoms. Attention to upper airway congestion, secretions, and irritation should be included, particularly since these may predispose not only to worsened nocturnal bronchospasm but also to sleep-related obstructive apnea. Aside from this, the timing and duration of pharmacologic therapy for asthma must be considered, since both sleep and circadian variations appear to play a

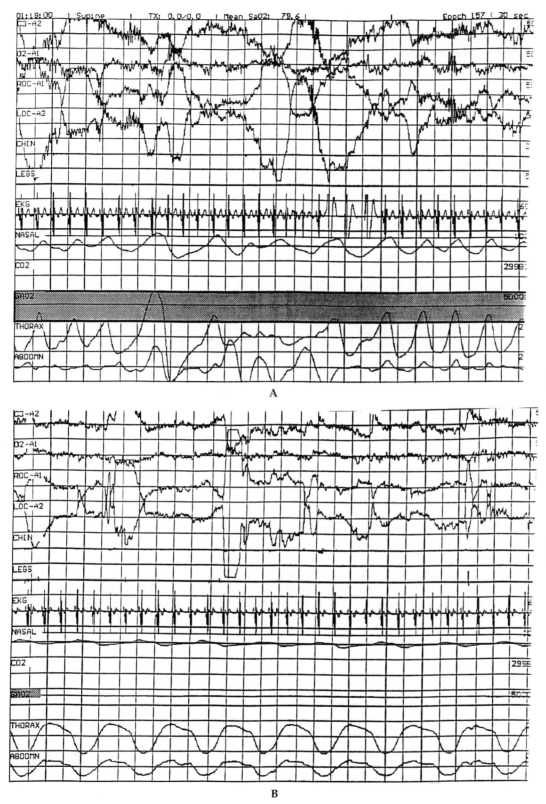

FIGURE 14-3 (*A*) Severe hypoxemia during rapid eye movement (REM) sleep in a 40-year-old woman with a severe restrictive ventilatory defect secondary to neuromuscular disease. C3-A2, O2-A1, central and occipital referential EEGs; ROC-A1, LOC-A2, right and left electrooculograms; NASAL, nasal/oral airflow; THORAX, thoracic respiratory effort; ABDOMN, abdominal respiratory effort. Mean oxygen saturation of hemoglobin (Sa$_{O_2}$) is less than 80 percent for this 30-s epoch. Note the markedly irregular respiratory effort and wide, complex ectopy. (*B*) Same patient in REM sleep during nasal intermittent positive pressure ventilation. Abbreviations are the same as for (*A*). Respiration is regular at the backup rate of 16 per minute; mean Sa$_{O_2}$ is 94 percent for this epoch.

role in the tendency for bronchospasm and airways resistance to worsen at night.[108] Nocturnal asthma may be associated with significant oxygen desaturation,[109,110] and there is evidence that asthma fatalities are most likely to occur during the night.[111,112] The use of inhaled bronchodilators immediately before bedtime is recommended for nocturnal worsening of asthma, and systemic steroids should be used when necessary. Inhaled steroids have efficacy in controlling both diurnal and nocturnal asthma and may be inherently less sleep disruptive than other therapies. There are also studies suggesting that afternoon dosing of prednisone may be the most efficacious method of using oral steroids in patients with nocturnal asthma.[113] If these interventions do not suffice, longer-acting bronchodilators, both inhaled and oral, may be more efficacious than standard preparations, although high doses of such agents have the potential of being sleep-disruptive.[114] Some authors have found that different long-acting theophylline preparations have varying efficacies in controlling nocturnal decreases in airflow as well as symptoms, and in particular, regimens that allow higher theophylline levels during the night may be most effective in treating asthma-related sleep-disordered breathing without causing added sleep disruption. This again demonstrates that the pharmacokinetics of each medication used must be taken into account when treating nocturnal asthma.[115] It has been suggested that supplemental oxygen may benefit patients with nocturnal hypoxemia due to asthma, but there are few data to judge overall efficacy and safety of oxygen therapy in this setting. Nasal CPAP has not been found to be of benefit in nocturnal asthma without concommitant OSA (see below). Other disorders of sleep that may be present and mimic nocturnal asthma should be considered in patients with difficult-to-control nocturnal asthma, such as OSA, disorders of nocturnal hypoventilation (see above), sleep-related laryngospasm, sleep-choking syndrome, and gastroesophageal reflux.[37,38] The clinician should be aware that the medications most commonly effective for nocturnal asthma are in fact likely to themselves be sleep-disruptive. Further, the sleep of patients with nocturnal asthma often shows a pattern of idiopathic arousals and/or paroxysmal EEG alpha, or awake, activity that may be associated with nonrestorative sleep despite the clinician's success in treating nocturnal bronchospasm and hypoxemia.[109]

ASTHMA AND OSA OVERLAP

Asthma and OSA may be coexistent causes of sleep-disordered breathing. Asthmatic breathing during sleep can mimic OSA, even in the sleep laboratory. Recognition of the coexistence of these two entities in a given patient may be difficult, but it is important to do so; the successful treatment of one cannot be ensured without treatment of the other. Sleep disruption due to nocturnal asthma may lead to respiratory periodicity and decreased upper airway muscle dilator activity, each of which may predispose to OSA. At the same time, irritation of the upper airways, mouth breathing, and hypoxemia occurring in OSA could predispose to increased bronchial reactivity. Apart from the general treatment considerations of nocturnal asthma described above, nasal CPAP has been shown to improve nocturnal symptoms as well as to improve daytime pulmonary function up to 2 weeks after initiating therapy in a small group of patients with OSA and asthma.[116] Conversely, when CPAP has been attempted in patients with nocturnal asthma without OSA, there has been a decrement in sleep quality.[117] CPAP should be used with caution during acute expiratory airflow obstruction because barotrauma is a potential risk. Warm air humidification in conjunction with the CPAP circuit may benefit the asthmatic patient by preventing airway cooling and desiccation that may otherwise occur with this therapy.

CHRONIC OBSTRUCTIVE PULMONARY DISEASE

Nocturnal Oxygen and Nocturnal Ventilation

Chronic obstructive pulmonary disease (COPD) commonly contributes to significant sleep-disordered breathing. Sleep fragmentation is common, likely contributing to further overall worsening of respiratory function as well as quality of life. A typical (though by no means inclusive) pattern in patients with COPD is awake-sleep transitions associated with respiratory periodicity and decreases in airflow (obstructive and central), non-REM sleep fragmentation with arousals that may be associated with cough or secondary to increased work of breathing and chemoresponses to fluctuations in Pa_{O_2} and Pa_{CO_2}, and markedly irregular breathing with significant and sometimes severe hypoxemia in REM sleep.[118] The particular tendency to impaired respiration in REM sleep in patients with COPD is likely multifactorial and similar in pathophysiology to patients with neuromuscular and other restrictive defects: hypoventilation due to blunted respiratory drive and responsiveness, increased upper airway resistance, loss of accessory muscles of respiration, and exaggerated ventilation-perfusion mismatching due to decreased functional residual capacity, bronchospasm, and decreased clearance of airway secretions. Do such potential abnormalities in respiration require additional identification and treatment in COPD patients other than the supplemental oxygen they may already be receiving for awake hypoxemia? Studies have demonstrated the benefits of including nocturnal O_2 in the regimen of patients with awake hypoxemia,[106,107] and to the extent that asleep Sa_{O_2} nadirs in COPD patients have been found to decrease linearly, and thus predictably, according to mean daytime levels,[119] the degree of nocturnal hypoxemia is generally correlated with nocturnal hypoxemia. Furthermore, the degree of sleep-related hypoxemia has not been found to be more sensitive than the levels of awake hypoxemia in predicting mortality.[119] Therefore, sleep studies have not been routinely recommended in COPD patients,[119,120] and specific levels and duration of sleep-related hypoxemia are commonly ignored in favor of treating patients with 24-h levels of supplemental O_2 based on O_2 flows that maintain Sa_{O_2} above 90 percent awake, perhaps increasing the flow rate slightly during sleep compared with awake rates. However, there are numerous problems with such an approach to therapy in patients with COPD, particularly in a growingly aggressive environment in which lung-reduction surgery and lung transplant are being offered as treatment options in patients with severe COPD.[121] There is considerable variation in the general correlation between awake Sa_{O_2} and REM Sa_{O_2} nadirs, and patients who may desaturate most severely may not be identified by awake Sa_{O_2} levels.[122] Studies have not necessarily addressed REM sleep; further, it is often observed that REM periods themselves may be different in terms of REM density and degree of REM-related sleep-disordered breathing in the same patient on a given night of study. There are not sufficient data regarding these patterns of hypoxemia in sleep to rule out an additive effect of REM hypoxemia on mortality in COPD; further, not only volume and density of REM but also CO_2 and pH levels during sleep are issues that have received little attention in patients with COPD. Even the long-term effects of identifying and treating coexisting upper airway obstruction during sleep in COPD patients has not been fully investigated (see "COPD/OSA Overlap" below). Additionally, oxygen alone in COPD patients is not likely to completely resolve nocturnal hypoxemia, does not tend to improve sleep quality or overall gas exchange, and in fact may worsen nocturnal hypoventilation.[86] Further, decreased mortality is only one of several legitimate end points in treating sleep-disordered breathing in COPD patients; effects on dyspnea, lung function, and exercise tolerance, as well as daytime sleepiness and mood, have received little attention in this regard. Because the sleep-disordered breathing of patients with COPD is, to some extent, a disorder of hypoventilation, it seems reasonable to examine attempts at nocturnal ventilation in this disorder, in a fashion analogous to the treatment of nocturnal hypoventilation discussed earlier. In fact, noninvasive ventilatory support has been attempted in both acute and chronic respiratory failure in patients with COPD. Negative pressure cannot be considered in many patients due to diathesis toward upper airway obstruction[123]; however, there are data to document that such ventilation in COPD patients with severe hypercapnia can improve respiratory function.[124] Recent randomized, controlled data have demonstrated improved quality of life and awake and sleeping gas exchange at 3-month follow-up in hypercapnic COPD patients treated with nasal nocturnal bilevel positive pressure ventilation and oxygen compared with oxygen alone; tolerance of the equipment was generally good.[125] Additionally, nasal positive-pressure ventilation has been found to improve gas exchange and result in lower complications, hospital days, and mortality in patients admitted to the intensive care unit with acute worsening of respiratory function as compared with standard therapy in similar patients.[126] Opposing data also have been published, including failure to achieve improved awake or asleep gas exchange or sleep quality after 3 months of nasal pressure-support ventilation,[127] along with inability to tolerate the treatment in many patients. Similarly, such ventilatory support was not found to be superior to oxygen alone in improving sleep quality or nocturnal Sa_{O_2}, nor was there improvement in awake gas exchange at 2 weeks in similarly ventilated patients.[86] Of note, all the above-referenced studies used nasal pressure support from a bilevel positive-pressure device using a maximal inspiratory pressure of 20 cmH_2O. Such a regimen is not ideally suited to provide ventilation in all patients, and it may be that pressure- or volume-cycled support with a ventilator may be more effective in some patients. Newer bilevel devices, as mentioned earlier, are now available that give the option of providing up to 35 cmH_2O inspiratory support. At the present time, from these studies it appears that COPD patients most likely to achieve improvement in awake or asleep gas exchange and/or quality of life from nocturnal ventilatory support are those with severe awake hypercapnia ($Pa_{CO_2} \geq 55$ mmHg) and/or with a demonstrably deteriorating clinical course.[128,129] Improvement in long-term survival with any nocturnal ventilatory mode, including use of a tracheostomy tube to accomplish nocturnal positive-pressure ventilation, remains to be demonstrated in this patient population. Nasal CPAP itself may improve work of breathing and concomitant dyspnea but has no significant role in the treatment of sleep-disordered breathing in patients with COPD without demonstrated upper airway obstruction during sleep. When embarking on nasal ventilation in COPD patients, one must be vigilant regarding bronchospasm, secretions, and cardiac function. Even when such therapy can be demonstrated to be effective under conditions of close supervision, such as in the sleep laboratory or ICU, long-term success with such a regimen at home is likely to be limited by discomfort with the mask and pressure, the tendency for leak via the mask or mouth to occur, and patient motivation and compliance.

Other Therapies

Numerous pharmacologic agents have been used in the treatment of sleep-disordered breathing related to COPD. Tricyclic antidepressants, just as in OSA, would appear rational in terms of decreasing REM sleep, but there are no compelling data to show significant improvement in gas exchange or survival with this therapy, and side effects remain limiting.[130] Similarly, there are few studies documenting efficacy of respiratory stimulant agents in improving nocturnal gas exchange or long-term survival or quality of life, and these agents also generally have significant side effects.[131] The roles of lung transplant and lung-reduction surgery in ameliorating sleep-disordered breathing related to COPD remain to be investigated.

Summary

While up to now supplemental O_2 has been the mainstay of treatment for sleep-disordered breathing in patients with COPD, the therapeutic imperatives are likely more complicated than previously thought, and more comprehensive treatment of hypoxemia and hypoventilation during sleep, as well as sleep disruption, not only may be feasible but indeed may be more beneficial than oxygen supplementation alone for some patients. The indications for and efficacy of nocturnal noninvasive ventilation should be considered in the assessment of COPD patients, particularly in the case of severe hypercapnia or clinical deterioration.

COPD/OSA OVERLAP

As with asthma and OSA, there is overlap between OSA and COPD. Although the overall prevalence of OSA in COPD is not known, in a recent trial of noninvasive nocturnal ventilation in COPD patients with a forced expiratory volume in 1 s (FEV_1) of less than 1 L, 4 of 23 patients were found to have OSA such that they were not randomized.[127] Prospective trials of CPAP and/or other positive-pressure modalities in this situation are not currently available and need to be done, but the significant prevalence of OSA/COPD overlap argues for considering polysomnography in patients with COPD, since treatment of the OSA with CPAP presumably would be beneficial in this situation. Further, when OSA coexists with COPD, the use of supplemental O_2 alone during sleep may be associated with prolongation of apneas and / or with a greater rise in sleep-related Pa_{CO_2} than that occurring in COPD alone.[132,133]

References

1. Rosen RC, Rosekind M, Rosevear C, et al: Physician education in sleep and sleep disorders: a national survey of U.S. medical schools. *Sleep* 16:249, 1993.
2. Dement WC (chairman): *Wake up America: A National Sleep Alert,* vol I: *Executive Summary and Report of the National Commission on Sleep Disorders Research.* Washington: U.S. Government Printing Office, 1993.
3. Phillipson EA: Control of breathing during sleep. *Am Rev Respir Dis* 118:909, 1978.
4. Önal E, Lopata M: Periodic breathing and the pathogenesis of occlusive sleep apneas. *Am Rev Respir Dis* 126:676, 1982.
5. Lopes JM, Tabachnik E, Muller NL, et al: Total airway resistance and respiratory muscle activity during sleep. *J Appl Physiol* 54: 773, 1983.
6. Young T, Palta M, Dempsey J, et al: Occurrence of sleep-disordered breathing among middle-aged adults. *N Engl J Med* 328: 1230, 1993.
7. Olson LG, King MT, Hensley MJ, Saunders NA: A community study of snoring and sleep-disordered breathing. *Am J Respir Crit Care Med* 152:711, 1995.
8. He J, Kryger MH, Zorick FJ, et al: Mortality and apnea index in obstructive sleep apnea: Experience in 385 male patients. *Chest* 94:9, 1988.
9. Partinen M, Jamieson A, Guilleminault C: Long-term outcome for obstructive sleep apnea syndrome patients: Mortality. *Chest* 94:1200, 1988.
10. Lavie P, Herer P, Peled R, et al: Mortality in sleep apnea patients: A multivariate analysis of risk factors. *Sleep* 18:149, 1995.
11. Aldrich MS: Automobile accidents in patients with sleep disorders. *Sleep* 12:487, 1989.
12. Findley LJ, Levinson MP, Bonnie RJ: Driving performance and automobile accidents in patients with sleep apnea. *Clin Chest Med* 13:427, 1992.
13. Findley LJ, Unverzagt ME, Suratt PM: Automobile accidents involving patients with obstructive sleep apnea. *Am Rev Respir Dis* 138:337, 1988.
14. Findley L, Fabrizio M, Thommi G, Suratt PM: Severity of sleep apnea and automobile crashes. *N Engl J Med* 320:868, 1989.
15. Carskadon MA, Dement WC, Mitler MM, et al: Guidelines for the Multiple Sleep Latency Test (MSLT): A standard measure of sleepiness. *Sleep* 9:519, 1986.
16. Strobel RJ, Rosen RC: Obesity and weight loss in obstructive sleep apnea: A critical review. *Sleep* 19:104, 1996.
17. Guilleminault C, Tilkian A, Dement WC: The sleep apnea syndromes. *Ann Rev Med* 27:465, 1976.
18. Issa FG, Sullivan CE: Alcohol, snoring, and sleep apnea. *Neurol Neurosurg Psychiatry* 45:353, 1982.
19. Scrima L, Broudy M, Nay K, Cohn MA: Increased severity of obstructive sleep apnea after bedtime alcohol ingestion: Diagnostic potential and proposed mechanisms of actions. *Sleep* 5: 318, 1982.
20. Bonora M, St John WM, Bledsoe TA: Differential elevation by protriptyline and depression by diazepam of upper airway respiratory motor activity. *Am Rev Respir Dis* 13:41, 1985.
21. Hishikawa Y, Furuya E, Wakamatsu H: Hypersomnia and periodic respiration: Presentation of two cases and comment on the physiopathogenesis of the pickwickian syndrome. *Folia Psychiatr Neurol Jpn* 24:163, 1970.
22. Catlin G: *The Breath of Life.* London, Trubner, 1862, p 72.
23. Lavie P: Rediscovering the importance of nasal breathing in sleep or, shut your mouth and save your sleep. *J Laryngol Otol* 101:558, 1987.
24. Basner RC, Ringler J, Berkowitz S, et al: Effect of inspired air temperature on genioglossus activity during nose breathing in awake humans. *J Appl Physiol* 69:1098, 1990.
25. Gleeson K, Zwilich CW, Braier K, White DP: Breathing route during sleep. *Am Rev Respir Dis* 134:115, 1986.
26. Olsen KD, Kern EB: Nasal influences on snoring and obstructive sleep apnea. *Mayo Clin Proc* 65:1095, 1990.
27. Sher AE: The upper airway in obstructive sleep apnea syndrome: Pathology and surgical management, in Thorpy MJ (ed): *Handbook of Sleep Disorders.* New York, Marcel Dekker, 1990, pp 311–335.
28. Cartwright RD: Effect of position on sleep apnea therapy. *Sleep* 110:7, 1984.
29. Sullivan CE, Berthon-Jones M, Issa FG: Remission of severe obesity-hypoventilation syndrome after short-term treatment during sleep with nasal continuous positive airway pressure. *Am Rev Respir Dis* 128:177, 1983.
30. Sullivan CE, Issa FG, Berthon-Jones M, et al: Home treatment of obstructive sleep apnea with continuous positive airway pressure applied through a nose mask. *Bull Eur Physiopathol Respir* 20:49, 1984.
31. Rajagopal KR, Bennett LL, Dillard TA, et al: Overnight nasal CPAP improves hypersomnolence in sleep apnea. *Chest* 90: 172, 1986.
32. Kribbs NB, Pack AI, Kline LR, et al: Effects of one night without nasal CPAP treatment on sleep and sleepiness in patients with obstructive sleep apnea. *Am Rev Respir Dis* 147:1162, 1993.
33. Kribbs NB, Pack AI, Kline LR, et al: Objective measurement of patterns of nasal CPAP use by patients with obstructive sleep apnea. *Am Rev Respir Dis* 147:887, 1993.
34. Stepanski EJ, Dull R, Basner RC: CPAP titration protocols among accredited sleep disorders centers. *Sleep Res* 25:374, 1996.
35. Lamphere J, Roehrs T, Wittig R, et al: Recovery of alertness after CPAP in apnea. *Chest* 96:1364, 1989.
36. Berthon-Jones M: Feasibility of a self-setting CPAP machine. *Sleep* 16:S120, 1993.
37. Basner RC, Önal E: Dealing with the differential diagnosis of obstructive sleep apnea syndrome. *Comp Ther* 20:273, 1994.
38. Thorpy MJ (chair), Diagnostic Classification Steering Committee: *International Classification of Sleep Disorders: Diagnostic and Coding Manual.* Lawrence, Kansas, Allen Press, 1990.
39. Sanders MH, Moore SE: Inspiratory and expiratory partitioning of airway resistance during sleep in patients with sleep apnea. *Am Rev Respir Dis* 127:554, 1983.
40. Reeves-Hoche MK, Hudgel D, Meck R, Zwillich CW: Continuous versus bilevel positive airway pressure for obstructive sleep apnea. *Am J Respir Crit Care Med* 151:443, 1995.
41. Tilkian AG, Guilleminault C, Schroeder JS, et al: Hemodynamics in sleep induced apnea. *Ann Intern Med* 85:714, 1976.
42. Buda AJ, Schroeder JS, Guilleminault C: Abnormalities of pulmonary artery wedge pressures in sleep-induced apnea. *Int J Cardiol* 1:67, 1981.
43. Ringler J, Basner RC, Shannon R, et al: Hypoxemia alone does not explain blood pressure elevations after obstructive apneas. *J Appl Physiol* 69:2143, 1990.
44. Fletcher EC, Munafo DA: Role of nocturnal oxygen therapy in obstructive sleep apnea. When should it be used? *Chest* 98: 1497, 1990.
45. Chan CS, Grunstein RR, Bye PTP, et al: Obstructive sleep apnea with severe chronic airflow limitation: Comparison of hypercapnic and eucapnic patients. *Am Rev Respir Dis* 140:1274, 1989.
46. Bonora M, St John WM, Bledsoe TA: Differential elevation by protriptyline and depression by diazepam of upper airway respiratory motor activity. *Am Rev Respir Dis* 13:41, 1985.
47. Smith PL, Haponik EF, Allen RP, Bleecker ER: The effects of

protriptyline in sleep disordered breathing. *Am Rev Respir Dis* 127:8, 1983.

48. Hanzell DA, Proia NG, Hudgel DW: Response of obstructive sleep apnea to fluoxetine and protriptyline. *Chest* 100:416, 1983.

49. Brownell LG, Perez-Padilla R, West P, Kryger MH: The role of protriptyline in obstructive sleep apnea. *Bull Eur Physiopathol Respir* 19:621, 1983.

50. Cook WR, Benich J, Wooten SA: Indices of severity of obstructive sleep apnea syndrome do not change during medroxyprogesterone therapy. *Chest* 96:262, 1989.

51. Fairbanks DNF: Tracheostomy for obstructive sleep apnea. Indications and techniques, in Fairbanks DNF, Fujita S (eds): *Snoring and Obstructive Sleep Apnea.* New York, Raven Press, 1994, pp 169–177.

52. Partinen M, Guilleminault C: Daytime sleepiness and vascular morbidity at seven-year follow-up in obstructive sleep apnea patients. *Chest* 97:27, 1989.

53. Rojewski TE, Schuller DE, Clark RW, et al: Videoendoscopic determination of the mechanism of obstruction in obstructive sleep apnea. *Otolaryngol Head Neck Surg* 92:127, 1984.

54. Sher AE, Thorpy MJ, Shprintzen RJ, et al: Predictive value of Mueller's maneuver in selection of patients for uvulopalatopharyngoplasty. *Laryngoscope* 95:1483, 1985.

55. Ryan CF, Dickson RI, Lowe AA, et al: Upper airway measurements predict response to uvulopalatopharyngoplasty in obstructive sleep apnea. *Laryngoscope* 100:248, 1990.

56. Sher AE, Schechtman KB, Piccirillo JF: The efficacy of surgical modifications of the upper airway in adults with obstructive sleep apnea syndrome. *Sleep* 19:156, 1996.

57. Fairbanks DN: UPPP complications and avoidance strategies. *Otolaryngol Head Neck Surg* 102:239, 1990.

58. Waldhorn RE, Herrick TW, Nguyen MC, et al: Long-term compliance with nasal continuous positive airway pressure therapy of obstructive sleep apnea. *Chest* 97:33, 1990.

59. Riley RW, Powell NB, Guilleminault C: Obstructive sleep apnea syndrome: A review of 306 consecutively treated surgical patients. *Otolaryngol Head Neck Surg* 108:117, 1993.

60. Waite PD, Wooten V, Lachner J, Guyette RF: Maxillo-mandibular advancement surgery in 23 patients with obstructive sleep apnea syndrome. *J Oral Maxillofac Surg* 47:1256, 1989.

61. Kamami YV: Laser CO_2 for snoring: Preliminary results. *Acta Otorhinolaryngol Belg* 44:451, 1990.

62. An American Sleep Disorders Association Report: Practice parameters for the use of laser-assisted uvulopalatoplasty. *Sleep* 17:744, 1994.

63. Miljeteig H, Mateika S, Haight JS, et al: Subjective and objective assessment of uvulopalatopharyngoplasty for treatment of snoring and obstructive sleep apnea. *Am J Respir Crit Care Med* 150:1286, 1994.

64. Schmidt-Nowara W, Lowe A, Wiegand L, et al: Oral appliances for the treatment of snoring and obstructive sleep apnea: A review. *Sleep* 18:501, 1995.

65. Clark GT, Blumenfeld I, Yoffe N, et al: A crossover study comparing the efficacy of continuous positive airway pressure with anterior mandibular positioning devices on patients with obstructive sleep apnea. *Chest* 109:1477, 1996.

66. Eveloff SE, Rosenberg CL, Carlisle CC, Millman RP: Efficacy of a Herbst mandibular advancement device in obstructive sleep apnea. *Am J Respir Crit Care Med* 149:905, 1994.

67. Miki H, Hida W, Chonan T, et al: Effects of submental stimulation during sleep on upper airway patency in patients with obstructive sleep apnea. *Am Rev Respir Dis* 140:1285, 1989.

68. Podzus T, Peter JH, Hochban W, et al: Electrical hypoglossal (HG) nerve stimulation in obstructive sleep apnea (OSA). *Am J Respir Crit Care Med* 151:538, 1995.

69. Guilleminault C, Powell N, Bowman B, Stoohs R: The effect of electrical stimulation on obstructive sleep apnea syndrome. *Chest* 107:67, 1995.

70. Ancoli-Israel S, Kripke DF, Klauber MR, et al: Morbidity, mortality, and sleep-disordered breathing in community dwelling elderly. *Sleep* 19:277, 1996.

71. Ancoli-Israel S, Klauber MR, Kripke DF, et al: Sleep apnea in female patients in a nursing home: Increased risk of mortality. *Chest* 96:1054, 1989.

72. Guilleminault C, Stoohs R, Clerk A, et al: A cause of excessive daytime sleepiness: The upper airway resistance syndrome. *Chest* 104:781, 1993.

73. Bradley TD, Phillipson EA: Central sleep apnea. *Clin Chest Med* 13:493, 1992.

74. Bonnet MH, Dexter JR, Arand DL: The effect of triazolam on arousal and respiration in central sleep apnea patients. *Sleep* 13:31, 1990.

75. White DP, Zwillich CW, Pickett CK, et al: Central sleep apnea: Improvement with acetazolamide therapy. *Arch Intern Med* 142:1816, 1982.

76. Issa F, Sullivan CE: Reversal of central sleep apnea using nasal CPAP. *Chest* 90:165, 1986.

77. Findley LJ, Zwillich CW, Ancoli-Israel S, et al: Cheyne-Stokes breathing during sleep in patients with left ventricular heart failure. *South Med J* 78:11, 1985.

78. Hoffstein V, Slutsky AS: Central sleep apnea reversed by continuous positive airway pressure. *Am Rev Respir Dis* 135:1210, 1987.

79. Alex CG, Önal E, Lopata M: Upper airway occlusion during sleep in patients with Cheyne-Stokes respiration. *Am Rev Respir Dis* 133:42, 1986.

80. Takasaki Y, Orr D, Popkin J, et al: Effect of nasal continuous positive airway pressure on sleep apnea in congestive heart failure. *Am Rev Respir Dis* 140:1578, 1989.

81. Naughton MT, Liu PP, Benard DC, et al: Treatment of congestive heart failure and Cheyne-Stokes respiration during sleep by continuous positive airway pressure. *Am J Respir Crit Care Med* 151:92, 1995.

82. Hanly PJ, Millar TW, Steljes DG, et al: The effect of oxygen on respiration and sleep in patients with congestive heart failure. *Ann Intern Med* 111:777, 1989.

83. Steens RD, Millar TW, Xialong S, et al: Effect of inhaled 3% CO_2 on Cheyne-Stokes respiration in congestive heart failure. *Sleep* 17:61, 1994.

84. Gastaut M, Tassinari CA, Duron B: Polygraphic study of the episodic diurnal and nocturnal manifestations of the Pickwick syndrome. *Brain Res* 2:167, 1966.

85. Lopata M, Önal E: Mass loading, sleep apnea, and the pathogenesis of obesity hypoventilation. *Am Rev Respir Dis* 126:640, 1982.

86. Lin C-C: Comparison between nocturnal nasal positive pressure ventilation combined with oxygen therapy and oxygen monotherapy in patients with severe COPD. *Am J Respir Crit Care Med* 154:353, 1996.

87. Guilleminault C, Cummiskey J: Progressive improvement of apnea index and ventilatory response to CO_2 after tracheostomy in obstructive sleep apnea syndrome. *Am Rev Respir Dis* 126:14, 1982.

88. Sullivan CE, Berthon-Jones M, Issa FG: Remission of severe obesity-hypoventilation syndrome after short-term treatment during sleep with nasal continuous positive airway pressure. *Am Rev Respir Dis* 128:177, 1983.

89. Van de Graaf WB: Thoracic influences on upper airway patency. *J Appl Physiol* 65:2124, 1988.

90. Bye PT, Ellis ER, Issa FG, et al: Respiratory failure and sleep in neuromuscular disease. *Thorax* 45:241, 1990.

91. Braun NMT: Respiratory muscle dysfunction. *Heart Lung* 13:327, 1984.

92. Hill NS: Noninvasive ventilation: Does it work, for whom, and how? *Am Rev Respir Dis* 147:1050, 1993.

93. Curran FJ: Night ventilation by body respirators for patients in chronic respiratory failure due to late stage Duchenne muscular dystrophy. *Arch Phys Med Rehabil* 62:270, 1981.

94. Garay SM, Turino GM, Goldring RM: Sustained reversal of chronic hypercapnia in patients with alveolar hypoventilation syndromes: Long-term maintenance with noninvasive mechanical ventilation. *Am J Med* 70:269, 1981.

95. Kerby GR, Mayer LS, Pingleton SK: Nocturnal positive pressure ventilation via nasal mask. *Am Rev Respir Dis* 135:738, 1987.

96. Ellis RE, Bye PTP, Bruderer JW, Sullivan CE: Treatment of respiratory failure during sleep in patients with neuromuscular disease: Positive-pressure ventilation through a nose mask. *Am Rev Respir Dis* 135:148, 1987.

97. Vianello A, Bevilacqua M, Salvador V, et al: Long-term nasal intermittent positive pressure ventilation in advanced Duchenne's muscular dystrophy. *Chest* 105:445, 1994.

98. Bach JR, Alba AS, Saporito LR: Intermittent positive pressure ventilation via the mouth as an alternative to tracheostomy for 257 ventilator users. *Chest* 103:174, 1993.

99. Meduri GU, Turner RE, Abou-Shala N, et al: Noninvasive positive pressure ventilation via face mask: First-line intervention in patients with acute hypercapnic and hypoxemic respiratory failure. *Chest* 109:179, 1996.

100. Moxham J, Shneerson JM: Diaphragmatic pacing. *Am Rev Respir Dis* 148:533, 1993.

101. Ellis ER, Grunstein RR, Chan S, et al: Noninvasive ventilatory support during sleep improves respiratory failure in kyphoscoliosis. *Chest* 94:811, 1988.

102. Mezon BL, West P, Israels J, Kryger M: Sleep breathing abnormalities in kyphoscoliosis. *Am Rev Respir Dis* 122:617, 1980.

103. Bye PTP, Issa F, Berthon-Jones M, Sullivan CE: Studies of oxygenation during sleep in patients with interstitial lung disease. *Am Rev Respir Dis* 129:27, 1984.

104. Shea SA, Winning AJ, McKenzie E, Guz A: Does the abnormal pattern of breathing in patients with interstitial lung disease persist in deep, non-rapid eye movement sleep? *Am Rev Respir Dis* 139:653, 1989.

105. Perez-Padella R, West P, Lertzman M, Kryger MH: Breathing during sleep in patients with interstitial lung disease. *Am Rev Respir Dis* 132:224, 1985.

106. Nocturnal Oxygen Therapy Trial Group: Continuous or nocturnal oxygen therapy in hypoxemic chronic obstructive lung disease: A clinical trial. *Ann Intern Med* 93:391, 1980.

107. Medical Research Council Working Party Report: Long-term domiciliary oxygen therapy in chronic hypoxic cor pulmonale complicating chronic bronchitis and emphysema. *Lancet* 1:681, 1981.

108. Ballard RD, Saathoff MC, Patel DK, et al: Effect of sleep on nocturnal bronchoconstriction and ventilatory patterns in asthmatics. *J Appl Physiol* 67:243, 1989.

109. Catterall JR, Douglas NJ, Calverley PMA: Irregular breathing and hypoxaemia during sleep in chronic stable asthma. *Lancet* 1:301, 1982.

110. Montplaisir J, Walsh J, Malo JL: Nocturnal asthma: Features of attacks, sleep and breathing patterns. *Am Rev Respir Dis* 125:18, 1982.

111. Cochrane GM, Clark TJH: A survey of asthma mortality in patients between ages 35 and 65 in the greater London hospitals in 1971. *Thorax* 30:300, 1975.

112. Robertson CF, Rubinfeld CR, Bowes G: Deaths from asthma in Victoria: A 12-month survey. *Med J Aust* 152:511, 1990.

113. Beam WR, Weiner DE, Martin RJ: Timing of prednisone and alterations of airways inflammation in nocturnal asthma. *Am Rev Respir Dis* 146:1524, 1992.

114. Fitzpatrick MF, Mackay T, Driver H, Douglas NJ: Salmeterol in nocturnal asthma: A double-blind, placebo-controlled trial of a long-acting inhaled beta 2 agonist. *Br Med J* 301:1365, 1990.

115. Martin RJ, Cicutto LC, Ballard RD: Circadian variations in theophylline concentrations, and the treatment of nocturnal asthma. *Am Rev Respir Dis* 139:475, 1989.

116. Chan CS, Woolcock AJ, Sullivan CE: Nocturnal asthma: Role of snoring and obstructive sleep apnea. *Am Rev Respir Dis* 137:1502, 1988.

117. Martin RJ, Pak J: Nasal CPAP in non-apneic nocturnal asthma. *Chest* 100:1024, 1991.

118. Fleetham J, West P, Mezon B, et al: Sleep, arousals, and oxygen desaturation in chronic obstructive pulmonary disease. *Am Rev Respir Dis* 126:429, 1982.

119. Connaughton JJ, Catterall JR, Elton RA, et al: Do sleep studies contribute to the management of patients with severe chronic obstructive pulmonary disease? *Am Rev Respir Dis* 138:341, 1988.

120. American Thoracic Society: Indications and standards for cardiopulmonary sleep studies. *Am Rev Respir Dis* 137:1502, 1989.

121. Dantzker DR, Scharf SM: Surgery to reduce lung volume (editorial). *N Engl J Med* 334:1128, 1994.

122. Fletcher EC, Miller J, Divine GW, et al: Nocturnal oxyhemoglobin desaturation in COPD patients with arterial oxygen tensions above 60 mmHg. *Chest* 92:604, 1987.

123. Hyland RH, Hutcheon MA, Perl A, et al: Upper airway occlusion induced by diaphragm pacing for primary alveolar hypoventilation: Implications for the pathogenesis of obstructive sleep apnea. *Am Rev Respir Dis* 124:180, 1981.

124. Gigliotti F, Spinelli A, Duranti R, et al: Four-week negative pressure ventilation improves respiratory function in severe hypercapnic COPD patients. *Chest* 105:87, 1994.

125. Meecham Jones DJ, Paul EA, Jones PW, Wedzicha JA: Nasal pressure support ventilation plus oxygen compared with oxygen therapy alone in hypercapnic COPD. *Am J Respir Crit Care Med* 152:538, 1995.

126. Brochard L, Mancebo J, Wysocki M, et al: Noninvasive ventilation for acute exacerbations of chronic obstructive pulmonary disease. *N Engl J Med* 333:817, 1995.

127. Strumpf DA, Millman RP, Carlisle CC, et al: Nocturnal positive-pressure ventilation via nasal mask in patients with severe chronic obstructive pulmonary disease. *Am Rev Respir Dis* 144:1234, 1991.

128. Elliot MW, Simonds AK, Carroll MP, et al: Domiciliary nocturnal nasal intermittent positive pressure ventilation in hypercapnic respiratory failure due to chronic obstructive lung disease: Effects on sleep and quality of life. *Thorax* 47:342, 1992.

129. Meecham Jones DJ, Marino W: Intermittent volume cycled mechanical ventilation via nasal mask in patients with respiratory failure due to COPD. *Chest* 99:681, 1991.

130. Series F, Cormier Y: Effects of protriptyline on diurnal and nocturnal oxygenation in patients with chronic obstructive pulmonary disease. *Ann Intern Med* 113:507, 1990.

131. Connaughton JJ, Douglas NJ, Morgan AD, et al: Almitrine improves oxygenation when both awake and asleep in patients with hypoxia and carbon dioxide retention caused by chronic bronchitis and emphysema. *Am Rev Respir Dis* 132:206, 1985.

132. Goldstein RS, Ramcharan V, Bowes G, et al: Effect of supplemental nocturnal oxygen on gas exchange in patients with severe obstructive lung disease. *N Engl J Med* 310:425, 1984.

133. Guilleminault C, Cumminskey J, Motta J: Chronic obstructive airflow disease and sleep studies. *Am Rev Respir Dis* 122:397, 1980.

Chapter 15
COUGH EFFECTIVENESS

SUZANNE C. SMELTZER
MARC H. LAVIETES

An effective cough facilitates sputum removal. Cough does not appear to be necessary for sputum removal in normal subjects. Mucociliary clearance is sufficient to clear airway secretions. By contrast, patients with excessive secretions, such as those with pneumonia or cystic fibrosis, and patients with malfunctioning mucociliary apparatus, such as those with airway disease or congenitally nonfunctioning cilia, rely on cough to expectorate and thus to maintain patent airways. Clinicians have long recognized a relationship between failure to cough and recurrent respiratory tract infections. The literature of pulmonary medicine, however, has failed both to define cough effectiveness and to quantify cough effectiveness in any specific patient population. This chapter discusses some of the approaches that have been used to study the effectiveness of cough. These include (1) the study of maximal expiratory airflow during cough, (2) the use of subjective questionnaires regarding patients' perceptions of the effectiveness of their cough, and (3) the evaluation of sputum removal as inferred from the removal of inhaled radiolabeled particles from the lung.

Phases of Cough

A *cough* is a sudden explosive exhalation of air that occurs immediately following rapid opening of the glottis. Cough may be initiated by a variety of afferent stimuli. There are three phases of cough: (1) an initial inspiratory phase, during which time air is inspired through an opened glottis, (2) glottal closure, when high intrathoracic pressure is generated as expiratory muscles contract against the closed glottis, and (3) expiratory, during which the glottis opens rapidly and a brief (≤ 50 ms) period of supramaximal expiratory flow occurs.

A schematic representation of a supramaximal flow transient is shown in Fig. 15-1.[1] In this example, supramaximal flow has been created experimentally by a normal subject exhaling forcefully against a closed shutter. Peak expiratory flow of this transient occurs within 20 ms of the shutter's opening. Within 40 ms, expiratory flow has returned to that flow rate seen on the subject's own maximal expiratory flow-volume curve, a flow designated as Vmax in the figure. Much of the air expelled during this cough transient resides in the trachea during the compressive phase. The rate of exhalation of that tracheal air is effort-dependent. By contrast, the remainder of air expired during the supramaximal flow transient originates within the lung; its maximal rate of expiration is effort-independent. It is likely that the height of this peak flow is related to muscle strength and that this peak is therefore diminished in patients with neuromuscular diseases. It is widely held that development of this supramaximal flow transient is critical for the expectoration of sputum.

The term *effectiveness* refers to the capability of producing a result. Coughs may serve many purposes. Cough preceded by inspiration may clear the airways of excessive secretions. Cough preceded by little or no inspiration may serve to defend the airways against inhalation of noxious airborne agents. Finally, cough may accompany a variety of tracheal, intrathoracic, and/or intraabdominal lesions. Teleologically, the purpose of cough in these circumstances is unclear. Possibly, cough in these cases is a premonitory sign or warning of illness for the patient. While there appear to be many functions of cough, the function most easily explored experimentally is that of mucus removal. This chapter will review the literature regarding effectiveness of cough in the removal of airway secretions.

Assessment of the mechanical effectiveness of cough first appeared in the British literature.[2,3] These articles suggested that cough effectiveness would depend on the "scrubbing action" of rapid expiratory airflow passing over the compressed walls of proximal airways. A flow versus time trace from these studies appears in Fig. 15-2. The authors defined the duration of one cough, that is, an individual cough occurring within a volley of coughs, as the time between peak flows of two successive coughs. Thus this assessment would envision the entirety of forced exhalation rather than the brief transient of supramaximal flow alone as being critical for sputum removal. Their mathematical expression for scrubbing action depends, in part, on the extent of compression of the trachea during the forced exhalation phase of cough. This is compatible with the notion that effective sputum removal depends on both development of the supramaximal flow transient and achievement of high linear velocity of airflow during the entire cough. Of interest, patients with tracheostomies and laryngectomies who cannot close their glottis may nevertheless have effective cough. By achieving tracheal compression without glottal closure, presumably by making a compressive effort against a closed mouth, they may generate linear flow velocity sufficient to clear secretions from central airways in the absence of a supramaximal flow transient.[4]

The idea of scrubbing action, which has not been developed in the clinical literature, would seem to be of interest, especially in the consideration of cough effectiveness in muscular dystrophy patients. These patients may generate transients of supramaximal airflow when coughing at low lung volumes but may fail to sustain maximal expiratory flow between coughs within volleys of coughs.[5]

A large body of literature has evaluated airway clearance by quantifying the removal of inhaled radiolabeled particles over time. As we shall see later, this technique is not ideal for the evaluation of cough effectiveness because enhanced clearance and improvement in lung function are not directly related. Improvement in clearance as measured in the laboratory may coincide with deterioration in lung function in patients whose mucus production increases in volume. To date, technology to quantify mucus production is unavailable.

The use of a subjective scoring system for analysis of cough effectiveness has been proposed recently.[6] This system requires the subject to rate on a numerical scale his or her perception of the frequency, severity, and discomfort associated with his or her cough. Preliminary data show a correlation between increased gas trapping and increasing symptoms as judged from estimates of chronic bronchitis

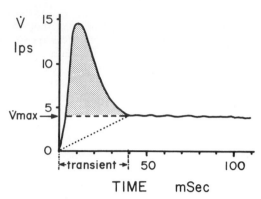

FIGURE 15-1 A triggered flow transient, flow plotted versus time. The stippled area represents volume displaced from airways during tracheal compression. The dashed line represents parenchymal flow if the migration of the equal pressure point (EPP) were instantaneous. The dotted line represents parenchymal flow if EPP migration were slow. (Reprinted, with permission, from Knudson et al.[1])

patients' perception of their own discomfort.[7] Much investigation remains to be done, however, before subjective scales that quantify the patients' perceptions of the severity of cough may be used to quantify cough effectiveness.

What We May Learn from Studies of Airway Clearance

The literature is replete with studies measuring the distribution of inhaled radiolabeled particles within the lung and their subsequent elimination, or clearance, from the lung. An often repeated protocol has required the subject to inhale an aerosol of labeled particles until the label has distributed evenly throughout the lung fields. Lung imaging has then been repeated hourly after the inhalation maneuver. From these sequential images, clearance is computed as "percentage of original label retained." A graphic illustration of data from one such experiment appears in Fig. 15-3. This article suggested that normal persons clear 90 percent of particles inhaled in no more than 600 min.[8] This clearance process occurred in two discrete phases. In the first phase, label could be shown to clear steadily from the lung periphery, while for the first half hour label increased slightly in the trachea. After 1 h, however, a second phase was identified, one in which the trachea was nearly free of aerosol. The trachea remained aerosol-free over the next 24 h, while the remainder of the lung periphery continued to empty. This observation

would suggest that mucociliary clearance from the trachea is quite rapid, an observation that has been confirmed by many recent studies.[9–12] In fact, the rate of transport of a particle through the trachea is shown to be approximately 5 mm/min; through the large airways distal to the trachea, 1 mm/min.[13] Transport rates in more peripheral airways are slower still. It would appear that these slow transport rates in the periphery prevent mucus accumulation in the major airways. Since normal subjects cough as little as once per hour, it is presumed that clearance rates derived from the removal of radiolabeled particles reflect the rate of sputum removal by the ciliary apparatus alone.[14]

There does not appear to be agreement on clearance rates for normal subjects among laboratories.[15,16] This is due in part to great variability even among normal persons. In addition, clearance rates are affected by inhaled particle size.[8] Large particles (e.g., 4.9 μm) distribute centrally and are removed during the first phase. By contrast, small particles (e.g., 1.3 μm) distribute peripherally. Their clearance patterns are slow; no first phase of clearance can be seen.

Other variables that may influence aerosol penetration into the lung include inspiratory flow rate and airway caliber.[17] These variables would appear to affect particle distribution and elimination in patients with lung disease more than in normal subjects.

Common inhaled toxins, for example, cigarette smoke, impair mucociliary clearance. Data suggest that ciliary dysfunction in distal airways may be the earliest and most subtle abnormality to occur with cigarette smoking. One study has shown that young, healthy smoking subjects with normal spirometry whose smoking histories do not exceed 10 pack-years may nevertheless exhibit delay in the second phase of mucociliary clearance.[18] In a complementary study, similar young smoking subjects, when asked to inhale a small dose of a radiolabel by tidal breathing, show reduction of that label deposited into the lung periphery. While airway clearance appears to have been normal in the smokers of that study, this is so because label fails to distribute to the periphery so that there is no prolonged second phase of clearance.[19] Normalization of aerosol clearance often occurs months after cessation of smoking.[20]

The Study of Cough with the Techniques of Radiolabeled Particle Elimination

The studies cited earlier describe the removal of radiolabeled particles by mucociliary clearance from the airways of healthy noncoughing subjects. Cough is a second mechanism

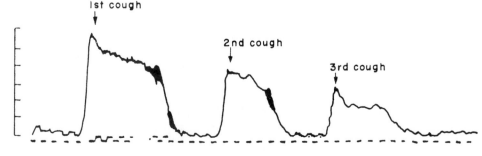

FIGURE 15-2 A tracing of flow (ordinate) versus time (abcissa) in the study of mechanical assessment of cough. Each marking repesents 0.04 s. (Reprinted, with permission, from Lawson and Harris.[2])

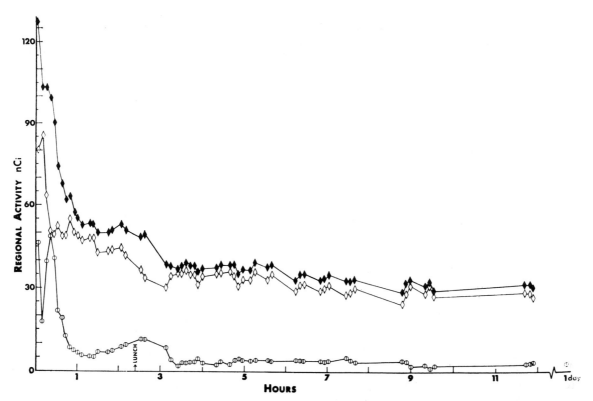

FIGURE 15-3 Clearance curves from a healthy nonsmoking subject following inhalation of 3.9-μm ^{98}Au-tagged particles for the whole lung. Note the initial accumulation of label in the trachea that coincides with the rapid initial emptying of the lung. Closed triangles, whole lung; open triangles, lung periphery; circles, trachea. (Reprinted from *Arch Environ Health*, 18:738–755, 1969. Reprinted with permission of the Helen Dwight Reid Educational Foundation. Published by Haldraf Publications, 1319 Eighteenth St., NW, Washington DC, 20036-1802. Copyright 1969).

for removal of inhaled particles, as well as removal of sputum, from airways. To be complete, there is yet a third mechanism for the removal of inhaled particulate matter from the lung, namely, alveolar clearance by macrophages. This mechanism is slow and not assessed by the techniques described in this chapter.

Cough effectiveness can be assessed by the radiolabeled particle elimination technique. To assess cough, subjects are coached to produce two clearance curves: one curve during which time the subject coughs and the other while the subject breathes quietly but avoids coughing. Acceleration of clearance by cough would indicate both heightened sputum removal and effective cough.

To study the effect of cough on sputum removal in normal individuals, volunteer subjects have been coached to cough regularly during the first few hours following the inhalation of a radiolabeled marker.[21] While the rate of particle and/or sputum removal during the first few hours is accelerated by coughing, the clearance of labeled particles over a 24-h period in coughing normal subjects was no different from that in noncoughing controls. This would suggest that in normal subjects, cough may enhance particle removal briefly following the inhalation of particulate matter but that mucociliary clearance is the major determinant of airway clearance. Of note, voluntary bursts of rapid shallow inspirations, known as *inspiratory huffing*, in the absence of cough also brought about accelerated particle removal during the first few hours of a 24-h observation period. This accelerated expectoration occurred when the voluntary bursts were performed shortly after inhalation of the radiolabel. The fact that both huffing and cough could accelerate the rate of particle removal during the first 2 h (but not the entire 24 h) of the experiment suggested that either maneuver may stimulate the first phase of mucus removal by enhancing tracheal mucociliary clearance. To support the notion that coughing is not a requisite for sputum removal in normal individuals, it can be shown that coughing is in fact disruptive to the orderly clearance of mucus from the airways of experimental animals.[22] Of interest, neither coughing nor inspiratory huffing could enhance the 1- or 2-h clearance rates in asymptomatic smokers with otherwise normal lung function.[23] This is further evidence that disruption of mucociliary clearance is the earliest abnormality of airway function induced by smoking.

Chronic airway obstruction is accompanied by the impairment of mucociliary clearance from central airways.[24] This is most pronounced in patients with severe airway obstruction, whose rate of expiratory flow during tidal breathing approximates their maximal flow as seen on their maximal expiratory flow-volume curve. This would imply that the formation of sites of flow limitation within large airways during tidal breathing interferes with orderly mucociliary clearance. Coughing is known to enhance clearance of particulate matter in patients with chronic airway obstruction, while forced exhalation alone does not.[25–27] In fact, coughing in patients with airway obstruction facilitates movement of secretions toward central airways even in the absence of copious sputum expectoration.[28]

By what mechanism might cough enhance sputum removal in these patients? In airway obstruction patients as in normal individuals, the compressive phase of cough allows for the development of a proximal site of flow limitation at the glottis. Expansion rather than flattening of the large airways immediately distal to the glottis must occur during this phase. The rapid exhalation immediately following glottal opening may facilitate sputum removal, at least until a regimen of flow limitation is reestablished throughout the lung. Most likely, coughing does not enhance sputum removal in normal individuals because such individuals do not demonstrate a regimen of flow limitation during tidal breathing. From a teleologic perspective, it is thus not surprising that patients with airway obstruction cough more frequently than do normal individuals. New data showing that cough is suppressed in chronic airway obstruction patients during sleep are somewhat surprising, given the fact that patients often complain that their sleep is disturbed by coughing.[14,29]

There is no consensus in the literature as to whether or not bronchodilators, adrenergic or anticholinergic, enhance sputum clearance in patients with airway obstruction.[30,31] There may be many explanations for this. Bronchodilation is accompanied by movement of flow-limiting segments downstream and thus reduces the volume of airway compressed during the cough process. Alternately, bronchodilators may alter the physical properties of sputum so as to interfere with mucus clearance. To this end, Pavia and colleagues[32] described a group of chronic bronchitis patients for whom ipratropium caused bronchodilation, as measured by serial lung function tests. At the same time, these subjects showed both slowing of lung mucus clearance when compared with subjects free from airway obstruction and a decrease in the volume of sputum expectorated over a 6-h period after ipratropium.

In summary, clearance studies show that cough is effective in that it enhances label (and presumably sputum) removal in patients with airway obstruction. Serial studies in patients receiving bronchodilator therapy are difficult to interpret, however. Therapy may relieve airway obstruction and reduce symptoms. At the same time, it diminishes the effect of cough on particle removal. Thus, while there is some relationship between cough and radiolabel clearance in airway obstruction patients, there is poor correlation between clearance, lung function, and clinical well-being. There are no studies examining the frequency and/or robustness of cough in such patients. Clearly, the issue of effectiveness of cough is not addressed by studies of removal of an inhaled radioactive label alone.

Tracheal Flexibility and Cough Efficiency

While the importance of glottal closure, airway compression, and supramaximal peak expiratory airflow for cough effectiveness has been discussed in the literature, little attention has been given to the fact that cough efficiency is related to the flexibility of proximal airway walls. Experimental data suggest that clearance of mucus along the cartilaginous surface of an airway is reduced in a rigid (as opposed to a collapsible) tracheobronchial tree.[33] The fact that muscular constriction diminishes both the distensibility

and compressibility of an airway suggests that bronchospasm would impair cough effectiveness.[34] It is also conceivable that the trachea in chronic bronchitis is rigid and thus not conducive to expectoration. To date, the compliance of the tracheobronchial tree in chronic bronchitis has not been studied.

By contrast, clinical and experimental studies of tracheal mechanics in emphysema are available.[35,36] Of interest, the notch separating effort-dependent from non-effort-dependent flow, characteristic of the spirogram in emphysema, is a reflection of the abrupt collapse of the trachea during forced exhalation. It is not difficult to imagine that this transient flow limitation in the upper airway interferes with sputum removal.

Finally, certain physicochemical characteristics of sputum may be important for effective, productive cough. Sputum that is nonviscous and nonadherent is easily removed from airway walls and thus more easily expectorated than viscous, adherent sputum.

Cough in Patients with Neuromuscular and Neurologic Disorders

Respiratory muscle function is affected in many neurologic disorders.[37] It is generally acknowledged that ineffective cough is a consequence of respiratory muscle weakness and is responsible, at least in part, for the frequent respiratory tract complications associated with neurologic and neuromuscular disorders. These include spinal cord injury (SCI), multiple sclerosis (MS), and muscular dystrophy, to name a few. Ineffective cough is different from respiratory failure per se and thus may be overlooked in some patients because of life-threatening respiratory failure.

There are many mechanisms or reasons that cough might become ineffective in patients with neuromuscular disorders. One set of conditions, including MS or quadriplegia, is characterized by expiratory muscle weakness.[38] SCI patients, for example, have been shown to be unable to generate adequate esophageal or gastric pressure during voluntary cough.[39] Here, dynamic airway compression is limited. This results in a decrease in maximal linear airflow through large airways during the expiratory phase of cough and an inability to remove airway secretions.[40] In another set of conditions exemplified by the muscular dystrophies or amyotrophic lateral sclerosis, expiratory muscle weakness may be closely related in time to impairment of inspiratory muscles. In these patients, hypercapnia and respiratory failure may occur with or without cough failure, retention of secretions, and respiratory tract infection.

Rigidity of the chest wall also has been suggested as a contributing factor to cough ineffectiveness in patients with neurologic disorders such as Parkinson's disease.[40] The diminished chest wall compliance associated with many chronic neuromuscular disorders may affect cough by interfering with thoracic excursion during both the inspiratory and the expiratory phases of cough. Finally, the accumulation of airway secretions may be particularly problematic for patients whose neurologic disorders are characterized by pharyngeal paralysis. While the possibility of effective cough in tracheostomized patients was noted earlier, nevertheless, patients who are unable to close their glottis tightly have difficulty in developing adequate intrathoracic pressure during the compressive phase of cough.

Whether or not cough effectiveness can be improved by training expiratory muscles is not known. Of interest, tetraplegic patients with cervical cord lesions may be taught to develop positive or expiratory intrathoracic pressure by using the pectoralis major as a respiratory muscle.[41] Training has been shown to increase expiratory muscle strength in both SCI and MS patients.[42,43] Whether or not this training may improve the clinical course of these patients is unclear.

Alternate Methods for Sputum Removal

Chest physical therapy is a traditional method to assist with the removal of sputum. Review of the literature suggests that postural drainage and/or chest percussion improves mucus clearance and lung function only in those conditions characterized by voluminous sputum production, e.g., chronic bronchitis and cystic fibrosis.[44] Forced expirations without glottal closure and airway compression may promote expectoration more than does cough in these patients.[45,46] This may be so because forced exhalations must increase airflow velocity without creating sites of flow limitation within proximal airways.

Other less popular methods are described in the literature and are used by some clinicians. Sputum removal may be enhanced by the mechanical production of rapid expiratory flow. This is accomplished by the application of positive, followed by negative, pressure at the mouth by means of a pressure generator and face mask. This venerable method is still used in the treatment of patients with neuromuscular disorders.[47] Chest wall vibration has been shown to enhance mucus removal in animal model studies but has yet to be tested widely in clinical practice.[48]

Recent laboratory experiments show the development of positive airway pressure in anesthetized dogs when electrical stimulation is applied to the lower thoracic spinal cord.[49] This approach may offer an improved method for sputum removal in patients with spinal cord lesions.

New Avenues of Study

Little has been written on the efferent limb of the cough reflex. How is the central command to cough distributed to the efferent limb of the reflex, namely, the respiratory muscles? How is the pressure generated by muscular contraction coupled to supramaximal expiratory cough flow? And what is the relationship between effort (measured as flow or intrathoracic pressure) and sputum removal? Will training respiratory muscles enhance the effectiveness of cough? One promising avenue for exploration has been presented by Beardsmore and colleagues,[50] who have proposed the ratio of peak cough flow to maximal expiratory flow as seen on the maximal expiratory flow-volume curve as an index of airway function relevant to the study of cough. This ratio may provide a helpful tool for testing of interesting hypotheses relating to cough effectiveness. First, what is the relationship between effort (esophageal pressure) and flow, as given by this ratio? Second, what is the relationship between this ratio and the effectiveness of sputum removal, as measured by studies of the elimination of radiolabeled aerosols?

References

1. Knudson RJ, Mead J, Knudson DE: Contribution of airway collapse to supramaximal expiratory flow. *J Appl Physiol* 36:653, 1974.
2. Lawson TV, Harris RS: Assessment of the mechanical efficiency of coughing in healthy young adults. *Clin Sci* 33:209, 1967.
3. Harris RS, Lawson TV: The relative mechanical effectiveness and efficiency of successive voluntary coughs in healthy young adults. *Clin Sci* 34:569, 1968.
4. Young S, Abdul-Sattar N, Caric D: Glottic closure and high flows are not essential for productive cough. *Bull Eur Physiopathol Respir* 23:11S, 1987.
5. Szeinberg A, Tabachnik E, Rashed N, et al: Cough capacity in patients with muscular dystrophy. *Chest* 94:1232, 1988.
6. Petty TL: The national mucolytic study. *Chest* 97:75, 1990.
7. Tomkiewicz RP, Albers GM, Ramirez OE, et al: Relationship between a scoring system for respiratory symptoms, lung function, and properties of sputum in patients with chronic bronchitis and cystic fibrosis. *Chest* 108(3):148S, 1995.
8. Albert RE, Lippmann M, Briscoe W: The characteristics of bronchial clearance in humans and the effects of cigarette smoking. *Arch Environ Health* 18:738, 1969.
9. Mortensen J, Groth S, Lange P, et al: Bronchoscintigraphic visualization of the acute effect of tobacco exposure and terbutaline on mucociliary clearance in smokers. *Eur Respir J* 2:721, 1989.
10. Groth S, Mortensen J, Lange P, et al: Imaging of the airways by bronchoscintigraphy for the study of mucociliary clearance. *Thorax* 43:360, 1988.
11. Yeates DB, Aspin N, Levison H, et al: Mucociliary tracheal transport rates in man. *J Appl Physiol* 39:487, 1975.
12. Goodman RM, Yergin BM, Landa JF, et al: Relationship of smoking history and pulmonary function tests to tracheal mucous velocity in nonsmokers, young smokers, ex-smokers, and patients with chronic bronchitis. *Am Rev Respir Dis* 117:205, 1978.
13. Yeates DB, Pitt BR, Spektor DM, et al: Coordination of mucociliary transport in human trachea and intrapulmonary airways. *J Appl Physiol* 51:1057, 1981.
14. Hsu JY, Stone RA, Logan-Sinclair RB, et al: Coughing frequency in patients with persistent cough: Assessment using a 24-hour ambulatory recorder. *Eur Respir J* 7:1246, 1994.
15. Lourenco RV, Klimek MF, Borowski CJ: Deposition and clearance of 2-micron particles in the tracheobronchial tree of normal subjects: Smokers and non-smokers. *J Clin Invest* 50:1411, 1971.
16. Thomson ML, Short MD: Mucociliary function in health, chronic obstructive airway disease, and asbestosis. *J Appl Physiol* 26:535, 1969.
17. Dolovich M, Eng P, Ryan G, Newhouse MT: Aerosol penetration into the lung. *Chest* 80(suppl):834, 1981.
18. Foster WM, Langenback EG, Bergofsky EH: Disassociation in the mucociliary function of central and peripheral airways of asymptomatic smokers. *Am Rev Respir Dis* 132:633, 1985.
19. Isawa T, Teshima T, Hirano T, et al: Mucociliary clearance mechanism in smoking and non-smoking normal subjects. *J Nucl Med* 25:352, 1984.
20. Camner P, Philipson K, Arvidsson T: Withdrawal of cigarette smoking. *Arch Environ Health* 26:90, 1973.
21. Bennett WD, Foster WM, Chapman WF: Cough-enhanced mucus clearance in the normal lung. *J Appl Physiol* 69:1670, 1990.
22. Smaldone GC, Itoh H, Swift DL, et al: Effect of flow-limiting segments and cough on particle deposition and mucociliary clearance in the lung. *Am Rev Respir Dis* 120:747, 1979.
23. Bennett WD, Chapman WF, Gerrity TR: Ineffectiveness of cough for enhancing mucus clearance in asymptomatic smokers. *Chest* 102:412, 1992.
24. Smaldone GC, Foster WM, O'Riordan TG, et al: Regional impairment of mucociliary clearance in chronic obstructive pulmonary disease. *Chest* 103:1390, 1993.

25. Oldenburg FA, Dolovich MB, Montgomery JM, et al: Effects of postural drainage, exercise, and cough on mucus clearance in chronic bronchitis. *Am Rev Respir Dis* 120:739, 1979.

26. Mortensen J, Jensen C, Groth S, et al: The effect of forced expirations on mucociliary clearance in patients with chronic bronchitis and in healthy subjects. *Clin Physiol* 11:439, 1991.

27. Camner P, Mossberg B, Philipson K, et al: Elimination of test particles from the human tracheobronchial tract by voluntary coughing. *Scand J Respir Dis* 60:56, 1979.

28. Hasani A, Pavia D, Agnew JE, et al: Regional mucus transport following unproductive cough and forced expiration technique in patients with airways obstruction. *Chest* 105:1420, 1994.

29. Power JT, Stewart IC, Connaughton JJ, et al: Nocturnal cough in patients with chronic bronchitis and emphysema. *Am Rev Respir Dis* 130:999, 1984.

30. Mossberg B, Strandberg K, Philipson K, et al: Tracheobronchial clearance in bronchial asthma: Response to beta-adrenergic stimulation. *Scand J Respir Dis* 57:119, 1976.

31. Bennett WD, Chapman WF, Mascarella JM: The acute effect of ipratropium bromide bronchodilator therapy on cough clearance in COPD. *Chest* 103:488, 1993.

32. Pavia D, Bateman JRM, Sheahan NF: Clearance of lung secretions in patients with chronic bronchitis: Effect of terbutaline and ipratropium bromide aerosols. *Eur J Respir Dis* 61:245, 1980.

33. Soland V, Brock G, King M: Effect of airway wall flexibility on clearance by simulated cough. *J Appl Physiol* 63:707, 1987.

34. Olsen CR, Stevens AE, McIlroy MB: Rigidity of trachea and bronchi during muscular constriction. *J Appl Physiol* 23:27, 1967.

35. Turino GM, Lourenco RV, McCracken GH: Role of connective tissues in large pulmonary airways. *J Appl Physiol* 25:645, 1968.

36. Gandevia B: Spirogram of gross tracheobronchial collapse in emphysema. *Q J Med* 32:23, 1963.

37. Epstein SK: An overview of respiratory muscle function. *Clin Chest Med* 15(4):619, 1994.

38. Smeltzer SC, Skurnick JH, Troiano R, et al: Respiratory function in multiple sclerosis: Utility of clinical assessment of respiratory muscle function. *Chest* 101:479, 1992.

39. Siebens AA, Kirby NA, Paulos DA: Cough following transection of spinal cord at C6. *Arch Phys Med Rehabil* 45:1, 1964.

40. De Troyer A, Pride NB: The respiratory system in neuromuscular disorders, in Roussos C, Macklem PT (eds): *The Thorax*, part B. New York, Marcel Dekker, 1986, p 1089.

41. Estenne M, VanMuylem A, Gorini M, et al: Evidence of dynamic airway compression during cough in tetraplegic patients. *Am J Respir Crit Care Med* 150:1081, 1994.

42. Estenne M, Knopp C, Vanvaerenbergh L, et al: The effect of pectoralis muscle training in tetraplegic subjects. *Am Rev Respir Dis* 139:1218, 1989.

43. Smeltzer SC, Lavietes MH, Cook SD: Expiratory training in multiple sclerosis. *Arch Phys Med Rehabil* 77:909, 1996.

44. Kirilloff LH, Owens GR, Rogers RM, et al: Does chest physical therapy work? *Chest* 88:436, 1985.

45. Hasami A, Pavia D, Agnew JE, et al: Regional lung clearance during cough and forced expiration technique (FET): Effects of flow and viscoelasticity. *Thorax* 49:557, 1994.

46. Sutton PP, Parker RA, Webber BA, et al: Assessment of the forced expiration technique, postural drainage and directed coughing in chest physiotherapy. *Eur J Respir Dis* 64:62, 1983.

47. Barach AL, Beck GJ, Smith W: Mechanical production of expiratory flow rates surpassing the capacity of human coughing. *Am J Med Sci* 226:241, 1953.

48. King M, Phillips DM, Gross D, et al: Enhanced tracheal mucus clearance with high frequency chest wall compression. *Am Rev Respir Dis* 128:511, 1983.

49. DiMarco AF, Romaniuk JR, Supinski GS: Electrical activation of the expiratory muscles to restore cough. *Am J Respir Crit Care Med* 151:1466, 1995.

50. Beardsmore CS, Wimpress SP, Thomson AH, et al: Maximum voluntary cough: An indication of airway function. *Bull Eur Physiopathol Respir* 23:465, 1987.

Chapter 16

MECHANISMS OF DYSPNEA

RICHARD M. SCHWARTZSTEIN

HAROLD L. MANNING

Patients with chronic pulmonary disease are often disabled because of shortness of breath. Our ability to design interventions that will improve their functional capacity depends in large part on the degree to which we can identify the specific pathophysiologic mechanisms that produce *dyspnea*. This task is complicated by several considerations. Since respiratory sensations originate from a number of receptors stimulated simultaneously, including the peripheral and central chemoreceptors and receptors in the upper airways, lungs, and chest wall, dyspnea should be viewed as a "synthetic" experience analogous to hunger.[1] As yet, no single receptor has been identified that, when stimulated, produces dyspnea. Furthermore, we must appreciate the difference between a *sensation*, the neural activity that results when a receptor is stimulated, and a *perception*, the reaction of the individual after the neural activity has been processed. The behavior manifest by the patient reflects this perception and may be colored by emotional aand psychological factors as well. A sensation experienced by a patient who is relaxed and in familiar surroundings may elicit a very different response than the same sensation experienced under conditions in which the patient feels anxious and vulnerable.

Studies of the language used by patients to describe their dyspnea demonstrate that both normal individuals performing a variety of respiratory tasks and patients with different pulmonary abnormalities experience a range of respiratory sensations and can distinguish among them.[2-5] Furthermore, a single patient may have several conditions, for example, chronic obstructive pulmonary disease (COPD) and congestive heart failure (CHF), each of which can independently lead to dyspnea. While the basic pathology of some diseases, such as emphysema, may not be amenable to therapy, complications such as hypoxia, hyperinflation, and deconditioning may be treatable. Thus an understanding of the specific pathophysiologic principles applicable to a given patient is critical in the design of a therapeutic program. The assessment of the patient must be sufficiently broad to identify comorbid conditions and physiologic abnormalities contributing to the breathing discomfort.

To understand the mechanisms of dyspnea in a way that will be relevant for those engaged in pulmonary rehabilitation programs, we will outline the physiology of dyspnea in two broad contexts. First, we will review the basic physiology of dyspnea and describe general mechanisms that may be present in one or more disease states and which contribute either to a specific quality of dyspnea or to its intensity. Second, we will examine the clinical physiology of dyspnea, an approach that focuses on dyspnea at the level of organ systems. This approach is useful in generating differential diagnoses when faced with a patient suffering from dyspnea

and aids in the search for multiple causes of an individual's breathlessness. However, before embarking on this discussion, one should be cognizant of some of the limitations and problems associated with studies of the mechanisms of dyspnea.

Problems in the Study of Dyspnea

WHAT IS THE SENSATION?

What is dyspnea? Is it "difficult or labored breathing"?[6] Is it a sensation of "feeling breathless or experiencing air hunger"?[7,8] Is it a sensation of "chest tightness"?[3] Is it the sense of "effort" to breathe?[9,10] Dyspnea encompasses these and other sensations as well. Thus it may be unclear what one is measuring if one merely asks a patient to rate his or her "shortness of breath," and it may be misleading if one "guides" the subject in a particular direction by asking the individual to rate "breathing difficulty"; that is, the patient will likely describe sensations that seem relevant to the notion of "difficult" such as the "effort" to breathe but may not comment on a sensation such as "chest tightness." Physiologic parameters such as pressure or tension may predict the intensity of dyspnea in a subject whose respiratory system is subject to resistive or elastic loads,[9] but these parameters have much less to do with the dyspnea associated with acute hypercapnia in individuals being passively ventilated[7,8] or with dyspnea caused by an acute pulmonary embolism.

Studies of the language of dyspnea demonstrate that dyspnea, like pain, is comprised of several qualitatively distinct sensations.[2-5] Using questionnaires that list a range of descriptive phrases (Table 16–1), investigators can more accurately assess the specific sensation experienced by the subject. Since many cardiopulmonary disorders are characterized by an increased mechanical load, the sense of respiratory "effort," which is believed to arise from a corollary discharge transmitted from the brain stem to the sensory cortex during reflex or automatic breathing and from the motor cortex to the sensory cortex during voluntary respiratory movements,[11] is a relatively common finding.[5] Nevertheless, it is important when performing or evaluating studies on dyspnea to be specific about the sensations that are being examined. When asking patients or experimental subjects to describe their dyspnea, we prefer to use the phrases "uncomfortable breathing," or "breathing discomfort" that we believe convey as broad a notion as possible to the individual and do not generate a bias toward a particular sensation.

WHAT IS THE STIMULUS?

Unlike investigations of many sensory phenomena involving heat, light, or sound in which the stimulus provoking the sensation is well defined and easily measured, studies of dyspnea, especially those involving patients, must deal with a more complex array of physiologic variables that can contribute to the respiratory discomfort. For example, in a patient with COPD, information from the chemoreceptors, chest wall, and airways may all be integrated to produce dyspnea. In a patient exercising, one also must consider the metabolic demands of the activity. Thus, in a patient with emphysema who becomes short of breath walking up a flight of stairs, is the stimulus for dyspnea the low oxygen saturation, the

TABLE 16-1 Descriptive Phrases Used to Establish the Quality of Dyspnea

My breath does not go in all the way.
My breathing requires effort.
I feel that I am smothering.
I feel a hunger for more air.
My breathing is heavy.
I cannot take a deep breath.
I feel out of breath.
My chest feels tight.
My breathing requires more work.
I feel that I am suffocating.
I feel that my breath stops.
I am gasping for breath.
My chest is constricted.
I feel that my breathing is rapid.
My breathing is shallow.
I feel that I am breathing more.
I cannot get enough air.
My breath does not go out all the way.
My breathing requires more concentration.

SOURCE: From Simon et al.[2]

increased airways resistance, the dynamic hyperinflation and intrinsic positive end-expiratory pressure (PEEPi), or the level of oxygen consumption? Many factors are likely to play a role. Thus, defining the "mechanism" is challenging as one attempts to isolate each element of the system to elucidate its contribution to respiratory discomfort.

WHAT IS THE NEURAL PATHWAY?

While we know that information transmitted from the lungs to the brain via the vagus nerve plays a role in determining the pattern of breathing[12] and may be important in producing the respiratory discomfort associated with breath holding[13] and bronchoconstriction,[14] there is no specific receptor in the lungs, airways, or chest wall that when stimulated produces a respiratory sensation that would be characterized as dyspnea. This is part of the reason why it is difficult to define the stimulus for the sensations as described above. In the end, dyspnea is best viewed as a set of sensations that arises from the integration of information from a variety of sources.

LABORATORY INVESTIGATIONS AND CLINICAL DYSPNEA

In an effort to isolate and study discrete physiologic mechanisms contributing to dyspnea, investigators often create models of pathophysiologic abnormalities applied to normal subjects. While this approach has helped us to understand the role of abnormalities such as hypoxia, hypercapnia, and resistive and elastic loads in producing respiratory sensations, it is not clear how well these experimental constructs represent actual disease states. For example, airway obstruction in asthma may be simulated with external resistive loads, but the sensations associated with such loads can be quite different from what is experienced by patients with acute bronchoconstriction, in whom the load is internal and likely associated with stimulation of pulmonary irritant receptors.[14,15] Nevertheless, these studies, many of which are cited below, provide valuable insight into the physiology of dyspnea.

Basic Physiology of Dyspnea

RESPIRATORY SYSTEM RECEPTORS AND BREATHING DISCOMFORT

CHEMORECEPTORS

Most conditions that provoke dyspnea are associated with increases in ventilation caused by either increased metabolic demand (e.g., exercise), gas-exchange abnormalities resulting from ventilation-perfusion mismatching, or stimulation of receptors in the lungs, chest wall, or upper airways. Dyspnea generally has been attributed to this increased ventilation, especially in patients in whom there is increased respiratory system impedance and in whom the act of breathing does not satisfy the "urge to breathe."[6] However, recent evidence suggests that stimulation of the chemoreceptors may lead to breathing discomfort independently of increases in respiratory muscle output that raise ventilation.

Hypercapnia

Acute elevations in P_{CO_2} have been used experimentally for many years to produce dyspnea.[2,16–19] Initial reports of two individuals who were unable to increase their ventilation in response to the elevated level of CO_2, a normal subject who was paralyzed[20] and a patient with quadriplegia,[21] suggested that ventilatory muscle activity was necessary for the dyspnea associated with CO_2. However, other studies have produced a preponderance of evidence to indicate that CO_2 can lead to respiratory discomfort to a greater degree than would be expected from the level of ventilation[19] and can even do so in the absence of any reflex increase in ventilatory muscle activity. For example, Banzett and colleagues[18] found that ventilator-dependent C1–2 quadriplegics who lacked functioning respiratory muscles experienced "air hunger" with a 7-mmHg increase in end-tidal CO_2. This work was followed by the demonstration that normal subjects completely paralyzed with neuromuscular blocking agents developed a sense of breathing discomfort with relatively small, that is, 5 to 10 mmHg, increases in P_{CO_2}.[7,22] The unpleasant sensation associated with acute hypercapnia is generally described as a sense of an "urge or need to breathe" or a sense of "air hunger."[2,7,18]

The exact neural pathway by which acute hypercapnia produces dyspnea has not been established. Three hypotheses have been proposed, including (1) CO_2-sensitive neurons in the forebrain or midbrain, (2) direct projection to the forebrain from the chemoreceptors, and (3) corollary discharge, that is, a neural discharge to the sensory cortex that is generated simultaneously with and in proportion to the brain stem output to the respiratory muscles.[23] Patients with congenital central hypoventilation syndrome, individuals who lack a ventilatory response to hypercapnia, experience no respiratory discomfort even when P_{CO_2} is markedly elevated.[24] While the defect in this condition is poorly characterized, the behavior of these subjects argues against the first hypothesis, that is, that there are CO_2-sensitive neurons in the forebrain. Current knowledge does not allow us to distinguish between the remaining two hypotheses. Regardless of the neural pathway by which hypercapnia leads to dyspnea, it seems likely that changes in pH at the level of the central chemoreceptor are important in generating the breathing discomfort. Patients with chronic hypercapnia who have undergone metabolic compensation for the respiratory acidosis do not manifest the same symptoms as the acutely hypercapnic subject.

Hypoxia

As with hypercapnia, acute hypoxia has been thought to produce dyspnea as a consequence of the reflex increase in ventilation. In a study by Lane and associates[25] in which dyspnea during exercise was compared with dyspnea during exercise plus hypoxia at matched ventilation, there was no additional respiratory discomfort attributable to the hypoxia, indicating that either hypoxia did not contribute independently to dyspnea or the contribution could not be distinguished from the level of ventilation. Studies of the effect of supplemental oxygen in hypoxic patients also have supported this hypothesized relationship between ventilation and dyspnea. For example, the improvement in exertional dyspnea in hypoxic patients with COPD who were given oxygen was shown to correlate with the reduced ventilation associated with a higher P_{O_2}.[26]

Other investigators, however, have produced conflicting results that support an independent role for hypoxia in the generation of breathing discomfort. Chronos and colleagues[27] demonstrated that normal subjects experience more dyspnea when exercising under hypoxic conditions and less dyspnea when breathing 100% oxygen than they do when breathing room air.[27] Similarly, patients with COPD exercising under hypoxic conditions rate the intensity of dyspnea higher than in the normoxic state,[28] and progressive hypoxia in normal individuals is associated with greater breathing discomfort than comparable degrees of ventilation resulting from exercise.[29] In addition, sudden changes in oxygenation during exercise lead to abrupt increases and decreases in breathing discomfort that precede the full ventilatory response to the change in oxygen saturation.[27]

Clinically, patients often report that they have less dyspnea when using supplemental oxygen even if their baseline oxygen saturation is greater than 90 percent. However, given the possibility of a placebo effect in patients who commonly equate breathing discomfort with insufficient oxygen levels, one must be cautious in interpreting these findings, especially if oxygen is administered by nasal prongs or transtracheal catheter. Moreover, some of the effect may be mediated by receptors in the large airways (see below), which, when stimulated, may reduce ventilation and ameliorate dyspnea.[30–32]

MECHANORECEPTORS

There are a variety of receptors that assist the body in monitoring changes in pressure, flow, and volume in the respiratory system and that respond to the inhalation of noxious materials. Information from these receptors appears to play a role in modulating the intensity of dyspnea, and in some cases, such as the discomfort associated with acute bronchoconstriction,[14,15] the receptors may be the primary cause of the patient's dyspnea.

Upper Airway Receptors

Dyspneic patients often describe relief when they open a window and feel air on their face or when they sit in front of a fan. It is possible that this effect is mediated by a decrease in output from the respiratory centers, a hypothesis consistent with the observation that cold air directed against the face increases breath-holding time.[33] Alternatively, there may

be an effect on respiratory sensation that is independent of changes in central respiratory output. In normal subjects made breathless with external inspiratory resistive loads, cold air directed onto the face reduced dyspnea with minimal changes in ventilation.[34] These areas of the face are innervated by the trigeminal nerve, which also carries sensory information from the buccal mucosa. Inhalation of cold air during exercise by patients with COPD reduced both exertional dyspnea and ventilation,[35] whereas in normal subjects blunting of the response from these receptors with topical lidocaine or the inhalation of warm, humidified air worsened dyspnea.[36] It remains uncertain whether the receptors that mediate these effects respond to the mechanical changes associated with airflow or to the temperature changes that accompany it.

Pulmonary Receptors

There are three major categories of receptors in the airways and lung parenchyma that transmit information relevant to respiratory sensation via the vagus nerve to the brain.[37] *Slowly adapting receptors (SARs),* also known as *pulmonary stretch receptors,* are activated as lung volume increases. The primary stimulus for activation appears to be an increase in tension in the airway wall. These receptors are believed to be responsible for the Hering-Breuer reflex that terminates a deep inflation.

Rapidly adapting receptors (RARs), also known as *irritant receptors,* are found in the airway epithelium and respond to a variety of mechanical and chemical stimuli. These receptors are activated by large and rapid changes in lung volume, particulate matter, histamine, and direct mechanical stimulation. In contrast to the inhibitory effect of the SARs, the RARs in the distal airways are felt to have a stimulatory effect on breathing. RARs may play a role in the ventilatory changes observed in asthma.

The third major category of pulmonary receptors consists of *C-fibers* (also known as *J-receptors*), which are unmyelinated afferent nerve fibers located in small airways and near alveolar capillaries. As with rapidly adapting receptors, C-fibers appear to be stimulated by both mechanical and chemical factors. A number of endogenous chemicals such as histamine, bradykinin, serotonin, and prostaglandins activate these receptors and may mediate the body's response to asthma, pulmonary embolism, and edema or inflammation within the interstitium.

Individuals whose tidal volume is limited or constrained experience significant respiratory discomfort.[38,39] While chest wall receptors may play a role in monitoring thoracic expansion (see below), pulmonary receptors are sufficient to detect changes in lung volume. Patients with high cervical spinal cord injury who have interruption of sensory pathways from the chest wall can still detect changes in tidal volume as small as 100 mL and note a sensation of air hunger when tidal volumes are reduced.[8,40] Over 40 years ago, Fowler demonstrated that the dyspnea associated with breath holding was relieved with a single breath taken from a bag containing a gas mixture similar to what was in the alveoli.[41] The relief of the breath-holding discomfort was attributed to afferent information arising in the lungs or chest wall. However, when these experiments were repeated in patients with lung transplants who have fewer intact pulmonary receptors than normal individuals, the relief from the first breath after the breath hold was less dramatic, a finding suggesting a particularly important role for lung receptors in the relief of breath-holding discomfort.[42]

Although airway obstruction leads to increased resistance to flow and dynamic hyperinflation, both of which increase the work of breathing, there is increasing evidence that a component of the dyspnea of asthma arises from stimulation of pulmonary receptors. At comparable degrees of airway resistance, bronchoconstriction produces a greater intensity of dyspnea than do external resistive loads.[14,15] Furthermore, the quality of the breathing discomfort is different. External resistive loads lead to a sense of increased "effort or work of breathing," while mild degrees of bronchoconstriction are associated with a sense of "chest tightness of constriction."[2,3,15] When airway receptors are blunted by the inhalation of lidocaine, the dyspnea of bronchoconstriction is alleviated, whereas the respiratory discomfort secondary to external resistive loads is not affected.[14] Additional investigations designed to stimulate C-fibers have produced related sensations of choking and chest pressure.[43]

Emphysema is characterized by the loss of lung elastic recoil. Small airways, lacking the support of the surrounding lung parenchyma, are compressed during exhalation when pleural pressure exceeds the pressure within the airway. Receptors in the airway walls may be stimulated by this compression and may contribute to the dyspnea of COPD. When dynamic compression of the airways is accentuated in patients with COPD by the application of a negative pressure at the mouth, respiratory discomfort is increased.[44] Conversely, the beneficial effect of pursed-lips breathing and continuous positive airway pressure (CPAP) on dyspnea in individuals with emphysema may, in part, be a consequence of reduced dynamic airway compression.

Given the variety of receptors in the lungs, it is not surprising that one sees a range of effects on respiratory sensation. Stimulation of irritant receptors in the airways appears to contribute to the discomfort of asthma. In contrast, activation of SARs reduces the dyspnea associated with states of increased respiratory drive such as is seen with acute hypercapnia.

Chest Wall Receptors

Information from the chest wall relevant to respiratory sensation is believed to arise primarily from muscle spindles and tendon organs.[45,46] Muscle spindles function as length or stretch receptors. Passive lengthening of the muscles, as occurs with a patient on a ventilator, also activates the spindles. Tendon organs are believed to serve as force receptors. While costovertebral joints contain movement receptors, little is known about their role in respiratory sensation.

Under experimental conditions, when an individual is forced to constrain tidal volume below that which would otherwise be dictated by the ventilatory stimulus (usually acute hypercapnia), dyspnea is increased.[17,38,39] While stretch receptors in the lungs are sufficient to mediate this effect,[8] information from chest wall receptors also may play a role.[42,47]

A number of investigators have used chest wall vibration to examine the effect of chest wall receptors on respiratory sensation. The rationale behind these experiments is the assumption that mechanical vibrators applied over the intercostal muscles stimulate muscle spindles. In studies of normal subjects made breathless with resistive loads and CO_2,[48]

and in patients with COPD at rest[49] and while breathing CO_2,[50] vibration of the intercostal muscles during inspiration relieved dyspnea. In this last study, however, it appeared that there might be a "threshold" of dyspnea intensity beyond which the effect of vibration might not be seen. Patients with COPD made breathless with acute hypercapnia reported a decrease in dyspnea with chest wall vibration, but during cycle ergometry, a stimulus that provoked a more rapid rise in and greater severity of dyspnea, the vibration did not have a significant effect[50] (Figs. 16–1 and 16–2). While these experiments utilized "in phase" vibration, that is, vibration of inspiratory muscles during inspiration, "out of phase" vibration, that is, vibration of the inspiratory muscles during expiration, has been shown to provoke dyspnea.[51] In each of these studies, it is possible that chest wall vibration also stimulated pulmonary receptors, which could have accounted for some of the effect observed.

SENSE OF EFFORT

Breathing is unique among the vital functions of the body in that it is subject to both volitional (cortical) and automatic (brain stem) control. Activation of the respiratory muscles is associated with conscious awareness of the outgoing motor command that is perceived as a "sense of effort." This sensation is believed to arise from activation of the sensory cortex by a corollary discharge from either the respiratory neurons in the brain stem or the motor cortex simultaneously with the initiation of the motor command.[52] The sense of effort appears to be a function of the ratio of the pressure generated by the ventilatory muscles on a given breath to the maximal pressure-generating capacity of the muscles.[53] Thus, when the respiratory muscles are called on to generate a greater pressure because of an increase in airway resistance and/or decrease in respiratory system compliance, or when the capacity of the respiratory muscles is reduced by neuromuscular disease, the muscles operate closer to their maximal capacity, and the sense of effort is increased. Effort is also accentuated when the neural output to the respiratory muscles is heightened by chemical stimuli such as acute hypercapnia.

Since a large number of cardiopulmonary conditions are characterized by increased respiratory system impedance, inspiratory muscle fatigue or weakness, or increased drive to breathe, the sense of effort is common to a range of pathophysiologic states.[5] However, there are other conditions, such as acute pulmonary embolism, in which the sense of effort appears not to play a significant role. Moreover, Demediuk and colleagues[19] demonstrated that subjects who maintained a constant ventilation by following a visual target experienced greater air hunger and less respiratory effort with acute hypercapnia than they did while breathing room air. This study suggests that a corollary discharge arising solely from the automatic respiratory centers in the medulla produces a different sensory experience than when it accompanies voluntary ventilatory commands originating in the motor cortex.

INTEGRATIVE ASPECTS OF BASIC PHYSIOLOGY

To this point, we have focused on the role of specific receptors located throughout the respiratory system in producing and modulating respiratory discomfort. However, the nature of

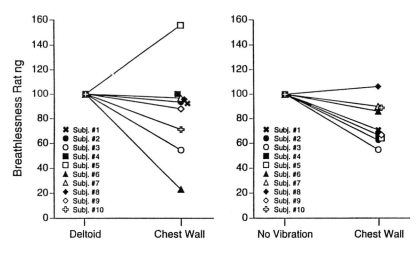

FIGURE 16-1 Breathlessness ratings in patients with COPD during a period of acute steady-state hypercapnia with in-phase chest wall vibration expressed as a percentage of ratings during deltoid (D) and no vibration (NV) controls. Chest wall vibration significantly reduced sensations of breathlessness compared with deltoid ($p < .05$) and no vibration ($p < .01$) controls. (Used, with permission, from Cristiano and Schwartzstein.[50])

cardiopulmonary disease is such that it is uncommon in a given patient complaining of dyspnea for only one type of receptor to be stimulated. For example, in a patient with acute bronchospasm, there may be stimulation of irritant receptors in the lung, and if the individual is hypoxic, the peripheral chemoreceptors will be activated as well. In addition, there is an increased mechanical load on the ventilatory muscles. Thus, to fully appreciate the complexity of dyspnea, one must view it in an integrated fashion and examine the consequences of multiple stimuli interacting simultaneously.

NEUROMECHANICAL DISSOCIATION

The notion that dyspnea may reflect an inadequate mechanical response to the motor commands sent to the respiratory muscles was first put forth by Campbell and Howell[54] as the concept of "length-tension inappropriateness." Under conditions of increased mechanical impedance, the respiratory muscles develop a tension that is out of proportion to the degree of shortening of the muscles; there is less volume displacement of the lungs than "expected." This "inappropriateness" was felt to be the source of the respiratory discomfort associated with many clinical disorders.

In recent years, this concept has been broadened to include afferent information arising from a range of sites in the respiratory system, including receptors in the upper airway, lungs, and chest wall.[39,55] As neural impulses from the respiratory neurons reach the ventilatory muscles, they are translated into changes in pressure, flow, and volume from the pharynx to the distal airways, along with changes in the length and tension of the chest wall muscles. Pressure and flow receptors in the airways, stretch and irritant receptors in the lungs, and muscle spindles and tendon organs in the chest wall are stimulated and transmit information back to the brain. If this afferent information matches what would be expected under normal conditions given the efferent signals from the brain, dyspnea is minimized. If there is dissociation between the outgoing motor command and the incoming sensory information, respiratory discomfort increases. This concept has been termed *efferent-reafferent dissociation*[55] or *neuromechanical dissociation*[56] and can explain the modulation of dyspnea observed under a range of experimental and clinical conditions. For example, larger tidal volumes with increased stimulation of pulmonary and chest wall receptors reduce the dyspnea associated with acute hypercapnia.[8,17,38,39] Chest wall vibration and the presumed increased stimulation of chest wall and/or pulmonary receptors reduce the breathlessness of resistive loads,[48–50] whereas decreasing inspiratory flow below that desired by the individual can increase the breathing discomfort associated with mechanical ventilation.[57]

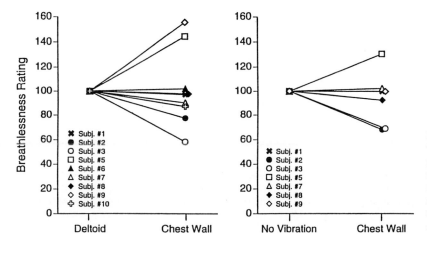

FIGURE 16-2 Breathlessness ratings in patients with COPD during steady-state exercise with in-phase chest wall vibration expressed as a percentage of ratings during deltoid (D) and no vibration (NV) controls. The change in breathlessness was not significantly different during chest wall vibration compared with controls. (Used, with permission, from Cristiano and Schwartzstein.[50])

EXERCISE

Most individuals, both normal subjects and patients with cardiopulmonary disease, experience breathing discomfort if they engage in vigorous physical activity. Exertional dyspnea is probably the most common reason a patient is referred to pulmonary rehabilitation. Yet, despite the frequent occurrence of this problem, our understanding of exercise-related breathing discomfort remains limited.

In healthy subjects, dyspnea during exercise increases in concert with increasing ventilation,[58] and after cessation of the activity, dyspnea decreases as ventilation returns to normal.[59] However, the level of ventilation alone cannot fully explain the breathing discomfort associated with exercise because we know that at matched levels of ventilation, exercise[60] as well as hypercapnia[19,29] and hypoxia[29] produce greater dyspnea than voluntary hyperventilation (isocapnic hyperpnea). Exercise, hypoxia, and hypercapnia are all characterized by increased activity in the "reflex" or automatic respiratory centers and are generally associated with a sensation of an "urge to breathe," a sense of "air hunger," or "need to breathe."[8,18,61] While the increased ventilation and dyspnea accompanying hypoxia and hypercapnia are likely mediated through stimulation of chemoreceptors, the mechanism by which exercise produces these changes remains obscure. In normal individuals, exercise is characterized by a normal (or slightly increased) P_{O_2} and normal to low levels of P_{CO_2}. Some data suggest that activation of locomotor areas in the brain can account for the increase in ventilation and the breathing discomfort associated with exercise,[62] but the persistence of both for at least several minutes following cessation of activity argues against this being the sole explanation.[59] Studies of young individuals with congenital central hypoventilation syndrome have yielded conflicting results regarding the role of the medullary respiratory centers in the dyspnea and hyperpnea of exercise. While one demonstrated hypoventilation and the absence of breathing discomfort with exercise,[63] others have found an appropriate increase in ventilation as well as dyspnea in these patients.[24,64]

Well-conditioned individuals are able to perform vigorous physical activity with relatively little breathing discomfort. What sets them apart from the poorly conditioned person? Fitness is characterized by enhanced ability to deliver oxygen to the muscles and to utilize that oxygen to perform aerobic metabolism. A well-conditioned individual is able to generate a higher cardiac output during exercise and has skeletal muscles with higher concentrations of mitochondria and oxidative enzymes, attributes that maximize aerobic metabolism. When the aerobic capacity of the individual is exceeded, anaerobic metabolism ensues and results in the production of lactic acid. In addition to placing an increased demand on the respiratory system as one hyperventilates to compensate for the accumulation of acid, the onset of anaerobic processes also may be associated with stimulation of mechanoreceptors in the muscles. These receptors, termed *ergoreceptors*, may contribute to the hyperpnea of exercise, at least in patients with chronic congestive heart failure.[65–67] The activity of the ergoreceptors may be blunted by exercise training.[67] The role of these receptors in exertional dyspnea in normal subjects and patients with chronic lung disease has not been studied.

TABLE 16-2 Clinical Physiology of Dyspnea

Cardiovascular system dyspnea
   Cardiac disease
   Anemia
   Deconditioning
Respiratory system dyspnea
   The respiratory controller
   The ventilatory pump
   The gas exchanger

Clinical Physiology of Dyspnea

When confronted with a patient complaining of breathing discomfort, the physician usually tries to determine whether a disorder of the cardiovascular or respiratory system is primarily responsible for the symptom. From the standpoint of the basic physiologic mechanisms discussed earlier, this distinction is somewhat artificial. Interstitial lung disease and pulmonary edema may both result in stimulation of C-fibers in the lungs as well as peripheral chemoreceptors if hypoxia is present; respiratory muscle dysfunction may be a characteristic of both COPD and chronic congestive heart failure (CHF). Nevertheless, as one begins to formulate a therapeutic plan for a patient and to decide if an exercise program will be beneficial in improving functional capacity, this construct can be useful.

Each of the major categories, cardiovascular and respiratory system dyspnea, can be further divided into three subcategories (Table 16–2). Much of our understanding of the mechanisms of dyspnea in cardiovascular disorders is speculative,[68] since relatively few studies have directly examined dyspnea in these conditions. Nonetheless, we will attempt to weave physiologic mechanisms into the fabric of these clinical pictures.

CARDIOVASCULAR SYSTEM DYSPNEA

The cardiovascular system must pump oxygenated blood to the tissues to meet the metabolic needs of the body at rest and during exercise. In order to perform aerobic metabolism, the tissues must be able to acquire oxygen bound to hemoglobin and have an adequate level of oxidative enzymes to utilize the oxygen. For the purposes of this discussion, we will consider *cardiovascular system dyspnea* in a broad sense as any breathing discomfort that occurs in the absence of pulmonary disease and that arises from a derangement in the body's ability to deliver and/or use oxygen. These derangements can be secondary to primary cardiac disease, anemia, and/or impaired utilization of oxygen by the tissues.

CARDIAC DISEASE

There are many forms of cardiac disease, a detailed discussion of which is beyond the scope of this chapter. However, regardless of the type of cardiac disease, we can consider three general mechanisms by which heart disease may cause or contribute to dyspnea: (1) a reduction in cardiac output, leading to reduced oxygen delivery to the periphery (including the respiratory muscles), (2) increased pulmonary venous pressure, and/or (3) chemoreceptor stimulation by hypoxia and, rarely, hypercapnia.

Left ventricular end-diastolic pressure and hence pulmonary venous pressure often rise in the setting of ischemic and/or valvular heart disease. Acute myocardial ischemia is well recognized as a cause of breathing discomfort, and dyspnea on exertion may be an early warning sign of underlying coronary artery disease. Over one-third of men between the ages of 40 and 59 who had severe exertional dyspnea in the absence of signs of coronary disease were found to have a myocardial infarction during a 5-year follow-up compared with only 8.1 percent in those without breathing discomfort.[69,70] During transient ischemia, the left ventricle becomes less compliant, resulting in an increase in left ventricular end-diastolic pressure. Pulmonary venous and capillary pressures rise, and there may be transudation of fluid into the pulmonary interstitium. Similar elevations in pulmonary venous and capillary pressures may occur in patients with hypertensive cardiomyopathy or valvular heart disease. This increase in lung water has a number of effects on pulmonary mechanics and gas exchange that likely contribute to dyspnea in patients with CHF. Fluid in the interstitium causes a decrease in lung compliance, and edema of the bronchial walls narrows the airway by passively reducing cross-sectional area and by stimulating airway receptors that lead to bronchoconstriction.[71] The presence of interstitial or alveolar edema also leads to worsening ventilation-perfusion mismatch, which increases the minute ventilation necessary to achieve adequate CO_2 elimination and may cause hypoxia. These factors in concert may cause a substantial increase in the work of breathing, thereby heightening the sense of respiratory effort. Additionally, C-fibers in the lung are believed to be stimulated by interstitial liquid,[72] and this may be another factor contributing to dyspnea in CHF.

The reduction in cardiac output that accompanies many types of cardiac disease affects the function of both the ventilatory and the limb muscles. Reduced blood flow to the respiratory muscles may lead to fatigue, especially in the setting of an increased mechanical load.[73] Respiratory muscle weakness is a common finding in CHF,[74,75] and although the exact mechanism remains uncertain, reduced blood flow to the respiratory muscles may be a key factor. As noted earlier, both muscle fatigue and weakness heighten the sense of respiratory effort, and the increased sense of effort may be an important mechanism of dyspnea in patients with CHF. A reduction in cardiac output also may affect respiratory control. For any given level of exercise, ventilation is increased in patients with CHF compared with normal controls,[76] and in CHF, the relationship between ventilation and carbon dioxide production is characterized by a steeper slope than normal.[77] One hypothesis for the exaggerated ventilatory response to exercise is that there are mechanoreceptors in limb muscles that are sensitive to the accumulation of metabolites that occurs when the muscle is working beyond the ability of the cardiovascular system to provide oxygen,[65–68] and these receptors may contribute to both the increase in ventilation[78] and dyspnea observed in CHF.

Finally, we have already discussed in some detail the role of chemical stimuli in the pathogenesis of dyspnea. Some but not all patients with cardiac disease are hypoxic, and patients with severe pulmonary edema may become hypercapnic. To the extent that hypoxia and/or hypercapnia are present in a patient with cardiac disease, they represent yet another potential stimulus for dyspnea.

ANEMIA

When the hematocrit drops below 30 percent, exertional dyspnea is seen frequently. The oxygen-carrying capacity of the blood is reduced, and the body compensates by increasing cardiac output. The mechanism by which anemia produces dyspnea is unknown. To generate a higher than normal cardiac output, the heart may require a greater left ventricular end-diastolic pressure, which results in elevated pulmonary vascular pressures. Such pressures may lead to dyspnea by stimulating C-fibers in the pulmonary capillaries (as discussed earlier). However, tachycardia is often the first response of the heart when an increased cardiac output is needed, and it is unclear to what extent intracardiac and pulmonary vascular pressures rise. Alternatively, reduced oxygen delivery to the skeletal muscles may lead to the early development of metabolic acidosis and stimulation of ergoreceptors.[66,67]

DECONDITIONING

Most normal individuals develop breathing discomfort with vigorous activity. Those with a very sedentary existence experience dyspnea with relatively modest exercise. If obesity is superimposed on the picture, the functional limitation becomes even more pronounced. Sedentary individuals are distinguished from well-conditioned athletes by a lesser ability to increase cardiac output during exercise and by decreased utilization of oxygen by the skeletal muscles. Thus, in the sedentary or deconditioned individual, maximal oxygen consumption is reduced, and anaerobic metabolism begins at lower levels of physical work. While the development of metabolic acidosis results in a greater minute ventilation for any given workload than would be seen in the absence of acidosis, this in and of itself is unlikely to be a major cause of dyspnea in the deconditioned patient because even highly trained athletes do not have a ventilatory limit to exercise.[79] Rather, we believe it is more likely that changes in the local milieu of the skeletal muscle resulting from anaerobic metabolism and the deconditioned state are the cause of the discomfort that is often characterized as "heavy breathing" or "breathing more."[80] It is important to remember that deconditioned individuals, even those with significant underlying lung disease, often will indicate on close questioning that they are limited in their activity more by fatigue than by dyspnea.[81]

RESPIRATORY SYSTEM DYSPNEA

When considering dyspnea arising from abnormalities of the respiratory system, it is useful to think of the three components of the system, each of which is necessary to move oxygen from the environment down to the alveoli and pulmonary capillaries and carbon dioxide back out to the atmosphere: the respiratory controller, the ventilatory pump, and the gas exchanger. In many patients, there are derangements of more than one component, such as a patient with COPD, who has airways obstruction and a hyperinflated chest (ventilatory pump) as well as increased dead space (gas exchanger). Nevertheless, as one assesses a patient and considers possible treatment strategies for breathing discomfort, identifying the elements that may contribute to the discomfort is an important first step.

THE RESPIRATORY CONTROLLER

Many stimuli can cause increases in ventilation, including acute hypoxia and hypercapnia, metabolic acidosis, hormonal changes such as increased progesterone levels during pregnancy, drugs (e.g., aspirin in large quantities), stimulation of pulmonary receptors, and exercise. While increases in ventilation require the individual to perform greater work with the respiratory muscles, studies have demonstrated that voluntary hyperpnea produces less intense dyspnea than does a comparable level of ventilation resulting from reflex stimulation of the respiratory centers from acute hypercapnia[19] or exercise.[60] A component of dyspnea associated with hypoxia appears to be secondary to a direct effect of hypoxia (i.e., not simply a consequence of the increase in ventilation), although there are conflicting data in this regard.[25-29] Metabolic acidosis appears to produce an intensity of dyspnea comparable with levels of exercise resulting in similar ventilation.[82]

Additional evidence that stimulation of the respiratory controller produces dyspnea that is separate from the mechanical work of achieving the increased ventilation comes from studies assessing the quality of the respiratory discomfort. While the sense of effort is associated with increased mechanical work,[2-5,9] conditions that cause a reflex increase in ventilation commonly produce a sensation of air hunger or a need to breathe.[3-5,7,8] We believe that these varying sensations represent different physiologic mechanisms.

While stimulation of the respiratory centers leads to dyspnea, one also should note that respiratory discomfort may alter the pattern of breathing.[83] Subjects breathing through an external resistance tend to adopt a slow, deep breathing pattern, whereas individuals breathing with an elastic load typically have a rapid respiratory rate with small tidal volumes. The acute onset of severe respiratory discomfort may be associated with intense respiratory efforts.[84] On the other hand, more chronic changes in pulmonary mechanics can lead to adjustments in the controller that reduce ventilatory effort.[85] Whether or not the respiratory controller adapts with time to minimize respiratory discomfort remains unclear, but the data support a primary role for stimulation of the controller as a source of dyspnea.

THE VENTILATORY PUMP

The ventilatory pump is comprised of those structures necessary for the movement of air into and out of the lungs. The ventilatory muscles, the bones of the chest wall, the upper and lower airways, the pleura, and the peripheral nerves that connect the respiratory centers to the ventilatory muscles are all essential for the normal functioning of the ventilatory pump. Derangements of any of these components lead to an increased mechanical load on the system or to reduced efficiency in the movement of gases into and out of the lung. In these settings, a greater neural output from the controller is required to achieve a given level of ventilation, and the individual experiences breathing discomfort characterized as a sense of "effort or work of breathing."[61]

Patients with airways obstruction from asthma experience a range of sensations as their forced expiratory volume in 1 s (FEV_1) declines. At very mild degrees of bronchoconstriction,

chest tightness, which we believe emanates from stimulation of pulmonary receptors (see earlier discussion of pulmonary receptors), predominates, whereas greater degrees of airway obstruction are characterized by an increased sense of effort and eventually "air hunger."[15,61,86] In addition to the increased mechanical work needed to overcome airways obstruction, patients with asthma are often hyperinflated, a condition that places the inspiratory muscles in a shortened position and reduces their mechanical efficiency. These factors probably account for the observation that patients with asthma complain to a greater extent about the discomfort associated with inspiration than that with expiration.[86,87]

COPD, like asthma, is characterized by a combination of increased airways resistance and dynamic hyperinflation. In patients with emphysema, hyperinflation may be dramatic, and positive pressure may persist in the alveoli throughout expiration (intrinsic or auto-PEEP). The presence of intrinsic PEEP places a further load on the respiratory muscles at the onset of inspiration; i.e., the muscles must overcome the PEEP before inspiratory flow can be initiated. These mechanical factors likely account for the finding that, like patients with asthma, patients with COPD also complain of more breathing difficulty during inspiration than during expiration.[53,88,89] These factors presumably also account for the prevalence of the "sense of effort" and "work of breathing" as the qualitative descriptors most characteristic of the breathing discomfort reported by patients with COPD[3,5,61] and for the fact that treatment with continuous positive airway pressure (CPAP), which assists the inspiratory muscles in overcoming the threshold inspiratory load imposed by intrinsic PEEP, reduces dyspnea in these individuals.[90,91] By breathing at an elevated end-expiratory lung volume, patients with COPD operate along a relatively flat portion of their pressure-volume curve; that is, the compliance of the respiratory system is reduced. This further increases the work of breathing, contributes to the sense of respiratory effort, and may lead to the additional discomfort, recently described by patients with COPD as feeling as if one cannot get an adequate or satisfying breath.[92]

Chest wall abnormalities such as kyphoscoliosis reduce the compliance of the chest wall, thereby leading to increased work of breathing and a heightened sense of effort. Patients with neuromuscular disease, for example, myasthenia gravis, have difficulty generating a sufficient inspiratory pressure. Neural output from the respiratory centers in the brain increases, and the patient also experiences a breathing discomfort described as "effort."[3-5]

THE GAS EXCHANGER

The ultimate purpose of the respiratory system is to add oxygen to and remove carbon dioxide from the blood. This requires an intact "gas exchanger" comprised of alveoli and the associated pulmonary capillaries. Conditions that reduce the surface area of this interface (e.g., emphysema or pulmonary fibrosis), retard diffusion of gases across it (e.g., interstitial inflammation or fluid), or block movement of gas into the alveoli (e.g., pneumonia, pulmonary edema, or mucus plugging) result in hypoxia and/or hypercapnia. Acute derangements in P_{O_2} and P_{CO_2} generally lead to increased ventilation and a sense of air hunger or need to breathe[2,7,18,25-28] (see "Chemoreceptors" above). Patients with pulmonary embolism are frequently hypoxic, although the intensity of their

TABLE 16-3 Change in Quality of Dyspnea in Asthmatic Patients with Acute Bronchospasm during Treatment with Albuterol

Descriptor of Dyspnea	Before Bronchodilator	After First Bronchodilator Dose	After Second Bronchodilator Dose	After Third Bronchodilator Dose
Tight	16	8	5	6
Breathing more	1	11	12	6
Work	7	3	5	4
Effort	6	5	4	3
Breath does not go out	7	5	4	4

NOTE: Number of patients ($n = 25$) selecting each descriptor of dyspnea on presentation to an emergency department with acute bronchoconstriction and following each of three doses of nebulized albuterol administered at 20-min intervals. There was a significant decrease ($p < .05$) in the number of patients experiencing "tightness" and increase in the number perceiving that they were "breathing more" after the inhaled bronchodilator. In contrast, the number of patients experiencing a sensation of increased "effort" or "work" of breathing did not change significantly with bronchodilator therapy.

SOURCE: Adapted from Moy et al.[93]

dyspnea is often out of proportion to any gas-exchange abnormality. Anecdotal reports of very rapid resolution of dyspnea in association with thrombolytic therapy (J Markis, personal communication) suggest that stimulation of pressure receptors in the pulmonary vasculature or right atrium may play a role in the respiratory discomfort experienced by patients with pulmonary embolism. Pulmonary emboli also lead to the release of various mediators, for example, kinins, that may have an additional impact on irritant receptors within the lung.

Many of the problems that lead to abnormalities of the gas exchanger also affect the ventilatory pump. Thus it is common for a patient to experience several qualitatively distinct types of dyspnea[3,5] and for the treatment of one abnormality to alleviate one sensation but not another.[93] Asthma provides one of the best examples of this principle. Chest tightness is present at mild degrees of bronchoconstriction, whereas the sense of effort becomes prominent at greater degrees of airways obstruction.[15] The sense of air hunger also may be present, especially if leukotrienes are triggering the bronchospasm.[86] When patients with acute flares of their asthma are treated with beta agonists in an emergency department, they experience relief of their chest tightness, possibly by decreasing stimulation of irritant receptors in the airways, yet they continue to feel a sense of increased effort to breathe, presumably secondary to persistent obstruction (and the resulting mechanical load) produced by airways inflammation[93] (Table 16-3).

As this discussion demonstrates, the basic physiology of dyspnea is important in understanding respiratory discomfort in various clinical conditions. It is common for more than one mechanism to contribute to dyspnea in a given patient (Table 16-4). These insights, however, form the basis for a rational approach to the treatment of patients with breathing discomfort.

Behavioral Aspects of Dyspnea

An understanding of the way a patient reacts to respiratory discomfort requires that we make a distinction between the actual *sensation*, that is, the neural activation of a receptor, and the *perception*, or response of the individual to the sensation. Since it is difficult to isolate and quantify the specific stimulus or stimuli that lead to dyspnea, we have a poor understanding of the relationship between a given respiratory sensation and the perception of that sensation. Predicting how a particular person will function with a given degree of respiratory discomfort is even more problematic. For example, while there is a general relationship between FEV_1 and dyspnea (Fig. 16-3), at any given level of airways obstruction there is tremendous interindividual variability in dyspnea. Some of this variability probably reflects the fact that no single number or measurement fully characterizes the respiratory system, but some of the variability also may be due to differences in the central neurologic processing of the signals emanating from receptors throughout the respiratory system. Alternatively, psychological factors and previous experiences inherent within the individual may play a dominant role in the perception of the sensation.

The context in which the sensation occurs is important in

TABLE 16-4 Possible Mechanisms of Dyspnea in Selected Conditions

Condition	Mechanism
Asthma	Increased sense of effort
	Stimulation of irritant receptors in airways
Neuromuscular disease	Increased sense of effort
COPD	Increased sense of effort
	Hypoxia
	Hypercapnia
	Dynamic airway compression
Mechanical ventilation	Afferent mismatch
	Factors associated with the underlying condition
Pulmonary embolism	Stimulation of pulmonary receptors in pulmonary vasculature or right atrium (?)
Deconditioning	Stimulation of ergoreceptors (?)
Congestive heart failure	Stimulation of J-receptors
	Stimulation of pulmonary receptors in pulmonary vasculature (?)
	Hypoxia
	Stimulation of ergoreceptors

SOURCE: Modified from Manning HL, Schwartzstein RM: Pathophysiology of dyspnea. *N Engl J Med* 333:1547, 1995.

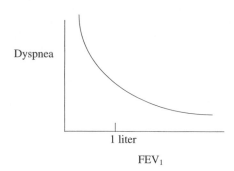

FIGURE 16-3 Dyspnea as a function of FEV$_1$. While there is great variability in the correlation between FEV$_1$ and breathlessness for any given patient, one generally begins to see significant increases in dyspnea as FEV$_1$ approaches 1 L.

determining the perception of the discomfort as "normal" or "abnormal." When engaging in very vigorous physical exercise, most healthy individuals will experience breathing discomfort but will not be distressed by it. This is an expected sensation in the context of heavy activity. On the other hand, the same sensation felt while walking several blocks on flat ground would likely be viewed as pathologic and provoke anxiety and concern in the individual.

Depression and anxiety also may affect the perception of respiratory sensations. The association of these emotional states with chronic lung disease has been observed in several studies.[94-96] While it is not clear whether the presence of the chronic disease predisposes to the development of anxiety or depression or whether these conditions, as preexisting states, merely make the perception of any discomfort more pronounced, it is apparent that the emotional or affective condition of the patient can influence the reaction of the patient to breathing discomfort.[97] Adaptive, independent patients appear to be more tolerant of mechanical loads on the respiratory system, whereas those who are dependent and anxious perceive great discomfort with relatively small loads.[98,99] To the extent that anxiety may lead to hyperventilation, the patient with emotional distress can develop a spiral of increasing dyspnea when the cardiorespiratory system is stressed; for example, increased airways resistance leads to increased work of breathing and a sense of effort that cause anxiety, leading to increasing ventilation, increased mechanical work, greater sense of discomfort, more anxiety, and so on (Fig. 16–4). In many ways, perception is the product of mind and body, of physical sensations and emotional responses.

Implications for Pulmonary Rehabilitation

Pulmonary rehabilitation has been shown to improve exercise performance in many patients with chronic lung disease. Among the potential mechanisms for the observed increase in exercise capacity are enhanced cardiovascular fitness, increased respiratory muscle strength and endurance, improved efficiency of breathing pattern, and desensitization to respiratory discomfort. One of the challenges confronting a physician providing care for patients with chronic dyspnea is to determine the primary factor that is responsible for an individual's functional limitation, especially in patients with more than one pathophysiologic problem, for example, interstitial lung disease and asthma or COPD and cardiovascular deconditioning. Are hyperinflation and increased work of breathing the major problem, or is the patient experiencing chest tightness arising from stimulation of pulmonary irritant receptors by airway inflammation and bronchospasm? Ideally, if one can identify the pathologic process and the underlying physiologic mechanisms responsible for a patient's breathing discomfort, a treatment program can be designed to address specifically those issues, maximize functional status, and minimize respiratory symptoms.

Future advances in treatment of dyspnea are likely to arise from a better understanding of the mechanisms producing the discomfort. The use of CPAP to reduce the work of breathing and possibly the stimulation of airway receptors by dynamic compressed airway is one such example.[90,91] Chest wall vibration has been shown to reduce the dyspnea associated with hypercapnia and external resistive loads in normal subjects[48] and in patients with COPD,[49,50] presumably by increasing the afferent feedback from pulmonary and/or chest wall receptors and reducing neuromechanical dissociation. Inhaled lidocaine may be useful in reducing dyspnea in patients whose symptoms are due to stimulation of airway irritant receptors.[14]

Identification of the emotional responses to dyspnea that amplify the patient's discomfort is another important goal of the rehabilitation program. When a patient develops a sense of control or mastery over the symptom and the disease responsible for it, functional status is likely to improve.[100] An understanding of the behavioral response to the sensations produced by the cardiopulmonary disease is critical to a therapeutic program.

Summary

Dyspnea is comprised of a complex set of qualitatively distinct sensations arising from multiple physiologic mechanisms. Sensory input from receptors ranging from the upper airway to the pulmonary parenchyma and from the chemoreceptors to the chest wall plays an important role in modifying the quality and intensity of the respiratory discomfort associ-

FIGURE 16-4 Cycle of anxiety and dyspnea. Patients with lung disease and breathlessness often become anxious when attempting to perform a physical task. Anxiety leads to hyperventilation, which, in the presence of increased mechanical impedance, may lead to worsening dyspnea. This increased discomfort causes further anxiety, hyperventilation, and more dyspnea.

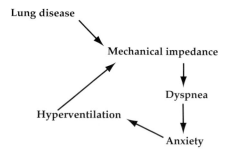

ated with cardiopulmonary diseases. In any given patient, there may be more than one type of dyspnea, and multiple mechanisms may be active. When evaluating a patient whose functional status is compromised by dyspnea, it is important to try to determine which factors are responsible for the exercise limitation. Furthermore, it is important to consider the individual's behavioral response to the sensation, the perception of the experience.

An understanding of the basic and clinical physiology of dyspnea helps guide the clinician in planning diagnostic and therapeutic strategies for patients with shortness of breath. Ultimately, new therapies as well as better application of established treatments may evolve as our knowledge of the physiology of this symptom grows.

References

1. Harver A, Mahler DA: The symptom of dyspnea, in Mahler DA (ed): *Dyspnea*. Mount Kisco, NY, Futura, 1990; pp 1–54.
2. Simon PM, Schwartzstein RM, Weiss JW, et al: Distinguishable sensations of the breathlessness induced in normal volunteers. *Am Rev Respir Dis* 140:1021, 1989.
3. Simon PM, Schwartzstein RM, Weiss JW, et al: Distinguishable types of dyspnea in patients with shortness of breath. *Am Rev Respir Dis* 144:826, 1990.
4. Elliott MW, Adams L, Cockroft A, et al: The language of breathlessness: Use of verbal descriptors. *Am Rev Respir Dis* 144:826, 1991.
5. Mahler DA, Harver A, Lentine T, et al: Descriptors of breathlessness in cardiorespiratory diseases. *Am J Respir Crit Care Med* 154:1357, 1996.
6. Wright GW, Branscomb BV: The origin of the sensations of dyspnea. *Trans Am Clin Climatol Assoc* 1966:116, 1954.
7. Banzett RB, Lansing RW, Brown R, et al: "Air hunger" arising from increased P_{CO_2} persists after complete neuromuscular block in humans. *Respir Physiol* 81:1, 1990.
8. Manning HL, Shea SA, Schwartzstein RM, et al: Reduced tidal volume increases air hunger at fixed P_{CO_2} in ventilated quadriplegics. *Respir Physiol* 90:19, 1992.
9. Killian KJ, Gandevia SC, Summer E, Campbell EJM: Effect of increased lung volume on perception of breathlessness, effort and tension. *J Appl Physiol* 57:686, 1984.
10. Supinski GS, Clary SJ, Bark H, Kelsen SG: Effect of inspiratory muscle fatigue on perception of effort during loaded breathing. *J Appl Physiol* 62:300, 1987.
11. McClosky DI: Kinesthetic sensibility. *Physiol Rev* 58:763, 1978.
12. Clark FJ, von Euler C: On the regulation of the depth and rate of breathing. *J Physiol* 222:267, 1972.
13. Guz A, Noble MIM, Eisele JH, Trenchard D: Experimental results of vagal blockade in cardiopulmonary disease, in Porter R (ed): *Breathing*. Hering-Breuer Centenary Symposium, London, J&A Churchill, 1970; pp 315–329.
14. Taguchi O, Kikuchi Y, Hida W, et al: Effects of bronchoconstriction and external resistive loading on the sensation of dyspnea. *J Appl Physiol* 71:2183, 1991.
15. Schwartzstein R, Lilly J, Israel E, et al: Breathlessness of asthma differs from that of external resistive loads. *Am Rev Respir Dis* 142:A596, 1991.
16. Hill L, Flack F: The effect of excess carbon dioxide and want of oxygen upon the respiration and the circulation. *J Physiol* 37:77, 1908.
17. Remmers JE, Brooks J, Tenney SM: Effect of controlled ventilation on the tolerable limit of hypercapnia. *Respir Physiol* 4:78, 1968.
18. Banzett RB, Lansing RW, Reid MB, et al: "Air hunger" from increased P_{CO_2} in mechanically ventilated quadriplegics. *Respir Physiol* 76:53, 1989.
19. Demediuk BH, Manning HL, Lilly J, et al: Dissociation between dyspnea and respiratory effort. *Am Rev Respir Dis* 146:1222, 1992.
20. Campbell EJM, Godfrey S, Clark TJH, et al: The effect of muscular paralysis induced by tubocurarine on the duration and sensation of breath-holding during hypercapnia. *Clin Sci* 36:323, 1969.
21. Noble MIM, Eisele JH, Trenchard D, Guz A: Effect of selective peripheral nerve blocks on respiratory sensations, in Porter R (ed): *Breathing*. Hering-Breuer Centenary Symposium. London, J&A Churchill, 1970; pp 233–251.
22. Gandevia SC, Killian K, McKenzie DK, et al: Respiratory sensations, cardiovascular control, kinaesthesia and transcranial stimulation during paralysis in humans. *J Physiol* 470:85, 1993.
23. Banzett RB, Lansing RW: Respiratory sensations arising from pulmonary and chemoreceptor afferents, in Adams L, Guz A (eds): *Respiratory Sensation*. New York, Marcel Dekker, 1996; pp 155–180.
24. Shea SA, Andres LP, Shannon DC, et al: Respiratory sensations in subjects who lack a ventilatory response to CO_2. *Respir Physiol* 93:203, 1993.
25. Lane R, Adams L, Guz A: The effects of hypoxia and hypercapnia on perceived breathlessness during exercise in humans. *J Physiol* 428:579, 1990.
26. Swinburn CR, Wakefield JM, Jones PW: Relationship between ventilation and breathlessness during exercise in chronic obstructive airways disease is not altered by the prevention of hypoxemia. *Clin Sci* 67:515, 1984.
27. Chronos N, Adams L, Guz A: Effect of hyperoxia and hypoxia on exercise-induced breathlessness in normal subjects. *Clin Sci* 74:531, 1988.
28. Lane R, Cockcroft A, Adams L, Guz A: Arterial oxygen saturation and breathlessness in patients with chronic obstructive airways disease. *Clin Sci* 72:693, 1987.
29. Adams L, Lane R, Shea SA, et al: Breathlessness during different forms of ventilatory stimulation: A study of mechanisms in normal subjects and respiratory patients. *Clin Sci* 69:663, 1985.
30. Liss HP, Grant BJB: The effect of nasal flow on breathlessness in patients with chronic obstructive lung disease. *Am Rev Respir Dis* 137:1285, 1988.
31. Couser JI, Make BJ: Transtracheal oxygen decreases inspired minute ventilation. *Am Rev Respir Dis* 139:627, 1989.
32. Scott GC, Hinson JM, Scott RP, et al: The effects of transtracheal gas delivery on central inspiratory neuromuscular drive. *Chest* 104:1199, 1993.
33. McBride B, Whitelaw WA: A physiological stimulus to upper airway receptors in humans. *J Appl Physiol* 51:1189, 1981.
34. Schwartzstein RM, Lahive K, Pope A, et al: Cold facial stimulation reduces breathlessness induced in normal subjects. *Am Rev Respir Dis* 136:58, 1987.
35. Spence DPS, Graham DR, Ahmed J, et al: Does cold air affect exercise capacity and dyspnea in stable chronic obstructive pulmonary disease? *Chest* 103:693, 1993.
36. Simon PM, Basner RC, Weinberger SE, et al: Oral mucosal stimulation modulates intensity of breathlessness induced in normal subjects. *Am Rev Respir Dis* 144:419, 1991.
37. Coleridge HM, Coleridge JCG: Reflexes evoked from tracheobronchial tree and lungs, in Cherniack NS, Widdicombe JG (eds): *Handbook of Physiology*, sec 3: *The Respiratory System*, vol 2: *Control of Breathing*. Bethesda, MD, American Physiological Society, 1986, pp 396–429.
38. Chonan T, Mulholland MB, Cherniack NS, Altose MD: Effects of voluntary constraining of thoracic displacement during hypercapnia. *J Appl Physiol* 63:1822, 1987.
39. Schwartzstein RM, Simon PM, Weiss JW, et al: Breathlessness induced by dissociation between ventilation and chemical drive. *Am Rev Respir Dis* 139:1231, 1989.

40. Banzett RB, Lansing RW, Brown R: High-level quadriplegics perceive lung volume change. *J Appl Physiol* 62:567, 1987.

41. Fowler WS: Breaking point of breath-holding. *J Appl Physiol* 6:539, 1954.

42. Flume PA, Eldridge FL, Edwards LJ, Houser JM: The Fowler breath-holding study revisited: Continuous rating of respiratory sensation. *Respir Physiol* 95:53, 1994.

43. Paintal AS: Sensations from J receptors. *NIPS* 10:283, 1995.

44. O'Donnell DE, Sanii R, Anthonisen NR, Younes M: Effect of dynamic airway compression on breathing pattern and respiratory sensation in severe chronic obstructive pulmonary disease. *Am Rev Respir Dis* 135:912, 1987.

45. Shannon R: Reflexes from respiratory muscles and costovertebral joints, in Cherniack NS, Widdicombe JG (eds): *Handbook of Physiology, sec 3: The Respiratory System, vol 2: Control of Breathing.* Bethesda, MD, American Physiological Society, 1986; pp 431–447.

46. Gandevia SC, Macefield G: Projection of low threshold afferents from human intercostal muscles to the cerebral cortex. *Respir Physiol* 77:203, 1989.

47. Altose MD, Syed I, Shoos L: Effects of chest wall vibration on the intensity of dyspnea during constrained breathing. *Proc Int Union Physiol Sci* 17:288, 1989.

48. Manning HL, Basner R, Ringler J, et al: Effect of chest wall vibration on breathlessness in normal subjects. *J Appl Physiol* 71:175, 1991.

49. Sibuya M, Yamada M, Kanamaru A, et al: Effect of chest wall vibration in patients with chronic respiratory disease. *Am J Respir Crit Care Med* 149:1235, 1994.

50. Cristiano LM, Schwartzstein RM: Effect of chest wall vibration on dyspnea during hypercapnia and exercise in chronic obstructive pulmonary disease. *Am J Respir Crit Care Med* 155:1552, 1997.

51. Homma I, Obata T, Sibuya M, Uchida M: Gate mechanism in breathlessness caused by chest wall vibration in humans. *J Appl Physiol* 56:8, 1984.

52. McCloskey DI: Corollary discharges: Motor commands and perception, in Brookhart JM, Mountcastle VB (eds): *Handbook of Physiology, sec 1: The Nervous System, vol 2: Control of Breathing.* Bethesda, MD, American Physiological Society, 1981; pp 1415–1447.

53. O'Connell JM, Campbell AH: Respiratory mechanics in airways obstruction associated with inspiratory dyspnea. *Thorax* 31:669, 1976.

54. Campbell EJM, Howell JBL: The sensation of breathlessness. *Br Med Bull* 19:36, 1963.

55. Schwartzstein RM, Manning HL, Weiss JW, Weinberger SE: Dyspnea: A sensory experience. *Lung* 168:185, 1990.

56. O'Donnell DE, Webb KA: Exertional breathlessness in patients with chronic airflow limitation. *Am Rev Respir Dis* 148:1351, 1993.

57. Manning HL, Molinary EJ, Leiter JC: Effect of inspiratory flow rate on respiratory sensation and pattern of breathing. *Am J Respir Crit Care Med* 151:751, 1995.

58. Adams L, Chronos N, Lane R, Guz A: The measurement of breathlessness induced in normal subjects. *Clin Sci* 69:7, 1985.

59. Stark RD, Gambles SA, Lewis JA: Methods to assess breathlessness in healthy subjects: A critical evaluation and application to analyse the acute effects of diazepam and promethazine on breathlessness induced by exercise or by exposure to raised levels of carbon dioxide. *Clin Sci* 61:429, 1981.

60. Lane R, Cockroft A, Guz A: Voluntary isocapnic hyperventilation and breathlessness during exercise in normal subjects. *Clin Sci* 73:519, 1987.

61. Schwartzstein RM, Cristiano LM: Qualities of respiratory sensation, in Adams L, Guz A (eds): *Respiratory Sensation.* New York, Marcel Dekker, 1996; pp 125–154.

62. Eldridge FL, Waldrop TG: Neural control of breathing during exercise, in Whipp BJ, Wasserman K (eds): *Exercise: Pulmonary*

63. Hyland RH, Jones NL, Powles ACP, et al: Primary alveolar hypoventilation treated with nocturnal electrophrenic respiration. *Am Rev Respir Dis* 117:165, 1978.

64. Shea SA, Andres LP, Shannon D, Banzett RB: Ventilatory response to exercise in humans lacking ventilatory chemosensitivity. *J Physiol (Lond)* 468:623, 1993.

65. Tallaride G, Baldoni F: Cardio-respiratory reflex from muscles during dynamic and static exercise in the dog. *J Appl Physiol* 58:844, 1985.

66. Clark AL, Piepoli M, Coats AJ: Skeletal muscle and the control of ventilation on exercise: Evidence for metabolic receptors. *Eur J Clin Invest* 25:299, 1995.

67. Clark A, Volterrani M, Swan JW, et al: Leg blood flow, metabolism and exercise capacity in chronic stable heart failure. *Int J Cardiol* 55:127, 1996.

68. Clark A, Poole-Wilson P: Breathlessness in heart disease, in Adams L, Guz A (eds): *Respiratory Sensation.* New York, Marcel Dekker, 1996; pp 263–283.

69. Cook DG, Shape AG: Breathlessness, lung function and risk of heart attack. *Eur Heart J* 9:1215, 1988.

70. Cook DG, Shaper AG: Breathlessness, angina pectoris and coronary artery disease. *Am J Cardiol* 63:921, 1989.

71. Lloyd TC: Reflex effects of left heart and pulmonary vascular distention on airways of dogs. *J Appl Physiol* 49:620, 1980.

72. Paintal AS: Mechanism of stimulation of type J pulmonary receptors. *J Physiol* 203:511, 1969.

73. Aubier M, Trippenback T, Roussos C: Respiratory muscle fatigue during cardiogenic shock. *J Appl Physiol* 51:449, 1981.

74. Hammond MD, Bauer KA, Sharp JT, Rocha RD: Respiratory muscle strength in congestive heart failure. *Chest* 98:1091–1094, 1990.

75. McParland C, Krishnan B, Wang Y, Gallagher C: Inspiratory muscle weakness and dyspnea in chronic heart failure. *Am Rev Respir Dis* 146:467–472, 1992.

76. Rubin SA, Brown HV: Ventilation and gas exchange during exercise in severe chronic heart failure. *Am Rev Respir Dis* 129:S63, 1984.

77. Clark AL, Poole-Wilson PA, Coats AJS: The relationship between ventilation and carbon dioxide production in patients with chronic heart failure. *J Am Coll Cardiol* 20:1326, 1992.

78. Asmussen E, Nielsen M: Experiments on nervous factors controlling respiration and circulation during exercise employing blocking of the blood flow. *Acta Physiol Scand* 60:103, 1964.

79. Mahler DA, Loke J: The physiology of endurance exercise: The marathon. *Clin Chest Med* 5:63, 1984.

80. Schwartzstein RM: The language of dyspnea, in Mahler DA (ed): *Dyspnea.* New York, Marcel Dekker 1998; pp 35–62.

81. Killian KJ, Summer E, Jones NL, Campbell EJM: Dyspnea and leg effort during incremental cycle ergometry. *Am Rev Respir Dis* 145:1339, 1992.

82. Lane R, Adams L: The effects of metabolic acidosis on perceived breathlessness during exercise in humans. *J Physiol* 461:47, 1993.

83. Cherniack N: Respiratory sensation as a respiratory controller, in Adams L, Guz A (eds): *Respiratory Sensation.* New York, Marcel Dekker, 1996; pp 213–230.

84. Gottfried SB, Altose MD, Kelsen SG, Cherniack NS: Perception of changes in airflow resistance in obstructive pulmonary disorders. *Am Rev Respir Dis* 124:566, 1981.

85. Oliven A, Cherniack NS, Deal EC, Kelsen SG: The effect of acute bronchoconstriction on respiratory activity in patients with chronic obstructive pulmonary disease. *Am Rev Respir Dis* 131:236, 1987.

86. Schwartzstein R, Carpenter E, Brughera A, et al: Quality of breathlessness during bronchoconstriction with different inhalational agents. *Am Rev Respir Dis* 145:A630, 1992.

87. Chapman KR, Rebuck AS: Inspiratory and expiratory resistive

loading as a model of dyspnea in asthma. *Respiration* 44:425, 1983.

88. O'Donnell DE, Webb KA: Exertional breathlessness in patients with chronic airflow limitation: The role of lung hyperinflation. *Am Rev Respir Dis* 148:1351, 1993.

89. Suero JT, Woolf CR: Alterations in the mechanical properties of the lung during dyspnea in chronic obstructive pulmonary disease. *J Clin Invest* 49:747, 1970.

90. O'Donnell DE, Sanii R, Giesbreht G, Younes M: Effect of continuous positive airway pressure on respiratory sensation in patients with chronic obstructive pulmonary disease during submaximal exercise. *Am Rev Respir Dis* 138:1185, 1988.

91. O'Donnell DE, Sanii R, Younes M: Improvement in exercise endurance in patients with chronic airflow obstruction using continuous positive airway pressure. *Am Rev Respir Dis* 138:1510, 1988.

92. O'Donnell DE, Bertley JC, Chau LK, Webb KA: Qualitative aspects of exertional breathlessness in chronic airflow limitation: pathophysiologic mechanisms. *Am J Respir Crit Care Med* 155:109, 1997.

93. Moy ML, Harver A, Lantin ML, Schwartzstein RM: Language of dyspnea in assessment of patients with acute asthma treated with nebulized albuterol. *Am J Respir Crit Care Med* (in press).

94. Gift AG, Plaut M, Jacox A: Psychological and physiological factors related to dyspnea in patients with chronic obstructive pulmonary disease. *Heart Lung* 15:595, 1986.

95. Gift AG, Cahill CH: Psycho-physiologic aspects of dyspnea in chronic obstructive pulmonary disease: A pilot study. *Heart Lung* 19:252, 1990.

96. Dudley DL, Martin CJ, Holmes TH: Dyspnea: Psychologic and physiologic observations. *J Psychosom Res* 11:325, 1968.

97. Guenard H, Gallego J, Dromer C: Exercise dyspnea in patients with respiratory disease. *Eur Respir Rev* 5:6, 1995.

98. Burns BH, Howell JBL: Disproportionately severe breathlessness in chronic bronchitis. *Q J Med* 38:277, 1969.

99. Hudgel DW, Cooperson DM, Kinsman RA: Recognition of added resistive loads in asthma: The importance of behavioral styles. *Am Rev Respir Dis* 126:121, 1982.

100. Carrieri-Kohlman V, Douglas MK, Gromley JM, Stulbarg MS: Desensitization and guided mastery: Treatment approaches for the management of dyspnea. *Heart Lung* 22:226, 1993.

PART III

ASSESSMENT OF THE PULMONARY REHABILITATION PATIENT

Chapter 17

ASSESSMENT OF LUNG MECHANICS

MELVIN LOPATA

This chapter focuses on indications, measurement, interpretation, and clinical application of pulmonary function testing as it relates to diseases affecting lung mechanics. I will include a brief review of the physiology and pathophysiology of lung mechanics.

Physiology of Lung Mechanics

For a chapter dealing with pulmonary function testing, a review of the nomenclature of lung volumes and capacities is in order, and these terms can be illustrated by the volume tracings generated by spirometry (Fig. 17-1). Conventionally, the lung is divided into four lung volumes, which are primary nonoverlapping subdivisions.[1,2] In addition, there are four lung capacities, which are comprised of two or more primary volumes. In this chapter I will focus on those volumes and capacities most relevant to basic function testing.

The amount of air that is inspired or expired during each respiratory cycle is the *tidal volume* (VT) (Fig. 17-1). When one inspires completely and then expires maximally, the amount of air that is expired after a maximal inspiration is the *vital capacity* (VC). After maximal expiration, there is still air remaining in the lung, and this volume of gas is the *residual volume* (RV). Combining the VC and RV derives the *total lung capacity* (TLC), the maximum amount of air in the lungs at full inspiration. After a maximal inspiration, if one relaxes and passively expires, the respiratory system (lungs and chest wall) will deflate to a stable level, which is termed the *functional residual capacity* (FRC). The FRC is the resting level of the respiratory system and is the amount of air in the lungs at end-expiration.

Lung (and chest wall) mechanics are the properties of the lung involved in lung inflation and deflation, that is, the movement of air in and out of the lung. In the breathing process, these so-called properties provide a mechanical barrier to air movement that requires energy expenditure to overcome. Simply stated, there are two broad lung components determining the mechanics of respiration, the airways and the parenchyma, and the mechanical properties they transduce are *airway resistance* and *lung elastic recoil*, respectively.

AIRWAY RESISTANCE

The principles governing airway resistance and airflow in the tracheobronchial tree are similar to but not the same as those in rigid tubes. *Resistance* is the pressure required to generate flow across a tube (R = pressure/flow), the units of measurement being centimeters of water per liter per second. Airway resistance depends on the length of the tube, the viscosity of the gas being moved, and the radius of the tube such that the longer the tube, the greater the viscosity, and the smaller the radius, the greater is the resistance (Poiseuille's law).[3] The fact that the airways are continuously branching and changing in size toward the periphery of the lung and are collapsible tubes exerts a profound influence on the resistive properties of the airways. The pattern of airflow in tubes, including airways, can be streamlined, such as laminar or turbulent, the former having a flow profile that is axial to the tube and the latter having a chaotic profile with movement both axial and radial in direction.[3] The latter profile consumes considerable energy, so a given flow under turbulent conditions will require a greater driving pressure than under laminar conditions. Thus airway resistance is greater with turbulent than with laminar flow. In addition, whereas flow is proportional to driving pressure with laminar flow, this relationship is curvilinear with turbulent flow; that is, exponentially more pressure is required to generate increasing flows. The pattern of flow in a given tubular or airway system depends on the airway size and the velocity, density, and viscosity of the gas being moved. The greater the air velocity, airway diameter, and gas density, the greater is the probability for turbulence. In the tracheobronchial tree, the flow in the proximal airways—trachea and mainstem and lobar bronchi—is turbulent because of their relatively large diameter and branching, which, along with the larynx, introduces mechanical obstructions that promote turbulence. As the branching airways narrow and their total cross-sectional area increases, gas velocity decreases and flow becomes laminar. In the small airways of less than 2 mm in diameter, flow is entirely laminar. In the intermediate airways, flow is both laminar and turbulent, the latter especially at sites of branching. As a result of the branching pattern of the airways and its effects on flow profiles of air movement, most of the resistance to airflow along the tracheobronchial tree is in the large airways.[4] Ninety percent of the pressure drop to generate airflow occurs in airways greater than 2 mm (50 percent occurring across the larynx and trachea), and only 10 percent occurs along the peripheral airways. Because measured airway resistance is predominantly due to the large airways, the periphery of the lung, airways less than 2 mm, is termed the *silent area* of the lung.[5]

Airway resistance depends on and is inversely proportional to lung volume. Resistance is high at low volumes and low at high inflations. This volume dependency of resistance is mediated by lung elastic recoil, which subtends a tethering effect on the intraparenchymal airways that supports their patency via direct radial traction to the

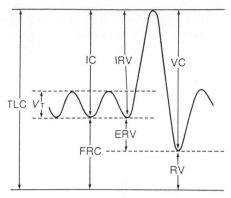

FIGURE 17-1 Divisions of lung volumes and capacities: TLC, total lung capacity; IC, inspiratory capacity; IRV, inspiratory reserve volume; FRC, functional residual capacity; ERV, expiratory reserve volume; VC, vital capacity; RV, residual volume.

bronchial walls. At high lung volumes, elastic recoil is high, and the resulting radial support of the airways maintains relatively high patency and thereby low resistance in the airways. The decrease in lung recoil at low volumes results in less traction, less patent airways, and higher resistance. Airway caliber and thus resistance also depends on bronchial smooth muscle tone, which is a function of the balance between bronchial sympathetic and parasympathetic activity. Epinephrine secreted from the adrenal medulla relaxes smooth muscle and decreases airway tone and resistance; parasympathetic discharge via vagal efferents to the bronchial wall constricts smooth muscle and increases tone and resistance.

LUNG ELASTIC RECOIL

The other component of lung mechanics is the property of elastic recoil, which, along with the elastic properties of the chest wall, determines the distensibility and pressure-volume characteristics of the respiratory system. The lungs and chest wall act like separate but interdependent elastic bodies, the classic analogy being two connected springs with opposing recoil characteristics. The lung spring recoils inward (deflation), its resting level being less than residual volume, whereas the chest wall spring recoils outward (inflation) for most of its volume, resting at about 60 percent of TLC. When these two opposing elastic forces are equal, the respiratory system is mechanically at rest and is at FRC. To inspire above FRC, the inspiratory muscles must generate pressure to overcome the recoil of the lung, while the outward recoil of the chest wall assists inspiration to 60 percent of TLC, when the muscles must work against both elastic systems to further inspire. When the inspiratory muscles can no longer generate the increasing pressure necessary for continued inspiration, maximal inflation or TLC is reached. To expire below FRC, the expiratory muscles must generate pressure to overcome the recoil of the chest wall, while lung recoil assists expiration. When the expiratory muscles can no longer generate the pressure against the increasing chest wall elastic recoil (and with the closure of small airways), maximal deflation (RV) is reached.[6] Thus the elastic-mechanical properties of the lung and chest wall determine in large part the state of inflation and the lung volumes and capacities that we measure in the clinical pulmonary function labora-

tory. Disease-induced alterations in lung elastic recoil may alter the inflation characteristics of the respiratory system, resulting in clinically definable and measurable changes in lung volumes and capacities, all to be discussed later in this chapter.

FLOW DYNAMICS

Integral to pulmonary function testing is the use of spirometry to test dynamic airway function. The hallmark of this testing methodology is the forced expiratory vital capacity (FVC) maneuver, in which the patient expires from TLC to RV as forcefully and as rapidly as possible. If, during this maneuver, one constructs an *xy* plot of change in flow measured at the mouth versus change in volume from TLC to RV, one develops an expiratory flow-volume loop (Fig. 17-2). This construct shows that at the beginning of expiration there is a brisk rise in airflow to an early peak followed by an abrupt drop-off and almost linear decline of flow until expiration is completed. The expiratory loop clearly contrasts with the pattern of flow versus volume seen during the forced inspiratory maneuver done from RV to TLC (Fig. 17-2). During forced expiration, after the initial increase, the continued rise in flow appears to be impeded, and flow rates for the last three-quarters of the FVC appear to be limited. This flow limitation is characteristic of the forced expiratory vital capacity and is inherent in the dynamics that result from collapsible airways that are subjected to forces generated within the thorax.

During the forced expiratory maneuver, pressures generated by maximum expiratory muscle contraction and by the elastic recoil of the lungs combine to provide a pressure head (alveolar pressure) to move air from the alveoli to the mouth, which is at atmospheric or zero pressure relative to the alveoli. As air moves along the airways, the original level of alveolar pressure will decrease progressively, due mostly to frictional pressure losses. At the same time, as lung volume is decreasing, lung recoil pressure is decreasing, thus decreas-

FIGURE 17-2 Inspiratory flow-volume loops plotting flow (*x* axis) versus volume (*y* axis) during a forced inspiratory and expiratory vital capacity. Abbreviations as in Fig. 17-1.

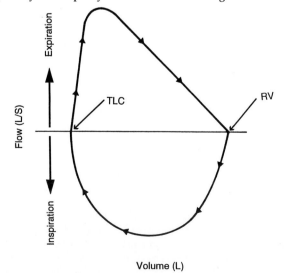

ing the alveolar driving pressure and the intraairway pressure as well. Because the expiratory muscle pressure is transmitted to the pleural space that surrounds the intrathoracic airways, a point will be reached where the decreasing intraairway pressure falls below the extraairway pleural pressure (negative intramural pressure), resulting in compression and critical narrowing of the airways, forming localized choke points that serve to limit expiratory flow.[7] Since it is the expiratory force acting through pleural pressure that mediates the airway collapse and flow limitation, increasing expiratory effort will only serve to increase the extramural pressure and will not increase flow rates; thus these limited but maximum attainable flows are in a sense independent of effort. Indeed, the expiratory flow rates after achievement of peak flow are referred to as *effort-independent*. As lung volume is decreasing during the forced expiration, the flow rates achieved along the descending slope of the loop are the maximum that can be developed at that lung volume due to the dynamics of flow limitation and are referred to as $\dot{V}max$. $\dot{V}max$ depends on lung volume; flow is greater the higher the volume at which it is generated. In addition, this maximum flow is derivative of the two components of lung mechanics, airway resistance and lung elastic recoil.[7] Lung recoil, which is also volume-dependent, generates the driving pressure for flow generation, whereas the intrinsic resistance of the airways between the alveoli and the site of compression determines the flow level for a given recoil driving pressure. Whatever the resulting flow, it is the maximum ($\dot{V}max$) that can be achieved during the forced expiratory maneuver and for a given individual is quite reproducible. Lung disease, by altering lung elastance and/or airway resistance, will modify the ability to generate $\dot{V}max$ and thereby can be detected, quantified, and assessed by means of pulmonary function testing.[8]

Pathophysiology of Lung Mechanics

Lung diseases can pathologically alter the mechanical properties of the lung by their effect on the airways and lung parenchyma. From a pathophysiologic perspective, lung disease can be divided into two components. Diseases that affect the airways, such as bronchitis (acute and chronic), asthma, and emphysema, result in increased airways resistance and are referred to as *obstructive lung diseases;* diseases that affect the lung parenchyma by diffuse inflammation (sarcoidosis, hypersensitivity pneumonitis, histiocytosis X) or fibrosis that result in increased lung elastance with stiff, noncompliant lungs that impair the ability to inflate the lung and maintain normal lung volumes are termed *restrictive lung diseases*. Extrapulmonary diseases such as obesity and kyphoscoliosis that have an impact on the chest wall and impair lung expansion or neuromuscular disease that involves the respiratory muscles also may cause restrictive disease. Diseases that affect lung elastic recoil also influence airway function. Emphysema, which destroys alveoli resulting in loss of lung elasticity and overdistensible lungs, has a profound effect on airway dynamics during an FVC maneuver. This loss of lung recoil decreases the driving pressure for $\dot{V}max$ and directly impairs expiratory flow generation.[9] Since lung elastic recoil provides a tethering function that supports the patency of the intraparenchymal airways by means of radial traction on the air-

TABLE 17-1 Pulmonary Function Testing: Indications

Assess complaint of breathlessness
Determine presence and degree of respiratory impairment
Determine the pathophysiology of respiratory disease
Assess prognosis of disease
Assess therapeutic response
Follow course of disease over time
Assess operative risk vis-à-vis respiratory disease
Assess disability

ways, loss of recoil in emphysema results in increased collapsibility of the airways and, again, decreased $\dot{V}max$ during a forced expiratory maneuver.[9] Thus emphysema causes airways obstruction due to its effect on lung elastic recoil.

Restrictive diseases, such as pulmonary fibrosis, that increase lung elastic recoil also may change airway dynamics. This increased recoil provides added radial traction and support to the airways such that they are less collapsible during an FVC maneuver. Thus expiratory flow rates, or $\dot{V}max$, will be preserved or possibly increased in some restrictive diseases.[10]

Emphysema and pulmonary fibrosis represent two opposite pathologic processes with contrasting effects on lung mechanics, pulmonary pathophysiology, and as will be evident later, pulmonary function tests.

Pulmonary Function Testing

INDICATIONS

The indications for pulmonary function tests (PFTs) are listed in Table 17-1. PFTs often demonstrate their utility in assessing patients with unexplained complaints of shortness of breath. Abnormal tests signal the presence of pulmonary disease and a pathologic process altering lung mechanics. Interpretation of the abnormal test results allows determination of the type of altered mechanics, whereas attention to the degree of the abnormality, especially over time, permits assessment of prognosis and natural history of the disease or the response to therapy.

I will discuss pulmonary function testing as it is commonly performed in clinical laboratories and which provides the basic data base from which clinical interpretations are made. I will first relate the nature of the test, the methodology of testing, and then interpretation of the tests, particularly as it relates to altered lung mechanics.

METHODOLOGY

LUNG COMPLIANCE
It is appropriate to begin a discussion on methods of assessing lung mechanics with a review of the one method of testing that directly describes the static mechanical properties of the lung, that is, lung compliance. Though not a method used routinely in clinical pulmonary function laboratories, it is a relatively straightforward procedure that can supply exact data on the state of lung elasticity and compliance.

Determining lung elastic recoil requires the measurement of lung recoil pressure using a catheter pressure manometer that records pressure changes in the lower third of the esoph-

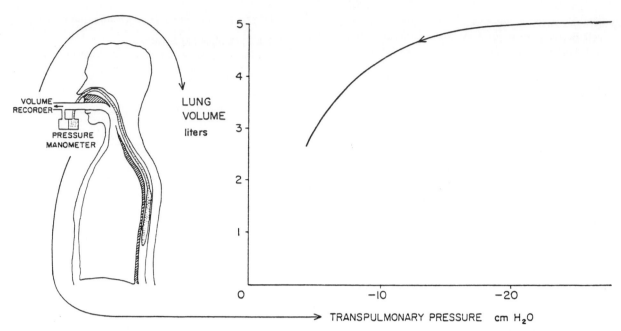

FIGURE 17-3 Static pressure-volume relationship in a normal subject. A deflation pressure-volume curve, from TLC to FRC, is constructed (see text) to assess the elastic characteristics of the lung. The static compliance, expressed in liters per centimeter of water, is the ratio of volume change (*y* axis) to pressure change (*x* axis) calculated over the linear part of the curve above FRC. Transpulmonary pressure is determined from measurements of pleural pressure with an esophageal catheter manometer. (Reprinted, with permission, from Bates et al.[11])

agus (Fig. 17-3). The change in esophageal pressure at this level directly reflects intrathoracic pleural pressure.[11] During a breath hold, pleural pressure subtracted from mouth pressure, which is equal to alveolar pressure under conditions of zero flow, and measured via a differential pressure transducer gives transpulmonary pressure (Ptp), which reflects lung recoil pressure. The elastic properties of the lung are determined by constructing a pressure-volume curve that plots the change in Ptp (abscissa) versus volume (ordinate) during an expiration from TLC to FRC. This expiratory maneuver is done stepwise with brief breath holds against a shuttered airway to ensure a stable lung volume during the breath hold. Ptp is recorded during the breath hold so that the measured pressure is obtained under static conditions and thereby represents true recoil pressure. Multiple expiratory trials and breath holds are performed to obtain sufficient data points to construct the *xy* plot of pressure versus volume. To account for different patient sizes, actual lung volume on the ordinate is normalized as percentage of predicted TLC (see Fig. 17-3).

The normal pressure-volume curve is curvilinear, being relatively linear above FRC but flattening at high lung volumes. Lung recoil depends on lung volume, increasing, though nonlinearly, as volume increases. At FRC, Ptp is about 5 cmH$_2$O, while it rises to 30 cmH$_2$O at TLC. Elasticity can be measured in a number of ways. The most common method is to determine lung compliance, which is a measurement of the slope ($\Delta V / \Delta P$) of the pressure-volume curve 0.5 L above FRC. Normal lung compliance is 0.2 L/cmH$_2$O, or stated differently, for every centimeter of water of distending pressure, the lung inflates 200 mL. An increase in this slope (increased lung compliance) indicates more distensible lungs, and a decrease in slope (decreased lung compliance)

means stiff, less distensible lungs. The position of the patient's pressure-volume curve compared with normal also assesses elasticity. A shift to the left shows that at a given lung volume, recoil pressure is diminished, whereas a shift to the right denotes increased Ptp, indicative of decreased and increased lung elastic recoil, respectively. A shift to the left of the curve is associated with high compliance and reduced elasticity; a right shift and low compliance are concordant and signify increased elasticity.

SPIROMETRY

Clinical PFTs for assessing lung mechanics can be divided into two categories that are listed in Table 17-2. I refer to the first category as *dynamic lung function testing* because the hallmark of this testing is spirometry and, along with the maximum voluntary ventilation (MVV), involves active effort on the part of the patient, and these tests assess airway function, which is a dynamic process. The performance of a forced expiratory vital capacity determination has been discussed earlier, and most laboratories will have the patient perform a forced inpiratory vital capacity test as well, inspiring from RV to TLC as forcefully and rapidly as possible.

Most of the data obtained from spirometry are derived

TABLE 17-2 Pulmonary Function Testing: Assessment of Lung Mechanics

Dynamic lung function
Spirometry
Maximum voluntary ventilation
Static lung function
Lung volumes/capacities

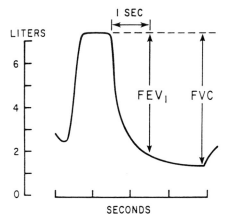

FIGURE 17-4 Spirometric measurement of the forced vital capacity (FVC) and forced expiratory volume in 1 s (FEV₁).

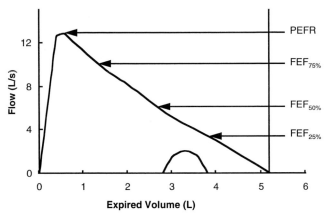

FIGURE 17-6 Expiratory flow-volume loop depicting the sites of instantaneous maximum flows. PEFR, peak expiratory flow rate. See text for definition of the FEFs.

from a single forced expiratory vital capacity maneuver, providing both volume and flow measures that are used to assess airway function. Classically, spirometry data were derived directly from the expiratory spirogram, the units of measure being volume (ordinate) versus time (abscissa) (Fig. 17-4). In the analysis of the spirometric data, the total FVC, reflecting the ventilatory capability of the patient, is measured. Then a timed vital capacity is measured, that is, the amount of air expired during the first second of the FVC, that being referred as the FEV₁. The FEV₁ is related to the FVC as a ratio or percentage, providing a measure of rate of expiration; normally, one should be able to forcefully expire at least 70 to 80 percent of one's vital capacity, depending on age and height, in 1 s.

It is now common in most clinical laboratories to display the forced vital capacity as a flow-volume loop, as was described earlier. Because the effort-independent component of this configuration that describes $\dot{V}$max is determined by the intrinsic lung mechanics, the qualitative presentation of the loop and the quantification of the actual $\dot{V}$max at various lung volumes are important factors in assessing lung mechanics and dynamic lung function. From the expiratory flow-volume loop, the FVC and FEV₁ can be determined as per standard spirometry (Fig. 17-5). In addition, specific flow

FIGURE 17-5 Expiratory flow-volume loop depicting the FVC and FEV₁ from the volume axis. The curved line is expiratory tidal volume.

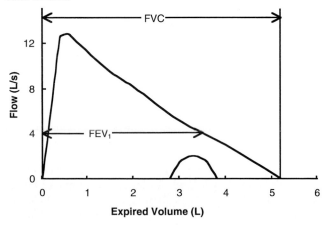

rates at specified volumes during the FVC are calculated (Fig. 17-6). The flow rates are designated as *forced expiratory flow* (FEF) measured at a given lung volume. The common flows measured and reported are FEF₇₅, FEF₅₀, FEF₂₅, and FEF₂₅₋₇₅, which reflect the forced expiratory flow (or $\dot{V}$max) at 75, 50, and 25 percent of the vital capacity and the mean flow at between 25 and 75 percent of the vital capacity, respectively.

The MVV is performed by the patient breathing in and out as deeply and rapidly as possible for about 10 s, and the total ventilation during this brief period is tabulated and extrapolated for a 1-min period. The MVV reflects the total ventilatory capability of the patient or, stated differently, the patient's ventilatory reserve. The unit of measurement for the FVC and FEV₁ is liters; for FEF, liters per second; and for the MVV, liters per minute.

LUNG VOLUMES

Since lung volumes and capacities are generally in a steady state, their measurement is that of a static function. The methodology of measurement is done with the patient breathing quietly, again consistent with a relatively static process. Thus I refer to lung volume testing as *static function testing.*

To assess all lung volumes and capacities, one has to be able to quantitate those components which cannot be measured by spirometry, particularly RV. The most common method for this task is that of helium dilution, whereby the patient breathes from a source with a known small concentration of helium[12] (Fig. 17-7). The helium is breathed until there is equilibration of the gas between the lungs and the source. If the original volume and concentration of helium at the source are known, the final, equilibrated helium concentration is measured, and the equilibrated volume of helium consists of the original volume plus lung volume; the latter can be determined by a simple algebraic equation in which lung volume is the unknown.[12] Since helium breathing is begun when the patient is at end-expiration, and since the equilibration is done during quiet tidal breathing, the actual lung volume/capacity measured is FRC. Subsequently, the expiratory reserve volume (ERV) can be measured with a spirometer by the patient maximally expiring from end-expiration (FRC) to RV. RV is then calculated by subtracting

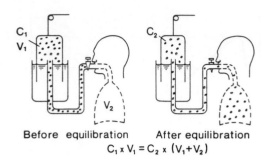

Before equilibration   After equilibration

$$C_1 \times V_1 = C_2 \times (V_1 + V_2)$$

FIGURE 17-7 Measurement of the FRC by helium dilution. Helium, of known volume (V_1) and concentration (C_1), is breathed by the subject until equilibration occurs between lungs and spirometer. The product $C_1 \times V_1$ will equal the final equilibrated concentration (C_2) times the new volume of helium, consisting of V_1 plus lung volume (V_2). Solving the algebraic equation for V_2 derives FRC. (Reprinted, with permission, from West JB: *Respiratory Physiology: The Essentials*, 5th ed. New York, Williams & Wilkins, 1995.)

TABLE 17-3 Pulmonary Function Tests

Dynamic lung function/spirometry
  FVC, liters
  FEV_1, liters
  FEV_1/FVC
  FEF_{25-75}, L/s
  FEF_{50}, L/s
  MVV, L/min
Static lung function/volumes and capacities
  TLC, liters
  VC, liters
  FRC, liters
  RV, liters

the ERV from the helium-measured FRC. By adding the spirometry-measured VC to the RV, TLC is determined. Generally, the VC used in these calculations is not the FVC but a VC performed slowly but completely. The unit of measurement for volumes and capacities is liters.

Accurate measurement of lung volumes with dilutional methods requires true equilibration between the test gas at its source and the lungs. Conditions such as airways obstruction that impair or limit gas distribution to peripheral lung units or bullae that are essentially noncommunicating with the airways may interdict the equilibration process necessary to correctly determine lung volumes. As such, the helium dilution measurement of volume tends to underestimate the true lung volume in patients with these conditions. Measurement of lung volume by the body plethysmographic (body box) method obviates this problem and provides an accurate measure of volume independent of the status of the airways. The body box is a sealed airtight chamber in which the patient sits, and it functions on the principle of Boyle's law, that in a closed system, pressure times volume is constant ($P_1 \times V_1 = P_2 \times V_2$).[12] Simply stated, as a patient breathes, or pants, inside the box, changes in volume displacement of the thorax are transduced to changes in pressure measurable within the box. From this change in pressure, the actual volume displacement of the thorax (and lungs) can be calculated. Again, this method directly measures FRC, which may be referred to as *intrathoracic gas volume*.

Pulmonary function testing involves considerable variability, in particular technical variation related to the equipment, performance of the procedure, and the patient and the technician. To ensure quality testing and results, this variability must be minimized by close adherence to the standards of performance published by the American Thoracic Society, the European Respiratory Society, and others.[13–17]

INTERPRETATION

The data obtained from spirometry and lung volume testing offer two groups of results (Table 17-3), all being absolute measures of that particular test. To determine whether a result is abnormal and, if so, to what degree, the patient's test value has to be compared with a normal reference. For each parameter, the predicted value for a given patient can

be derived from regression equations obtained from cross-sectional population studies of normal, nonsmoking men and women of all age groups.[18–21] Based on the patient's age, gender, and height, a predicted value is calculated. There are a number of commonly used reference equations, and a given laboratory should use the published equations derived from populations that best fit the populations tested in that laboratory. This calculated predicted value represents the normal function for the tested patient. To detect abnormal function, a lower limit of normal has to be determined, this being neither a simple nor universally agreed on process. The historical use of 80 percent predicted as the lower-limit threshold has incurred disfavor because its use is considered somewhat arbitrary, bearing no statistical validity.[20,22] However, its use is steeped in tradition and, I believe, has served its purpose rather well. Use of the 80 percent threshold is likely close to an acceptable lower limit but tends to misclassify those individuals whose demographics are at the ends of the reference population, such as short and old individuals. Using a fixed lower limit of normal is usually reliable when the result is well above or below this threshold but may become problematic for borderline values. In these instances, correct assumptions about the presence or absence of abnormality depend heavily on the prior probability of disease. Expectations of disease presence support an abnormal interpretation, whereas the probable absence of disease supports normalcy. Of importance, the 80 percent predicted threshold cannot apply to maximum expiratory flows. Because of the great variability of these parameters, lower limits of normal are 50 to 60 percent.[23,24] In addition, because the FEV_1/FVC ratio depends on age and height, defining a fixed ratio, such as 0.75, as a lower limit of normal, again a common practice, is probably not warranted.[22]

It is now felt that a lower limit of normal can be estimated from a regression model, that values below the fifth percentile are taken as the threshold, below which a result is considered abnormal. This normal limit can be calculated (lower limit of normal = predicted value − 1.645 × standard error of estimate) if the individual reference values are gaussian, as may be the case for FVC and FEV_1 but not for FEV_1/FVC and the maximum flow rates.[22] Indeed, this equation has been shown to be less of a predictor of lower limit than the fifth percentile.[25]

Since there is no generally applicable or accepted method to determine the lower limit of normal, I continue to find it useful to use 80 percent of predicted as the threshold for FVC, FEV_1, FEV_1/FVC, and lung volumes. For maximum flows, because of the variability, 60 percent of predicted is a reasonable alternative. One must realize that whatever threshold is used, the prior probability of disease and the clinical correlation should be considered if at all possible. In addition, there are no published data on the sensitivity, specificity, or predictive power (positive or negative) of any derived threshold. Thus defining abnormality as well as interpreting the abnormal results is as much an art as a science.

When an abnormality is present, the severity of the defect should be graded. Again, there is no universally accepted criterion for such grading, but generally the predicted values can be used to grade severity. Although also somewhat arbitrary, the following scheme has proved to be useful for grading impaired spirometry exclusive of maximum flows: mild—percent predicted < 100 and > 70 (or ≤80 percent and >70 percent if 80 percent of predicted is used as the lower limit threshold); moderate—percent predicted ≤ 70 and > 50; severe—percent predicted ≤ 50.[22]

Once an abnormality of pulmonary function is detected and quantified, the next step in the testing process is interpretation of the test results. Interpretation is based on characterizing the pathophysiology of the disease process in terms of its effect on lung mechanics. I prefer to characterize the interpretation of PFTs on the basis of the "law of twos" as follows. Anatomically, the lung consists of two components, the airways and the alveoli, or parenchyma. Similarly, there are two components to the physiology of lung mechanics, frictional resistance of the conducting airways and elastic "resistance" of the lung parenchyma. Pathologically, these two components are still quite evident; diseases that affect the airways and result in increased airways resistance cause *obstructive* lung disease; diseases that affect the lung parenchyma resulting in increased elastance cause *restrictive* lung disease. Pulmonary function interpretation involves determining which pathophysiologic process is present, that is, whether the patient has obstructive or restrictive (or both) lung disease. Of note, in interpreting abnormal PFTs, it is customary to characterize impaired lung mechanics as obstructive or restrictive ventilatory defects.

Taking each type of PFT category, dynamic and static, I will review the criteria and the decision process for interpreting the derived data.

INTERPRETATION OF SPIROMETRY

OBSTRUCTIVE LUNG DISEASE

Spirometry is the singular method for diagnosing obstructive lung disease. The effects of airways obstruction on the classic spirometric tracing or on the expiratory flow-volume loop usually are clearly recognizable (Fig. 17-8). In the presence of airways obstruction, expiratory flow rates are diminished, and expiration is slowed and prolonged. This diminished flow rate is qualitatively apparent as a decrease in the slope of the volume versus time spirometric tracing (see Fig. 17-8) and a decreased slope and concavity of the descending limb of the flow-volume loop (Fig. 17-9). Quantitatively, the total FVC may be decreased, but more important, and most consistent, the FEV₁ is decreased to a greater degree than the FVC so that the FEV₁/FVC is diminished. This low FEV₁/FVC is the hallmark of airways obstruction. In mild obstruction, the FVC may be in the normal range and only the FEV₁ decreased, but as obstruction worsens, the FVC will decrease, although less than the FEV₁, and the ratio is decreased. The FEV₁ is a consistent and reproducible parameter and is commonly

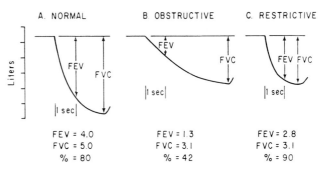

FIGURE 17-8 Forced expiratory spirogram depicting normal, obstructive, and restrictive patterns. See text for explanation. (Reprinted, with permission, from West JB: *Respiratory Physiology: The Essentials*, 4th ed. New York, Williams & Wilkins, 1992).

used, either the absolute measure or the percent predicted, to follow the course of the obstruction over time, especially in response to therapy. The severity of obstruction should be based more on the FEV₁ than on the FEV₁/FVC.

The FVC is decreased in obstruction in part as a result of increased collapsibility of the airways associated with the forced expiratory maneuver and the inability to fully expire during the rapid attempt at expiration. Indeed, if a patient with airways obstruction performs a slow VC, airway compression is lessened, and the time to expire is prolonged so that this measure may be significantly greater than that resulting from the FVC. This difference between the fast and slow VC is typical of airways obstruction and is referred to as *air trapping*.

Expiratory flows, be it the FEF₇₅, FEF₅₀, FEF₂₅, or FEF₂₅₋₇₅, are diminished in airways obstruction and reflect the effect of the pathologic process, increased airways resistance, and/or decreased lung elastic recoil to impair the ability to generate V̇max. The flow rates at low volumes are sensitive to the presence of early or mild obstruction. The slowing of flow rates at the terminal portion of the spirogram (FEF₇₅, FEF₂₅₋₇₅) is considered to signify the presence of small airways disease,[26] but though suggestive, it is not specific for such a process.[27]

If airways obstruction is present in a given patient, the response to acute bronchodilation should be assessed. After baseline spirometry, a short-acting beta₂ agonist (e.g., albuterol) is inhaled by the patient, and the test repeated in 15 to 30 min. Essentially, the change in FEV₁ is the most reliable parameter to determine the presence and degree of reversibility. The standard criterion for significant improvement in airways obstruction is an increase in FEV₁ of 12 to 15 percent of baseline.[22] Any and all of the other spirometric measures may increase with bronchodilation as well, but the consistency and reproducibility of the FEV₁ make it the parameter of choice. Reversible airways obstruction is the hallmark of asthma. However, patients with other types of obstructive lung disease such as chronic obstructive pulmonary disease (COPD) may show some degree of reversibility, whereas not all asthmatics will demonstrate reversibility, especially acutely in the laboratory.[22] Following the FEV₁ over time provides a vehicle to observe the long-term response to therapy or to use as a guide for changing therapy, such as instituting systemic steroids in patients with asthma.

The MVV is sensitive to airways obstruction because the high flow rates the procedure generates increase turbulent

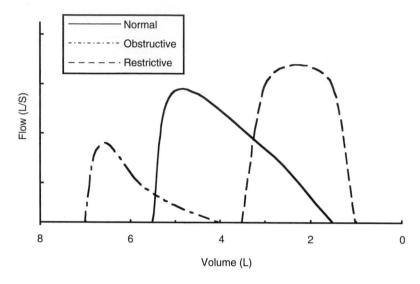

FIGURE 17-9 Expiratory flow-volume loops comparing normal, obstructive, and restrictive patterns. See text for explanation.

flow in the airways and worsen the obstruction. Thus the MVV is reduced early and falls in proportion to the degree of obstruction and the decrease in FEV_1. Actually, the expected MVV for a given degree of obstruction or ventilatory impairment can be calculated by multiplying the patient's FEV_1 by 40.[11] Generally, this calculated value matches the actual measured MVV. If the actual value is less than that calculated, the most common reason is suboptimal patient effort. The presence of upper airway obstruction or respiratory neuromuscular disease is rarely a cause of this MVV disparity.

RESTRICTIVE LUNG DISEASE

Restrictive diseases also can affect spirometric measures and can be diagnosed by spirometric testing. As discussed previously, restrictive processes alter spirometry by their tendency to increase lung elastic recoil, which decreases lung distensibility and changes airway dynamics. In restriction, the FVC may be reduced due ostensibly to the inability to fully inflate the stiff lungs. The FEV_1 will be reduced proportionately to the FVC so that the FEV_1/FVC will be normal, clearly differentiating this process from obstructive disease (see Fig. 17-8). Actually, because the increased lung recoil may generate increased $\dot{V}max$, expiratory flow rates may be increased, as evident by a high FEV_1/FVC.[21] Extending this state to the measures of maximum expiratory flow, the FEFs are preserved in restriction and may even increase relative to the volume change such that the slope of the expiratory flow-volume loop is increased[22] (see Fig. 17-9). As the restrictive process progresses and the FVC falls, at some point flow rates will decrease, but generally they will be reduced in proportion to the loss of lung volume.

Because airway function is preserved and patients can sustain rapid respirations in restrictive lung disease, the MVV generally will be maintained even though the VC is impaired. Eventually, as the disease progresses and volume generation becomes increasingly limited due to decreased lung compliance, the MVV will be reduced, typically occuring when the FVC falls to less than 50 percent of predicted.[11] A reduced FVC without evidence of obstruction is not invariably considered secure evidence of restriction, this interpretation requiring a reduction of TLC.[22]

The comparative effects of obstructive and restrictive disease on dynamic lung function are reviewed in Table 17-4. It provides a guide for distinguishing between obstruction and restriction based on the results of spirometry. In summary, obstructive disease is evident by impaired expiratory flow rates, particularly by a decreased FEV_1/FVC ratio, and diminished maximum flows. Restriction is characterized by a decreased FVC with a normal to increased FEV_1 ratio; expiratory flow rates also will be preserved.

STATIC LUNG VOLUMES

OBSTRUCTIVE LUNG DISEASE

Obstructive lung disease can have a profound effect on lung volumes. Both acute obstruction and chronic disease can alter the normal lung volume configuration. When presented with an acute impediment to airflow, such as an exacerbation of asthma, FRC will increase[11,12] (Fig. 17-10). This increase in end-expiratory lung volume is termed *hyperinflation* and represents an attempt by the respiratory system to compensate for the increase in airway resistance. Breathing at a higher volume will decrease airway resistance due to higher elastic recoil and radial traction on the airways that improves the patency of the airways, and the higher recoil will provide more driving pressure to generate airflow. However, breathing at increased FRC places the diaphragm at a disadvantaged length and configuration, diminishing its

TABLE 17-4 Pulmonary Function Testing: Interpretation of Spirometry

	PATHOPHYSIOLOGY[a]	
Test	Obstruction	Restriction
FVC, liters	$\leftrightarrow \downarrow$	$\downarrow$
FEV_1, liters	$\downarrow \downarrow$	$\downarrow$
FEV_1/FVC	$\downarrow$	$\leftrightarrow$
FEF_{25-75}, L/s	$\downarrow$	$\leftrightarrow \downarrow$
FEF_{50}, L/s	$\downarrow$	$\leftrightarrow \downarrow$
MVV, L/min	$\downarrow$	$\leftrightarrow \downarrow$

[a] $\leftrightarrow$, No change; $\uparrow$, increase; $\downarrow$, decrease; $\leftrightarrow \downarrow$, no change early, decrease late in disease.

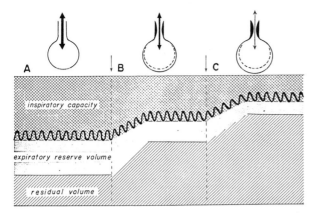

FIGURE 17-10 *A.* **Effects of increased airways resistance on functional residual capacity (expiratory reserve volume plus residual volume). Expiratory obstruction leads to increased FRC and RV.** *B* **and** *C* **represent application of two grades of resistance. (Reprinted, with permission, from Forster RE, et al:** *The Lung: Physiologic Basis of Pulmonary Function Tests.* **St. Louis, Mosby-Year Book, 1986.)**

contractility and efficiency. Along with the increase in FRC, RV also will increase, but TLC generally remains normal (see Fig. 17-10).

Patients with emphysema also may have an increase in FRC, but the mechanism of hyperinflation relates to the loss of lung elastic recoil that results from the emphysematous process. The FRC level is determined by the recoil forces of the lung and chest wall, with end-expiration occuring at the point at which the two opposing recoil pressures are equal and thus balanced. When lung elasticity is diminished, the lung recoil pressure is diminished, and a higher lung volume is necessary to generate the same pressure as when elastance was normal. Thus, in emphysema, a new equilibrium between the lungs and chest wall is established, but at a higher

lung volume. As in the acute situation, RV also increases with FRC. Because RV is also dependent on the ability to fully expire, which is limited with airways obstruction, RV usually increases to a relatively greater degree than FRC. Again, TLC generally remains in the normal range, although it may increase in patients with emphysema and, at times, in asthma as well.[11] Note that FRC increases at the expense of VC, which is diminished as hyperinflation progresses.

As noted previously, lung volumes measured by the helium dilution method may underestimate true volumes in patients with obstructive airways disease, especially emphysema. Determining the FRC with the body plethysmograph provides an accurate measure of resting lung volume that may be greater than that measured by helium dilution. When present, this difference between body box and helium dilution FRC also has been referred to as *air trapping.*

RESTRICTIVE LUNG DISEASE

The increased lung elastic recoil associated with restrictive diseases such as pulmonary fibrosis affects resting lung volume quite the opposite from that noted earlier for emphysema. With increased lung elastance, lung recoil pressure is increased, and a lower lung volume is necessary to generate the pressure that will balance the outward recoil of the chest wall. Thus respiratory system equilibrium and FRC are established at a reduced lung volume. Because the stiff, noncompliant lungs impede inspiration, VC and TLC are usually diminished along with FRC.[12] RV generally follows FRC and is also reduced. The reduction of all measured volumes and capacities in a proportionate manner is termed *concentric restriction* and is typical of many restrictive processes, especially fibrosis (Fig. 17-11). A nonconcentric restriction can be seen in patients with obesity, in whom the FRC is diminished due to abdominal adiposity elevating the diaphragm, but the VC and TLC remain close to or within normal range (see Fig. 17-11). On the other hand, patients with neuromuscular disease and inspiratory muscle weakness may demonstrate

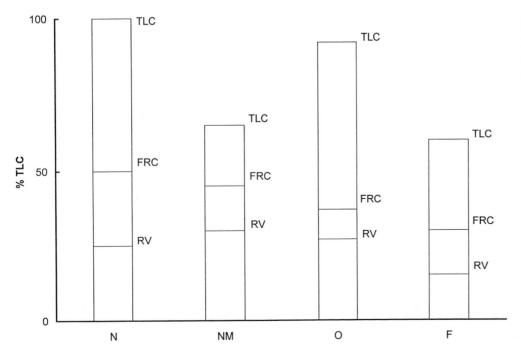

FIGURE 17-11 Subdivisions of lung volume in normal subjects (N) and in patients with neuromuscular disease (NM), obesity (O), and pulmonary fibrosis (F).

TABLE 17-5 Pulmonary Function Testing: Interpretation of Lung Volumes

Test	PATHOPHYSIOLOGY[a]	
	Obstruction	Restriction
TLC, liters	↔ ↑	↓
VC, liters	↓	↓
FRC, liters	↑	↓
RV, liters	↑ ↑	↓

[a] ↔, No change; ↑, increase; ↓, decrease ↔↑, no change early, increase late in disease.

a normal or slightly reduced FRC with a greater reduction in VC and TLC, representing a different pattern of nonconcentric restriction (see Fig. 17-11).

The comparative effects of obstruction and restriction on lung volumes are presented in Table 17-5. In summary, obstructive lung disease affects static lung volumes primarily with an increase in FRC (hyperinflation) and RV, a reduction in VC, and maintenance of a normal TLC. Restrictive lung disease results in loss of one or more components of lung volume or lung capacity.

LUNG COMPLIANCE

Measurement of lung compliance is the most specific method for assessing static lung mechanics, that is, lung elasticity. In patients with emphysema, the pressure-volume curve is shifted upward and to the left with an increase in slope (Fig. 17-12). The upward shift reflects the hyperinflation and increase in resting lung volume. The leftward movement directly demonstrates the loss of elastic recoil such that at FRC and TLC Ptp is reduced. The increased slope depicts the high compliance of the lungs.[11]

In patients with pulmonary fibrosis, the opposite situation occurs. The pressure-volume curve is shifted downward and to the right, and the slope is diminished, signifying reduced lung volume, increased recoil, and a decreased compliance, respectively (see Fig. 17-12).

FIGURE 17-12 Pressure-volume curves depicting normal subjects and patients with emphysema and pulmonary fibrosis. See text for explanation.

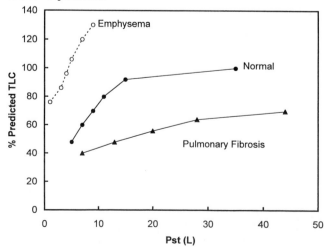

References

1. Kory RC: Clinical spirometry: Recommendation of the Section on Pulmonary Function Testing, Committee on Pulmonary Physiology, American College of Chest Physicians. *Dis Chest* 43:214, 1963.
2. Pappenheimer J, Comroe JH Jr, Counard A, et al: Standardization of definitions and symbols in respiratory physiology. *Fed Proc* 9:602, 1950.
3. Comroe JH: *Physiology of Respiration.* Chicago, Year Book Medical Publishers, 1974.
4. DuBois AG: Resistance to breathing, in Fenn WO, Rahn H (eds): *Handbook of Physiology: A Critical, Comprehensive Presentation of Physiological Knowledge and Concepts,* vol 1. Washington, American Physiological Society, 1995; pp 451–462.
5. Woolcock AJ, Vincent NJ, Macklem PT: Frequency dependence of compliance as a test for obstruction in small airways. *J Clin Invest* 48:1097, 1969.
6. Leith DE, Mead J: Mechanisms determining residual volume of the lungs in normal subjects. *J Appl Physiol* 23:221, 1967.
7. Hyatt RE: Forced respiration, in Macklem PT, Mead J (eds): *Handbook of Physiology,* vol 3. Bethesda, American Physiological Society, 1986.
8. Rodarte JR, Hyatt RE: Basics of RD: Respiratory mechanics. *Am Thorac Soc* 4:1, 1976.
9. Jones JG, Fraser RB, Nadel JA: Effect of changing airway mechanics on maximum expiratory flow. *J Appl Physiol* 38:1012, 1975.
10. Gibson GJ, Pride NB: Pulmonary mechanics in fibrosing alveolitis: The effects of lung shrinkage. *Am Rev Respir Dis* 116:637, 1977.
11. Bates DV, Macklem PT, Christie RV: *Respiratory Function in Disease.* Philadelphia, Saunders, 1971.
12. Comroe JH, Foster RE, DuBois AB, et al: *The Lung: Clinical Physiology and Pulmonary Function Tests.* Chicago, Year Book Medical Publishers, 1962.
13. American Thoracic Society: Standardization of spirometry: 1987 update. *Am Rev Respir Dis* 136:1285, 1987.
14. Gardner JM, Clausen JL, Epler G, et al: Pulmonary function laboratory personal qualifications. *Am Rev Respir Dis* 134:623, 1986.
15. Gardner JM, Clausen JL, Crapo RO, et al: Quality assurance in pulmonary function laboratories. *Am Rev Respir Dis* 134:625, 1986.
16. Quanjer PhH, Helms P, Bjure J, et al: Standardization of lung function tests in paediatrics. *Eur Respir J* 2(suppl 4):121S, 1989.
17. Morris AH, Kanner RE, Crapo RO, et al: *Clinical Pulmonary Function Testing: A Manual of Uniform Laboratory Procedures,* 2d ed. Salt Lake City, Intermountain Thoracic Society, 1984.
18. Schoenberg JB, Beck GJ, Bouhuys A: Growth and decay of pulmonary function in healthy blacks and whites. *Respir Physiol* 33: 367, 1978.
19. Knudson RJ, Burrows B, Lebowitz MD: The maximal expiratory flow-volume curve: Its use in the detection of ventilatory abnormalities in a population study. *Am Rev Respir Dis* 114:871, 1976.
20. Crapo RO, Morris AH, Gardner JM: Reference spirometric values using techniques and equipment that meet ATS recommendations. *Am Rev Respir Dis* 123:659, 1981.
21. Miller A, Thornton JC, Warshaw R, et al: Mean and instantaneous expiratory rates, FVC, and FEV$_1$. Prediction equations from a probability sample of Michigan, a large industrial state. *Bull Eur Physiopathol Respir* 22:589, 1986.
22. American Thoracic Society: Lung function testing: Selection of reference values and interpretive strategies. *Am Rev Respir Dis* 144:1202, 1991.

23. Knudson RJ, Lebowitz MD, Holberg CJ: Changes in the normal maximal expiratory flow-volume curve with growth and aging. *Am Rev Respir Dis* 127:725, 1983.

24. Paoletti P, Pistelli G, Fazzi P, et al: Reference values for vital capacity and flow-volume curves from a general population study. *Bull Eur Physiopathol Respir* 22:451, 1986.

25. Lebowitz MD, Holberg CJ: Comparisons of spirometric reference values and the proportions of abnormals among male smokers and those symptomatic in a community population. *Am Rev Respir Dis* 141:1491, 1990.

26. Bates DV: *Respiratory Function in Disease*. Philadelphia, Saunders, 1989.

27. Flenley DC: Chronic obstructive pulmonary disease. *Dis Mon* 34:537, 1988.

Chapter 18

METHODS OF ASSESSING EXERCISE CAPACITY

LAWRENCE MARTIN

Patients referred for *pulmonary rehabilitation* usually have the opportunity to enter an aerobic exercise program. *Exercise training,* as such programs are generally called, connotes a wide variety of methods for both assessing exercise capacity and carrying out the program. In this chapter, *exercise* and *exercise training* refer to aerobic exercise, such as activity that sustains an elevated heart rate for at least several minutes. Exercises designed for chronic obstructive pulmonary disease (COPD) patients also can be nonaerobic, for example, to strengthen specific respiratory muscles. Nonaerobic exercise as part of a rehabilitation program is discussed elsewhere in this book. This chapter reviews the more commonly employed methods of assessing and carrying out aerobic exercise and also discusses aspects of basic physiology germane to the topic.

Although exercise training for pulmonary rehabilitation is the focus of this chapter, there are other reasons to test exercise capacity in patients with pulmonary disease. A formal exercise test is particularly helpful when symptoms seem out of proportion to information from resting pulmonary function tests. Often patients can do far more exercise under controlled conditions than they thought possible. Even in patients with significant pulmonary impairment, there is no way to predict the specific reason for exercise limitation, and a formal exercise assessment may provide the answer: for example, hypoxemia, early onset of metabolic acidosis, or simply poor motivation. Other reasons to test exercise capacity include evaluation for resectional lung surgery, assessing improvement from medical or surgical therapy, evaluation for disability, and testing for exercise-induced asthma.

Why Exercise Training?

Today it is universally recognized that regular aerobic exercise confers benefits. Apart from the subjective sensation of "feeling better," there are measurable cardiovascular benefits: lower heart rate and higher stroke volume at rest and exercise, higher cardiac output at the maximum level of exercise, higher arteriovenous oxygen extraction, elevation of high-density lipoprotein cholesterol, modest reduction of blood pressure in hypertensives,[1-3] and lowering of risk for non-insulin-dependent diabetes.[4] Indeed, for people with or without cardiovascular risk factors, exercise is now viewed as a nonspecific "common sense" activity, akin to eating balanced meals, losing excess weight, stopping smoking, etc.

In the 1950s and early 1960s it was recommended that COPD patients limit their exercise.[5] This recommendation now seems as inappropriate as the prolonged bed rest pre-scribed for myocardial infarction patients at the time. Because of its cardiovascular benefits, regular exercise became mainstream therapy for heart patients in the 1970s and early 1980s, well before it was commonly accepted for patients with lung disease.

There are several reasons for belated acceptance of exercise therapy in chronic lung disease. Cardiac exercise regimens are impractical in patients who, because of chronic dyspnea, often have profound deconditioning. Furthermore, depression, anxiety, and inappropriate fear of exercise are prevalent in patients with COPD.[6] In addition, it has been difficult to prove efficacy in this group of patients. The most widely available tests of pulmonary impairment—spirometry and resting arterial blood gases—do not improve with exercise training.[7-10] Nonetheless, a scientific basis for exercise training in chronic lung disease is now established, and in the last few years, many reviews on the subject have appeared.[5,8,11-23]

By far the lung condition most studied with exercise has been COPD. Over 40 years ago, Barach and colleagues[24] observed benefit of exercise in COPD. In a review paper on therapies for nontuberculous lung disease, they made the following brief comment:

> In two patients with pulmonary emphysema in whom dyspnea on exertion was relieved during inhalation of oxygen, an exercise program was instituted with subsequent marked improvement of capacity to exercise without oxygen. A flow of 10 liters/minute of oxygen through a double bent nasal tube was used while the patient strode back and forth across the room. The number of steps walked with oxygen was doubled each day, and the walking without oxygen increased gradually to the point of slight dyspnea. The progressive improvement in ability to walk without dyspnea suggested that a physiologic response similar to a training program in athletes may have been produced. Since the vital capacity did not change significantly as a result of exercise, it seemed likely that improvement in circulatory function was at least one factor in the benefit obtained [pp. 375–376].

It took another decade for more formal studies to appear. In the 1960s, Pierce and coworkers[25] put nine patients with stable, severe COPD through an exercise training program; the result was a decrease in heart rate, respiratory rate, and minute ventilation and an increase in exercise tolerance. A comprehensive care program for COPD patients was first described by Petty and colleagues in 1969.[26]

Since the 1960s, many studies have shown benefits of aerobic exercise for COPD patients. Casaburi summarized 36 reports of exercise training published through 1988, plus a study by the author and colleagues published in 1991; these 37 reports included 933 patients with COPD.[15] The patients' average age was 61 years and average FEV$_1$ was 1.1 L; 19 percent of them were women. A wide range of exercise parameters was employed (frequency, length of sessions, etc.), but 31 of 32 studies in which exercise performance was evaluated showed benefit.[15] The one study that did not show benefit included only 7 patients.[27]

Studies of exercise outcome in COPD can be broadly divided into two types, uncontrolled and controlled. In uncontrolled studies, the patients' baseline characteristics have been compared with postexercise results. Thirty of the stud-

TABLE 18-1 Controlled Studies on Exercise Training in COPD (Listed in Chronologic Order)

Reference	No. of Patients	Duration	IMPROVEMENT IN EXERCISE		
			Max. Level[a]	Endurance[a]	Dyspnea[a]
Sinclair, 1980[41]	17T 16C	Daily for 40 wks	NE	Yes	Yes
Cockcroft, 1981[52]	18T 16C	Daily for 6 mos	Yes	Yes	Yes
Busch, 1988[27]	20T 10C	Daily for 18 wks	NE	No	Yes
O'Donnell, 1993[36]	23T 13C	Daily for 8 wks	Yes	Yes	Yes
Goldstein, 1994[35]	45T 44C	3 times weekly for 24 wks	NE	Yes	Yes
Reardon, 1994[87]	10T 10C	Twice a week for 6 wks	No	Yes	Yes
Wykstra, 1994[82]	28T 15C	Daily for 12 wks	Yes	Yes	Yes
O'Donnell, 1995[10]	30T 30C	Daily for 6 wks	Yes	Yes	Yes
Toshima, 1990[88] and Ries, 1995[9]	57T 62C	12 4-h sessions for 8 wks	Yes	Yes	Yes
Berry, 1996[45]	17T 8C	3 times a week for 12 wks	Yes	No	[b]

[a] Statistically significant change compared with control group.
[b] Improved but not significantly different from control group.
NOTE: T = exercise-trained; C = controls, not exercise-trained; NE = not evaluated.

ies listed in Casaburi's review had no control group, and most of them were small (less than 20 patients each).[15] Several large uncontrolled studies of more than 100 patients each have been reported, with emphasis on various aspects of exercise training.[26,28,29] All have shown some benefit to patients.

In the controlled studies, one group of COPD patients received exercise training, and a comparable group did not; several of these studies are listed in Table 18-1. Compared with controls, patients in these studies generally showed an increase in maximum exercise level (as determined from the treadmill speed and grade or the attained workload on a bicycle ergometer) and/or in exercise endurance (e.g., walking a greater distance in a fixed period of time). Most patients also developed a lessening of dyspnea with exercise training.

In the largest controlled study to date, 57 patients completing an exercise program demonstrated a significant increase in exercise endurance (82 versus 11 percent in controls), maximal treadmill workload (32 versus 14 percent), and peak oxygen uptake (8 versus 2 percent).[9] They also experienced improvement in dyspnea and muscle fatigue with exercise.

Since exercise training has not been shown to improve resting pulmonary function tests or arterial blood gases, slow the natural progression of disease, or improve survival, these should not be the goals in patients with chronic lung impairment. Nor should the goal be some level of physiologic performance, such as target heart rate or level of oxygen consumption. The overriding goal—and an extremely important one—is simply to make the breathless patient feel better and live more comfortably: "to restore the patient to the highest possible level of independent function."[9]

As expected, the most common pulmonary condition for which anaerobic exercise is prescribed is COPD, a condition for which "exercise training" is now a recognized therapy (Table 18-2). There is also a growing body of literature on exercise training for other types of chronic lung disease,[30–33] and some studies of pulmonary rehabilitation have included a spectrum of lung diseases.[34]

For COPD patients, anaerobic exercise is often combined with education about lung disease, smoking cessation, diet control, chest physical therapy, breathing technique training, and psychological counseling into a comprehensive program of pulmonary rehabilitation (see Table 18-2). Rehabilitation programs, while under the direction of a physician, are typically carried out by ancillary personnel.

An exercise program for COPD or other pulmonary patients must address four questions:

• Can the patient exercise safely?
• Which mode of aerobic exercise should be used?
• How should exercise capacity be assessed?
• How should progress be monitored?

TABLE 18-2 Therapies for Chronic Obstructive Pulmonary Disease

Common, applicable to large numbers of patients
Medications
  Bronchodilators
  Corticosteroids
  Antibiotics
  Diuretics
Supplemental oxygen
Patient education[a]
Smoking cessation[a]
Diet control (weight reduction or gain)[a]
Chest physical therapy[a]
Breathing technique training, including inspiratory muscle strengthening[a]
Psychological counseling[a]
Exercise training[a]

Less common, applicable to selected patients only
Partial lung resection
Alpha₁-antitrypsin replacement therapy
Nighttime bilevel positive airway pressure ventilation
Continuous mechanical ventilation
Lung transplantation

[a] Components of a comprehensive pulmonary rehabilitation program.

Can the Patient Exercise Safely?

There is no purpose in recommending a patient for exercise training if there is a major limitation or contraindication. COPD patients are typically middle-aged and with a long smoking history and so are at risk for other smoking-related problems, such as peripheral vascular and coronary artery disease. Leg or chest pain from these conditions might make exercise training impossible until the cause is corrected. Other contraindications could include severe hypoxemia, orthopedic or neurologic impairment, anemia, psychiatric disorder, poor motivation, or simple inability to follow instructions. In two controlled studies with over 100 COPD patients each, 48 and 64 percent of patients considered for exercise training were excluded for a variety of reasons.[9,35]

Exercise evaluation for pulmonary patients begins with full assessment of the lung disease, including a thorough history and physical examination, chest x-ray, resting pulmonary function tests (including spirometry and diffusing capacity for carbon monoxide), arterial blood gases, hemoglobin measurement, and electrocardiogram (ECG). It is generally recommended that a formal cardiac stress test (12-lead ECG with a graded exercise protocol) be done to exclude significant coronary artery disease.[14,36] If a cardiac stress test is not performed, the patient should at least have an initial exercise assessment under medical supervision with monitoring of a single-lead ECG (usually V_5) and pulse oximetry.

Generally, an Sa_{O_2} less than 88 percent or that falls to less than 88 percent with exercise qualifies the patient for portable nasal oxygen.[37] If indicated, supplemental oxygen can be used during exercise training. Severe hypoxemia that persists with supplemental oxygen is a contraindication to exercise.

Note that CO_2 retention, an indicator of advanced lung disease, is not a contraindication to exercise training. In a study by Foster and colleagues,[28] both eucapnic and hypercapnic patients improved on a 6-min walk test that was part of a comprehensive rehabilitation program. The group with severe hypercapnia ($P_{CO_2} > 54$ mmHg) increased their 6-min walking distance from 336 to 597 ft.

Age is also not a contraindication to exercise training in general[38] or to an effective exercise program for patients with lung disease.[36,39] In one study of 28 COPD patients (average age 78 ± 3 years) the 12-min walking distance improved significantly after exercise training.[40] Several studies reporting benefit of exercise included patients above age 75.[34,41]

Once the patient is accepted for exercise training, a nonphysician therapist can monitor progress using an established protocol. There is a well-recognized learning curve for most patients, particularly when a motorized treadmill or bicycle is used, so two or more supervised exercise tests may be required before the formal program begins.

Which Mode of Aerobic Exercise?

The purpose of aerobic exercise is to achieve a certain energy expenditure that will lead to an improvement in well-being and less dyspnea on exertion. While an athlete or a cardiac patient without lung disease may use a variety of exercise modes for training (e.g., outdoor running, swimming, outdoor bicycling, pushups) and have a specific physiologic target (e.g., oxygen uptake or heart rate 85 percent of predicted maximum), goals for the pulmonary-impaired patient are more modest: some easily measured improvement in exercise endurance and/or tolerance and a decline in dyspnea with activity. Table 18-3 lists the most commonly employed modes of achieving these goals.

For lung disease patients, the goal of each exercise session is usually to the point of limiting symptoms. Most of the studies reviewed by Casaburi exercised patients to an intensity "as tolerated" or "according to ability"; specific physiologic goals (e.g., 75 percent of predicted maximum heart rate) were far less common.[15] Indeed, physiologic goals are generally impractical, since pulmonary patients often experience ventilatory or blood-gas limitation well before limitation in cardiac output or oxygen uptake.[7,23,42-44]

It is not the mode of exercise that is important, only that the result of each session achieves a sustained increase in heart rate and oxygen uptake over the resting state. Any mode of aerobic exercise may give this result, including low-intensity exercise that does not lead to an increase in peak oxygen uptake over the training period.[45]

The greatest aerobic activity is generated with use of the legs; running and bicycling are about equal and better for aerobic exercise than walking. For various reasons (orthopedic or peripheral vascular disease, inability to stay on a treadmill, loss of balance on a bicycle), some patients cannot exercise using their legs; for them, arm-only machines can be employed. In a nationwide survey of 283 pulmonary rehabilitation programs in 44 states, 235 reported the devices used for exercise stress tests: 37 percent used the treadmill, 23 percent used a cycle ergometer, and 40 percent used both. However, in programs using both devices, 73 percent reported using the treadmill the most, while 27 percent reported using the cycle the most.[46] (Other programs used free walking.)

Muscle conditioning is specific for the type of exercise used and is not transferred to other muscle groups.[2,47,48] Thus exercise tolerance for walking will not be improved with arm-only exercise. Similarly, a COPD patient with dyspnea on arm raising will not benefit if he or she trains only with the leg muscles. A comprehensive rehabilitation program should provide some flexibility, i.e., be able to provide for both leg and arm exercise.

MAINLY LEG EXERCISE

The motorized treadmill is perhaps the most common device used in pulmonary rehabilitation programs[46] (Fig. 18-1). In both cardiac and pulmonary rehabilitation, a graded program is commonly used during initial assessment of exercise tolerance. In the widely used Bruce protocol for the study

TABLE 18-3 Modes of Exercise for the Pulmonary-Impaired Patient

1. Mainly leg exercise
   a. Motorized treadmill
   b. Bicycle pedaling (including cycle ergometer)
   c. Free walking
   d. Stair-climbing machines
2. Mainly arm exercise
   a. Arm ergometer
   b. Weight lifting
   c. Miscellaneous (ball throwing, rope pulling)
3. Arm and leg exercise
   a. Cross-country skiing machine
   b. Rowing machine
   c. Swimming

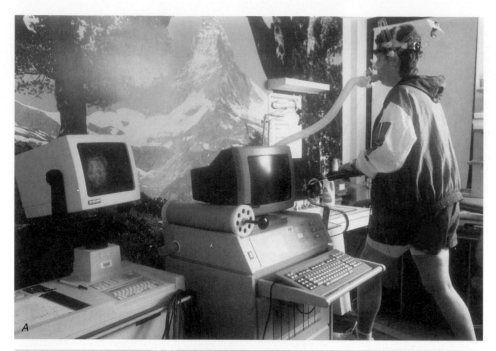

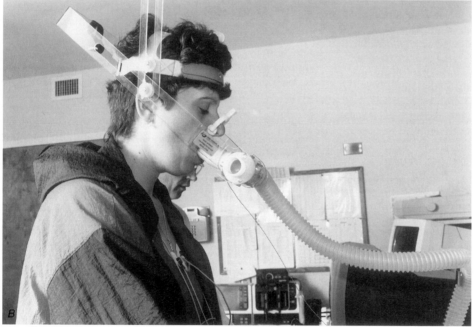

FIGURE 18-1 Subject and equipment for group 2 measurements on treadmill. (*A*) Subject is walking on treadmill and exhaling through mouthpiece and connecting hose to device that measures oxygen uptake and carbon dioxide output, respiratory rate, and tidal volume. To the right of the blow-up photo of the Matterhorn is a poster showing a dyspnea scale (see Fig. 18-8). (*B*) Close-up of subject. The ECG monitoring wires can be seen connected to her chest.

of patients with heart disease,[49] treadmill speed and/or elevation grade are increased at 3-min intervals, for a total of 27 min (Table 18-4). This and other graded protocols for heart patients are necessarily modified for pulmonary-impaired patients. For example, treadmill speed can start at 1.0 mi/h and be increased by 0.5-mi/h increments up to 3.0 mi/h; if this speed is tolerated, elevation can be added in increments of 2 to 5 percent.

There are several relative disadvantages of treadmill exercise.[50] It is an unnatural way to walk, and patients are often concerned about "falling off" or not being able to keep up. Compared with a stationary bicycle, it is more difficult for the patient to stop exercising if he or she develops limiting symptoms. Also, the treadmill sometimes presents difficulty

TABLE 18-4 Bruce Protocol for Treadmill Exercise Testing

Duration of Interval, min	Treadmill Speed, mi/h	Grade of Elevation, %
3	1.7	0
3	1.7	5
3	1.7	10
3	2.5	12
3	3.4	14
3	4.2	16
3	5.0	18
3	5.5	20
3	6.0	22

NOTE: Commonly modified for pulmonary-impaired patients; see text.

with the subject hooked up to a mouthpiece (for expired gas collection), monitoring wires, and a pulse oximeter. Finally, the learning curve associated with the machine may make it difficult to know if exercise tolerance is improving or if the patient is just getting used to walking on a treadmill.

Once the patient feels comfortable with treadmill walking, and after the initial graded exercise test, each training session can be conducted in a steady state, e.g., 10-min intervals at a fixed elevation and speed. The steady-state level can then be increased during a single session or at subsequent sessions, and in this way, exercise tolerance can be increased over time.

Stationary cycling is also a popular mode of exercise (Fig. 18-2). Because it is not motorized, bicycling is considered safer than a treadmill, although for some patients the technique may be less familiar. Compared with a treadmill, a stationary cycle is easier to use with multiple monitoring devices attached to the patient. For this reason, and also because a cycle (configured as an ergometer) allows precise calculation of workloads, research programs favor it over the treadmill. Also, most reference values for maximal exercise testing are based on cycle measurements.[50]

Repetitive stair climbing is practical with either stationary steps or a climbing machine that offers resistance to each step. Such machines, used to sufficient intensity, can confer similar aerobic benefits as the treadmill and stationary bicycle.

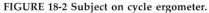

FIGURE 18-2 Subject on cycle ergometer.

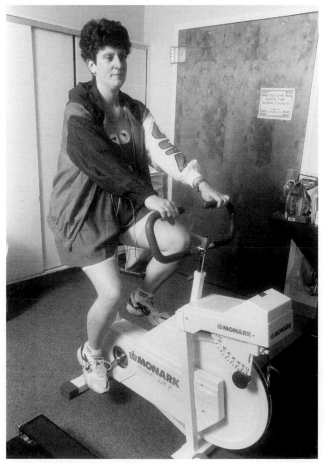

The simplest aerobic exercise is free walking, since all it requires is a comfortable pair of shoes and a place to walk; it is simple and natural, what patients do every day. Another advantage of free walking is that it gets often-sedentary patients out of the house. The 12-min walk test, first proposed by McGavin,[51] has since been widely employed as a means of monitoring progress, although the test is sometimes shortened to only 6 min. With either duration, exercise tolerance is assessed from the distance walked, whether or not the patient stops to catch his or her breath. This distance can then be monitored easily for progress.[41,52-54]

Free walking has two limitations for exercise training. One is that it takes much longer to achieve a given energy expenditure compared with motorized treadmill or bicycling. Notwithstanding the observation of Barach and associates[24] in the 1950s, patients are unlikely to develop a true training effect, since the level of intensity is too low. However, if walking achieves the same heart rate as the cycle or treadmill, a training effect may be achieved.[2] Another disadvantage of free walking is that outdoor exercise is not suitable during inclement weather (or, in many areas, during winter months), so an indoor venue must be found, such as a gym or shopping mall. While this is logically not a problem, the difficulty of "getting there" may be used as an excuse by poorly motivated patients to quit exercising.

ARM-ONLY EXERCISE

Upper extremity exercise is used increasingly for both exercise assessment and training and is of particular benefit in patients who, for whatever reason, cannot exercise with their legs (Fig. 18-3). One advantage of upper extremity exercise is that it works muscles used in other activities of daily living besides walking. Several studies have shown the efficacy of arm exercise in pulmonary rehabilitation.[16,47,48,55-57] One disadvantage is that the level of oxygen uptake (V_{O_2}) reached is lower than with leg exercise because of the smaller muscle mass employed.[58]

ARM AND LEG EXERCISE

Patients may use all limb muscles in swimming, rowing, and skiing. Swimming, while good aerobic exercise, adds a logistical problem to a rehabilitation program (finding a pool, ensuring patients can swim, providing a life guard, etc.). However, swimming may be ideal exercise for the motivated patient to do on his or her own. Stationary rowing and cross-country skiing devices are also good for aerobic exercise and may be used by selected patients.

How Should Exercise Capacity Be Assessed?

Table 18-5 lists the most common measurements made during initial assessment of exercise capacity, grouped according to equipment needed. Each succeeding group represents an increased level of complexity. Group 3 and 4 measurements are usually confined to a research setting or else used when testing is for a specific clinical problem, such as evaluation of pulmonary artery pressures during exercise.

As might be expected, many of the measurements in Table 18-5 will differ between ventilation-limited patients and a

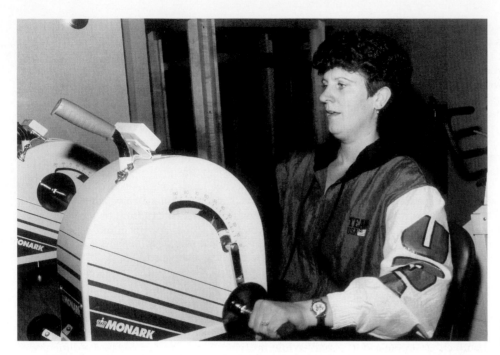

FIGURE 18-3 Subject using arm ergometer.

TABLE 18-5 Measurements during Exercise Testing

Group 1: No mouthpiece
Symptoms, particularly level of dyspnea (self-assessment based
  on numerical scale)
Heart rate
Respiratory rate
Sp_{O_2}
Single-lead electrocardiogram
12-lead electrocardiogram
Blood pressure
Group 2: Mouthpiece, oxygen and carbon dioxide analyzer
Tidal volume
Minute ventilation
Dead space ventilation
Alveolar ventilation
End-tidal P_{CO_2}
Carbon dioxide output (V_{CO_2})
Oxygen uptake (V_{O_2})
Respiratory quotient (V_{CO_2}/V_{O_2})
Anaerobic threshold[a]
Group 3: Arterial line
Arterial blood gases: Pa_{O_2}, Pa_{CO_2}, pH
HCO_3^-
Lactate
V_D/V_T
$P(A-a)_{O_2}$
Anaerobic threshold
Group 4: Right-sided heart catheter
Pulmonary artery pressure
Cardiac output
Mixed venous P_{O_2} and Sa_{O_2}

[a] Can be determined in various ways, either from exhaled gases or blood
measurements.[43,50,88]

healthy population (Table 18-6). Whereas a healthy population has fairly predictable physiology at submaximal and maximal levels of exercise, there is a variable and unpredictable response in ventilation-limited patients; indeed, perhaps the only predictable feature of this group is that they cannot exercise to maximum levels predicted for their age. How far they can exercise, why they stop, and their exercise physiology at the cessation of exercise are highly variable.

By definition, ventilation-limited patients cannot achieve predicted maximum minute ventilation with exercise. This limitation is illustrated by the flow-volume loops in Fig. 18-4 comparing exercise in a normal individual with a severe COPD patient.[5] Whereas the normal individual can increase exercise ventilation and comfortably breathe well within maximum flow rates, the patient with severe COPD cannot. In severe COPD, flows are limited by the patient's lung disease; furthermore, the patient with COPD breathes at a slightly higher lung volume (flow-volume loop is shifted to the left).

With an increase in the work of exercise there is a corresponding increase in the following physiologic parameters (Fig. 18-5): heart rate, minute ventilation, alveolar ventilation, oxygen uptake (V_{O_2}), and carbon dioxide output (V_{CO_2}). These parameters increase linearly with work rate up to the anaerobic threshold (AT), at which point their slopes begin to diverge (see Fig. 18-5).

In healthy subjects, Pa_{CO_2} and Pa_{O_2} stay fairly constant before anaerobic threshold (see Fig. 18-5). Pa_{CO_2} is a function of CO_2 production (V_{CO_2}) and alveolar ventilation (V_A), according to the equation

$$Pa_{CO_2} = \frac{V_{CO_2} \times 0.863}{V_A}$$

TABLE 18-6 Some Differences during Exercise between Sedentary Healthy People and Patients with Ventilatory Limitation from COPD[a]

	Healthy Sedentary	Ventilation-Limited (COPD)
AT	50–60% V_{O_2} max	Variable; may not occur
Pa_{O_2}	Constant before AT Increased after AT	Variable
Pa_{CO_2}	Constant before AT Decreased after AT	Normal or increased at any point
pH	Constant before AT Decreased after AT	Normal or decreased at any point
VEmax	Less than resting MVV	Equal or greater than resting MVV
Exercise limitation	Cardiac output, peripheral muscles	Minute ventilation
V_{O_2} max	Close to predicted value; reproducible result; may reach a plateau	Far from predicted value; varies from test to test; does not plateau
V_{O_2}/heart rate	>80% predicted max	Reduced
V_D/V_T	Reduced	Unchanged or increased
Exercise Rx	Target heart rate or V_{O_2}	Not clearly defined; usually to point of limiting dyspnea
Main reason for improvement over time	Physiologic training effect	Unclear; multifactorial

[a] Information from several sources, including refs. 1, 3, 19, and 50. See text for discussion of tests.

NOTE: AT = anaerobic threshold, point of increase in lactic acid production; MVV = maximal voluntary ventilation at rest; VEmax = maximal minute ventilation; V_{O_2}max = maximal oxygen uptake.

where VA is the total or minute ventilation (VE) minus the dead space ventilation (VD). Normally, Pa_{CO_2} stays constant before AT, since both V_{CO_2} and VA increase in tandem before anaerobic threshold. The increased VA is brought about by an increase in both respiratory rate (tachypnea) and tidal volume (hyperpnea). This physiologic state—normal Pa_{CO_2} with tachypnea and hyperpnea—reminds us that clinical assessment cannot be used to determine adequacy of alveolar ventilation in either the healthy subject or the COPD patient at rest or during exercise.

At AT, the supply of oxygen becomes insufficient to meet the metabolic requirement of working muscles, and metabo-

FIGURE 18-4 Flow-volume loops in healthy subject and patient with COPD during rest and exercise. In COPD, tidal breathing expiratory flow abuts the expiratory flow curve from forced vital capacity maneuver. During exercise (*Ex.*), the COPD patient breathes at a slightly higher lung volume (leftward shift of flow-volume loop). In the normal subject, there is a large venti- latory reserve during both rest and exercise. (From Olopade CO, Beck KC, Viggiano RW, Staats BA: Exercise limitation and pulmonary rehabilitation in chronic obstructive pulmonary disease: Subject review. *Mayo Clin Proc* 67:144–157, 1992. Used with permission.)

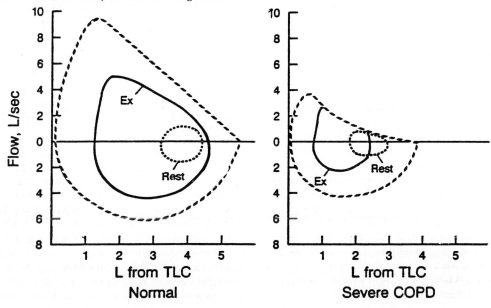

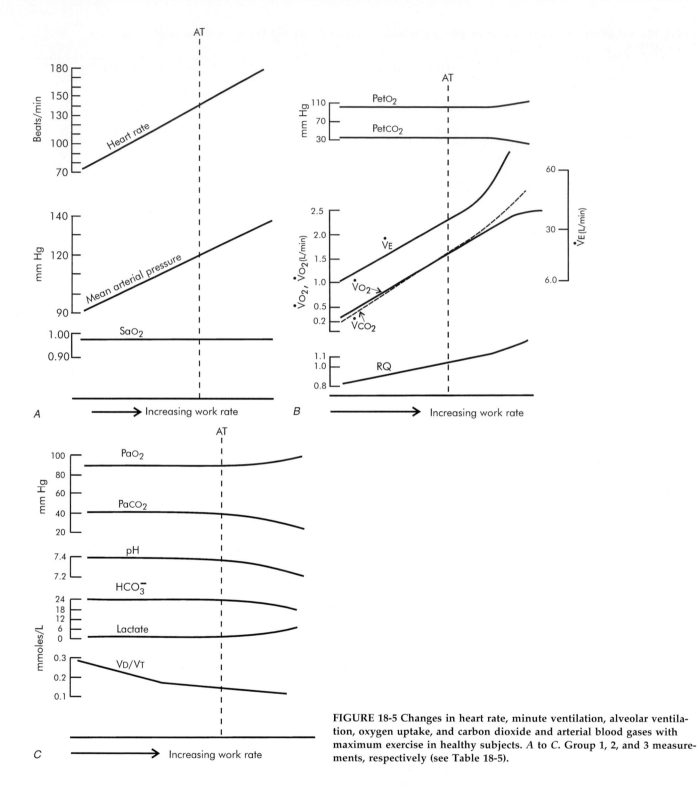

FIGURE 18-5 Changes in heart rate, minute ventilation, alveolar ventilation, oxygen uptake, and carbon dioxide and arterial blood gases with maximum exercise in healthy subjects. *A* to *C*. Group 1, 2, and 3 measurements, respectively (see Table 18-5).

lism shifts to an anaerobic mode, with production of lactic acid. Continued exercise beyond AT brings about several important changes (see Fig. 18-5):

1. Lactic acid begins to accumulate from anaerobic metabolism and with it a metabolic acidosis and fall in HCO_3^- and blood pH.
2. V_E and V_A increase out of proportion to V_{O_2} and V_{CO_2}.
3. Pa_{CO_2} decreases and Pa_{O_2} increases.

The "gold standard" for identifying AT is measurement of lactate levels, but this is impractical in most instances and is not used widely. More widely employed to identify AT are changes in the slopes of expired gas. Particularly popular for assessing AT in COPD patients is the V-slope method; when the slope of V_{CO_2} exceeds that of V_{O_2}, the assumption is that lactate is rising and producing more CO_2 for elimination.[59] However, the correlation of this and other expired gas techniques with measured lactate levels is not 100 percent.[43,50]

Normal resting V_{O_2} is about 300 mL O_2 per minute. V_{O_2} rises immediately with aerobic exercise and is considered the best measurement of the metabolic requirement of work. In healthy subjects, V_{O_2}max is the standard measurement of exercise capacity.[1] In middle-aged healthy people V_{O_2}max is 2.25 ± 0.43 L/min.[59] Anaerobic threshold—the point at which lactic acid increases—normally occurs at about 50 to 60 percent of the individual's V_{O_2}max.[1] Thus if an individual's V_{O_2}max is 2 L/min, AT will occur at a V_{O_2} of about 1.0 to 1.2 L/min. At the AT, exercising muscles need more oxygen than the lungs and heart can deliver, and additional energy needs are met by anaerobic metabolism. (Anaerobic metabolism is relatively inefficient, producing only 3 ATP molecules versus 36 when glucose is fully metabolized aerobically.) To compensate for the developing lactic acidosis, the healthy subject hyperventilates (lowers Pa_{CO_2}) and V_{CO_2} increases at a faster rate than before AT. At the same time, Pa_{O_2} goes up, as predicted by the alveolar gas equation (see Fig. 18-5).

Pa_{CO_2} BEYOND ANAEROBIC THRESHOLD

Discussion of Pa_{CO_2} beyond AT is germane to the topic of ventilation-limited patients. In healthy subjects, exercise is limited by cardiac output and the capillary capacity of the exercising muscles; when they can no longer deliver sufficient oxygen to the mitochondria, lactic acid is produced from anaerobic metabolism. Lactic acid is buffered by HCO_3^-, which then falls along with blood pH, signifying a state of metabolic acidosis. At the same time, the buffering reaction creates additional CO_2, beyond that continually produced by exercising muscles; this extra CO_2 also must be ventilated off and is one reason why minute ventilation increases out of proportion to oxygen uptake after AT. In health, Pa_{CO_2} never rises despite large increments in V_{CO_2} (unless there is an external impediment to ventilation).[60–62] Indeed, the normal ventilatory reserve is such that beyond AT, healthy subjects hyperventilate and *lower* Pa_{CO_2} (see Fig. 18-5) to compensate for the developing metabolic acidosis. Hyperventilation is the other reason for the increase in slope of V_E after AT.

In summary, beyond AT, the subject is faced with markedly increased ventilatory demands for three reasons. First is the increase in CO_2 production as the work of exercise increases beyond AT; if this was the only reason for the V_{CO_2} increase, V_E would continue to increase linearly with V_{O_2}. Second, the CO_2 load is increased further because of buffering of HCO_3^-, presenting an additional ventilatory demand. Third, the subject must hyperventilate (increase CO_2 output at a greater rate than called for by CO_2 delivered to the lungs) in order to compensate for metabolic acidosis. Healthy people respond very well to these demands and easily hyperventilate beyond AT; ventilation-limited patients cannot and frequently hypoventilate (Pa_{CO_2} goes up)[59,63,64] (Fig. 18-6).

A patient with reduced FEV_1 has a low maximum voluntary ventilation (MVV), which in turn limits minute and alveolar ventilation (V_A) with exercise. Because V_A does not rise commensurate with the increased level of V_{CO_2}, Pa_{CO_2} may increase at a level of exercise where it would normally remain constant or go down. Hypercapnia accentuates the sensation of dyspnea and leads to early cessation of exercise. In Fig. 18-6 this is shown to occur despite the rise in lactate

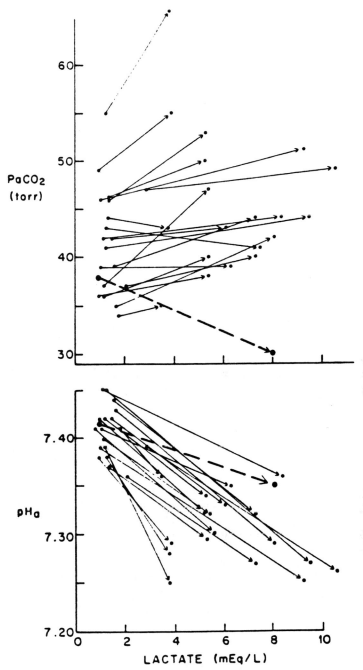

Figure 18-6 Rise in Pa_{CO_2} with rise in lactate in COPD patients subject to heavy exercise (*unbroken arrows*). The dashed arrow in each figure represents the average response of 10 normal subjects who developed the same degree of lactic acidosis. Normal subjects hyperventilate (lower Pa_{CO_2}) and develop only metabolic acidosis. The COPD patients in this study developed metabolic and respiratory acidosis. (From Casaburi R, Patessio A, Ioli R, et al: Reductions in exercise lactic acidosis and ventilation as a result of exercise training in patients with obstructive lung disease. *Am Rev Respir Dis* 143:9–18, 1991. Used with permission.)

levels (i.e., Pa_{CO_2} should be going down). The rise in Pa_{CO_2} adds a respiratory acidosis to the metabolic acidosis, and pH falls more than would be expected from a given rise in blood lactate.[64]

HYPOXEMIA WITH EXERCISE

Pa_{O_2} normally remains unchanged before anaerobic threshold, at which point it rises along with the fall in Pa_{CO_2}. However, the alveolar-arterial P_{O_2} difference rises significantly with exercise. A typical normal change with exercise would be a 3-mmHg decline in Pa_{O_2} (93 to 90), a 19-mmHg increase in $P(a-a)_{O_2}$ (9 to 28), and a 6-mmHg decline in Pa_{CO_2} (40 to 34).[65] Since Pa_{O_2} does not decrease, the increase in $P(A-a)_{O_2}$ must be due to increase in alveolar P_{O_2}.

Pa_{O_2} is a function of the inspired partial pressure of oxygen ($P_{I_{O_2}}$), Pa_{CO_2}, and respiratory exchange ratio, as shown by the alveolar gas equation:

$$PA_{O_2} = P_{I_{O_2}} - (PA_{CO_2}) \left[F_{I_{O_2}} + \frac{(1 - F_{I_{O_2}})}{R} \right]$$

$P_{I_{O_2}}$ is a function of the fraction of inspired oxygen, the barometric pressure, and the airway water vapor pressure, all constant during exercise. R is the respiratory exchange ratio, V_{CO_2}/V_{O_2}. With exercise, PA_{O_2} increases because of the decline in Pa_{CO_2} and increase in R, which goes from a baseline 0.8 at rest (e.g., V_{CO_2} 240 mL/min, V_{O_2} 300 mL/min) to 1.11 (V_{CO_2} 4000 mL/min, V_{O_2} 3600 mL/min), crossing 1.0 at the anaerobic threshold.[65]

Decline in Pa_{O_2} is common in patients with lung disease and may occur from any of the principal physiologic causes: elevation of Pa_{CO_2}, ventilation-perfusion imbalance, diffusion impairment, low mixed venous oxygen saturation (from increased peripheral oxygen extraction) in the presence of low V/Q lung units, and shunts.[65–67] Normal pulmonary diffusing capacity has sufficient reserve that there is adequate oxygen transfer no matter how vigorous the exercise. However, if there is alveolar membrane thickening, destruction of capillaries (as in emphysema), or anemia, pulmonary diffusing capacity will be reduced, and the shorter pulmonary circulation transit time during exercise may then reduce oxygen transfer (Fig. 18-7).

Although ventilation-limited patients frequently manifest hypoxemia with exercise, its occurrence cannot be reliably predicted from pulmonary function studies.[68] In the study by Ries and colleagues,[68] an $FEV_1/FVC \geq 0.50$ or a single-breath diffusing capacity for carbon monoxide (DLCOsb) $\geq$ 20 mL/min/mmHg was 100 percent predictive in *excluding* a fall in Pa_{O_2} with exercise (see Fig. 18-7). In another study, a DLCOsb above 55 percent of predicted was 100 percent specific in excluding oxygen desaturation with exercise.[69]

Apart from ventilatory limitation or blood-gas abnormalities, other factors may account for early cessation of exercise: lack of motivation, leg pain, chest pain, overall poor physical fitness. The initial exercise test is essential to determine exercise capacity and specific reason(s) for limitation. Detailed discussion of exercise test interpretation can be found in several sources.[1,70,71]

PULSE OXIMETRY

Apart from measurement of heart rate, probably the most commonly measured exercise variable is oxygen saturation by pulse oximetry (Sp_{O_2}). This is so because exercise oximetry is so widely used to assess need for supplemental oxygen in patients with dyspnea, whether or not they are being considered for exercise training. Such a test may consist of

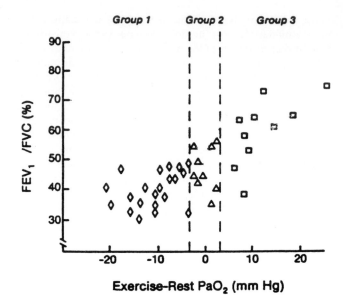

Figure 18-7 Hypoxemia during exercise cannot be predicted from baseline lung function studies. Figure plots FEV_1/FVC versus change in Pa_{O_2} with exercise in 40 patients with COPD. Patients are grouped according to changes in Pa_{O_2} with exercise. Group 1 (*diamonds*) had more than 3 mmHg decrease in Pa_{O_2}. Group 2 (*triangles*) had no change (±3 mmHg). Group 3 had more than 3 mmHg increase in Pa_{O_2}. (From Ries AL, Farrow JT, Clausen JL: Pulmonary function tests cannot predict exercise-induced hypoxemia in chronic obstructive pulmonary disease. Chest 93:454–459, 1988. Used with permission.)

nothing more than walking the patient in the hospital corridor while measuring finger pulse oximetry.

Whatever the purpose for exercising a patient, it is essential to screen for exercise-induced hypoxemia because it may be the cause of symptoms and is treatable. Above 85 percent true oxygen saturation, Sp_{O_2} is accurate to within about ±3 percent of the blood oxygen saturation as measured with a cooximeter (Sa_{O_2}).[72] However, there are several potential pitfalls to using pulse oximetry for exercise testing, including improper capture of pulse, inaccuracy at very low levels of Sa_{O_2}, intravenous dyes, skin pigment, and poor signal response. In a review of 10 studies utilizing both ear and finger pulse oximetry during exercise, Mengelkoch and associates[73] found that only 67 percent of the pulse oximeters studied were considered accurate when Sa_{O_2} was more than 85 percent in nonsmokers. However, the current generation of finger pulse oximeters appears to be more accurate than the older ear probe–equipped models.[73] It is interesting that most of the studies reviewed used cycle ergometry, since it produces less oximetry artifact than a treadmill.

An avoidable pitfall of pulse oximetry can occur when there is excess carboxyhemoglobin. In contrast to blood cooximeters, which utilize four wavelengths of light to separate out oxyhemoglobin from reduced hemoglobin, methemoglobin (MetHb), and carboxyhemoglobin (COHb), pulse oximeters utilize only two wavelengths of light.[74,75] As a result, pulse oximeters measure COHb and part of any MetHb along with oxyhemoglobin and combine the three into a single reading, the Sp_{O_2}. (MetHb absorbs both wavelengths of light emitted by pulse oximeters so that Sp_{O_2} is not affected as much by MetHb as for a comparable level of COHb.) Powers and colleagues[74] showed that in subjects who smoked and had COHb levels of more than 4 percent, pulse oximeters significantly overestimated Sa_{O_2}.

Whereas excess methemoglobin is an uncommon finding clinically, excess carboxyhemoglobin is present in all cigarette and cigar smokers. A resting Sp_{O_2} should be correlated with a measured Sa_{O_2} and (if a blood cooximeter is available) COHb and methemoglobin levels. If the measured Sa_{O_2} does not agree with Sp_{O_2}, the fact should be noted, reason(s) sought, and then accounted for during the exercise test. If a measured Sa_{O_2} cannot be correlated with Sp_{O_2}, exercise testing should not be done in current smokers so as to avoid falsely high Sa_{O_2} readings. (The half-life of CO breathing ambient air is about 6 h, so 24 h after smoking cessation the CO level should be normal, i.e., less than 2.5 percent.)

Carbon monoxide also can be measured in exhaled air as parts per million (ppm) and correlated with a blood carboxyhemoglobin level (e.g., 10 ppm roughly equals 2% COHb). Also, if a cooximeter is available, carboxyhemoglobin can be reliably measured on a venous blood sample; the value is the same as arterial. If venous COHb is elevated, its value can be subtracted from the Sp_{O_2} to get a truer reading of the patient's Sa_{O_2}. Attention to CO is important if one is to obtain accurate estimation of the patient's blood oxygen status.

OTHER MEASUREMENTS

Space does not permit detailed discussion of all potential measurements, and the reader is referred to other sources for additional information.[1,43,50,76,77] Note that measurement of oxygen consumption and carbon dioxide production requires a method to continually collect and analyze exhaled air; this in turn requires a mouthpiece be kept in place during exercise (see Fig. 18-1). An indwelling arterial line is necessary for arterial blood gases; a postexercise arterial blood gas—even 20 to 30 s after exercise—may show values very different from those obtained during exercise.[78] Certainly, collecting exhaled gases and arterial blood adds to the complexity of any test, the latter more so than the former. Fortunately, neither set of measurements is necessary for an effective exercise program. Simplicity and accurate measurements are more important than complexity and a plethora of measurements. At minimum, initial testing should monitor heart rate and pulse oximetry and assess the level of dyspnea.

Finally, note that the list in Table 18-5 includes a scale to measure dyspnea, since this may be the best way to follow progress of COPD patients. A commonly used rating scale is the one by Borg.[79] However, any dyspnea scale may be useful as long as the patient understands it. The scale used in our laboratory, modified after Borg and with simple pictorials, is shown in Fig. 18-8.

How Should Progress Be Monitored?

Nationwide, there is tremendous variation in how exercise capacity is assessed and progress monitored.[11,15,23,46] The methods range from the distance covered in a 6-min walk test, without any other measurement, all the way to graded exercise with indwelling arterial line and continuous measurement of exhaled gases. There is general consensus that when used for clinical purposes, methodology should not drive the program but should instead by driven by the experience and interest of the personnel involved.[23,80] As might be expected, it has not been shown that more measurements lead to better compliance by the patient or improvement in subjective and objective outcome parameters.[36] Absent accepted standards for exercise training, the only essential stipulation is that *some* measurement be made to demonstrate improvement, even if it is only a subjective dyspnea questionnaire.

Since the COPD population is also heterogeneous in terms of impairment, one would expect a range of physiologic responses to exercise. Whereas patients with only mildly diminished FEV_1 are often able to exercise beyond anaerobic threshold (as in the normal population), more severely impaired patients will be limited by minute ventilation and quit exercising before lactic acid is produced.[44] Nonetheless, patients at all levels of impairment can benefit from aerobic training. In a study of 33 patients with COPD, asthma, pulmonary fibrosis, and a wide range of FEV_1 values (0.33 to 3.8 L; 17 had an $FEV_1 < 1.0$ L), Niederman and colleagues[34] found that the percentage of change in exercise endurance was similar at all levels; degree of improvement was not correlated with baseline lung function. Other studies exercising severely impaired patients also have shown benefit.[28,81]

The nonresearch pulmonary rehabilitation program should not be concerned about making sophisticated measurements during exercise. Instead, it is important to understand the patient's limitations and work gradually to build up exercise capacity. Monitoring can be limited to charting the patient's level of dyspnea and duration of exercise. Furthermore, exercise can take place in a hospital, outpatient facility, or the patient's home. Studies have shown that exercise training can be successful in the home, providing the patient is highly motivated.[26,27,31,82] However, at all times the initial screening exercise test should be done under supervision.

How *much* exercise is defined by session duration, session frequency, duration of the program, and intensity.[11,14] All these parameters are variable, but there are some rough guidelines. Each session should last at least 20 min, but 30 to 60 min is preferable.[2,3] However, in severely limited patients, exercise may only be tolerable for a few minutes. Alternating brief periods of exercise with rest (e.g., 5 min each) may allow the patient to build up tolerance for continuous 20- or 30-min exercise sessions.

As to frequency, there should be from 3 to 5 sessions a week.[2,3,64] Most published studies have run programs for 5 to 10 weeks before releasing patients to continue on their own.[64] However, in the national survey by Bickford and colleagues[46] of 283 pulmonary rehabilitation programs, there was a significant variation in number of program sessions per week (1 to 7) and program duration (1 to 52 weeks); this and other information in the survey (e.g., a variety of exercise testing methods) indicate that no uniform or standard exercise protocol is currently employed.

As to intensity, the American College of Sports Medicine (ACSM) recommends four separate exercise strategies to choose from: (1) at 50 percent of peak V_{O_2}, (2) at an intensity above anaerobic threshold, (3) at a near-maximal intensity, and (4) at a specific level of dyspnea.[3] All four strategies are predicated on measurements made during an initial graded exercise test.

Exercise to a specific level of dyspnea (ACSM strategy 4) seems best suited for ventilation-limited patients. During a

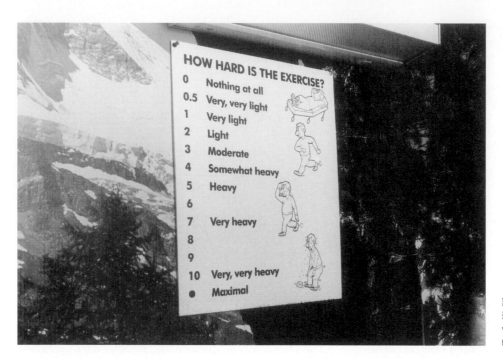

Figure 18-8 Dyspnea scale used during exercise. The chart is easily viewed by the patients during the test (see Fig. 18-1).

graded exercise test, V_{O_2} can be measured and correlated with the patient's perception of dyspnea (Fig. 18-9). For example, at 50 percent of the patient's peak V_{O_2}, the perceived dyspnea rating may be 3. In subsequent training sessions, this level of dyspnea becomes the target and presumably will correlate with 50 percent peak V_{O_2}.[83] To be most accurate and effective, the reference should be rechecked during the training program.

Notwithstanding the four strategies for intensity based on an initial graded exercise test, a fifth strategy seems most commonly practiced: to a level of dyspnea "as tolerated," without any correlative measurements.[15,46] Of 283 programs surveyed by Bickford and colleagues,[46] 232 recommended that patients monitor their heart rate while exercising and 267 that they monitor level of dyspnea. However, when asked to choose, 181 programs favored level of dyspnea and 35 programs favored heart rate.

Clearly, there is tremendous latitude in executing an exercise program. Provided the patient is motivated, some exercise regimen should be able to improve exercise performance. An hour or two of low-intensity exercise as little as three times a week can show measurable benefit.[12] Although achievement of a training effect would be desirable, emphasis to date has been on making the primary goal an improvement in breathlessness, not a specific physiologic change. Thus, in current practice, clinical assessment is more emphasized than physiologic measurement.

To be useful (and justify the program's existence), there should be some standard measurement of exercise endurance before the program begins and at its completion, e.g., time and speed on the treadmill or distance walked in 12 min and a scalar assessment of dyspnea by the patient (see Fig. 18-8). However, as with initial assessment of exercise capacity, what parameters should be monitored and how often are best determined by the interest and experience of the program personnel.

Why Do Patients Improve?

Improvement in exercise level and endurance with training could be explained by nonphysiologic effects, for example, improved motivation or adaptation to the exercise testing method over time, called a *learning effect*. A true physiologic response from anaerobic exercise is called a *training effect*, meaning a physiologic improvement that could only occur from the exercise.

From measurements made at the beginning and end of an exercise program, a physiologic training effect can be shown in one of several ways: a reduced ventilatory requirement and heart rate for the same level of exercise, an increase in aerobic muscle enzymes and capillary density, a delay in onset of lactic acidosis, or a decreased production of lactate with a corresponding decrease in minute ventilation for the same level of exercise.[5,15,42,64]

While virtually all studies show improved exercise tolerance (either in maximum level attained or in endurance), a true training effect has been infrequently demonstrated. Belman and Kendregan[42] showed no increase in muscle enzymes despite improved exercise tolerance. In a study not yet duplicated, Casaburi and associates[64] showed decreased lactate and minute ventilation in a group of subjects with mild to moderate COPD (mean FEV_1 of 1.70 to 1.87 L) after both high (above AT) and low (below AT) levels of exercise. The high-level-exercise group achieved a reduction in lactic acid of 32 percent versus 12 percent in the low-level-exercise group. A letter critical of the study's conclusion suggested that the patients were significantly less impaired than most subjects in a pulmonary rehabilitation program, and that is why they were able to achieve a training effect.[84]

It appears that with sufficiently intense exercise, ventilation-impaired patients can show an anaerobic training effect, at least when the impairment is mild to moderate. It may

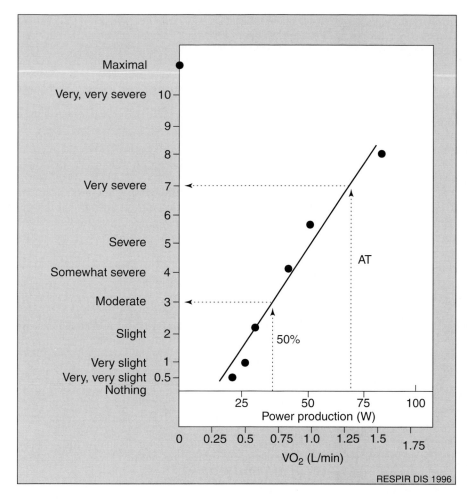

Figure 18-9 Correlation of V_{O_2} with patient's perception of dyspnea during a graded exercise test. This graph is from a 67-year-old man with severe COPD exercising on a cycle ergometer. At 50 percent of peak V_{O_2} the corresponding dyspnea rating was 3; at the anaerobic threshold (AT), the corresponding dyspnea rating was 7. (Reproduced with permission from Scott JA, Mahler DA: How to prescribe exercise for patients with COPD. *J Respir Dis* 17:527–536, 1996.)

well be, however, that most patients who enter pulmonary rehabilitation (the majority of whom have COPD) do not exercise to sufficient intensity to develop a training effect. It is also likely that more severely impaired patients are not able to reach sufficient intensity because of limiting dyspnea. In any case, while perhaps desirable, a training effect is not a requirement for patients with lung disease to benefit from aerobic exercise.[5,34]

Thus the question remains. Several controlled studies show that aerobic exercise improves exercise performance (see Table 18-1), but we still do not know *why*. As cogently pointed out by Belman,[13] investigators have claimed success for their respective programs despite the fact that training modes, intensity, and frequency have varied widely. Since a true aerobic training effect seems unlikely for most patients, and lung function and gas exchange do not improve with exercise, there must be other reasons.

Normally, respiratory muscles do not limit exercise tolerance, so specific respiratory muscle training (often offered in rehabilitation programs along with exercise training) should not improve exercise ability.[23] In line with this observation, a meta-analysis of extant studies found that respiratory muscle training does not benefit patients with chronic airflow limitation.[85] A controlled study comparing exercise training with and without inspiratory muscle training came to the same conclusion.[45]

It also has been suggested that some patients improve their "technique of exercising" and thereby achieve better endurance, but this seems an unlikely explanation for the improvement seen in so many studies. "Enhanced mechanical efficiency" is an explanation offered by O'Donnell and colleagues,[10] who found that patients were able to reduce their ventilatory demand for a given level of exercise after exercise training when there was no change in anaerobic threshold.

A major factor accounting for increased exercise endurance is probably increased patient motivation spurred by the attention of the program personnel. Patients do more because they are encouraged and, in a sense, "rewarded" for better performance. Thus after several sessions they exercise at capacity, knowing their success will meet with approval. (An analogy would be someone who improves an IQ score when the testers have a direct, personal interest in the outcome. The subject's native intelligence has not changed, but his or her motivation to do better has.)

Another plausible explanation is "desensitization" to the sensation of dyspnea.[13,42,86] Patients exercising in a controlled environment can learn to overcome the anxiety and apprehension associated with dyspnea and hence become desensitized to the symptom; they still have dyspnea, but it does not bother them as much, so they are able to continue exercising.

Whatever the reason(s), exercise training seems to help most ventilation-limited patients, young and old, and with mild, moderate, or severe impairment. There is wide latitude in how a program should be carried out, and the details seem less important than that the patient be encouraged to perform some type of symptom-limited aerobic exercise on a regular basis; this means several times a week for at least a few weeks. Aerobic exercise training should be part of a comprehensive program of pulmonary rehabilitation, with emphasis on patient education, particularly the importance of continuing exercise long after the formal program has ended.

References

1. Jones NL, Campbell EJM: *Clinical Exercise Testing*. Philadelphia Saunders 1988.
2. Casaburi R: Physiologic responses to training. *Clin Chest Med* 15:215–228, 1994.
3. *American College of Sports Medicine's Guidelines for Exercise Testing and Prescription*, 5th ed. Baltimore, Williams & Wilkins, 1995.
4. Lynch J, Helmrich SP, Lakka TA, et al: Moderately intense physical activities and high levels of cardiorespiratory fitness reduce the risk of non-insulin-dependent diabetes mellitus in middle-aged men. *Arch Intern Med* 156:1307–1314, 1996.
5. Olopade CO, Beck KC, Viggiano RW, Staats BA: Exercise limitation and pulmonary rehabilitation in chronic obstructive pulmonary disease: Subject review. *Mayo Clin Proc* 67:144–157, 1992.
6. Dudley DL, Glaser EM, Jorgenson BN, Logan DL: Psychosocial concomitants to rehabilitation in chronic obstructive pulmonary disease: 1. Psychosocial and psychological considerations. *Chest* 77:413–420, 1980.
7. Belman MJ: Exercise in chronic obstructive pulmonary disease. *Clin Chest Med* 7:585–597, 1986.
8. Celli BT: Pulmonary rehabilitation in patients with COPD. *Am J Respir Crit Care Med* 152:861–864, 1995.
9. Ries AL, Kaplan RM, Limberg TM, Prewitt LM: Effects of pulmonary rehabilitation on physiologic and psychosocial outcomes in patients with chronic obstructive pulmonary disease. *Ann Intern Med* 122:823–832, 1995.
10. O'Donnell DE, McGuire M, Samis L, Webb KA: The impact of exercise reconditioning on breathlessness in severe chronic airflow limitation. *Am J Respir Crit Care Med* 152:2005–2013, 1995.
11. American Thoracic Society: Standards for the diagnosis and care of patients with chronic obstructive pulmonary disease. *Am J Respir Crit Care Med* 152:S77–S120, 1995.
12. Belman MJ: Exercise in patients with chronic obstructive pulmonary disease. *Thorax* 48:936–946, 1993.
13. Belman MJ: Exercise training in patients with chronic obstructive pulmonary disease, in Bach JR (ed): *Pulmonary Rehabilitation*. Philadelphia, Hanley & Belfus, 1996; chap 8.
14. Casaburi R: Principles of exercise training. *Chest* 101:263S–267S, 1992.
15. Casaburi R: Exercise training in chronic obstructive lung disease, in Casaburi R, Petty TL (eds): *Principles and Practice of Pulmonary Rehabilitation*. Philadelphia, Saunders, 1993; chap 16, pp 204–224.
16. Celli BT: The clinical use of upper extremity exercise. *Clin Chest Med* 15:339–349, 1994.
17. Epstein SK, Celli BR: Cardiopulmonary exercise testing in patients with chronic obstructive pulmonary disease. *Cleve Clinic J Med* 60:119–128, 1993.
18. Folgering H, von Herwaarden C: Exercise limitation in patients with pulmonary diseases. *Int J Sports Med* 15:107–111, 1994.
19. Gallagher CG: Exercise limitation and clinical exercise testing in chronic obstructive pulmonary disease. *Clin Chest Med* 15:305–326, 1994.
20. Hodgkin JE: Pulmonary rehabilitation. *Clin Chest Med* 11:447–454, 1990.
21. Marciniuk DD, Gallagher CG: Clinical exercise testing in chronic airflow limitation. *Med Clin North Am* 80:565–587, 1996.
22. Ries AL: Position paper of the American Association of Cardiovascular and Pulmonary Rehabilitation: Scientific basis of pulmonary rehabilitation. *J Cardiopulmonary Rehabil* 10:418–441, 1990.
23. Ries AL: The importance of exercise in pulmonary rehabilitation. *Clin Chest Med* 15:327–337, 1994.
24. Barach AL, Bickerman HA, Beck G: Advances in the treatment of non-tuberculous pulmonary disease. *Bull NY Acad Med* 28:353–384, 1952.
25. Pierce AK, Taylor HF, Archer RK, Miller WF: Responses to exercise training in patients with emphysema. *Arch Intern Med* 113:28–36, 1964.
26. Petty TL, Nett LM, Finigan MM, et al: A comprehensive care program for chronic airway obstruction: Methods and preliminary evaluation of symptomatic and functional improvement. *Ann Intern Med* 70:1109–1120, 1969.
27. Busch AJ, McClements JD: Effects of a supervised home exercise program on patients with severe chronic obstructive pulmonary disease. *Phys Ther* 68:469–474, 1988.
28. Foster S, Lopez D, Thomas HM III: Pulmonary rehabilitation in COPD patients with elevated P_{CO_2}. *Am Rev Respir Dis* 138:1519–1523, 1988.
29. Carlson DJ, Ries AL, Kaplan RM: Prediction of maximum exercise tolerance in patients with COPD. *Chest* 100:307–311, 1991.
30. Cypcar D, Lemanske RF Jr: Asthma and exercise. *Clin Chest Med* 15:351–368, 1994.
31. deJong W, Grevink RG, Roorda RK, et al: Effect of a home exercise training program in patients with cystic fibrosis. *Chest* 105:463–468, 1994.
32. Emter M, Herala M, Stalenheim G: High-intensity physical training in adults with asthma. *Chest* 109:323–330, 1996.
33. Foster S, Thomas HM: Pulmonary rehabilitation in lung diseases other than chronic obstructive pulmonary disease. *Am Rev Respir Dis* 141:601–604, 1990.
34. Niederman MS, Clemente PH, Fein AM, et al: Benefits of a multidisciplinary pulmonary rehabilitation program: Improvements are independent of lung function. *Chest* 99:798–804, 1991.
35. Goldstein RS, Gort EH, Stubbing D, et al: Randomised controlled trial of respiratory rehabilitation. *Lancet* 344:1394–1397, 1994.
36. O'Donnell DE, Webb KA, McGuire MA: Older patients with COPD: Benefits of exercise training. *Geriatrics* 48:59–66, 1993.
37. Nocturnal Oxygen Therapy Trial Group: Continuous or nocturnal oxygen therapy in hypoxemic chronic obstructive lung disease: A clinical trial. *Ann Intern Med* 92:391–398, 1980.
38. Hagberg JM, Graves JE, Limacher M, et al: Cardiovascular responses of 70- to 79-year-old men and women to exercise training. *J Appl Physiol* 66:2589–2594, 1989.
39. Rooney EM: Exercise for older patients: Why it's worth your effort. *Geriatrics* 48:68–77, 1993.
40. Couser JI, Guthmann R, Hamadeh MA, Dane CS: Pulmonary rehabilitation improves exercise capacity in older elderly patients with COPD. *Chest* 107:730–734, 1995.
41. Sinclair DJM, Ingram CG: Controlled trial of supervised exercise training in chronic bronchitis. *Br Med J* 280:519–521, 1980.
42. Belman MJ, Kendregan BA: Exercise training fails to increase skeletal muscle enzymes in subjects with chronic obstructive pulmonary disease. *Am Rev Respir Dis* 123:256–261, 1981.
43. Belman MJ, Epstein LJ, Doornbos D, et al: Non-invasive determinations of the anaerobic threshold: Reliability and validity in patients with COPD. *Chest* 102:1028–1034, 1992.
44. Punzal PA, Ries RL, Kaplan RM, Prewitt LM: Maximum intensity exercise training in patients with chronic obstructive pulmonary disease. *Chest* 100:618–623, 1991.
45. Berry MJ, Adair NE, Sevensky KS, et al: Inspiratory muscle training and whole-body reconditioning in chronic pulmonary disease: A controlled randomized trial. *Am J Respir Crit Care Med* 153:1812–1816, 1996.

46. Bickford L, Hodgkin JE, McInturff SL: National pulmonary rehabilitation survey: Update. *J Cardiopulmonary Rehabil* 15:406–411, 1995.

47. Lake FR, Henderson K, Briffa T, et al: Upper-limb and lower-limb exercise training in patients with chronic airflow obstruction. *Chest* 97:1077–1082, 1990.

48. Couser JI, Martinez FJ, Celli BR: Pulmonary rehabilitation that includes arm exercise reduces metabolic and ventilatory requirements for simple arm elevation. *Chest* 103:37–41, 1993.

49. Bruce RA, Kusumi F, Hosmer D: Maximal oxygen intake and nomographic assessment of functional aerobic impairment in cardiovascular disease. *Am Heart J* 85:546–562, 1973.

50. Zeballos RJ, Weisman IM: Behind the scenes of cardiopulmonary exercise testing. *Clin Chest Med* 15:193–214, 1994.

51. McGavin CR, Gupta SP, McHardy GJR: Twelve-minute walking test for assessing disability in chronic bronchitis. *Br Med J* 1:822–823, 1976.

52. Cockcroft AE, Saunders MJ, Berry G: Randomized controlled trial of rehabilitation in chronic respiratory disability. *Thorax* 36:200–203, 1981.

53. Sassi-Dambron D, Eakin EG, Ries AL, Kaplan RM: Treatment of dyspnea in COPD: A controlled trial of dyspnea management strategies. *Chest* 107:724–729, 1995.

54. ZuWallack RL, Patel K, Reardon JZ, et al: Predictors of improvement in the 12-minute walking distance following a six-week outpatient pulmonary rehabilitation program. *Chest* 99:805–808, 1991.

55. Ries AL, Ellis B, Hawkins RW: Upper extremity exercise training in chronic obstructive pulmonary disease. *Chest* 93:688–692, 1988.

56. Ellis B, Ries AL: Upper extremity exercise training in pulmonary rehabilitation. *J Cardiopulmonary Rehabil* 11:227–231, 1991.

57. Martinez FJ, Vogel PD, Dupont DN, et al: Supported arm exercise vs. unsupported arm exercise in the rehabilitation of patients with severe chronic airflow obstruction. *Chest* 103:1397–1402, 1993.

58. Martin TW, Zeballos RJ, Weisman IM: Gas exchange during maximal upper extremity exercise. *Chest* 99:420–425, 1991.

59. Sue DY, Wasserman K, Moricca RB, Casaburi R: Metabolic acidosis during exercise in patients with chronic obstructive pulmonary disease: Use of the V-slope method for anaerobic threshold determination. *Chest* 94:931–938, 1988.

60. Kerem D, Melamed Y, Moran A: Alveolar P_{CO_2} during rest and exercise in divers and non-divers breathing O_2 at 1 ATA. *Undersea Biomed Res* 7:17–26, 1980.

61. Lally DA, Zechman FW, Tracy RA: Ventilatory responses to exercise in divers and non-divers. *Respir Physiol* 20:117–129, 1974.

62. Goff LG, Bartlett RG Jr: Elevated end-tidal CO_2 in trained underwater swimmers. *J Appl Physiol* 10:203–206, 1957.

63. Nery LE, Wasserman K, French W, et al: Contrasting cardiovascular and respiratory responses to exercise in mitral valve and chronic obstructive pulmonary diseases. *Chest* 83:446–453, 1983.

64. Casaburi R, Patessio A, Ioli F, et al: Reductions in exercise lactic acidosis and ventilation as a result of exercise training in patients with obstructive lung disease. *Am Rev Respir Dis* 143:9–18, 1991.

65. Wagner PD: Ventilation-perfusion matching during exercise. *Chest* 101:192S–198S, 1992.

66. Augusti AGN, Barbera JA, Roca J, et al: Hypoxic pulmonary vasoconstriction and gas exchange during exercise in chronic obstructive pulmonary disease. *Chest* 97:268–275, 1990.

67. Barbera JA, Roca J, Ramirez J, et al: Gas exchange during exercise in mild chronic obstructive pulmonary disease. *Am Rev Respir Dis* 144:520–525, 1991.

68. Ries AL, Farrow JT, Clausen JL: Pulmonary function tests cannot predict exercise-induced hypoxemia in chronic obstructive pulmonary disease. *Chest* 93:454–459, 1988.

69. Owens GR, Rogers RM, Pennock BE, Levin D: The diffusing capacity as a predictor of arterial oxygen desaturation during exercise in patients with chronic obstructive pulmonary disease. *N Engl J Med* 310:1218–1221, 1984.

70. Sue DY: Exercise testing in the evaluation of impairment and disability. *Clin Chest Med* 15:369–388, 1994.

71. Weisman IM, Zeballos JZ: An integrated approach to the interpretation of cardiopulmonary exercise testing. *Clin Chest Med* 15:421–445, 1994.

72. Escourrou PJL, Delaperche MF, Visseaux A: Reliability of pulse oximetry during exercise in pulmonary patients. *Chest* 97:635–638, 1990.

73. Mengelkoch LJ, Martin J, Lawler J: A review of the principles of pulse oximetry and accuracy of pulse oximeter estimates during exercise. *Phys Ther* 74:40–49, 1994.

74. Powers SK, Dodd S, Freeman J, et al: Accuracy of pulse oximetry to estimate HbO_2 fraction of total Hb during exercise. *J Appl Physiol* 67:300–304, 1989.

75. *Principles of Pulse Oximetry.* Clinical monograph, Nellcor Corp., Pleasanton, CA, 1991.

76. Ortega F, Montemayor T, Sanchez A, et al: Role of cardiopulmonary exercise testing and the criteria used to determine disability in patients with severe chronic obstructive pulmonary disease. *Am J Respir Crit Care Med* 150:747–751, 1994.

77. Zimmerman MI, Miller A, Brown LK, et al: Estimated vs. actual values for dead space/tidal volume ratios during incremental exercise in patients evaluated for dyspnea. *Chest* 106:131–136, 1994.

78. Ries AL, Fedullo PF, Clausen JL: Rapid changes in arterial blood gas levels after exercise in pulmonary patients. *Chest* 83:454–456, 1983.

79. Borg GAV: Psychophysical bases of perceived exertion. *Med Sci Sports Exerc* 14:377–381, 1982.

80. Clark CJ: Setting up a pulmonary rehabilitation programme. *Thorax* 49:270–278, 1994.

81. Mall RW, Medeiros M: Objective evaluation of results of a pulmonary rehabilitation program in a community hospital. *Chest* 94:1156–1160, 1988.

82. Wykstra PJ, Van Altens R, Kraan J, et al: Quality of life in patients with chronic obstructive pulmonary disease improves after rehabilitation at home. *Eur Respir J* 7:269–273, 1994.

83. Scott JA, Mahler DA: How to prescribe exercise for patients with COPD. *J Respir Dis* 17:527–536, 1996.

84. Belman MJ, Mohsenifar Z: Reductions in exercise lactic acidosis and ventilation as a result of exercise training in patients with obstructive lung disease (letter). *Am Rev Respir Dis* 144:1220–1221, 1991.

85. Smith K, Cook D, Guyatt GH, et al: Respiratory muscle training in chronic airflow limitation: A meta-analysis. *Am Rev Respir Dis* 145:533–536, 1992.

86. Belman MJ, Brooks LR, Ross DJ, Mohsenifar Z: Variability of breathlessness measurement in patients with chronic obstructive pulmonary disease. *Chest* 99:566–571, 1991.

87. Reardon J, Awad E, Normandin E, et al: The effect of comprehensive outpatient pulmonary rehabilitation on dyspnea. *Chest* 105:1046–1052, 1994.

88. Toshima MT, Kaplan RM, Ries AL: Experimental evaluation of rehabilitation in chronic obstructive pulmonary disease: Short-term effects on exercise endurance and health status. *Health Psychol* 9:237–252, 1990.

Chapter 19

RESPIRATORY MUSCLE TESTING

GERALD SUPINSKI

The purpose of this chapter is to review the various techniques that are currently available to assess respiratory muscle function in patients. To achieve this goal, we will review a number of commonly used tests of muscle "strength," of muscle "endurance," and of specific, more advanced forms of measurement that may be suitable for selected patients and/or research situations.

Since pulmonary rehabilitation has a goal of optimizing patient functional capacity, it seems logical that various objective monitors of performance should be assessed periodically to gauge the response to therapeutic interventions. Incorporation of tests of respiratory muscle function as part of such a global assessment strategy is commonly employed. This approach assumes, however, that the capabilities of these muscles are an important determinant of overall patient well-being. While such a relationship appears clear for some diseases (e.g., respiratory muscle functional status clearly limits respiratory performance in patients with neuromuscular diseases), in other conditions (e.g., chronic obstructive lung disease) such a relationship is less well established. Specifically, some data exist to suggest that respiratory muscle functional capabilities are reasonably well maintained in many patients with severe but stable obstructive lung disease.[1] In addition, a few reports suggest that some aspects of respiratory muscle function may even be better than normal in the typical patient with some respiratory diseases (e.g., stable asthmatics and some patients with cystic fibrosis), a finding that may reflect an adaptive response to repeated exacerbations of disease in these individuals (i.e., exacerbations may act as a training stimulus).[2,3]

A good argument can be made, however, that improvement in respiratory muscle function, to even "supernormal" levels, is theoretically desirable as part of a rehabilitation strategy in patients with lung disease. It is reasonable to believe that muscles that are stronger and/or have enhanced endurance capabilities should allow individuals to better maintain respiratory performance if a pulmonary disease exacerbation should occur. Moreover, recent work suggests that a number of stresses that are commonly present in sick patients (e.g., electrolyte abnormalities, infection, heart failure) can produce large, acute reductions in muscle capabilities. One would think that the impact of such acute systemic alterations on respiratory function in general would be diminished in patients with good "baseline" respiratory muscle strength and endurance. Taking all these considerations together, it is my opinion that measures designed to improve muscle function and tests designed to monitor muscle capabilities should play an important role in rehabilitation efforts.

Physiologic Principles of Respiratory Muscle Testing

A brief review of muscle physiologic principles should help to place the use of tests of respiratory muscle function into a broader perspective and should help the reader better understand the rationale for the specific "controls" used for various tests. It is important to first point out that the force generated by a muscle is a function of its level of excitation, its initial length, and its mode of contraction (i.e., whether contracting isometrically at a constant length or shortening against a load).[4] I will review the manner in which each of these factors modulates force output in turn.

When a muscle is stimulated by a single electrical stimulus, this is referred to as a muscle *twitch*. As muscle stimulation frequency is increased from a single "twitch" stimulus to 20 impulses per second (i.e., 20 Hz), there is a concomitant nearly linear increase in muscle force generation. At still higher stimulus frequencies (i.e., 20 to 50 Hz), force rises more slowly as frequency is increased and, for human muscles, reaches a plateau at firing frequencies above 50 Hz. This dependence of muscle force generation on neural stimulus frequency is referred to as the *force-frequency relationship* (Fig. 19-1). Under normal physiologic conditions, muscles are stimulated by electrical impulses delivered via motor nerves, with motor neurons in these nerves typically activated at 5 to 20 Hz. During a normal contraction, firing frequency varies over time for a given motor neuron and varies among motor neurons. Under extreme circumstances (e.g., for the respiratory system, when carbon dioxide levels rise and cause a chemoreceptor-reflex-mediated increase in motor outflow), firing frequencies of motor neurons can rise to much higher levels (i.e., to 50 to 100 Hz), but these high rates are only sustained transiently.[5]

At a given stimulation frequency, muscle force generation is highly dependent on muscle length. Each muscle has a "length" of optimal force generation (at this length, termed *Lo*, the individual sarcomeres within the muscle are so aligned that optimal contact between actin and myosin cross-bridges is achieved), and increases in length above or decreases in length below this optimal length tend to decrease force output (Fig. 19-2). Most muscles are constructed so that the normal "resting" length is close to Lo. For the respiratory muscles, the inspiratory muscles, as a group, appear to be close to Lo at lung volumes below functional residual capacity (FRC). In contrast, the expiratory muscles as a group have a length near Lo when lung volume is close to total lung capacity (TLC) and shorten to lengths below Lo as lung volume falls to FRC and thence to residual volume (RV). This particular aspect of muscle function has important implications for respiratory muscle testing, as will be explained in the section on assessment of respiratory muscle strength.

A final determinant of muscle force output is the mode of muscle contraction. The term *isometric contraction* refers to a muscle contracting at a constant length against, typically, a rigid support, whereas an *isotonic contraction* is a contraction in which the muscle shortens while working against a submaximal, fixed load (e.g., a fixed mass attached to one end of the muscle). The force developed by a muscle contracting isometrically at maximum activation and at an optimal length (Lo) is termed the *muscle Po*; this parameter is frequently

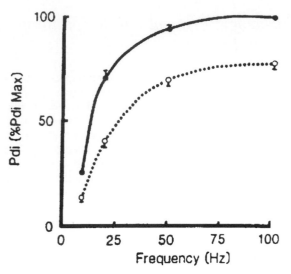

FIGURE 19-1 The effect of altering muscle stimulation frequency on an index of muscle force output. In this case, the diaphragm is stimulated with phrenic impulses at different stimulus frequencies (x axis), and transdiaphragmatic pressure (y axis) is taken as the index of force output. The solid curve reflects force output of a fresh muscle, whereas the dashed line represents the pressure-frequency relationship after a period of fatiguing contractions. (From DiVito and Grassino,[77] with permission.)

measured in experimental situations and provides a defined index of muscle force-generating capacity, such as muscle strength. When, on the other hand, a muscle contracts against an external load (e.g., a resistance or a weight), the muscle will shorten if this load is less than Po; the lower the level of load, the faster the muscle will shorten. During such isotonic contractions, it is the speed of muscle shortening that provides an index of muscle contractility, since the force generated during such contractions is simply a function of the

FIGURE 19-2 The effect of altering muscle length on muscle force output during isometric contraction. Note that Lo, the length at which force generation is maximal, for this muscle is close to the measured resting length of this muscle. (From Goldberg and Roussos,[75] with permission.)

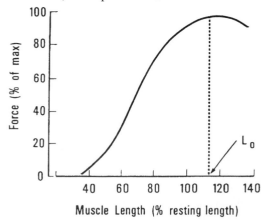

magnitude of the external load and not of an intrinsic property of the muscle itself.

As indicated in the preceding paragraph, the best way to precisely define the strength of a muscle (or muscle group) is to activate the muscles at a defined stimulation frequency, at a defined length, and under isometric conditions. It should be clear that it is difficult to achieve these conditions in patients, and certain compromises must be made to obtain a usable parameter of respiratory muscle function. When making these compromises, we usually have to accept several trade-offs. For example, although it is possible to precisely define the level of activation of the diaphragm by electrically stimulating the phrenic nerve, such stimulation is often uncomfortable and requires specialized equipment. It is easier to simply ask subjects to perform a "maximal" muscle contraction, but such contractions are highly effort-dependent and often impossible to achieve reproducibly in ill patients. The fact that a number of different tests of respiratory muscle strength have been developed is based on such compromises. Common "compromises" that are made are (1) to assume that maximal volitional contractions of the respiratory muscles result in maximal muscle activation, (2) to assume that respiratory muscle contractions made with the airway occluded occur with these muscles contracting in a quasi-isometric fashion, and (3) to assume that respiratory muscle length is a simple function of lung volume and that we can constrain inspiratory or expiratory muscle length by performing contractions at defined lung volumes.

The factors that influence muscle endurance and fatigability are even more complex than those which influence muscle strength. As a corollary, it is even more difficult, when performing tests to assess muscle "endurance" or "fatigability," to adequately control for all the potential variables affecting these measurements than it is to control for the factors that influence measurements of muscle strength. In general, muscle *endurance* (i.e., the time that a specific work task can be sustained) and muscle *fatigability* (i.e., the rate at which its force-generating or shortening capacity declines over time during strenuous contraction) are influenced by the following factors: (1) muscle strength, (2) the oxidative capacity of muscle, (i.e., the capillary and mitochondrial density), (3) substrate availability (i.e., glucose, glycogen stores, fatty acids, and blood-borne substrates), (4) the capacity of the central circulation to supply adequate blood to the muscle capillary bed, and (5) the nature of the endurance task a given muscle is asked to perform.[4]

Muscle *strength* influences endurance by determining the stimulation frequency at which a muscle must be driven to achieve a given level of force generation. A weak muscle will need to be driven at a relatively higher stimulation frequency relative to a strong muscle, and higher-frequency stimulation can tax the sarcolemmal machinery involved in propagation of action potentials along the outer muscle membrane and down muscle t-tubules. As a result, additional "sites" of muscle fatigue may develop in weak muscles compared with stronger muscles when such weak muscles are required to take on the same endurance task.

Traditionally, muscle oxidative capacity has been considered the major determinant of endurance. While older texts argue that greater oxidative machinery improves endurance by permitting greater rates of ATP generation and hence better maintenance of muscle energy stores during contraction, more recent data would suggest that muscle endurance is not so simply determined. It appears that a number of different "types" of fatigue can develop simultaneously, and to differing degrees, in a contracting muscle, including failure of action potential propagation (alluded to in the preceding paragraph) and muscle failure due to accumulation of "toxic" by-products of contraction (e.g., ATP hydrolysis increases cell phosphate concentrations, and phosphate interacts directly with and interferes with contractile protein function).[6] Surprisingly little data exist to indicate that global muscle energy store depletion is a cause of fatigue, and ample ATP concentrations remain in muscle at the point of task failure in nuclear magnetic resonance (NMR) studies that have examined this issue.[7,8] It is possible, however, that regional ATP depletion may occur in some contracting muscles and that some degree of force reduction may result from such regional ATP deficiency.

Systemic factors also influence muscle endurance, since a given muscle will receive less oxygen delivery, all other factors being equal, if the blood pressure is low or significant systemic hypoxemia exists. Under certain circumstances, availability of blood-borne substrates and/or muscle glycogen stores can be a limiting factor in muscle function during exercise.[9] It is known, for example, that limb muscle endurance at moderate levels of exercise is a function of muscle glycogen concentrations, with the limits of endurance coinciding with depletion of internal muscle glycogen stores.[9]

Endurance is also a function of the specific task a muscle is asked to perform. Very high-intensity maneuvers (e.g., for the respiratory muscles, repeated efforts to generate maximal inspiratory pressures) may primarily tax action potential transmission. In contrast, more moderate, more sustained forms of exercise may tax intracellular processes to a greater degree, resulting in a fatigue state more determined by metabolic by-product accumulation than by neuromuscular transmission failure.

These various factors must be kept in mind when assessing respiratory muscle endurance with currently available tests. It is also important to remember that endurance testing is even more critically dependent on patient cooperation than is strength measurement. The forms of maximal respiratory maneuvers commonly used to assess strength require only brief efforts and cooperation on the part of patients (i.e., only a few seconds), whereas assessment of endurance over time requires a sustained patient effort.

Tests of Respiratory Muscle Strength

Determination of inspiratory and expiratory pressure development to assess respiratory muscle strength has long been a component of the standard evaluation of patients with breathing disorders. Recent work has established new normative values for these measurements and has more clearly defined the clinical scenarios in which this information can be helpful. In addition, advances in our understanding of respiratory muscle physiology have led to an appreciation of previously unrecognized limitations in the acquisition and application of these measurements. This section will review, in turn, (1) measurement and interpretation of maximum inspiratory pressure (MIP or PImax) and maximum expiratory pressure (MEP or PEmax) and (2) measurement and use of transdiaphragmatic pressure generation (Pdi).

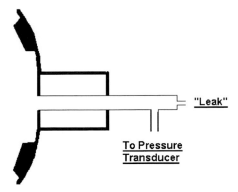

FIGURE 19-3 Mouthpiece used for determination of inspiratory pressure generation. The flanged portion on the left is placed in the mouth, and the stopcock on the right (marked by the large X) is attached to calibrated pressure transducer via its sidearm. Note that the stopcock is attached, in turn, to a small opening that serves the purpose of preventing mouth artifacts.

MEASUREMENT OF MAXIMUM INSPIRATORY PRESSURE (MIP OR PIMAX) AND MAXIMUM EXPIRATORY PRESSURE (MEP OR PEMAX)

The usual approach to measurement of inspiratory pressure generation requires a subject to generate a maximal inspiratory effort while attempting to inhale through a large-bore, rigid mouthpiece (typically having an internal diameter of 2–3 cm) attached to a calibrated pressure transducer.[10] These measurements are typically made with subjects in a seated position, with a noseclip in place to prevent nasal air leakage, and with the mouthpiece placed firmly against the lips (Fig. 19-3). Several types of pressure transducers have been used for these measurements, including standard differential transducers that generate an electrical signal proportional to the pressure gradient developed across a flexible metal diaphragm held in metal chamber. The subject is generally asked to generate as large an inspiratory effort as possible and to attempt to sustain this pressure generation for 2 to 3 s.

Inspiratory pressures are usually measured at one of two lung volumes, FRC (i.e., the airway is occluded, and the inspiratory effort initiated at a lung volume of FRC), or RV (i.e., for these latter maneuvers, subjects are instructed to slowly and completely exhale to RV prior to sealing the lips around the mouthpiece). To prevent measurements of artifactual pressure "overshoots" (i.e., signal "ringing"), the "maximal" pressure recorded for a given inspiratory effort is taken as the highest that was sustained for at least a 0.5-s period. Traditionally, a minimum of three to five maneuvers are performed, with the requirement that some degree of reproducibility in maximal pressure generation is achieved (typically, generating maximal pressures that are within 10 percent of each other on serial maneuvers). A short rest is generally provided between maneuvers to avoid the development of muscle fatigue. Vigorous coaching by the technician supervising the test appears to facilitate obtaining "accurate" and reproducible measurements. Visual feedback of pressure signals also aids performance, and demonstration of the maneuver by a technician prior to testing speeds achievement of reproducibility by subjects. As should be apparent, a hard copy or computer display readout during these maneuvers is useful in ensuring that the pressures

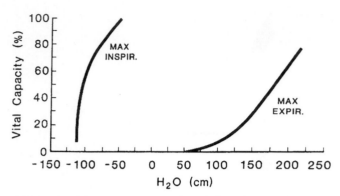

FIGURE 19-4 The pressure-generating ability of the respiratory muscles varies with the lung volume, as shown in this figure. Maximum inspiratory pressure is greatest (i.e., most negative) at low lung volumes, as shown by the left-hand curve, whereas expiratory pressure is most positive at high lung volumes, as shown by the curve on the right. Note that this figure presents the actual pressures measured at the mouth as a function of lung volume. (From Goldberg and Roussos,[75] with permission.)

reported were, in fact, sustained for a sufficient period of time.

Maximal expiratory pressure measurements are performed in a fashion analogous to inspiratory pressure determinations save that subjects are asked to make "expiratory" efforts against an occluded airway, with measurements traditionally made at FRC and TLC (i.e., for this latter determination, subjects slowly inhale to "maximal" lung volumes prior to initiating expiratory efforts).

It is important to note that it is commonplace to provide a 1-mm hole placed in the mouthpiece or in the pressure-measuring circuit when performing either inspiratory or expiratory pressure measurements.[10] This hole results in a small, controlled "leak" during performance of maneuvers, minimizing artifactual negative and positive pressure development by the orofacial muscles during maximal pressure measurements. In my experience, such a leak is especially important for expiratory pressure measurements. One can easily close the glottis and generate extremely high expiratory pressures using the cheek muscles alone in the absence of such a leak in the expiratory circuit. In the presence of a small leak, the oral cavity rapidly deflates when an attempt is made to generate expiratory pressures with the oropharyngeal musculature and a closed glottis, preventing pressure generation and eliminating this artifact. Of course, it is also important when instructing subjects that it be made clear that maneuvers are to be performed with the glottis open and while using only the chest cage muscles to generate pressure.

INTERPRETATION OF MIP (PiMAX) AND MEP (PeMAX) MEASUREMENTS

Several physiologic factors other than the intrinsic force-generating capacity of the inspiratory and expiratory muscles influence measurements of inspiratory and expiratory pressures.[11] Both inspiratory and expiratory pressure generation varies with lung volume (Fig. 19-4), with inspiratory pressures growing as lung volume decreases and expiratory pressures increasing as lung volume becomes larger (hence the traditional recommendation to measure inspiratory pressure

at RV and to measure expiratory pressure at TLC). Several factors contribute to this lung volume dependency. First, as lung volume increases, the inspiratory muscles move down their length-tension curves, reducing their force and inspiratory pressure-generating capacity. Moreover, alterations in the geometric configuration of the diaphragm and inspiratory intercostals also may act to reduce the mechanical "advantage" of the inspiratory muscles as lung volume increases, reducing the pressures achieved for a given level of intrinsic muscle force development and further causing a reduction in muscle pressure generation as lung volume increases.

In addition, the "mouth" pressures recorded during inspiratory and expiratory pressure generation at different lung volumes are influenced by the static recoil pressure of the lung and chest wall. For example, if an individual inhales to maximal lung volume, places a closed airway against his or her mouth, and then relaxes, a positive pressure will be recorded from the mouthpiece reflecting the inward recoil of the respiratory system. The mouth pressure generated during a maximal expiratory pressure at TLC therefore should represent the "sum" of the pressures generated due to respiratory system recoil and the "actual" pressure generated by the expiratory muscles.

These relationships are shown diagramatically in Fig. 19-5. As mentioned earlier, reducing lung volume increases the length and the intrinsic pressure-generating ability of the inspiratory muscles, whereas increasing lung volume lengthens the expiratory muscles and increases intrinsic expiratory muscle pressure-generating capacity. The respiratory system recoils inward at high lung volumes (i.e., generates a positive pressure during relaxation against an occluded airway) and

FIGURE 19-5 Inspiratory and expiratory pressure generation as a function of lung volume. As also displayed in Figure 19–4, the measured maximal inspiratory pressure (MIP) is shown as a solid curved line on the left, whereas the measured maximal expiratory pressure (MEP) is shown as a solid curved line on the right. I also subtracted the elastic recoil pressure of the respiratory system to obtain the actual pressures generated by the respiratory muscles (Pmus curves); the Pmus curve for the expiratory muscles is displayed as a dotted line on the right, and the Pmus curve for the inspiratory muscles is displayed as a dotted line on the left.

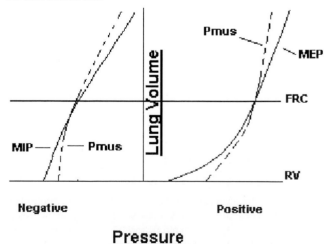

recoils outward at volumes below FRC (i.e., generates a negative pressure during relaxation against an occluded airway). This recoil acts to increase the magnitude of the expiratory pressure recorded at TLC during maximal expiratory muscle efforts (Pmouth = PEmus + Prs, where Prs represents the relaxation pressure generated by the passive elements of the respiratory system). Conversely, respiratory system recoil makes the inspiratory pressures recorded at the mouth more "negative" for inspiratory efforts generated at an occluded airway at RV (Pmouth = PImus + Prs, with all these parameters representing negative numbers). Note that at FRC, Prs = 0, so the pressures measured at the mouth during either inspiratory or expiratory efforts made at FRC represent the "true" pressure-generating capacity of these respective muscle groups and are independent of the static elastic recoil properties of the respiratory system.

This discussion brings to question the relative merit of measuring inspiratory pressures at RV instead of FRC and of measuring expiratory pressures at TLC instead of FRC. As indicated earlier, measurements made at TLC and RV can be influenced by the elastic properties of the respiratory system. On the other hand, one problem associated with measurements made at FRC is the fact that FRC is often dynamically determined in patients with lung disease (i.e., these patents may not reach true equilibrium conditions of zero airflow throughout the lungs between breaths), and as a result, "resting" FRC can vary substantially over time.

As an additional complicating factor, note that an initial expiratory muscle contraction is required (to exhale completely) for inspiratory muscle pressure generation to be measured at RV. If the expiratory muscles are extremely weak, this factor per se will affect the level of the RV achieved, influencing the length of the inspiratory muscles and altering the inspiratory pressure generated during the subsequent inspiratory maneuver.

Generally, however, the magnitude of the effect on pressure generation due to alterations of respiratory compliances and variation in the lung volumes achieved in a cooperative subject during performance of inspiratory pressure measurements at RV and expiratory pressure measurements at TLC are not great. As a result, measurement of these pressures in this fashion can still be recommended for most clinical work, and the determination as to whether or not significant intrinsic respiratory muscle weakness is present is usually straightforward. In complex clinical cases, however, consideration of the physiologic complexities just reviewed may be required to accurately interpret inspiratory and expiratory pressure measurements.

Normal values for PImax/MIP and PEmax/MEP determinations have been reported in several recent studies,[9,12–14] and one group of these is presented in Table 19-1. Generally speaking, the MIP and/or MEP are considered to be significantly reduced when below 50 percent of their predicted values.

CLINICAL USE OF MIP (PIMAX) AND MEP (PEMAX) MEASUREMENTS

Traditionally *both* MIP and MEP are determined when trying to assess respiratory muscle function. It is of interest that it is the usual clinical practice to assess both indices when assessing respiratory muscle strength in patients sent to a

TABLE 19-1 Predicted Normal Values for PImax (MIP) and PEmax (MEP) (in cmH$_2$O)

	9–18 Years	19–49 Years	50–69 Years	70 Years
Females				
MIP	90 ± 25	91 ± 25	77 ± 18	66 ± 18
MEP	136 ± 34	138 ± 39	124 ± 37	108 ± 28
Males				
MIP	96 ± 35	127 ± 28	112 ± 20	76 ± 27
MEP	170 ± 32	216 ± 45	196 ± 45	133 ± 42

SOURCE: From Rochester and Arora,[78] with permission.

pulmonary function laboratory but only to examine inspiratory pressures when doing bedside examination of critically ill patients in the intensive care unit or in the hospital ward. A good argument can be made, however, that omission of either test hampers the interpretation of measurement of the other.

As an example of this, consider interpretation of a "low" measured value for MIP in a patient with obstructive lung disease. One possible explanation for such a reduction could be that the patient in question has hyperinflated lungs and that this increased lung volume so alters the coupling between inspiratory muscle force generation and pressure generation that the latter is reduced while the former is unaffected (i.e., this patient has no intrinsic abnormality of muscle function). It would therefore be difficult to determine if a given reduction in inspiratory pressure generation in such a patient reflected simply an alteration in lung volume, the development of a superimposed myopathy, or some combination of the two. If, however, alterations in pressure generation were simply due to alterations in lung volume, then expiratory pressure generation should be "normal" in such an individual, while a global myopathy would reduce both inspiratory and expiratory pressure generation. As a result, measurement of both MIP and MEP in such a patient allows detection of respiratory muscle disturbance in the presence of concomitant obstructive lung disease.

Combined MIP and MEP measurements are also helpful in patients with disorders that selectively "knock out" particular groups of respiratory muscles while sparing others. For example, isolated diaphragmatic paralysis will reduce the MIP, but MEP measurements will be normal. In contrast, midthoracic spinal cord injuries cause some reduction in MIP but produce far greater reductions in MEP measurements. Lower spinal cord injuries, i.e., those which affect the abdominal muscles but leave the upper rib cage muscles intact, will leave the MIP normal. Since, however, maximal generation of MEP requires both abdominal and rib cage muscles, MEP will be severely reduced in these patients. In contrast, global muscle disturbances usually reduce both indices of pressure generation.

There are several specific situations in which measurements of respiratory muscle strength may be useful. Perhaps the most common situation in which this testing is important is in refining the differential diagnosis in patients receiving screening pulmonary function tests. A typical situation to consider would be the evaluation of a patient sent for testing because of nonspecific respiratory symptoms (e.g., dyspnea, altered exercise tolerance, hypoxia of unknown etiology, etc.) in whom either no previous lung disease was defined or whose symptoms seemed excessive for a previously known form of lung disease. If, for example, lung volume measurements indicate the presence of a significant restrictive ventilatory defect, then respiratory muscle testing is important to exclude the possibility that the defect is on the basis of muscle weakness.

Measurements of MIP and MEP are also obviously useful in patients with a suspected systemic myopathy in whom there is concomitant evidence of limb muscle weakness.[15] In these patients these tests can be an additional clue to the existence of disease or an indication of disease severity (e.g., measurement of inspiratory pressures in the Guillain-Barré syndrome is used to determine the point at which mechanical ventilatory support is necessary). MIP and MEP determinations are therefore useful in evaluating patients with myasthenia gravis, muscular dystrophies, the Guillain-Barré syndrome, the Eaton-Lambert syndrome, polymyositis, and other connective tissue disease–related myopathies. When measuring respiratory pressure-generating capacity in patients with limb muscle disease, it is important to remember that a recent study found that the magnitude of the respiratory weakness present in these patients correlates poorly with the severity of limb muscle weakness.[16] As a result, MIP and MEP should be assessed routinely in patients with systemic neuromuscular disorders. Severe respiratory muscle weakness in these patients may be an indication for therapy (e.g., nocturnal ventilatory noninvasive support), and the need for this and the degree to which the respiratory muscles may be afflicted in these disorders can be underestimated based on assessment of limb muscle strength alone.

A third indication for the measurement of MIP and MEP is to evaluate patients with acute respiratory failure of unknown etiology. In these patients, respiratory muscle testing may provide the first and sometimes only evidence of the presence of a systemic myopathy. I have seen patients with respiratory insufficiency due to myasthenia gravis, acid maltase deficiency, and carnitine deficiency in whom peripheral muscle involvement appeared to be minimal by the usual manual clinical testing. Such patients require additional testing to establish the diagnosis of a myopathy (e.g., muscle biopsies, muscle electromyography, and nerve conduction testing). Other disorders that have been reported to cause selective respiratory muscle weakness include polymyositis, mononeuritis multiplex, and polio.

Assessment of respiratory muscle strength also can be useful in several clinical conditions in which respiratory muscle weakness accompanies a systemic disease process (i.e., diseases not considered traditionally to produce "myopathic" changes). An example of this is the muscle dysfunction associated with infection.[17,18] Significant reductions in respiratory muscle strength can occur during the development of even minor respiratory infections, including the common "cold,"[17] and some recent animal studies indicate that the development of frank sepsis may induced life-threatening reductions in diaphragmatic contractility.[18] Other conditions that are associated with reductions in respiratory muscle contractile function include congestive heart failure, respiratory muscle fatigue due to sustained ventilatory loading by disease, electrolyte disturbances (hypokalemia, hypocalcemia, hypomagnesemia, and hypophosphatemia), prolonged use of neuromuscular blocking agents, sustained steroid use, hypothyroidism, and uremia.[19–21]

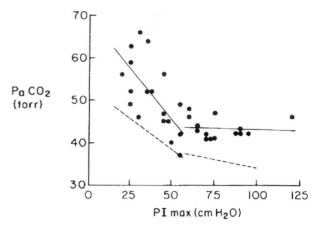

FIGURE 19-6 Display of inspiratory pressure (Pimax) versus arterial carbon dioxide concentration for a group of patients with COPD. Every dot represents data from an individual patient. Carbon dioxide retention was not seen until Pimax fell below 50 cmH$_2$O for this patient population. (From Rochester and Braun,[22] with permission.)

Respiratory muscle strength testing also can provide prognostic information for patients with known myopathies or obstructive lung disease. In these groups of patients, there appears to be a stereotypical relationship between disease-related reductions in respiratory muscle strength and the evolution of changes in vital capacity and carbon dioxide retention over time. For example, in patients with chronic obstructive pulmonary disease (COPD), carbon dioxide retention is usually not seen until the MIP falls to values below 50 cmH$_2$O.[22] Below this level, there appears to be a relatively linear increase in carbon dioxide tensions with further decrements in inspiratory pressure-generating capacity (Fig. 19-6). A similar relationship also has been described between respiratory muscle strength and carbon dioxide levels in patients with "pure" neuromuscular disease.[23] As might be expected, patients with neuromuscular diseases have less carbon dioxide retention for a given level of muscle dysfunction than patients with COPD (Fig. 19-7). The break point for carbon dioxide retention in neuromuscular disease appears to occur when the respiratory muscle strength is less than 50 percent of its predicted value (in this latter study, *respiratory muscle strength* was defined as the average of MIP and MEP, with each of these parameters expressed as a percentage of its expected value). Of interest, respiratory muscle strength may be a better predictor of disability in patients with neuromuscular disease than other indices of respiratory function. In keeping with this possibility, there appears to be little relationship between alterations in vital capacity (VC), total lung capacity (TLC), or the FEV$_1$/FVC ratio and patient functional capacity (i.e., whether patients are ambulatory, wheelchair-bound, or bedridden) but a good correlation between the degree of functional capacity and both MIP and MEP.

Yet another use of respiratory muscle strength measurements is to provide information that can be used in determining the weanability of patients receiving mechanical ventilation. In one recent study, patients with an MIP of less than −20 cmH$_2$O were found to be extremely difficult to wean (i.e., with the approach and duration of weaning attempted in this study, no patient with an MIP below this value was

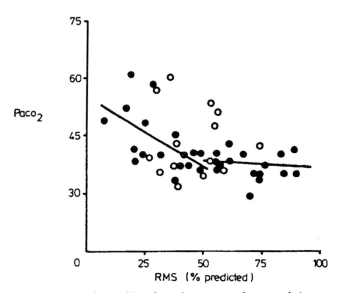

FIGURE 19-7 Relationship of respiratory muscle strength (on the *x* axis) versus arterial carbon dioxide concentration (on the *y* axis) for patients with neuromuscular diseases. Carbon dioxide retention is not seen until RMS (respiratory muscle strength, the average of MIP and MEP as a percent of predicted values) falls below 50 percent. (From Braun et al.,[76] with permission.)

weaned).[24] While the negative predictive value of this index was found to be good, this index only had a 60 percent positive predictive value at the -20 cmH_2O level (the sensitivity of an MIP value more negative than -20 cmH_2O as a predictor of successful weaning was 1.00, and the specificity was 0.14). The good negative predictive value of this index indicates that weaning is not likely to be possible unless some minimum level of muscle strength is present. The low positive predictive value of this index is also not surprising because successful weaning depends on the balance between respiratory capacity and respiratory requirements. While strength is an index of capacity, the work required of these muscles depends on lung mechanics, pulmonary gas exchange, and the required levels of oxygen use and carbon dioxide production.

One therefore would expect an integrative index that takes both respiratory system capacity and work requirements into account to provide a better prediction of weaning success or failure. Several integrative indices have been described and tested, and they appear to be reasonably good. For example, Yang and colleagues[24] found that the ratio of breathing frequency (f) to tidal volume (TV), assessed during a brief spontaneous breathing trial performed prior to weaning, provides an especially good indicator of weaning success or failure. In this study, a value of less than 105 for this f/TV ratio predicted successful weaning with a 97 percent sensitivity and a 64 percent specificity.

Another integrative index described is the $P_{100}/P_{I}max$ ratio.[25] P_{100} (i.e., the pleural pressure generated within the first 100 ms of a spontaneous breathing effort and measured during a respiratory occlusion) may provide an indication of ventilatory requirements, whereas $P_{I}max$ provides an indication of muscle capacity. One might expect that the lower the requirement/capacity or $P_{100}/P_{I}max$ ratio, the greater would be the weaning success and that high ratios would be associ-

ated with a failure to wean. In fact, one recent study found that a $P_{100}/P_{I}max$ ratio of less than 0.08 was associated with an extremely high likelihood of success and values in excess of this a high likelihood of failure.[25]

One therefore could view measurement of $P_{I}max$ (i.e., MIP) as useful in two respects when assessing weanability. First, this parameter can used as part of an initial assessment when predicting weaning success or failure. For this purpose, it appears that measurements of $P_{I}max$ should be combined with measurement of the P_{100} to determine the $P_{100}/P_{I}max$ ratio, since this ratio provides a better discrimination of patients than measurement of the $P_{I}max$ (MIP) alone. Second, measurement of muscle strength is an important follow-up assessment in patients who fail weaning. In this situation, this assessment provides a means of detecting previously undiagnosed diseases and determining *why* weaning has failed.

LIMITATIONS OF CURRENT TECHNIQUES TO MEASURE MIP AND MEP

MIP and MEP assessment has well-defined limitations. There are three issues that must be taken into account when interpreting these tests: (1) as described earlier, these parameters depend on lung volume, (2) reproducibility can be a problem, with a mean coefficient of variation of up to 20 percent in normal cooperative subjects and even higher in other patient populations, and (3) these tests measure only maximum muscle force output and not low-frequency force-generating capacity or muscle endurance.

The first problem should be understood by all interpreting these tests; MIP values fall as lung volume increases, and MEP values increase with increasing lung volumes. As explained in an earlier section, measurement of both MIP and MEP can provide some help in some circumstances in determining whether or not intrinsic muscle weakness is present (reductions in both MIP and MEP cannot be ascribed simply to a change in lung volume, since a given change in volume could reduce one but not both of these parameters).

Reproducibility can be improved by careful testing, making sure that several consecutive measurements achieve similar levels of pressure development. Even so, wide variation sometimes can be seen.[26] Studies also have shown that there is a significant learning effect when testing subjects with a progressive increase in both MIP and MEP from the first to fifth effort in the average patient.[13] As a result, the number of efforts required to train an individual to achieve reproducible levels may be large. To further complicate matters, it is possible that an element of fatigue may set in with excessively large numbers of maneuvers, reducing reliability. Thus, even when carefully employing the "standard" approach to measuring MIP and MEP, reproducibility is a problem.

The third problem listed earlier relates to the fact that both MIP and MEP measure muscle strength during maximal muscle recruitment. Normal breathing results in levels of respiratory motor drive and patterns of respiratory muscle fiber recruitment that are quite different from those achieved during the maximal ballistic effort required to generate a maximal level of pressure development. The latter maneuver results in high-frequency stimulation of muscle fibers and, when done properly, is associated with the recruitment of both fast and slow fibers within the respiratory muscles. In contrast, regular breathing usually activates muscle fibers at low motor neuron firing frequencies (e.g., 5 to 15 Hz) and involves selective recruitment of primarily slow muscle fibers. It is important to recognize that recent experiments have indicated that it is possible for muscles to develop a form of fatigue that is associated primarily with reductions in muscle force development during low-frequency muscle stimulation (i.e., in the 5 to 15 Hz range) with relatively unimpaired force development in response to high-frequency stimulation.[19] Moreover, it has been suggested that such low-frequency fatigue may be present in clinical conditions in which the respiratory muscles are overloaded. Such low-frequency fatigue would not be expected to be measured by either MIP or MEP assessments but could seriously reduce the ability of the respiratory muscles to generate normal levels of ventilation. This constitutes a major limitation of the use of MIP and MEP measurements to assess respiratory muscle function.

In addition, both MIP and MEP are only indices of muscle strength, and muscle strength and endurance are not equivalent. Breathing may, in fact, be the most extreme example of an "endurance" event. It could be argued that measurement of respiratory muscle strength alone is irrational, since this assessment fails to test the capacity of these muscles to perform the specific task (i.e., breathing against a respiratory workload for a protracted time) for which these muscles are used.

It is worth noting that these problems have spurred efforts to devise new ways of testing the respiratory muscles to overcome problems of testing reproducibility and to provide measures of low-frequency force development and muscle endurance. Several of these newer techniques will be reviewed in the sections that follow. Many of these newer approaches require appreciable investments in equipment and the development of significant expertise.

One recently described approach that is both relatively simple to use and also may improve reproducibility is the assessment of respiratory muscle pressure generation during a sniff maneuver.[27] When performing this assessment, patients are asked to sniff, and during this maneuver, measurements are made of either esophageal, transdiaphragmatic, or mouth pressure generated.[27-31] Studies have suggested that there is a good correlation between sniff Pmax and the conventional MIP/Pimax measurement. Moreover, and more important, most reports suggest that the reproducibility and ease of performing the sniff Pmax may be superior to that of the MIP/Pimax.

MEASUREMENT OF TRANSDIAPHRAGMATIC PRESSURE (Pdi)

In some clinical situations (e.g., suspected diaphragmatic paralysis), specific assessment of the pressure-generating capacity of the diaphragm may be indicated. When the diaphragm contracts, it normally moves downward, increasing subdiaphragmatic pressure (i.e., abdominal pressure) and reducing pleural pressure, and as a result, it is possible to specifically assess diaphragmatic pressure generation by measuring these changes in abdominal and pleural pressure. It is customary to estimate the abdominal pressure swings resulting from diaphragmatic contraction by measuring changes in gastric pressure and to estimate changes in pleural pressure from esophageal pressure swings during maximal "static" diaphragmatic contractions. These two pressures can be determined by passing small balloon-tipped catheters into the esophagus and stomach and connecting these catheters, after balloon inflation, to differential pressure transducers[32,33] (Fig. 19-8). If these catheters are placed through the nose, the esophageal balloon usually will need to be placed approximately 45 cm from the nares and inflated with 0.4 mL of air in a typical adult patient (this distance will vary depending on body habitus, and correct placement can be assessed by examining the esophageal waveform during inspiratory efforts; esophageal pressures should fall during spontaneous inspiration). The gastric balloon generally needs to be placed 60 cm from the nares in an adult and inflated with 4 mL of air (again, correct placement is confirmed by examining pressure swings during inspiratory efforts). After balloon placement, the transdiaphragmatic pressure (Pdi) generated during a maximal diaphragmatic contraction is calculated as Pdi = Pg − Ppl, where Pg represents gastric pressure and Ppl represents pleural pressure. As an example,

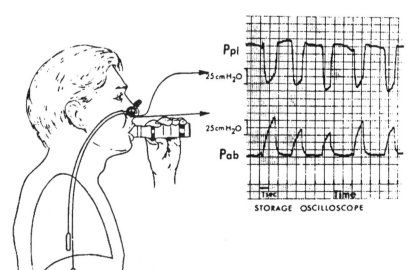

FIGURE 19-8 Transdiaphragmatic pressure is being measured in this individual. Swallowed balloons are attached to pressure transducers, and the recorded pressures are displayed on an oscilloscope face (the esophageal balloon is taken to represent pleural pressure, Ppl, whereas gastric pressure is taken as a representation of abdominal pressure, Pab). The subject uses visual feedback to achieve maximal deflection of the pressure waveforms during inspiratory maneuvers. (From Laporta and Grassino,[33] with permission.)

a diaphragmatic contraction that raises gastric pressure by 30 cmH_2O (i.e., Pg = +30 cmH_2O) and lowers pleural pressure by 50 cmH_2O (i.e., Ppl = −50 cmH_2O) would result in a Pdi of 80 cmH_2O (i.e., Pdi = +30 − (−50) cmH_2O = 80 cmH_2O).

When interpreting these measurements, it is important to recognize the fact that both the manner in which the other respiratory muscles are used and the properties of the chest cage will influence the magnitude of the abdominal and pleural pressures that can be generated during a given diaphragmatic contraction. If, for example, the abdominal wall is prevented from moving outward either by a static contraction of the abdominal wall musculature or by placement of a restricting band around the abdomen, then diaphragmatic shortening during contraction will be reduced and high abdominal pressure swings will result. As another example, if the rib cage muscles are not or cannot be activated during diaphragmatic contraction (as would occur with a low cervical spinal cord injury that spares the spinal roots innervating the diaphragm but paralyzes the intercostal muscles), inward displacement of the upper rib cage will result during diaphragmatic contraction, reducing the pleural pressure swings achieved.

It is therefore important that diaphragmatic contractions be carried out in a standardized manner when measuring transdiaphragmatic pressure generation so that one can control, as much as possible, the pattern of contraction of the other respiratory muscles. Several approaches to generating such "standardized" contractions have been reported, and it is clear that the measured Pdi will vary depending on the precise fashion in which such maneuvers are performed (see Laporta and Grassino[33] for a more complete description of this issue). One commonly used maneuver involves having subjects make an inspiratory effort against an occluded airway (i.e., subjects try to inhale with noseclips and a mouthpiece placed after the inspiratory limb of the mouthpiece circuit is occluded) and, while doing so, try to expand the rib cage while simultaneously pushing out the abdomen.[33] Training and use of feedback (i.e., having the subject observe a visual feedback of pressure values and strive to optimize this index with repeated attempts) appear to facilitate attainment of reproducible, maximal Pdi values.[33] Pdi values normally should be greater than 50 cmH_2O during such a maneuver, and values below 25 cmH_2O should raise suspicion that diaphragmatic paralysis may be present.

Tests of Respiratory Muscle Endurance and Fatigability: Rationale

One may ask why determination of respiratory muscle endurance is important, since endurance measurements are not currently part of the routine assessment of pulmonary function. It is clear, however, that in some clinical conditions there is a clear dissociation between muscle strength and endurance.[7,34,35] Patients with asthma have been reported to show elevations of endurance relative to strength,[2] whereas steroid-treated individuals show marked reductions in endurance relative to strength.[35] I have recently observed a profound reduction in respiratory muscle endurance in a patient with a mitochondrial myopathy at a time when strength was selectively well preserved.

Strength and endurance of limb muscles are very separate muscle properties. It is apparent that weight lifters have very strong leg muscles yet may be poor distance runners, whereas world-class distance runners usually have leg muscles far weaker than those of a power lifter. One would not choose an Olympic marathon team by testing athletes for leg strength, and by the same token, one might think measurement of muscle endurance would be a better means of determining the ability of the respiratory muscles to sustain breathing than would a measurement of respiratory muscle strength.

It is important that energetic principles be considered when performing endurance testing of muscles. It is clear that the rate at which a skeletal muscle uses energy during contraction is a function of the force or tension achieved per unit time, the frequency of muscle activation, and the speed of muscle shortening.[36] The reason for this relationship is apparent on examining types of cellular energy use during contraction. The largest portion of the energy used during contraction is for cross-bridge cycling necessary to develop force. For a given level of force, however, energy use rates are higher when a muscle shortens than when it contracts isometrically (the Fenn effect). Energy use for both force development and muscle shortening is a consequence of hydrolysis of ATP by the myosin ATPase of the contractile proteins. Calcium cycling by the sarcoplasmic reticulum represents yet another energy-requiring cellular process (i.e., energy is used to pump calcium back into the sarcoplasmic reticulum at the end of a contraction, a process that can consume up to 30 percent of the energy required for muscle work).

Based on these considerations, it has been suggested that the workload placed on the respiratory muscles by a given physiologic challenge may best be quantitated by measuring either the pressure-time index of muscle contraction (i.e., the integral of pressure over time; this should provide a rough index of the mean tension developed by the respiratory muscles) or the power generated by the respiratory muscles (i.e., power is the product of the pressure generated and the tidal volume moved during a respiratory muscle contraction; this index takes both force generation and muscle shortening into account).[37,38]

Unfortunately, it is not clear that muscle endurance is simply a function of energy use rates, and most experimental studies have suggested that the development of muscle fatigue is largely the result of accumulation of by-products of muscle metabolism (i.e., increases in cellular inorganic phosphate ion concentrations, increases in hydrogen ion concentrations, formation of reactive oxygen species).[39] The relationship of tension or power generation to accumulation of these latter substances during contraction is incompletely delineated. Thus, while the pressure-time index or the power output is useful conceptually in quantifying muscle energy use rates (and will be used in the discussion below), muscle endurance is probably not just a function of these parameters. One also should consider the fact that muscle endurance depends on systemic as well as local muscle properties (this was reviewed earlier) when testing muscle endurance. The amount and type of food intake over the days preceding testing, the use of drugs that affect cardiac or vascular function, and the presence of significant cardiovascular disease each may affect the response to testing.

For the purpose of respiratory muscle testing, it is commonplace to test endurance in one of several ways: (1) determination of the time that an individual can sustain a given level of ventilation, (2) the time that a patient or subject can sustain breathing against a given inspiratory resistive load, (3) the time that an individual can sustain breathing against a given inspiratory threshold load, and (4) determination of the highest pressure that a subject can achieve during an incremental threshold loading trial. In a few studies, endurance also has been measured using isoflow techniques and by assessing the rate of decline of pressure over time during a series of maximum inspiratory pressures. I will review each of these techniques in turn in the next subsection.

SPECIFIC TESTS OF RESPIRATORY MUSCLE ENDURANCE

One of the earliest tests described to evaluate respiratory muscle endurance was the determination of *maximum sustainable ventilation* (MSV), defined, for practical reasons, as the maximal ventilation that can be maintained for more than 15 min.[40] This traditionally was determined by having subjects perform a series of several breathing trials, separated by rest periods, with each trial performed at a different level of ventilation. After completion of this series of trials, a graph of time versus ventilation was then constructed, and the MSV was determined graphically as the plateau of the ventilation-time curve (Fig. 19-9).

When performing MSV testing, the test apparatus should be constructed to permit isocapnia during hyperpneic maneuvers and should permit feedback to allow a target level of ventilation to be attained continuously. Numerous publications have provided descriptions of equipment set-ups to achieve these goals.[40,41] Previous work suggests that the sustainable ventilation that can be achieved during such testing is approximately 65 percent of the MVV (i.e., MVV is the maximum voluntary ventilation, a parameter determined by measuring the level of ventilation achieved during a maximal effort over 12 s and multiplying this latter number by 5).

Recently, investigators have described an incremental testing procedure to estimate MSV by rapidly (every 3 min)

FIGURE 19-9 Display of ventilation versus endurance time for isocapneic hyperventilation trials. The higher the target ventilation, the shorter is the time that the level of ventilation can be sustained. The plateau of the ventilation-time curve is the maximal sustainable ventilation (MSV). (From Aldrich,[19] with permission.)

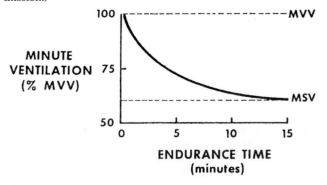

increasing the target ventilation a subject is asked to attain.[42] In this incremental testing, the MSV is taken as the level of ventilation achieved over the final breaths at the highest target ventilation level achieved (this has been reported to approximate the MSV recorded during traditional testing). A number of series have reported MSV values in normal subjects and, as is standard practice, have reported the MSV as a fraction of a given individual's MVV.[40–42]

As should be apparent, determination of the MSV is a measure that is beyond the capabilities of most pulmonary function laboratories. In addition, the work performed by the respiratory muscles during isocapneic hyperventilation is obviously highly dependent on chest wall and lung mechanical characteristics (i.e., resistive and compliance relationships). One might expect this index to be highly influenced by these mechanical parameters, making it difficult to separate changes in endurance attendant on alterations in muscle function per se from changes due to alterations in respiratory mechanical properties.

In theory, a more muscle-specific method of testing endurance is the use of external loads to test respiratory system capabilities. The pressure gradient across these external devices represents the effective load applied to the respiratory system; the magnitude of this load is therefore relatively independent of lung/chest wall mechanics and provides a better test of intrinsic muscle function than isocapneic hyperventilation. It should be understood, however, that the magnitude of the workload resulting from an external resistive load is a function of breathing pattern. If an individual breathes slowly (achieving a long inspiratory time), the pressure gradient and pressure-time index attendant on breathing against a given resistance is much lower than when inspiratory flow is high. Both experimental subjects and patients quickly learn, in my experience, when breathing on a resistive circuit, to alter their breathing pattern to minimize respiratory muscle work.

For this reason, most investigators now use threshold loading to test inspiratory muscle endurance. The first described inspiratory threshold load consisted of a breathing circuit connected to a cylinder containing a weighted plunger.[43] When using such a plunger, no airflow occurs until a critical threshold pressure is achieved, and once this pressure is reached, the plunger opens, allowing (in theory) unlimited airflow, provided that the inspiratory threshold pressure is maintained. The magnitude of pressure required to open the load and initiate airflow can be varied by changing the weight applied to the plunger. With this device, it is much easier to constrain the pressure achieved during breathing to a set target and thereby control the respiratory workload.

In my experience, however, some subjects nevertheless still find ways to "cheat" when breathing against threshold loads by shortening inspiratory time and adopting a rapid inspiratory airflow. This strategy reduces the pressure-time index that must be generated to breath against a given load, resulting in an artifactual prolongation of threshold load time. As a result, some measure to control inspiratory timing and inspiratory airflow is still advisable if one wishes to obtain relatively reliable and reproducible measurements when using inspiratory threshold loading.

As originally described, patient endurance during threshold loading was determined by applying a series of inspiratory threshold loads (with suitable periods of rest between

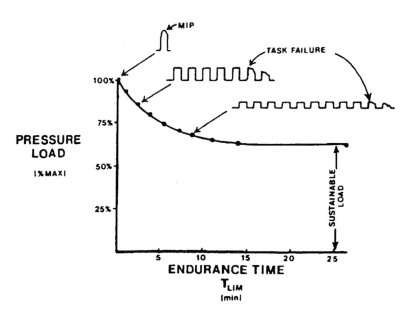

FIGURE 19-10 Display of pressure versus endurance time for a series of breathing trials. The higher the pressure load, the shorter is the time that the loaded breathing trial can be sustained. The level of pressure generation that can be sustained indefinitely is determined as the plateau of the pressure-time curve. (From DiVito and Grassino,[77] with permission.)

them) and calculating the sustainable inspiratory pressure from plots of load magnitude versus load time (Fig. 19-10); see Nickerson and Keens[43] for an example of this determination. As should be apparent, such multiple load testing requires a great deal of effort and laboratory time and is not suitable for everyday use. Several reasonable alternatives exist, however. One option is to test subjects at a single level of threshold load (e.g., at a load chosen so that the pressure achieved is 70 percent of the MIP and with airflow constrained so that inspiration is confined to 40 percent of the respiratory cycle). In motivated individuals, repeated testing over time could be used to gauge responses to various therapeutic interventions (e.g., muscle training).

Another approach to make threshold testing more clinically practical is incremental threshold loading during a single testing trial.[44] This form of testing is performed in a fashion analogous to the testing traditionally used to incrementally increase exercise levels during whole-body exercise testing in cardiac and pulmonary laboratories. Specifically, subjects are initially placed on a low level of threshold load (i.e., 30 percent of the MIP), and the load is increased by 5 to 10 cmH$_2$O every 2 min until the subject reaches a level of load that can no longer be sustained. The highest achieved load is taken as the peak pressure reached, and this pressure is taken as an index of muscle function. While this incremental method of threshold load testing has the appeal of ease of use, one potential drawback may be that the peak pressures achieved during such incremental trials may be more a function of muscle strength than of muscle endurance.

Yet another test that has been described is to have subjects perform repeated sustained MIP maneuvers.[45] Specifically, patients are asked to generate a series of MIPs (e.g., 12 in a row) of prescribed duration (e.g., 15 s) and with a set rest period (i.e., 7.5 s) between adjacent MIP maneuvers. This type of testing has the appeal of being a relatively pure test of muscle function, of being relatively simple to do, and of requiring little equipment. I have found it difficult, however, for the average patient to carry out the complex maneuvers required for this form of testing.

ASSESSMENT OF RESPIRATORY MUSCLE FATIGUE

It is commonplace to describe a patient going into respiratory failure as "tiring out" and to place such patients on various forms of mechanical ventilation to prevent respiratory arrest. Surprisingly few objective data are available, however, to support the concept that respiratory muscle fatigue is actually occurring in such situations. The purpose of this subsection is to describe methods by which the development of fatigue can, in theory, be measured objectively. It should be emphasized, however, that these approaches are largely research-based and are not a part of current clinical practice.

It is important to recognize that *fatigue* is defined as a loss of skeletal muscle force and/or velocity that is accompanied by recovery during rest.[46] As a result, a single measurement of force is inadequate to assess fatigue, and muscle force-generating or shortening capability must be demonstrated to fall during serial measurements over time to determine if a fatigue state is present. It has proven useful to classify fatigue into different types: (1) central fatigue, (2) peripheral high-frequency fatigue, and (3) peripheral low-frequency fatigue. *Central fatigue* refers to a condition in which muscle force generation is limited by an inability to generate sufficient neural output to fully activate the muscle.[47] On the other hand, *peripheral fatigue* refers to failure at the neuromuscular junction or within the muscle machinery.[19] Peripheral fatigue can be subclassified into *high-* and *low-frequency fatigue* based on the shape of the postfatigue muscle force-frequency relationship. If fatigue results in depression of the forces generated by a muscle in response to high-frequency electrical stimulation (e.g., in humans, 50 to 100 Hz), then high-frequency fatigue is present, whereas a reduction in the force generated in response to low-frequency stimuli (i.e., 1 to 20 Hz) indicates the presence of low-frequency fatigue. Loss of force at low frequencies is thought to represent an impairment of muscle excitation-contraction coupling, whereas a reduction in high-frequency force generation is thought to indicate an alteration in neuromuscular junction transmission or a reduction in sarcolemmal membrane excitability.[19]

While it is convenient to discuss the characteristics of central, high-frequency peripheral, and low-frequency fatigue separately, it is likely that all three forms of fatigue can develop simultaneously. Moreover, since these forms of fatigue have different physiologic characteristics, a test well suited to detect one form may be incapable of detecting another form. As an example, consider the utility of using serial measurements of MIP to detect respiratory muscle fatigue (i.e., reductions in inspiratory pressure generation could be taken as a sign of fatigue). This parameter is highly dependent on effort, and time-dependent reductions could represent lack of motivation, central fatigue, high-frequency peripheral fatigue, or simply an alteration in lung volume. In addition, failure of the MIP to change does not exclude the development of fatigue, since this test is not suitable to detect low-frequency fatigue.

Several tests have been proposed to permit detection of fatigue: (1) serial assessment of MIP or Pdi measurements over time, (2) serial measurements of muscle relaxation rates, (3) serial assessments of diaphragmatic force generation over time using phrenic stimulation techniques, and (4) use of diaphragm electromyographic characteristics (Pdi/EMG ratios and/or centroid frequency assessment) to detect fatigue. While serial assessments of MIP and/or Pdi over time appear to be an obvious approach to assessing fatigue development, the limitations described earlier are so pronounced that this cannot be recommended as a truly reliable means of detecting fatigue development. On the other hand, phrenic nerve stimulation techniques and electromyographic analysis hold much promise (these will be discussed in detail later) but require significant investments in equipment and are currently used primarily in research settings. Relaxation rates also have been used to provide an index of fatigue development, and assessment of inspiratory muscle relaxation can be done with substantially less equipment than that required for EMG or phrenic nerve stimulation techniques.

Assessment of relaxation rates as an index of fatigue makes use of the fact that the rate of relaxation of muscle force after cessation of contraction typically slows as fatigue develops.[48] Rate of relaxation of the respiratory muscles typically is determined by examining the rate of decay of the pressure waveform generated by contraction of a particular muscle group (Fig. 19-11). For example, relaxation rate for the diaphragm can be determined by examining the rate of fall of Pdi at the end of a given diaphragmatic contraction. This rate of fall can be quantitated in several ways: (1) by drawing a tangent to the steepest portion of the declining pressure-time curve and determining the rate of pressure fall dp/dt, also known as the MRR, or (2) by plotting the natural logarithm or pressure as a function of time (this plot is nearly linear over the lower 70 percent of the pressure-time relationship during muscle relaxation) and calculating the reciprocal of the slope of this line (this reciprocal represents the time constant of the monoexponential decay of pressure with time and is termed τ). Because MRR varies with the amplitude of the pressure waveform, this value is usually normalized by expressing this parameter as the percentage fall in pressure over 10 s. A slowing of relaxation is manifest as a decline in the MRR or an increase in τ.

This approach has been used to assess the relaxation rate of pressure in a variety of settings, including (1) assessment of the relaxation of esophageal (Pes) or transdiaphragmatic (Pdi) pressure during sniffs with and without airway occlusion,[48,50] (2) measurement of Pes or Pdi pressure relaxation rates following phrenic nerve stimulation, (3) detection of changes in Pes or Pdi relaxation rates during breathing against inspiratory resistive loading,[48,49,51] or (4) estimation of MRR of nasopharyngeal or mouth pressures during sniff maneuvers (the former is termed the *sniff nasal inspiratory pressure*, or SNIP, maneuver).[50,52] Of note, transmission of brief pressure swings from the alveoli to the upper airways can be distorted in patients with lung disease, raising potential problems for the use of the SNIP maneuver in such patients.

While a number of experiments have demonstrated a qualitative relationship between the development of muscle fatigue and a slowing of respiratory muscle relaxation in a variety of circumstances (e.g., during loaded breathing), it should be understood that there is no exact, quantitative relationship between changes in relaxation and alterations in force-generating capacity during fatigue. In fact, in certain experimental conditions it is possible to produce fatigue without changes in relaxation rate, and vice versa. Nevertheless, one recent study found that slowing or relaxation of the respiratory muscles predicted failure during weaning from mechanical ventilation,[53] suggesting that this index may

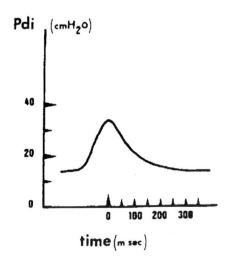
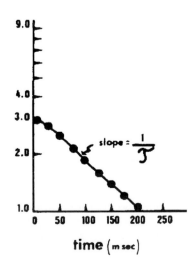

FIGURE 19-11 The manner in which the relaxation constant of a pressure waveform can be determined. The left panel displays the raw tracing of transdiaphragmatic pressure versus time, whereas the right panel displays the natural logarithm of pressure versus time for the relaxation portion of the pressure waveform. The relaxation constant ς is the inverse of the slope of the linear portion of the right-hand curve. (From Aubier et al.,[58] with permission.)

have some clinical value in specific, well-defined applications.

Tests of Special Utility

In this section I provide a description of two forms of testing (assessment of thoracoabdominal motion and lung volume measurements) that can provide useful information about muscle function under certain specific circumstances. These two forms of testing have the advantage of simplicity and widespread applicability, but they suffer because the information obtained by these techniques is more qualitative than that garnered with the other techniques described in this chapter. Often the information obtained by these techniques provides the impetus for more direct and quantitative forms of testing (e.g., an observation that abdominal paradox is present can lead to measurement of transdiaphragmatic pressure gradients).

THORACOABDOMINAL MOTION

Evaluation of the pattern of motion of the chest wall can provide useful information in several clinical situations. In patients with selective diaphragmatic weakness, one usually can see inward motion of the abdominal wall during inspiration (i.e., *abdominal paradox*), providing an important clue that diaphragmatic dysfunction is present. Conversely, patients who rely on the diaphragm as the sole muscle of inspiration (e.g., patients with low cervical cord lesions) often will demonstrate paradoxical inward motion of the upper chest during diaphragmatic contraction.

Motion of the chest wall and abdomen often can be assessed for sufficient qualitative accuracy for clinical uses simply by inspecting and palpating these structures during breathing efforts. More quantitative assessment of body surface movements now can be done with a number of techniques. Perhaps the most commonly used of these is inductive plethysmography,[54] which uses the principles of magnetic inductance to measure body cross-sectional areas. When using this technique, elastic bands containing insulated wire coils are placed around the body structure to be assessed (in the case of the respiratory system, around the chest cage and abdomen). These coils are connected to oscillators, and the magnetic inductance of the coil-band assembly is assessed continuously. Changes in the cross-sectional area contained within a given band result in measurable changes in magnetic inductance that can be calibrated and expressed as volumetric changes for the compartment the bands are placed around. With this approach it is possible to monitor changes in inspiratory volume and thoracoabdominal configuration over time, partitioning inspired volumes into chest and abdominal components. These devices are available commercially, and this technique has been employed extensively in a number of clinical settings (e.g., it can be used for monitoring respiratory parameters during weaning from mechanical ventilation).

LUNG VOLUME MEASUREMENTS

Lung volume measurements sometimes can provide information regarding respiratory muscle function. Severe worsening of muscle function can produce significant alterations in lung volume measurements, with reductions in inspiratory muscle strength causing a decrease in the inspiratory capacity and hence a smaller total lung capacity. Similarly, reductions in expiratory muscle strength reduce the capacity to exhale to low lung volumes, thereby decreasing expiratory reserve volumes. Since FRC is determined by the elastic recoil of the chest wall and lung and acute muscle weakness produces only small reductions in chest wall elastic recoil, FRC is relatively normal in disorders that cause pure muscle weakness. As a result, muscle disorders that weaken both inspiratory and expiratory muscles cause a restrictive ventilatory defect characterized by reductions in TLC, inspiratory capacity, and expiratory reserve volume with maintenance of a relatively normal FRC and an increase in RV and the RV/TLC ratio. This pattern differs from that observed with restrictive ventilatory disorders due to lung disease, which typically reduce all components of lung volume (i.e., TLC, FRC, and RV are each reduced). I also should point out that there is a curvilinear relationship between alterations in muscle strength and changes in VC. Because of the shape of lung and chest wall elastic recoil curves, relatively large reductions in muscle strength occur before VC falls and changes in lung volumes become manifest. In addition, one should recognize that there are secondary changes in chest wall and lung compliance that can occur with long-standing muscle disorders that also will influence lung volume measurements.[55] As a result, measurements of respiratory muscle strength (i.e., MIP and MEP) are more sensitive and reliable indices of developing muscle weakness than are measurements of lung volume.

Assessment of lung volume also can be useful in another very specific clinical condition. Patients with diaphragmatic paralysis (e.g., resulting from bilateral phrenic nerve lesions) often present with complaints of difficulty breathing on lying down and demonstrate marked reductions in inspiratory capacity when moving from an upright to a recumbent posture. When recumbent, the paralyzed diaphragm cannot effectively prevent movement of the abdominal contents into the chest cage during inspiration in these patients, resulting in a low inspired volume. When these patients are upright, however, gravity prevents movement of the abdominal contents into the chest during inspiration, preserving inspiratory capacity.

Newer Approaches of Assessing Muscle Function

A common problem attendant to many, if not all, of the measurements made in the preceding sections of this chapter is the requirement that a subject volitionally perform difficult breathing maneuvers in order to obtain reliable data. Several approaches are now available to assess certain aspects of respiratory muscle function in a more objective manner, and the two most prominent of these newer techniques (phrenic nerve stimulation and analysis of respiratory muscle electromyography) will be discussed in this section. As will be apparent, these latter techniques require much more complex equipment and user training than the simpler approaches discussed in preceding sections and are currently used largely in research settings.

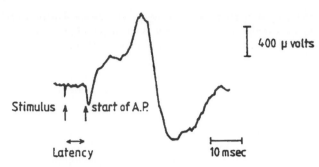

FIGURE 19-12 Recording of a diaphragm electromyographic mass action potential elicited in response to electrical stimulation of the phrenic nerve. The time delay between the phrenic stimulation and the onset of the action potential represents the conduction time (i.e., latency). (From DiVito and Grassino,[77] with permission.)

PHRENIC NERVE STIMULATION

The phrenic nerves are fairly superficial in the neck and amenable to electrical or magnetic stimulation by placement of suitable electrodes (Fig. 19-12). Electrical stimulation can be and has been performed both transcutaneously, using electrode pads, and percutaneously, using needles or wires placed below the skin surface.[56-58] Magnetic stimulation can be carried out using devices placed over either the cervical spine posteriorly or anteriorly over the phrenic nerves.[59] Percutaneous electrode placement carries the risks associated with placement of any needle in the neck region (e.g., infection, carotid puncture, etc.), but percutaneous electrodes are more stable and often are desirable in research settings where reproducible nerve stimulation over time is essential. Transcutaneous electrodes are used more commonly, have fewer potential risks, but also result in much less reproducibility stimulation.

For the usual clinical applications, the phrenic nerves are stimulated with single impulses (sometimes termed *twitch stimulation* because it elicits a twitch of the ipsilateral hemidiaphragm) that are relatively well tolerated.[57,58] In some research reports, stimulation of the phrenic nerve with trains of electrical impulses has been carried out, and these investigations have contributed greatly to our understanding of respiratory muscle physiology.[56] High-frequency stimulation, however, is fairly painful and currently has little clinical application.

Several different parameters can be monitored when performing phrenic nerve stimulation, including (1) the time required for conduction of electrical impulses from the site of stimulation in the neck to the diaphragm, (2) the magnitude and characteristics of the diaphragm electromyographic waveform (mass action potential) elicited by stimulation of the phrenic nerve, and (3) the transdiaphragmatic pressure elicited by phrenic nerve stimulation. It is commonplace to perform phrenic nerve stimulation as a clinical tool to examine these nerves for damage; for this purpose, nerve conduction times and the elicited electromyographic impulse (1 and 2) are examined.[60] When performing such an assessment, the diaphragm mass action potential is recorded using electrodes generally placed over the seventh to ninth intercostal spaces in the anterior axillary line. Normally, phrenic stimulation elicits an action potential within 6 to 10 ms (see Fig. 19-12),

and a longer conduction time generally indicates phrenic nerve damage.

Assessment of transdiaphragmatic pressure generation in response to phrenic nerve stimulation is a far more difficult procedure to perform (Fig. 19-13). It is generally believed that bilateral stimulation is required to obtain reproducible measurements,[57,58] and great care must be taken to ensure that activation is achieved and maintained during this form of assessment. Care also must be taken to characterize or control thoracoabdominal configuration, lung volume, and the use of other muscles during stimulation trials, since each of these variables can greatly influence the transdiaphragmatic pressures elicited during phrenic nerve stimulation.[61] Despite these difficulties and drawbacks, which currently limit use of this technique to a few research centers around the world, the fact that this approach permits a nonvolitional assessment of muscle function provides an enormous advantage over current clinical methods. It is possible that a variation of this approach eventually will provide the "gold standard" method of clinically assessing respiratory muscle strength.

RESPIRATORY MUSCLE ELECTROMYOGRAPHY

Diaphragm electromyography has been used in several ways to facilitate the measurement of various aspects of muscle

FIGURE 19-13 Diagramatic display of the monitors commonly used when measuring transdiaphragmatic pressure in response to electrical stimulation of the phrenic nerves. Bilateral neck electrodes are employed for nerve stimulation. The gradient between mouth and esophageal pressure is taken as an index of transpulmonary pressure Ppl, whereas the gradient between esophageal and gastric pressures is taken as transdiaphragmatic pressure (Pdi). Maximality of diaphragm activation is monitored using electromyographic electrodes placed over the right (EdiR) and left (EdiL) hemidiaphragms. Rib cage and abdominal respibands can be used to monitor thoracoabdominal configuration during diaphragmatic contractions. (From Aubier et al.,[58] with permission.)

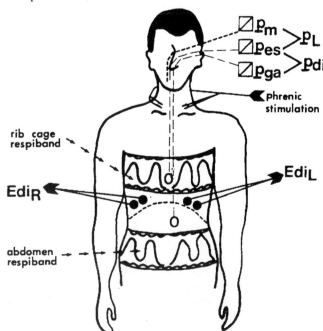

function.[60-64] Recordings of the diaphragm electromyographic signal evoked by phrenic nerve stimulation or used to assess nerve conduction by the phrenic nerve are used to detect nerve damage. Note that this form of nerve stimulation causes simultaneous activation of all the motor nerve fibers, resulting in the mass activation of all diaphragmatic motor units and simultaneous depolarization of all motor fibers within the ipsilateral hemidiaphragm. The resulting electromyographic potential is therefore termed the *mass action potential*. The size and shape of this potential provide some information about the muscle, since myopathic processes tend to reduce the size and may change the shape of the elicited waveform. Evidence of such alterations therefore may suggest the presence of a myopathic process, but it is difficult, when examining the diaphragm in this fashion, to be sure that technical artifacts are not contributing to alterations (since one does not have precise control of the electrode-muscle interface in the diaphragm).

In addition, the diaphragm electromyogram can be recorded during spontaneous respiratory muscle contractions, and the resulting signal can be analyzed in several ways to provide physiologic information. Recent research has suggested that recording artifacts in the diaphragm electromyogram can be reduced by employing esophageal electrodes (these electrodes are in close approximation to the crural portion of the diaphragm and provide a more constant signal than do electrodes placed over the chest wall near the diaphragmatic insertion.[65-68] When using electromyographic recording in this fashion, it is also important to take steps to minimize artifact due to movement and ECG contamination, and recent publications have described computer techniques to largely eliminate these problems.[68] Once recorded in this fashion, the resulting electromyographic activity can be analyzed in two ways: (1) an integration technique can be employed to provide a moving time average of the total level or "power" of the electrical signal being recorded, and (2) an analysis can be made of the frequency components of the recorded signal, with an attempt made to determine the amplitude or relative power of the different frequency components making up the entire signal. To understand these two uses, one must recognize that a muscle electromyogram represents a composite of all the action potentials being generated in the muscle underlying the electrode. A large fiber activated by the brain at a low neural firing rate will generate large but infrequent muscle action potentials, whereas a slow fiber activated frequently will generate smaller but more frequent action potentials. As more fibers are activated or fibers are activated more frequently, the total number of action potentials recorded will increase, and the amplitude or power of the integrated signal will rise. In addition, if a change occurs in the distribution of muscle fibers being used or more fibers are activated at a given firing frequency, then a shift will occur in the amplitude of the different frequency components making up the diaphragm electromyogram. As an example, if the activation frequency of a given group of fibers increases from 20 to 30 Hz (and all other factors remain constant), then the total number of action potentials recorded (and the integrated amplitude or power) at 20 Hz will decrease, and the integrated amplitude of action potentials recorded at 30 Hz will rise.

Several techniques have been described to determine either (1) total diaphragmatic EMG amplitude or "power" as a function of time or (2) frequency analysis of the diaphragmatic EMG at a given time to provide a graph of integrated amplitude (EMG power) as a function of action potential firing frequency. Such forms of analysis can be carried out both by employing computer techniques and by using various forms of analog equipment that make use of multiple bandpass filters and RC circuits.[63,64,69]

Studies have suggested that the moving-time average of integrated electromyographic activity correlates well with oxygen consumption and muscle force development for nonfatigued muscles.[70] It also has been suggested that an assessment of the ratio of transdiaphragmatic pressure to integrated EMG activity may provide a means of determining the onset of muscle fatigue, since the force generated per unit activation should, in theory, fall as fatigue develops.

A number of studies also have described useful applications for the analysis of electromyographic amplitude as a function of action potential frequency (this is referred to as a *power-frequency spectrum*). Numerous reports have indicated that the development of muscle fatigue usually is associated with a shift in the power-frequency spectrum of the muscle electromyogram, with a reduction in high-frequency power and an increase in the power present at low frequencies[62-64,69,71] (see Fig. 19-14 for an example of such use). Often such a shift is quantitated by reporting a decrease in the "centroid frequency" of the electromyogram, where the term *centroid frequency* refers to a weighted average of the amplitude of action potential waveforms recorded at different frequencies (the lower this number, the larger is the proportion of EMG amplitude at lower action potential frequencies).

Implications for Rehabilitation: Assessment of Training Responses

Many, if not most, rehabilitation programs make use of pulmonary muscle training programs to improve the function of these muscles.[71] As mentioned earlier, improved function could, in theory, allow patients with various forms of lung disease to better tolerate episodes of decompensation (e.g., induced by the development of infections or other disorders).

Several forms of respiratory training have been employed in clinical studies, including the use of inspiratory resistive loading for varying periods each day, use of inspiratory threshold loading for various times per day, and other more eclectic techniques (e.g., periods of daily hyperpnea, repeated maximal static inspiratory efforts each day).[72,73] Some studies show such training to be useful in eliciting increases in respiratory muscle function (i.e., increases in muscle strength and endurance), whereas others do not. Additional studies will be needed to properly define the ultimate utility of such training programs. Nevertheless, several of the tests described earlier should be useful in monitoring the response to respiratory training efforts.

When assessing the response to various forms of training, it should be remembered that there is a degree of specificity in the training response. Training regimens that employ endurance forms of exercise have been shown to elicit increases in muscle endurance. In contrast, strength-training regimens (e.g., the generation of repeated maximal pressures) appear to selectively increase respiratory muscle strength without altering muscle endurance capacity.[74]

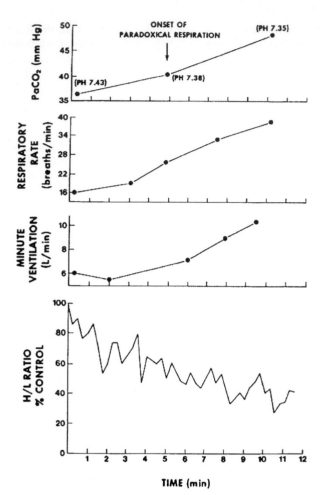

FIGURE 19-14 Recordings of (from top to bottom) arterial carbon dioxide level, respiratory rate, minute ventilation, and the diaphragm electromyographic high-low ratio (H/L ratio) over time in a patient with lung diseases during a trial of weaning from mechanical ventilation. This patient "failed" weaning and had to be placed back on mechanical ventilation. Note that the diaphragm H/L ratio (a ratio of high-frequency to low-frequency power of the diaphragm electromyogram), an index of muscle fatigue, decreased over time during this trial. (From Cohen et al.,[62] with permission.)

Final Recommendations

Of the various forms of assessment reviewed herein, MIP and MEP measurements remain the primary tests used to assess respiratory muscle function. These measurements should be used for the workup of patients with restrictive ventilatory defects, in determination of the presence and severity of respiratory myopathic processes, as a tool in the evaluation of patients with respiratory failure of unknown etiology, in providing prognostic information for patients with known myopathies and COPD, and as a component to evaluation of patients being weaned from mechanical ventilation. Interpretation of the MIP and MEP should take into account test reproducibility, the dependence of these measures on lung volumes, and the fact that these tests measure only one aspect of muscle function.

Measurement of maximal transdiaphragmatic pressure remains a useful technique for specific patients (e.g., suspected diaphragmatic paralysis) and may provide quantitative data that corroborate more qualitative assessments in this patient group.

Of the techniques used for assessment of respiratory endurance, the use of incremental threshold load testing appears to have the greatest promise, since this approach permits a form of reproducible, relatively rapid testing of endurance. Assessment of muscle fatigue remains a difficult problem clinically, and while assessment of muscle relaxation rate may reach a point of clinical utility in the future, all tests of this parameter of muscle function remain experimental at the present time.

Assessment of thoracoabdominal movement is a good way of qualitatively evaluating other conditions in which specific respiratory muscle groups are altered. Lung volume measurements often can provide a clue as to the existence of a muscle disorder and may provide the impetus for additional testing.

Phrenic nerve stimulation remains an accepted method of determining the integrity of the phrenic nerve and of detecting unilateral and bilateral alterations in nerve function that can cause hemi- and total diaphragm paralysis and paresis.

A number of investigational techniques (e.g., sniff assessments of muscle function, electrical and magnetic stimulation of the phrenic nerves with concomitant measurement of transdiaphragmatic pressure generation, and various forms of electromyographic recording) are being developed and provide the possibility of more objectively measuring respiratory muscle function. Some of these techniques (e.g., assessment of maximal respiratory pressure generation during sniffs) are well enough established, whereas others (e.g., magnetic stimulation of the phrenic nerves) require additional testing to better define the exact clinical circumstances in which these forms of assessment should be used.

References

1. Similowski T, Yan S, Gauthier AP, et al: Contractile properties of the human diaphragm during chronic hyperinflation. *N Engl J Med* 325:917–923, 1991.
2. McKenzie DK, Gandevia SC: Strength and endurance of inspiratory, expiratory and limb muscles in asthma. *Am Rev Respir Dis* 134:999–1004, 1986.
3. Szeinberg A, England S, Mindorff C, et al: Maximal inspiratory and expiratory pressures are reduced in hyperinflated, malnourished, young adult male patients with cystic fibrosis. *Am Rev Respir Dis* 132:766–769, 1985.
4. Edwaards RHT: Human muscle function and fatigue, in Porter R, Whelan J (eds): *Human Muscle Fatigue: Physiological Mechanisms.* London, Pitman Medical (Ciba Foundation Symposium 82), 1981; pp 1–18.
5. Sieck GC: Diaphragm muscle: Structural and functional organization. *Clin Chest Med* 9:195–210, 1988.
6. Jones DA: Muscle fatigue due to changes beyond the neuromuscular junction, in Porter R, Whelan J (eds): *Human Muscle Fatigue: Physiological Mechanisms.* London, Pitman Medical (Ciba Foundation Symposium 82), 1981; pp 178–190.
7. Dawson MJ, Gadian DG, Wilkie DR: Studies of the biochemistry of contracting and relaxing muscle by the use of ^{31}P NMR in conjunction with other techniques. *Phil Trans R Soc Lond [B]* 289:445–455, 1980.
8. Gadian DG, Radda GK, Brown TR, et al: The activity of creatine

kinase in frog skeletal muscle studied by saturation-transfer nuclear magnetic resonance. *Biochem J* 194:215–228, 1981.

9. Neufer PD, Costill DL, Flynn MG: Improvements in exercise performance: Effects of carbohydrate feedings and diet. *J Appl Physiol* 62:983–988, 1987.

10. Black LF, Hyatt RE: Maximal respiratory pressures: Normal values and relationship to age and sex. *Am Rev Respir Dis* 99:696–702, 1969.

11. Ringvist T: The ventilatory capacity in healthy subjects: An analysis of causal factors with special reference to the respiratory forces. *Scand J Clin Lab Invest* 18:5–179, 1966.

12. Hyatt RE, Black LF: Maximal static respiratory pressures in generalized neuromuscular disease. *Am Rev Respir Dis* 103:641–650, 1971.

13. Enright PL, Kronmal RA, Manolio TA, et al: Respiratory muscle strength in the elderly. *Am J Respir Crit Care Med* 149:430–438, 1994.

14. Wilson SH, Cooke NT, Edwards RHT, Spiro SG: Predicted normal values for maximal respiratory pressures in Caucasian adults and children. *Thorax* 39:535–538, 1984.

15. DeTroyer A, Pride NB: The respiratory system in neuromuscular disorders, in Roussos C, Macklem PT (eds): *The Thorax*, part B. New York, Marcel Dekker, 1985; pp 1089–1121.

16. Vincken W, Elleker MG, Cosio MG: Determinants of respiratory muscle weakness in stable chronic neuromuscular disorders. *Am J Med* 82:53–58, 1987.

17. Mier-Jedrzejowicz A, Brophy C, Green M: Respiratory muscle weakness during upper respiratory tract infections. *Am Rev Respir Dis* 138:5–7, 1988.

18. Hussain SNA, Simkus G, Roussos C: Respiratory muscle fatigue: A cause of ventilatory failure in septic shock. *J Appl Physiol* 58:2033–2040, 1985.

19. Aldrich TK: Respiratory muscle fatigue. *Clin Chest Med* 9:225–236, 1988.

20. Ferguson GT: Corticosteroids and respiratory muscles. *Chest* 104:1649–1650, 1993.

21. Laroche CM, Cairns T, Moxham J, Green M: Hypothyroidism presenting with respiratory muscle weakness. *Am Rev Respir Dis* 138:472–478, 1988.

22. Rochester DF, Braun NMT: Determinants of maximal inspiratory pressure in chronic obstructive pulmonary disease. *Am Rev Respir Dis* 132:42–47, 1985.

23. Braun NM, Arora NS, Rochester DF: Respiratory muscle and pulmonary function in polymyositis and other proximal myopathies. *Thorax* 38:616–623, 1983.

24. Yang KL, Tobin MJ: A prospective study of indexes predicting the outcome of trials of weaning from mechanical ventilation. *N Engl J Med* 324:1445–1450, 1991.

25. Capdevila XJ, Perrigault PF, Perey PJ, et al: Occlusion pressure and its ratio to maximum inspiratory pressure are useful predictors for successful extubation following T-piece weaning trial. *Chest* 108:482–489, 1995.

26. Multz AS, Aldrich T, Prezant D, et al: Maximal inspiratory pressure is not a reliable test of inspiratory muscle strength in mechanically ventilated patients. *Am Rev Respir Dis* 142:529–532, 1990.

27. Miller JM, Moxham J, Green M: The maximal sniff in the assessment of diaphragm function in man. *Clin Sci* 69:91–96, 1985.

28. Laroche CM, Mier AK, Moxham J, Green M: The value of sniff esophageal pressures in the assessment of global inspiratory muscle strength. *Am Rev Respir Dis* 138:598–603, 1988.

29. Heritier F, Rahm F, Pasche P, Fitting JW: Sniff nasal inspiratory pressure: A noninvasive assessment of inspiratory muscle strength. *Am J Respir Crit Care Med* 150:1678–1683, 1994.

30. Heritier F, Perret C, Fitting JW: Maximal sniff mouth pressure compared with maximal inspiratory pressure in acute respiratory failure. *Chest* 100:175–178, 1991.

31. Uldry C, Fitting JW: Maximal values of sniff nasal inspiratory pressure in healthy subjects. *Thorax* 50:371–375, 1995.

32. Gibson GJ, Clark E, Pride NB: Static transdiaphragmatic pressures in normal subjects and in patients with chronic hyperinflation. *Am Rev Respir Dis* 124:685–690, 1981.

33. Laporta D, Grassino A: Assessment of transdiaphragmatic pressure in humans. *J Appl Physiol* 58:1469–1476, 1985.

34. Weiner P, Suo J, Fernandez E, Cherniack R: The effect of hyperinflation on respiratory muscle strength and efficiency in healthy subjects and patients with asthma. *Am Rev Respir Dis* 141:1501–1505, 1990.

35. Weiner L, Azgod L: Inspiratory muscle training during treatment with corticosteroids in humans. *Chest* 107:1041–1044, 1995.

36. Homsher E, Kean CJ: Skeletal muscle energetics and metabolism. *Annu Rev Physiol* 40:93–131, 1978.

37. Bellemare F, Grassino A: Effect of pressure and timing of contraction on human diaphragm fatigue. *J Appl Physiol* 53:1190–1195, 1982.

38. Bellemare F, Grassino A: Evaluation of human diaphragm fatigue. *J Appl Physiol* 53:1196–1206, 1982.

39. Westerblad H, Lannergren J, Allen DG: Fatigue of striated muscles: Metabolic aspects, in Roussos C (ed): *The Thorax*, 2nd ed. New York, Marcel Dekker, 1995.

40. Belman MJ, Mittman C: Ventilatory muscle training improves exercise capacity in chronic obstructive pulmonary disease patients. *Am Rev Respir Dis* 121:273–280, 1980.

41. Freedman S: Sustained maximum voluntary ventilation. *Respir Physiol* 8:230–240, 1970.

42. Mancini DM, LaMance D: Evidence of reduced respiratory muscle endurance in patients with heart failure. *J Am Coll Cardiol* 24:972–981, 1994.

43. Nickerson BG, Keens TG: Measuring ventilatory muscle endurance in humans as sustainable inspiratory pressure. *J Appl Physiol* 52:768–772, 1982.

44. Martyn JB, Moreno RH, Pare PD, Pardy RL: Measurement of inspiratory muscle performance with incremental threshold loading. *Am Rev Respir Dis* 135:919–923, 1987.

45. Mckenzie DK, Gandevia SC: Strength and endurance of inspiratory, expiratory, and limb muscles in asthma. *Am Rev Respir Dis* 134:999–1004, 1986.

46. NHLBI Workshop: Respiratory muscle fatigue: Report of the Respiratory Muscle Fatigue Workshop Group. *Am Rev Respir Dis* 142:474–480, 1990.

47. Bellemare F, Bigland-Ritchie B: Central components of diaphragmatic fatigue assessed by phrenic nerve stimulation. *J Appl Physiol* 62:1307–1316, 1987.

48. Esau SA, Bellemare F, Grassino A, et al: Changes in relaxation rate with diaphragmatic fatigue in humans. *J Appl Physiol* 54:1353–1360, 1983.

49. Esau SA, Bye PTP, Pardy RL: Changes in rate of relaxation of sniffs with diaphragmatic fatigue in humans. *J Appl Physiol* 55:731–735, 1983.

50. Koulouris N, Vianna LG, Mulvey DA, et al: Maximal relaxation rates of esophageal, nose, and mouth pressures during a sniff reflect inspiratory muscle fatigue. *Am Rev Respir Dis* 193:1213–1217, 1989.

51. Mador MJ, Kufel TJ: Effect of inspiratory muscle fatigue on inspiratory muscle relaxation rates in healthy subjects. *Chest* 102:1767–1773, 1992.

52. Kyroussis D, Mills G, Hamnegard CH, et al: Inspiratory muscle relaxation rate assessed from sniff nasal pressure. *Thorax* 49:1127–1133, 1994.

53. Goldstone JC, Green M, Moxham J: Maximum relaxation rate of the diaphragm during weaning from mechanical ventilation. *Thorax* 49:54–60, 1994.

54. Sackner JD, Nixon AJ, Davis B: Non-invasive measurement of ventilation during exercise using respiratory inductive plethysmography. *Am Rev Respir Dis* 122:867–871, 1980.

55. DeTroyer A, Berenstein S, Cardier R: Analysis of lung volume

restriction in patients with respiratory muscle weakness. *Thorax* 35:603–610, 1980.

56. Aubier M, Farkas G, DeTroyer A: Detection of diaphragmatic fatigue in man by phrenic stimulation. *J Appl Physiol* 50:538–544, 1981.

57. Bellemare F, Bigland-Ritchie B: Assessment of human diaphragm strength and activation using phrenic nerve stimulation. *Respir Physiol* 58:263–277, 1984.

58. Aubier M, Murciano D, Lecocguic Y, et al: Bilateral phrenic stimulation: A simple technique to assess diaphragmatic fatigue in humans. *J Appl Physiol* 58:58–64, 1985.

59. Similowski T, Fleury B, Launois S, et al: Cervical magnetic stimulation: A new painless method for bilateral phrenic nerve stimulation in conscious humans. *J Appl Physiol* 67:1311–1318, 1989.

60. McKenzie DK, Gandevia SC: Electrical assessment of respiratory muscles, in Roussos C (ed): *The Thorax*, part B, 2nd ed. Lung Biology in Health and Disease Series, vol 85. New York, Marcel Dekker, 1996; pp 1029–1048.

61. Gandevia SC, McKenzie DK: Human diaphragmatic EMG: Changes with lung volume and posture during supramaximal phrenic stimulation. *J Appl Physiol* 60:1420–1428, 1986.

62. Cohen C, Zagelbaum G, Gross D, et al: Clinical manifestations of inspiratory muscle fatigue. *Am J Med* 73:308–316, 1982.

63. Gross D, Grassino A, Ross WRD, Macklem PT: Electromyogram pattern of diaphragmatic fatigue. *J Appl Physiol* 46:1–7, 1979.

64. Moxham J, Edwards RHT, Aubier M, et al: Changes in EMG power spectrum (high/low ratio) with force fatigue in man. *J Appl Physiol* 53:1094–1099, 1982.

65. Beck J, Sinderby C, Weinberg J, Grassino A: Effects of muscle-to-electrode distance on the human diaphragm electromyogram. *J Appl Physiol* 79:975–985, 1995.

66. Sinderby C, Lindstrom L, Comtois N, Grassino AE: Effects of diaphragm shortening on the mean action potential conduction velocity in canines. *J Physiol (Lond)* 490:207–214, 1996.

67. Sinderby CA, Comtois AS, Thomson RG, Grassino AE: Influence of the bipolar electrode transfer function on the electromyogram power spectrum. *Muscle Nerve* 19:290–301, 1996.

68. Sinderby C, Lindstrom L, Grassino AE: Automatic assessment of electromyogram quality. *J Appl Physiol* 79:1803–1815, 1995.

69. DeLuca CJ: Myoelectric manifestations of localized muscular fatigue in humans. *Crit Rev Biomed Eng* 11:251–279, 1984.

70. Bigland-Ritchie B, Woods JJ: Integrated EMG and oxygen uptake during dynamic contractions of human muscles. *J Appl Physiol* 36:475–479, 1974.

71. Harver A, Mahler DA, Daubenspeck JA: Targeted inspiratory muscle training improves respiratory muscle function and reduces dyspnea in patients with chronic obstructive pulmonary disease. *Ann Intern Med* 111:117–124, 1989.

72. Pardy RL, Rivington RN, Despas PJ: The effects of inspiratory muscle training on exercise performance in chronic airflow limitation. *Am Rev Respir Dis* 123:426–433, 1981.

73. Aldrich TK, Karpel JP: Inspiratory muscle resistive training in respiratory failure. *Am Rev Respir Dis* 131:461–462, 1985.

74. Leith DE, Bradley M: Ventilatory muscle strength and endurance training. *J Appl Physiol* 41:508–516, 1976.

75. Goldberg P, Roussos C: Assessment of respiratory muscle dysfunction in chronic obstructive lung disease. *Med Clin North Am* 74:643–660, 1990.

76. Braun NM, Arora NS, Rochester DF: Respiratory muscle and pulmonary function in polymyositis and other proximal myopathies. *Thorax* 38:616–623, 1983.

77. DiVito J, Grassino A: Respiratory muscle fatigue, in Roussos C (ed): *The Thorax*, New York, Marcel Dekker, 1995; pp 1861–1890.

78. Rochester DF, Arora NS: Respiratory muscle function. *Med Clin North Am* 67:576, 1983.

Chapter 20

SLEEP QUALITY

DAVID W. HUDGEL

Many patients with chronic lung disease complain of difficulty sleeping. There are several possible causes of this. Bronchospasm, mucus plugging of airways, or arterial blood-gas changes (e.g., hypoxia and hypercapnia) due to nocturnal worsening of the chronic lung disease may interrupt sleep.[1] In the Tucson Epidemiologic Study,[2] 39 to 53 percent of subjects with respiratory symptoms reported insomnia compared with 28 percent of subjects without respiratory symptoms. Excessive daytime sleepiness was present in 12 to 23 percent of respiratory patients compared with 9 percent of controls.[2] In this prospective, community-based study, the presence of respiratory symptoms, in addition to obesity, age, and gender, was a predictor of sleep-related symptoms. In another survey, sleep-related symptomatology was the third most commonly reported symptom after dyspnea and fatigue in patients with chronic obstructive pulmonary disease (COPD).[3] Of course, the symptom of fatigue also could be caused by a sleep disturbance, but it could be due to other factors such as deconditioning, overexertion, and secondary affective disorders such as mental depression. When polysomnography has been performed on patients with chronic lung disease, very frequent arousals have been found.[1] This same pattern of disturbed sleep also has been demonstrated in patients with asthma[4] and cystic fibrosis.[5]

It is possible that sleep-related symptoms in individuals with chronic pulmonary disease such as COPD could be due to the presence of a primary sleep disorder unrelated to the respiratory illness, since COPD patients are usually in the age range in which primary sleep disorders such as sleep apnea and periodic leg movements occur.[6] In combination with pulmonary disease, such sleep disorders likely would potentiate sleep-related symptomatology or add to the general sensations of physical fatigue and mental depression. Most likely, recognition and treatment of sleep complications of a lung disease or a primary sleep disorder will improve the overall sense of well-being of a respiratory disease patient, even lessen respiratory symptoms, and improve the patient's quality of life. Thus the physician must be sensitive to the possible sleep-related complications of chronic respiratory diseases, and he or she also must be aware of the possible presence of a primary sleep disorder in patients with chronic lung diseases. Specific therapy for a sleep disorder may be needed in addition to enhanced therapy for the lung disease during the sleeping hours.

Types of Sleep Disorders Found in Patients with Chronic Lung Disease

Insomnia surely can occur in patients with chronic lung diseases.[2] Insomnia can be secondary to the disease state itself[1]; the medications prescribed to treat the lung disease, such as theophylline[7]; anxiety about issues related to health status; or unrelated to the lung condition. The time sequence of the insomnia related to progression of the lung disease or in the prescription of certain medications will help determine the cause of the insomnia. Preexisting anxiety or anxiety related to the lung disease surely might produce enough anxiety to disturb sleep. The cause of the insomnia, as determined by these historical variables, will indicate the type of treatment needed. For instance, if insomnia accompanies worsening of the lung disease, enhancement of the lung disease treatment may help the insomnia. However, use of certain medications, such as theophylline or corticosteroids, may improve lung function but worsen the insomnia. If so, hopefully, a compromise can be found that will result in improvement in both conditions.

Hypoxemia is a major factor that may affect sleep in patients with chronic lung diseases.[8-13] Oxygenation during sleep and subsequent sleep quality may be affected by the underlying lung disease but also by other factors. For instance, obstructive sleep apnea (OSA) is common in the fifth to the seventh decades of life and can occur in patients with chronic lung disease.[6] In addition, a decrease in lung volume may occur especially in rapid eye movement (REM) sleep because of accessory respiratory muscle hypotonia and further worsen sleep oxygenation by disturbing the matching ventilation to perfusion.[14] It is also possible that ventilatory drives may influence the degree of sleep-related hypoxemia. For example, hypercapnic COPD patients had more sleep-related hypoxemia than nonhypercapnic patients even though the level of oxygenation was similar in the two groups of patients.[6,15,16] Cough rarely produces arousal in that most nocturnal coughing occurs following arousal from sleep.[17] Of course, continued coughing or repetitive coughing spells throughout the night may prevent resumption and maintenance of sleep. Airway mucus accumulation may produce increased work of breathing and blood-gas changes, either one of which or both may result in the arousal, which is then followed by coughing.

Diagnosis of Sleep Disorders

Chronic sleepiness has obvious consequences on cognitive and affective functioning. Sleep disruption and daytime sleepiness will contribute to impairment of the sense of well-being and happiness. Diagnosis and treatment for a sleep disorder will greatly improve the clinical status of such a patient. The health care provider should keep this area of the patient's functioning in mind along with concerns about such issues as nutrition, exercise, and socialization.

The most useful diagnostic method for determining the presence of sleep-related complications of lung disease is the clinical history. Often, the history is better obtained from a spouse or family member than from the patient. The presence of inappropriate sleepiness while driving a vehicle, in meetings, in social gatherings, and in conversations, is often an indication that a significant sleep disorder exists. Heavy snoring or frequent nocturnal awakenings also may be indicative of such a problem. The appearance of cognitive or affective abnormalities without obvious cause might indicate that poor sleep is present. The physical examination is helpful in gauging the patient's overall appearance and mood. The finding of cor pulmonale when the arterial oxygen tension is above 60 mmHg during wakefulness without deterioration of airflow obstruction suggests that the nocturnal oxygenation may be significantly low. Overnight finger pulse oximetry can be used to determine the presence of sleep hypoxemia. When done in the hospital, this test is often inconclusive because of the sleep disruption that commonly occurs in this setting. Two nights of oximetry are often needed to obtain enough sleep for analysis. One should examine a full night's recording of arterial oxygen saturation. Alarms should not be used during these tests to detect sleep hypoxemia. The alarms will disturb sleep and defeat the purpose of the whole test. Polysomnography, along with evening and morning spirometric assessments of lung function, often can determine the specific cause of nocturnal hypoxemia. Polysomnography that records sleep stage, body position, breathing pattern, and oxygenation will distinguish between obstructive sleep apnea and ventilatory insufficiency as the cause of a patient's sleep hypoxemia. Once a diagnosis is made, specific treatment can be initiated.

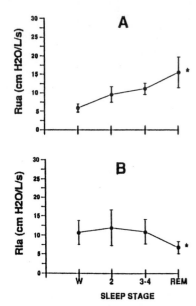

FIGURE 20-1 Upper airway resistance, Rua, and lower airway resistance, Rla, in wakefulness and different sleep stages. (Reprinted with permission from Ballard et al.[18])

Specific Sleep Disorders Related to Specific Pulmonary Diseases and Their Mechanisms

CHRONIC OBSTRUCTIVE LUNG DISEASE

Hypoxemia is the most common abnormality found during sleep in COPD patients. As might be expected, the degree of daytime hypoxemia is predictive of the extent of worsening nocturnal hypoxemia.[13] The lower the ventilatory response to hypercapnia, the greater is the degree of nocturnal hypoxemia. However, neither the degree of airflow obstruction nor the awake P_{CO_2} is significantly related to the extent of the sleep hypoxemia.[13] Hypoxemia in COPD patients usually is found in REM rather than in non-REM sleep and is usually oscillatory in nature.[8] In a very comprehensive study, Ballard and colleagues[18] examined the physiology of the sleep-related hypoxemia in COPD. Interestingly, lung volume and airway resistance did not worsen during sleep, as measured in a horizontal body plethysmograph; in fact, lung resistance was lower (but upper airway resistance higher) in REM sleep than in wakefulness or stage 2 non-REM sleep (Fig. 20-1). Tidal volume and minute ventilation fell progressively through the sleep stages, the lowest values being recorded in REM sleep. The decreased ventilation and hypoxemia could be related to the increase in upper airway resistance and the decrease in respiratory muscle output, as measured by the mouth occlusion pressure. Thus the REM-specific hypoxemia in these patients was more likely related to sleep apnea/hypopnea and not worsening in lung function. When data were evaluated over time instead of by sleep stage, there was an increase in lung resistance over the night, consistent with the common finding of decreased flow rates present on arising in the morning. However, the hypoxemia associated with this deterioration in lung mechanics is usually not as severe as that seen in REM sleep. The results from these studies suggest that airway function per se does not worsen oxygenation significantly during sleep but that there is a REM sleep stage–related decrease in ventilatory muscle compensation for the increased load to breathing produced by a combination of two variables: the increase in upper airway

resistance that normally occurs in REM sleep and the baseline physiologic abnormalities resulting from the lung disease itself.

If the upper airway closes during REM sleep in COPD patients, treatment for obstructive sleep apnea may be needed. If oxygen administration alone corrects the hypoxemia and reduces the number of nocturnal arousals, then this is adequate treatment.[19] Persistent sleep hypoxemia, sleep disruption secondary to the upper airway obstruction, or the presence of excessive daytime sleepiness indicates that specific treatment for sleep apnea may be indicated. Noninvasive ventilatory support will alleviate the upper airway occlusion, the REM-related hypoxemia, sleep disruption, and daytime sleepiness. Nasal continuous positive airway pressure (nCPAP) may be helpful, but one has to be careful with nCPAP in COPD patients because the nCPAP loads expiratory muscles and can contribute to respiratory failure. The use of bilevel pressure devices may alleviate this potential complication of noninvasive ventilatory support in COPD because lower levels of expiratory pressure often can be used with bilevel pressure support.

ASTHMA

In asthmatic patients, a worsening of bronchoconstriction often occurs overnight whether or not sleep occurs.[20] However, sleep-dependent physiologic changes in lung function do occur. Sleep is associated with a decrease in accessory chest wall muscle tonic activity,[21] and a subsequent significant drop in functional residual capacity (FRC) then occurs[22] (Fig. 20-2). The reduction in lung volume results in a decrease in airway caliber, increasing airflow resistance and potentiating the maldistribution of ventilation. Both variables may contribute to subsequent hypoxemia. Often the worsening asthma awakens asthmatic patients, usually in the early morning hours, classically at approximately 4 A.M.[23] This awakening is not specific to the sleep stage.

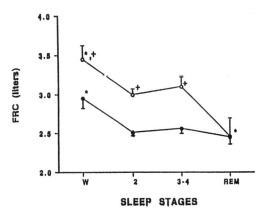

FIGURE 20-2 Decrease in functional residual capacity, FRC, from wakefulness to different sleep stages. Open circles, asthmatics; closed circles, controls. (Reprinted with permission from Ballard et al.[20])

The etiology of nocturnal asthma has received much attention, but to date, no single cause has been identified. Likely multiple factors are involved. Interestingly, a greater amount of airway inflammation has been found in the early morning hours at the time the bronchoconstriction worsens.[24] Other variables that may be important are the circadian fluctuations in catecholamines and corticosteroids, which are at their nadir in the early morning hours.[25] The balance between cholinergic and adrenergic neural activities may be altered in sleep, especially in REM sleep, a state in which cholinergic activity predominates. This relative increase in cholinergic activity may worsen bronchoconstriction.[26] Gastroesophageal reflux[27] and nocturnal allergen exposure[24] also may play a role in some patients. When recurrent, this early morning awakening surely produces daytime sleepiness and associated symptoms.

Some asthmatic patients also may have obstructive sleep apnea (OSA). In fact, systemic corticosteroids may potentiate this problem by increasing central, truncal obesity. Control of the asthma may become difficult when sleep apnea is present. Treatment with nCPAP can lead to an improvement in asthma control and a reduction in airway hyperreactivity.

INTERSTITIAL LUNG DISEASE

Patients with interstitial lung disease (ILD) may experience sleep disruption and nocturnal hypoxemia.[28] Similar to patients with COPD, the hypoxemia usually occurs in REM sleep.[29] Snorers with ILD may have OSA.[30] Interestingly, the hypoxemia seen in these patients during sleep may not be as severe as that seen during exercise.[31] The mechanism of the sleep disturbances and hypoxemia in these patients has not been defined except to note that relative hypoventilation may occur during sleep.[29] This hypoventilation may be caused by an increase in upper airway resistance, as noted earlier in COPD and asthma.

CHEST WALL DISEASES

Hypoxemia, especially during REM sleep, can be seen in patients with chest wall deformities such as kyphoscoliosis.[32] Respiratory muscle mechanical disadvantage, muscle weakness, and hypoventilation may be the most important etiologic factors.[33] Often, paradoxical motion of the respiratory muscles occurs in these patients in the supine position, especially during sleep. This produces inefficient ventilation, and despite the increased work of breathing, subsequent hypoventilation occurs. The role of the upper airway in producing the hypoventilation in these patients is unknown.

Consequences of Sleep Disorders in Patients with Lung Diseases

EFFECT OF SLEEP DISORDER ON CLINICAL STATUS

As stated earlier, symptoms of fatigue, sleepiness, and an overall feeling of poor health are worsened by the presence of a sleep disorder in patients with chronic pulmonary diseases. In a questionnaire study of patients with chronic airflow limitation and control subjects, it was found that patients, most of whom experienced no worsening of their lung function during sleep, had a longer sleep-onset time, shorter total sleep time, more awakenings, less satisfying sleep, were less refreshed on awakening, and had more excessive daytime sleepiness.[34] The severity of the patients's lung disease was not correlated with these symptoms, except that there was a relationship between more abnormal baseline lung function and a lower perception of daytime functioning. One major problem with this study is the lack of lung function measurements before, during, or following the sleep period and a lack of objective confirmation of poor sleep quality. The role of medications was not considered. Of course, it is possible that other related entities such as gastroesophageal reflux may have contributed to poor sleep in these patients.[35] However, it is logical to conclude that more severe lung disease is associated with more sleep disruption.

An unanswered question is whether or not poor sleep worsens lung function. Evidence suggests that respiratory muscle performance may be affected by sleep. Rest sometimes improves the performance of the respiratory muscles. If respiratory muscle rest occurs in sleep, as presumably it does in healthy individuals, then daytime respiratory muscle function might be improved in COPD, and dyspnea might be lessened. However, in many COPD patients, the work of breathing during sleep is higher than during wakefulness, and so muscle rest does not occur. Chronic respiratory muscle fatigue prevails in these individuals, leading to inefficient ventilation and dyspnea, which, in turn, would worsen sleep quality.

Treatment of Sleep Disorders and Sleep Quality

MEDICATIONS

Optimization of bronchodilator therapy has been the primary method used in the past for improving the status of COPD or asthma and thereby improving the associated poor sleep quality. Long-acting theophylline preparations administered at bedtime have been shown to be more useful in improving nocturnal oxygenation and overnight airflow limitation in COPD than inhaled beta$_2$ agonists given at bedtime.[36-38] In studies evaluating the effect of theophylline on sleep quality, it has been found that sleep may or may not be disturbed by theophylline administration.[7,36,38] However, theophylline has not been shown to improve the abnormal sleep pattern in these patients. Inhaled ipratropium bromide has been shown to be helpful in COPD patients with nocturnal desaturation.[39] Oral long-acting salbutamol improved morning lung function in asthmatics but not COPD patients compared with placebo, and it did not improve oxygenation or sleep pattern in either disease state.[40] Oral sustained-release albuterol (8 mg) added to already established medication programs did not improve lung function, oxygenation, or sleep pattern in asthma or COPD patients.[41] Thus improvement of the nocturnal pulmonary status may or may not improve sleep quality. If sleep quality is not improved, either the lung condition was not improved enough by the medication(s) given, or the sleep disruption was not due to the presence of the lung disease. The sleep disruption also could be due to medication side effects.

An attempt has been made to improve nocturnal oxygenation in COPD patients with ventilatory stimulants. Almitrine bismesylate increased awake arterial oxygen tension and thereby improved the extent of arterial oxygen desaturation seen in COPD patients.[42] Similar effects were seen with progesterone[43] and protriptyline.[44] However, significant side effects limit the usefulness of these agents.

Benzodiazepine use in patients with chronic lung disease is hazardous because of the possible decrease in ventilatory drive produced by the sedative nature of these compounds. Although when evaluated objectively, this does not appear to be a major problem with benzodiazepine use in COPD.[45] However, the potential suppression of ventilation by these drugs limits their use by clinicians in patients with chronic airflow limitation. A nonbenzodiazepine, zolpidem, reduced the number of nocturnal awakenings and increased sleep time in COPD patients.[46] Therefore, for those patients with stable mild to moderately severe COPD, hypnotic agents can be given safely to improve sleep quality. As in a healthy population, one must be concerned about possible adverse effects on wakefulness function and about the potential development of tolerance.

OXYGEN

Oxygen supplementation is known to reverse hypoxemic end-organ damage only during COPD.[47] However, even COPD patients were shown to have elevated pulmonary artery pressures only during hypoxemia.[48] In a placebo-controlled 3-year trial of COPD patients whose daytime resting arterial oxygen tension was equal or greater than 60 mmHg but who experienced sleep arterial oxygen desaturation, oxygen therapy decreased pulmonary artery pressure, whereas the pulmonary artery pressure increased in patients treated with compressed air.[49] Mortality was higher in sleep-desaturating patients versus those without nocturnal desaturation. Sleep quality also was better in the COPD patients who did not experience sleep-induced arterial oxygen desaturation, but surprisingly, although oxygen supplementation improved oxygenation, it did not improve sleep stage distribution in those patients with sleep-induced arterial oxygen desaturation. Thus oxygen therapy improves cardiovascular function and survival in COPD patients, but it may not improve sleep quality in these patients.

NONINVASIVE MECHANICAL VENTILATION

Several studies have examined the short-term impact of noninvasive pressure-assisted nocturnal ventilation on sleep quality and quality of life in patients with COPD. Since the work of breathing is elevated in COPD patients during wakefulness and sleep, it was reasoned that ventilatory muscle rest provided by mechanical assistance devices such as nCPAP would improve daytime muscle strength and endurance as well as sleep quality. Respiratory muscle performance, but not sleep quality, was improved in a study conducted by Mezzanotte and associates[50] in eight COPD patients given low levels of nCPAP (5 to 8 cmH$_2$O pressure) during sleep for 7 to 20 days compared with five COPD controls. These investigators found that if nCPAP pressures were taken too high, sleep disruption occurred. At these higher pressures, nCPAP would be expected to increase the work of breathing and produce hypercapnia, making the device less tolerable and less beneficial for COPD patients. This problem is partially resolved with the use of bilevel pressure noninvasive ventilatory support. This type of device delivers a higher pressure during inspiration than in expiration and thereby provides more of a ventilatory assist than nCPAP. Jones and colleagues[51] showed that arterial blood gases and overall quality-of-life variables were improved in chronically hypercapnic COPD patients with bilevel pressure support during sleep plus oxygen therapy compared with oxygen supplementation alone. Total sleep time and sleep efficiency increased with this pressure-support ventilatory assist device. Likely this improvement in sleep contributed to the improved quality-of-life data. In contrast, Gay and associates[52] did not find an improvement in sleep quality or in overall comfort in a group of hypercapnic COPD patients given bilevel noninvasive pressure support nightly for 3 months compared with a sham-treated patient group. Both these latter two studies used a run-in period to ensure stability of disease prior to beginning the trial. Thus the role of noninvasive pressure-assisted ventilatory support in sleep quality is unclear at this time. It may be especially useful for the COPD patients with respiratory muscle weakness or the patient with severe airways obstruction, both of whom might benefit from a period of ventilatory muscle rest. In these types of patients, volume-assisted ventilatory support may be considered. However, this type of ventilatory support has not been studied in a longitudinal fashion in COPD.

Summary

Worsening of the pulmonary physiology or the existence of a separate sleep disorder may produce disturbed sleep and subsequent daytime fatigue, sleepiness, and cognitive and/or affective abnormalities. Enhanced treatment of the lung disease, supplemental oxygen, and noninvasive ventilatory support all improve abnormal physiology and may improve sleep quality. Sedative-hypnotics can be used successfully, but care must be taken to make certain that these medications do not suppress ventilatory control, leading to nocturnal hypoxemia. Hopefully, clinicians will be concerned about the quality of sleep in patients with chronic lung diseases and be cognizant of the improvement in quality of life that a good night's sleep can provide these patients.

References

1. Cormick W, Olson LG, Hensley MJ, Saunders NA: Nocturnal hypoxemia and quality of sleep in patients with chronic obstructive pulmonary disease. *Thorax* 41:846–854, 1986.

2. Klink M, Dodge R, Quan SF: The relation of sleep complaints to respiratory symptoms in a general population. *Chest* 105:151–154, 1994.

3. Kinsman RA, Yaroush RA, Fernandez E, et al: Symptoms and experiences in chronic bronchitis and emphysema. *Chest* 83:755–761, 1983.

4. Montplaisir J, Walsh J, Malo JL: Nocturnal asthma: Features of attacks, sleep and breathing patterns. *Am Rev Respir Dis* 125:18–22, 1982.

5. Stokes DC, McBride JT, Wall MA, et al: Sleep hypoxemia in young adults with cystic fibrosis. *Am J Dis Child* 134:741–745, 1980.

6. Catterall JR, Douglas NJ, Calverley PMA, et al: Transient hypoxemia during sleep in chronic obstructive pulmonary disease is not a sleep apnea syndrome. *Am Rev Respir Dis* 128:24–29, 1983.

7. Mulloy E, McNicholas WT: Theophylline improves gas exchange during rest, exercise, and sleep in severe chronic obstructive pulmonary disease. *Am Rev Respir Dis* 148:1030–1036, 1993.

8. Hudgel DW, Martin RJ, Capehart M, et al: Contribution of hypoventilation to sleep oxygen desaturation in chronic obstructive pulmonary disease. *J Appl Physiol* 55(3):669–677, 1983.

9. George CF, West P, Kryger MH: Oxygenation and breathing pattern during phasic and tonic REM in patients with chronic obstructive pulmonary disease. *J Appl Physiol* 57:234–243, 1987.

10. Wynne JW, Block AJ, Hemenway J, et al: Disordered breathing and oxygen desaturation during sleep in patients with chronic obstructive lung disease (COLD). *Am J Med* 66:573–579, 1979.

11. Fleetham J, West P, Mezon B, et al: Sleep, arousals, and oxygen desaturation in chronic obstructive pulmonary disease: The effect of oxygen therapy. *Am Rev Respir Dis* 126:429–433, 1982.

12. Fletcher EC, Miller J, Divine GW, et al: Nocturnal oxyhemoglobin desaturation in COPD patients with arterial oxygen tensions above 60 mmHg. *Chest* 97:604–608, 1987.

13. Vos PJ, Folgering HT, van Herwaarden CL: Predictors for nocturnal hypoxaemia (mean $Sa_{O_2} < 90\%$) in normoxic and mildly hypoxic patients with COPD. *Eur Respir J* 8:74–77, 1995.

14. Johnson MW, Remmers JE: Accessory muscle activity during sleep in chronic obstructive pulmonary disease. *J Appl Physiol* 57:1011–1017, 1984.

15. Tirlapur VG, Mir MA: Nocturnal hypoxemia and associated electrocardiographic changes in patients with chronic obstructive airways disease. *N Engl J Med* 306:125–130, 1982.

16. Tatsumi K, Kimura H, Kunitomo F, et al: Sleep arterial oxygen desaturation and chemical control of breathing during wakefulness in COPD. *Chest* 90:68–73, 1986.

17. Power JT, Stevard IC, Connaughton JJ, et al: Nocturnal cough in patients with chronic bronchitis and emphysema. *Am Rev Respir Dis* 130:999–1001, 1984.

18. Ballard RD, Clover CW, Suh BY: Influence of sleep on respiratory function in emphysema. *Am J Respir Crit Care Med* 151:945–951, 1995.

19. Calverley PMA, Brezinova V, Douglas NJ, et al: The effect of oxygenation on sleep quality in chronic bronchitis and emphysema. *Am Rev Respir Dis* 126:206–210, 1982.

20. Ballard RD, Saathoff MC, Patel DK, et al: Effect of sleep on nocturnal bronchoconstriction and ventilatory patterns in asthmatics. *J Appl Physiol* 67:243–249, 1989.

21. Ballard RD, Clover CW, White DP: Influence of non-REM sleep on inspiratory muscle activity and lung volume in asthmatic patients. *Am Rev Respir Dis* 147:880–886, 1993.

22. Ballard RD, Irvin CG, Martin RJ, et al: Influence of sleep on lung volume in asthmatic patients and normal subjects. *J Appl Physiol* 68:2034–2041, 1990.

23. Catterall JR, Calverley PMA, Brezinova V, et al: Irregular breathing and hypoxaemia during sleep in chronic stable asthma. *Lancet* 1:301–304, 1982.

24. Martin RJ, Cicutto LC, Ballard RD, Szefler SJ: Airway inflammation in nocturnal asthma. *Am Rev Respir Dis* 137:284A, 1988.

25. Barnes P, FitzGerald G, Brown M, Dollery C: Nocturnal asthma and changes in circulating epinephrine, histamine and cortisol. *N Engl J Med* 303:263–267, 1986.

26. Catterall JR, Rhind GB, Whyte KF, et al: Is nocturnal asthma caused by changes in airway cholinergic activity? *Thorax* 43:720–724, 1988.

27. Pack AI: Acid: A nocturnal bronchoconstrictor? (editorial). *Am Rev Respir Dis* 141:1391–1392, 1990.

28. McNicholas WT, Coffey M, FitzGerald MX: Ventilation and gas exchange during sleep in patients with interstitial lung disease. *Thorax* 41:777–782, 1986.

29. Tatsumi K, Kimura H, Kunitomo F, et al: Arterial oxygen desaturation during sleep in interstitial pulmonary disease: Correlation with chemical control of breathing during wakefulness. *Chest* 95:962–967, 1989.

30. Bye PTP, Issa F, Berthon-Jones M, Sullivan CE: Studies of oxygenation during sleep in patients with interstitial lung disease. *Am Rev Respir Dis* 129:27–32, 1984.

31. Midgren B, Hansson L, Eriksson L, et al: Oxygen desaturation during sleep and exercise in patients with interstitial lung disease. *Thorax* 42:353–356, 1987.

32. Midgren B, Petersson K, Hansson K, et al: Nocturnal hypoxaemia in severe scoliosis. *Br J Dis Chest* 82:226–236, 1988.

33. Sawicka EH, Branthwaite MA: Respiration during sleep in kyphoscoliosis. *Thorax* 42:801–808, 1987.

34. van Keimpema ARJ, Ariaansz M, Nauta JJP, Postmus PE: Subjective sleep quality and mental fitness in asthmatic patients. *J Asthma* 32(1):69–74, 1995.

35. Ducolone A, Vandevenne A, Jouin H, et al: Gastroesophageal reflux in patients with asthma and chronic bronchitis. *Am Rev Respir Dis* 135:327–332, 1987.

36. Man GCW, Chapman KR, Ali SH, Darke AC: Sleep quality and nocturnal respiratory function with once-daily theophylline (Uniphyl) and inhaled salbutamol in patients with COPD. *Chest* 110:648–653, 1996.

37. Zwillich CW, Neagley SR, Cicutto L, et al: Nocturnal asthma therapy: Inhaled bitolterol versus sustained-release theophylline. *Am Rev Respir Dis* 139:470–474, 1989.

38. Martin RJ, Pak J: Overnight theophylline concentrations and effects on sleep and lung function in chronic obstructive pulmonary disease. *Am Rev Respir Dis* 145:540–544, 1992.

39. Martin RJ, Smith P, Hudgel D, et al: Ipratropium bromide (Atrovent) improves arterial oxygen saturation (Sa_{O_2}) in patients with COPD during sleep. *Am J Respir Crit Care Med* 153:A126, 1996.

40. Veale D, Cooper BG, Griffiths CJ, et al: The effect of controlled-release salbutamol on sleep and nocturnal oxygenation in patients with asthma and chronic obstructive pulmonary disease. *Respir Med* 88:121–124, 1994.

41. Van Keimpema Anton RJ, Ariaansz M, Raaijmakers Jan AM, et al: Treatment of nocturnal asthma by addition of oral slow-release albuterol to standard treatment in stable asthma patients. *J Asthma* 33(2):119–124, 1996.

42. Gothe B, Cherniack NS, Bachand RT Jr, et al: Long-term effects of almitrine bismesylate on oxygenation during wakefulness and sleep in chronic obstructive pulmonary disease. *Am J Med* 84:436–444, 1988.

43. Skatrud JB, Dempsey JA, Iber C, Bessenbrugge A: Correction of CO_2 retention during sleep in patients with chronic obstructive pulmonary disease. *Chest* 91:688–692, 1987.

44. Series F, Cormier Y: Effects of protriptyline on diurnal and noctur-

nal oxygenation in patients with chronic obstructive pulmonary disease. *Ann Intern Med* 113:507–511, 1990.

45. Block AJ, Dolly FR, Slayton PC: Does flurazepam ingestion affect breathing and oxygenation during sleep in patients with chronic obstructive lung disease? *Am Rev Respir Dis* 129:230–233, 1984.

46. Steens RD, Pouliot Z, Millar TTW, et al: Effects of zolpidem and triazolam on sleep and respiration in mild to moderate chronic obstructive pulmonary disease. *Sleep* 16(4):318–326, 1993.

47. Fulmer JD, Snider GL: ACCP-NHLBI National conference on oxygen therapy. *Chest* 86:234–247, 1984.

48. Fletcher ED, Luckett RA, Miller T, et al: Cardiopulmonary hemodynamics in lung disease patients with and without nocturnal oxyhemoglobin desaturation and arterial oxygen tensions above 60 torr. *Chest* 95:757–764, 1989.

49. Fletcher ED, Luckett RA, Goodnight-White S, et al: A double-blind trial of nocturnal supplemental oxygen for sleep desaturation in patients with chronic obstructive pulmonary disease and a daytime Pa_{O_2} above 6.0 mmHg. *Am Rev Respir Dis* 145:1070–1076, 1992.

50. Mezzanotte WS, Tangel DJ, Fox AM, et al: Nocturnal nasal continuous positive airway pressure in patients with chronic obstructive pulmonary disease. *Chest* 106:1100–1108, 1994.

51. Jones DJM, Paul EA, Jones PW, Wedzicha JA: Nasal pressure support ventilation plus oxygen compared with oxygen therapy alone in hypercapnic COPD. *Am J Respir Crit Care Med* 152:538–544, 1995.

52. Gay PC, Hubmayr RD, Stroetz RW: Efficacy of nocturnal nasal ventilation in stable, severe chronic obstructive pulmonary disease during a 3-month controlled trial. *Mayo Clin Proc* 71:533–542, 1996.

Chapter 21

NEUROPSYCHOLOGICAL ASSESSMENT OF CHRONIC OBSTRUCTIVE PULMONARY DISEASE

NANCY L. ADAMS

The American College of Chest Physicians (ACCP) and American Association of Cardiovascular and Pulmonary Rehabilitation (AACVPR) *Evidence-Based Guidelines*[1] note that "several studies have documented impairment on tests of cognitive or neuropsychological functioning among hypoxemic patients with chronic obstructive pulmonary disease (COPD),"[2-4] but no guidelines for intervention are presented. However, the evidence of cognitive changes in COPD discussed below suggests that this is a disease that affects the brain as well as cardiopulmonary function.[5] Chronic hypoxemia affects metabolism and thus affects neurotransmission, but it also may affect other cellular processes.[3,13] Second, psychological disturbance documented in many patients[6-9] suggests that depression and anxiety frequently affect those with COPD "but are not necessary concomitants" of the disease.[5] Behavioral interventions are used frequently in pulmonary rehabilitation programs; however, the guidelines'[1] review of this literature suggests that results are equivocal. Anxiolytics and antidepressants are often prescribed, but evidence-based guidelines are lacking.[1]

The literature suggests partial answers to these questions. This chapter reviews the type and extent of cognitive deficits and psychological complaints found in COPD patients. Based on this evidence, a psychologist should be part of the pulmonary rehabilitation screening process examining both cognitive and emotional status. Patients with responses below recommended cutoff scores on screening tests or who have additional medical or cognitive complaints should be considered for further medical or cognitive evaluations. Such data hopefully will be useful in designing individualized training and compensation strategies in pulmonary rehabilitation programming for patients and families. An individualized approach is recommended for several reasons: Cognitive and emotional deficits do not affect all COPD patients, deficits may improve with oxygen therapy but often do not fully clear, deficits are more likely to occur with older and less educated patients, and deficits may be affected by other sociocultural factors[5] and by disease duration.[2]

Cognitive Deficits

Cognitive deficits associated with hypoxemia in COPD patients were first described by Westlake and Kaye.[10] This work languished until Krop and colleagues[11] in 1973 demonstrated improved cognitive test scores for 10 subjects with severe COPD ($Pa_O \leq 55$ mmHg) after receiving a month of oxygen therapy compared with 12 controls with similar airway obstruction but $Pa_O > 55$ mmHg who received no oxygen therapy. The designs and small sample sizes limit the utility of these early studies.

The combined sample[12-15] of the Nocturnal Oxygen Therapy Trial (NOTT) and the Intermittent Positive Pressure Breathing (IPPB) study replicated and extended the work of Krop and colleagues.[11] These 302 patients are the largest group of patients studied to date and are drawn from multiple centers in the United States and Canada (six for NOTT and two for IPPB). Patients in the NOTT and IPPB studies were recruited from hospital clinic centers and private practices and studied before they began oxygen therapy. Nonpatient controls were selected by a standardized neighborhood search strategy beginning with the residence of the patient. Controls were matched to patients on age, sex, race, education, and occupation. Using the two-factor Hollingshead index of social position, patients and controls were in the lower-middle-class range and were of average intelligence [estimated from Wechsler Adult Intelligence Scale (WAIS) vocabulary subtest scores[23]]. Patients were excluded who had other causes for cognitive impairment. Sociodemographic characteristics and respiratory function values of the subjects are presented in Table 21-1.[3]

Pre- and posttesting was done while the patients were on room air. Tests assessed attention, language, abstracting, complex perceptual motor, simple sensory, simple motor, and memory functioning. Although subjects exhibited comparable levels of premorbid ability, pretreatment scores across the 27 tests showed that patients scored significantly worse than controls on most measures. Many of the individual tests showed a gradient of deterioration according to severity of hypoxemia, although groups did not vary significantly on age, education, or verbal intelligence test scores. No respiratory function measure predicted test scores except hypoxemia, although all patients had significant airway obstruction. To evaluate the incidence of cognitive impairment, scores on a summary cognitive test measure were compared between patient groups. After the effects of age were removed, 6 percent of the mildly hypoxemic patients, 26 percent of the moderately hypoxemic patients, and 41 percent of the severely hypoxemic patients were judged cognitively impaired.

The neuropsychological data were factor analyzed to reduce the number of variables.[4] A four-factor solution accounted for 58 percent of the variance. Factor scores for each patient were standardized so that they would have a mean of 0 and a standard deviation of 1, and the results are illustrated in Fig. 21-1. When scores were adjusted for age, the factor solution was essentially unchanged.

Multivariate analysis revealed that patients with increasing hypoxemia scored worse on three of the four factors. There were no differences between any patient group and controls on factor 1; tests that entered factor 1 came from tasks comprising verbal intelligence and memory measures. Factor 2 is a perceptual learning and problem-solving factor containing tests that are most sensitive to brain functioning; this factor most effectively separated the groups. Moderately hypoxemic subjects were significantly worse than controls and mildly hypoxemic patients but significantly better than the severely hypoxemic group.

Factor 3 was based primarily on tests that measure alertness and psychomotor speed. These skills appeared to be

TABLE 21-1 Basic Demographic and Pulmonary Characteristics of Combined NOTT/IPPB Patients and Controls: Means and Standard Deviations (SD)

	Group 1 Controls (N = 99)	Group 2 Mildly Hypoxemic COPD (N = 86)	Group 3 Moderately Hypoxemic COPD (N = 155)	Group 4 Severely Hypoxemic COPD (N = 61)
Age[a]	63.1 (10.3)	61.6 (7.5)	64.3 (8.2)	65.9 (8.3)
Education	10.2 (3.6)	9.7 (3.0)	9.8 (3.7)	9.4 (3.4)
Sex–male	75 (76%)	76 (88%)	119 (77%)	48 (77%)
Pa_{O_2} (mmHg) (resting, room air)		67.8 (6.3)	54.4 (2.7)	44.4 (4.1)
Pa_{CO_2} (mmHg) (resting, room air)		34.9 (4.1)	42.1 (7.4)	45.8 (8.4)
FEV_1, % predicted (prebronchodilator, best value)	38.0 (12.1)	29.3 (12.5)	30.9 (14.9)	
FVC_1, % predicted (prebronchodilator, best value)	68.2 (17.5)	53.2 (16.9)	54.3 (18.0)	

[a] ANOVA ($P < .05$); group 4 is significantly older than group 2 (Neuman Keuls).
SOURCE: Grant et al,[14] with permission.

preserved, even with moderate hypoxemia. Patients with severe hypoxemia, however, appeared to have significant difficulty with these tasks.

Factor 4 was comprised of scores on two measures of hand motor functioning. Mildly hypoxemic patients' scores were lower than those of controls but not significantly so. Moderate and severely hypoxemic patients showed approximately equal functional difficulties. Skills comprising factor 4 may exhibit a threshold effect.

Grant and coworkers[3] then explored what medical or demographic descriptors predict cognitive test performance.

Education played its largest role in predicting factor 1, accounting for 33 percent of the variance. Age and Pa_{O_2} accounted for 21 percent of the variance in factor 2, with education and other respiratory variables explaining an additional 9 percent of the variance. Education and respiratory rate accounted for 21 percent of the variance in factor 3, with age and Pa_{O_2} accounting for an additional 5 percent of the variance. Age and exercise level accounted for 18 percent of the variance in factor 4, with hemoglobin, education, and Pa_{O_2} accounting for an additional 5 percent of the variance.

Of perhaps more importance, a combination of age and

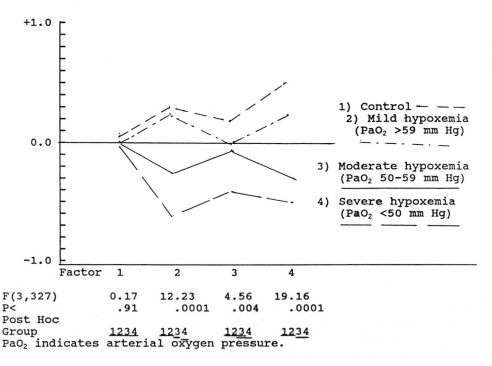

FIGURE 21-1 Factor analytically derived ability scores for controls and patients with COPD at three levels of hypoxemia.

Pa_{O_2} accounted for most of the variance in factor 2, the factor most sensitive to brain disease. Hypoxemia is the one medical variable that contributes reliably to explaining performance deficits. After reviewing the neuroscience literature, Grant and coworkers[3,13] suggested that hypoxemia affects the biosynthetic pathways that produce neurotransmitters, especially acetylcholine.

Della Sala and colleagues[16] questioned whether COPD patients with mild to moderate hypoxemia and who qualify for oxygen therapy would demonstrate deficits on focused and divided attention tasks. On such tasks, patients and controls scored essentially at ceiling on accuracy, but patients, as predicted, had significantly longer reaction times than controls. Patients were close to 5 years younger than the subjects studied by Grant and coworkers.[3,12-15] The study needs to be replicated with a larger U.S. sample but shows promise as a method sensitive to cognitive effects in COPD patients exhibiting mild hypoxemia.

Do cognitive deficits improve with oxygen therapy? Krop and colleagues[11] reported mild improvements for 10 patients tested on oxygen compared with 12 controls with an equal degree of COPD after 1 month of therapy. Finger Tapping, a test of motor speed, increased by roughly a third bilaterally; other changes in test scores were statistically significant but minor in degree. Heaton and coworkers[12] suggested that these changes reflect short-term effects of oxygen that have a rapid onset, probably relating to improvement in functioning of hypoxic neurons from stimulation of oxygen-dependent enzyme systems involved in the synthesis of neurotransmitters.[16-21]

Heaton and coworkers[12] reported follow-up cognitive and personality test data on 150 NOTT patients 6 months after they were randomized to continuous oxygen treatment (COT) or nocturnal oxygen treatment (NOT). After 6 months of treatment, patients were retested after stabilization on room air; 42 percent showed very modest improvement in comparison with normal controls, and the rates on COT and NOT were indistinguishable. Heaton and colleagues[12] suggested that more improvement was seen by Krop and coworkers[11] in their patients because they were tested on oxygen. Twenty COT and 17 NOT patients were retested on room air after 12 months of therapy. COT patients scored significantly higher than NOT patients on three of five standardized summary test measures. Although statistically significant, these changes were minor in degree. Heaton and colleagues[12] speculated these beneficial effects of oxygen therapy, evident when tested on room air after a year of treatment, reflect renewed synthesis of macromolecules critical to the neuron's physicochemical integrity, formation of neurotransmitters, or other metabolic needs. There were no changes on personality test or quality-of-life measures over the 6- or 12-month treatment periods. Heaton and colleagues[12] speculated that their measures may not be sufficiently sensitive or the patients may be insufficiently sensitive to life changes, consistent with Dudley's observation[22] that their lives are in an "emotional straightjacket."

Cognitive abilities were found to deteriorate significantly in patients who received maximum oxygen and medical therapies over an average of 10-year disease duration by Incalze and coworkers.[2] This was a carefully designed study limited, however, to a small sample from a lower socioeconomic class of Italian background. It needs to be replicated with U.S.

patients. Subjects had episodes of decompensated COPD with chronic respiratory failure during the previous 2 years and were diagnosed with hypoxic-hypercapnic COPD despite receiving maximal oxygen and medical therapies. The study first compared performance of COPD patients with that of normal controls, normal elderly, and samples of patients with multi-infarct and Alzheimer's dementias. The study protocol included more verbal measures and measures with some easier items than in the studies by Grant and coworkers.[3,12-15] Among COPD patients, lower scores were obtained by those with longer disease duration and those who were older. Patients with less education tended to score lower. Stage of COPD and arterial blood-gas measures did not discriminate between patient groups.

The group profiles of COPD patients, normal elderly (10 years older), and those with multi-infarct dementia were similar. On average, patients with COPD performed slightly worse than older normal individuals. COPD patients studied by Grant and coworkers[3,12-15] responded closely to normal elderly, suggesting that COPD leads to diffuse brain impairment. Data obtained by Incalze and colleagues[16] suggested that some additional process, not understood, compromises verbal memory, verbal generativity, and expressive skills in this older COPD sample, areas that are intact in the work of Grant and coworkers.[3,12-15] This mild verbal impairment was significant in comparisons of COPD patients and normal controls.

The second principal finding of the work of Incalze and colleagues[16] was that with increasing disease duration, patients with COPD showed increasingly different cognitive profiles. Using discriminate analysis, the cognitive profile described earlier classified approximately half the COPD patients. The scores of 12 percent in the remainder were comparable with those of normal controls and 15 percent comparable with those of the normal elderly (not showing the verbal deficits noted). Twelve percent also were comparable with those in the multi-infarct sample and 12 percent comparable with the Alzheimer's sample. No further diagnostic work was done, however, to determine whether some of the Incalze and coworkers' COPD patients might meet multiple neurologic diagnostic criteria.

Summary and Recommendations

Cognitive test profiles of COPD patients do not fit a simple pattern. When patients first come to medical attention cognitive deficits are usually most evident on perceptual learning and problem-solving tasks with verbal intelligence intact. Deficits are usually mild. Age, Pa_{O_2}, and education may predict up to 25 percent of the variance in neuropsychological test performance. Reaction times may be more sensitive to mild cognitive impairment. Initially, there is evidence of worse deficits in subjects with lower Pa_{O_2}. However, as the disease progresses, there is likely to be further cognitive deterioration and no relationship between mental status and physical parameters of COPD is apparent. This may be because, as COPD progresses, exacerbations are marked by other factors, including hypercapnia, acidosis, or hypocapnia secondary to hypoxemia-induced hyperventilation or transient oxyhemoglobin desaturation.

There are no studies evaluating what cognitive deficits are

predictive of difficulty in pulmonary rehabilitation programs. Based on cognitive rehabilitation studies, the following suggestions may prove useful.

I suggest that a clinical psychologist be considered as part of the evaluation team. The psychologist can screen patients to answer whether any emotional distress can be addressed in educational or psychological groups or whether referrals for further diagnosis or medication are needed. The psychologist also can screen patients' cognitive abilities. This information will be useful in individualizing the programming and deciding whether a neuropsychological referral is needed. The cognitive screening should examine whether the patient can read with comprehension the written material used in the program. My experience at my own hospital with informed consent procedures is that patients in clinical trials need material written at a fourth- to fifth-grade level. The role of the neuropsychologist is to serve as a consultant to the clinical psychologist, evaluate patients with significant cognitive deficits, interpret the results to the patient and family, and teach pulmonary rehabilitation staff compensation strategies that may be useful to particular patients or that might be considered for general program strategies.

Selection of tests for a neuropsychological screening battery and remediation aids that will be most useful will depend on when patients are referred. If they are referred earlier in their disease course when cognitive deficits are absent or milder they may learn more easily. If they are referred as part of a final intervention effort they are more likely to have cognitive symptoms, be less able to learn, and suffer from more emotional distress.

Results of a simple reaction time test may be useful in identifying patients with mild to moderate disease who qualify for oxygen therapy and who need longer to process new information. No cognitive deficit is usually suspected by medical staff in this group. The longer response time may not make a significant difference in programming. However, these patients may be more vulnerable to cognitive decline as their disease progresses; this is a question for further research.

Based on the results of the NOTT and IPPB trials, patients with moderate and severe hypoxemia also may need some additional time to process information or perform tasks. This is the group of patients studied by Incalzi and colleagues,[2] who found some patients with cognitive functioning comparable with patients with multi-infarct or Alzheimer's dementia. These patients are also more likely to have other significant cognitive deficits.

Trail Making B can be used to evaluate problem solving skills. The Ray Auditory Verbal Learning Test[23] can be used to evaluate learning and prose recognition memory portion to evaluate exaggeration of deficits. Premorbid intellectual ability as well as reading ability can be estimated from the WAIS vocabulary subtest or the North American Adult Reading Test.[23] Premorbid ability level can be estimated from the WAIS vocabulary subtest or the North American Adult Reading Test.[23] Patients who score more than 2 standard deviations below their estimated premorbid ability level are likely to have significant cognitive deficits.[23] The Mattis Dementia Rating Scale and the CERAD Behavior Rating Scale for Dementia[23] may be more useful with more seriously ill patients.

Patients with significant deficits are likely to benefit from

program modifications borrowed from the neuropsychological rehabilitation literature.[24,25] Other pulmonary rehabilitation patients also may benefit from these techniques when anxiety or depression interfere with performance.

Executive function (problem-solving) deficits are common in patients with compromised frontal brain functioning. Following Luria, problem solving includes these steps[24,25]:

1. Motivational difficulties that may be independent of depression, anxiety, or other personality disturbance
2. Ability to restrain impulsivity, investigate the problem, and analyze its features
3. Selection of possible solutions and creation of a plan of action
4. Choice of appropriate methods for executing the plan
5. Solving the problem
6. Evaluating the solution and making appropriate corrections

Many programs focus first on training the patient to be aware of his or her difficulties and using positive-reinforcement methods to motivate activity and self-awareness. Program structuring is used to identify problems and implement solutions. Specific recommendations can be found in Meier and coworkers[24] and the program by the Florida Society of Neurology.[25]

Language deficits should be suspected in patients with severe hypoxemia. Identifying language deficits[23] and structuring the program to accommodate them are crucial. The most important issues include identifying how much information a patient can process (one versus two or more clauses) at a time and whether the patient understands more complex grammatical structures. Second, the examination evaluates naming ability. Third, the examination evaluates the patient's ability to organize and express her or his thoughts. Subtests from the Benton Multilingual Aphasia Examination[23] may be used; these subtests have adequate norms and results can be obtained in approximately a half hour.

Memory deficits[23–27] can be addressed in several ways:

1. *Use of memory aids.* These include presenting the patient with written information and having the patient write information in memory notebooks, calendars, etc. This is particularly useful for patients with prospective memory deficits (trouble recalling to do something in the future). It is crucial that the patient learn to consistently use the memory aid. Procedures need to be rehearsed as part of the training program. When patients question what to do, they need to be directed to where the information can be found rather than being told the answer. For more severely compromised patients, caregivers need to be trained in the same skills.

2. *Use routines.* As much as possible, make the rehabilitation program routine. It may be helpful to allow patients to help plan the less structured portions of the day (e.g., educational or psychotherapy sessions) to improve motivation, teach them that problems can be specified (to help overcome catastrophising), and encourage participation.

3. *Include patients in instruction roles.* Doing this on a rotating basis in presentation of information or in leading portions of exercises or programs may facilitate learning.

4. *Using spaced retrieval,*[28] a modification of repetition of information. This may be more useful with patients who

have more severe cognitive deficits. Essentially patients are cued to recall the information with increasingly longer delay intervals between cuing (e.g., 1 min, 5 min). When the patient fails, cuing returns to the lower level of success and continues until the patient has no difficulty recalling the task in the future. This is a labor-intensive method that is quite successful and may be useful to teach caregivers.

Lezak,[23] Meier,[24] the Florida Society of Neurology,[25] Brandimonte and coworkers,[26] and Wilson[27] give additional suggestions for working with memory deficits. The screening memory test suggested earlier may provide trainers with the information they need to decide what compensation strategies to use. Patients who perform poorly on the screening tests are more likely to need more detailed neuropsychological assessment. Information from rehabilitation personnel and families may help target the evaluation so that it can be briefer and provide more specific recommendations.

Deficits in motor dexterity or motor strength were common in NOTT and IPPB patients. This may be judged in current patients by the physical therapist or can be tested for quickly by the neuropsychologist with the instruments used in the NOTT and IPPB trials. These deficits may mean that these patients fatigue more easily and need breaks and will hopefully respond to more physical therapy. Implicit memory techniques may assist motor learning.

Quality of Life

The quality-of-life literature is complex because it reflects so many different perspectives. Schipper and coworkers[29] define quality of life as including (1) physical functioning, (2) occupational functioning, (3) psychological functioning, (4) social interaction, and (5) somatic sensation. Pulmonary rehabilitation programs often use instruments from the quality-of-life literature to identify goals of rehabilitation and determine whether a given patient warrants treatment for emotional distress. Quality of life measures may correlate more highly with patient complaints than physical function measures.[34] Instruments are also used in program evaluation. This section will review the literature on instrumentation and implications that can be drawn for an integrated biopsychosocial model of quality of life for COPD.

Quality-of-life studies in COPD often include one or more of these instruments: the Sickness Impact Profile, Quality of Well-Being Scale, McMaster Health Index Questionnaire, Medical Outcomes Study Short Form 36, and Nottingham Health Profile. These instruments all contain items covering multiple domains of functioning. They vary in length but generally can be completed in under 30 minutes. This practice provides evidence of convergent validity and allows comparisons with other chronic diseases. Studies generally show that COPD produces disability comparable with other chronic diseases.[30] The disadvantage of the general instruments is that too little information may be provided about the specific qualities of a disease. COPD patients are not wheelchair-bound and can get around their homes, so their mobility measures are relatively good on most scales. However, the general measures do not take into account the extreme effort patients may make to achieve this mobility. This omission seems to have led to denials of disability claims.[30,32] A few

TABLE 21-2 Sleep Hygiene Rules for Trouble with Sleep onset or Difficulty Maintaining Sleep

1. Go to bed at the same time every night. Set aside an area outside your bedroom where you will not be disturbed. Include a comfortable chair and a reading light. Select material to read that you enjoy but can put down easily. Avoid material that will make you want to stay awake to finish. Read for 30 min or so, until you feel sleepy, and then go to bed. The goal of this rule is to mentally and emotionally disengage from daily activities. Second, it may help you become more sensitive to internal cues of sleepiness so that you will be more likely to fall asleep when you go to bed.

2. Do not use your bed for anything except sleep; i.e., do not read, watch television, eat, or worry in bed. Sexual activity is the only exception to this rule. This rule is designed to place activities associated with arousal away from the bedroom and to break up behavioral patterns or aversive conditioning associated with the bedroom.
    a. If bedtime is the time you have for thinking about the day's events and planning the next day, stop this behavior and set aside a period of time during the day prior to bedtime to worry and plan.
    b. Many people without sleep problems read or listen to music or television in bed without disturbing their sleep. This may not be the case for those with sleep disorders. This instruction is designed to establish new routines to facilitate sleep onset.

3. If you find yourself unable to fall asleep, get up and return to reading. Stay up until you feel sleepy, and then return to the bedroom to sleep. Younger people should get up after 10 min in bed and older persons after 20 min.

4. If you awaken during the night, repeat rule 3. Do this as often as necessary throughout the night.
    Rules 3 and 4 are intended to help you dissociate bed from any frustration associated with not falling asleep easily or awakening during the night. By getting out of the bedroom and engaging in sleep-promoting activities, you are taking control of the problem, which is likely to make the sleep disorder more manageable, reduce any distress associated with sleeping, and weaken any negative feelings associated with the bedroom.

5. Set your alarm and get up at the same time every morning irrespective of how much sleep you got during the night. This will help your body to acquire a consistent sleep rhythm.
    People with insomnia often have irregular sleep habits because they try to make up for a short night of sleep by sleeping later in the morning or napping during the day. It is important to break this cycle by sticking to a regular sleep schedule. Initially, you may feel somewhat sleep deprived as you start this program. However, feeling tired may increase the chances you will fall asleep earlier the following night and strengthen the cues of bed and bedroom for sleep.
    Often patients with insomnia are used to following a different sleep schedule on weekends or nights off work than they do during the week. It is important to have as consistent a schedule for all seven nights as possible. However, a deviation of no more than an hour in wake times has not been found to interfere with establishing a consistent routine.

6. Do not nap during the day. However, one brief nap that takes place regularly does not seem to interfere with bedtime sleepiness. Many people have a habit of napping 30 to 45 min or of relaxing for 20 to 30 min as a nap substitute. The nap should not, however, reduce the chance you will feel sleepy in the evening.

SOURCE: From Bootzin and Rider,[39] with permission.

instruments specific to COPD are now available, and these would be more appropriate to use in program evaluation and individualized patient planning. The best known is the Chronic Respiratory Disease Questionnaire (CRDQ).[33] McSweeny and Labuhn[30] mention other measures and review the quality-of-life literature.

Assessing emotional disturbance is a quality-of-life issue and is important in designing pulmonary rehabilitation programs and treating patients.[34] Depression, characterized by pessimism, self-dislike, and feelings of sadness, is reported in almost all studies of COPD in this country and in Europe. Incidence rates range from 2 percent to over 70 percent;

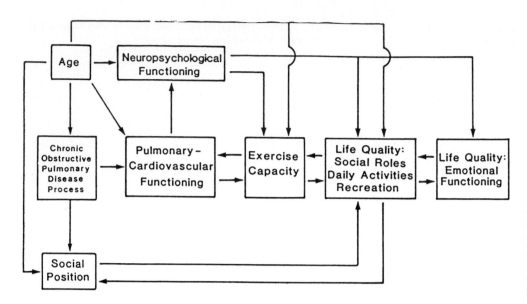

FIGURE 21-2 Heuristic model for the interrelation of COPD and other variables affecting life quality. (From McSweeny et al.[39] Copyright by the American Medical Association. Reprinted with permission.)

baseline incidence of major depression in men (who comprise most of the COPD population) ranges from 5 to 12 percent and for dysthymic disorder is approximately 3 percent. The latter rate is somewhat higher for women. Studies generally concur[30] that depression is higher than base rates in COPD and that the cause is reactive to losses associated with the chronic condition. Borak and coworkers[31] found that a majority of 48 COPD patients reported high degrees of anxiety, depression, and psychological tension; had low self-esteem; and did not believe that long-term oxygen therapy would be effective. Kaptein and colleagues[32] reported significant partial correlations among depression, anxiety, and social stigma with the presence of dyspnea and absence from work. However, damage to the limbic system by the disease process may contribute to affective symptoms.[30] A few COPD patients require treatment for psychotic symptoms, supporting the view that COPD has caused some compromise in brain function. Patients should be evaluated for the presence of a major depression or an anxiety disorder. There is also a higher incidence of personality disorders and abuse of alcohol, which patients may be using to minimize their emotional distress. Medications suggested for either depression or anxiety need to be selected in cooperation with pulmonary physicians, minimizing side effects and complications with pulmonary medications.

In an education or group psychotherapy program, patients should have the opportunity to discuss the losses they have suffered from COPD and the relationship between anxiety and increased dyspnea, as well as adaptations they have made in their lives because of these reactions. The goal is to promote some external validation for their feelings as well as explore alternatives to their choices. Patients may need to learn that it is acceptable to ask for help, and they may need information to mobilize such resources as home health aids and other community assistance. The program should include training in both cognitive and behavioral coping strategies. By carefully organizing their activities, patients can conserve energy and accomplish more. Learning to effectively intervene in their lives should help patients feel a sense of mastery and self-efficacy.

Patients should be evaluated for sleep disorders because many COPD patients have sleep complaints, as discussed below; in addition, there is a high incidence of depression among patients with sleep apnea. The psychotherapy group is also a good setting to learn relaxation methods for emotional control. Progressive relaxation,[37] diaphragmatic breathing, autogenic training, meditation, yoga, hypnosis, and electromyographic biofeedback are effective nonpharmacologic treatments for anxiety and for sleep disorders.

Patients with COPD have a variety of sleep complaints, including disruptions of sleep with cough, dyspnea, or restlessness. Patients with sleep apnea are at increased risk for COPD.[37] They are prone to develop poor sleep hygiene due to the sleep disruption. Recommendations by Bootzin and coworkers[38] include a combination of stimulus-control instructions and relaxation training, as well as general sleep education. Relaxation therapy should be taught in class rather than by a tape so that instructions are not conditioned to the recorder.[39] The role sleep disorders play in the illness should be covered in patient education (see Table 21-2).

Emphasize steps 3 and 4 of Table 21-2 for patients who have difficulty with sleep maintenance. Use sleep logs to track areas of difficulty and progress. Sleep rehabilitation therapy may be done in group sessions. However, development of each patient's treatment plan should be individualized. Compliance is likely to be higher and areas of confusion identified and clarified when instructions and rationale are discussed individually with patients for each treatment rule.

Quality-of-life studies of COPD patients[30,35] show that social role functioning, especially outside the home, and sexual functioning are limited. Hobbies and recreational activities are limited. Patients who are older, have less education, have lower socioeconomic status, and have fewer psychosocial assets and economic security show poorer quality of life. Data show a strong correlation between improved exercise capacity and quality of life.[36] McSweeny and coworkers[40] and Prigatano and colleagues[41] examined the relationship between neuropsychological functioning and quality of life [measured by the Sickness Impact Profile (SIP) total score] using correlation coefficients and regression analyses. They found moderate but significant differences between neuropsychological functioning (reflected in a summary measure of cognitive abilities) and SIP total score. Clinician ratings of neuropsychological impairment significantly contributed to a multiple regression analysis including age, socioeconomic status, and COPD severity as predictors, with SIP total score as the dependent variable. Twenty-five percent of the quality-of-life variance was accounted for by the overall equation. McSweeny's heuristic model explaining these interrelationships of COPD and other variables affecting quality of life is explained in Fig. 21-2.

The American Thoracic Society[42] maintains a web site to provide information about quality of life and functional status instruments used in assessment of patients with pulmonary disease: http://www.thoracic.org/qol/qcrit.html

References

1. ACCP/AACVPR Pulmonary Rehabilitation Guidelines Panel: Pulmonary rehabilitation: Joint ACCP/AACVPR evidence-based guidelines. *J Cardiopulmonary Rehabil* 7:371–405, 1997.
2. Incalzi RA, Gemma A, Marra C, et al: Chronic obstructive pulmonary disease: An original model of cognitive decline. *Am Rev Respir Dis* 148:418–424, 1993.
3. Grant I, Heaton RK, McSweeny AJ, et al: Neuropsychologic finding in hypoxemic chronic obstructive pulmonary disease. *Arch Intern Med* 142:1470–1476, 1982.
4. Fix AJ, Golden CJ, Daughton D, et al: Neuropsychological deficits among patients with chronic obstructive pulmonary disease. *Int J Neurosci* 16:99–105, 1982.
5. Griffith DE, Kronenberg RS: Psychologic, neuropsychologic, and social aspects of COPD, in Cherniack NS (ed): *Chronic Obstructive Pulmonary Disease.* Philadelphia, Saunders, 1991.
6. Agle DP, Baum GL, Chester EH, et al: Multidiscipline treatment of chronic pulmonary insufficiency: I. Psychological aspects of rehabilitation. *Psychosom Med* 35:41–49, 1973.
7. Borak J, Sliwinski P, Piasecki A, et al: Psychological status of COPD patients on long-term oxygen therapy. *Eur Respir J* 4:59–62, 1991.
8. Light RW, Merrill EJ, Despares JA, et al: Prevalence of depression and anxiety in patients with COPD. *Chest* 87:35–38, 1985.
9. Morgan AD, Peck DF, Buchanan DR, et al: Effect of attitudes and beliefs on exercise tolerance in chronic bronchitis. *Br Med J* 286:171–173, 1983.
10. Westlake L, Kaye M: Raised intracranial pressure in emphysema. *Br J Med* 1:302–304, 1954.
11. Krop H, Block AJ, Cohen E: Neuropsychologic effects of continuous oxygen therapy in chronic obstructive pulmonary disease. *Chest* 64:317–322, 1973.
12. Heaton RK, Grant I, McSweeny AJ, et al: Psychologic effects of continuous and nocturnal oxygen therapy in hypoxemic chronic obstructive pulmonary disease. *Arch Intern Med* 143:1941–1947, 1983.
13. Prigatano GP, Parsons O, Wright E, et al: Neuropsychological test performance in mildly hypoxemic patients with chronic obstructive pulmonary disease. *J Consult Clin Psychol* 51:108–116, 1983.
14. Grant I, Prigatano G, Heaton R, et al: Progressive neuropsychologic impairment and hypoxemia. *Arch Gen Psychiatry* 44:999–1006, 1987.
15. Rourke S, Adams KM: The neuropsychological correlates of acute and chronic hypoxemia, in Grant I, Adams KM (eds): *Neuropsychological Assessment of Neuropsychiatric Disorders.* New York, Oxford University Press, 1996.
16. Della Sala S, Donner CF, Sacco C, Spinnler H: Does chronic lung failure lead to cognitive failure? *Arch Suiss Neurol Psych* 143:343–354, 1992.
17. Davis JN, Carlson A, MacMillan V, et al: Brain tryptophan hydroxylation: Dependence on arterial oxygen tension. *Science* 182:72–74, 1973.
18. Gibson GE, Pulsinelli W, Blass JP, et al: Brain dysfunction in mild to moderate hypoxia. *Am J Med* 70:1247–1254, 1981.
19. MacMillan V: Cerebral monoamine and energy metabolism during recovery from hypoxia-oligemia. *Can J Physiol Pharmacol* 58:147–152, 1980.
20. Salford LG, Plum F, Siesjo BK: Graded anoxia-oligemia in rat brain: I. Biochemical alterations and their implications. *Arch Neurol* 29:227–233, 1973.
21. Siesjo BK: Brain energy metabolism and catecholaminergic activity in hypoxia, hypercapnia, and ischemia. *J Neural Transm Suppl* 14:17–22, 1978.
22. Dudley DL: *Psychophysiology of Respiration in Health and Disease.* New York, Appleton-Century-Crofts, 1969.
23. Lezak MD: *Neuropsychological Assessment,* 3d ed. New York, Oxford University Press, 1995.
24. Meier MJ, Benton AL, Diller L: *Neuropsychological Rehabilitation.* New York, Guilford Press, 1987.
25. Florida Society of Neurology: Treatment of behavioral disorders, 22d annual course in behavioral neurology and neuropsychology, 1996. Orlando, FL.
26. Brandimonte M, Einstein GO, McDaniel MA (eds): *Prospective Memory: Theory and Applications.* Mahwah, NJ, Lawrence Erlbaum and Associates, 1996.
27. Wilson BA: *Rehabilitation of Memory.* New York, Guilford Press, 1987.
28. McKittrick L, Camp C, Black FW: Prospective memory intervention in Alzheimer's disease. *J Gerontol* 47:337–343, 1992.
29. Schipper H, Clinch J, Power V: Definitions and conceptual issues, in Spiker B (ed): *Quality of Life Assessments in Clinical Trials.* New York, Raven Press, 1990.
30. McSweeny AJ, Labuhn KT: The relationship of neuropsychological functioning to health-related quality of life in systemic disease: The example of chronic obstructive pulmonary disease, in Grant I, Adams KM (eds): *Neuropsychological Assessment of Neuropsychiatric Disorders.* New York, Oxford University Press, 1996.
31. Borak J, Sliwinski P, Piasecki Z, Zielinski J: Psychological status of COPD patients on long-term oxygen therapy. *Eur Respir J* 4:59–61, 1991.
32. Kaptein AA, Brand PLP, Dekker FW, et al: Quality-of-life in a long-term multicentre trial in chronic nonspecific lung disease: Assessment at baseline. *Eur Respir J* 6:1479–1484, 1993.
33. Guyatt GH, Berman LB, Townsend M, et al: A measure of quality of life for clinical trials in chronic lung disease. *Thorax* 42:773–778, 1987.
34. Kaplan RM, Eakin EG, Ries AL: Psychosocial issues in the rehabilitation of patients with chronic obstructive pulmonary disease, in Casaburi R, Petty TL (eds): *Principles and Practice of Pulmonary Rehabilitation.* Philadelphia, Saunders, 1993.
35. Williams SJ: Chronic respiratory illness and disability: A critical review of the psychosocial literature. *Soc Sci Med* 28:791–803, 1989.
36. Lacasse Y, Wong E, Guyatt GH, et al: Meta-analysis of respiratory rehabilitation in chronic obstructive pulmonary disease. *Lancet* 348:1115–1119, 1996.
37. Rourke SB, Adams KM: The neuropsychological correlates of acute and chronic hypoxemia, in Grant I, Adams KM (eds): *Neuropsychological Assessment of Neuropsychiatric Disorders.* New York, Oxford University Press, 1996.
38. Bernstein DA, Borkovec T: *Progressive Relaxation Training: A Manual for the Helping Professions.* Champaign, Ill.: Research Press, 1973.
39. Bootzin R, Rider S: Behavioral techniques and biofeedback for insomnia, in Pressman M, Orr W (eds): *Understanding Sleep: The*

Evaluation and Treatment of Sleep Disorders. Washington, American Psychological Association, 1997.
40. McSweeny AJ, Grant I, Heaton RK, et al: Life quality of patients with chronic obstructive pulmonary disease. *Arch Intern Med* 142:473–478, 1982.

41. Prigatano GP, Wright EC, Levin D: Quality of life and its predictors with mild hypoxemia and chronic obstructive pulmonary disease. *Arch Intern Med* 144:1613–1619, 1984.
42. American Thoracic Society: Health-Related Quality of Life Research: Measuring Patient Centered Outcomes. Chicago, 1998.

Chapter 22

ASSESSMENT OF PSYCHOSOCIAL STATUS

AUDREY G. GIFT

GEORGIA L. NARSAVAGE

Assessment of the chronic obstructive pulmonary disease (COPD) patient needs to be comprehensive, including a history and physical examination, pulmonary function tests, laboratory tests, and measures of psychosocial status. This is important because psychosocial status has been shown to be linked to other parameters, for instance, to blood-gas changes such as hypoxia and hypercapnia. Hypoxemia has been shown to bring about changes in neurophysiologic functioning and to be associated with depression.[1] Administration of oxygen, however, has been shown to have no effect on the depression seen in COPD.[2] Even those on long-term oxygen therapy have been shown to have high levels of depression and low self-esteem.[3] Depression may be related to dyspnea level as well as the actual level of oxygenation. Depression levels have been shown to be higher, plasma oxygen levels lower, and plasma carbon dioxide levels higher at times of high dyspnea when compared with times of low dyspnea.[4] Others have proposed that carbon dioxide levels are related to the decreased ventilation seen with increased depression.[5] Low carbon dioxide levels have been associated with high levels of depression, especially when the severity of airway obstruction is taken into consideration.[6] Thus the many changes that occur with COPD may influence the evaluation of depression in these patients.

Psychosocial status also must be considered in light of the medications the patient is taking. Research suggests that the higher levels of depression, characterized by a pessimistic outlook, with feelings of hopelessness and worthlessness, found in COPD patients when compared with normal individuals may be due to the use of systemic steroids.[7] Depression in COPD has been found to be higher than in those with spinal cord injuries but similar to that in those with multiple sclerosis or rheumatoid arthritis who also take systemic steroids.[8] Other medications that have been implicated as contributing to psychological changes are antihypertensives, hormones, H_2 receptor blockers, antibiotics, and others.

Another factor found to be related to the psychological status of the COPD patient and that should be considered in a comprehensive assessment is the smoking history of the patient. In a study of 3213 adults in a community, depression was found to occur in 2.9 percent of the nonsmokers and in 6.6 percent in those who did smoke.[9] Those with depression also were found to be 40 percent less likely to quit when compared with nondepressed individuals.[9a] This relationship between smoking and an increase in psychiatric symptomatology has been reported in other diseases as well, with those who smoke reported to have greater depression.[10]

The assessment of the psychological status of the patient is important to integrate into a comprehensive assessment of the COPD patient. In a study of 600 adults, it was found that those with more psychological symptoms were more likely to report respiratory symptoms than those without psychological symptoms.[11] Since the psychological state of the patient also has been linked with their level of functioning, a comprehensive assessment of the patient should include an assessment of his or her functional status, especially performance. While such a comprehensive assessment of the patient is desirable, it is beyond the scope of this chapter. This chapter focuses only on that portion of the assessment related to psychological status. First, several comprehensive psychological assessment instruments will be described, followed by a presentation of each of the psychological dimensions implicated in the care of the COPD patient. Each psychological dimension will be defined, the effect on rehabilitation discussed, and tools for measurement presented. While it is understood that the clinician would not want to administer a battery of instruments to assess all psychological dimensions in every patient, multiple measures are presented to give the clinician a comparison of the tools available for use when a patient's history would indicate such a need. Others may wish to adopt a comprehensive screening tool for wider use. These will be discussed first.

Multidimensional Assessment of Psychological Status

There are a number of psychological assessment tools designed to evaluate a battery of psychological symptom dimensions. It is important to remember that these batteries are designed to screen patients most likely to suffer from psychological symptoms and to identify those in need of further evaluation from a mental health provider.

The *Minnesota Multiphasic Personality Inventory* (MMPI) was designed to assess the personality of older adults. It consists of 550 true-false items organized into 10 dimensions of personality: hypochondriasis, depression, hysteria, psychopathic-deviate, masculinity-femininity, paranoia, psychasthenia, schizophrenia, hypomania, and social introversion. Scores are also obtained on four validity scales: question, lie, validity, and defensiveness. An examiner is required to administer and score the inventory. It is available in 45 languages, making it one of the most widely used psychological tests in the world. It is also available in a revised version, known as the MMPI-2. The depression scale consists of 15 items and takes about 5 minutes to administer.

The *Symptom Checklist 90, Revised* (SCL-90-R) is a psychological screening test that has been normed for adult medical patients, adult psychiatric patients, and adolescents. It consists of 90 items assessing current psychological status along 9 symptom dimensions that include depression, anxiety, somatization and hostility, obsessive-compulsive, interpersonal sensitivity, phobic anxiety, paranoid ideation, and psychoticism. There are three global indices of distress (the global severity index, positive symptom index, and positive symptom total). Each item on the SCL-90-R is rated on a five-point scale of distress ranging from "not at all" at one pole to "extremely" at the other. An average score is obtained for the items on each scale and converted to a T score from the appropriate normative group.[12] Concurrent validity was established with the MMPI as the criterion. Internal consistency has been established using Cronbach's alpha at .87 for the total inventory and range from .72 to .81 for the subscales. The short form of this scale is called the *Brief Symptom Inventory* (BSI). It consists of 53 items measuring the same 9 symptom dimensions as the long form.

Another screening tool that measures a battery of psychiatric symptoms is the *Profile of Mood States* (POMS). Subjects are asked to indicate their feelings for the past week by responding to 65 one-word or short-phrase items naming an emotion. Each emotion is rated on a five-point scale from not at all to extremely. The scale can be self-administered or delivered orally. The Profile of Mood States has been used widely in research. It takes approximately 20 min to administer. The POMS measures six affective or emotional dimensions: tension (9 items), depression (15 items), anger (12 items), vigor (8 items), fatigue (7 items), and confusion (7 items).[13] The scoring ranges from 0 to 60, with norms provided for college students and psychiatric patients.[14] Internal consistency for the six scales ranges from .84 to .95.[13] Disadvantages include its length and the difficulty that some subjects have with the Likert format.

The *Multiple Affect Adjective Checklist* (MAACL) was designed originally to measure the three negative moods of anxiety, depression, and hostility.[15] The original MAACL consisted of 132 affect-connoting adjectives with instructions asking subjects to check all the words that describe the feelings that apply. It was the first test designed to measure affects as states as well as traits. The MAACL is easy to administer and has an eighth grade reading level. Each item is scored as either checked or not checked and takes approximately 5 min to complete. Scoring was bipolar, with negative items being reversed to contribute to the scoring. Across the scales, the median internal reliability estimate over eight samples was reported as .85 (range .69 to .95). The internal consistency reliability of the MAACL when used with mothers of very low birth weight infants was .85 for the anxiety scale and .87 for the depression scale.[16] Concurrent validity was supported by the correlation in anxiety scores between the MAACL and Spielberger's State-Trait Anxiety Inventory (r = .66).[16]

In 1985, Zuckerman and Lubin[17] revised the MAACL using a factor analysis in an effort to eliminate the high correlation seen among the subscales that resulted in a lack of discriminant validity. The new scale continues to have all 132 items but is scored in a unipolar manner, with only the negative items contributing to the score for the negative moods. The other items contribute to two additional scales labeled as *positive affect* and *sensation seeking*.[17] The trait scale is standardized using a national probability sample. This scoring system, however, has resulted in extremely skewed distributions with little variability.[18] Some have questioned the ability of this new scoring system to be responsive to change.[19]

Depression

Depression has been estimated to affect from 42 to 76 percent of COPD patients. It is perhaps the most devastating psychological aspect to be considered during evaluation.[20,21] The only known study of pulmonary patients in which the different kinds of depressive disorders were considered separately is a study of lung transplant applicants that found that 6 percent of the patients had one episode of major depression,

6 percent had recurrent major depressions, 2 percent had dysthymic disorder, 6 percent had adjustment disorder with depressed mood, and 2 percent had organic mood disorder with depression.[22]

DEFINITION

There is much confusion in the literature regarding depression in the patient with COPD. Much of this is due to a lack of understanding of the differences among the depressive disorders. The American Psychiatric Association (APA), in their compendium of psychological symptoms, the *Diagnostic and Statistical Manual IV*, differentiates among clinical depression, dysthymia, and an adjustment disorder with depressed mood (the usual diagnosis given to someone with depressive symptoms due to pulmonary disease). The APA recommends that to assess depression, patients must be evaluated by a trained clinician who can match their symptoms to the criteria for the diagnostic categories and arrive at a diagnosis.

The diagnosis of *major depression* is characterized by the presence of five or more of the following symptoms for a 2-week period and represents a change from previous functioning. At least one of the first two symptoms must be present: having a depressed mood most of the day nearly every day or having a markedly diminished interest or pleasure in all or almost all activities most of the day nearly every day. Other symptoms include a significant increase or decrease in weight, sleep disturbance, insomnia or hypersomnus, agitation or retardation nearly every day, loss of interest in usual activities, fatigue or loss of energy, feelings of worthlessness or inappropriate guilt, diminished ability to think or concentrate, and recurrent thoughts of death. These symptoms are not due to physiologic effects or bereavement. Depression can occur in a single episode or recurrent episodes separated by at least 2 months. The criteria for a diagnosis of *minor depression* is the presence of two to five of these symptoms.

DYSTHYMIA

The essential feature of dysthymia is a chronically depressed or irritable mood for most of the day, more days than not. These characteristics must be present for at least 2 years. Other criteria for a diagnosis of dysthymia include at least two of the following: poor appetite or overeating, insomnia or hypersomnia, low energy or fatigue, low self-esteem, poor concentration or difficulty making decisions, and feelings of hopelessness. Once again, it is important that the symptoms not be due to physiologic effects or bereavement.

ADJUSTMENT DISORDER WITH DEPRESSED MOOD (REACTIVE DEPRESSION)

The classification of adjustment disorder with depressed mood is identified by a reaction to an identifiable stressor that occurs within 3 months of the onset of the stressor(s). The maladaptive nature of the reaction is indicated by either impairment in occupational functioning, usual social activities, or relationships with others. The person may exhibit symptoms that are in excess of the normal or expected reaction to the stressor(s), such as a trauma or being diagnosed with a fatal disease. The disturbance is not merely one instance but rather a pattern of overreaction to stress that has persisted for not longer than 6 months after the stressor disappears. If it lasts more than 6 months, it is considered chronic.

For the clinician to arrive at a diagnosis requires a complete understanding of the depression categories and a skill in interviewing patients to obtain the appropriate information. This can be time-consuming. There are, however, screening tools that have been developed to determine those most at risk for a depressive episode. These screening tools are not indicative of the depressive diagnostic category but rather are used to screen for patients most likely to be depressed and in need of therapeutic interventions. The term *depression* will be used in this chapter, even though in most of the studies only depressive symptoms were measured.

EFFECT ON REHABILITATION

Depression also has been linked to disability.[23] Borson and colleagues,[24] in a study of 406 patients from a Veterans Administration primary care clinic, found disability, defined as days in bed or away from one's usual activities, to correlate with depressive symptoms and not with pulmonary function test results. Those who were depressed reported that they were unable to work because of medical disability. In our studies of depression in COPD, we found that when COPD patients who reported exercising regularly were compared with patients with comparable pulmonary function test results who did not exercise, the exercisers were found to have significantly less depression.[25] Since the exercisers chose to participate in group exercises, it may be that those who were most severely depressed were unable to follow an exercise regime. Jones and colleagues[26] examined the factors predicting functioning and found that depression and dyspnea accounted for 62 percent of the variance in functioning. Moody and colleagues,[27] using a convenience sample of 45 COPD patients, also found a relationship between self-reported functional ability and depression. The authors proposed that COPD resulted in dyspnea and depression that diminished functional status and quality of life. Yellowlees[28] supports this model in his presentation of four case studies in which the subjects demonstrated a decrease in social and occupational functioning made more severe by depression than would be expected from their physiologic state.

Although one would expect depression to be improved with improved functioning after a pulmonary rehabilitation program, this has not always been the case. Toshima and associates[28a] randomly assigned 119 COPD patients to an 8-week comprehensive rehabilitation program or an 8-week education-only control program. They found significantly better improvement in exercise endurance ($F = 12.11$, $P < .001$) and self-efficacy for walking in those receiving the rehabilitation program but no differences between the groups in depression. This is similar to the findings of Ries and colleagues.[29] Others have reported an improvement in depression after an education-only program, but unfortunately, the measure used to evaluate depression was not indicated in this report.[30] In an evaluation of the effectiveness of a 4-week inpatient pulmonary rehabilitation program involving graduated exercise, along with other therapies, Agle and colleagues[30a] found improvement in depression in only 8 of the 16 who began with noticeable symptoms of depression. Depression was evaluated using psychiatric interviews, with an independent observer concurring in 77 percent of the clinical judgments as to presence or absence of symptoms. Success in the rehabilitation program came from those who had begun with less severe symptoms of depression. Others, however, have found that depression was not predictive of success in pulmonary rehabilitation.[3]

ASSESSMENT OF DEPRESSION

There are a number of screening instruments designed to identify potential cases of depression quickly, inexpensively, and with a minimum of psychometric time or training.[31] Many of these instruments measure depressive symptoms that are not appropriate for the older adult or overlap the symptoms expected with COPD. This may explain why few have observed changes in depression after pulmonary rehabilitation.

The *Beck Depression Inventory* is one of the first to be developed for the study of depression. It is available in long and short forms. The items on the scale were derived from clinical observations of symptoms and attitudes. It measures the intensity or "depth of depression" by having the subject report his or her feelings during the past week based on a Likert scale from 0 (not at all) to 3 (intensely). The long form consists of 21 items and takes from 10 to 15 min to complete. A score from 0 to 9 indicates normal, from 10 to 15 indicates mild depression, from 16 to 19 indicates mild to moderate depression, from 20 to 29 indicates moderate to severe depression, and from 30 to 63 indicates severe depression. A split-half reliability coefficient of $r = .93$ was found in a mixed sample of 409 inpatients and outpatients. Test-retest reliability has been reported as $r = .74$ for 30 subjects tested at a 3-month interval.[32] Criterion validity was demonstrated by a correlation of .66 with clinical ratings of depression in a sample of 409 inpatients and outpatients and by high correlations with other self-report inventories of depression. The Beck Depression Inventory is brief, widely used, discriminates subtypes of depression, and has been shown to be appropriate cross-culturally.[33] The disadvantages include the fact that some of the items are somatic in nature and create false-positive results, especially in patients with chronic lung disease. The tool does not detect mild depression well. Also, the scale was not designed for older adults, who may find the Likert scale confusing and some of the items inappropriate to their age group.

The short form of the Beck Depression Inventory consists of the 13 items found to have the highest factor loadings from the long form and with less emphasis on somatic items. The subject is asked to indicate his or her feelings that day. A score from 0 to 4 indicates minimal or no depression, 4 to 7 indicates mild depression, 8 to 15 indicates moderate depression, and 16 or greater indicates severe depression. Scores on the short form correlate well with the long form, but the reliability of this form of the scale is lower than that for the long form. This is most likely due to the fact that subjects are asked to indicate their feelings at the moment for the short form and for the past week on the long form. The scale takes approximately 5 min to administer.

The *Center for Epidemiological Studies Depression Scale* is a 20-item self-report scale that was developed at the National Institute of Mental Health to be used in epidemiologic studies of depressive symptomatology in the general population. It was partially derived from the Beck Depression Inventory but strongly emphasizes the psychological component rather than somatic complaints (17 of 20 items) such as depressed mood, guilt, worthlessness, hopelessness, and helplessness. Four of the items ask about positive feelings. It focuses on current emotional experiences. Scoring consists of the number of symptoms of depression weighted by the frequency and duration of each symptom. Total scores range from 0 to 60, with a score of 15 or greater indicating depression. The scale is brief, taking only 10 min to administer. It includes few somatic items.[34] This scale has been found to be appropriate for use with a wide variety of cultures, geographic locations, and age groups. Reliability coefficients have been reported as .90 for a clinical population and .85 for a general population.[35] Validity was established by patterns of correlations with other self-report measures, by correlations with clinical ratings of depression, and by relationships with other variables that support its construct validity.[35] Disadvantages include the fact that the Likert scaling can be confusing to older adults. With the low cutoff score, there are many false-positive results with this scale.

The *Geriatric Depression Scale* is a depression scale that was developed for the older population. This is a self-report scale asking subjects to indicate their feelings during the past week using a yes/no format. The long form consists of 30 items that avoid the somatic area. It was normed on older adults, who took approximately 8 to 10 min to complete it. A score of 18 items indicates major depression, 11 to 18 indicates minor depression, and under 11 indicates no depression. Using these cutoff scores, the scale was found to have a sensitivity of 92 percent, a specificity of 89 percent, and a negative predictive value of 99 percent.[36] The scale has good internal consistency, with an alpha of .94 and a test-retest reliability of .86.[37] Construct validity was established by the scale being able to differentiate between healthy and ill older adults, while concurrent validity was established by comparing it with the Hamilton Depression Inventory and the Zung Self-Rating Depression Scale.[38] Disadvantages include the fact that the scale has been found to be insensitive to mild depression and has not been tested for sensitivity to change with treatment in patients with chronic lung disease.[36]

The short form of the Geriatric Depression Scale consists of 15 items selected because of their high correlation with depressive symptoms. Similar to the long form, there are few somatic items. Subjects are asked to indicate their feelings for the past week using a yes/no format. A score of over 16 indicates severe depression, 8 to 16 indicates moderate depression, and 5 to 7 indicates mild depression. The short form takes approximately 5 min to administer. A disadvantage of the short form is its low reliability compared with the long form ($r = .66$). There is no known study using this form with the COPD population.

The *Hamilton Depression Rating Scale* was designed to measure the severity and pattern of depression in patients already diagnosed rather than as a screen for the presence of depression. This scale measures a unitary dimension of depression using a 17-item semistructured interview format. Symptom severity is rated, preferably by two clinicians, as 0 to 2 or 0 to 4, with half-point increments possible for experienced raters. The total score ranges from 0 to 100 and is the sum of the ratings.[39]

The Hamilton Depression Rating Scale is the most widely used instrument for psychiatric patients. It has been translated into many languages and validated cross-culturally.[40] Older adults, however, have been found to have difficulty with some of the items. The scale has not been demonstrated to be appropriate for those not already diagnosed with depression. Internal consistency of the scale has been reported at .78.[32] Correlations between the total scores of two experienced raters for the same interview ranged from .84 to .90 on 70 depressed male patients.[39] Validity has been demonstrated by its correlation with the Beck Depression Inventory and the Zung Self-Rating Depression Scale.[32] It was able to discriminate among psychiatric inpatients, outpatients, and those in a general practice.

The *Self-Rating Depression Scale* measures depression as withdrawal from the functions of life with concomitant disturbances in the whole organism. It is a 20-item self-report scale using a Likert format to measure four dimensions of depression: self-esteem, well-being, depression, and optimism. Scores over 60 indicate major depression, whereas those from 50 to 59 indicate lesser forms of depression. The scale takes 15 to 20 min to administer. It is widely used with older adults but has poor reliability with adults over age 70, who tend to have difficulty with the Likert format. When compared with a clinical interview, the accuracy of this scale in detecting depression is suspect, especially for detection of mild depression. This is most likely due to the higher noncompletion rate than the Geriatric Depression Scale and is confounded by somatic and cognitive items.

Anxiety

Anxiety and panic have been associated with COPD in from 2 to 96 percent of patients.[21,41] Wells and colleagues[42] found that those with chronic lung disease had a higher incidence of anxiety than that found in general medical patients without a chronic condition. In a comparison between patients with COPD and those with other diagnoses coming to a family practice, those with COPD were found to be significantly more anxious, as measured on the anxiety subscale of the SCL-90 and a yes/no questionnaire, the Symptom Questionnaire.[43] The authors state that the scores for COPD patients were similar to those of psychiatric patients. Others have noted that women are more likely to report anxiety than are men.[44] Additionally, it has been suggested that the dyspnea experienced by those with COPD, rather than gender, leads to more anxiety.[45]

DEFINITION

The group of psychological disorders referred to as the *anxiety disorders* includes anxiety, panic, and fear. Anxiety is a state of heightened awareness or an unpleasant emotional state. Spielberger and colleagues[46] differentiate between the temporary state of anxiety at a particular point in time and the more permanent trait or tendency to face life events with anxiety. Fear is generally regarded as a reaction to an event, whereas panic is an exaggeration of that reaction. The DSM-IV defines anxiety as the apprehensive anticipation of future danger or misfortune accompanied by a feeling of dysphoria or somatic symptoms of tension. The focus of anticipated danger may be external or internal and is usually specified in the definition of anxiety. For instance, if COPD patients experience anxiety as a direct physiologic consequence of their medical condition, it is referred to as *anxiety disorder* due to a general medical condition. Anxiety disorders also include obsessive-compulsive disorder, which is characterized by obsessions, the uncontrollable need to dwell on an idea that causes anxiety, and compulsions, which are repetitive acts performed to relieve the fear connected with obsession. These behaviors have been noted by clinicians caring for COPD patients and may be related to their high anxiety level.

EFFECT ON REHABILITATION

Light and colleagues[21] found no relationship between anxiety, as measured by the Spielberger Anxiety Scale, and functioning, as measured by the 12-min walk distance. Others, however, have found such a relationship. Morgan[47] used the Multiple Affect Adjective Checklist (MAACL) and found that anxiety was significantly related to the 12-min walk distance. Anxiety also has been shown to affect functioning when the Sickness Impact Profile was used as the measure of functioning.[26,48] Anxiety also has been shown to be related to respiratory symptoms in a cyclic relationship with an increase in anxiety producing an increase in the sensation of dyspnea, which in turn precipitates more anxiety.

ASSESSMENT OF ANXIETY

The *Spielberger State-Trait Anxiety Inventory* consists of two 20-item scales assessing an anxiety state and trait. *State* is the current level of anxiety experienced at the moment, whereas *trait* anxiety measures how a person generally feels. This scale is designed to be used by both adults and adolescents. Both forms are self-administered using a four-point Likert scale ranging from "not at all" to "very much so" for the state measure and "almost never" to "almost always" for the trait measure. Both scales have positive and negatively worded items. Scores for each item are totaled (with negatively worded items reversed), resulting in scale totals that range from 20 to 80. Norms have been established for each age group and for disease groups of psychiatric or medical-surgical patients. Reliability has been demonstrated, with internal consistencies all above .90. Stability of the trait anxiety scale was demonstrated after 1 h and ranged from .73 to .86. Validity has been established using the contrasted-groups approach, comparing scores before and after exposure to stressful events. Scores on this scale also have been shown to be comparable with scores on other anxiety scales.[46]

The *Jalowiec Coping Scale* (JCS) lists 60 coping behaviors that subjects rank according to the degree to which they have used the behavior to deal with a specific stressor.[49] The JCS was developed using the Lazarus framework of coping and first reported by Jalowiec and Powers[50] in 1981. The scale was revised and tested in 1984 and again in 1989.[49] Sixty coping behaviors representing problem or emotion-focused coping behaviors are self-rated on a scale from zero to three to indicate the extent of use. Internal consistency, indicated by Cronbach's alpha, for the total scale ranges from .88 to .96. Studies have supported construct validity by factor analysis.[49,51,52]

Self-Efficacy

DEFINITION

Self-efficacy, based in social learning theory, is perceived to be a psychological mechanism that mediates and explains psychobiologic functioning in specific situations when individuals have the ability to exercise control.[52a] Two components of self-efficacy theory have been proposed: (1) self-efficacy expectations or judgments about one's capability to perform the behavior itself and (2) outcome expectations or beliefs that specific consequences will follow performance of the behavior. The primary focus of research into achieving health behavior change has been examining the efficacy expectation component of self-efficacy theory.[53]

Strecher and colleagues[54] examine how self-efficacy has been differentiated from, although linked to, a number of other concepts. Having an internal "health locus of control" or belief that one's own behavior affects outcomes can increase self-efficacy if the capability exists to perform the behavior but may decrease self-efficacy if the skills or information needed to perform the behavior are lacking. Similarly, effects of high "hardiness" in people who have perceptions of control, are committed to achievement, and are challenged by change can be postulated.[55] Strecher and colleagues[54] differentiate self-efficacy and self-esteem as evaluation of one's capability to perform versus evaluation of one's worth obtained from performance in specific situations. The concepts of anxiety and depression are not components of self-efficacy, but both may influence it. Performance anxiety may result from perceived inefficacy.[54] Similarly, Kavanagh[56] argues that "reductions in self-efficacy and performance appear to be both consequences of depression and determinants of it; low self-efficacy predicts depressive episodes."

Self-efficacy expectations can be recognized as a determinant of secondary appraisal within Lazarus and Folkman's "coping theory" in that belief that one can accomplish a behavior affects how one evaluates what could and should be a response to a threat or challenge.[57] Finally, Seligman's "learned helplessness theory" suggests that people do not respond because they have failed before and feel they cannot succeed, although others can (personal helplessness), or that no one can succeed (universal helplessness).[57a] Learned helplessness has been characterized as related to low self-efficacy.

EFFECT ON REHABILITATION

Self-efficacy expectancies, or judgments about an individual's own capabilities to perform specified behaviors, can be developed and changed through mastery experiences, modeling, social persuasion, and (re)interpretation of physiologic responses. *Mastery experiences* occur when an individual actually performs a desired behavior successfully, *modeling* refers to viewing another similar individual performing the desired behavior, and *social persuasion* involves verbally describing how and why one should perform the desired behavior. Pulmonary rehabilitation programs are designed to provide mastery experiences, modeling, and social persuasion through interaction of the individual with health care personnel and other patients with similar problems. Interpretation of physiologic responses results from an individual's perception of the positive or negative aspects of performing the behavior. For example, the increased breathing rate and dyspnea resulting from the initial exercise in a pulmonary rehabilitation program may cause anxiety. This may be interpreted as an inability to perform activities unless individuals can be helped to reinterpret this physiologic aspect and feel safe by recognizing their own ability to deal with this as a normal response.

Self-efficacy theory links behavioral performance with patients' beliefs in their ability to perform in varied situations and disease states. The influence of self-efficacy before and after exercise training in predicting exercise compliance in cardiac patients has been documented.[57b] Preoperative self-efficacy has been related significantly to performance of postoperative behaviors.[58] Self-efficacy problem-solving strategies served as mediators on intention to smoke in a study of over 4000 sixth, eighth, and tenth graders.[59] A review of 10 health behavior studies noted that pre- and posttreatment self-efficacy has been found to be predictive of smoking reduction and cessation.[54] These findings suggest that programs designed to change health-related behaviors could be supported by attending to participants' self-efficacy expectations.

Self-efficacy expectations in patients with COPD have been investigated by Kaplan and colleagues.[60,61] In a study of 60 older adults with COPD randomly assigned to control or experimental exercise training groups, those who received specific exercise compliance support significantly increased walking activity after 3 months, but this change was mediated by changes in perceived efficacy for walking.[60] Greater perceived self-efficacy for walking increased in the experimental group ($F_1, 56 = 16.08, P < .001$). Also, there was a significant correlation of exercise tolerance with walking self-efficacy in those subjects who had an internal health locus of control ($r = .45, P < .05$). These data suggest that individuals who feel that they can affect their own behavior will increase self-efficacy expectations for walking in an structured exercise program and thus improve exercise performance.

In a study of 119 patients with COPD randomly assigned to a comprehensive rehabilitation program or a control education-only group, self-efficacy for walking was not significantly increased by the pulmonary rehabilitation exercise program alone. Patients needed help to interpret behaviors to increase self-efficacy. Nevertheless, high self-efficacy for walking at the beginning of the program did predict treadmill endurance and maintenance of performance. Also, patients in the comprehensive rehabilitation program with initially low self-efficacy demonstrated the greatest improvements in endurance when compared with the education-only group.[28a] Kaplan and colleagues[61] later reported on this same sample, that self-efficacy was a significant predictor of survival 5 years after participation in the study. Self-efficacy expectations for walking had the highest validity for these patients with significant univariate predictive ability ($P < .01$). However, when controlling for the physiologic variable FEV_1, statistically significant in a multivariate model ($P < .0001$), self-efficacy was only marginally significant ($P = .1$). Although it might be argued that self-efficacy is merely a reflection of physiologic status, this study does demonstrate the value of an easily administered self-report scale when repeated and costly laboratory testing may not be desired or feasible.

ASSESSMENT OF SELF-EFFICACY

Multiple measures of self-efficacy have been reported,[54] because efficacy expectations and thus measures of those expectations need to relate to the specific behavior being studied. Self-efficacy scales measure the individual's perception of ability to perform rather than the actual performance of a behavior. In general, the behavior must be modifiable in order to be affected by self-efficacy. A unidimensional questionnaire that has been useful in measuring self-efficacy related to ability to refrain from smoking has been described by Condiotte and Lichtenstein.[62] Self-efficacy scales related to cardiac stress have been developed and used by Ewert and colleagues. Also, an asthma self-efficacy scale has been described by Tobin and colleagues.

Toshima and associates[28a] adapted Ewert's cardiac self-efficacy scales to measure functional disabilities associated with COPD using a 46-item questionnaire. Each of the seven behavior scales includes statements describing increasingly difficult behaviors, such as walking 1 block to walking 3 miles. Subjects rate whether or not they can do the activity and then indicate their level of certainty or confidence (0 to 100 percent) that they can do it. The highest level that is listed as 100 percent confidence is the scale score. A sample of this measure can be found in Schwarzer[63] on page 354.

A 34-item COPD Self-Efficacy Scale has been developed by Wigal and colleagues[64] incorporating a five-factor structure: negative affect, emotional arousal, breathing difficulty related to physical exertion, difficulty associated with weather/environment, and behavioral risk factors that lead to breathing difficulty. Respondents report their degree of confidence that they could manage or avoid breathing difficulty using a five-point Likert-type scale from "not at all confident" to "very confident." Psychometric analysis supports both validity and reliability with a test-retest reliability of .77 ($P < .001$) and internal consistency with a Cronbach's alpha of .95. A sample of the questionnaire is provided in the article (page 1195), but scoring instructions must be obtained directly from the authors.

In summary, measures of self-efficacy directly related to behaviors that are the focus of pulmonary rehabilitation have been developed. Research suggests that they can be used to identify areas of potential difficulty for participants as well as areas that already have a high level of efficacy. Thus programs can be targeted efficiently toward areas most in need of development, promoting cost-effective use of the limited time available for rehabilitation programs.

Hardiness

DEFINITION

The concept of hardiness, rooted in existential psychology that rejects the notion of constant personality characteristics, postulates that individuals can turn stress into an opportunity for growth. *Hardiness* is theorized to be an internal personality factor influencing patients' responses to stressful events such as symptoms of pulmonary disease by motivating them to resist or increase resistance to debilitating effects, thus promoting adaptation to the illness.[55,65–67] Three components of hardiness have been proposed: (1) *control* is described as the feeling that a course of events can be influenced by involvement, (2) *commitment* is thought to promote involvement in what is happening rather than avoidance of a situation, and (3) *challenge* is thought to allow an individual to see potential for change, recognize change as a normal part of life, and tolerate ambiguity.[67]

EFFECT ON REHABILITATION

Magnani[68] and Lee[69] reported that hardiness related to self-perceived health and activity among independently functioning older adults and rural adults. Descriptive research has shown a significant relationship between high hardiness and increased physiologic functioning in patients with diabetes,[70] as well as in patients with COPD.[55] Researchers have shown high hardy people to have improved psychosocial functioning,[55,68,71] more frequent use of social support,[72] and involvement in health promotion activities.[73] Conversely, low hardy individuals report poor health practices[74] and more neurotic symptoms.[75] Hardy patients with COPD demonstrate more problem-solving coping skills and a healthy attributional style.[76] Research has likewise demonstrated that outcomes of rehabilitation have been related to hardiness levels. Patients with COPD who are lower in hardiness have demonstrated disproportionate disability in a measured 12-min walk test.[77] Psychoneuroimmunology researchers have demonstrated the affect of psychological aspects of personality on the immune system. Hardiness in fostering an attitude of not "giving up" can enhance a patient's prospects for recovery and successful completion of pulmonary rehabilitation indicated by outcomes such as increased pulmonary functional status.[55]

ASSESSMENT OF HARDINESS

Three survey tools have been developed to measure hardiness. Tool development has progressed from a general focus on hardiness as a personality factor in well individuals promoting illness resistance to a specific focus on health-related hardiness promoting resistance of debilitation from chronic illness.[67]

Kobasa's Personal Views Survey is a 36-item four-point Likert scale with lower scores indicating the presence of hardiness.[75] Analysis of reliability resulted in a Cronbach's alpha coefficient of .86; 3-week test-retest correlated at .74; convergent and discriminant validity were supported for the control and commitment subscales.[78]

Pollock's Health Related Hardiness Scale (HRHS) is a 34-item six-point Likert scale, originally developed with lower scores indicating the presence of hardiness.[79] Research conducted since 1990 converts scoring such that higher scores indicate higher levels of hardiness. Two-week test-retest Pearson r was .92; the alpha coefficient was .84; and content and convergent validity were demonstrated[79] with two subscales: control and commitment/challenge.

Wallston's Health Hardiness Inventory (HHI-31) incorporates an 11-item "perceived health control" subscale within a 31-item five-point Likert-type scale ranging from "strongly disagree" to "strongly agree."[79a] This subscale has been used to identify subjects who are low and high in hardiness. Reliability and validity are acceptable, with Cronbach's alpha coefficient of .87 for the total scale; control, commitment, and challenge subscales were .86, .83, and .74, respectively. Total scores for hardiness can range from 31 to 155, with a median

norm of 115 based on prior research samples of patients with arthritis. In a study of 124 patients with COPD, hardiness scores ranged from 62 to 146, with a mean of 115.2 (SD 15.2) with control, commitment, and challenge subscores, and high hardiness was evident in 46 percent of the subjects.[80]

Hardiness measures may be useful in identifying subjects who should be most likely to benefit from a pulmonary rehabilitation program, especially when age or severe physiologic status would make entry into a program questionable. Although physiologic indicators such as FEV_1 cannot be ignored, the demonstrated ability to function in individuals with severe disease states but high hardiness supports its consideration in pulmonary rehabilitation selection.

Coping

DEFINITION

Coping is usually defined as the efforts taken to master stressors. Cohen and Lazarus[81] state that people routinely examine events to determine if they are threatening or challenging and, if so, what the magnitude of the threat or challenge might be. They then evaluate their own resources for dealing with the threat or challenge. Coping includes the behaviors and thinking that the person does to alleviate the stressor and has been categorized as being problem-focused or emotion-focused. Problem focused strategies can be behavioral, such as seeking help from family and friends or reducing illness risk factors. Cognitive coping activities, such as changing the meaning of the situation by minimizing the seriousness of the illness, are also considered problem-focused. Emotion-focused strategies are intrapsychic in nature and serve to regulate stressful emotions by means of defensive thought processes.

EFFECT ON REHABILITATION

The first known qualitative studies that dealt with coping in COPD patients, published by Fagerhaugh[82] and Barstow, described strategies patients with emphysema used to maintain functional status within the confines of the illness. Similar findings in emphysema-bronchitis subjects were noted by Carrieri and Janson-Bjerklie.[83] In their study, Lazarus' coping model was used to examine management of dyspnea in 68 patients with chronic lung disease. Thematic analysis of structured interviews suggested that subjects used both problem-focused and emotion-focused coping to manage dyspnea, although problem-focused strategies were described more frequently in response to the physical symptom of dyspnea. Gift and Austin[25] similarly found that COPD patients who participated in a systematic exercise program ($N = 10$) used fewer emotion-focused coping strategies than did nonexercisers ($N = 10$). The positive relationship of problem-focused coping in COPD to increased 12-min walking distance has been suggested using quantitative measures in a sample of 104 COPD outpatients.[55]

Coping has multiple interactive factors, including biological, psychological, and social components. The McSweeney and colleagues[84] study of 203 patients with COPD noted that functional status, as represented by scores on the Sickness Impact Profile Scale, was more related to age ($r = .31$, $P < .001$), sociocultural factors ($r = .26$, $P < .002$), neurologic functioning ($r = .22$, $P < .005$), and interrelationships between factors than to the severity of COPD ($r = .16$, $P = .04$). Prigatano and colleagues,[48] examining a 100-patient subset of a large sample of people with COPD, found that pulmonary function tests (FEV$_1$) correlated only with physical functioning ($r = -.26$, $P < .05$), whereas personality measures correlated with both physical ($r = .46$, $P < .001$) and psychosocial functioning ($r = .68$, $P < .001$). These and other studies[47,85,86] suggest that positive outcomes relate to differences in both physiologic and psychological coping.

In examining the process of coping within the context of a particular stressful situation, Folkman and Lazarus[87] suggest that positive outcomes depend on both personal and situational factors. They suggest that all coping strategies can relate to positive outcomes. Problem-focused strategies are used for potentially solvable problems to eliminate or decrease the effect of a stressor. Emotion-focused strategies are used when there is little prospect for positive change to manage anxiety and restore or maintain self-esteem. Mixed-focus strategies change both the meaning and the effect. Conversely, Billings and Moos[88] suggest that problem-focused strategies relate to positive outcomes, whereas emotion-focused strategies relate to more negative outcomes. There is evidence that because the process of coping is transactional, measurement of the coping strategies used actually reflects coping interacting with other factors such as personality.[81] This interaction could account for some of the inconsistent results found in coping research. Nevertheless, assessing the barriers and available supportive factors that can hinder or help patients cope with the stress of disease and pulmonary rehabilitation can provide worthwhile information, especially when "dropouts" are encountered.

ASSESSMENT OF COPING

The *Ways of Coping Scale* consists of 66 coping strategies divided into eight coping subscales indicating patterns of coping. The Confronting Coping subscale consists of items such as "Tried to get a person responsible to change his or her mind." The Distancing Coping subscale consists of items such as "Went on as if nothing had happened." "Tried to keep my feelings to myself" is an example of the Self-Controlling subscale, whereas "Asked relatives and friends who I respected for advice" is an example of the Seeking Social Support subscale. The Accepting Responsibility subscale consists of items such as "Criticized or lectured myself," whereas the Escape-Avoidance subscale consists of items such as "Hoped a miracle would happen." An example of the Positive Reappraisal subscale is "Found new faith," whereas an example of the Planful Problem-Solving subscale is "Made a plan of action and followed it." Subjects respond to each item on a scale from 1 to 5 indicating the usefulness of each strategy (with 1 being the least useful and 5 being the most useful). A higher score on each of the scales indicates that the coping strategy was used more frequently.

The *Jalowiec Coping Scale* is a 40-item instrument that assesses problem-focused coping strategies (15 items) and emotion-focused coping strategies (25 items) on a five-point Likert-type scale indicating degree of use. Construct validity has been demonstrated.[52] Internal consistency in emergency department patients ranged from .75 to .86.[50]

Family Assessment

To this point, all psychosocial assessment has been focused on assessment of the individual, but patients usually do not function in isolation to others but rather in relationship to others in their family. Understanding family interactions in terms of functioning, communicating, and supporting each other can be a key to understanding why some patients do or do not benefit from pulmonary rehabilitation. Function, communication, and support are evidenced in family interaction patterns in terms of the roles each member assumes. Assessment would include examining the relationships between husband and wife or parent and child or other caregiver. Patients and families should be questioned on their actual and perceived roles, including occupational and other duties in their life situations. Patients with pulmonary disease may express satisfaction or disturbances in family, work, or social relationships; responsibilities related to these roles also should be assessed.[89]

While performing the physical assessment, signs of abuse or neglect may be observed. Weight loss, fatigue, and impaired cognitive function could indicate reactions to stress as well as disease. Injuries or bruises may indicate physical abuse; an enlarged liver could relate to chronic alcoholism; track marks often indicate intravenous drug injection; and nasal inflammation can be symptoms of cocaine abuse.[89]

In addition to a physical examination, objective data for family assessment include observations of family interactions and behaviors.[89] Signs that may indicate family dysfunction include labile emotions, withdrawal, irritability, difficulty sleeping and eating, inability to concentrate, and increased feelings of dependency. Communication observations include who does the talking and who remains silent, who is listening to whom, how disagreements are handled, who is involved in making decisions, what nonverbal communication is apparent, and how a participant responds to success and failure.

Family coherence is a "fundamental coping strategy families employ in the management of family problems."[90] *Family Assessment Inventories for Research and Practice*[90] provides a variety of tools that can be used by the practitioner to assess and provide support in deficit areas. Family stressors, family strengths, and the family appraisal of the situation are all important components of addressing the need to support family functioning if the patient is to derive maximum benefit from a program of rehabilitation. Risk identification at the family level as well as at the individual level can assist in setting appropriate goals, can reduce dissatisfaction engendered by unrealistic expectations for the pulmonary rehabilitation program, and can use family strengths to reinforce the individual's adaptation to living with pulmonary disease.

References

1. McSweeney AJ, Heaton RK, Grant I, et al: Chronic obstructive pulmonary disease: Socioemotional adjustment and life quality. *Chest* 77:309–311, 1980.
2. Lahdensuo A, Ojanen M, Ahonen A, et al: Psychosocial effects of continuous oxygen therapy in hypoxaemic chronic obstructive pulmonary disease patients. *Eur Respir J* 2:977–980, 1989.
3. Ojanen M, Lahdensuo A, Laitinen J, Karvonen J: Psychosocial

changes in patients participating in a chronic obstructive pulmonary disease rehabilitation program. *Respiration* 60:96–102, 1993.

4. Gift AG, Cahill CA: Psychophysiologic aspects of dyspnea in chronic obstructive pulmonary disease: A pilot study. *Heart Lung* 19:252–257, 1990.

5. Matthews AW: The relationship between central carbon dioxide sensitivity and clinical features in patients with chronic airways obstruction. *Q J Med* 46:179–195, 1987.

6. Gordon GH, Michiels TM, Mahutte CK, Light RW: Effect of desipramine on control of ventilation and depression scores in patients with severe chronic obstructive pulmonary disease. *Psychiatr Res* 15:25–32, 1985.

7. Gift AG, Wood RM, Cahill CA: Depression, somatization and steroid use in chronic obstructive pulmonary disease. *Int J Nurs Stud* 26:281–286, 1989.

8. DeCencio DV, Leshner M, Leshner B: Personality characteristics of patients with chronic obstructive pulmonary emphysema. *Arch Phys Med Rehabil* 471–475, 1968.

9. Glassman AH, Helzer JE, Covey LS, et al: Smoking, smoking cessation, and major depression. *JAMA* 264:1546–1549, 1990.

9a. Anda RF, Williamson DF, Escobedo LG, et al: Depression and the dynamics of smoking. *JAMA* 264:1541–1545, 1990.

10. Haire-Joshu D, Heady S, Thomas L, et al: Depressive symptomatology and smoking among persons with diabetes. *Res Nurs Health* 17:273–282, 1994.

11. Dales RE, Spitzer WO, Schechter MT, Suissa S: The influence of psychological status on respiratory symptom reporting. *Am Rev Respir Dis* 139:1459–1463, 1989.

12. Derogatis LR: *The Symptom Checklist-90-Revised (SCL-90-R) Manual.* Towson, MD, Clinical Psychometric Research, 1986.

13. McNair DM, Lorr M, Dropplemen LF: *Manual for the Profile of Mood States.* San Diego, Educational and Industrial Testing Service, 1993.

14. Kaye JM, Lawton MP, Gitlin LN, et al: Older peoples' performance on the Profile of Mood States (POMS). *Clin Gerontol* 7(3/4):35–55, 1988.

15. Zuckerman M, Lubin B: *Manual for the Multiple Affect Adjective Check List.* San Diego, Educational and Industrial Testing Service, 1965.

16. Gennaro S: Postpartal anxiety and depression in mothers of term and preterm infants. *Nurs Res* 37:82–85, 1988.

17. Zuckerman M, Lubin B: *Manual for the MAACL-R: The Multiple Affect Adjective Check List—Revised.* San Diego, Educational Testing Service, 1985.

18. Zuckerman M, Lubin B, Rinck C: Construction of new scales for the Multiple Affect Adjective Check List. *J Behav Assess* 5:119–129, 1983.

19. Jacobsen BS, Munro BH, Brooten DA: Comparison of original and revised scoring systems for the Multiple Affect Adjective Check List. *Nurs Res* 45:57–60, 1996.

20. Burnum JF: Diagnosis of depression in a general medical practice. *Postgrad Med* 72:71–76, 1982.

21. Light RW, Merrill EJ, Despars JA, et al: Prevalence of depression and anxiety in patients with COPD. *Chest* 87:35–38, 1985.

22. Craven JL, Bright J, Dear CL: Psychiatric, psychosocial, and rehabilitative aspects of lung transplantation. *Clin Chest Med* 11:247–257, 1990.

23. Gift AG, McCrone SH: Depression in patients with COPD. *Heart Lung* 22:289–297, 1993.

24. Borson S, Barnes RA, Kukull WA, et al: Symptomatic depression in elderly medical outpatients: Prevalence, demography and health service utilization. *J Am Geriatr Soc* 34:341–347, 1986.

25. Gift AG, Austin DJ: The effects of a program of systematic movement on COPD patients. *Rehab Nurs* 17:6–10, 1992.

26. Jones PW, Bayerstock CM, Littlejohns P: Relationship between general health measured with the Sickness Impact Profile and respiratory symptoms, physiological measures, and mood in patients with chronic airflow limitation. *Am Rev Respir Dis* 140:1538–1543, 1989.

27. Moody L, McCormick K, Williams AR: Psychophysiologic correlates of quality of life in chronic bronchitis and emphysema. *West J Nurs Res* 13:336–352, 1991.

28. Yellowlees PM: The treatment of psychiatric disorders in patients with chronic airways obstruction. *Med J Aust* 147:349–352, 1987.

28a. Toshima MT, Kaplan RM, Ries AL: Experimental evaluation of rehabilitation in chronic obstructive pulmonary disease: Short-term effects on exercise and health status. *Health Psych* 9:237–252, 1990.

29. Ries AL, Kaplan RM, Limberg TM, Prewitt LM: Effects of pulmonary rehabilitation on physiologic and psychosocial outcomes in patients with chronic obstructive pulmonary disease. *Ann Intern Med* 122:823–832, 1995.

30. Sahn SA, Nett LM, Petty TL: Ten-year follow-up of a comprehensive rehabilitation program for severe COPD. *Chest* 77(suppl):311–314, 1980.

30a. Agle DP, Baum GL, Chester EH, Wendt M: Multidiscipline treatment of chronic pulmonary insufficiency: Psychological aspects of rehabilitation. *Psychosomatic Medicine* 35:41–49, 1973.

31. Yesavage JA: Depression in the elderly. *Postgrad Med* 91:255–261, 1992.

32. Mayer JM: Assessment of depression, in McReynolds P (ed): *Advances in Psychological Assessment*, vol 4. San Francisco: Jossey-Bass, 1978.

33. Marsella AJ, Sanborn KO, Kameoka V, et al: Cross-validation of self-report measures of depression among normal populations of Japanese, Chinese, and Caucasian ancestry. *J Clin Psychol* 31:281–287, 1975.

34. Gallagher D, Thompson LW, Levy SM: Clinical psychological assessment of older adults, in Poon LW (ed): *Aging in the 1980s: Psychological Issues.* Washington, American Psychological Association, 1980; pp 19–40.

35. Radloff LS: The CES-D scale: A self-report depression scale for research in the general population. *Appl Psychol Measure* 1:385–401, 1977.

36. Koenig HG, Meador KG, Cohen HJ, Blazer DG: Self-rated depression scales and screening for major depression in the older hospitalized patient with medical illness. *J Am Geriatr Soc* 36:699–706, 1988.

37. Brink TL, Yeasavage JA, Lum O, et al: Screening tests for geriatric depression. *Clin Gerontol* 1:37–43, 1982.

38. Yesavage JA, Brink TL, Rose TL, et al: Development and validation of the geriatric depression screening scale: A preliminary report. *J Psychiatr Res* 17:37–49, 1983.

39. Hamilton M: A rating scale for depression. *J Neurol Neurosurg Psychiatry* 23:56–62, 1960.

40. Fava GA, Kellner R, Munari F, Pavan L: The Hamilton Depression Rating Scale in normals and depressives. *Acta Psychiatr Scand* 66:26–32, 1982.

41. Karajgi B, Rifkin A, Doddi S, Kollie R: The prevalence of anxiety disorders in patients with chronic obstructive pulmonary disease. *Am J Psychiatry* 147:200–201, 1990.

42. Wells KB, Golding JM, Burnam MA: Affective, substance use, and anxiety disorders in persons with arthritis, diabetes, heart disease, high blood pressure, or chronic lung condition. *Gen Hosp Psychiatry* 11:320–327, 1989.

43. Kellner R, Samet J, Pathak D: Dyspnea, anxiety, and depression in chronic respiratory impairment. *Gen Hosp Psychiatry* 14:20–28, 1992.

44. Kinsman RA, Yaroush RA, Fernandez E, et al: Symptoms and experiences in chronic bronchitis and emphysema. *Chest* 83:755–761, 1983.

45. Rosser R, Guz A: Psychological approaches to breathlessness and its treatment. *J Psychosom Res* 25:439–447, 1981.

46. Spielberger CD, Gorsuch RL, Lushene R, et al: *Manual for the*

State-Trait Anxiety Inventory (Form Y). Palo Alto, Consulting Psychologists Press, 1983.

47. Morgan A: Chronic bronchitis, disability and the attitudes and beliefs of patients. *Midwife Health* 23:104–108, 1987.

48. Prigatano G, Wright E, Levin D: Quality of life and its predictors in patients with mild hypoxemia and chronic obstructive pulmonary disease. *Arch Intern Med* 144:1613–1619, 1984.

49. Jalowiec A: Revision and testing of the Jalowiec Coping Scale. Presented at the Midwest Nursing Research Society Conference, Cincinnati, April 4, 1989.

50. Jalowiec A, Powers M: Stress and coping in hypertensive and emergency room patients. *Nurs Res* 30:10–15, 1981.

51. Jalowiac A, Murphy SP, Powers MJ: Psychometric assessment of the Jalowiac Coping Scale. *Nurs Res* 33:157–161, 1984.

52. Jalowiec A: Confirmatory factor analysis of the Jalowiec Coping Scale, in Waltz C, Strickland O (eds): *Measurement of Nursing Outcomes, Measuring Client Outcomes*. New York, Springer, 1988; pp 287–308.

52a. Bandora A: Self-efficacy mechanism in psychobiologic functioning, in Schwarzer R (ed): *Self-Efficacy: Thought Control of Action*. Philadelphia, Hemisphere, 1992; pp 355–394.

53. Jensen K, Banwart L, Venhaus R, et al: Advanced rehabilitation nursing care of coronary angioplasty patients using self-efficacy theory. *J Adv Nurs* 18:926–931, 1993.

54. Strecher VJ, DeVellis BM, Becker MH, Rosenstock IM: The role of self-efficacy in achieving health behavior change. *Health Educ Q* 13:73–91, 1986.

55. Narsavage GL, Weaver TE: Physiological status, coping, and hardiness as predictors of outcomes in chronic obstructive pulmonary disease. *Nurs Res* 43:90–94, 1994.

56. Kavanagh DJ: Self-efficacy and depression, in Schwarzer R (ed): *Self-Efficacy: Thought Control of Action*. Philadelphia, Hemisphere Publishing, 1992; pp 177–193.

57. Lazarus R, Folkman S: *Stress, Appraisal and Coping*. New York, Springer, 1984.

57a. Abramson LY, Garber J, Seligman ME: Learned helplessness in humans: An attributional analysis, in Garber J, Seligman ME (eds): *Human Helplessness Theory and Applications*. New York, Academic Press, 1980.

57b. Stewart KJ, Kelemeen MH, Ewart CK: Relationships between self efficacy and mood before and after exercise training. *J Cardiopulm Rehabil* 14:35–42, 1994.

58. Oetker-Black SL, Hart F, Hoffman J, Geary S: Preoperative self-efficacy and postoperative behaviors. *Appl Nurs Res* 5:134–139, 1992.

59. Covington MV, Omelich CL: The influence of expectancies and problem-solving strategies on smoking intentions, in Schwarzer R (ed): *Self-Efficacy: Thought Control of Action*. Philadelphia, Hemisphere Publishing, 1992; pp 263–283.

60. Kaplan RM, Atkins CJ, Reinsch S: Specific efficacy expectations mediate exercise compliance in patients with COPD. *Health Psychol* 3:223–242, 1984.

61. Kaplan RM, Ries AL, Prewitt LM, Eakin E: Self-efficacy expectations predict survival for patients with chronic obstructive pulmonary disease. *Health Psychol* 13:366–368, 1994.

62. Condiotte MM, Lichtenstein E: Self-efficacy and relapse in a smoking cessation program. *J Consult Clin Psychol* 49:648–658, 1981.

63. Schwarzer R (ed): *Self-Efficacy: Thought Control of Action*. Philadelphia, Hemisphere Publishing, 1992.

64. Wigal JK, Creer TL, Kotses H: The COPD self-efficacy scale. *Chest* 99:1193–1196, 1991.

65. Kobasa SC: Stressful life events, personality and health: An inquiry into hardiness. *J Person Soc Psychol* 37:1–11, 1979.

66. Pollock SE: The stress response. *Crit Care Q* 6:1–14, 1984.

67. Pollock SE: The hardiness characteristic: A motivating factor in adaptation. *Adv Nurs Sci* 11:53–62, 1989.

68. Magnani L: Hardiness, self-perceived health, and activity among independently functioning older adults. *Scholar Inquiry Nurs Pract* 4:171–183, 1990.

69. Lee H: Relationship of hardiness and current life events to perceived health in rural adults. *Res Nurs Health* 14:351–359, 1991.

70. Pollock SE: Adaptive responses to diabetes mellitus. *West J Nurs Res* 11:265–280, 1989.

71. Pollock SE: Adaptation to chronic illness: A program of research for testing nursing theory. *Nurs Sci Q* 6:86–92, 1993.

72. Boyle A, Grap M, Younger J: Personality hardiness, ways of coping, social support, and burnout in critical care nurses. *J Adv Nurs* 16:850–857, 1991.

73. Pollock S, Christian B, Sands D: Responses to chronic illness: Analysis of psychological and physiological adaptation. *Nurs Res* 39:300–304, 1990.

74. Wiebe D, McCallum D: Health practices and hardiness as mediators in the stress-illness relationship. *Health Psychol* 5:425–438, 1986.

75. Kobasa S: The hardy personality: Toward a social psychology of stress and health, in Sulo J, Sanders G (eds): *Social Psychology of Health and Illness*. Hillsdale, NJ, Erlbaum, 1982.

76. Narsavage GL, Weaver TE: Causal attribution and hardiness related to coping with COPD. *Am Rev Respir Dis* 145:A477, 1992.

77. Narsavage G, Weaver T: Coping and hardiness related to functioning with COPD. *Am Rev Respir Dis* 143:A806, 1991.

78. Hull J, Von Treuren R, Virnelli S: Hardiness and health: A critique and alternative approach. *J Person Soc Psychol* 53:518–530, 1987.

79. Pollock S, Duffy M: The Health Related Hardiness Scale: Development and psychometric analysis. *Nurs Res* 39:218–222, 1990.

79a. Wallston KA, Stein MJ, Smith CA: Form C of the MHLC scales: A condition-specific measure of locus of control. *J Pers Assess* 63:534–553, 1994.

80. Narsavage GL: Pulmonary functional outcomes after home care nursing: Phase I (abstract). *Eur Respir J* 9:35S, 1996.

81. Cohen F, Lazarus RS: Coping and adaptation in health and illness, in Mechanic D (ed): *Handbook of Health, Health Care and the Health Professions*. New York, Free Press, 1983.

82. Fagerhaugh S: Getting around with emphysema. *Am J Nurs* 73:94–99, 1973.

83. Carrieri VK, Janson-Bjerklie S: Strategies patients use to manage the sensation of dyspnea. *West J Nurs Res* 8:284–305, 1986.

84. McSweeney A, Grant I, Heaton R, et al: Life quality of patients with COPD. *Arch Intern Med* 142:473–478, 1982.

85. Postma D, Burema J, Gimeno F, et al: Prognosis in severe chronic obstructive pulmonary disease. *Am Rev Respir Dis* 119:357–367, 1979.

86. Freedberg P, Hoffman L, Light W, Kreps M: Effect of progressive muscle relaxation on the objective symptoms and subjective responses associated with asthma. *Heart Lung* 16:24–30, 1987.

87. Folkman S, Lazarus R: The relationship between coping and emotion: Implications for theory and research. *Soc Sci Med* 26:309–317, 1988.

88. Billings A, Moos R: Coping, stress, and social resources among adults with unipolar depression. *J Person Soc Psychol* 46:877–891, 1984.

89. Narsavage GL: Families and their relationships, in Craven R, Hirnle C (eds): *Fundamentals of Nursing: Human Health and Function*, 2d ed. Philadelphia, Lippincott, 1996; pp 1441–1464.

90. McCubbin HI, Thompson AI (eds): *Family Assessment Inventories for Research and Practice*. Madison, WI, University of Wisconsin, 1987.

Chapter 23

IMPAIRMENT AND DISABILITY EVALUATION

THEODORE G. LIOU
RICHARD E. KANNER

Physicians play a key role in the medicolegal evaluation of impairment and disability and ultimately the disbursement of disability insurance payouts. Physicians gather medical information and perform consultative examinations for governmental and private disability programs. The information gathered directly determines the presence or absence of impairments. Following the determination of impairment, a primarily medical evaluation, physicians also may participate in the determination of disability, which involves both medical and legal considerations. Finally, in disputed claims of disability, physicians are frequently called on to be expert witnesses before administrative law and higher-ranking judges.

In 1992, the Social Security Administration provided payments to 3,473,330 disabled workers through its Old Age, Survivors and Disability (OASDI) program. Approximately 640,000 of these workers were added during 1992, chosen out of a pool of 1.3 million new applicants for disability payments. Payments were made to these disabled workers amounting to more than $2 billion, of which 4.1 percent was for diseases of the respiratory system.[1] While these figures are already substantial, even larger sums are involved when one considers all federal programs along with state and private insurance programs. Approximately $30 billion in benefits from all these sources were paid to about 20,000,000 disabled workers in 1993.[2] A breakdown of specific amounts by disease types is not yet available, but a reasonable estimate is that more than a billion dollars was paid to sufferers of respiratory diseases.

The determination of disability and any payments depends directly on information provided by physicians following thorough evaluation. A careful history and physical examinations and appropriate pulmonary and exercise testing constitute the core of objective data gathering. However, the data gathered do not lead directly to a determination of disability. Rather, the data can directly support a finding of impairment due to respiratory disease.

The definition of impairment is distinct from the definition of disability. *Impairment* involves loss or abnormality of an anatomic structure, physiologic function, or mental or emotional functioning.[3] Using this definition, impairment can be determined to exist solely on the basis of medical evaluation.

Disability does not have a simple definition, and what it is interpreted to be varies widely in scope depending on the agency, private or public, that determines the presence or absence of disability. For example, the Social Security Disability Insurance Program considers people disabled if they are "unable to engage in substantial gainful activity."[4] In con-

trast, the Americans with Disabilities Act of 1990 (ADA) determines that a person is disabled if he or she has a physical or mental impairment that substantially limits one or more of the major life activities, has a record of such an impairment, or is regarded as having such an impairment.[5]

The judicial system continues to interpret the definitions of disability and their relationships to impairment as a result of the review of multiple cases brought under the various acts. For example, under the ADA, the courts have established that some impairments automatically constitute disability, such as insulin-dependent diabetes[6] and cystic fibrosis.[7] Other impairments that limit the ability to perform one job but not the performance of other jobs do not constitute a disability under the ADA.[8] These decisions have altered the meaning of disability under the ADA but not necessarily under other parts of the law. Unfortunately, the continuing changes brought about by case law have increased the difficulties for physicians in understanding disability.

The confusion over terminology also has been increased because the World Health Organization (WHO) has defined *impairment* and *disability* somewhat differently from U.S. laws.[9] WHO defines *impairment* as the physiologic loss of function. *Disability* is defined as the impact of the physiologic loss. For example, a decrease in forced expiratory volume in 1 s (FEV_1) is an impairment by WHO terminology that results in a decrease in exercise ability, which is a disability. Under U.S. terminology, both the decrease in FEV_1 and the decrease in exercise ability are impairments. WHO has added the term *handicap* in this context to mean social and occupational disadvantage, a term analogous to the American idea of disability.[9,10] It is important to understand these distinctions when evaluating claimants from the many countries, especially in Europe, where the WHO definitions generally have been accepted.

In addition to the basic concept of disability, there is also the concept of occupational disability or job-specific disability. The same impairment to one worker may be annoying but to another can mean a catastrophic loss of income. For example, baker's asthma is vocation ending for an apprentice baker but is inconsequential to a musician. At the same time, a hand tremor secondary to bronchodilating agents that completely control asthma may be a minor annoyance to a baker but may be devastating to a musician.

In an attempt to clarify what is meant by disability, the WHO handicap guidelines for evaluation have been created. These guidelines aim at standardizing the evaluation procedures and criteria for determining the severity of an impairment, which can then be used in assessing disability. However, several sets of guidelines are in common use, and certain agencies have unique guidelines. Thus it is crucial that an evaluating physician consult with the governmental or private insurance agency requesting the evaluation and use the guidelines preferred or mandated.

The physician is expected to prepare an objective report of his or her evaluation of a claimant's impairment. For the pulmonary physician, the report must provide all the elements required in the preferred guidelines including the results of history and physical evaluation and the results, with interpretations, of objective testing. When a test, such as exercise testing, is optional under the guidelines used, the physician who chooses to perform such a test should state his or her rationale and provide an easily understandable and concise interpretation of the results. Clearly stated indications and interpretations for an optional test may help avoid delaying a claim because the test was unusual or unexpected by the processing agency. Impairment/disability evaluation guidelines frequently specify not only the required and optional content of an impairment evaluation report but also the format of presentation. It is clearly helpful to the applicant and the agency to conform as much as is possible to all the requirements and suggestions. Finally, it is important to avoid statements concerning the presence or absence of impairments outside the scope of the request.

Guidelines for Evaluation

Given the differing guidelines and definitions of disability among agencies, evaluating physicians should follow the specific guidelines recommended by the particular governmental agency or private insurance company. Nonetheless, there are general guidelines that are published and in widespread use, and these include the American Medical Association *Guides to the Evaluation of Permanent Impairment*[11] and, for pulmonary disorders, several statements from the American Thoracic Society (ATS).[12-14] Governmental programs usually have sets of guidelines that are frequently tailored to the needs of a specific piece of legislation.

AMERICAN MEDICAL ASSOCIATION GUIDELINES

The American Medical Association (AMA) *Guides to the Evaluation of Permanent Impairment* is mandated or recommended for use in 55 percent of workers' compensation jurisdictions and is in frequent use in many of the remaining jurisdictions in the United States.[11] These guidelines were first published in 1971 and have been revised and updated at regular intervals. The guidelines include general suggestions about impairment evaluation and the preparation of physician reports and chapters on the evaluation of impairments due to disease in specific organ systems. These guidelines review the history and physical examination process and, for pulmonary physicians, briefly discuss the use of chest x-rays, spirometry, diffusion measurements, exercise studies, and arterial blood-gas determinations. The guidelines also include classification systems that identify levels of impairment and levels of work. These classifications are used widely and frequently are useful in judging the impact of respiratory impairment with regard to disability.

The AMA also has recently published a companion book entitled *Disability Evaluation*.[15] This book also provides a synopsis of the impairment evaluation and provides classification systems for impairments (Table 23-1). It extends the previous AMA publication by providing a larger overview of the disability determination process. It also discusses the difficult questions of temporary impairment and asthma-induced impairments by including the ATS recommendations of 1993.[14]

AMERICAN THORACIC SOCIETY GUIDELINES

The American Thoracic Society has published a series of statements that are used widely for the evaluation of impairment and disability due to respiratory diseases. An initial statement was published in 1982 and was revised in 1986.[12,13] An additional statement addressing the approach for claim-

ants with asthma was published in 1993.[14] Most of the standards and suggestions included in these statements have been adopted by the AMA and appear in both AMA publications.[11,15] However, there are a few subtle differences that are pointed out in the most recent AMA publication.[15]

SOCIAL SECURITY ADMINISTRATION GUIDELINES

While most private insurance firms mandate use of the AMA impairment guidelines,[11] the Social Security Administration (SSA) uses its own guidelines[4] for administration of its two disability programs. The SSA covers more people with disability than any other agency. Disability insurance benefits are provided under Title II of the Social Security Act. Persons or dependents and widows of persons who have worked and made Social Security payments are eligible for disability insurance benefits. The Supplemental Security Income program covers disabled individuals of all ages who are disabled and have limited income and resources under Title XVI of the Social Security Act. A description of each program, the process of disability determination under Social Security, brief suggestions for the medical report format, and listings of impairments with specific evidentiary requirements are included in a single volume.[4]

BLACK LUNG BENEFITS

Other disability programs use their own guidelines. For example, the Black Lung Program provides for separate disability benefits for coal miners and is administered by the Department of Labor. The program is authorized under Title IV of the federal Coal Mine Health and Safety Act of 1969, as amended by the Black Lung Benefits Act of 1972, the Federal Mine Safety and Health Amendments Act of 1977, the Black Lung Benefits Reform Act of 1977, the Black Lung Benefits Revenue Act of 1977, the Black Lung Benefits Amendments of 1981, and the Black Lung Benefits Revenue Act of 1981. The current regulations for the Black Lung Program are found in the *Code of Federal Regulations*.[16] The act covers self-employed miners, workers employed in or around a coal mine or preparation facility in the extraction or preparation of coal, and transportation and construction workers who work or have worked in or around coal mines to the extent that they were exposed to coal dust.

Following the filing of a disability claim through a local Social Security office, the applicant receives a packet including specific instructions for an examining physician. The wording of the current act allows each applicant to have a "complete pulmonary evaluation," which includes history, physical examination, chest x-ray, and spirometry but may include other pulmonary laboratory testing as judged by the physician to be needed to determine the presence of an impairment. The act includes specific guidelines on performance, interpretation, and quality control of testing. Chest radiography guidelines are based on the latest revision of the *Classification of the Pneumoconioses of the Union Internationale Contra Cancer/Cincinnati*, which has been incorporated in the International Labor Office guidelines.[17] Pulmonary function testing guidelines are based on the original ATS guidelines for performance of spirometry,[18] and they include a table showing 60 percent of predicted normal FEV_1 and forced vital capacity (FVC) depending on sex and height but based on older standard values.[19] With modern pulmonary function

TABLE 23-1 Ratings Schemes of AMA and ATS[a]

	FVC	FEV$_1$	FEV$_1$/FVC	DLCO	V$_{O_2}$	Comment
Class 1 (none)	≥80% pred.	≥80% pred.	≥0.70	≥70% pred.	≥25	Must meet all
	(≥80% pred.)	(≥80% pred.)	(≥0.75)	(≥80% pred.)	(—)	criteria
Class 2 (mild)	60–79% pred.	60–79% pred.	—	60–79% pred.	20–25	Must meet one
	(60–79% pred.)	(60–79% pred.)	(0.60–0.74)	(60–79% pred.)	(—)	criterion
Class 3 (moderate)	51–59% pred.	41–59% pred.	—	41–59% pred.	15–20	Must meet one
	(51–59% pred.)	(41–59% pred.)	(0.41–0.59)	(41–59% pred.)	(—)	criterion
Class 4 (severe)	≤50% pred.	≤40% pred.	—	≤40% pred.	≤15	Must meet one
	(≤50% pred.)	(≤40% pred.)	(≤0.40)	(≤40% pred.)	(—)	criterion
Prediction equation	Crapo, 1980			Crapo, 1981	Units: mL/O$_2$/min/kg weight	

[a] Classification schemes recommended by the AMA and ATS (in parentheses). % pred. = percentage of predicted value. The ratio FEV$_1$/FVC is expressed as an *absolute* number, not as percentage of predicted; to emphasize this and to avoid confusion, the ratio is expressed as a decimal in this table.
SOURCE: Modified from Demeter et al,[15] with permission of the American Medical Association.

testing equipment, any standard set of predicted normal values can be requested by a physician and may be provided directly on the spirometry report.

OTHER PROGRAMS

Other special governmental programs and numerous different private and state-managed disability programs provide benefits to disabled persons. Many of these programs use the AMA or ATS guidelines; however, many use guidelines that are unique. The examining physician should be aware of the specific requirements of each program to which a claimant applies and should not hesitate to contact the administrator who oversees a particular program, especially when questions arise about the admissibility of particular pulmonary tests.

All the different guidelines have a common goal—to determine whether the patient applicant has an impairment and whether the impairment constitutes a disability. To achieve this, nearly all the guidelines require a history and physical examination. Most also require spirometry and chest radiographs. Some additionally allow measurement of arterial blood gases and exercise testing. When tests that are considered necessary are outside the scope of the guidelines or of a specific program, the physician usually can contact the program administrator to ascertain whether the test would be allowed.

Objective Testing

There is an array of pulmonary tests that may be helpful in the complete evaluation of disability due to respiratory disease. Under most guidelines, the examining physician is asked to judge the appropriateness of each test and to give medical interpretations of results.

PULMONARY FUNCTION TESTING

SPIROMETRY
Most useful data obtained with spirometry result from measurements of the forced expiratory volume in 1 s (FEV$_1$), forced vital capacity (FVC), and a calculation of the FEV$_1$/FVC ratio before and after the administration of bronchodilators. Although a few disability programs request measure-

ment of the FEF$_{25–75}$ and maximal voluntary ventilation (MVV) for evaluation of impairment, they are not essential or requested under ATS,[12] AMA,[11] or Social Security Administration[4] guidelines.

Each of the spirometric measurements must be carried out in accordance with accepted performance procedures. In the United States, the standards for performing spirometry are maintained and regularly reviewed and revised by the American Thoracic Society.[20] Specific guidelines and quality control for performance have been written for the four measurements, FEV$_1$, FVC, FEF$_{25–75}$, and MVV. General recommendations on spirometry interpretation are also published by the American Thoracic Society.[21] Other standards that agree for the most part with the ATS recommendations and that are used widely in disability evaluation include the recommendations of the Intermountain Thoracic Society.[22] Several sets of normal values beside those used by the American and Intermountain Thoracic Societies are in common use in interpreting the results of spirometric measurements.[23]

The AMA, ATS, and Social Security guidelines recommend spirometry with bronchodilators if clinically indicated. For the AMA guidelines, the presence of wheezing is an indication for bronchodilator testing.[11] These three most widely used guidelines[4,11,12] each recommend testing bronchodilators when obstructive disease is present, as defined by an FEV$_1$/FVC of less than 0.70. The best results for FEV$_1$ and FVC regardless of bronchodilator use are to be reported. It must be documented that at least three maximal efforts with at least two results with 5 percent or less reproducibility were obtained.

In addition to the interpretations of spirometry that are important for diagnosis and management of respiratory disease, additional statements directly addressing impairment should be made when impairment/disability evaluation is the purpose of testing. If a specific threshold is identified that defines an impairment, a statement should be included explicitly identifying the threshold crossed and the level of impairment identified. For example, if an FVC of 55 percent of predicted is found under the ATS guidelines for impairment,[12] one might report, "The claimant has a moderately impaired level of lung function that is correlated with a diminishing ability to meet the physical demands of many jobs based on an FVC of 55 percent of predicted normal." Under the classification system used in the AMA guidelines,[11] one might say that the same applicant "... has a class 3 impairment that is 26 to 50 percent or moderate impairment of the whole person." In these examples, the 55 percent of predicted figure is based on the reference values for FVC from Crapo and colleagues,[24] as specified in both the ATS and AMA guidelines.

DIFFUSING CAPACITY MEASUREMENTS

The single-breath carbon monoxide diffusing capacity (DLCOsb) measures the ability of the lung to transfer carbon monoxide from inspired gas to pulmonary capillary blood. The factors that influence the results include distribution of alveolar ventilation, alveolar volume, alveolar–capillary wall characteristics, capillary size, and the concentration and reactivity of hemoglobin in the blood.

There are several single-breath methods, but in addition, there are rebreathing and steady-state methods of evaluating gas transfer. Efforts have been made to standardize the single-breath test so that interlaboratory differences are minimized. The latest recommendations for diffusing capacity measurements of the ATS in 1995[25] are not substantially different from previous recommendations.[26] The techniques for performing the measurement are well described in the Intermountain Thoracic Society guidelines for pulmonary function testing.[22]

Measurement of the DLCOsb is not always necessary in the evaluation or management of impairment or disability, and the physician must judge the need of the test. For example, the hypothetical applicant with an FVC of 55 percent of predicted has an established impairment regardless of DLCOsb measurement results. If the goal is to establish whether an impairment exists without regard to severity, then measuring the DLCOsb does not add to the evaluation. The DLCOsb may be of use to document impairment of gas exchange in a applicant with no measurable defect in spirometry but whose clinical history or physical examination suggests the presence of respiratory disease.

The diffusing capacity is also useful in grading the severity of an impairment. Under both AMA and ATS guidelines, severity of respiratory impairment is graded using the most abnormal single result of FEV_1, FVC, and DLCOsb (see Table 23-1). Thus a class 2 or mild impairment of the whole person can be based on an FVC of 75 percent and an FEV_1 of 60 percent of predicted; however, if the same claimant also has a DLCOsb of 35 percent, then the impairment is class 4, or severe impairment of the whole person.

In contrast to other disability programs, the Social Security Administration is very specific regarding the performance and use of diffusion measurements. In addition to specific guidelines for performance of the DLCOsb measurement, the Social Security Administration publication for disability evaluation[4] also includes recommendations on the appropriateness of ordering the test. Under the Social Security Disability evaluation guidelines, the DLCOsb measurement should be ordered when chronic respiratory impairment is already documented, but previous testing, including spirometry, has not established the level of impairment.

LUNG VOLUME MEASUREMENTS

Measurements of lung volumes, particularly the total lung capacity (TLC), are frequently helpful in clinical pulmonary medicine but not in impairment/disability evaluation. Clini-

cally, the TLC can help distinguish severe obstructive disease with a markedly decreased FVC due to air trapping, severe restrictive disease, or a combined obstructive and restrictive disease. In the evaluation of impairment and disability, TLC measurement is not helpful because the primary question is whether impairments are present or not. Carefully describing or naming the respiratory disease process itself is in fact not essential. For example, an FVC of 50 percent of predicted constitutes an AMA or ATS class 4 (see Table 23-1) severe impairment of the whole person. However, applicants with either severe obstruction or severe restriction or both can have an FVC of 50 percent.

ARTERIAL BLOOD-GAS MEASUREMENTS

Arterial blood-gas (ABG) measurements [i.e., arterial pH, partial pressure of carbon dioxide (Pa_{CO_2}), partial pressure of oxygen (Pa_{O_2}), and oxygen saturation (Sa_{O_2})] may be useful in the evaluation of impairment/disability. ABG measurements must be carried out by a laboratory that is certified by a governmental agency or participates in a satisfactory manner in a nationally recognized proficiency program. One widely used reference set of guidelines and standards is published and updated on a continuing basis by the National Committee for Clinical Laboratory Standards (NCCLS).[27] Their standards and guidelines are accepted and approved by the American National Standards Institute. Careful observation of the guidelines on specimen handling, collection, and analysis helps to ensure that ABG measurements will be acceptable to a disability agency.[28]

In the evaluation of impairment, the primary goal of an ABG measurement is to establish arterial hypoxemia. Hypoxemia by itself is not evidence of impairment. However, it can support the finding of impairment and provide information about the severity of impairment when specific conditions such as cor pulmonale are present. In the presence of normal spirometry, abnormal ABG results can confirm the presence of gas-exchange defects due to respiratory disease.

Caution must be employed when ABG measurements are used to establish hypoxemia because nonrespiratory factors caused by the altitude at which the ABG measurement is made must be taken into account. Tables are provided, for example, by the Social Security guidelines that assist in determining hypoxemia for three altitude ranges: 0 to 3000 ft, 3000 to 6000 ft, and greater than 6000 ft above sea level. Voluntary or involuntary hypoventilation also may cause an apparent hypoxemia and must be excluded by evaluation of the ventilatory status of the applicant. The tables for the three altitude ranges in the Social Security guidelines provide minimum Pa_{O_2} thresholds. Below these thresholds, hypoxemia is considered in the table to depend on the Pa_{CO_2}. The varying threshold for hypoxemia based on the Pa_{CO_2} is designed to correct hypoventilation.

The report of ABG results should include the actual measured results, a diagnosis of the acid-base status, and a diagnosis of the oxygenation status. A statement identifying the proficiency standards used by the blood-gas laboratory, the concentration or fraction of inspired oxygen, the claimant's status when the sample was drawn (resting, walking, etc.), and the altitude and the barometric pressure in the laboratory at the time of the test also must be included. When the disability guidelines identify a specific minimum arterial partial pressure for hypoxemia, that threshold should be identified along with the abnormal value. It also may be helpful to include a statement briefly justifying the use of ABG measurements.

A sample report might read, "ABG measurement at 1500 m elevation and at P_B 640 while the applicant was breathing room air at rest showed pH 7.37, Pa_{CO_2} 37, Pa_{O_2} 55, and Sa_{O_2} 88 percent. The test was performed in accordance with all applicable current guidelines and standards of the National Committee for Clinical Laboratory Standards. The results reveal normal acid-base, normal ventilatory status, and moderate hypoxemia based on low Pa_{O_2} and low Sa_{O_2}. This test confirms the moderate impairment of gas exchange suggested by the moderately low DLCOsb previously performed and reported."

PULMONARY EXERCISE TESTING

Pulmonary exercise testing is helpful. Clinically, it is used to distinguish exercise limitation due to pulmonary causes from cardiac or other causes such as obesity, voluntary deconditioning, or perhaps malingering. In the setting of rehabilitation, exercise testing is helpful in identifying the potential for recovery of work ability and in formulating an exercise prescription. The general opinion[11,12,15,34] is emerging that exercise testing can be of great use in many potentially impaired claimants.

Exercise testing should be performed in compliance with nationally recognized standards. The American College of Sports Medicine publishes the most widely used set of guidelines.[29] While the guidelines are thorough and provide an in-depth framework for performing exercise testing, they recognize that the needs of individual claimants may require some modification of the exercise test. The evaluating physician should be familiar with the risks, indications, contraindications, and actual techniques of exercise testing.

The Social Security Administration[4] has very specific guidelines and measurements that are to be followed in the performance of exercise testing for an evaluation for impairment. It remains the responsibility of the physician to decide whether testing is appropriate and to follow the guidelines as closely as possible.

There have been changes in ideas concerning the usefulness of exercise testing in the evaluation of impairment. The 1986 ATS guidelines[12] stated that exercise testing was not required because earlier literature demonstrated a reliable relationship between FEV_1 and DLCOsb[30–33] and exercise ability. The 1993 AMA guidelines[11] agreed that exercise testing was not mandatory but recognized that exercise testing is helpful in differentiating cardiac from pulmonary causes of impairment. In addition, these guidelines stated that exercise testing might be useful in the assessment of applicants whose daily activities require moderately strenuous and sustained exertion or heavy and frequent exertion and whose complaints are inconsistent with the results of testing at rest.[12]

A number of publications support the most recent AMA position.[15] Using cycle ergometry, Oren and colleagues[35] evaluated 348 workers who claimed to have or were suspected of having exercise limitation on the basis of history, physical examination, and resting studies. Their results showed that 46 (31 percent) of 148 workers predicted to have a normal work capacity by resting measurements actually had low measured work capacities. Thirty-six of the 46 (78 percent) had previously unsuspected cardiac disease, 7 had lung disease, and 3 had noncardiopulmonary disease. Their results with workers judged to have low exercise capacity were equally striking.[35] Of 66 applicants predicted to have low work capacities, fully a third were thought to be normal after exercise testing. In a British study of 119 men referred with confirmed or suspected work-related pulmonary disorders, Cotes and colleagues[10] presented data that showed that loss of exercise capacity cannot be predicted reliably on the basis of FEV_1, FVC, FEV_1/FVC ratio, or DLCOsb.

The current literature suggests then that exercise testing may be valuable in at least two settings. First, in applicants judged to be normal, exercise testing may reveal unanticipated reductions in exercise capacity. The majority of these applicants will have occult cardiac disease[35] that results in the presence of respiratory symptoms with relatively normal resting pulmonary studies. From the narrow technical view of evaluation for impairment due to respiratory disease, the finding of cardiac disease does not often alter the normal results of resting pulmonary evaluation. However, for a physician, identification of the exercise impairment from any nonpulmonary cause is still important both from a disability viewpoint and from a patient care viewpoint. The applicant may have a nonpulmonary impairment that still qualifies as a disability, and the evaluation may proceed along different but more relevant lines. The applicant also may have new opportunities for treatment or rehabilitation based on a better understanding of his or her previously occcult disease.

Second, in a significant number of claimants who have abnormal pulmonary function tests, exercise testing may reveal that their capacity to do work is in fact undiminished. For some claimants, this may bolster their confidence to return to work. For those who continue with their disability claims, the legal implication is uncertain, since the single worst indicator in many evaluation schemes determines the level of impairment. For example, an FEV_1 of 63 percent of predicted with a measured V_{O_2} of 26 mL O_2 per minute per kilogram still qualifies as a class 2 or mild impairment under AMA and ATS guidelines despite the normal V_{O_2} measurement (see Table 23-1). In this hypothetical example, the exercise test did not add to the evaluation of the claimant's impairment, and current standards require that every measurement made be in the normal range before classifying a claimant as normal. However, a normal exercise test in this setting may allow a claimant to proceed with rehabilitation or retraining for work that requires an exercise intensity that is not anticipated by abnormal resting studies.

Exercise testing also may provide information that can help to identify claimants who have strong secondary gains and possibly fictitious complaints. Using standard exercise protocols and measuring V_{O_2}, dead space ventilation, alveolar-arterial oxygen gradient, and the arterial–end-tidal CO_2 gradient, a diagnosis of poor effort can be made.[36] Whether poor effort is due to true malingering or some other cause such as extreme anxiety will still need to be determined by the evaluating physician.

In practice, any applicant who has respiratory symptoms out of proportion to resting pulmonary testing results or who complains of general inability to work due to unexplained fatigue should be strongly considered for exercise testing to confirm otherwise occult impairment. Additionally, any applicant contemplated for a rehabilitation or retraining program should undergo exercise testing because knowledge of maximal sustainable exercise capacity can be used to guide the design and level of intensity of the rehabilitation or retraining.

The physician's report of exercise testing should include a technical description of the testing performed. The testing must comply with the evaluation guidelines and/or applicable nationally recognized practice, and a statement should be included stating that the testing was technically acceptable. A concise description of the actual protocol, the grades of exercise, and the performance of the exercise must be included. Actual measurements that comply with the specific requirements of the disability agency must be reported.

The physician usually also must provide an interpretation of the examination. There should be a simple statement of the level of exercise achieved and whether this was normal. Statements should follow for abnormal test results delineating which organ system or what particular etiology or etiologies are responsible for the abnormal test.

A sample report might read, "Exercise testing was performed in accordance with the guidelines of the American College of Sports Medicine and was technically acceptable. Using cycle ergometry, the patient pedaled at 60 rev/min with no load for 5 min. The work rate was then increased by 15 watts per minute. Arterial blood was sampled before, every other minute during, and after exercise, and intraarterial pressure was continuously measured via a percutaneous radial arterial line. Exercise was stopped due to generalized fatigue. The patient exercised past his anaerobic threshold and achieved a maximal V_{O_2} of 19 mL O_2/min per kilogram. Dead space ventilation was unusually high, but the heart rate reserve also was high. Twelve-lead ECG monitoring during exercise revealed no abnormalities. The results indicate mild to moderate exercise limitation consistent with respiratory limited exercise. This constitutes a class 3 or moderate impairment due to respiratory causes according to the ATS guidelines."

POLYSOMNOGRAPHY

Sleep-related disordered breathing may cause temporary or permanent impairment. Sleep-disordered breathing is found in 9 percent of women and 24 percent of men of middle age.[37] Two percent of women and 4 percent of men in the same study were found to have occult sleep apnea.[37]

There are two categories of sleep apnea, obstructive and central, with common associated morbidities. Obstructive sleep apnea is the predominant type. Both categories result in periodic cessation of breathing during sleep with resulting recurrent episodes of hypoxemia and arousal from sleep.[38] Early symptoms may be limited to excessive daytime drowsiness, decreased alertness, restlessness, fatigue, and unsatisfying sleep without measurable abnormalities of gas exchange or blood pressure. Other findings may include aggravation of chronic alveolar hypoventilation with chronic blood-gas abnormalities,[39] pulmonary hypertension, right or left heart failure,[40] and systemic hypertension.[41] Sleep apnea may impair an applicant's cognitive ability[42] to do useful work of any type and may result in a personal and public hazard, as with an applicant who operates heavy machinery or drives despite overwhelming daytime drowsiness.[43-46]

Given the high incidence of sleep-disordered breathing and apnea and the common sequelae of daytime drowsiness, it should be anticipated that a significant number of impairment evaluations will require sleep studies.

The diagnosis and distinction between the two types of sleep apnea as well as the treatment depend on proper testing with polysomnography and multiple sleep latency testing. Guidelines for the performance of polysomnography are published by the American Electroencephalographic Society[47] and the American Thoracic Society.[48] Polysomnography may be followed by a multiple sleep latency test, which is a standardized measure of daytime sleepiness.[49,50]

While technical performance of sleep testing is well standardized, the assessment of degree of impairment in claimants with abnormal tests is not. Cognitive dysfunction, excessive sleepiness, fatigue, and other daytime symptoms of sleep-disordered breathing can all severely impair an individual's ability to perform useful work. Unfortunately, the physician must judge the severity of impairment without the benefit of recognized grading guidelines. This may not be difficult in some cases; musicians cannot perform with greatly decreased dexterity, physicians cannot treat patients to the best of their ability with severe cognitive impairments, and commercial drivers or pilots cannot perform their functions safely with even brief but overwhelming episodes of daytime sleepiness. In other cases, when the sleep disturbance is mild and the daytime deficits are subtle, the evaluating physician must use his or her best judgment on a case-by-case basis.

Presentation of testing results should be in accordance with the recommendations of recognized guidelines and standards.[47-50] The report should include a summary of technical findings followed by a concise interpretive section. Clear statements stating the normality or abnormality of the study or studies and justifications of the impressions should be included. For impairment/disability examinations, as concise a statement as possible should be added stating the estimated degree of impairment. Unlike interpreters of spirometry, arterial blood gases, and exercise studies, reporters of sleep testing must specifically qualify to perform and interpret sleep testing under the guidelines already cited. If the impairment/disability evaluating physician is not qualified, then testing needs to be requested of and performed by a qualified physician and sleep laboratory. In this case, impairment statements should be requested of the interpreting physician.

TESTING FOR SPECIAL CONDITIONS AND CIRCUMSTANCES

ASTHMA

The presence of cough, sputum production, wheeze, chest tightness, or breathlessness by history with episodic and possibly nocturnal worsening suggests the diagnosis of asthma. Symptoms may be triggered by any of a large number of triggering stimuli from exposure to specific allergens to emotional or physical stress or to environmental conditions such as cold air. The presence of completely or partially reversible and variable airflow obstruction or increased responsiveness to methacholine or histamine completes the diagnosis. When specific allergens or environmental conditions can be identified as triggers of asthma, spirometric

TABLE 23-2 Postbronchodilator FEV$_1$

Score	FEV$_1$ % Predicted
0	>Lower limit of normal
1	70–Lower limit of normal
2	60–69
3	50–59
4	<50

SOURCE: From Chan-Yeung et al,[14] with permission.

TABLE 23-3 Reversibility of FEV$_1$ or Degree of Airway Hyperresponsiveness[a]

Score	% FEV$_1$ Change	PC$_{20}$ mg/mL or Equivalent
0	<10	>8
1	10–19	8–>0.5
2	20–29	0.5–>0.125
3	≥30	≤0.125
4	—	—

[a] When FEV$_1$ is above the lower limit of normal, PC$_{20}$ should be determined and used for rating of impairment; when FEV$_1$ is <70% predicted, the degree of reversibility should be used; when FEV$_1$ is between 70% predicted and the lower limit of normal, either reversibility or PC$_{20}$ can be used.

Reversibility with bronchodilator is calculated as

$$\frac{\text{FEV}_1 \text{ postbronchodilator} - \text{FEV}_1 \text{ prebronchodilator}}{\text{FEV}_1 \text{ prebronchodilator}} \times 100\%$$

Airway responsiveness is expressed as that concentration of agent that will provoke a fall in FEV$_1$ of 20% from the lowest postsaline value. Plot the concentration of methacholine/histamine against the fall in FEV$_1$ using a logarithm scale for the doubling concentrations. The PC$_{20}$ is obtained by interpolation between the last two points. The formula for linear interpolation of the PC$_{20}$ from the log dose-response curve is as follows:

$$\text{PC}_{20} = \text{antilog } C1 + \frac{(\log C2 - \log C1)(20 - R1)}{(R2 - R1)}$$

where C1 = second-last concentration (<20% FEV$_1$ fall)
C2 = last concentration (>20% FEV$_1$ fall)
R1 = % fall FEV$_1$ after C1
R2 = % fall FEV$_1$ after C2

SOURCE: From Chan-Yeung et al,[14] with permission.

testing before and after exposure to the trigger can be very helpful. The reversible nature of asthma frequently complicates efforts to confirm the presence of asthma, while the variability of disease, whether treated or untreated, makes assessments of impairment severity difficult.

The variable nature of asthma over time has created a need to address both temporary and permanent impairment from asthma. Initial evaluation of impairment for asthma should address whether optimal, meaning maximally effective, therapy has been instituted. If not, then the evaluation should proceed to assign a temporary impairment rating. However, if optimal therapy has been instituted and the disease is stable, then an evaluation of permanent impairment can be performed. It is important to note that optimal therapy does not equate to all therapies but rather that optimal therapy has been instituted when any additional therapy or therapies are not likely to help. Since not all therapies are tolerated by all patients, avoidance of a potentially beneficial therapy because of demonstrated unacceptable side effects does not make a patient's treatment regimen suboptimal.

The American Thoracic Society has published guidelines specific to impairment evaluation for asthma.[14] Within these guidelines, suggestions are made for the diagnostic workup of asthma. In the absence of symptoms, asthma is not present. The results of spirometry in any one of three circumstances is used to confirm the diagnosis:

1. Airflow obstruction (FEV$_1$/FVC < 0.7) with an improvement in FEV$_1$ ≥ 12 percent or 200 mL after bronchodilators
2. Airflow obstruction with an improvement in FEV$_1$ ≥ 20 percent after a steroid trial
3. No airflow obstruction but a provocation concentration to cause a 20 percent drop in FEV$_1$ ≤ 8 mg/mL methacholine or histamine.

The ATS guidelines provide a scoring system to assess the severity of asthma based on (1) the FEV$_1$ as a percentage predicted (Table 23-2), (2) the reversibility of FEV$_1$ or the degree of hyperresponsiveness (Table 23-3), and (3) the minimum medication required (Table 23-4). The total score is then translated into an impairment class, 0 to V (Table 23-5). Class 0 is not impaired, whereas class V is total impairment due to asthma that is not adequately controlled despite maximal treatment (e.g., with prednisone ≥20 mg PO qd, the FEV$_1$ remains less than 50 percent of predicted).

The evaluating physician should still include additional statements about asthma-caused impairments. Due to the variability of disease, it is important to determine a time for reevaluation. For claimants deemed to have temporary impairment, this time period essentially correlates with the time required to reach optimal therapy. For claimants with

permanent impairment due to asthma, this time period may be yearly in recognition that asthma occasionally improves spontaneously or that newer therapies may provide relief of symptoms. Physicians also should include statements judging what impact the impairment has on the claimant's quality of life and especially the claimant's ability to perform his or her chosen occupation. The assessment of impact may be further complicated because asthma may precede a claimant's employment in a particular occupation, but occupationally related exposures may cause exacerbations in a claim-

TABLE 23-4 Minimum Medication Need[a]

Score	Medication
0	No medication
1	Occasional bronchodilator, not daily, and/or occasional cromolyn, not daily
2	Daily bronchodilator and/or daily cromolyn and/or daily low-dose inhaled steroid (<800 μg beclomethasone or equivalent)
3	Bronchodilator on demand and daily high-dose inhaled steroid (>800 μg beclomethasone or equivalent) or occasional course (1–3/yr) systemic steroid
4	Bronchodilator on demand and daily high-dose inhaled steroid (>1000 μg beclomethasone or equivalent) and daily systemic steroid

[a] The need for minimum medication should be demonstrated by the treating physician (e.g., previous records of exacerbation when medications have been reduced).
SOURCE: From Chan-Yeung et al,[14] with permission.

TABLE 23-5 Summary Impairment Ratings Classes[a]

Impairment Class	Total Score
0	0
I	1–3
II	4–6
III	7–9
IV	10–11
V	Asthma not controlled despite maximal treatment; i.e., FEV$_1$ remaining <50% despite use of ≥20 mg prednisone/day.

[a] The impairment rating is calculated as the sum of the patient's scores from Tables 23-2, 23-3, and 23-4.
SOURCE: From Chan-Yeung et al,[14] with permission.

ant's asthma and thus have a significant additional impact on that patient. Finally, factors that alter the ability to treat asthma such as intolerance to medication or other health problems such as heart disease that requires treatment with beta-adrenergic blocking agents should be included in the physician's report.

OCCUPATIONAL ASTHMA

The symptoms and clinical findings of occupational asthma can be identical to those of nonoccupational asthma; however, in occupational asthma, the variable airflow obstruction is caused by a specific agent in the workplace. Occupational asthma may take two forms, variable airflow obstruction that is a result of (1) exposure to a workplace stimulus without sensitization to the stimulus and (2) sensitization and reexposure to a specific workplace stimulus.

Workers without sensitization-induced asthma may have *irritant-induced asthma* (IIA). IIA is typically induced by repeated exposure to an environmental irritant such as smoke, sulfur dioxide, or ammonia fumes. The reactive airways dysfunction syndrome may be a part of IIA where a single exposure results in lung disease. Thereafter, exposure to other allergens or to irritant gases in the workplace at concentrations much lower than present governmental safety standards can cause exacerbations of airflow obstruction that can be severe. These patients are similar to patients with asthma not associated with a specific occupation and may have symptoms occurring away from the workplace.

Workers who inhale organic dusts may develop variable airflow obstruction without sensitization. One well-known condition is *byssinosis,* in which workers are exposed to the dusts of flax, hemp, cotton, and perhaps sisal. These workers typically have symptoms of chest tightness, wheezing, and cough most severely early in a work week with gradual but incomplete improvement during the work week and resolution on days away from work. This condition is variously classified as asthma, an asthma-like syndrome, or airway bronchoconstriction.

A large number of sensitizing agents have been identified[51] that may be intrinsic to an occupation (e.g., western red cedar dust for carpenters) or may be incidental (e.g., river fly antigens for workers at power plants along waterways). High-molecular-weight compounds result in occupational asthma in atopic workers, whereas low-molecular-weight compounds such as TDI and cobalt can cause problems in both atopic and nonatopic individuals. Careful history taking

may reveal possible antigens, and a history of atopy may be helpful in narrowing the list of likely compounds. Specific testing using spirometry before and after exposure to suspected agents may be confirmatory. For some workers, a specific antigen may not be identifiable. Nevertheless, historical findings, such as coworkers exhibiting similar symptoms, and additional special testing can support the idea that asthma is occupational in nature. Spirometry before and after a work shift can be helpful. Spirometry done immediately before and after a vacation can show improvement in pulmonary function; further testing after return to work showing a decrease in pulmonary function can be additional confirmatory data. Additional testing that is not standardized but may be of some value includes serial peak expiratory flow rates performed every 2 h during the day by the patient for 2 to 3 weeks followed by continued measurements during a vacation of 10 days or more. Serial bronchoprovocation testing during a period of work and a period of vacation also may be helpful, although standards for interpretation do not exist.

The physician evaluation of impairment in occupational asthma is similar to the evaluation of asthma in general except that a specific link between the impairment and the workplace is sought. When such a link is confirmed, the physician should include statements in his or her report specifying the link and the implications. For many patients, occupational asthma will require vocational retraining because removal from the exposure often will require leaving the occupation. These workers can be considered 100 percent impaired for that particular occupation. For other workers, it is practical to change jobs within a company to avoid the exposure; in this instance, it is crucial that the agent triggering the asthma be identified clearly in the medical report. For some workers, changing occupations may represent an especially severe hardship. For these, efforts at minimizing exposures, special personal protective equipment, and desensitization may make sense. The evaluating physician can include recommendations specifically tailored to the specific patient that consider the impact on quality of life and the risks of different options. For example, for a patient who cannot leave his or her occupation because of severe family disruption, recommendations on minimizing exposure and the use of special masks should be accompanied by a statement of the risk of developing a permanent asthmatic condition.

HYPERSENSITIVITY PNEUMONITIS

Also known as *extrinsic allergic alveolitis,* hypersensitivity pneumonitis is an immunologically derived disorder due to exposure to any of a number of organic dusts that affect the distal lung. Patients with the acute disease suffer fever, cough, and dyspnea 4 to 6 h after exposure to the antigen. Patients exposed to smaller amounts of antigen or for longer periods can develop a chronic condition characterized by malaise, anorexia, and weight loss in addition to cough and dyspnea. Airflow obstruction, restriction, and diffusion defects can all be seen on pulmonary function testing.

A large number of antigens associated with a variety of occupations have been identified as the causative agents of hypersensitivity pneumonitis. Thermophilic actinomycetes produce a variety of proteins that can be encountered by farmers in moldy hay (farmer's lung), sugar cane field workers in bagasse (bagassosis), mushroom workers in compost (mushroom worker's lung), and numerous other workers in a variety of materials. Other mold species, including *Aspergillus, Penicillium,* and *Cephalosporium* also can cause hypersensitivity pneumonitis. Avian antigens are well documented to cause hypersensitivity pneumonitis. Antigens from other species, including bacteria, amoebas, insects, and mammals, as well as a few chemicals, also have been implicated.

For evaluation of impairment/disability, the physician's goal is to make the diagnosis of hypersensitivity pneumonitis and identify the causative antigen. A careful history is often enough to help distinguish this condition from asthma and to narrow the list of possible tests of antigens. Pulmonary function during an acute exacerbation usually shows decreased lung volumes. Challenge testing can establish that disease is occupationally related. After a 72-h absence from the workplace, pulmonary function testing before and during the 24 h after return to the workplace may establish that there is an antigen in the workplace. Inhalation challenges in the laboratory with possible antigens collected from the workplace will be needed to determine the actual antigen, however. Pulmonary functions as well as the physical examination and white blood cell count are used in monitoring for 24 h following the inhalational challenge. Multiple repetitions of testing are frequently needed before a specific antigen is identified. Unfortunately, there are no standardized antigens to assist in this process.

Gradation of impairment is usually not needed in the evaluation of impairment/disability with hypersensitivity pneumonitis. Since the best treatment is avoidance of all known causative antigens, and since the potential of continued exposure is permanent lung injury and disease, all patients with this diagnosis are 100 percent impaired and should be considered completely disabled for occupations where the patient is likely to come into contact with known causative antigens.

OCCUPATIONALLY SPECIFIC DISABLEMENT

There are selected jobs for which patients are disabled despite a mild or even subclinical degree of pulmonary disease. Examples include jobs that require underwater submersion and exposure to hyperbaric conditions for patients with asthma, emphysema, and probably cystic fibrosis and patients who have had a spontaneous pneumothorax. These same patients and others who have previously had acute respiratory distress syndrome may be disabled for jobs that require frequent ascents or descents of more than 2500 m with or without supplemental oxygen (exclusive of altitude changes associated with passenger status in commercial aircraft). Other patients with mild or even moderate diffusion defects may be perfectly capable of working at sea level but are completely disabled doing any work at high altitudes without supplemental oxygen. For example, a rancher seen in our clinic with chronic bronchitis was examined at 1500 m elevation, where he has normal oxygenation, but his ranch is located at 3000 to 4000 m elevation, where he was found on field testing to be markedly hypoxemic without supplemental oxygen.

Unfortunately, no general guidelines for evaluation or testing can be established easily for occupationally specific disablements such as those discussed here. A history and physical examination should be performed in all patients. Upon consideration of the initial findings, the evaluating physician can chose objective tests that may include none, any, or all of the objective testing methods discussed earlier. The physician must carefully discover and then consider the conditions, requirements, and environments of an occupation in deciding whether an occupationally specific disablement exists once a patient has reported pulmonary symptoms and testing has revealed some degree of abnormality.

Preparation of the Physician Report of Impairment/Disability

The physician report plays a key role in the determination of compensation for a patient demonstrated to have an impairment and a disability. Certain elements must be contained within each report, including patient identification, statements of findings and diagnoses, an estimate of degree of impairment, and recommendations for retraining. In addition, the report must conform with legal standard definitions of specific diseases when such definitions exist and must conform with specific agency guidelines. It should be kept in mind that the report will be treated as a legal rather than a strictly medical document and that the report may be used during any appeal processes in the case of denied claims.

IDENTIFYING INFORMATION

The report must include identifying information. Basic information such as name and address must be included. Other information that is helpful includes date of evaluation and dates of follow-up visits, referral source or sources, and specific reason for evaluation.

FINDINGS AND DIAGNOSIS STATEMENTS

The findings and diagnosis statements may encompass a number of elements. There should be a section on previous evaluations that are directly relevant to the impairment/disability evaluation. A section summarizing the physician's history and physical examination should follow along with a section listing the objective tests obtained, their dates, places of performance, and their results. A summary section detailing the diagnostic assessment should conclude the statements of findings and diagnosis.

A listing of records of previous evaluations reviewed should be included in the physician report. Medical records from other practitioners along with the dates of visits and hospitalization and the dates of the records themselves (if different) should be included. Pertinent objective tests and their results from other practitioners or facilities along with the dates performed should be listed.

The history findings section should include all pertinent historical and physical examination findings for the specific impairment or disability claimed. Historical data sources should be identified, such as the patient, relatives, coworkers, and/or previous medical charts. If there are discrepancies between sources that are substantive and pertinent, a comment should be included.

The physical findings section should include all pertinent positives and negatives from a thorough physical examination. Special attention should be given to the respiratory system examination.

A listing of objective tests performed should be included. Each test performed, the dates performed, the performer, the result, and the interpretation of each result should be listed. Additional comments detailing patient compliance with testing procedures also may be added. Where results seem discrepant, statements either resolving the discrepancy or explaining why one test is more credible than another should be included.

A section summarizing the findings and giving a clinical impression of the medical condition must be included with the physician report. The key pieces of historical, physical examination, and objective testing results may be represented briefly in support of an overall diagnosis. For impairment/disability evaluations, it should be stated whether the final diagnosis results in an impairment.

DEGREE-OF-IMPAIRMENT ESTIMATION

For patients in whom a diagnosis is made that confirms an impairment, the physician should make an estimate of the degree of impairment. For patients in whom the impairment is documented with spirometry, diffusion measurements, or exercise studies, this may be relatively easy, since scoring systems have been devised.[11,12] In patients with asthma, a scoring system has been created, but the variable nature of asthma may make it difficult to simply score a patient's impairment. For these patients, and for patients with impairments without scoring systems, a statement from the physician with a best estimate of degree of impairment with rationale should be provided.

RESULTS OF PREVIOUS THERAPY AND PROGNOSIS OF PROPOSED THERAPY

For patients who have already undergone some form of treatment for their impairment, the details of therapy and the responses should be provided. Comments about compliance or noncompliance with therapy and an assessment of the reasons for noncompliance may be included. Success or failure of therapy is usually of interest to the disability agency along with the reasons for failure. For patients who have not been treated previously, suggested therapies, if any, should be included in this section, along with an opinion about the potential for success of any proposed therapy or the potential for residual impairment following successful therapy.

RECOMMENDATIONS FOR RETRAINING AND ASSESSMENT OF RETRAINABILITY

The physician who completes an evaluation of impairment is in a good position to assess the potential for retraining of an impaired worker. On the basis of the patient's occupational history supplemented by educational history, the physician may well be able to identify the intellectual ability of the worker for retraining. The intellectual challenges presented by the former occupation and educational status should give a reasonable estimate of the ability of the impaired worker to handle the challenges of other occupations. Knowledge of the physical limitations imposed by a worker's impairment may allow an employer to make reasonable changes in work conditions to allow continued work at the same occupation or may guide in selecting what types of occupations are reasonable goals of retraining. For example, a mail room worker with asthma induced by cold air from the nearby loading dock could be accommodated by warming his or her workplace and limiting the entrance of cold air. Also,

for example, a bread baker in a hotel kitchen with baker's asthma could be counseled not to retrain as a confectionary cook, where flour exposure may be substantial, but he or she could be encouraged to retrain to work preparing meal entrees, where the exposure to flour can be minimized.

CONFORMITY WITH LEGAL STANDARD DEFINITIONS OF SPECIFIC DISEASES

In evaluating an impairment, the physician must take into account legal definitions of diseases that may exist. When precisely worded definitions of a disease are available under a specific disability program, the physician should state the actual definition as published and state that the claimant's condition fulfills the definition. Using the actual language of the legal definition is helpful in clarifying whether a condition qualifies under that legal definition.

CONFORMITY WITH SPECIFIC AGENCY GUIDELINES

In general, disability agencies do not require that physician reports adhere to a specific or rigid format in providing a medical report. The Social Security Administration, for example, provides a general guideline that specifies that medical history, clinical findings, laboratory findings, diagnosis, treatment prescribed with response and prognosis, and a statement giving an assessment of the claimant's residual abilities should all be included.[4] Other disability agencies are similar in requiring only that enough information is provided to make a determination of impairment and disability. Commonly, however, a physician will be asked to respond to specific questions. Such questions should be answered to the best of the physician's ability. If, for some questions, an answer cannot be provided, then an explanation for the lack of an answer must be provided. Sometimes these questions are asked by nonmedical persons who do not know the subleties of particular diseases. A thorough, well-organized, easily understandable report that addresses all specific questions and minimizes medical jargon is essentially the only requirement needed to satisfy nearly all disability agencies.

Legal Considerations

USE OF PHYSICIAN REPORT FOR APPEAL OF IMPAIRMENT/DISABILITY HEARING

Claimants often may not be satisfied with the outcome of a disability hearing. In all disability programs, some appeals process exists. For example, under Social Security, an administrative appeals process can be initiated within 60 days of a decision.[4] Usually this process starts with the local disability determination service. Further appeals may be heard by administrative law judges and may proceed before an administrative appeals council. An applicant who exhausts the administrative appeals process may file suit in federal district court and pursue appeals up to the Supreme Court of the United States.

During an appeals process, the physician report plays as significant a role in providing information as during the initial hearing. This role underscores the importance of clear organization of the relevant historical information, the objective data, and the physician's diagnoses, plans, and opinions. Every statement that is made in the physician report must be clearly stated and supported by objective data and clear, understandable reasoning. Medical jargon or slang should be avoided as much as possible in the report. Inclusion in a physician report of citations of guidelines, standards, or other published relevant literature can be extremely helpful in supporting a physician's opinion. It is helpful to remember when preparing the initial report that a possible appeals process will involve mainly legal personnel and that an easily understood medical report may help speed the process.

ROLE OF PHYSICIAN AS EXPERT WITNESS

Physicians are frequently asked to act as expert witnesses. Physicians may be called on by the claimant (plaintiff), the disability agency (defendant), or occasionally an administrative law judge. When asked to provide expert testimony, it is crucial for the physician to remember that medical and legal terminology are quite different. When working with an attorney, it is helpful to meet prior to formal testimony in order for both attorney and physician to come to a common understanding about the particular regulations and laws involved and the medical evidence and opinions to be presented. A physician may teach the attorney the pertinent medical terms and their meanings while learning what aspects of the law are applicable to the case being decided. Ideally, a common understanding between attorney and physician will help to guide attorney questioning and focus and clarify physician presentation of technical medical data.

References

1. U.S. Department of Health and Human Services SSA: OASDI benefits awarded: Disabled workers. *Social Security Bulletin Annual Statistical Supplement*, SSA Publication No 13-11700:262, 1993.
2. U.S. Bureau of the Census: *Statistical Abstract of the United States: 1995*, 115th ed. Washington, U.S. Government Printing Office, 1995.
3. McNeil JM: *Americans with Disabilities: 1991–1992*. U.S. Bureau of the Census, Current Population Reports, P70-33. Washington, U.S. Government Printing Office, 1993.
4. Social Security Administration: *Disability Evaluation under Social Security*, SSA Publication No. 64-039. Washington, U.S. Department of Health and Human Services, 1995.
5. Americans with Disabilities Act, 42 U.S.C. paragraph 12102(2)(A–C); 29 C.F.R. paragraph 1630.2(g)(1–3).
6. *Sarsycki v. United Parcel Service* (1994, WD Okla.), 862 F. Supp. 336, 6 ADD 1126, 3 AD case 1039.
7. *Emery v. Caravan of Dreams* (1995, ND Tex.), 879 F. Supp. 640, 9ADD 278, 4 AD case 409.
8. *Sharp v. Abate* (1995, SD NY), 887 F. Supp. 695, 10 ADD 612, 4 AD case 902.
9. World Health Organization: *International Classification of Impairments, Disabilities, and Handicaps*. Geneva, WHO, 1980.
10. Cotes JE, Zejda J, King B: Lung function impairment as a guide to exercise limitation in work-related lung disorders. *Am Rev Respir Dis* 137:1089, 1988.
11. American Medical Association: *Guides to the Evaluation of Permanent Impairment*, 4th ed. Chicago, American Medical Association, 1993.
12. Renzetti AD Jr, Bleecker ER, Epler GR, et al: Evaluation of impairment/disability secondary to respiratory disorders: A statement of the American Thoracic Society. *Am Rev Respir Dis* 133:1205, 1986.
13. Kass I, Bell CW, Epler GE, et al: Evaluation of impairment/disability secondary to respiratory disease: A statement of the American Thoracic Society. *Am Rev Respir Dis* 126:945, 1982.
14. Chan-Yeung M, Harber P, Bailey W, et al: Guidelines for the evaluation of impairment/disability in patients with asthma: A statement of the American Thoracic Society. *Am Rev Respir Dis* 147:1056, 1993.
15. Demeter SL, Andersson GBJ, Smith GM (eds): *Disability Evaluation*. St Louis, Mosby-Year Book, 1996.
16. 20 C.F.R. part 718: Standards for determining coal miners' total disability or death due to pneumoconiosis.
17. International Labor Office: *Guidelines for the Use of the ILO International Classification of Radiographs of Pneumoconioses*. Geneva, International Labor Office, 1980.
18. Gardner RM, Baker CD, Broennle AM, et al: ATS statement—Snowbird Workshop on Standardization of Spirometry. *Am Rev Respir Dis* 119:831, 1979.
19. Knudson RJ, Slatin RC, Lebowitz MD, Burrows B: The maximal expiratory flow-volume curve. *Am Rev Respir Dis* 113:587, 1976.
20. Crapo RO, Hankinson JL, Irvin C, et al: Standardization of spirometry. *Am J Respir Crit Care Med* 152:1107, 1995.
21. Becklake M, Crapo RO, Buist S, et al: Lung function testing: Selection of reference values and interpretative strategies. *Am Rev Respir Dis* 144:1202, 1991.
22. Morris AH, Kanner RE, Crapo RO, Gardner RM (eds): *Clinical Pulmonary Function Testing: A Manual of Uniform Laboratory Procedures*, 2d ed. Salt Lake City, Intermountain Thoracic Society, 1984.
23. Ghio AJ, Crapo RO, Elliott CG: Reference equations used to predict pulmonary function at institutions with respiratory disease training programs in the United States and Canada: A survey. *Chest* 63:136, 1990.
24. Crapo RO, Morris AH, Gardner RM: Reference spirometric values using techniques and equipment that meet ATS recommendations. *Am Rev Respir Dis* 123:659, 1981.
25. Crapo RO, Hankinson JL, Irvin C, et al: Single-breath carbon monoxide diffusing capacity (transfer factor): Recommendations for a standard technique—1995 update. *Am J Respir Crit Care Med* 152:2185, 1995.
26. Crapo RO, Gardner RM, Clausen JL, et al: Single breath carbon monoxide diffusing capacity (transfer factor): Recommendations for a standard technique—An official statement of the American Thoracic Society. *Am Rev Respir Dis* 136:1299, 1987.
27. National Committee for Clinical Laboratory Standards: *NCCLS pH and Blood Gas*, NCCLS Document SC5-L (ISBN 1-56238-193-8). Villanova, PA, NCCLS, 1993.
28. National Committee for Clinical Laboratory Standards: *Blood Gas Pre-Analytical Considerations: Specimen Collection, Calibration, and Controls: Approved Guideline*, NCCLS Document C27-A (ISBN 1-56238-190-3). Villanova, PA, NCCLS, 1990.
29. Mahler DA, Froelicher VF, Miller NH, York TD: *ACSM's Guidelines for Exercise Testing and Prescription*, 5th ed. Baltimore, Williams & Wilkins, 1995.
30. Armstrong BW, Workman JN, Holcombe HH Jr, Roemmich WR: Clinicophysiologic evaluation of physical working capacity in persons with pulmonary disease. *Am Rev Respir Dis* 93:90, 1966.
31. Roemmich W, Blumenfeld HL, Moritz H: Evaluating remaining capacity to work in minor applicants with simple pneumoconiosis under 65 years of age under Title IV of Public Law 91–173. *Ann NY Acad Sci* 200:608, 1972.
32. Wehr KL, Johnson RL Jr: Maximum oxygen consumption in patients with lung disease. *J Clin Invest* 58:880, 1976.
33. Cotes JE, Poser V, Reed JW: Estimation of exercise ventilation and oxygen uptake in patients with chronic lung disease. *Bull Eur Physiopathol Respir* 18:221, 1982.
34. Carlson DJ, Ries AL, Kaplan RM: Prediction of maximum exercise tolerance in patients with COPD. *Chest* 100:307, 1991.
35. Oren A, Sue D, Hansen J, et al: The role of exercise testing in impairment evaluation. *Am Rev Respir Dis* 135:230, 1987.

36. Wasserman K, Hansen JE, Sue DY, et al: *Principles of Exercise Testing and Interpretation,* 2d ed. Malvern, PA, Lea & Febiger, 1994.

37. Young T, Palta M, Dempsey J, et al: The occurrence of sleep-disordered breathing among middle-aged adults. *N Engl J Med* 328:1230, 1993.

38. Strollo PJ Jr, Rogers RM: Obstructive sleep apnea. *N Engl J Med* 334:99, 1996.

39. Martin TJ, Sanders MH: Chronic alveolar hypoventilation: A review for the clinician. *Sleep* 18:617, 1995.

40. Bonsignore MR, Marrone O, Insalaco G, Bonsignore G: The cardiovascular effects of obstructive sleep apnoeas: Analysis of pathogenic mechanisms. *Eur Respir J* 7:786, 1994.

41. Hla KM, Young TB, Bidwell T, et al: Sleep apnea and hypertension. *Ann Intern Med* 120:382, 1994.

42. Naëgelé B, Thouvard V, Pépin J-L, et al: Deficits of cognitive executive functions in patients with sleep apnea syndrome. *Sleep* 18:43, 1995.

43. George CF, Nickerson PW, Hanly PJ, et al: Sleep apnoea patients have more automobile accidents. *Lancet* 8556:447, 1987.

44. Findley LJ, Unverzagt ME, Suratt PM: Automobile accidents involving patients with obstructive sleep apnea. *Am Rev Respir Dis* 138:337, 1988.

45. Aldrich MS: Automobile accidents in patients with sleep disorders. *Sleep* 12:487, 1989.

46. Strohl KP, Bonnie RJ, Findley L, et al: Sleep apnea, sleepiness, and driving risk: An official statement of the American Thoracic Society. *Am J Respir Crit Care Med* 150:1463, 1994.

47. American Electroencephalographic Society: Guideline fifteen: Guidelines for polygraphic assessment of sleep-related disorders (polysomnography). *J Clin Neurophysiol* 11:116, 1994.

48. Phillipson EA, Remmers JE, Cohn MA, et al: Indications and standards for cardiopulmonary sleep studies. *Am Rev Respir Dis* 139:559, 1989.

49. Carskadon MA, Dement WC, Mitler MM, et al: Guidelines for the Multiple Sleep Latency Test (MSLT): A standard measure of sleepiness. *Sleep* 9:519, 1986.

50. Thorpy MJ: Report from the American Sleep Disorders Association: The clinical use of the Multiple Sleep Latency Test. *Sleep* 15:268, 1992.

51. Chan-Yeung M: Occupational asthma. *Chest* 98(suppl):148S, 1990.

PART IV
GENERAL TREATMENT CONSIDERATIONS

Chapter 24
REVERSIBLE OBSTRUCTIVE AIRWAY DISEASE

LEONARD BIELORY

JOHN OPPENHEIMER

Asthma therapy has undergone tremendous evolution over the past decade. The concept of change has been captured in several publications, including publications by the National Heart Lung and Blood Institute, the International Consensus, and *World Health Organization Guidelines on the Diagnosis and Management of Asthma*. Pivotal to this evolution has been acknowledgment of the importance of inflammation in asthma. Asthma has been redefined from an episodic bronchospastic disease to one of chronic inflammation with resulting expiratory obstruction and bronchial hypperresponsiveness. Even patients diagnosed with mild disease may be found to have inflammation of their bronchial mucosa. More disconcerting information has been gleaned from research demonstrating that should anti-inflammatory therapy be delayed, a component of lung remodeling may occur[1] that ultimately may result in fixed lung obstruction. Chronic care of the asthmatic patient involves knowledge of the available agents and the appropriate timing for their use, which is based on disease severity.

Bronchodilators

This group of drugs provides bronchodilitation via smooth muscle relaxation of the bronchial tubes. This group includes the beta$_2$ agonists, phosphodiesterase / adenosine receptor inhibitors, and anticholinergic agents.

BETA AGONISTS

These agents have been used increasingly over the past 30 years as the bronchodilator of choice in asthma, but treatment with adrenergic substances was noted as early as the late 1800s. During the past 20 years, modifications of the basic sympathomimetic amines' structural nucleus have resulted in more specificity for the beta$_2$-adrenergic receptor. Modifications also have resulted in slower metabolism and thus longer duration of efficacy. Beta-adrenergic agonists exert direct bronchodilating effects on the airway including smooth muscle G-protein–linked receptors and also may provide additional indirect antiasthma effects via stabilization of the mast cell, inhibition of cholinergic neurotransmission, release of protective epithelial factors, and increase in mucociliary clearance.[2-5]

Beta$_2$ agonists are available in additional forms (inhaled, oral, and injectable). It should be noted that the oral route provides no additional significant benefit except perhaps improved "compliance," while it is associated with more adverse side effects. In almost all cases, the same can be said for the injectable route. In rare cases of severe exacerbation of disease in which patients have severe respiratory compromise and may not be able to receive inhalation, beta-agonist therapy via the intravenous route may be needed.[6]

Short-acting inhaled beta$_2$ agonists such as albuterol and terbutaline show efficacy within 5 min with peak effect at 30 to 90 min and duration of 4 to 6 h. Their role in the management of asthmatic patients is currently being reevaluated. With the evolution of asthma's definition from bronchospasm to inflammation, experts are no longer recommending the use of these agents on a regular "round-the-clock basis" and are now recommending their use solely on an as-needed basis. There is an evolving literature that points to prolonged regular use of such agents resulting in subsensitivity to these agents[19-22] (see below).

Improvement in lung function with increasing doses of beta$_2$ agonists appears to follow a logarithmic cumulative dose-response curve.[7] Studies have demonstrated that when comparing the metered-dose inhaler (MDI) with the nebulized route of administration of beta$_2$ agonists, 8- to 10-fold greater doses with nebulization are required for equivalent efficacy.[8] This disparity in dose is secondary to continuous delivery of nebulized material during both inspiration and expiration, as well as the fact that the nebulizer is quite inefficient, with only 40 to 50 percent of drug being available.[9] Interestingly, beyond added inefficiency and longer time required for treatment with nebulization, the nebulizer has been associated with an increase in beta-agonist side effects. Even in the setting of severe disease, a recent study in asthma exacerbation requiring emergency room visits demonstrated no significant bronchodilating effects when comparing nebulized beta$_2$ agonists with delivery through an MDI with spacer.

Inhaled beta$_2$-agonist therapy is felt to be the most superior bronchodilator. There is some controversy in the literature regarding its additive effects with theophylline or with anticholinergics. In one study, when beta$_2$ agonists were delivered at customary doses, the addition of theophylline resulted in additive bronchodilatation.[10] On the other hand, several studies have demonstrated a lack of significant additive bronchodilating effects in the emergent setting.[11] In studies comparing beta$_2$ agonist therapy with ipatroprium, no superiority was seen with ipatroprium with regard to acute symptom control. Added to this, beta$_2$ agonists demonstrated a faster onset of action (see below).

LONG-ACTING BETA AGONISTS

In the United States, the only available long-acting beta$_2$ agonist is salmeterol. This agent provides prolonged bronchodilatation, demonstrating significant effect for 12 h. This characteristic makes this agent extremely attractive in the treatment of nocturnal asthma.[12,13] Studies comparing salmeterol given twice daily head to head with albuterol given four times daily have demonstrated that salmeterol is more effective in patients with asthma requiring maintenance therapy.[14] A major concern regarding this drug is the fact that efficacy is slower in onset, generally requiring minutes; thus it is recommended that all patients using this agent also should have a short-acting beta$_2$-agonist inhaler for rescue. Like short-acting agents, concern regarding subsensitivity has been raised.

Beyond discussions regarding beta-agonist subsensitivity, concerns have been spurred by deaths in asthma patients using salmeterol.[14] In a pivotal 16-week nationwide surveillance study comparing 16,787 patients using salmeterol and 8,393 patients using albuterol, there was a small but not statistically significant excess mortality in the group using salmeterol.[16] Using bronchial hyperresponsiveness as an endpoint, Booth and colleagues[17] demonstrated that salmeterol provided significant protection against methacholine-induced bronchoconstriction for even 12 h after administration. Methacholine challenges were performed after 8 weeks of use of salmeterol, and after withdrawal of drug, no rebound increase in airway hyperresponsiveness was demonstrated. However, Cheung and colleagues[18] demonstrated that following 8 weeks of chronic salmeterol use, the significant increases in FEV$_1$ were maintained throughout the study period; however, with prolonged use of salmeterol, the initial 10-fold increase in the dose of methacholine needed to result in a 20 percent drop in FEV$_1$ was significantly attenuated.

Greening and colleagues,[19] as well as Woolcock's group,[20] have demonstrated that when examining clinical end points such as symptom control and spirometric measures, the addition of salmeterol to inhaled steroid therapy was found to be more effective than doubling the dose of inhaled steroids. Thus a review of the literature with regard to the topic of short and long-acting beta$_2$ agonists is all but clear. Clear consensus does include aggressive use of anti-inflammatory therapy (see below). Frequent use of short-acting beta$_2$-agonist therapy represents a marker of lack of disease control. Patients who despite high doses of anti-inflammatory therapy are having continued breakthrough of symptoms are candidates for long-acting beta$_2$-agonist therapy, especially for treatment of nocturnal exacerbation of symptoms. One thing is clear, use of long-acting beta$_2$-agonist therapy should not be begun until anti-inflammatory therapy has been started.[21]

SUBSENSITIVITY

Subsensitivity, a reduction in the effect of beta$_2$ agonists following continued use, is a potential sequela of the chronic use of these agents. Theories abound regarding the cause, which include uncoupling of the beta$_2$-adrenergic receptor from its G protein, as well as reduction in synthesis of new receptors. Interestingly, corticosteroids appear to reverse these processes when examined in vitro.[22,23]

Beyond the aforementioned theoretical concerns, several studies have intimated that at least a component of the rise in asthma mortality may be secondary to overuse of beta$_2$-agonist therapy.[24] Although the opinion of a direct cause-and-effect link between beta$_2$ agonist use and an increase in mortality is not held by many, most experts do believe that increased use of beta$_2$ agonists, prescribed and over the counter, is a marker of disease in poor control and may be responsible indirectly for death in asthmatics by resulting in delay in more aggressive anti-inflammatory therapy.[25-27]

ANTICHOLINERGICS

Ipatropium bromide is the only anticholinergic bronchodilator approved for inhalation in the United States. This drug, which is a quaternary derivative of atropine, is absorbed poorly from airway mucosal surfaces when inhaled, thus resulting in bronchodilation with amelioration of systemic antimuscarinic side effects seen from atropine.[28,29] The action of this class of drugs stems from blockade of the resting parasympathetic-induced bronchial tone. Anticholinergics also can inhibit reflex cholinergic bronchoconstriction following such stimuli as cold air and various gases. In contrast to beta$_2$-agonist therapy, which appears to exert its effects mainly on small airways, most investigators believe that anticholinergic agents predominantly affect the large, central airways in asthmatic patients.[30,31] On the whole, inhaled anticholinergic drugs provide less bronchodilation and are slower in onset than beta$_2$-agonist therapy.[31,32] In light of the slower onset of action, these drugs are not generally used in the treatment of acute asthma.

In the treatment of chronic asthma, studies have demonstrated an additive effect of anticholinergics in conjunction with beta$_2$ agonists.[34,35] Also, the combination of anticholinergics with theophylline demonstrated better bronchodilitation than either agent alone.[36] Overall, anticholinergic agents have been relegated in general practice to use in patients unable to tolerate beta$_2$-agonist or theophylline preparations. Although they receive mention in the international consensus report for asthma, they are not approved for use in the treatment of asthma in this country.

Anticholinergic compounds have been demonstrated to be most efficacious in the chronic obstructive pulmonary disease (COPD) patient. They appear to be best suited for the patient with a significant bronchitic component in light of the fact that beyond providing bronchodilating effects, they also provide a decrease in mucous production.

THEOPHYLLINE PREPARATIONS

Methylxanthine theophylline has been described in the literature since the 1920s. Initially, research was being undertaken for the drug's diuretic potential. In the 1970s, this drug gained popularity. This occurred largely due to the development of sustained-release preparations and a method of measuring serum levels. Beyond theophylline, other methylxanthines such as caffeine and theobromine share a bronchodilatory effect. Despite theophylline's long history, controversy abounds with regard to its mechanism of action. Proposed mechanisms include phosphodiesterase inhibitor, adenosine receptor antagonist, stimulation of endogenous catecholamine release, inhibition of prostaglandin E$_2$ decrease in smooth muscle free calcium levels, mast cell stabilizer, and stimulant to diaphragmatic contractility.[37-46]

THEOPHYLLINE LEVELS

Work performed by Weinberger and colleagues[47] demonstrated that side effects from theophylline were noted with levels greater than 20 μg/mL. Parameters of pulmonary function, such as FEV$_1$, were shown to increase linearly in relation to the rise in the logarithm of the plasma theophylline

TABLE 24-1 Theophylline Levels Are Affected by a Variety of Agents

Increase	Decrease
Beta-blocking agents	Barbiturates
Calcium channel blockers	Beta agonists
Cimetidine, rantitidine	Rifampin
Corticosteroids	Phenytoin
Ephedrine	Cigarette smoking
Influenza virus vaccine	
Mexiliitine	
Quinolones	
Hepatitis	
Cirrhosis	
Congestive heart failure	
Pneumonia	
Renal failure	

concentration.[48] It should be noted that an increase in concentration from 0 to 10 μg/mL is associated with a 30 percent increase in lung function compared with baseline, whereas an increase from 10 to 20 μg/mL results in only a 10 percent further improvement. As a result of such data, the most recent WHO asthma guidelines have recommended theophylline levels between 5 to 15 μg/mL.

Theophylline preparations had been first-line therapy in asthma, but with our recent shift of the definition, this therapy has been relegated to a more subservient role. This change has been reinforced with concern regarding the drug's narrow therapeutic window. Following Weinberger's demonstration of drug side effects including seizure and even death with levels greater than 20 μg/mL, there have been large legal settlements regarding toxicity.[50] In addition, our understanding that clearance can be altered when theophylline is used with other drugs or even viral illness (Table 24-1) has led physicians to be more hesitant to use this class of agents.

Despite concerns regarding theophylline preparations, asthma specialists have found this a very useful agent for control of the nocturnal component of asthma. Much of this has stemmed from the development of newer theophylline preparations that are able to demonstrate prolonged bronchodilation, for as long as 24 h, even when dosing is only once in the evening.[49] Added to this, there has been literature demonstrating that patients are more compliant with oral agents than with those administered via the inhaled route.[51] Thus, with once-daily dosing and a patient preferred route of administration, one of the contributing causes of bad outcome, i.e., poor compliance, from asthma could be resolved.

Theophylline preparations have been demonstrated to inhibit exercise-induced bronchoconstriction even at low doses with resulting levels of 6.7 μg/mL. Unfortunately, protection appears to be afforded in a dose-dependent fashion.[52] When comparing theophylline with albuterol or a combination of both as a maintenance asthma therapy over a 3-month period, Joad and colleagues[53] demonstrated that theophylline and/or combination therapy was superior to albuterol when examining nocturnal control, interference with activity or frequency of wheeze. Revington and colleagues[54] performed a study with similar stratification of therapy in a group of asthmatics requiring fairly high doses of inhaled steroids

(mean 1100 μg/day). They demonstrated that morning peak flows were similarly improved in the group receiving theophylline or combination, whereas albuterol provided similar morning flows to the group on placebo. When examining evening peak flows, combination therapy resulted in greater flows than theophylline alone, which resulted in better flows than albuterol or placebo.[54] Studies have demonstrated similar efficacy between theophylline preparations and sodium cromolyn or nedocromil sodium when examining parameters such as symptom control and lung function. Interestingly, in both cases, theophylline was noted to result in more side effects.[55,56] When comparing theophylline with inhaled steroids in children, Tinkelman and coworkers[57] demonstrated that inhaled beclomethasone resulted in comparable symptom control with less rescue bronchodilator use and fewer exacerbations requiring systemic steroids. Although theophylline resulted in greater complaints of side effects, beclomethasone at 332 μg per day has resulted in a reduction in growth velocity even though no reductions in serum cortisols were detected.[57]

Theophylline has seen a recent renaissance secondary to its potential anti-inflammatory effects. This is by no means a new concept. Pauwels and colleagues[58] demonstrated that theophylline had the ability to ablate the late phase of the allergic response. They attributed this to its potential anti-inflammatory effects. Several years later, Cockroft[59] was unable to demonstrate theophylline's ability to block allergen-induced hyperresponsiveness, whereas cromolyn sodium use prior to challenge did reduce bronchial hyperresponsivess. In 1994, with Sullivan's bronchoscopy study demonstrating that the chronic use of theophylline was associated with a reduction in total eosinophils as well as actived eosinophils (EG₂ positive) in the bronchial basement membrane, there was renewed interest in theophylline's potential anti-inflammatory effects.[60]

Anti-Inflammatory Agents

With our better understanding of the pathophysiologic changes in asthma being of an inflammatory nature, there has been a significant change in therapeutic focus, with anti-inflammatory agents being used earlier in the algorithm of care. Anti-inflammatory agents can be separated into two categories: nonsteroidal and steroidal agents. Nonsteroidal agents include cromolyn sodium, nedocromil sodium, and possibly theophylline preparations (see above).

Cromolyn sodium has demonstrated efficacy in controlling asthma symptoms, improving spirometric measures, and reducing bronchial hyperresponsiveness in some patients.[61–63] It has been shown to reduce both the immediate and the late phase of the allergic response.[64] Cromolyn has been demonstrated to stabilize the mast cell[65]; however, it is believed that this is not its only mechanism of action in light of its effect of reducing the late phase.[66,67] A major limitation of this drug is that it requires three to four times a day dosing. Also, research has demonstrated that it is less efficacious than inhaled steroids. This agent, when added to a regimen of inhaled steroids, has not been shown to be steroid-sparing.[68]

Nedocromil sodium has been shown to reduce asthma symptoms. It too reduces the immediate as well as late allergic response. With chronic use of this agent, Manolitsas and

TABLE 24–2 Guidelines for the Treatment of Asthma

Stage	Clinical Symptoms	Medications
Step 1: Intermittent	1 time a week Brief exacerbations Nighttime asthma symptoms Asymptomatic and normal lung function between exacerbations PEF or FEV_1 >80% predicted; variability >20%	None needed
Step 2: Mild persistent	>1 time a week but <1 time per day Exacerbations may affect activity and sleep Nightmare asthma symptoms >2 times a month PEF or FEV_1 >80% predicted; variability 20–30%	Either low-dose inhaled corticosteroid, leukotriene antagonists, cromoglycate, nedocromil, or sustained-release theophylline If needed, increase inhaled corticosteroids or add long-acting bronchodilator (especially for nighttime symptoms); either long-acting inhaled β_2-agonist, sustained-release theophylline, or long-acting oral β_2-agonist
Step 3: Moderate persistent	Symptoms daily Exacerbations affect activity and sleep Nighttime asthma symptoms >1 time a week Daily use of inhaled short-acting β_2-agonist PEF for FEV_1 >60%–<80% predicted; variability 30%	Inhaled corticosteroid, moderate to high dose or possibly leukotriene antagonists +1-inhaled anti-inflamatory agents Long-acting bronchodilator, especially for nighttime symptoms; either long-acting inhaled β_2-agonist, sustained release theophylline, or long-acting oral β_2-agonist
Step 4: Severe persistent	Continuous symptoms Frequent exacerbations Frequent nighttime asthma symptoms Physical activities limited by asthma symptoms PEF or FEV_1 >60% predicted variability >30%	Inhaled corticosteroid, high dose Long-acting bronchodilator; either long-acting β_2-agonist, sustained-release theophylline, and/or long-acting oral β_2-agonist, and Oral corticosteroid long term if not maintained on above therapy

colleagues[69] were able to demonstrate a significant reduction in the number of activated eosinophils present in the bronchial mucosa. Nedocromil has been shown to reduce symptom scores and improve spirometric measures as well as peak flow with chronic use.[69,70] Although this agent appears to be more potent than cromolyn sodium and can be dosed less frequently, it too is less potent than inhaled steroid agents.[72] When this agent is added to a regimen of inhaled steroids, it has demonstrated steroid-sparing effects.[72]

In our better understanding of the inflammation in asthma, several mediators have been implicated. Included in this list is the product of the 5-lipoxygenase pathway: LTA_4, LTB_4, LTC_4, LTD_4, and LTE_4.[73,74] These inflammatory mediators are largely produced by the mast cell and eosinophil. Studies have demonstrated the efficacy of the antagonists of these mediators in exercise, allergy, and aspirin challenges.[75–81] These agents provide an attractive alternative due to their oral delivery. Kelloway and colleagues[51] have demonstrated that patients are more likely to be compliant with therapy if it is ingested orally compared with the inhaled route.

Inhaled steroids are the most potent of the inhaled anti-inflammatory agents. Their mode of action has not been characterized clearly; however, they probably act at several sites of the inflammatory component of asthma through binding of a glucocorticoid receptor.[82,83] Steroids have been shown to inhibit release of mediators from inflammatory cells such

as macrophages and eosinophils but not from mast cells.[84–86] Interestingly, with prolonged use, steroids do cause a decrease in mast cell numbers within the airway.[87] Steroids also have been shown to reduce the influx of inflammatory cells into the lung following allergen challenge and to further reduce the microvascular leakage caused by these cells' inflammatory mediators.[88,89]

Inhaled steroids are considered to be the most potent of the inhaled anti-inflammatory agents. They have been demonstrated to reduce bronchial hyperresponsiveness,[90–93] improve lung function, reduce symptoms including need for rescue beta$_2$-agonist therapy, and reduce oral steroid requirements.[94–96] Inhaled steroids, beyond providing the aforementioned improvements in asthma, also have been demonstrated to reduce the number of asthma exacerbations requiring oral steroid rescue therapy.[91]

Interestingly, a clear dose-response has not been demonstrated in the literature, and several studies demonstrate no such association,[97,98] whereas others clearly do.[99,100] Much controversy has been expressed in the literature regarding steroid side effects, including adrenal suppression,[101–104] cataracts,[105,106] bone resorbtion,[106–112] and retardation in childhood growth.[113–115] It is, however, clear that delivery of corticosteroids through the inhaled route will result in less potential side effects compared with delivery via the oral route. Side effects may be potentially reduced with the use of spacer devices.[113-118] With such attachments, less drug will be deposited in the oropharynx and be available to the gastrointestinal tract. Unfortunately, no specific threshold dose is known with regard to side effects, but as Kamada and colleagues[119] point out in their recent review, clinicians should be aware of potential side effects and strive for attaining the lowest effective dose. This also must be weighed against recent data demonstrating that delay in glucocorticoid therapy may result in reduced effect of medicine, possibly due to lung remodeling following chronic inflammation.[114,120] In the treatment of COPD patients with inhaled steroids, efficacy has not been demonstrated consistently.[121,122]

Algorithm of Care: A Stepwise Approach

Much like the standard of care for hypertension, asthma is treated in a stepwise approach. This tact has been used since the initial asthma guidelines of 1991[20,123,124] but has been refined with the most recent guidelines, the *Global Initiative for Asthma* (GINA), by the World Health Organization. In all the asthma guidelines, asthma severity is stratified based on symptoms (frequency, duration) as well as objective measures (spirometry and variability in peak flows). In these newest GINA guidelines, asthma is stratified into four categories: intermittent, mild persistent, moderate persistent, and severe persistent (Table 24-2). Prior to treatment, the clinical features of *intermittent disease* include occurrence of asthma symptoms less than once per week with brief duration of symptoms and nocturnal exacerbation less than twice per month. Patients stratified to this category of disease demonstrate an FEV_1 that is greater than 80 percent of predicted with a low diurnal variation in peak flow of less than 20 percent. Prior to treatment, the clinical features of *mild persistent disease* include occurrence of asthma symptoms greater than once per week but less than once daily with nocturnal exacerbations greater than twice per month. Patients stratified to this category of disease demonstrate an FEV_1 that is greater than 80 percent of predicted with a diurnal variation in peak flow between 20 and 30 percent. In contrast, the clinical features of *moderate persistent disease* include occurrence of asthma symptoms requiring short-acting beta$_2$ agonists on a daily basis with nocturnal exacerbations greater than once per week. Patients stratified to this category of disease demonstrate an FEV_1 that is greater than 60 percent but less than 80 percent of predicted with a diurnal variation in peak flow of greater than 30 percent. Finally, patients with *severe persistent disease* suffer from continuous symptoms prior to therapy and suffer from frequent nighttime asthma symptoms. These patients demonstrate significant reduction in spirometry (<60 percent) and significant diurnal variability in peak flows (>30 percent). Overall, it is quite apparent that this stratification is based on an increase in symptoms with associated decrement in lung function when comparing milder with more severe disease.

The GINA guidelines recommend that in patients suffering solely from mild intermittent disease, beta$_2$ agonists should be used on an "as needed" basis. Patients stratified to mild persistent disease should start on a chronic anti-inflammatory regimen (nonsteroidal or low-dose inhaled steroid). In patients suffering from moderate persistent disease, experts recommend higher doses of inhaled anti-inflammatory ther-

apy. Should this not be enough to control symptoms (specifically nocturnal symptoms), long-acting beta$_2$ agonists or a theophylline preparation should be added. Finally, in patients with severe disease, high doses of inhaled steroids are generally required. Should this not be enough to control disease, oral steroids can be added (GINA). In patients not controlled despite aggressive therapeutic intervention as outlined above, physicians should consider concomitant illnesses that may complicate asthma control, such as sinusitis, gastroesophogeal reflux, and masqueraders of asthma such as vocal cord dysfunction. One also should consider the patient's environment. Research has demonstrated that with aggressive environmental control, in appropriate patients, reductions in symptoms, bronchial hypperresponsiveness, and medication requirements and improved peak flows can be achieved.[125]

Conclusions

With our greater understanding of the basic pathophysiology of asthma has come a change in our care of the asthmatic patient. Since inflammation of the bronchial mucosa is the underlying defect in asthma, anti-inflammatory agents have become the cornerstone of therapy. The clinician also should be careful to consider environmental triggers. Following dispensing of medicines, the physician's job is not complete, since added to this the patient should receive education about the illness in an attempt to better develop a partnership of care. Also, it is imperative that the asthmatic be instructed in proper metered-dose inhaler technique to ensure drug deposition to the lower respiratory tract.

References

1. Agertoft L, Pedersen S: Effects of long-term treatment with an inhaled corticosteroid on growth and pulmonary function in asthmatic children. *Respir Med* 88:373–381, 1994.
2. Tattersfield AC, Britton JR: *Beta-Andrenergic Agonists: Basic Mechanisms and Clinical Management.* London, Academic Press, 563–590, 1988.
3. McFadden ER: Beta–G-receptor antagonist: Metabolism and pharmacology. *J Allergy Immunol* 68:91–97, 1981.
4. Reed CE: Adrenergic bronchodilators: Pharmacology and toxicology. *J Allergy Immunol* 76:335–341, 1985.
5. Barnes PJ: Neural mechanisms in asthma. *Br Med Bull* 48:179–168, 1991.
6. Larsson S, Svedmyr N: Bronchodilating effects and side effects of beta-adrenergic stimulants by different modes of administration. *Am Rev Respir Dis* 861–866, 1977.
7. Weber RW, Petty WE, Nelson HS: Aerosolized terbutaline in asthmatics: Comparison of dosage strength, schedule and method of administration. *J Allergy Clin Immunol* 63:116–121, 1979.
8. Nelson HS, Spector SL, Whitsett TL, et al: The bronchodilator response to inhalation of increasing doses of aerosolized albuterol. *J Allergy Clin Immunol* 72:371–375, 1983.
9. Clay MM, Pavia D, Newman SP, et al: Assessment of jet nebulizers for lung aerosol therapy. *Lancet* 2:592–594, 1983.
10. Wolfe JD, Tashkin DP, Calvarese B, Simmons M: Bronchodilator effects of terbutaline and aminophylline alone and in combination in asthmatic patients. *N Engl J Med* 298:363–367, 1978.
11. Sacker MA, Kim CS: Auxiliary MDI aerosol delivery systems. *Chest* 88(suppl 2):161, 1985.
12. Fitzpatrick MF, Mackay T, Driver H, Douglas NJ: Salmeterol in

nocturnal asthma: A double-blind placebo-controlled trial of a long acting inhaled β_2 agonist. *Br Med J* 301:1365–1368, 1990.

13. Pearlman DS, Chervinsky P, LaForge C, et al: A comparison of salmeterol with albuterol in the treatment of mild to moderate asthma. *N Engl J Med* 327:1420–1425, 1992.

14. D'Alonzo GE, Nathan RA, Henochowicz S, et al: Salmeterol xinafoate as maintenance therapy compared with albuterol in patients with asthma. *JAMA* 271:1412–1416, 1994.

15. Finkelstein FN: Risks of salmeterol? (letter). *N Engl J Med* 331:1314, 1994.

16. Castle W, Fuller R, Hall J, Palmer J: Serevent nationwide surveillance study: Comparison of salmeterol with salbutamol in asthmatic patients who require regular bronchodilator treatment. *Br Med J* 306:1034, 1993.

17. Booth H, Fishwick K, Harkawat R, et al: Changes in methacholine induced bronchostriction with the long acting β_2 agonist salmeterol in mild to moderate asthmatic patients. *Thorax* 48:1121, 1993.

18. Cheung D, Timmers MC, Zwinderman AH, et al: Long-term effects of a long-acting β_2-adrenoceptor agonist, salmeterol, on airway hyperresponsiveness in patients with mild asthma. *N Engl J Med* 327:1198–1203, 1992.

19. Greening AP, Wind P, Northfield M, et al: Added salmeterol verses higher-dose corticosteroid in asthma patients with symptoms on existing inhaled corticosteroid. *Lancet* 344:219, 1994.

20. Woolcock A, Lundback B, Ringdal N, Jacques LA: Comparison of addition of salmeterol to inhaled steroids with doubling of the dose of inhaled steroids. *Am J Respir Crit Care Med* 153:1481, 1996.

21. National Heart, Lung and Blood Institute, National Institutes of Health: *International Consensus Report on Diagnosis and Management of Asthma*. NIH Publication No 92-3091. Bethesda, MD, U.D. Department of Health and Human Services, 1992.

22. Bai TR: Beta-2 adrenergic receptors in asthma: A current perspective. *Lung* 170:125, 1992.

23. Sears MR: The short and long-term effects of B-2 agonists, in Holgate ST, Austen KF, Lichtenstein LM, Kay AB (eds): *Asthma: Physiology, Immunopharmacology and Treatment*, 4th ed. London, Academic Press, pp 359–374, 1993.

24. Spitzer WO, Suissda S, Ernst P, et al: The use of β-agonist and the risk of death and near death from asthma. *N Engl J Med* 326:501, 1992.

25. Grainger J, Atkinson M, et al: Case-control study of prescribed fenoterol and death from asthma in New Zealand, 1977–81. *Thorax* 45:170, 1990.

26. Grainger J, Woodman K, Pearce N, et al: Prescribed fenoterol and death from asthma in New Zealand, 1981–7: A further case control study. *Thorax* 46:105, 1991.

27. Inhaled β_2-adrenergic agonist in asthma: Position statement. *J Allergy Clin Immunol* 91:1234, 1993.

28. Pakes GE, Brogden RN, Heel RC, et al: Ipratropium bromide: A review of its pharmacologic properties and therapeutic efficacy in asthma and chronic bronchitis. *Drugs* 20:237, 1980.

29. Gross NJ, Skorodin MS: Anticholinergic antimuscarinic bronchodilators. *Am Rev Respir Dis* 129:856, 1984.

30. McFadden ER, Ingram RH, Wellman JJ: Predominant site of flow and mechanisms of post-exertional asthma. *J Appl Physiol* 42:746, 1977.

31. Ashutosh K, Mead G, Dickey JC, et al: Density dependence of expiratory flow and brochodilator response in asthma. *Chest* 77:68–75, 1980.

32. Gross NJ: Ipratropium bromide. *N Engl J Med* 319:486, 1988.

33. Chapman KR: Anticholinergic bronchodilators for adult obstructive airway disease. *Am J Med* 91(suppl 4A):13s–16s, 1991.

34. Shenfield GM: Combination bronchodilator therapy. *Drugs* 24:414, 1982.

35. Laitinen LA, Poppius H: Combination of oxitropium bromide and salbutamol in the treatment of asthma with pressurized aerosols. *Br J Dis Chest* 80:179, 1986.

36. Kreisman H, Cohen H, Ghezzo E, et al: Combined therapy with ipritropium and theophylline in asthma. *Ann Allergy* 52:90, 1984.

37. Bergstrand H: Phosphodiestersase inhibition and theophylline. *Eur J Respir Dis* 61(suppl 109):37, 1980.

38. Polson JB, Kazanowski JJ, Goldman AL, Szentivanyi A: Inhibition of human pulmonary phosphodiesterase activity by therapeutic levels of theophylline. *Clin Exp Pharmacol Physiol* 5:535, 1978.

39. Cushley MJ, Tattersfield AE, Holgate ST: Adenosine induced bronchoconstriction in asthma: Antagonism by inhaled theophylline. *Am Rev Respir Dis* 129:380, 1984.

40. Mann JS, Holgate ST: Specific antagonism of adenosine induced brochoconstriction in asthma by oral theophylline. *Br J Clin Pharmacol* 19:85, 1985.

41. Higbee MD, Kumar M, Galant SP: Stimulation of endogenous catacholamine release by theophylline: A proposed additional mechanism of thoephylline effects. *J Allergy Clin Immunol* 70:377, 1982.

42. Fox C, Wolf E, Kagey-Sobotka A, et al: Comparison of human lung and intestinal mast cells. *J Allergy Clin Immunol* 81:89, 1988.

43. Horrobin DF, Manku MS, Franks DJ, Hamet P: Methylxanthine phosphodiesterase inhibitors behave as prostaglandin antagonists in a perfused rat mesenteric artery preparation. *Prostaglandins* 13:33, 1977.

44. Kolbeck RC, Speir WA, Carrier GO, Bransome ED: Apparent irrelevance of cyclic nucleotides to the relaxation of trachael smooth muscle induced by theophyline. *Lung* 156:173, 1979.

45. Orange RP, Kaliner MA, Laraia PJ, Austen KG: Immunological release of histamine and slow reacting substance of anaphylaxis from human lung: II. Incluence of cellular levels of cyclic AMP. *Fed Proc* 30:1725, 1971.

46. Aubier M, De Troyer A, Sampson M, et al: Aminophylline improves diaphragmatic contractility. *N Engl J Med* 305:249, 1981.

47. Hendclcs L, Bighley L, Richardson RH, et al: Frequent toxicity from IV aminophylline in critically ill patients. *Drug Intell Clin Pharmacol* 11–12, 1977.

48. Mitenko PA, Ogilvie RI: Rational intravenous doses of theophylline. *N Engl J Med*. 289:600, 1973.

49. Pedersen S: Treatment of nocturnal asthma in children with a single dose of sustained-release theophylline taken after supper. *Clin Allergy* 15:79, 1985.

50. *Wall Street Journal*, November 13, 1990.

51. Kelloway JS, Wyatt RA, Adlis SA: Comparison of patient's compliance with prescribed oral and inhaled asthma medication. *Arch Intern Med* 154:1349, 1994.

52. Magnussen H, Reugs G, Jorres R: Methylxanthines inhibit exercise-induced brochoconstriction at low serum theophylline concentration and in a dose dependent fashion. *J Allergy Clin Immunol* 81:531, 1988.

53. Joad JP, Ahren RC, Lindgren SD, Weinherger MM: Relative efficacy of maintenance therapy with theophylline inhaled albuterol and the combination for chronic asthma. *J Allergy Clin Immunol* 79:78, 1987.

54. Revington RN, Boulet LP, Cote J, et al: Efficacy of uniphyl, albuterol and their combination in asthmatic patients on high-dose inhaled steroids. *Am J Respir Crit Care Med* 151:325, 1995.

55. Furukawa CT, Shapiro GG, Bierman CW, et al: A double-blind study comparing the effectiveness of cromolyn sodium and sustained-release theophylline in childhood asthma. *Pediatrics* 4:453, 1984.

56. Crimi E, Orefice U, De Bendetto F, et al: Nedocromil sodium versus theophylline in the treatment of reversible obstructive airway disease. *Ann Allergy Asthma Immunol* 74:501, 1995.

57. Tinkelman DG, Reed CE, Nelson HS, Clifford KP: Aerosol beclomethasone dipropionate compared with theophylline a primary treatment of chronic, mild to moderately severe asthma in children. *Pediatrics* 92:64, 1993.

58. Pauwels R, Van Renterghem D, Vand Der Straeten, et al: The

effect of theophylline and enprofylline on allergen-induced bronchoconstriction. *J Allergy Clin Immunol* 76:583, 1985.

59. Cockroft D: Theophylline does not inhibit allergen-induced increase in airway responsiveness to methacholine. *J Allergy Clin Immunol* 83:913, 1989.

60. Sullivan P, Bekir S, Jaffar Z, et al: Anti-inflammatory effects of low dose oral theophylline in atopic asthma. *Lancet* 343:1006, 1994.

61. Bromptom Hospital and Medical Research Council Collaborative Trial: Long-term study of disodium cromoglycate in treatment of severe extrinsic or intrinsic bronchial asthma in adults. *Br Med J* 4:383, 1972.

62. Godfrey S, Balfour-Lynn L, Loenig P: The place of cromolyn sodium in the long-term management of childhood asthma based on 3–5-year follow-up. *J Pediatr* 87(3):465, 1975.

63. Cockroft DW, Murdock KY: Protective effect of inhaled albuterol cromolyn, beclomehtasone and placebo on allergen-induced increase in bronchial responsiveness to inhaled histamine (abstr). *J Allergy Clin Immunol* 77(suppl):122, 1986.

64. Barnes PJ: A new approach to the treatment of asthma. *N Engl J Med* 321:1517, 1989.

65. Cox JSG: Disodium cromoglycate: A specific inhibitor of reagenic antigen-antibody mechanisms. *Nature* 81:1328, 1967.

66. Skedinger MC, Augustine NH, Morris EZ, et al: Effect of disodium cromoglycate on neutrophil movement and intracellular calcium mobilization. *J Allergy Clin Immunol* 80:573, 1987.

67. Roy AC, Warren BT: Inhibition of cAMP phosphodiesterase by disodium cromoglycate. *Biochem Pharmacol* 23:917, 1974.

68. Barnes PJ: Inhaled glucocorticoids for asthma. *N Engl J Med* 332:868, 1995.

69. Monolitsas N, Wang J, Devalia J, et al: Regular albuterol, nedocromil sodium and bronchial inflammation in asthma. *Am J Respir Crit Care Med* 151:1925, 1995.

70. Cherniack R, Wasserman S, Ramsdell J, et al: A double-blind multicenter group comparative study of the efficacy and safety of nedocromil sodium in the management of asthma. *Chest* 97:1299, 1990.

71. Van As A, Chick T, Bodman S, et al: A group comparative study of the safety and efficacy of nedocromil sodium in reversible airways disease: A preliminary report. *Eur J Respir Dis* 69:143, 1986.

72. de Jong J, Teengs J, Postma D, et al: Nedocromil sodium versus albuterol in the management of allergic asthma. *Am J Respir Crit Care Med* 149:91, 1994.

73. Henderson WR: The role of leukotrienes in inflammation. *Ann Intern Med* 121:684, 1994.

74. Busse WW: The role of leukotrienes in asthma and allergic rhinitis. *Clin Exp Allergy* 26:868, 1996.

75. Finnerty JP, Wood-Baker R, Thomson H, Holgate ST: Role of leukotriences in exercise-induced asthma: Inhibitory effect of ICI 204219, a potent leukotriene D_4 receptor antagonist. *Am Rev Respir Dis* 145:746, 1992.

76. Makker IIK, Lau LC, Thomson HW, et al: The protective effect of inhaled leukotriene D_4 receptor antagonist ICI204219 against excercise-induced asthma. *Am Rev Respir Dis* 147:1413, 1993.

77. Taniguchi Y, Tamura G, Honma M, et al: The effect of an oral leukotriene antagonist ONO-1078 on allergen-induced immediate bronchostrition in asthmatic subjects. *J Allergy Clin Immunol* 92:507, 1993.

78. Findaly SR, Barden JM, Easley CB, Glass M: Effect of the oral leukotriene antagonist ICI 204,219 on antigen-induced bronchonstriction in subjects with asthma. *J Allergy Clin Immunol* 89:1040, 1992.

79. Nathan RA, Glass M, Minkwitz MC: Inhaled ICI 201,219 blocks antigen-induced bronchoconstriction in subjects with bronchial asthma. *Chest* 105:483, 1994.

80. Dahlen B, Margolskee DJ, Zetterstrom O, Dahlen SE: Effect of leukotriene receptor antagonist MK-0679 on baseline pulmonary function in aspirin-sensitive asthmatic subjects. *Thorax* 48:1205, 1993.

81. Holgate ST, Bradding P, Sampson A: Leukotriene antagonists and synthesis inhibitor: New directions in asthma therapy (review article). *J Allergy Clin Immunol* 98:1, 1996.

82. Gonzalez JP, Brogden RN: Nedocromil sodium: A preliminary review of its pharmacodynamic and pharmacokinetic properties and therapeutic efficacy in the treatment of reversible obstructive airways disease. *Drugs* 34:560, 1987.

83. Morris HG: Mechanisms of action and therapeutic role of coricosteroids in asthma. *J Allergy Clin Immunol* 75:1, 1985.

84. Barnes PJ, Adocock I: Anti-inflammatory actions of steroids: molecular mechanisms. *Trends Pharmacol Sci* 14:436, 1993.

85. Schleimer RP: Effects of glucocorticoids on inflammatory cells relevant to their therapeutic applications in asthma. *Am Rev Respir Dis* 141:S59, 1990.

86. Schleimer RP, Schulman ES, MacGlashan DW Jr, et al: Effects of dexamethasone on mediator release from human lung fragment and purified human lung mast cells. *J Clin Invest* 71:1830, 1983.

87. Latinen LA, Laitinen A, Haahtela T: A comparative study of the effects of an inhaled corticosteroid, budesonide and a β_2-agonist, terbutaline on airway inflammation in newly diagnosed asthma: A randomized, double-blind, parallel-group controlled trial. *J Allergy Clin Immunol* 90:32, 1992.

88. Boschetto P, Fabbri IM, Zocca E, et al: Prednisone inhibits late asthmatic reactions and airway inflammation induced by toluene diisocyanate in sensitized subjects. *J Allergy Clin Immunol* 80:261, 1987.

89. Erjefalt I, Persson CG: Anti-asthma drugs attenuate inflammatory leakage of plasma into airway lumen. *Acta Physiol Scand* 128:653, 1986.

90. Effect of inhaled triamcinolone on bronchial hyperreactivity and airway obstruction in asthma. *Ann Allergy* 64:207, 1990.

91. Juniper ER, Kline PA, Vanzieleghem MA, et al: Effect of long-term treatment with an inhaled corticosteroid on airway hyper-responsiveness and clinical asthma in nonsteroid-dependent asthmatics. *Am Rev Respir Dis* 142:832, 1990.

92. Vathenen AS, Know AJ, Wisniewski A, Tattersfield AE: Time course of change in bronchial reactivity with an inhaled corticosteroid in asthma. *Am Rev Respir Dis* 143:1317, 1991.

93. Haahtela T, Jarvinen M, Kava T, et al: Comparison of β_2-agonist terbutaline with an inhaled corticosteroid, budesonide, in newly detected asthma. *N Engl J Med* 325:388, 1991.

94. Salmeron S, Guerin J, Godard P, et al: High doses of inhaled corticosteroids in unstable chronic asthma: A multicenter, double-blind, placebo-controlled study. *Am Rev Respir Dis* 140:167, 1989.

95. Toogood JH: High-dose inhaled steroid therapy for asthma. *J Allergy Clin Imunol* 83:528, 1989.

96. Lacronique J, Renon D, Georges D, et al: High-dose beclomethasone: Oral steroid-sparing effect in severe asthmatic patients. *Eur Respir J* 4:807, 1991.

97. Hummel S, Lehtonen L, and Study Group: Comparison of oral steroid-sparing by high-dose inhaled steroid in maintenance treatment of severe asthma. *Lancet* 340:1483, 1992.

98. Grimfield A, Baculard A, Barbbier P, et al: Dose-effect relationship of beclomethasone dipropionate in moderate to severe childhood asthma (abstract). *Eur Respir J* 17(suppl):358s, 1993.

99. Gaddie J, Reid C, Skinner GR, et al: Aerosol beclomethasone dipropionate: A dose-response study in chronic bronchial asthma. *Lancet* 2:280, 1973.

100. Toogood JH, Lefcoe NM, Haines B, et al: A graded dose assessment of the efficacy of beclomethasone dipropionate aerosol for severe chronic asthma. *J Allergy Clin Immunl* 59:298, 1977.

101. Prahl P, Jensen T, Bjerregaard-Andersen H: Adrenocortical function in children on high-dose steroid aerosol therapy. *Allergy* 42:541, 1987.

102. Sherman B, Weinberger, Chen-Walden, Wendt H: Further studies of the effects of inhaled glucorticoids on pituitary adrenal function in healthy adults. *J Allergy Clin Immunol* 69:208, 1982.

103. Smith MJ, Hodson M: Effects of long-term inhaled high-dose beclomethasone dipopionate on adrenal function. *Thorax* 38:676, 1983.

104. Brown P, Blundell G, Greening AP, Crompton G: Hypothalomo-pituitary-adrenal axis suppression in asthmatics inhaling high-dose corticosteroids. *Respir Med* 85:501, 1991.

105. Toogood JH, Markov AE, Baskervill J, Dyson C: Association of ocular cataracts with inhaled and oral steroid therapy during long-term treatment of asthma. *J Allergy Clin Immunol* 91:571, 1993.

106. Ghanchi F: Young patients on inhaled steroids and cataract (letter). *Lancet* 342:671, 1993.

107. Reid DM: Methods of measurement of bone turnover and clinical evaluation of osteoporosis: Relevance to asthma and corticostroid therapy. *Respir Med* 87:9, 1993.

108. Puw EM, Prumel MF, Oosting H, et al: Beclomethasone inhalation decreases serum osteocalcin concentrations. *Br Med J* 302:627, 1991.

109. Teelucksingh SP, Padfield PL, Tibi L, et al: Inhaled corticosteroids, bone formation and osteocalcin. *Lancet* 338:60, 1991.

110. Leech J, Hodder R, Ooi D, Gay J: Effects of short-term inhaled budesonide and beclomethasone dippropionate on serum osteocalcin in premenopausal women. *Am Rev Respir Dis* 148:113, 1993.

111. Konig P, Hillman L, Cervantes, et al: Bone metabolism in children with asthma treated with inhaled beclomethasone dipropionate. *J Pediatr* 122:219, 1993.

112. Ali N, Capewell S, Ward M: Bone turnover during high-dose inhaled corticosteroid treatment. *Thorax* 46:160, 1991.

113. Wolthers OD, Pedersen S: Controlled study of linear growth in asthmatic children during treatment with inhaled corticorsteroids. *Pediatrics* 89:839, 1992.

114. Wolthers OD, Pedersen: Growth of asthmatic children during treatment with budesonide: A double-blind trial. *Br Med J* 303:163, 1991.

115. Wolthers OD, Pedersen: Short-term linear growth in asthmatic children during treatment with prednisolone. *Br Med J* 301:145, 1990.

116. Bisgaard H: Systemic activity of inhaled topical steroid in toddlers studied by knemometry. *Acta Paediatr Scand* 82:1066, 1993.

117. Prahl P, Jensen T: Decreased adreno-cortical suppression utilizing the Nebuhaler for inhalation of steroid aerosols. *Clin Allergy* 17:393, 1987.

118. Brown P, Blundell G, Greening A, et al: Do large volume spacer devices reduce the systemic effects of high dose inhaled corticosteroids? *Thorax* 45:736, 1990.

119. Kamada AK, Szefler SJ, Martin RJ, et al: Issues in the use of inhaled glucocorticosteroids. *Am J Repsir Crit Care Med* 153:1739, 1996.

120. Haahtela T, Jarvinen M, Kava T, et al: Effects of reducing or discontinuing inhaled budesonide in patients with mild asthma. *N Engl J Med* 331:700, 1994.

121. Watson A, Lim T, Joyce H, et al: Failure of inhaled corticosteroids to modify bronchonstrictor or bronchodilator responsivess in middle aged smokers with mild airflow obstruction. *Chest* 101:350, 1992.

122. Kerstijens HAM, Brand PLP, Hughes MD, et al: A comparison of bronchodilator therapy with or without inhaled coricostroid therapy for obstructive airways disease. *N Engl J Med* 327:1413, 1992.

123. National Asthma Education Program, Expert Panel on the Management of Asthma, National Heart Lung and Blood Institute: Guidelines for the diagnosis and management of asthma. *J Allergy Clin Immunol* 88:425, 1991.

124. National Heart, Lung and Blood Institute, National Institutes of Health: *Global Initiative for Asthma: Global Strategy for Asthma Management and Prevention,* NHLBI/WHO Workshop Report Publication No 95-3659. Bethesda, MD, U.S. Department of Health and Human Services, 1992.

125. Platts-Mills TAE, Mitchell EB, Nock P, et al: Reduction of bronchial hyperreactivity during prolonged allergen avoidance. *Lancet* 2:675, 1982.

Chapter 25 _____

MUCOLYTIC AGENTS, AGENTS FOR THE RELIEF OF DYSPNEA, AND RESPIRATORY STIMULANTS

MATTHEW G. MARIN
MARC H. LAVIETES

This chapter considers a number of disparate pharmacologic and nonpharmacologic approaches that may be useful in rehabilitating the patient with pulmonary disease. Some of these approaches may be beneficial in an individual patient. This chapter delineates the scientific background for the use of these approaches and their efficacy.

Mucolytic Agents

A productive cough is a characteristic common to a number of different pulmonary diseases, including pneumonia, acute and chronic bronchitis, tuberculous and fungal infections, cystic fibrosis, and lung neoplasms. A common treatment of this symptom involves drugs that serve to mobilize and assist in sputum expectoration. These medications have been variously termed *expectorants, mucokinetic, mucolytic, mucotropic,* or *mucoevacuant agents*. These terms are essentially synonymous, and for the purpose of this chapter, we will employ the term *mucolytic agent*. Unfortunately, the clinical use of mucolytic agents has enjoyed limited success in the treatment of productive cough.[1] In the sections that follow, we delineate (1) causes of productive cough, (2) mechanism of action and evidence for effectiveness of mucolytic agents, and (3) suggestions for the management of a productive cough.

CAUSES OF PRODUCTIVE COUGH

The underlying cause of a cough productive of mucus is a failure of mucociliary clearance, a mechanism that protects the lungs from inhaled noxious particles.[2] Mucociliary clearance depends on the effective interaction of ciliary beating of surface epithelial cells of the airways and the overlying mucus. Mucus, secreted by both submucosal gland cells and goblet cells,[2,3] lines the airways and is moved out of the airways by mechanical coupling to the tips of the beating cilia. Factors that are likely to be of importance in failure of mucociliary clearance include hypersecretion of mucus secondary to hypertrophy or hyperplasia of mucous glands and goblet cells, an increase in the secretory activity of individual mucus-secreting cells,[4–8] altered mucous rheology,[9–11] mechanical uncoupling of ciliary beating from the overlying mucous layer, and ineffective or absent ciliary beating.[2,3,9] Which of these factors contributes to a productive cough in a specific disease entity is not well known. With failure of mucociliary clearance, mucus accumulates in the airways. Cough serves to shear mucus from the airways and to propel it out of the lungs. Cough, then, is a backup mechanism that largely comes into play when the normal mucociliary cleansing apparatus fails.

MECHANISM OF ACTION AND EVIDENCE FOR EFFECTIVENESS OF MUCOLYTIC AGENTS

Because many pulmonary diseases are characterized by an increased volume of tenacious expectorated sputum, it is not surprising that clinicians have sought agents that liquefy and ease evacuation. Despite little confirmatory evidence,[12] it is presumed that this action will be of benefit to the patient. Table 25-1 summarizes the primary types of mucolytic agents that have been employed in clinical practice. The mechanism of action of mucolytics is variable.[12] Many of the agents have a thiol group that reduces disulfide bonds and breaks the mucous glycoproteins into smaller molecules. This results in less viscous molecules, facilitating expectoration.[13] Iodides and iodine-containing agents have been used for many years as mucolytic agents. The mechanism of action of these drugs is unknown but is presumed to relate to the induction of bronchorrhea, which serves to facilitate the evacuation of mucus.[14] More recently, recombinant human DNase has been introduced as a mucolytic agent.[15] DNA is released by dying inflammatory cells and adds considerably to the viscosity of the mucous secretion.[15] DNase functions to reduce the size of DNA in the sputum and thereby decrease sputum viscosity. Recombinant human DNase circumvents the problem of allergic reactions related to the use of DNases derived from animal species.[15]

A number of animal studies have explored the effects of agents that contain thiol groups. Some of these studies have concentrated on ultrastructural changes in the airway secretory cells, as well as the secretory product.[16-18] These studies have yielded conflicting results. For instance, L-cysteine methyl ester in dogs seemed to act both as a secretogogue and as a stimulator for increased mucus synthesis.[16] In rabbits, oral ingestion of *N*-acetylcysteine, carbocysteine, and Na-2-mercaptoethane sulfonate was demonstrated to cause degeneration of goblet cells and injury to ciliated epithelial cells.[18] Rogers and Jeffery[17] were able to inhibit cigarette smoke–induced hyperplasia of mucous cells in rats by treatment with 1% *N*-acetylcysteine in the drinking water. More recently, Livingstone and colleagues[19] studied the effects of thiol group agents on the rheologic properties of secretions obtained from pigs. They failed to demonstrate any significant alteration in the rheology of mucus due to either acetylcysteine or carboxymethylcysteine.

Several studies have explored the clinical effects of *N*-acetylcysteine in human patients.[20-24] Again, evidence for efficacy is conflicting and in general, provides minimal support for the clinical utility of *N*-acetylcysteine. Olivieri and colleagues[20] measured tracheal mucociliary transport in 12 bronchitic patients and demonstrated a modest but statistically significant increase in transport following oral *N*-acetylcysteine (600 mg/day). However, Millar and colleagues,[24] studying 9 bronchitic patients in a controlled, double-blind, cross-over trial employing the same dose of oral *N*-acetylcysteine, were unable to demonstrate any significant difference in mucociliary clearance, lung function, or viscosity of expectorated

Two pharmacologic qualities of almitrine may render this agent useful for treatment of COLD patients. First, as a stimulant of peripheral chemoreceptors, both the aortic and carotid bodies, almitrine may stimulate ventilation briefly during exacerbations of chronic bronchitis. Second, as a constrictor of the pulmonary vasculature, almitrine might enhance hypoxic pulmonary vasoconstriction in regions with low ventilation-perfusion ratios, thereby preserving an adequate arterial oxygen tension. Relief of hypoxia and, concomitantly, reduction of hypoxic ventilatory drive conceivably would lessen dyspnea. Alternatively, the increase of respiratory drive might worsen dyspnea.

Clinical trials in patients with severe but stable COLD appear mostly in the European literature. An improved arterial oxygen tension with no change in carbon dioxide was found in all studies. However, improvement in life span or in quality of life of COLD patients did not invariably accompany this improvement in gas exchange. Furthermore, a lessening of dyspnea occured for some patients; a worsening of dyspnea was reported by others.[64–67]

Progesterone has been proposed as a stimulant to respiration. When given on a long-term basis to obesity-hypoventilation patients, progesterone stimulates ventilation and improves gas exchange as well.[68] However, this therapy has not retained favor in current practice. Similarly, intravenous doxapram has been proposed as a respiratory stimulant to be administered briefly to COLD or obesity-hypoventilation patients during episodes of acute illness.[69,70] This therapy is intended to sustain adequate ventilation during acute illness and thereby avoid respiratory failure. Side effects, such as hypertension, tachycardia, and arrhythmia, have limited the usefulness of this agent.

References

1. Celli BR, Snider GL, Heffner J, et al: Standards for the diagnosis and care of patients with chronic obstructive pulmonary disease. *Am J Respir Crit Care Med* 152:S78, 1995

2. Wanner A: Clinical aspects of mucociliary transport. *Am Rev Respir Dis* 116:73, 1977.

3. Lucas AM, Douglas LC: Principles underlying ciliary activity in the respiratory tract: II. A comparison of nasal clearance in man, monkey and other animals. *Arch Otolaryngol* 20:518, 1934.

4. Coles SJ, Reid L: Glycoprotein secretion in vitro by human airway: Normal and chronic bronchitis. *Exp Mol Pathol* 29:326, 1978.

5. Reid L, Bhaskar K, Coles S: Clinical aspects of respiratory mucus. *Adv Exp Med Biol* 144:369, 1982.

6. Lamb D, Reid L: Mitotic rates, goblet cell increase and histochemical changes in mucus in rat bronchial epithelium during exposure to sulphur dioxide. *J Pathol Bacteriol* 96:97, 1968.

7. Lopez-Vidriero MT, Reid L: Pathophysiology of mucus secretion in cystic fibrosis. *Mod Probl Paediatr* 19:120, 1977.

8. Reid L: Chronic bronchitis and hypersecretion of mucus. *Lect Sci Basic Med* 8:235, 1959.

9. Litt M: Mucus rheology: Relevance to mucociliary clearance. *Arch Intern Med* 126:417, 1970.

10. Lethem MI, James SL, Marriott C: The role of mucous glycoproteins in the rheologic properties of cystic fibrosis sputum. *Am Rev Respir Dis* 142:1053, 1990.

11. Lopez-Vidriero MT, Charman J, Keal E, et al: Sputum viscosity: Correlation with chemical and clinical features in chronic bronchitis. *Thorax* 28:401, 1973.

12. Marin MG: Update: Pharmacology of airway secretion. *Pharmacol Rev* 46:35, 1994.

13. Moratalla R, Romera R, Galiano A: Pharmacological study of the new mucolytic drug N-guanyl-cysteine. *Arzneimittelforschung* 36:918, 1986.

14. Pavia D, Agnew JE, Glassman JM, et al: Effects of iodopropylidene glycerol on tracheobronchial clearance in stable, chronic bronchitic patients. *Eur J Respir Dis* 67:177, 1985.

15. Shak S, Capon DJ, Hellmiss R, et al: Recombinant human DNase I reduces the viscosity of cystic fibrosis sputum. *Proc Natl Acad Sci USA* 87:9188, 1990.

16. Yanaura S, Takeda H, Misawa M: Behavior of mucus glycoproteins of tracheal secretory cells following L-cysteine methyl ester treatment. *J Pharmacobiodyn* 5:603, 1982.

17. Rogers DF, Jeffery PK: Inhibition by oral N-acetylcysteine of cigarette smoke–induced "bronchitis" in the rat. *Exp Lung Res* 10:267, 1986.

18. Konradova V, Vavrova V, Sulova J: Comparison of the effect of three oral mucolytics on the ultrastructure of the tracheal epithelium in rabbits. *Respiration* 48:50, 1985.

19. Livingstone CR, Andrews MA, Jenkins SM, et al: Model systems for the evaluation of mucolytic drugs: Acetylcysteine and S-carboxymethylcysteine. *J Pharm Pharmacol* 42:73, 1990.

20. Olivieri D, Marsico SS, Del Donno M: Improvement of mucociliary transport in smokers by mucolytics. *Eur J Respir Dis* 66:142, 1985.

21. Millar AB, Pavia D, Agnew JE, et al: Effect of oral N-acetylcysteine on mucus clearance. *Br J Dis Chest* 79:262, 1985.

22. British Thoracic Society Research Committee: Oral N-acetylcysteine and exacerbation rates in patients with chronic bronchitis and severe airways obstruction. *Thorax* 40:832, 1985.

23. Rasmussen JB, Glennow C: Reduction in days of illness after long-term treatment with N-acetylcysteine controlled-release tablets in patients with chronic bronchitis. *Eur J Respir Dis* 1:351, 1988.

24. Dueholm M, Nielsen C, Thorshauge H, et al: N-Acetylcysteine by metered dose inhaler in the treatment of chronic bronchitis: A multi-centre study. *Respir Med* 86:89, 1992.

25. Petty TL: The National Mucolytic Study: Results of a randomized, double-blind, placebo-controlled study of iodinated glycerol in chronic obstructive bronchitis. *Chest* 97:75, 1990.

26. Zahm JM, Girod de Bentzmann S, Deneuville E, et al: Dose-dependent in vitro effect of recombinant human DNase on rheological and transport properties of cystic fibrosis respiratory mucus. *Eur Respir J* 8:381, 1995.

27. Heijerman HG, van Rossem RN, Bakker W: Effect of rhDNase on lung function and quality of life in adult cystic fibrosis patients. *Neth J Med* 46:293, 1995.

28. Shah PL, Scott SF, Fuchs HJ, et al: Medium-term treatment of stable stage cystic fibrosis with recombinant human DNase I. *Thorax* 50:333, 1995.

29. Fuchs HJ, Borowitz DS, Christiansen DH, et al: Effect of aerosolized recombinant human DNase on exacerbations of respiratory symptoms and on pulmonary function in patients with cystic fibrosis: The Pulmozyme Study Group. *N Engl J Med* 331:637, 1994.

30. Ranasinha C, Assoufi B, Shak S, et al: Efficacy and safety of short-term administration of aerosolised recombinant human DNase I in adults with stable stage cystic fibrosis. *Lancet* 342:199, 1993.

31. Ramsey BW, Astley SJ, Aitken ML, et al: Efficacy and safety of short-term administration of aerosolized recombinant human deoxyribonuclease in patients with cystic fibrosis. *Am Rev Respir Dis* 148:145, 1993.

32. Aitken ML, Burke W, McDonald G, et al: Recombinant human DNase inhalation in normal subjects and patients with cystic fibrosis: A phase 1 study. *JAMA* 267:1947, 1992.

33. Shah PL, Scott SF, Geddes DM, et al: Two years experience with recombinant human DNase I in the treatment of pulmonary disease in cystic fibrosis. *Respir Med* 89:499, 1995.

34. Shah PI, Bush A, Canny GJ, et al: Recombinant human DNase I in cystic fibrosis patients with severe pulmonary disease: A short-

term, double-blind study followed by six months open-label treatment. *Eur Respir J* 8:954, 1995.

35. Ferguson GT, Cherniack RM: Management of chronic obstructive pulmonary disease. *N Engl J Med* 328:1017, 1993.

36. Lakshminarayan S, Sahn SA, Hudson LD, et al: Effect of diazepam on ventilatory responses. *Clin Pharmacol Ther* 20:178, 1976.

37. Clergue F, Desmonts JM, Duvaldestin P, et al: Depression of respiratory drive by diazepam as premedication. *Br J Anaesth* 53:1059, 1981.

38. Kronenberg RS, Cosio MG, Stevenson JE, et al: The use of oral diazepam in patients with obstructive lung disease and hypercapnia. *Ann Intern Med* 83:83, 1975.

39. Mitchell-Heggs P, Murphy K, Minty K, et al: Diazepam in the treatment of dyspnea in the "pink puffer" syndrome. *Q J Med* 49:9, 1980.

40. Man GCW, Hsu K, Sproule BJ: Effect of alprazolam on exercise and dyspnea in patients with chronic obstructive pulmonary disease. *Chest* 90:832, 1986.

41. Santiago TV, Johnson J, Riley DJ, et al: Effects of morphine on ventilatory response to exercise. *J Appl Physiol* 47:112, 1979.

42. Bellofiore S, DiMaria GU, Privitera S, et al: Endogenous opioids modulate the increase in ventilatory output and dyspnea during severe acute bronchoconstriction. *Am Rev Respir Dis* 142:812, 1990.

43. Harris-Eze AO, Sridhar G, Clemens RE, et al: Low-dose nebulized morphine does not improve exercise in interstitial lung disease. *Am J Respir Crit Care Med* 152:1940, 1995.

44. Supinski G, Dimarco A, Bark H, et al: Effect of codeine on the sensations elicited by loaded breathing. *Am Rev Respir Dis* 141:1516, 1990.

45. Woodcock AA, Gross ER, Gellert A, et al: Effects of dihydrocodeine, alcohol, and caffeine on breathlessness and exercise tolerance in patients with chronic obstructive lung disease and normal blood gases. *N Engl J Med* 305:1611, 1981.

46. Johnson MA, Woodcock AA, Geddes DM: Dihydrocodeine for breathlessness in "pink puffers." *Br Med J* 286:675, 1983.

47. Light RW, Muro JR, Sato RI, et al: Effects of oral morphine on breathlessness and exercise tolerance in patients with chronic obstructive pulmonary disease. *Am Rev Respir Dis* 139:126, 1989.

48. Light RW, Stansbury DW, Webster JS: Effect of 30 mg of morphine alone or with promethazine or prochlorperazine on the exercise capacity of patients with COPD. *Chest* 109:975, 1996.

49. Greenberg HE, Scharf SM, Green H: Nortriptyline-induced depression of ventilatory control in a patient with chronic obstructive pulmonary disease. *Am Rev Respir Dis* 147:1303, 1993.

50. Schiffman GL, Stansbury DW, Fischer CE, et al: Indomethacin and perception of dyspnea in chronic airflow obstruction. *Am Rev Respir Dis* 137:1094, 1988.

51. Petty TL, O'Donohue WJ Jr: Further recommendations for prescribing, reimbursement, technology development, and research in long-term oxygen therapy. *Am J Respir Crit Care Med* 150:875, 1994.

52. Anthonisen NR: Long-term oxygen therapy. *Ann Intern Med* 99:519, 1983.

53. Dewan NA, Bell CW: Effect of low flow and high flow oxygen delivery on exercise tolerance and sensation of dyspnea. *Chest* 106:1061, 1994.

54. Dean NC, Brown JK, Himelman RB, et al: Oxygen may improve dyspnea and endurance in patients with chronic obstructive pulmonary disease and only mild hypoxemia. *Am Rev Respir Dis* 146:941, 1992.

55. O'Donnell DE, McGuire M, Samis L, et al: The impact of exercise reconditioning on breathlessness in severe chronic airflow limitation. *Am J Respir Crit Care Med* 152:2005, 1995.

56. Ries AL, Kaplan RM, Limberg TM, et al: Effects of pulmonary rehabilitation on physiologic and psychosocial outcomes in patients with chronic obstructive pulmonary disease. *Ann Intern Med* 122:823, 1995.

57. Sibuya M, Yamada M, Kanamaru A, et al: Effect of chest wall vibration on dyspnea in patients with chronic respiratory disease. *Am J Respir Crit Care Med* 149:1235, 1994.

58. Mohsenifar Z, Rosenberg N, Goldberg HS, et al: Mechanical vibration and conventional chest physiotherapy in outpatients with stable chronic obstructive lung disease. *Chest* 87:483, 1985.

59. Piquet J, Brochard L, Isabey D, et al: High-frequency chest wall oscillation in patients with chronic airflow obstruction. *Am Rev Respir Dis* 136:1355, 1987.

60. Carrieri-Kohlman V, Douglas MK, Gormley JM, et al: Desensitization and guided mastery: Treatment approaches for the management of dyspnea. *Heart Lung* 22:226, 1993.

61. Garner SJ, Eldridge FL, Wagner PG, et al: Buspirone, an anxiolytic drug that stimulates respiration. *Am Rev Respir Dis* 139:946, 1989.

62. Mendelson WB, Martin JV, Rapoport DM: Effects of buspirone on sleep and respiration. *Am Rev Respir Dis* 141:1527, 1990.

63. Rapoport DM, Greenberg HE, Goldring RM: Differing effects of the anxiolytic agents buspirone and diazepam on control of breathing. *Clin Pharmacol Ther* 49:394, 1991.

64. Bardsley PA, Howard P, Tang O, et al: Sequential treatment with low-dose almitrine bismesylate in hypoxaemic chronic obstructive airways disease. *Eur Respir J* 5:1054, 1992.

65. Bakran I, Vrhovac B, Stangl B, et al: Double-blind, placebo-controlled clinical trial of almitrine bismesylate in patients with chronic respiratory insufficiency. *Eur J Clin Pharmacol* 38:249, 1990.

66. Riberio SA, Jardim JRB, Romaldini H, et al: Effects of almitrine on the ventilatory control, breathing pattern and maximal exercise tolerance in hypoxemic patients with chronic obstructive pulmonary disease. *Braz J Med Biol Res* 28:859, 1995.

67. Winkelmann BR, Kullmer TH, Kneissl DG, et al: Low-dose almitrine bismesylate in the treatment of hypoxemia due to chronic obstructive pulmonary disease. *Chest* 105:1383, 1994.

68. Sutton FD, Zwillich CW, Creagh E, et al: Progesterone for outpatient treatment of pickwickian syndrome. *Ann Intern Med* 83:476, 1975.

69. Moser KM, Luchsinger PC, Adamson JS, et al: Respiratory stimulation with intravenous doxapram in respiratory failure. *N Engl J Med* 288:427, 1973.

70. Houser WC, Schlueter DP: Prolonged doxapram infusion in obesity-hypoventilation syndrome. *JAMA* 239:340, 1978.

Chapter 26
OXYGEN THERAPY

HUGO D. MONTENEGRO

This chapter reviews the rationale, indications, prescription guidelines, and methods and equipment currently available for the administration of long-term oxygen therapy. Therapeutic benefits of long-term oxygen therapy have been documented mainly for hypoxemic patients with chronic obstructive pulmonary disease (COPD). However, similar beneficial effects also should be expected in patients with hypoxemia secondary to other pulmonary disorders.

Beneficial Effects

Although the use of oxygen as a therapeutic agent in the management of patients with pulmonary disorders has long been advocated,[1] it is only recently that multicenter longitudinal studies in hypoxemic COPD patients have demonstrated improved survival with the long-term administration of supplemental oxygen. In addition, oxygen therapy also has been shown to improve exercise performance, pulmonary hemodynamics, sensation of dyspnea, and neuropsychological derangements.

Survival

Two landmark studies convincingly demonstrated that long-term oxygen therapy improves survival. In the Nocturnal Oxygen Therapy Trial (NOTT),[2] patients receiving nocturnal oxygen therapy (12 h/day) had an annual death rate of 20 percent; patients on continuous oxygen therapy (19 h/day) had an annual death rate of 11 percent.[2] In the British Medical Research Council (MRC) trial, patients receiving no oxygen had a 5-year survival of approximately 20 percent with an annual death rate of about 40 percent; patients on oxygen therapy (15 h/day) had a 40 percent 5-year survival rate with an annual death rate of approximately 18 percent.[3] The MRC study reported a reduced mortality after only 500 days of therapy, mostly in men, and a very high mortality rate in women who received no oxygen therapy. Other studies have reported equal survival rates in men and women,[4] better survival in women,[5] or worse survival in women receiving oral steroids.[6]

Exercise Performance

In COPD patients with hypoxemia at rest or during exercise, the administration of supplemental oxygen has been shown to improve endurance and exercise performance during cycle ergometry, treadmill exercise, or timed walking.[7-9] In these patients, supplemental oxygen reduced minute ventilation and respiratory frequency for a given workload,[10] increased oxygen delivery and oxygen utilization by muscles during exercise,[11] improved ventilatory capacity by postponing the onset of respiratory muscle fatigue,[12] and reduced lactate levels.[13,14] The reduction in minute ventilation may be due in part to a reduction in chemoreceptor activity,[15,16] although estimation of hypoxic drive does not seem to predict which patients may improve with the administration of supplemental oxygen.[17]

Pulmonary Hemodynamics

Pulmonary artery hypertension and cor pulmonale are significant variables known to affect mortality in patients with COPD.[18,19] Uncontrolled studies have shown improvement in survival in hypoxemic COPD patients who received supplemental oxygen.[20-23] One study[24] showed a yearly decrease in mean pulmonary artery pressure of 2.15 ± 4.4 mmHg during long-term oxygen therapy compared with a yearly increase of 1.47 ± 2.3 mmHg before the administration of oxygen in the same group. Multicenter controlled studies have confirmed the beneficial effects of long-term oxygen in pulmonary hemodynamics. In the NOTT study,[2] the group of patients who received continuous oxygen therapy showed improvement in pulmonary vascular resistance, pulmonary artery pressure, and both baseline and exercise stroke volume index; the group receiving only nocturnal oxygen therapy showed stable hemodynamic variables. For both groups, changes in pulmonary hemodynamics during the first 6 months were associated with survival. Conversely, the removal of supplemental oxygen for several hours in patients with COPD receiving long-term oxygen therapy has been shown to have adverse effects on gas exchange, cardiac function, and pulmonary hemodynamics.[25]

Some studies have suggested that survival in hypoxemic COPD patients was related to the acute effect of oxygen on pulmonary hemodynamics; that is, changes in pulmonary artery pressure greater than 5 mmHg predicted 2-year survival.[26] Others, however, have not been able to confirm these findings.[27] Noninvasive evaluation of pulmonary hemodynamics, such as radionuclear assessment of left and right ventricular ejection fractions[11,26] and measurement of peak V_O,[28] may be helpful in predicting the responsiveness of pulmonary artery pressure to oxygen in hypoxemic COPD patients and also may be more clinically accessible than invasive methods.

Sensation of Dyspnea

The administration of oxygen in patients with COPD has been shown to improve the sensation of breathlessness, as measured by a visual analogue scale.[29,30] Improvement may be significant even in the absence of exercise-induced oxygen desaturation.[31] Because the administration of air via nasal cannula also has been shown to decrease the sensation of breathlessness, an effect on nasal receptors has been postulated as a mechanism of improvement achieved by the administration of oxygen.[32] Some studies have suggested that the burden of carrying portable oxygen equipment may abolish the beneficial effects of breathing supplemental oxygen on walking distance[33]; others have shown no deleterious effects.[34,35]

Neuropsychological Effect

Impairment in perceptual and motor abilities has been reported in hypoxemic COPD patients. In one study, tests suggestive of cerebral dysfunction were found in 42 percent of patients as compared with 14 percent of controls.[36] Higher cognitive functions such as abstracting ability and complex perceptual motor integration were more affected, although motor skills, speed, strength, and coordination also were abnormal. Depression and lack of motivation to perform the tests did not account for the results.

As part of the NOTT study, hypoxemic patients with COPD were given detailed neuropsychological and life quality examinations before and after receiving 6 months of supplemental oxygen. Patients receiving continuous oxygen therapy showed better neuropsychological performance than those receiving nocturnal oxygen therapy. Despite these improvements, however, there was no demonstrable change in emotional status or quality of life.[37] In a smaller group of hypoxemic COPD patients, the administration of continuous oxygen therapy for only 1 month improved motor integration and simple motor speed, both of which were abnormal before oxygen was administered.[38]

Adverse Effects

Two potential adverse effects of supplemental oxygen therapy include worsening of hypercapnia and oxygen toxicity.

HYPERCAPNIA

Worsening of hypercapnia following the uncontrolled administration of supplemental oxygen to COPD patients who are both hypoxemic and hypercarbic has been documented during acute exacerbations.[39,40] Severe hypoxemia and acidosis represent a higher risk.[41] Although depression of the hypoxic respiratory drive has been suggested as the main mechanism for this side effect,[39,40,42] there are no clinical data to support this statement. Clinical studies and data generated from a computer model of pulmonary circulation indicate that other important mechanisms include increased dead space and the Haldane effect.[43,44] Worsening of hypercapnia can be minimized by the administration of controlled oxygen therapy using air-entrapment masks.[40,41,45,46]

In stable patients with COPD, however, the administration of oxygen has not been shown to have the same effects on hypercapnia as in patients with acute exacerbations; in a group of awake COPD patients, the rise in arterial P_{CO_2} averaged 2 mmHg.[47] In another group studied during sleep, the rise in transcutaneous P_{CO} averaged 6 mmHg.[48]

OXYGEN TOXICITY

Although anatomic lesions suggestive of oxygen toxicity have been reported in patients who received long-term continuous oxygen therapy,[49] their clinical significance and impact on therapeutic outcome were never clear. In the NOTT study, indices of possible oxygen toxicity were graded during autopsy. There was a trend toward more interstitial fibrosis and type II alveolar cell hyperplasia in patients who received nocturnal oxygen. Because there was no matched control group available, the authors could not conclude whether the observed lesions actually were due to oxygen toxicity.[50]

Oxygen Therapy Prescription

The clinical guidelines for prescribing long-term oxygen therapy are based on the NOTT study and are shown in Table 26-1. According to Medicare guidelines, reimbursement will not be approved unless the patients meet the physiologic criteria in Table 26-1. Most private insurance carriers and the Department of Veterans Affairs follow the Medicare guidelines for reimbursement for long-term oxygen therapy. As per the guidelines, those patients who are in stable condition with a Pa_O of less than 55 mmHg and an Sa_O of less than 88 percent should receive long-term oxygen therapy.

To prescribe long-term oxygen therapy, a certificate of medical necessity (Health Care Finance Administration, HCFA Form 484) must be completed. The certificate of medical necessity requires the following information: patient's name, address, and HIC number; supplier's name, address, and identification number; pertinent diagnosis (ICD-9-CM codes and findings); estimated length of need; results of most recent arterial blood gases and/or oxygen saturation tests while the patient is breathing room air (if the test is performed under conditions other than room air, explanation should be attached); the oxygen flow rate in liters per minute; the need for either continuous (24 hours per day) or noncontinuous administration of oxygen either during walking, sleeping, or during exercise programs; the equipment required, including the supply and delivery systems; and if the prescription is for a portable or ambulatory system, a description of the activities/exercise that the patient regularly pursues that require that particular system.

Patients being discharged from a hospital after an acute exacerbation who have not received previous long-term oxygen therapy and who at the time of discharge qualify for home oxygen therapy need to be reevaluated 30 to 90 days after discharge when the patient is clinically more stable. Once the need for long-term oxygen therapy has been established, repeat measurements of arterial blood gases or oxygen saturation are not medically necessary or justifiable for recertification.[51] Initial documentation of the need for long-term oxygen therapy should be based on arterial blood gas measurements performed under stable conditions and analyzed by an appropriate laboratory. Oximetry is an appropriate and acceptable technique for documenting hypoxemia during activity and sleep, as well as for follow-up for evaluating and monitoring long-term oxygen therapy. If there are any major changes in the oxygen delivery system, the patient's oxygenation should be checked both at rest and during usual exercise to ensure that the hypoxemia has been corrected.

TABLE 26-1 Indications for Long-Term Oxygen Therapy

- $Pa_{O_2} \leq 55$ mmHg
- Pa_{O_2} 55–59 mmHg plus
  Erythrocytosis (hematocrit $\geq 55\%$)
  "P" pulmonale on electrocardiogram (P wave ≥ 3 mm)
  Peripheral edema

TABLE 26-2 Comparison of Gas, Liquid, and Concentrator Oxygen Systems

Characteristic	Gas	Liquid	Concentrator
Availability	Common	Limited	Common
Reliability	Generally good; Bourdon gauges may become inaccurate	Possible inaccurate setting, freezing of connector	Good, but needs regular service
Cost	Moderate	High	Low
Weight + use time, 2 L/m	H cylinder: 200 lb, 2.5 d	Reservoir: 120 lb, 8.9 d	Stationary 35-lb unit; no storage capability
Portable	E cylinder: 20 lb, 5 h	Portable: 6 lb, 4 h	
Portable + OCD (O$_2$-conserving device)	Fiber/alum: 4.5 lb, 12 h	OCD system: 5.5 lb, 8 h	
Transfill	Limited	Excellent	N/A
Power	None	None	110 volts ac
Ambulatory use	Good with conserver	Good alone and with conserver	Portable, but not suitable for ambulatory use

SOURCE: American Thoracic Society,[58] by permission.

Oxygen Equipment

There are two key components to be considered regarding oxygen equipment: supply systems and delivery systems.

SUPPLY SYSTEMS

Oxygen supply equipment (Table 26-2) can be categorized as[52]

1. Stationary oxygen equipment, including any large reservoir of oxygen that cannot be moved easily or carried by the patient (K cylinder containing compressed oxygen, oxygen concentrator, liquid oxygen reservoir)
2. Portable equipment, i.e., equipment that can be moved or transported by the patient but not carried by the patient during daily activities (E cylinder mounted on a cart or stroller, battery-operated oxygen concentrator)
3. Ambulatory oxygen, which includes any equipment that can be carried by most patients during activities of daily living (a small liquid oxygen canister, a small, lightweight cylinder)[52]

Based on the need for any of these oxygen supply systems, patients receiving long-term oxygen therapy may fall into one of the following groups:

1. Sedentary patients, for whom oxygen concentrator with a backup oxygen cylinder may be sufficient
2. Ambulatory or mobile patients who occasionally go out of the house for essential medical care or visits, for whom oxygen concentrator and supplemental cylinders on a stroller may be required
3. Ambulatory patients who leave home several times a week, for whom liquid oxygen with lightweight ambulatory units may be required[51]

DELIVERY SYSTEMS

NASAL CANNULA
The most commonly used delivery system is the nasal cannula. For a typical patient, a flow of 1 liter of oxygen per minute adds 3 to 4 percent to the fraction of inspired oxygen (F_{IO_2}). Because oxygen is delivered during inspiration and expiration, however, there may be substantial waste. In addition, the oxygen flow can induce nasal irritation, and the oxygen tubing may induce tenderness in the ears and cheeks.

OXYGEN-CONSERVING DEVICES
To minimize the waste of supplemental oxygen, a number of oxygen-conserving devices have been reported.[53–55] These devices are listed in Table 26-3; comparison of their characteristics is shown in Table 26-4.

Reservoir Cannulas
Both the oxygen-conserving nasal cannula and the pendant consist of a reservoir that expands and fills with dead-space gas during exhalation. Early in inhalation, the reservoir collapses, and a high concentration of oxygen is delivered. Oxygen savings under controlled conditions are from 50 to 75 percent at rest and 66 percent during exercise.[53]

Demand-Flow Oxygen Delivery Systems
These devices are designed to sense inhalation and cause a flow of oxygen to be delivered only during the inspiratory

TABLE 26-3 Oxygen-Conserving Devices

Reservoir cannulas
- Oxygen-conserving nasal cannulas (Oxymizer, Chad Therapeutics, Inc., Chatsworth, CA)
- Oxygen-conserving pendant (Oxymizer pendant, Chad Therapeutics, Inc., Chatsworth, CA)

Demand oxygen delivery systems
- Companion Oxygen Saver (Puritan Bennett, Inc., Lenexa, KS)
- Conservator (Penox Technologies, Inc. Pittston, PA)
- Pulsair (Pulsair, Inc., Ft. Pierce, FL)
- Oxymatic (Chad Therapeutics, Inc., Chatsworth, CA)
- Aluminum and fiber-wrapped cylinders
    Oxylite, Oxylite Mini (Chad Therapeutics, Inc., Chatsworth, CA)
    Walkabout, Walkabout Mini, Walkabout 2 (Pulsair, Inc., Ft. Pierce, FL)

Transtracheal oxygen catheters
- SCOOP (Transtracheal System, Englewood, CO)
- Heimlich Microtrach (Inmedco, Salt Lake City, UT)

TABLE 26-4 Oxygen-Conserving Devices

Characteristic	Reservoir	Demand Pulse	Transtracheal
Mechanism of conservation	Store during exhalation	Early inspiratory delivery	Store at end-exhalation; bypass dead space
Savings	2:1 to 4:1	3:1 to 7:1	2:1 to 3:1
Cosmetics	Obtrusive	Adequate	Best
Comfort	Adequate	Adequate	Good
Reliability	Good; simple	Mechanical	Mucus plug possible
Cost	Low	Significant	Significant
Specific advantages	Inexpensive, easily initiated, reliable	Highest savings, programmable delivery possible with alarms	Cosmetics, lack of nasal/ear irritation, good compliance, may reduce minute ventilation
Specific disadvantages	Bulky on face	Mechanically complicated, failure possible	Special care and training surgical complications

SOURCE: American Thoracic Society,[58] by permission.

phase. They can be driven by pressure, flow, or pressure and flow. With the companion Oxygen Saver, the delivery of oxygen ends within the first 25 percent of inspiration. With the Conserve Air, the flow starts at the beginning of the inspiratory cycle and is shut off at the end of inspiration. The Pulse Air delivers a fixed volume per breath according to preselected settings. With the Oxymatic, the pulse of oxygen is timed to interrupt flow during late inspiration. This unit can be set to deliver oxygen pulses during one of four breaths, two of four breaths, three of four breaths, or at almost every breath.[52] When compared with continuous-flow systems, the demand-flow oxygen delivery systems have shown oxygen savings of 50 to 86 percent.[53] One of the potential disadvantages of demand oxygen delivery systems is poor inspiration tracking. There is no information as to whether these devices will deliver oxygen during reduced inspiratory efforts, such as during sleep; because of this limitation, demand delivery devices are suggested for daytime use only.[55]

Some companies have designed lightweight cylinders for use in combination with demand-flow oxygen delivery systems. A list of some of these cylinders is included in Table 26-3. Their weight varies from 4.5 to 8.3 lb. The oxygen supply lasts from 10.5 to 28 h, with an oxygen flow of 2 L/min.

Transtracheal Oxygen Delivery
The administration of oxygen transtracheally was first introduced by Heimlich.[57] Since then, two types of transtracheal catheters are commonly used (see Table 26-3). Several factors are believed to alter the requirement of oxygen with a transtracheal oxygen system, mostly related to reduction of dead space. It also has been postulated that the breathing pattern may be affected with transtracheal oxygen administration.[58] Savings in oxygen requirements have ranged from 37 to 58 percent at rest and 30 percent during exercise.[53] Major potential disadvantages of the transtracheal oxygen system include the high cost, the increased risk of infections, and complications. Some absolute contraindications include subglottic stenosis, vocal cord paralysis, severe coagulopathy, and inability to practice self-care. Relative contraindications include processes in which healing may be altered, for example, patients using corticosteroids or immunosuppressive agents or those with uncontrolled diabetes.[59]

The overall goal of oxygen-conserving devices should include increased patient mobility and comfort. These devices can reduce the overall cost of oxygen therapy at home not necessarily by reducing the cost of the oxygen but by reducing the number of deliveries per month to the home.[58] Further studies are required to determine the true cost-effectiveness of all these devices.

Traveling with Oxygen

Recreational travel, including traveling on ground, water, and air, is possible for patients with COPD who require long-term oxygen therapy. Adequate and advanced preparation for a trip should allow most patients to travel without significant problems.

TRAVEL BY AIR

International aviation regulations recommend that aircraft flying at maximum altitude should maintain cabin pressure at a range of 8000 ft or 2438 m.[60] At this cabin pressure level, a normal individual would have a Pa_{O_2} of 65 to 68 mmHg; in contrast, a patient with COPD would develop significant hypoxemia.[61] Although it has been estimated that 5 percent of commercial air travelers are under medical care,[62] the frequency of adverse medical events during commercial traveling is low, but the data are scanty.[62,63] Because supplemental oxygen should be administered to a patient with COPD with a Pa_{O_2} of less than 55 mmHg, various equations have been developed to estimate a patient's Pa_{O_2} value.[63] Based on some of these equations, a sea-level Pa_{O_2} of less than 72 mmHg will predict a Pa_{O_2} of less than 50 mmHg at 8000 feet cabin altitude in 87 percent of subjects.[61,62] In patients who are already receiving long-term oxygen, it is recommended that in-flight oxygen be increased by 2 L above the flow use at sea level.

In planning commercial air travel for patients with COPD, advance arrangements are recommended.[62]

1. Interaction with physicians to determine whether there is a need for in-flight oxygen; submission of letters describing the condition and duration of in-flight oxygen.
2. Interaction with air carrier and travel agent. Notification of the need for oxygen at least 48 h before flight; choosing nonstop flights if possible; traveling during business hours

when vendors are available; considering the use of an agent who specializes in travel for patients with medical needs.

3. Interaction with oxygen vendor; dealing with a company that can arrange nationwide coverage.

4. Personal planning for travel date; early arrival to the airport; bringing nasal cannula.

CAR, BUS, AND RAIL TRAVEL WITH OXYGEN

The type of oxygen supplied during travel by car, motor home, bus, or rail is usually dictated by the patient's requirements. When the patient is traveling by car, he or she can have access to large-volume liquid reservoirs that can be secured in the car. For patients requiring only nocturnal oxygen, an oxygen concentrator can be rented and carried in the car for use when needed. An extensive list of the types of reservoirs and the names of the companies that produce them has been published recently[63] and is also available from manufacturing companies.

Support and encouragement by health care providers to pursue travel should be an important aspect of overall patient care.[56]

References

1. Barach AL: The therapeutic use of oxygen. *JAMA* 79:693–698, 1922.

2. Nocturnal Oxygen Therapy Trial Group: Continuous or nocturnal oxygen therapy in hypoxemic chronic obstructive lung disease. *Ann Intern Med* 93:391–398, 1980.

3. Medical Research Council Working Party: Long-term domiciliary oxygen therapy in chronic hypoxic cor pulmonale complicating chronic bronchitis and emphysema. *Lancet* 1:681–685, 1981.

4. Cooper CB, Waterhouse J, Howard P: Twelve-year clinical study of patients with hypoxic cor pulmonale given long-term domiciliary oxygen therapy. *Thorax* 42:105–110, 1987.

5. Miyamoto K, Aida A, Nishimora M, et al: Gender effect on prognosis of patients receiving long-term home oxygen therapy. *Am J Respir Crit Care Med* 152:972–976, 1995.

6. Ström K: Survival of patients with chronic obstructive pulmonary disease receiving long-term domiciliary oxygen therapy. *Am Rev Respir Dis* 147:585–591, 1993.

7. Zack MB, Palange AV: Oxygen supplemented exercise of ventilatory and nonventilatory muscles in pulmonary rehabilitation. *Chest* 88:669–675, 1985.

8. Bradley BL, Garner AE, Billiu D, et al: Oxygen-assisted exercise in chronic obstructive lung disease. *Am Rev Respir Dis* 118:239–243, 1978.

9. McKeon J, Murree-Allen K, Saunders N: Effects of breathing supplemental oxygen before progressive exercise in patients with chronic obstructive lung disease. *Thorax* 43:53–56, 1988.

10. Bye PT, Esau SA, Levy RD, et al: Ventilatory muscle function during exercise in air and oxygen in patients with chronic airflow limitation. *Am Rev Respir Dis* 132:236, 1985.

11. Morrison DA, Stovall JR: Increased exercise capacity in hypoxemic patients after long-term therapy. *Chest* 102:542–550, 1992.

12. Criner GH, Celli BR: Ventilatory muscle recruitment in exercise with O_2 in obstructed patients with mild hypoxemia. *J Appl Physiol* 63:195–200, 1987.

13. Stein DA, Bradley BL, Miller WC: Mechanisms of oxygen effects on exercise in patients with chronic obstructive pulmonary disease. *Chest* 81:6, 1982.

14. King AJ, Cooke NJ, Leitch AG, Flenley DC: The effects of 30% oxygen on the respiratory response to treadmill exercise in chronic respiratory failure. *Clin Sci* 44:151–162, 1973.

15. Berry RB, Mahulte CK, Kirsch JI, et al: Does the hypoxic ventilatory response predict the oxygen induced falls in ventilation in COPD? *Chest* 103:820–824, 1993.

16. Scano GA, Van Meerhaeghe A, Willeput R, et al: Effect of oxygen on breathing during exercise in patients with chronic obstructive lung disease. *Eur J Respir Dis* 63:23–30, 1982.

17. Light RW, Mahutte CK, Stransburg DW, et al: Relationship between improvement in exercise performance with supplemental oxygen and hypoxic ventilatory drive in patients with chronic airflow obstruction. *Chest* 95:751–756, 1989.

18. Dallari R, Barozzi G, Pinelli G, et al: Predictors of survival in subjects with chronic obstructive pulmonary disease treated with long-term oxygen therapy. *Respiration* 61:8–13, 1994.

19. Oswald-Mammosser M, Weitzenblum E, Quoix E, et al: Prognostic factors in COPD patients receiving long-term oxygen therapy. *Chest* 107:1193–1198, 1995.

20. Levine S, Bigelow DB, Hamstra RD, et al: The role of long-term continuous oxygen administration in patients with chronic airways obstruction with hypoxemia. *Ann Intern Med* 66:639–650, 1967.

21. Abraham AS, Cole RB, Bishop JM: Reversal of pulmonary hypertension by prolonged oxygen administration to patients with chronic bronchitis. *Circ Res* 23:147–157, 1968.

22. Leggett RJ, Cooke NJ, Clancy L, et al: Long-term domiciliary oxygen therapy in cor pulmonale complicating chronic bronchitis and emphysema. *Thorax* 31:414–416, 1976.

23. Neff TA, Petty TL: Long-term continuous oxygen therapy in chronic airway obstruction. *Ann Intern Med* 72:621–626, 1970.

24. Weitzenblum E, Sautegeau A, Ehrhart M, et al: Long-term oxygen therapy can reverse the progression of pulmonary hypertension in patients with chronic obstructive pulmonar disease. *Am Rev Respir Dis* 131:493–498, 1985.

25. Selinger SR, Kennedy TP, Buescher P, et al: Effects of removing oxygen from patients with chronic obstructive pulmonary disease. *Am Rev Respir Dis* 136:85–91, 1987.

26. Ashutosh K, Mead G, Dunsky M: Early effects of oxygen administration and prognosis in chronic obstructive pulmonary disease and cor pulmonale. *Am Rev Respir Dis* 127:399–404, 1983.

27. Sliwinski P, Hawrylkiewicz I, Gorecka D, Zielinski J: Acute effect of oxygen on pulmonary arterial pressure does not predict survival on long-term oxygen therapy in patients with chronic obstructive pulmonary disease. *Am Rev Respir Dis* 146:665–669, 1992.

28. Ashutosh K, Dunsky M: Noninvasive tests for responsiveness of pulmonary hypertension to oxygen. *Chest* 92:393–399, 1987.

29. Waterhouse JC, Howard P: Breathlessness and portable oxygen in chronic obstructive airways disease. *Thorax* 38:302–306, 1983.

30. Swinburn C, Mould H, Stone T, et al: Symptomatic benefit of supplemental oxygen in hypoxemic patients with chronic lung disease. *Am Rev Respir Dis* 143:913–915, 1991.

31. Dean NC, Brown JK, Himelman RB, et al: Oxygen may improve dyspnea and endurance in patients with chronic obstructive pulmonary disease and only mild hypoxemia. *Am Rev Respir Dis* 146:941–945, 1992.

32. Liss HP, Grant BJB: The effects of nasal flow on breathlessness in patients with chronic obstructive pulmonary disease. *Am Rev Respir Dis* 137:1285–1288, 1988.

33. Leggett RJE, Flenley DC: Portable oxygen and exercise tolerance in patients with chronic hypoxic cor pulmonale. *Br Med J* 2:84–86, 1977.

34. Woodcock A, Gross E: Oxygen relieves breathlessness in "pink puffers." *Lancet* 1:907–909, 1981.

35. Davidson A, Leach P, George R, Geddes D: Supplemental oxygen and exercise ability in chronic obstructive airways disease. *Thorax* 43:965–971, 1988.

36. Grant I, Heaton RK, McSweeny J, et al: Neuropsychologic findings in hypoxemic chronic obstructive pulmonary disease. *Arch Intern Med* 142:1470–1476, 1982.

37. Heaton RK, Grant I, McSweeny J, et al: Psychologic effects of continuous and nocturnal oxygen therapy in hypoxemic chronic obstructive pulmonary disease. *Arch Intern Med* 143:1941–1947, 1983.

38. Krop HD, Block AJ, Cohen E: Neuropsychologic effects of continuous oxygen therapy in chronic obstructive pulmonary disease. *Chest* 64:317–322, 1973.

39. Arnold WH, Grant JL: Oxygen-induced hypoventilation. *Am Rev Respir Dis* 95:255–261, 1967.

40. Campbell EJM: The J. Burns Amberson before: The management of acute respiratory failure in chronic bronchitis and emphysema. *Am Rev Respir Dis* 96:626–639, 1967.

41. Bone RC, Pierce AK, Johnson RL: Controlled oxygen administration in acute respiratory failure in chronic obstructive pulmonary disease. *Am J Med* 65:896–890, 1978.

42. Hutchison DCS, Flenley DC, Donald KW: Controlled oxygen therapy in respiratory failure. *Br Med J* 2:1159–1166, 1964.

43. Aubier M, Murciano D, Milic-Emili J, et al: Effects of the administration of O$_2$ on ventilation and blood gases in patients with chronic obstructive pulmonary disease during acute respiratory failure. *Am Rev Respir Dis* 122:747–756, 1980.

44. Hanson CW, Marshall BE, Frasch HF, Marshall C: Causes of hypercarbia with oxygen therapy in patients with chronic obstructive pulmonary disease. *Crit Care Med* 24:23–28, 1996.

45. Campbell EJM: A method of controlled oxygen administration which reduces the risk of carbon-dioxide retention. *Lancet* 2:12–14, 1960.

46. Warrell DA, Edwards RHT, Godfrey S, Jones NL: Effect of controlled oxygen therapy on arterial blood gases in acute respiratory failure. *Br Med J* 2:452, 1970.

47. Schiff MM, Massaro D: Effect of oxygen administration by a venturi apparatus on arterial blood gase values in patients with respiratory failure. *N Engl J Med* 277:950–953, 1967.

48. Goldstein RS, Ramaharan V, Bowes G, et al: Effect of supplemental nocturnal oxygen on gas exchange in patients with severe obstructive lung disease. *N Engl J Med* 310:425–429, 1984.

49. Petty TL, Stanford RE, Neff TA: Continuous oxygen therapy in chronic airway obstruction: Observations on possible oxygen toxicity and survival. *Ann Intern Med* 75:361–369, 1971.

50. Jacques J, Cooney TP, Silvers GW, et al: The lungs and causes of death in the nocturnal oxygen therapy trial. *Chest* 86:230–233, 1986.

51. Summary of the Third Consensus Conference held in Washington DC, March 15–16, 1990: New problems in supply, reimbursement, and certification of medical necessity for long-term oxygen therapy. *Am Rev Respir Dis* 142:721–724, 1990.

52. Summary of the Fourth Oxygen Consensus Conference, Washington DC, October 15–16, 1993: Further recommendations for prescribing, reimbursement, technology development, and research in long-term oxygen therapy. *Am J Respir Crit Care Med* 150:875–877, 1994.

53. Hoffman LA: Novel strategies for delivering oxygen: Reservoir cannula, demand flow, and transtracheal oxygen administration. *Respir Care* 39:363–377, 1994.

54. Tiep BL, Lewis MI: Oxygen conservation and oxygen-conserving devices in chronic lung disease: A review. *Chest* 92:263–272, 1987.

55. Corsello DR, Make BJ: Which oxygen-conserving device is best for your patient? *J Respir Dis* 13:27–42, 1992.

56. Hanaford M, Kraft M, Make BJ: Long-term oxygen therapy in patients with chronic obstructive pulmonary disease. *Semin Respir Med* 14:496–516, 1993.

57. Heimlich HJ: Respiratory rehabilitation with transtracheal oxygen system. *Ann Otol Rhinol Laryngol* 91:643–647, 1982.

58. Couser JI, Make BJ: Transtracheal oxygen decreases inspired minute ventilation. *Am Rev Respir Dis* 139:627–631, 1989.

59. American Thoracic Society: Standards for the diagnosis and rate of patients with chronic obstructive pulmonary disease. *Am J Respir Crit Care Med* 152:S77–S120, 1995.

60. Smeets F: Travel for technology-dependent patients with respiratory disease. *Thorax* 49:77–81, 1994.

61. Cottrell JJ: Altitude exposures during aircraft flight. *Chest* 92:81–86, 1988.

62. Gong H, Tashkin DP, Lee EY, Simmons MS: Hypoxia-altitude simulation test. *Am Rev Respir Dis* 130:980–986, 1984.

63. Stoller JK: Travel for the technology-dependent individual. *Respir Care* 39:347–362, 1994.

64. Schwartz JS, Bencowitz HZ, Moser KM: Air travel hypoxemia with chronic obstructive pulmonary disease. *Ann Intern Med* 100:473–477, 1984.

Chapter 27

PREVENTION OF PULMONARY INFECTIONS

LISA L. DEVER

WALDEMAR G. JOHANSON, JR.

Respiratory tract infection is a common cause of morbidity and mortality in patients with underlying lung disease. Although patients with acute or chronic lung conditions and/or respiratory failure constitute a heterogeneous group, they share one characteristic that predisposes them to respiratory infection—disruption of host defenses, particularly those which protect the epithelial surface. This leads to abnormal microbial colonization patterns and, in some instances, invasive infection. Other host defenses are similarly impaired in most patients with chronic respiratory disease. Exposure of the respiratory tract to microbial agents and the mobilization of defenses to counteract those exposures result in a balance that is usually tipped in favor of host defenses (Fig. 27-1). However, a variety of factors can unbalance these relationships. Understanding these concepts is fundamental to further discussion of strategies aimed at preventing infection.

Colonization

Colonization can be defined as the persistence of microorganisms at a body site without evidence of a host response. Colonization is often normal but may be abnormal when organisms are found at sites that normally are sterile or when organisms that are not normal inhabitants are found in a region of the body. The mouth and oropharynx are heavily colonized by certain species of bacteria. The anterior nares and nasal passages are less heavily contaminated but are universally colonized with bacteria. Microorganisms commonly isolated from the upper respiratory tract include viridans streptococci, *Neisseria* spp., *Micrococcus* spp., staphylococci, *Hemophilus* spp., and obligate anaerobes. Potentially pathogenic bacteria, such as *Streptococcus pneumoniae* and group A streptococci, also may colonize the upper respiratory tract of normal hosts. There are a number of determinants of the microbial flora of an anatomic area, including the physicochemical environment, host defenses, and specific bacterial properties. However, selective adherence of only some bacterial species to regional epithelial cells is probably the most important factor.

Host Defenses

The normal lung is sterile distal to the central carina.[1] The mechanisms that maintain sterility of these regions are known collectively as *host defenses*. Host defense mechanisms include mechanical factors (aerodynamic filtration, mucociliary flow, cough), mucus, soluble secretory factors, immuno-globulins, complement, plasma proteins, and phagocytic cells.[2]

The structure of the respiratory system protects it against airborne particles. Inspired particles that exceed 10 to 15 μm in diameter are deposited by inertial impaction in the nose and pharynx due to sharp angulations at these sites.[3] Smaller particles may reach respiratory bronchioles and even alveoli. Aspiration of liquids is prevented by reflex closure of the glottis following stimulation of receptors in the larynx and trachea and by the vigorous coughing that such stimulation evokes. Particulates that are deposited in the airways are removed by the mucociliary system. Effective function of this complicated system requires that the layers of the mucus blanket be maintained at a constant depth so that ciliary action can propel it toward the mouth. Ciliary beat frequency, normally 10 to 12 beats per second, may be influenced by many factors, including oxygen tension, humidity, and a variety of drugs. Effective function also requires that ciliary action proceed in wavelike fashion from the periphery toward the oropharynx.

Bacteria that are deposited in peripheral airways or alveoli are usually phagocytosed and killed in situ.[4] Species with limited virulence for the respiratory tract are phagocytosed and killed swiftly by resident alveolar macrophages. In contrast, inoculation of the lung with highly virulent bacteria, such as *S. pneumoniae*, elicits a prompt migration of neutrophils into the airways and alveoli as well as mobilization of the resident alveolar macrophage population. Even though they multiply quickly in the lung, these organisms are killed even more rapidly, so they are cleared promptly under normal circumstances. However, if some factor unbalances this response, such as inhibition of neutrophil migration (e.g., diabetes, alveolar edema), or interferes with intracellular killing (e.g., hypoxia, acidosis), bacterial killing may occur more slowly than bacterial multiplication. Tissue inflammation results, histologically recognized as pneumonia. Bacteria presented to the lung in a liquid bolus, such as contaminated upper airway secretions, are cleared more slowly than bacteria presented as aerosols, presumably because of the greater local concentration of bacteria in the former and the possible protective effect of the fluid itself.[5]

Alterations in Disease

UNDERLYING LUNG DISEASE

Colonization patterns of the upper respiratory tract are frequently abnormal in patients with chronic respiratory disease, probably more related to chronic illness and debility than to any specific effect of individual diseases. For example, chronic illness and malnutrition are associated with the emergence of gram-negative bacilli in the oropharyngeal flora. This phenomenon is apparently due to increased affinity for gram-negative bacilli by receptors on the surface of the respiratory epithelium.[6,7] Inoculation of bacteria into the lung occurs by aspiration of oropharyngeal secretions. Huxley and colleagues[8] showed that aspiration of oropharyngeal secretions during sleep is common in healthy adults. A number of factors promote aspiration in patients with chronic respiratory disease. The presence of devices in the upper air passages, for example, endotracheal tubes, tracheostomies, and nasogastric tubes, impairs swallowing and increases the like-

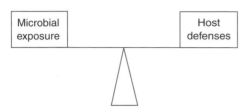

Microbial exposures are balanced
by host antibacterial defenses

FIGURE 27-1 Microbes are introduced into the respiratory tract in several ways, some of which are altered in patients with chronic respiratory diseases. Counteracting organisms introduced into the respiratory system are a variety of host defenses. The balance of these forces determines whether or not clinical infection will occur.

lihood of aspiration, as does marked shortness of breath and an ineffectual cough. Impaired consciousness is a major risk factor for aspiration. It is important to understand that the type of aspiration associated with most lung infections is *microaspiration,* referring to the inhalation of minute quantities of upper respiratory secretions. Since the bacterial concentration in such secretions is in the range of 10^8 per milliliter, aspiration of very small volumes produces a very substantial inoculum in the lung; that is, aspiration of 0.001 mL typically introduces 10,000 organisms. The lungs of patients with chronic respiratory disease are exposed to this level of bacterial challenge on a daily basis, often including highly pathogenic organisms due to the abnormal colonization patterns.

Lung defense mechanisms are impaired in multiple ways in patients with chronic obstructive pulmonary disease (COPD) and other chronic lung conditions. Abnormal viscosity or volume of secretions, impaired ciliary function, or even loss of ciliated epithelium leads to reduced mucociliary clearance and mucus plugging.[2] The effectiveness of cough is diminished by reduced airflow and respiratory muscle fatigue. These abnormalities lead to pooling of secretions in the airways, markedly impaired bacterial clearance, and increased risk of infection. Certain bacteria, notably, *Pseudomonas aeruginosa,* are most likely to cause infections in patients with retained secretions, probably because they adhere to receptors in respiratory mucus.[9,10]

Patients with chronic bronchitis may demonstrate a persistent bacterial flora in distal airways, a normally sterile region. The mechanisms underlying this observation have received little attention. It seems likely that adherence of the colonizing organisms to sites in distal airways is involved, but this is an unproven hypothesis. The most frequent bacterial pathogens isolated from these patients are *S. pneumoniae,* nontypable *H. influenzae, Moraxella (Branhamella) catarrhalis,* and to a lesser extent, *Chlamydia pneumoniae.*[11,12] Mucus hypersecretion in patients with COPD is closely associated with pulmonary infection and death.[13] Jenne and colleagues[14] demonstrated that the presence of untypable *H. influenzae* in the sputum of patients with COPD was accompanied by increased sputum volume and purulence; suppression by short courses of antibiotics was of transient benefit, whereas eradication by intensive therapy was followed by remissions lasting many months or even years. In experimental animals, persistence of bacteria in distal airways by incorporation into agarose beads results in extensive inflammation, mucus secretion, and airway injury.[15] These observations suggest that bacterial secretory products may be responsible for much of the inflammation and lung injury. Thus excessive mucus secretion and/or retention leads to bacterial colonization, which is, in turn, associated with further mucus hypersecretion and airway damage.

Colonization of the lower airways is common in patients with cystic fibrosis and may persist for extended periods of time. The airways of cystic fibrosis patients are most frequently colonized with *P. aeruginosa, Staphylococcus aureus,* and, to a lesser extent, by nontypable *H. influenzae. Burkholderia cepacia* has been found in up to 20 percent of cystic fibrosis patients and recently has been recognized as an important pathogen.[16–18] The pathophysiologic basis for selective colonization and subsequent infection with these microorganisms in cystic fibrosis is not well understood. However, it is likely that adherence properties and virulence factors play an important role.[18]

In all patients with a persistent bacterial flora in the distal airways, episodes of acute symptoms occur occasionally, typically about three to five times per year. These episodes, usually diagnosed as an exacerbation of chronic bronchitis, are characterized by increasing sputum volume, increased sputum viscosity, and worsening shortness of breath. High fever and marked leukocytosis are uncommon, but modest elevations in both are the rule. Viruses are a frequent, and probably underappreciated, cause of these acute infections in patients with chronic respiratory illness. Up to one-half of acute exacerbations of COPD are related to viral infections. Influenza viruses A and B, parainfluenza virus, respiratory syncytial virus (RSV), rhinovirus, coronavirus, and adenovirus may all be responsible for this syndrome. Increased rates of hospitalization for pneumonia, acute bronchitis, exacerbations of chronic respiratory illness, and congestive heart failure are observed during periods of influenza outbreaks.[19] This is particularly true for older adults and those who are chronically ill with cardiovascular and pulmonary diseases.[20] A recent prospective study of adult patients hospitalized with pneumonia found serologic evidence of influenza virus types A and B infection in 5.4 percent of patients and RSV infection in 4.4 percent.[21] Although usually regarded as an important cause of severe lower respiratory tract disease in infants and children, RSV has been associated with community-acquired pneumonia and exacerbations of chronic bronchitis in adults.[22] It also has been shown to cause severe lower respiratory tract disease in immunocompromised adult patients and institutionalized elderly people.[23–25] Viral infections are usually seasonal, occurring most frequently in winter, and can be acquired nosocomially. Such infections can lead to alterations in lung function such as increased airway resistance and reactivity following infection.[26–28] Patients with COPD may have more pronounced and prolonged deterioration of pulmonary function, although most eventually recover.[26]

Contaminated respiratory equipment or aerosols is another potential source of infection in patients with underlying pulmonary diseases. Outbreaks of respiratory infections have been associated with contamination of aerosol medications, mainstream nebulizers, and bedside spirometers.[29,30] Infec-

TABLE 27-1 Microbial Exposures in Normal Individuals and Individuals with Respiratory Disease

Colonization	Features	Examples
Normal	Restricted flora	"Normal flora"
	Restricted range	Oropharynx
Acute or chronic respiratory disease	Acquisition of new flora	Pathogens, i.e., *S. aureus, P. aeruginosa,* other GNBs
	Extended range colonized	Often includes distal airways

Inoculation of the Lungs	Mechanisms	Characteristics
Normal	Microaspiration	Daily, very small volumes
	Airborne organisms	Infrequent pathogens, predominantly viruses, e.g., influenza
Acute or chronic respiratory disease	Microaspiration increased	Presence of tubes, impaired upper airway reflexes, increased secretions
	Airborne organisms	Contaminated aerosols

tions due to respiratory therapy equipment contaminated by gram-negative bacilli such as *P. aeruginosa, Acinetobacter* spp., and *Enterobacter aerogenes* have been reported.[31–33] An outbreak of respiratory colonization and infection with *B. cepacia* in 42 mechanically ventilated patients was linked with contaminated multiple-dose vials of albuterol. In-use albuterol solutions were found to have unstable pH values and concentrations of benzalkonium chloride, a commonly used medical preservative, that allowed the growth of *B. cepacia*.[34] Potable water contaminated with *Legionella pneumophila* has been associated with an outbreak of Legionnaire's disease in 10 patients at a rehabilitation center.[35] Contaminated tap water used in jet nebulizers to humidify oxygen administered by face mask also has been implicated as the cause of legionellosis.[36]

Infections caused by contaminated respiratory therapy equipment are uncommon in hospitals in this country due to the widespread use of disposable equipment, but they pose a significant risk for patients using this equipment at home. The principal risk factor in these infections is the presence of water, especially if allowed to stand for many hours. Distilled water or even initially sterile water may be more of a hazard than tap water because the latter contains chlorine, whereas the former do not.

COLONIZATION OF TRACHEOSTOMY SITES

Chronic tracheostomy sites are always colonized with pathogenic bacteria. *S. aureus* is a common first colonizer, but gram-negative bacilli become prevalent after a week or two. Niederman and colleagues[37] observed 15 patients with long-term tracheostomies (mean of 25 months) who were admitted to the hospital. Three never had gram-negative bacilli isolated from the tracheostomy site, 7 were persistently colonized with *P. aeruginosa*, whereas 5 were transiently colonized with *P. aeruginosa* or another gram-negative bacilli. Gram-negative bacilli were isolated more frequently from the tracheostomy site than from the oropharynx. Repeated isolation of gram-negative bacilli was associated with the use of steroids, antibiotics, and mechanical ventilation. Three of the 7 patients (43 percent) persistently colonized developed pneumonia, versus only 1 of the 8 patients without persistent colonization. Aspirates from the level of the carina yielded an average of 6 isolates per specimen, mostly gram-

negative bacilli, in 16 patients with long-term tracheostomies. Organisms present in these aspirates were different from those obtained from the oropharynx, suggesting that the flora of a chronic tracheostomy are distinct from those of the oropharynx.

In addition to being colonized, a tracheostomy obviously alters host defenses in other ways as well. The mechanical protection provided by the angulated structure of the nose and upper airways is lost, as are the humidification and warming functions of the nose. Mucociliary transport is diminished to varying degrees depending on the preceding factors as well as on changes in the viscosity of tracheal mucus. For patients with continuing production of large volumes of mucus, especially if cough is ineffectual, suctioning through the tracheostomy is necessary, adding an additional risk of infection. As a practical matter, chronic tracheostomies should be regarded as a contaminated site for which the long-term aim is to minimize the occurrence of acute exacerbations of distal infection or invasive local infection, much like the management of an in-dwelling urinary catheter. Sterility is an unrealistic goal and cannot be accomplished by antibiotic therapy. Attempts to do so merely select an increasingly resistant bacterial population. The alterations in colonization and host defenses that predispose patients to infection are summarized in Tables 27-1 and 27-2.

TABLE 27-2 Antibacterial Defenses in Normal Individuals and in Chronic Respiratory Disease

Defense Mechanism	Impairment in Respiratory Disease
Mucociliary clearance	Decreased by excessive mucus secretion, epithelial cell injury, abnormally viscous mucus, effects of bacterial products
Cough	Decreased effectiveness due to airway obstruction, abnormal secretions, respiratory muscle weakness
Phagocytic cell function	Decreased airway recruitment and bacterial killing capacity
Humoral and cell-mediated immunity	Decreased by malnutrition and coexisting diseases

CLINICAL DISTINCTIONS BETWEEN COLONIZATION AND INFECTION

A common clinical problem in the care of patients with both acute and chronic lung disease is distinguishing colonization of the airways from infection. Recall that *colonization* is defined as the presence of bacteria *without* a host response. Thus the key clinical finding is the presence or absence of a host response. This distinction is often complicated by the occurrence of colonization on the background of an acute infection. Gram-negative bacilli appear in tracheobronchial secretions in at least 50 percent of patients who are intubated for ventilatory support.[38] Similarly, colonization of the respiratory tract by new pathogens, usually gram-negative bacilli, occurs in at least 20 percent of patients undergoing treatment for pneumococcal pneumonia or other specific infections. In these circumstances, the clinician must decide whether the appearance of new organisms represents a significant superinfection or merely colonization. Well-validated criteria for this decision making are not available. As a general rule, it is wise to remember the axiom that patients, not laboratory results, are being treated, and if the patient is doing well, the new culture findings should not be acted on. On the other hand, a rising white cell count, the presence of purulent secretions, or the appearance of redness and tissue inflammation spreading from a tracheostomy site would constitute strong evidence of a host response and therefore evidence of infection. Our approach is to limit our concern to patients who seem likely to have superinfections on clinical grounds and to investigate such patients by appropriate culture techniques if the causative organisms are unclear and if specific antimicrobial therapy is likely to make a significant difference in the patient's outcome.

Prevention of Infection

The aims underlying attempts to prevent bronchopulmonary infections in patients with chronic respiratory disease are to reduce the frequency and magnitude of inoculation of the lungs with infectious agents and at the same time to enhance the lungs' defense mechanisms. Accomplishing these aims requires a multipronged attack, as summarized in Table 27-3.

RESPIRATORY THERAPY

PULMONARY TOILET

Adequate removal of secretions is a critical factor in preventing infections. Bronchodilators are helpful in most patients with airway disease because, in addition to improving airflow, the adrenergic agonists also enhance mucociliary function.[39,40] Terbutaline is particularly effective in this regard.[40] Theophylline also stimulates ciliary motility and can improve mucociliary clearance.[41] Although ipratroprium does not directly increase mucociliary clearance, it is effective in reducing the volume of sputum without altering its viscosity.[42] Oral expectorants and other mucokinetic agents such as saturated iodide are of limited clinical usefulness.[39,43] Nebulized acetylcysteine, a potent mucolytic agent, can reduce the volume and viscosity of sputum and may be helpful in some patients.[39,43] Inhaled recombinant human DNase reduces the viscoelastic properties of sputum in patients with cystic fibrosis[44] and has been shown to be effective in reducing respiratory exacerbations and improving FEV_1.[45] Such therapy is extremely costly, however, limiting widespread use.[46] Further studies are needed to determine its effectiveness in patients with COPD or bronchiectasis from causes other than cystic fibrosis.

Postural drainage and chest percussion are time-honored techniques to assist patients in the evacuation of secretions. Countless studies have been performed, although very few have used suitable controls or precise endpoints. These techniques often have been shown to result in greater sputum volume than coughing alone, but presumably this would be only a transient difference. However, for patients with excessive secretions and an ineffectual cough, postural drainage with or without chest percussion can be very helpful. The optimal position is that which mobilizes the greatest volume of secretions, which is often manifested as that bodily position causing the greatest amount of coughing and patient discomfort. The duration of treatment should be determined by the tolerance of the patient.

BODY POSITION

For bedridden patients, body position is important for other purposes as well. Aspiration of gastric contents is a clear

TABLE 27-3 Strategies for the Prevention of Infection

Strategy	Techniques	Examples
Enhance systemic immunity	Immunization	Influenza and pneumococcal vaccines
	Improve nutritional status	Nutritional supplements and/or enteral feedings
	Immunomodulators[a]	*Cytokines (growth factors, interferon)*
	Immunotherapy	*Hyperimmune globulin*
Enhance mucociliary clearance	Removal of secretions and prevention of atelectasis	Postural drainage and percussion, mucolytics, bronchodilators
		Rotational therapy, subglottic secretion aspiration, recombinant DNase
Reduce microbial inoculation of the lungs	Decrease microaspiration	Body positioning, avoid upper airway instrumentation
	Avoid contaminated aerosols	Proper care of respiratory therapy devices
Alter colonization patterns	Eliminate colonizing pathogens in airways	Chronic oral antibiotic therapy, inhaled antibiotics
		Topical antibiotics (SDD)[b]
Early antimicrobial therapy	Inhibit or kill specific pathogens	Amantadine for influenza *Antibiotics for undefined upper respiratory infections*

[a] Italicized entries represent those of uncertain value.
[b] Selective digestive decontamination.

risk factor for pneumonia,[47] and minimizing aspiration is an important goal in patients who are at risk. In mechanically ventilated patients, Torres and coworkers[48] showed that the probability of aspiration increased with the length of time the patient was kept in the supine position. Placing patients in a semirecumbent position (45-degree angle) by elevating the head of the bed reduced aspiration of gastric contents. Although their study was not designed to determine the effects of body positioning on development of pneumonia, they suggest that elevating the head of the bed may be a simple and inexpensive approach to prevent respiratory tract infections.

When bedridden patients remain in one position for prolonged periods, dependent lung zones tend to develop atelectasis and retained secretions. Continuous lateral rotational therapy, or *kinetic therapy* as it is also called, involves continuous movement of bedridden patients by means of a specially designed rotating bed that turns at about eight rotations per hour along its longitudinal axis. This therapy is aimed at using gravity to prevent atelectasis and subsequent infection in patients with prolonged immobilization due to critical illnesses, stroke, spinal cord injury, mechanically assisted ventilation, head injury, or blunt chest trauma. Theoretical advantages include improved drainage of respiratory tract secretions, expansion of all lung regions, increased tidal volume, and reduction of pulmonary embolization. Although some studies have demonstrated the efficacy of such an approach in preventing infection, others have been less convincing.[49-52] Because of the expense of the beds and the inability of some patients to tolerate the confinement and continuous rotation of the bed, the use of such therapy is somewhat limited, particularly outside the hospital setting.

CARE OF RESPIRATORY THERAPY EQUIPMENT AND TRACHEOSTOMY STOMA CARE

It is reasonable to assume that the patient at home is at less risk for infection than when in the hospital or other health care facility. Proper training and adherence to decontamination techniques can minimize the risk of infection associated with respiratory therapy devices. Most airway procedures such as tracheostomy-tube cleaning, stomal cleaning, and suctioning can be carried out using "clean" rather than sterile techniques. This requires good handwashing and the use of clean, but not sterile, disposable gloves. Sterile suction catheters should be used only once and discarded. Sterile and draped conditions should be used for tracheostomy-tube changes in the home. Inner cannula cleansing of the tracheostomy tube can be performed as a clean technique using a solution of one part hydrogen peroxide to one part distilled water.[53] Distilled water is recommended as a suction catheter rinse and for use in all humidification devices. When possible, patients should use sterile water rather than distilled water for suction catheter rinses and when cleaning respiratory therapy equipment because of the possibility of contamination of the latter with organisms such as *P. aeruginosa* or *Legionella* spp.

Decontamination of all reusable respiratory therapy equipment such as ventilator circuitry, nebulizers, aerosol tubing, and peak flow meters should be performed twice weekly. The device should be disassembled and washed in a non-residue-forming detergent, rinsed with sterile or distilled water, and then soaked for 15 to 20 min in a white vinegar and distilled or sterile water solution (one part vinegar to

two parts water).[53] Nebulizers may be reused for a period of up to 2 weeks but should then be discarded. Quaternary ammonium compounds are more effective against gram-negative and gram-positive organisms than a vinegar solution and have been recommended as preferred disinfectants.[53] It cannot be overemphasized that all cleaned devices must be allowed to air dry thoroughly before reassembling for use. Moisture trapped in the devices can serve as a potential reservoir for organisms. All ventilator filters should be cleaned and changed at the frequency recommended by the manufacturer. Medications should be dispensed as single-dose vials to reduce the possibility of contamination of multidose vials.

In patients with cuffed tracheostomy tubes, oropharyngeal secretions accumulate above the cuff. Several techniques can be used to remove them. The easiest is to deflate the cuff and quickly suction via the tracheostomy; secretions that drop around the deflated cuff are thus removed. Obviously, removal by this approach may not be complete, but it is less traumatic for the patient. The alternative approach is to pass a suction catheter through the nose or mouth into the trachea above the cuff of the tracheostomy tube. This avoids intentionally contaminating the trachea with oropharyngeal secretions but is uncomfortable for the patient. A new style of endotracheal tube incorporates a separate suction channel ending above the cuff, allowing for the continuous aspiration of secretions collecting at that site. Use of this device reduced the incidence of nosocomial pneumonia compared with conventional endotracheal tubes.[54] Similar devices are not yet available on tracheostomy tubes but probably will be soon.

The tracheostomy stoma is a contaminated wound. In its early stages, daily cleaning with peroxide to remove crusted secretions is advisable. Neither topical nor systemic antibiotics are necessary unless evidence of soft-tissue infection develops. The tracheostomy tube should not be changed for the first week due to the possibility of dissecting the soft tissues of the neck during reinsertion. The track is well formed after a week, and this complication becomes rare. The stoma epithelializes with squamous epithelium over time, and the likelihood of local infection diminishes greatly. Gentle cleansing with saline-moistened gauze is all that is required for most patients.

ANTIBIOTIC THERAPY

PROPHYLACTIC ANTIBIOTICS

Antimicrobial therapy has been used in attempts to prevent colonization of the respiratory tract and prevent infection for over 40 years.[55] Prophylactic agents are successful in preventing colonization with specific organisms, such as penicillin preventing colonization and infection of the pharynx by group A streptococci. However, neither oral nor systemic drugs given prophylactically are efficacious in preventing colonization of the respiratory tract; they merely alter the colonizing flora. Antimicrobial agents delivered topically into the respiratory tract achieve very high concentrations in local secretions. Limitations on this type of use have included local tissue reactions, bronchospasm, and systemic absorption.

DECONTAMINATION OF THE DIGESTIVE TRACT

Selective digestive decontamination (SDD) is the ultimate prophylactic antibiotic regimen. This technique originally included application of topical antimicrobial agents (e.g., colistin, tobramycin, and amphotericin B) to the buccal mucosa and instilled into the stomach with the addition of a systemic antibiotic (cefotaxime).[56,57] Many differing antibiotic regimens have been studied since the original description. The rationale for this approach is that colonization precedes infection in critically ill patients and that high concentrations of antimicrobial agents at the mucosal surface will eliminate existing microorganisms and prevent the acquisition of new microorganisms. A number of studies have demonstrated that this technique is, in fact, effective in reducing respiratory infections in seriously ill patients.[56,58-60] However, despite the reductions of infection, mortality was not reduced in most of these studies. Meta-analysis has suggested that SDD is followed by a 10 percent reduction in mortality in intensive care unit patients, a magnitude of reduction that is difficult or impossible to demonstrate in a single study.[61] This benefit must be weighed against the real and potential harm caused by the administration of antibiotics in this fashion. Perhaps the greatest risk associated with attempts at manipulating the flora with topical antimicrobials is the selection for colonization and infection with antibiotic-resistant microorganisms. Increased rates of enterococcal and methicillin-resistant *S. aureus* colonization and infection have occurred in some intensive care units where SDD has been used.[56,58,62] SDD has never been widely advocated in the United States, although it is still used by its devotees in some intensive care units in Europe.

Antibiotic Prophylaxis in COPD
Many trials have examined the efficacy of prophylactic antibiotics in preventing or reducing the frequency of exacerbations of COPD, as reviewed by Murphy and Sethi.[12] Antibiotics studied have included tetracyclines, sulfonamides, trimethoprim-sulfamethoxazole, amoxicillin, penicillin, and erythromycin. Some studies have shown reductions in the frequency of exacerbations,[63-66] whereas others have not.[67-69] A recent meta-analysis of nine clinical trials found a small but statistically significant benefit associated with antibiotic therapy in patients with exacerbations of COPD.[70] Further, for studies in which pulmonary functions were monitored, treatment with antibiotics was associated with a significant improvement in peak flow, suggesting that such therapy might be particularly important for patients with markedly reduced lung function.[71] It appears that the patients most likely to experience a benefit were those with frequent exacerbations (four or more per year). In patients with bronchiectasis, chronic tetracycline therapy reduced the frequency and severity of lower respiratory illnesses; chronic penicillin therapy was no more efficacious than placebo.[72] Chronic therapy did not alter sputum purulence or volume but did decrease the isolation of *S. pneumoniae.*

Antibiotic Prophylaxis in Cystic Fibrosis
Prophylactic or "maintenance" antibiotics are frequently used in patients with cystic fibrosis in an attempt to reduce the frequency of exacerbations of pulmonary infections and prevent further deterioration in pulmonary function.[46] The oral antibiotics that have been used commonly include cephalosporins, macrolides, penicillins, trimethoprim-sulfamethoxazole, and quinolones. Recent studies,[46,73] however, have not confirmed that this practice is beneficial, at least not when

antistaphylococcal drugs are used. Others have suggested that there are sufficient clinical data to support this approach.[74] Intravenous antibiotics administered quarterly have been reported to slow the loss of pulmonary function and improve survival in cystic fibrosis patients[75] but subsequently resulted in an increased incidence of resistant organisms.[76] Further well-done clinical trials are needed to determine the role of antibiotic prophylaxis in the management of patients with cystic fibrosis and the selection of antibiotic-resistant organisms. Fluoroquinolone antibiotics should be used with particular caution because they are unique in providing an option for oral therapy of *Pseudomonas* infection.

INHALED ANTIBIOTICS
In 1954, Lepper and colleagues[55] introduced the concept of instilling aerosolized polymyxin B into the tracheobronchial tree in an attempt to prevent pneumonia in patients with poliomyelitis. Inhaled antibiotics have the theoretical advantage of delivering the antibiotic to the site of infection or colonization, as the case may be, and minimizing systemic effects of antibiotics. In 1973, Greenfield and coworkers[77] reported that aerosolized polymyxin was effective in reducing colonization of the upper respiratory tract with gram-negative bacilli in patients hospitalized in an intensive care unit at the Beth Israel Hospital in Boston. A later study in this same institution found that aerosolized polymyxin was effective in preventing *P. aeruginosa* pneumonia.[78] Investigators subsequently found that continuous administration of polymyxin B aerosol to all patients in the intensive care unit resulted in selection for polymyxin-resistant organisms.[79] During the 7-month study period, 11 patients acquired pneumonia, 10 due to polymyxin-resistant organisms. With publication of this study, the use of aerosolized antibiotics to prevent colonization or pneumonia in hospitalized patients was largely abandoned.

Aerosolized antibiotics are now used primarily to treat or prevent *Pseudomonas* colonization and infection in patients with cystic fibrosis, although conflicting data as to the efficacy of such therapies have been reported.[80-83] There is no evidence that inhaled antistaphylococcal antibiotics have an advantage over orally administered drugs. The efficacy of aerosolized antibiotics is influenced by a number of variables, including the type of nebulizer device used, the drug's physical properties and dosages used, the carrier, and patient characteristics.[84] A number of antibiotics including beta-lactams, polymyxins, colistin, and aminoglycosides have been used. A recent multicenter, double-blind, placebo-controlled trial found that short-term administration of aerosolized tobramycin was associated with improved pulmonary function and a decrease in the density of *P. aeruginosa* in sputum in patients with cystic fibrosis.[82] Neither ototoxicity nor nephrotoxicity occurred, and the frequency of isolation of tobramycin-resistant bacteria was not increased. A Danish investigation found that the combination of oral ciprofloxacin and aerosolized colistin for 3 weeks was more effective than no antipseudomonal therapy in preventing chronic colonization with *P. aeruginosa.*[81] Seven of 12 (58 percent) untreated patients became chronically colonized with *P. aeruginosa* (defined as the presence in monthly routine sputum specimens for 6 consecutive months and/or the development of precipitating serum antibodies against *P. aeruginosa*) versus 2 of 14 (14 percent) who received ciprofloxacin and colistin.

Other than in cystic fibrosis, inhaled antibiotics are infrequently used for several reasons. Inhaled colistin and polymyxin have been associated with bronchospasm and respiratory failure.[85] The routine use of inhaled antibiotics is expensive, and selection of antibiotic-resistant organisms represents a real problem. Nevertheless, inhaled antibiotics also may be useful in patients with bronchiectasis not associated with cystic fibrosis who are colonized with *P. aeruginosa* or other gram-negative bacilli and who have persistently purulent sputum. This clinical syndrome represents a chronic infection that is often not eradicated by systemic therapy alone. In selected patients, we prefer to use a combination of a systemic agent (or oral ciprofloxacin) plus inhaled polymyxin for an acute phase of treatment followed by chronic inhalation treatment for a period of months with the goal of long-term suppression of inflammation and sputum purulence.

IMMUNIZATION

PREVENTION OF INFLUENZA

There are two potential measures to prevent influenza infection: immunoprophylaxis with inactivated (killed) virus or chemoprophylaxis with an antiviral drug. Vaccination of patients at increased risk for infection before the influenza season is the single most important and cost-effective method for reducing the impact of influenza.[86] The efficacy and safety of the vaccine has been convincingly demonstrated repeatedly in both healthy adults and patients at increased risk for disease.[20,87–89] Overall efficacy rates have ranged from 30 to 85 percent. Differences in efficacy are due in part to patient groups studied, annual variations in the virulence of circulating viruses, and study methodologies used. Although many studies have been retrospective and observational, a randomized, double-blinded, placebo-controlled study of the efficacy of influenza vaccination in the elderly done in the Netherlands found approximately a twofold reduction in the risk of respiratory illness in vaccine recipients.[87] Furthermore, in a recent meta-analysis by Gross and coworkers[88] of 20 cohort studies, the pooled estimates of vaccine efficacy in elderly persons was 56 percent. Unfortunately, despite all the data available showing reductions in morbidity and mortality, hospitalizations, and medical care costs,[90,91] many patients at high risk for disease go unvaccinated each year.

Influenza vaccine typically contains antigens from three different virus subtypes (two type A and one type B) representing influenza strains circulating in the United States and around the world in the preceding year. Commercial preparations of vaccine are made from purified egg-grown viruses that are rendered noninfectious (inactivated). Vaccines can be whole virus, split virus (subvirion), or purified surface antigen. In adults, any of these preparations can be used safely with minimal systemic or febrile reactions. Inactivated influenza vaccine should not be given to persons who have severe allergies to eggs. Protective antibodies generally are detected 2 weeks or more after vaccination and may persist for years. Antibody response may vary among patient groups and individual patients. Annual immunization is recommended because of antigenic drift of influenza viruses and falling antibody titers with time. Vaccine usually becomes available in September and ideally should be administered prior to December. Target groups for vaccination include adults and children with chronic disorders of the cardiovascular or pulmonary systems, residents of nursing homes and chronic care facilities, individuals over the 65 years of age, and physicians, nurses, and other personnel having extensive contact with high-risk patients.[92] Providers of care to high-risk persons in the home setting as well as all household members, whether or not they provide care, also should be vaccinated.

Amantadine and rimantidine are antiviral drugs that have been shown to interfere with replication of influenza A viruses. Amantadine has been shown to reduce the signs and symptoms of influenza A infection by 50 percent[92,93] and reduce virus shedding. It is 75 to 90 percent effective when used as a prophylactic agent.[92,94,95] The drug is not effective against influenza B virus. The major side effects of the drug are insomnia, light-headedness, nervousness, drowsiness, and difficulty in concentration. Rimantidine appears to be better tolerated. For treatment of influenza A illness, amantadine should be given within 24 to 48 h of onset of illness at a daily dosage of 100 to 200 mg. Patients 65 years of age or older should take no more that 100 mg daily, and dosages should be decreased for children, patients with seizure disorders, and those with renal impairment. The drug should be continued for 48 h after resolution of symptoms. Although not a substitute for vaccination, amantidine may be useful for patients who cannot tolerate the vaccine or as an adjunct if an outbreak occurs before or less than 2 weeks after vaccination or is caused by strains of influenza A not closely related to those present in the vaccine. It also may be used to supplement protection offered by vaccination in patients who might be expected to have a poor antibody response.

PNEUMOCOCCAL VACCINE

The first commercially available 14-valent pneumococcal vaccine was licensed in the United States in 1978. In 1983, a reformulated 23-valent vaccine became available and has replaced the 14-valent vaccine. Serotypes contained in the vaccine cause more than 85 percent of invasive infection.[96] Pneumococcal vaccine is recommended for use in persons over the age of 2 years at increased risk of infection and in adults over the age of 65 years. Conflicting data have been reported regarding the efficacy of the vaccine and the duration of protection.[89] Some vaccine studies have failed to show efficacy in patients at moderate risk for infection, including those with COPD.[97,98] An indirect cohort analysis of a large number of patients done by the Centers for Disease Control and Prevention (CDC) found that the overall efficacy of the vaccine was 57 percent.[99] Efficacy for immunocompetent persons older than 65 years was 75 percent, and for patients with chronic pulmonary diseases, 65 percent. The vaccine was not effective for patients with alcoholism and cirrhosis, sickle cell disease, chronic renal failure, lymphoma, leukemia, or multiple myeloma.

There are a number of difficulties encountered in interpreting data regarding efficacy of the vaccine in patients with underlying pulmonary diseases, particularly patients with COPD. To begin with, there are limited data regarding the actual incidence of pneumococcal pneumonia in patients with COPD. Additionally, many pneumococcal infections in patients with COPD or other chronic pulmonary diseases are not associated with bacteremia and may not be microbiologically confirmed. Studies that have used systemic infection as a measure of vaccine efficacy might not adequately measure the effect of the vaccine in noninvasive disease.[12] Alternatively, pneumonia due to other etiologic agents may be misclassified as pneumococcal, underestimating the efficacy of the vaccine. Limited data are available on the ability of pneumococcal vaccination to decrease the carrier state. This may be of particular importance in patients with COPD, who are frequently colonized with *S. pneumoniae.*

Revaccination after 6 years is now recommended for patients with a high risk of fatal complications from pneumococcal infection, such as those who are asplenic, and in other groups in whom antibody titers decrease more rapidly.[100] Immunogenicity studies have not answered the question of whether revaccination should be given routinely in other patient groups. The recent vaccine study done by the CDC found that greater age and longer intervals since vaccination were not associated with lower protective efficacy. Given the lack of adverse effects from revaccination and the potential efficacy, some authorities have recommended that revaccination after 6 years be strongly considered in all patients 65 years of age and older.[101]

Despite recommendations for widespread use of pneumococcal vaccine in individuals at increased risk for infection, the vaccine is woefully underutilized. Shapiro and colleagues[102] reported that only 20 percent of control patients who had risk factors for pneumococcal disease had received the vaccine. With the global emergence of multi-drug-resistant pneumococci, the role of vaccination takes on even greater importance. Trials are currently being conducted to assess the efficacy of newer conjugate vaccines in preventing pneumococcal disease. Conjugating pneumococcal polysaccharide to protein carriers, such as has been done with *H. influenzae* type b vaccine, may increase the immunogenicity and, it is hoped, the efficacy.[103] There is compelling evidence to support the efficacy, safety, and cost-effectiveness of the vaccine and the recommendation that it be used routinely in all patients at risk for infection.

AREAS FOR FURTHER INVESTIGATION

Other potential, but as yet unproven, strategies to prevent infection include the use of so-called biologic response modifiers, or immunomodulators. These substances have the ability to modify host defense mechanisms and in so doing may provide protection against invading pathogens. A number of cytokines are being evaluated for the prevention and treatment of infection. Thus far the best-studied cytokines in humans include the colony-stimulating factors, granulocyte colony-stimulating factor (G-CSF) and granulocyte-macrophage colony-stimulating factor (GM-CSF), and interferon-γ. G-CSF and GM-CSF stimulate the production and function of myeloid cells and have been useful in hastening the resolution of neutropenia in oncology patients. G-CSF has been effective in improving survival in animal models of bacterial pneumonia[104,105] and is currently being studied as an adjunctive treatment strategy in humans with community-acquired pneumonia. Until further data are available, it is uncertain what role G-CSF and GM-CSF might have in the prevention of pulmonary infection in nonneutropenic patients. Interferon-γ activates macrophages and has been shown to be effective in the prevention and treatment of opportunistic infections in animals and humans when administered systemically and

locally to the lung.[2,106,107] Aerosol administration to normal humans results in activation of alveolar macrophages without activation of systemic mononuclear cells.[108] Clinical trials of systemic and aerosolized interferon-γ for the prevention and treatment of respiratory infection are in progress.[2]

Prevention of infection by administration of parenteral immunoglobulin has been attempted. As might be anticipated, such immunotherapy is relatively limited in scope, whereas the infecting bacteria have no such limitation. Cryz and coworkers[109,110] demonstrated that passive immunization with a hyperimmune globulin directed against prevalent serotypes of *Klebsiella* spp. and *P. aeruginosa* and against exotoxin A provided protection against infection in animal models of infection with these organisms. A recent multicenter study compared intravenous hyperimmune globulin derived from donors immunized with a 24-valent *Klebsiella* capsular polysaccharide plus an 8-valent *P. aeruginosa* O-polysaccharide–toxin, a conjugate vaccine, versus albumin in patients admitted to intensive care units.[111] Although the overall incidence of infections with these organisms in the treatment group was not reduced, there was a trend toward reduction of the incidence and severity of vaccine-specific *Klebsiella* infections. Active immunization with *Pseudomonas*-specific vaccines demonstrated enhanced intrapulmonary killing of *Pseudomonas* and prevention of bacteremia in an animal model of pulmonary infection.[112] Human data are lacking, and the tolerability and applicability of such a vaccine are limited.

Conclusion

Respiratory infections are common in patients undergoing rehabilitation for chronic lung disease. Prevention takes many forms generally aimed at augmenting host defenses that are impaired in the presence of chronic lung disease.

References

1. Laurenzi GA, Potter RT, Kass EH: Bacteriologic flora of the lower respiratory tract. *N Engl J Med* 265:1273, 1961.
2. Skerrett SJ: Host defenses against respiratory infection. *Med Clin North Am* 78:941, 1994.
3. Newhouse M, Sanchis J, Bienenstock J: Lung defense mechanisms. *N Engl J Med* 295:990–998, 1976.
4. Green GM, Jakab GJ, Low RB, et al: Defense mechanisms of the respiratory membrane. *Am Rev Respir Dis* 115:479, 1977.
5. Harris GD, Woods DE, Fine R, et al: The effect of intraalveolar fluid on lung bacterial clearance. *Lung* 158:91, 1980.
6. Johanson WG Jr, Higuchi JH, Chaudhuri TR, et al: Bacterial adherence to epithelial cells in bacillary colonization of the respiratory tract. *Am Rev Respir Dis* 121:55, 1980.
7. Johanson WG Jr, Woods DE, Chaudhuri T: Association of respiratory tract colonization with adherence of gram-negative bacilli to epithelial cells. *J Infect Dis* 139:667, 1979.
8. Huxley EJ, Viroslav J, Gray WR, et al: Pharyngeal aspiration in normal adults and patients with depressed consciousness. *Am J Med* 64:565, 1978.
9. Ramphal R, Pyle M: Evidence for mucins and sialic acid as receptors for *Pseudomonas aeruginosa* in the lower respiratory tract. *Infect Immun* 41:339, 1983.
10. Reddy MS: Human tracheobronchial mucin: Purification and binding to *Pseudomonas aeruginosa. Infect Immun* 60:1530, 1992.
11. Monso E, Ruiz J, Rosell A, et al: Bacterial infection in chronic obstructive pulmonary disease: A study of stable and exacer-

bated outpatients using protected specimen brush. *Am J Respir Crit Care Med* 152:1316, 1995.

12. Murphy TF, Sethi S: Bacterial infection in chronic obstructive pulmonary disease. *Am Rev Respir Dis* 146:1067, 1992.

13. Prescott E, Lange P, Vestbo J: Chronic mucus hypersecretion in COPD and death from pulmonary infection. *Eur Respir J* 8:1333, 1995.

14. Jenne JW, MacDonald M, Lapinski EM, et al: The course of chronic *Haemophilus* bronchitis treated with massive doses of penicillin and penicillin combined with streptomycin. *Am Rev Respir Dis* 101:907, 1970.

15. Cash HA, Woods DE, McCullough B, et al: A rat model of chronic respiratory infection with *Pseudomonas aeruginosa*. *Am Rev Respir Dis* 119:453, 1979.

16. Tablan OC, Martone WJ, Doershuk CF, et al: Colonization of the respiratory tract with *Pseudomonas cepacia* in cystic fibrosis: risk factors and outcomes. *Chest* 91:527, 1987.

17. Spencer RC: The emergence of epidemic, multiple-antibiotic-resistant *Stenotrophomonas (Xanthomonas) maltophilia* and *Burkholderia (Pseudomonas) cepacia*. *J Hosp Infect* 30(suppl):453, 1995.

18. Govan JRW, Deretic V: Microbial pathogenesis in cystic fibrosis: Mucoid *Pseudomonas aeruginosa* and *Burkholderia cepacia*. *Microbiol Rev* 60:539, 1996.

19. McBean AM, Babish JD, Warren JL: The impact and cost of influenza in the elderly. *Arch Intern Med* 153:2105, 1993.

20. Barker WH, Mullooly JP: Pneumonia and influenza deaths during epidemics. *Arch Intern Med* 142:85, 1982.

21. Dowell SF, Anderson LJ, Gary HE Jr, et al: Respiratory synctial virus is an important cause of community-acquired lower respiratory infection among hospitalized patients. *J Infect Dis* 174:456, 1996.

22. Morales F, Calder MA, Inglis JM, et al: A study of respiratory infections in the elderly to assess the role of respiratory syncytial virus. *J Infect* 7:236, 1983.

23. Sorvillo FJ, Huie SF, Strassburg MA, et al: An outbreak of respiratory syncytial virus pneumonia in a nursing home for the elderly. *J Infect* 9:252, 1984.

24. Garvie DG, Gray J: Outbreak of respiratory syncytial virus infection in the elderly. *Br J Med* 281:1253, 1980.

25. Englund JA, Sullivan CJ, Jordan MC, et al: Respiratory syncytial virus infection in immunocompromised adults. *Ann Intern Med* 109:203, 1988.

26. Hegele RG, Hayashi S, Hogg JC, et al: Mechanisms of airway narrowing and hyperresponsiveness in viral respiratory tract infections. *Am J Respir Crit Care Med* 151:1659, 1995.

27. Omenaas E, Bakke P, Eide GE, et al: Serum respiratory virus antibodies: Predictor of reduced one-second forced expiratory volume (FEV$_1$) in Norwegian adults. *Int J Epidemiol* 25:134, 1996.

28. Krzyzanowski M, Sherrill DL, Lebowitz MD: Longitudinal analysis of the effects of acute lower respiratory illnesses on pulmonary function in an adult population. *Am J Epidermiol* 131:412, 1990.

29. Cross AS, Roup B: Role of respiratory assistance devices in endemic nosocomial pneumonia. *Am J Med* 70:681, 1981.

30. Sanders CV Jr, Luby JP, Johanson WG Jr, et al: *Serratia marcescens* infections from inhalation therapy medications: Nosocomial outbreak. *Ann Intern Med* 73:15, 1970.

31. Atik M, Hanson B: Gram-negative pneumonitis: A new postoperative menace. *Chest* 74:635, 1970.

32. Reinarz JA, Pierce AK, Mays BB, et al: The potential role of inhalation therapy equipment in nosocomial pulmonary infection. *J Clin Invest* 44:831, 1965.

33. Hovig B: Lower respiratory tract infections associated with respiratory therapy and anesthesia equipment. *J Hosp Infect* 51:516, 1981.

34. Harstein AI, Rashad AL, Liebler JM, et al: Multiple intensive care unit outbreak of *Acinetobacter calcoaceticus* subspecies *anitratus* respiratory infection and colonization associated with contaminated, reusable ventilator circuits and resuscitation bags. *Am J Med* 85:624, 1988.

35. Nechwatal R, Ehret W, Klatte OJ, et al: Nosocomial outbreak of legionellosis in a rehabilitation center: Demonstration of potable water as a source. *Infection* 21:235, 1993.

36. Arnow PM, Chou T, Weil D, et al: Nosocomial Legionnaires' disease caused by aerosolized tap water from respiratory devices. *J Infect Dis* 146:460, 1982.

37. Niederman MS, Ferranti RD, Zeigler A, et al: Respiratory infection complicating long-term tracheostomy. *Chest* 85:39, 1984.

38. Johanson WG Jr, Pierce AK, Sanford JP, et al: Nosocomial respiratory infections with gram-negative bacilli. *Ann Intern Med* 77:701, 1972.

39. Snider GL, Faling LJ, Rennard SI: Chronic bronchitis and emphysema, in Murray JF, Nadal JA (eds): *Respiratory Medicine*, 2d ed. Philadelphia, Saunders, 1994; p 1331.

40. Santa Cruz R, Landa J, Hirsch J, et al: Tracheal mucous velocity in normal man and patients with obstructive lung disease: Effects of terbutaline. *Am Rev Respir Dis* 109:458, 1974.

41. Ziment I: Theophylline and mucociliary clearance. *Chest* 92:38S, 1987.

42. Ghafouri MA, Patil KD, Kass I: Sputum changes associated with the use of ipratropium bromide. *Chest* 86:387, 1984.

43. Ziment I: Pharmacologic therapy of obstructive airway disease. *Clin Chest Med* 11:461, 1990.

44. Shak S, Capon DJ, Hellmiss R, et al: Recombinant human DNase I reduces the viscosity of cystic fibrosis sputum. *Proc Natl Acad Sci USA* 87:9188, 1990.

45. Fuchs HJ, Borowitz DS, Christiansen DH, et al: Effect of aerosolized recombinant human DNase on exacerbations of respiratory symptoms and pulmonary function in patients with cystic fibrosis. *N Engl J Med* 331:637, 1994.

46. Ramsey BW: Management of pulmonary disease in patients with cystic fibrosis. *N Engl J Med* 335:179, 1996.

47. Torres A, Aznar R, Gatell JM, et al: Incidence, risk, and prognosis factors of nosocomial pneumonia in mechanically ventilated patients. *Am Rev Respir Dis* 142:523, 1990.

48. Torres A, Serra-Batlles J, Ros E, et al: Pulmonary aspiration of gastric contents in patients receiving mechanical ventilation: The effect of body position. *Ann Intern Med* 116:540, 1992.

49. Kelley RE, Vibulsresth S, Bell L, et al: Evaluation of kinetic therapy in the prevention of complications of prolonged bed rest secondary to stroke. *Stroke* 18:638, 1987.

50. Gentilello L, Thompson DA, Tonnesen AS, et al: Effect of a rotating bed on the incidence of pulmonary complications in critically ill patients. *Crit Care Med* 16:783, 1988.

51. Fink MP, Helsmoortel CM, Stein KL, et al: The efficacy of an oscillating bed in the prevention of lower respiratory tract infection in critically ill victims of blunt trauma: A prospective study. *Chest* 97:132, 1990.

52. Summer WR, Curry P, Haponik EF, et al: Continuous mechanical turning of intensive care unit patients shortens length of stay in some diagnostic-related groups. *J Crit Care* 4:45, 1989.

53. Lucas J: Home ventilator care, in O'Ryan JA, Burns DG (eds): *Pulmonary Rehabilitation: From Hospital to Home*. Chicago, Year Book Medical Publishers, 1984; p 211

54. Valles J, Artigas A, Rello J, et al: Continuous aspiration of subglottic secretions in preventing ventilator-associated pneumonia. *Ann Intern Med* 122:179, 1995.

55. Lepper MH, Kofman S, Blatt N, et al: Effect of eight antibiotics used singly and in combination on the tracheal flora following tracheostomy. *Antibiot Chemother* 4:829, 1954.

56. Dever LL, Johanson WG Jr: An update on selective decontamination of the digestive tract. *Curr Opin Infect Dis* 6:744, 1993.

57. Cockerill FR: Indications for selective decontamination of the digestive tract. *Semin Respir Infect* 8:300, 1993.

58. Kollef MH: The role of selective digestive tract decontamination

on mortality and respiratory tract infections: A meta-analysis. *Chest* 105:1101, 1994.

59. Gastinne H, Wolff M, Delatour F, et al: A controlled trial in intensive care units of selective decontamination of the digestive tract with nonabsorbable antibiotics. *N Engl J Med* 326:594, 1992.

60. Hammond JMJ, Potgieter PD, Saunders GL, et al: Double-blind study of study of selective decontamination of the digestive tract in intensive care. *Lancet* 340:5, 1992.

61. SDD Trialists' Collaboration: Meta-analysis of randomized control trials on the effect of selective decontamination of the digestive tract. *Br Med J* 307:525, 1993.

62. Daschner F: Emergence of resistance during selective digestive decontamination. *J Hosp Infect* 22:172, 1992.

63. Tager I, Speizer FE: Role of infection in chronic bronchitis. *N Engl J Med* 292:563, 1975.

64. The Working Party on Trials of Chemotherapy in Early Bronchitis of the Medical Research Council: Value of chemoprophylaxis and chemotherapy in early bronchitis. *Br Med J* 1:317, 1966.

65. Pridie RB, Datta N, Massey DG, et al: A trial of continuous winter chemotherapy in chronic bronchitis. *Lancet* 2:723, 1960.

66. Francis RS, Spicer CC: Chemotherapy in chronic bronchitis: Influence of daily penicillin and tetracycline on exacerbations and their cost. *Br Med J* 1:297, 1960.

67. Davis AL, Grobow EJ, Tompsett R, et al: Bacterial infection and some effects of chemoprophylaxis in chronic pulmonary emphysema: I. Chemoprophylaxis with intermittent tetracycline. *Am J Med* 31:365, 1961.

68. Buchanan J, Buchanan WW, Melrose AG, et al: Long-term prophylactic administration of tetracycline to chronic bronchitics. *Lancet* 2:719, 1958.

69. Pines A: Controlled trials of a sulphonamide given weekly to prevent exacerbations of chronic bronchitis. *Br Med J* 3:202, 1967.

70. Saint S, Bent S, Vittinghoff E, et al: Antibiotics in chronic obstructive pulmonary disease exacerbations: A meta-analysis. *JAMA* 273:957, 1995.

71. Anthonisen NR, Manfreda J, Warren CPW, et al: Antibiotic therapy in exacerbations of chronic obstructive pulmonary disease. *Ann Intern Med* 106:196, 1987.

72. Cherniack NS, Vosti KL, Dowling HF, et al: Long-term treatment of bronchiectasis and chronic bronchitis: A controlled study of the effects of tetracycline, penicillin, and an oleandomycin-penicillin mixture. *Arch Intern Med* 103:345, 1959.

73. Beardsmore CS, Thompson JR, Williams A, et al: Pulmonary function in infants with cystic fibrosis: The effect of antibiotic treatment. *Arch Dis Child* 71:133, 1994.

74. Hodson ME, Smith AL, Ramsey B: Maintenance treatment with antibiotics in cystic fibrosis patients. Sense or nonsense? Aerosol administration of antibiotics. *Respiration* 62(suppl 1):19, 1995.

75. Szaff M, Hoiby N, Flensborg EW: Frequent antibiotic therapy improves survival of cystic fibrosis patients with chronic *Pseudomonas aeruginosa* infection. *Acta Paediatr Scand* 72:651, 1983.

76. Jensen T, Pedersen SS, Hoiby N, et al: Use of antibiotics in cystic fibrosis: The Danish approach. *Antibiot Chemother* 42:237, 1989.

77. Greenfield S, Teres D, Bushnell LS, et al: Prevention of gram-negative bacillary pneumonia using aerosol polymyxin B as prophylaxis: I. Effect on the colonization pattern of the upper respiratory tract of seriously ill patients. *J Clin Invest* 52:2935, 1973.

78. Klick JM, Du Moulin GC, Hedley-White J, et al: Prevention of gram-negative bacillary pneumonia using polymyxin aerosol as prophylaxis: Effect on the incidence of pneumonia in seriously ill patients. *J Clin Invest* 55:514, 1975.

79. Feeley TW, Du Moulin GC, Hedley-Whyte J, et al: Aerosol polymyxin B and pneumonia in seriously ill patients. *N Engl J Med* 293:471, 1975.

80. MacLusky I, Levison H, Gold R, et al: Inhaled antibiotics in cystic fibrosis: Is there a therapeutic effect? *J Pediatr* 108:861, 1986.

81. Valeruis NH, Koch C, Hoiby N: Prevention of chronic *Pseudomonas aeruginosa* colonisation in cystic fibrosis by early treatment. *Lancet* 338:725, 1991.

82. Ramsey BW, Dorkin HL, Eisenberg JD, et al: Efficacy of aerosolized tobramycin in patients with cystic fibrosis. *N Engl J Med* 328:1740, 1993.

83. Touw DJ, Brimicombe RW, Hodson ME, et al: Inhalation of antibiotics in cystic fibrosis. *Eur Respir J* 8:1594, 1995.

84. Smith AL, Ramsey B: Aerosol administration of antibiotics. *Respiration* 62(suppl 1):19, 1995.

85. Wilson FE: Acute respiratory failure secondary to polymyxin-B inhalation. *Chest* 79:237, 1981.

86. Centers for Disease Control and Prevention: Prevention and control of influenza: Recommendations of the Immunization Practices Advisory Committee. *Ann Intern Med* 107:521, 1987.

87. Govaert TME, Thijs CTMCN, Masurel N, et al: The efficacy of influenza vaccination in elderly individuals: A randomized double-blind placebo-controlled trial. *JAMA* 272:1661, 1994.

88. Gross PA, Hermogenes AW, Sacks HS, et al: The efficacy of influenza vaccine in elderly persons: A meta-analysis and review of the literature. *Ann Intern Med* 123:518, 1995.

89. Fiebach N, Beckett W: Prevention of respiratory infections in adults: Influenza and pneumococcal vaccines. *Arch Intern Med* 154:2545, 1994.

90. Fedson DS: Clinical practice and public policy for influenza and pneumococcal vaccination of the elderly. *Clin Geriatr Med* 8:183, 1992.

91. Nichols KL, Margolis KL, Wuorenma J, et al: The efficacy and cost-effectiveness of vaccination against influenza among elderly persons living in the community. *N Engl J Med* 331:778, 1994.

92. Centers for Disease Control and Prevention: Prevention and control of influenza: Recommendations of the Advisory Committee on Immunization Practices (ACIP). *MMWR* 44(RR-3):1, 1995.

93. Van Voris LP, Betts RF, Hayden FG, et al: Successful treatment of naturally occurring influenza A/USSR/77 H1N1. *JAMA* 245:1128, 1981.

94. Atkinson WL, Arden NH, Patriarca PA, et al: Amantadine prophylaxis during an institutional outbreak of type A (H1N1) influenza. *Arch Intern Med* 146:1751, 1986.

95. Monto AS, Gunn RA, Bandyk MG, et al: Prevention of Russian influenza by amantadine. *JAMA* 241:1001, 1979.

96. Jorgensen JH, Howell AW, Maher LA, et al: Serotypes of respiratory isolates of *Streptococcus pneumoniae* compared with the capsular types included in the current pneumococcal vaccine. *J Infect Dis* 163:664, 1991.

97. Fine MJ, Smith MA, Carson CA, et al: Efficacy of pneumococcal vaccination in adults: A meta-analysis of randomized controlled trials. *Arch Intern Med* 154:2666, 1994.

98. Simberkoff MS, Cross AP, Al-lbrahim M, et al: Efficacy of pneumococcal vaccine in high-risk patients: Results of a Veterans Administration Cooperative Study. *N Engl J Med* 315:1318, 1986.

99. Butler JC, Breiman RF, Campbell JF, et al: Pneumococcal polysaccharide vaccine efficacy: An evaluation of current recommendations. *JAMA* 270:1826, 1993.

100. Centers for Disease Control and Prevention: Pneumococcal polysaccharide vaccine. *MMWR* 38:64, 1989.

101. ACP Task Force on Adult Immunization and Infectious Diseases Society of America: *Guide for Adult Immunization*. Philadelphia, American College of Physicians, 1990.

102. Shapiro ED, Berg AT, Austrian R, et al: The protective efficacy of polyvalent pneumococcal polysaccharide vaccine. *N Engl J Med* 325:1453, 1991.

103. Klein DL: Pneumococcal conjugate vaccines: Review and update. *Microb Drug Res* 1:49, 1995.

104. Hebert JC, O'Reilly M, Garnelli RL: Protective effect of recombinant granulocyte colony-stimulating factor against pneumococcal infections in splenectomized mice. *Arch Surg* 125:1075, 1990.

105. Nelson S, Summer W, Bagby G, et al: Granulocyte colony-stimulating factor enhances pulmonary host defenses in normal and ethanol-treated rats. *J Infect Dis* 164:901, 1991.

106. Murray HW: Cytokines as antimicrobial therapy for the T-cell-defecient patient: Prospects for treatment of nonviral opportunistic infections. *Clin Infect Dis* 17(suppl):S407, 1993.

107. Skerrett SJ, Martin TR: Intratracheal interferon-gamma augments pulmonary defenses in experimental legionellosis. *Am J Respir Crit Care Med* 149:50, 1994.

108. Jaffe HA, Buhl R, Mastrangeli A, et al: Organ specific cytokine therapy: Local activation of mononuclear phagocytes by delivery of an aerosol or recombinant interferon-gamman to the human lung. *J Clin Invest* 88:297, 1991.

109. Cryz SJJ, Mortimer P, Cross AS, et al: Safety and immunogenicity of a polyvalent *Klebsiella* capsular polysaccharide vaccine in humans. *Vaccine* 4:15, 1986.

110. Cryz SJJ, Furer E, Cross AS, et al: Safety and immunogenicity of a *Pseudomonas aeruginosa* O-polysaccharide–toxin A conjuate vaccine in humans. *J Clin Invest* 80:51, 1987.

111. Donata ST, Peduzzi P, Cross AS, et al: Immunoprophylaxis against *Klebsiella* and *Pseudomonas aeruginosa* infections. *J Infect Dis* 174:537, 1996.

112. Pennington JE, Hickey WF, Blackwood LL, et al: Active immunization with lipopolysaccharide *Pseudomonas* antigen for chronic bronchopneumonia in guinea pigs. *J Clin Invest* 68:1140, 1981.

Chapter 28

SMOKING CESSATION
NORMAN HYMOWITZ

Background

In the past, the most popular forms of tobacco use in the United States were chewing and dipping snuff. Cigarette smoking grew in popularity in the late 1880s. James Buchanan Duke brought Eastern European Jews to the United States in 1867 to roll cigarettes, and he used advertising to market his products.[1] Cigarettes were first mass-produced in Durham, North Carolina, in 1884, when Washington Duke used a newly invented cigarette machine to produce 120,000 cigarettes per day, thus introducing the era of inexpensive, abundant tobacco products for smoking and setting the stage for lung cancer, chronic-obstructive pulmonary disease, and heart disease in the twentieth century.[1]

In 1900, the total consumption of cigarettes in the United States was approximately 2.5 billion.[2] Cigarette consumption increased to a peak of 640 billion in 1981. By 1935, 52.5 percent of adult American males smoked cigarettes.[2] In 1947, more than 70 percent of American males of peak smoking age (approximately 20 to 35 years) smoked cigarettes.[3]

Since the 1960s, the adult smoking rate in the United States has declined to less than 30 percent. The overall smoking rate in the United States in 1993 was 25.0 percent, 27.7 percent for men and 22.5 percent for women.[4] The rate for adults with fewer than 12 years of education was 29.7 percent; for those with more than 12 years of education, the rate was 19 percent. Of the major ethnic and racial groups, the highest rates of smoking were for Native Americans and Alaskans (38.7 percent), followed by African Americans (26.0 percent), whites (25.4 percent), Hispanics (20.4 percent), and Asians and Pacific Islanders (18.2 percent).[4]

The start of the "antismoking movement" in the United States occurred in 1964, with the publication of the landmark Surgeon General's Advisory Committee Report, *Smoking and Health*.[5] More recently, cigarette smoking was cited by former U.S. Surgeon General C. Everett Koop as the chief avoidable cause of death and morbidity in American society and the number one public health problem of this time.[2] According to the World Health Organization,[6] approximately 3 million people die worldwide each year as a result of smoking, more than 400,000 per year in the United States alone. In the United States, tobacco is responsible for 179,820 deaths from cardiovascular diseases, 119,920 from lung cancer, 31,402 from other cancers, and 84,475 from respiratory diseases.[7]

The 1964 Surgeon General's report recognized the habitual nature of tobacco use, but it stopped short of recognizing tobacco use as an addiction.[5] The 1988 Surgeon General's report was entitled *The Health Consequences of Smoking: Nicotine Addiction*.[8] Major conclusions from this report were (1) cigarettes and other forms of tobacco are addicting; (2) nicotine is the drug in tobacco that causes addiction; and (3) the pharmacologic and behavioral processes that determine tobacco addiction are similar to those that determine addiction to drugs such as heroin and cocaine.

Most adult smokers are aware of the dangers of cigarette smoking, and a majority would like to quit.[2] Approximately 2 percent per year succeed, most making a number of quit attempts before finally succeeding.[2] Nearly half of all living adults in the United States who ever smoked have quit,[2] and most quit smoking "on their own."[9]

Analysis of data from the 1986 *Adult Use of Tobacco Survey* showed that about 90 percent of successful quitters and 80 percent of unsuccessful quitters used individual methods of smoking cessation rather than organized programs.[10] Most used a "cold turkey" approach. Women, middle-aged persons, more educated persons, persons who had made the most quit smoking attempts, and heavier smokers were most likely to use a cessation program.[10] Among smokers who had attempted to quit on their own within the previous 10 years, 47.5 percent were successful. Only 23.6 percent of persons who used cessation programs were successful. Fiore and coworkers[10] concluded that formal cessation programs serve a small, but important, population of smokers that includes heavier smokers (i.e., 25 or more cigarettes per day), the smokers who are most at risk of tobacco-related morbidity and mortality.

Approaches to Smoking Cessation

The recognition that most smokers stop smoking on their own, the modest success often achieved with labor-intensive group and individual programs, and the need to accomodate millions of smokers nationwide has led to a shift during the past decade from clinical to public health smoking cessation strategies. Whereas labor-intensive group and individual counseling programs were quite popular in the 1960s and 1970s, the emphasis in the 1990s is on cost-effective self-help cessation aids, pharmacologic therapy, and cessation programs which can be readily placed in environments that reach large numbers of smokers. Examples of public-health-oriented approaches to smoking cessation include bibliotherapy, mass media campaigns, over-the-counter medications and aids, group programs led by nonprofessional therapists, "quit and win" contests, worksite programs and incentives for quitting smoking, computer-assisted instruction, and brief interventions for smoking cessation delivered by physicians, dentists, nurses, and other health professionals. Although clinical approaches, such as intensive group and individual counseling, generate relatively high quit rates in a small number of people, public health approaches achieve more modest quit rates in much larger numbers of smokers.[11,12]

Early group and individual programs for smoking cessation were carried out by skilled clinicians working intensively with hard core smokers. Attention to design issues, such as control groups and completeness of follow-up, often was lacking or largely inadequate, and little effort was made to verify verbal reports of smoking status. Because of these shortcomings, many of the initial reports of success in helping smokers stop smoking must be taken with a "grain of salt." Still, it is valuable to review these early attempts. The early approaches to cessation were creative and imaginative and often form the basis for what is done today.

Recent studies of smoking cessation are more likely to conform to acceptable scientific standards. Reasons for improvement in research design and methodology are many and varied, including authoritative reviews of the early literature which pointed out methodologic shortcomings and called for more careful experimentation.[13-15] Cigarette smoking, a quantifiable behavior, was seized on by students of conditioning and learning, behavior modification, and cognitive-behavior therapy for analog and other studies which took place in university laboratories, used students as subjects, and contributed to a good many doctoral dissertations.[16] Behavioral medicine became an established discipline within clinical and experimental psychology in the late 1970s, and the importance of well designed studies of smoking behavior grew as the behavioral, public health, and medical professions became more aware of the health effects of smoking and the need to help people quit.

Today, research on tobacco prevention and control is funded by the federal government, states, foundations, and voluntary agencies. New technologies permit biochemical verification of smoking status. The appreciation of smoking as a risk factor for disease and the new emphasis on pharmacologic therapies, alone or in combination with behavioral interventions, has brought insight and sophistication from the fields of pharmacology, public health, and epidemiology to the smoking cessation arena, contributing to enhanced quality and quantity of research.

Despite much progress, smoking modification still requires art as well as science, and the success of therapeutic endeavors often depends on such nonspecific factors as the therapist's warmth, empathy, and concern. Although it is important, as a country, to treat smoking as a public health problem, to mobilize legislative and political support, and to implement cost-effective interventions to stem the tide of tobacco-related disease, the question of how to help *this* patient stop smoking is as important today as it was in the 1960s. Depressed and emotionally ill patients who have an extremely difficult time stopping smoking, patients with chronic obstructive pulmonary disease who persist in smoking, and highly addicted smokers from every racial and ethnic group and walk of life merit special attention and assistance. Once smokers quit, as much energy and care must go into helping them remain abstinent as went into the initial cessation. The kinds of interventions which can be offered are limited only by imagination and resources. By taking note of what worked in the past, by staying abreast of advancements in the field, and by taking advantage of a society which is much more hospitable to people trying to quit smoking than it was in the 1960s, today's practitioners have opportunities for success which were unknown to interventionists a decade or two ago.

This chapter provides a comprehensive review of the smoking cessation literature beginning with the earliest studies. A historical perspective is maintained to illustrate major developments in the field as well as to underscore persistent problems and issues which remain. Considerable space is devoted to newer public-health-oriented approaches as well as to pharmacologic therapies. The success of pulmonary rehabilitation depends on a patient who is freed from smoking. The goal of this chapter is to enable practitioners of rehabilitative medicine to implement innovative self-help and minimal intervention programs which reach out to large numbers of their constituents.

Group Therapy

EARLY GROUP THERAPY PROGRAMS

The APA Steering Committee on Practice Guidelines[17] noted that the goals of educational and supportive groups are to teach patients the harms of smoking and benefits of cessation and to provide group reinforcement for not smoking. While the guidelines questioned the efficacy of such procedures without specific behavior change technology, the steering committee concluded that many smokers who wish to quit derive important benefits from group support. Thus, educative and supportive groups are considered a promising therapy.[17]

Lawton[18] published one of the first reports on group therapy for smoking cessation. In developing the group approach, the following assumptions about smoking were made:

1. Psychological factors are an important component of the smoking habit, though the relative strengths of the psychological and physiologic components may vary from individual to individual.
2. Although the deepest roots of the psychological component in smoking may be unconscious and closely related to major needs of the individual, it is also a consciously indulged habit. Therefore, it can be modified through the mediation of cognitive processes, and substitutions may be made in a more or less conscious fashion.
3. The action of the individual cognitive structure may be greatly enhanced by a group effort to achieve the same goal.
4. Since smoking is a habit, one of the means necessary to deal with it is to interrupt the pattern long enough to break the stimulus-response expectation. Therefore, major efforts should be devoted to the early stages of habit breaking.

Recruitment of volunteers for Lawton's group was accomplished via announcements in the newspaper, over local radio stations, and in the newsletters of community organizations.[18] The author spoke personally at nine meetings of community groups seeking volunteers who were confirmed smokers and had a sincere desire to quit. It took several months to recruit 19 members. Lawton had originally hoped to recruit 24 members.

On an *a priori* basis, it was decided to meet twice per week during the first 3 weeks, in 1½-h sessions. Weekly sessions were arranged for the last 3 weeks. The rationale for this schedule of sessions was that efforts to stop would come early and require extra support at that time.[18]

The group members were hard core smokers. All of them smoked more than a pack of cigarettes per day, and one smoked three packs per day. Only three members had quit in the past for an extended period of time.

At the first meeting, the group leader briefly described to the group his convictions about the psychological component of smoking and the importance of the first week of abstinence in breaking the habit. He also conveyed his general orientation toward the exploration of both feeling and content in group discussion and his wish to limit discussion to smoking specifically.[18]

Four members took the initial meeting of the group as the signal to stop smoking immediately, and they spoke at length about their anticipation of discomfort. The leader encouraged expression of reservations about quitting and lack of conviction about ability to stop. During week 2, seven members who were still smoking made a joint resolution to quit smoking. From about the sixth session on, the group concentrated on attempting to "hold its gains" and in giving support to members who continued to have trouble quitting.

By the final session, 12 of the active 17 members (two members dropped out) reported that they were not smoking, yielding an end-of-treatment reported quit rate of 71 percent (12 of 17) or, more conservatively, 63 percent (12 of 19). Three months later, four members relapsed, yielding a conservative reported quit rate of 42 percent. Eighteen months later, there were only three reported abstainers (16 percent quit rate), causing Lawton to conclude that the group should be open-ended to allow for periodic support for nonsmoking maintenance.[18]

In 1959, McFarland reported a 10-day program for individuals who wished to stop smoking. The program had proved effective with small groups of 15 to 30 individuals in New York City and with individual patients at the Battle Creek Health Center, Battle Creek, Michigan.[19] McFarland then joined forces with a clergyman, Elman J. Falkenberg. The program was modified so that it could be carried out in 5 days (the 5-day plan) and accommodate groups of 300 or more smokers. Since the Seventh-Day Adventist Church initiated the 5-day plan in 1960, more than 14 million smokers have entered the program in over 150 countries.[20]

The program consisted of five evenings of 1½- to 2-h sessions, which were held beginning on Sunday and running through and including Thursday evening. A follow-up meeting was arranged for the first of the next week to determine how well the new nonsmokers were doing. The sessions were a combination of lectures, films, and demonstrations, with question and answer periods each evening.

The program sought to provide the "tobacco addict" with all-out support in every facet of life, physically, mentally, morally, and socially. For this reason, the program included a good health and physical fitness program, motives other than fear to stop smoking, material on how to cope with social pressures, and information on how to obtain strength through a firm conviction of a Power greater than that of an individual person. Key aspects of the program are described briefly in the following paragraphs.

Physical aspects: The program emphasized sudden cessation and complete withdrawal of all tobacco. Key components of this aspect of the program included (1) "forcing fluids" and hydrotherapy (baths and showers); (2) bland and low-cholesterol diet with no alcohol- or caffeine-containing beverages, and the use of fruits for dessert; (3) a physical fitness program with outdoor walking and breathing deeply after a meal, and slow, rhythmic deep breathing when an overpowering urge to smoke strikes, along with a glass of water; (4) avoidance of smoking companions and undue stress; (5) a daily personal control booklet, outlining what was to be done practically every waking moment; and (6) referral to a family physician if untoward physical symptoms developed (i.e., gastric irritation caused by sensitivity to citrus fruits or extreme nervousness).

Psychological aspects: Psychological features of the program included (1) showing a film demonstrating the surgical removal of a cancerous lung the first evening; (2) dividing each evening between a discussion of psychological and physiologic problems; (3) freely using principles of group therapy and group dynamics; and (4) discussing strategies to cope with the "irresistible urge."

Spiritual aspects: These included (1) no doctrine, creed, or dogma of theological nature being given; (2) the strong belief that an overruling Providence will come to the aid of a person who is really serious about stopping the use of tobacco; (3) as with Alcoholics Anonymous, encouragement to call for and use divine aid to cope with craving.

Social aspects: Group discussion, support, and reinforcement were stressed, and a "buddy system" was introduced at the first session.

Medication: The program did not stress use of medication. However, very nervous individuals were referred to their own doctor for tranquilizers.

On September 8 through 12, 1963, the 5-day program was conducted at the Palliser Hotel Ballroom in Calgary.[20] One hundred ninety-two smokers signed up to take the course, and 144 finished by attending the majority of sessions (three of the five sessions). The number who reported that they stopped smoking was 104, 72.2 percent of the 144 who finished the course (54.2 percent of the 192 who started the program). At 3 months, 33.9 percent of those who completed the course reported that they still were abstinent.

Thompson and Wilson[21] specifically addressed the issue of long-term abstinence in people who stopped smoking during the 5-day plan to stop smoking program. Two hundred ninety-eight persons attended the first session. Two hundred one people completed the fifth session. One hundred fifty (75 percent) of the 201 persons had not smoked a cigarette for the 24 h prior to the fifth session (50 percent of those who started the group). Of the 298 who started the study, 287 were contacted by telephone 10 weeks after the fifth session. Eighty four (29.4 percent) reported that they had not smoked a cigarette for a minimum of 7 days prior to the telephone interview (28 percent of the original 298 participants; 36 percent of those who completed the program).

The 84 participants who were not smoking at 10 weeks were contacted again at 10 months posttreatment. Forty-five said they had not smoked a cigarette since the program ended, and one said that he had not smoked a cigarette since a month after the program (55 percent; 15 percent of 298 participants who attended the first session).

Schlegel and Kunetsky[22] compared the quit smoking performance of participants who attended the 5-day plan to the performance of matched controls (matched according to age, sex, and amount of smoking). At the end of the group, 19 of 28 (68 percent) participants in the quit smoking group reported that they quit smoking by the last session. During this time, only one of the 28 matched controls quit smoking (3.6 percent). Six weeks later, 13 group participants were abstinent (46.4 percent) compared with two matched controls (7.1 percent).

THERAPY PLUS MEDICATION

Bachman[23] developed a stop smoking clinic which featured an 8-week program, with a 1½-h evening session held each week. The first half of each session (45 min) was devoted to medical lecture and the last half to group discussion and therapy. The subjects of the lecture at each session were as follows:

1. An introduction, a survey of the diseases resulting from smoking, the nature of the smoking habit, the social and economic ecology of smoking, and the therapeutic methods to be used.
2. Smoking and lung cancer.
3. Smoking and heart disease.
4. Smoking, bronchitis, and pulmonary emphysema.
5. The nuisances of smoking and the pleasures of stopping and the mechanics of various drug addictions and habituations (alcohol, narcotics, tobacco).
6. Hidden toxins in tobacco, smoking in the young, and the iniquities of cigarette advertising.
7. Smoking and weight.
8. Smoking and sexual functions and a general review.

As part of the therapy program, the patients were instructed to carry out a series of measures designed to "wean" them away from cigarettes. These measures included the following:

1. Change cigarette brands.
2. Post a "poison" label on the cigarette package.
3. Carry a card that reads "Is smoking worth it?"
4. Temporarily avoid coffee and coffee breaks, cocktails and cocktail hours, smoking and "bull sessions."
5. Use prayer (if the patient derives a positive motivation from religion).

Each course was limited to a maximum of 30 patients. Applicants were screened for compliance with patient selection requirements. In addition to the director, the clinic personnel included a dietitian, secretary, coordinator, and five lay group leaders who assisted in conducting the discussions.

Bachman[23] presented outcome data for 110 patients seen in six groups. Half the patients were male, and the entire group was ages 22 to 65. Smokers averaged about 40 cigarettes per day. As the second course ended, a decision was made to add deterrent drug therapy to reinforce the group therapy program. They used a cherry-flavored pastille containing 0.5 mg of lobeline sulfate (Nikoban), a compound which is related to nicotine. After some experimentation with dose and usage schedules, the schedule resolved itself to one pastille every hour for the first 4 days, followed by a gradual decrease in frequency over the next 2½ weeks. By the fourth week of therapy, most patients were able to discontinue regular use of the drug.

Of the 110 patients, 57 (51.8 percent) reported that they stopped smoking completely at the end of their respective courses. Of those who attended at least six of the eight sessions, 69.8 percent stopped smoking at the end of the course. Of those who attended fewer than six sessions, 18.6 percent stopped smoking at the end of the course. A 2-month to 1-year follow-up revealed that 67.9 percent and 25 percent of those who attend six or more sessions and those who attended fewer than six sessions, respectively, were still not smoking. The evaluation did not permit assessment of the independent contributions to cessation of the group program or the lobeline sulfate.

Ross[24] reported on 24 smoking withdrawal research clinics conducted at the Roswell Park Memorial Institute ($n = 1473$). The most commonly used format was an evening meeting during which educational material was presented, a physical examination done, and medication distributed. Clinics were held one evening weekly for the subsequent 3 weeks, during which time educational material was again presented and medication dispensed.

Thirty-four percent of those attending the clinics reported that they were able to stop smoking by the end of 1 week, and 16 percent stated that they were not smoking at 6 months follow-up. Medication use was manipulated between clinics to provide "mini" studies of efficacy. Lobeline was found to be more effective than a placebo, especially when combined with 8 mg of amphetamine. Five milligrams of lobeline plus 8 mg of amphetamine produced an initial success rate of 39 percent. Lobeline alone had a success rate of 27 percent, and amphetamine alone a success rate of 30 percent. A double placebo produced a success rate of 31 percent.

Schwartz and Dubitzkey[25] specifically studied the effectiveness of tranquilizers, individual counseling, and group therapy in a complex factorial design. Success in the study was defined as an 85 percent reduction in smoking from the pretreatment level. For all conditions combined ($n = 252$), the end of treatment "success rate" was 33 percent; at 4 months follow-up, 20.6 percent; and at 1-year follow-up, 20.2 percent. Reported quit rates were 29.4, 19, and 19.4 percent at end of treatment, 4 months, and 12 months, respectively. At the end of treatment, individual counseling yielded a 41.7 percent "success rate"; group counseling, 34.3 percent; and tranquilizers alone, 22.2 percent. Placebo subjects were more successful than those assigned to tranquilizers.

At 4-month follow-up, the greatest attrition in rate of success occurred among group subjects on tranquilizers. Almost 60 percent of the initial successes resumed their high rate of smoking. Individual counseling showed more than 40 percent recidivism, and the group with no pill yielded 37.5 percent recidivism. Subjects in the group with placebo and prescription with placebo conditions were most likely to remain successful. Few changes took place between 4-month and 1-year follow-ups.

Schwartz[15] describes, reviews, and critiques numerous other group programs and withdrawal clinics conducted in the 1960s. These include 11 5-day plan programs conducted in the United States, Canada, and England and 12 group discussion and therapy programs conducted in the United States and England. The interested reader is referred to Schwartz's review for insight into the nature and outcome of these programs.

Lichtenstein and Keutzer[26] offered a number of suggestions from "laboratory" research on smoking cessation, which may add to the success of traditional group cessation programs. Among their suggestions were (1) use of deposit-refunds or behavioral contracts to counteract attrition; (2) greater use of the smoker in an active, participative, rather than passive role in the group or clinic program (e.g., divide the group into small groups with a designated leader to problem solve and discuss various issues, such as coping with barriers to success); (3) use of role playing to effect attitude and behavior change[27]; (4) use of fear arousal techniques only when smokers also are given methods to control their habit; (5) discussion of and dealing with "counterarguments" as well as arguments against smoking (e.g., discussion of the most appealing prosmoking "messages" may immunize the smokers against future persuasive effects of these seductive appeals); (6) utilization of relaxation training to reduce tension which might otherwise trigger smoking; (7) use of self-monitoring techniques to help smokers become aware of situational factors which control their smoking; (8) a focus on social support for stopping smoking (i.e., invite spouse to attend therapy session); (9) consideration of the use of aversive smoke and/or satiation therapy; (10) warning participants that most relapse occurs within 3 months of the termination of the program; smoking clinics and programs must devote as much attention to follow-up and maintenance as to initial cessation; (11) collection of outcome data, so necessary for critical evaluation and program modification and improvement.

Group programs continue to remain an important and vital component of the stop smoking armamentarium. The early studies reviewed here contain many elements and concepts which have been incorporated into more contemporary programs. Although medications such as lobeline, amphetamines, and tranquilizers are rarely used today, the tact of combining pharmacologic and behavioral therapies is still very much in vogue and is likely to grow in popularity and importance in the future.

CLINICAL TRIALS OF DISEASE PREVENTION

Large-scale prospective clinical trials for disease prevention have included comprehensive and innovative programs for smoking cessation.[28] These trials, which have been carried out in countries around the globe, typically feature long-term intervention and follow-up, enrollment of smokers at excessive risk of disease and ill health, a strong medical component, group and individual interventions for smoking cessation, and creative and effective approaches to follow-up and long-term nonsmoking maintenance.

Two of these trials, both of which were carried out in the United States, are described below. They feature, for the time in which they were carried out, state-of-the-art interventions, and they demonstrate that successful long-term abstinence in a fairly substantial portion of smokers under treatment is possible and feasible. Each utilized group therapy approaches, although they incorporated diverse behavioral techniques and strategies to go along with education, group interaction, and support. In many ways, they serve as a model for developing effective long-term smoking cessation programs in the future. Unfortunately, the resources available to these large-scale endeavors seldom are available in other settings. The success of these trials, however, does raise the question of how other settings, such as work sites, hospitals, and health clinics, which allow long-term access to large numbers of smokers, can be mobilized to provide comparable comprehensive long-term intervention for smoking cessation.

MULTIPLE RISK FACTOR INTERVENTION TRIAL (MRFIT)

The primary objective of the MRFIT was to determine whether for a group of men at high risk of death from coronary heart disease (CHD) a special intervention program directed simultaneously toward reduction of three risk factors (elevated serum cholesterol, hypertension, and cigarette smoking) will result in a significant reduction in mortality from coronary heart disease.[29] To achieve the objectives of the trial, the 22 clinical centers involved in the MRFIT screened 361,662 men ages 35 to 57 and identified 12,866 who (1) were in the upper 10 to 15 percent of coronary risk because of the presence of risk factors; (2) did not have preexisting clinical coronary heart disease, and (3) were willing to commit themselves to a randomized 6-year intervention program. Half of the participants received special intervention (SI) for lowering of coronary risk, and half were referred to their own doctor for usual care (UC).

The intervention program consisted of three phases: (1) initial intervention, (2) extended intervention, and (3) maintenance.[30] Initial intervention was accomplished primarily within an "integrated group" framework at the start of the trial. Participants and their partners were invited to participate in ten to twelve 2-h weekly sessions of a group aimed at lowering cholesterol (dietary modification), managing high blood pressure (weight loss, sodium restriction, medication), and stopping smoking.[31]

Participants who successfully lowered their risk factors entered "maintenance"; those who did not entered "extended intervention." More often than not, participants entered both categories, because they had been successful in one part of the program, but not in another. Extended intervention included individual counseling and "focal groups" dealing solely with either smoking cessation, cholesterol reduction, weight loss, or some other aspect of the intervention.[31]

Maintenance included a number of activities aimed at helping participants sustain reduction in risk.[30] Examples of maintenance activities included group reunions, individual counseling sessions, telephone follow-up, social events, cooking classes for participants and their spouses, "health fairs" for the entire family, and food demonstrations.[31] All SI participants returned to the clinical centers every 4 months for data collection and assessment. At least once per year, participants met with a physician to review the results of the annual physical examination and to discuss their risk factor status.

The smoking cessation program for MRFIT was developed on the basis of assumptions which were shaped by (1) the special characteristics of the prospective clinical trial (e.g., intervention simultaneously on three risk factors, high risk of CHD, minimum of 6 years of follow-up); (2) development and modification of smoking techniques from the existing scientific literature in the early 1970s; and (3) a standardized approach to smoking cessation at each MRFIT clinical center.[32]

Since, in 1973, there was no one obviously superior smoking cessation method available, a wide variety of cessation techniques were used, and an attempt was made to maximize nonspecific factors (therapist concern, warmth, etc.) which contribute to cessation. Aversive techniques were not used because of concern of risk of producing arrhythmias in men already at high risk of CHD. Hypnosis also was ruled out.

Serum thiocyanate and expired air carbon monoxide served as objective measures of cigarette smoking.

Intervention on smoking began with the trial screening visits and included a formal discussion with a MRFIT physician. The group program focused on the development of the group as a resource for the participant, cognitive and educational approaches, and behavior modification. Six films were used frequently during the initial group program.[32] *Ashes to Ashes* is a 20-min film produced by the American Cancer Society, and the other five films are 5- to 10-minute "trigger" films now available from the National Institutes of Health. Three focus on the process of quitting and two on maintenance of cessation.

Behavior modification techniques included self-monitoring of smoking behavior, contracts for specific behavior change, positive reinforcement, stimulus control techniques (e.g., limit cigarette smoking to specific locations or times), giving up activities associated with the onset of smoking (no coffee drinking, no alcohol, etc.), stress management and relaxation training, substitute behaviors, thought stopping, brainstorming, role playing, and behavioral rehearsal. Participants generally prepared for a specific quit date, some going "cold turkey" and others tapering to a low level of smoking before attempting to quit. Most groups practiced going through periods without smoking (e.g., 24-h no smoking day) prior to the actual group quit date.

The maintenance program was based on a series of scheduled contacts between staff and participants, with the frequency of contacts decreasing over time as the participant continued to remain a nonsmoker.[32] The 4-month follow-up visits to the center, group reunions, a newsletter, and opportunities to meet with former smokers during intervention on other risk factors provided a rich support structure. Buddy systems and a telephone hot line also were implemented at some of the centers.

Approximately 64 percent of SI and UC participants smoked cigarettes at the start of the study, and they smoked an average of 34 cigarettes per day.[32] The first data collection point for SI participants was at 4 months, which in most cases corresponded closely to the end of the 10-week intervention program. The reported quit rate for SI smokers at 4 months was 47 percent. However, thiocyanate "adjustment" yielded a lower and more conservative initial cessation rate of 31 percent.[32]

At year 1, the reported and thiocyanate adjusted quit rates for SI were 43.1 and 31.4 percent, respectively. Of the SI men who stopped smoking by the 4-month visit, 56.1 percent did not report smoking at any follow-up visit (including 4- and 8-month visits between annual visits) through 48 months.[33] Of the SI smokers who reported not smoking at the year 1 visit, 60 percent continued to report cessation through year 6.[34]

Data for UC were available only at the annual examinations. At year 1, the reported and thiocyanate-adjusted quit rates for UC were 13.5 and 11.7 percent, respectively. Of the UC men who reported not smoking at year 1, approximately 50 percent continued to report cessation through year 6.[34]

The reported quit rates for SI men were 44.1, 44.4, 45.9, and 50 percent at years 2, 3, 4, and 6, respectively. For UC, comparable quit rates were 18.4, 20.4, 23.9, and 29 percent.[35] By year 6, there was relatively little discrepancy between reported and thiocyanate-adjusted quit rates for SI (50 versus 46 percent) and for UC (29 versus 29 percent).

For both SI and UC, the quit rate during the final years of the trial included smokers who quit early (by year 1) and remained abstinent, others who quit early, relapsed, and quit again, and still others who quit for the first time late in the trial. Most of the smokers who quit smoking did so early in the trial, with those quitting for the first time after year 1, in both groups, representing a more labile cohort of former smokers. After a year of not smoking had been achieved, the likelihood of relapse was relatively low, although participants continued to relapse even after many years of cessation.[34]

Hymowitz and colleagues[36] studied baseline factors associated with smoking cessation and relapse in the MRFIT. The variables which were positively associated with smoking cessation in SI and UC groups included age, education, and past success in quitting; there was a negative association with the number of cigarettes smoked per day. The expectation of quitting was positively associated with cessation in the SI groups only, whereas life events, alcohol, and the presence of a wife who smokes were significant predictors of reduced cessation for the UC group. The special intervention program may have overcome obstacles which interfered with cessation among UC participants. For UC participants, multivariate analysis showed that education, past success in quitting smoking, alcohol, and life events were associated with higher relapse rates. For SI, only alcohol emerged as a significant predictor of relapse.

The MRFIT extended the group therapy approach to include many of the suggestions which were recommended by Lichtenstein and Keutzer.[26] Behavioral technologies were employed, maintenance and follow-up received a great deal of attention, partners were invited to attend the group program, and relaxation training, as well as other approaches to coping with relapse, were employed. Compared with other studies in the early 1970s, the MRFIT stands out because of its emphasis on experimental design and evaluation. Follow-up strategies were vigorously followed, and expired air carbon monoxide and serum thiocyanate served as objective measures of smoking. The MRFIT also pioneered the use of brief medical intervention for smoking cessation.

LUNG HEALTH STUDY

The Lung Health Study (LHS) was a randomized multicenter clinical trial carried out from October 1986 to April 1994 that was designed to test the effectiveness of intervention—smoking cessation and bronchodilator administration—in people thought to be in the early stages of chronic obstructive pulmonary disease (COPD).[37] Participants were randomly assigned to one of three groups; usual care, who received no intervention; smoking intervention and the inhaled bronchodilator, ipratropium bromide (Atrovent, Boehringer Ingelheim Pharmaceuticals Inc., Ridgefield, CT) (SIA); and smoking intervention and an inhaled placebo (SIP). The major endpoint was the rate of decline of FEV_1.[37]

To test the primary hypotheses of the trial (i.e., whether an intervention program incorporating smoking cessation and the use of an inhaled bronchodilator in middle aged male and female smokers could slow the decline of lung function), it was necessary to increase smoking cessation rates among smokers who were at elevated risk of development of lung disease and to follow their progress over time.[38] Because high relapse rates typically are observed among heavily dependent smokers who quit, it was presumed that high initial cessation rates would have to be achieved to reach the sustained abstinence goal of 24 percent by year 5. Approximately 400 smokers were enrolled in the SI group at each of the 10 LHS clinics.

The smoking intervention program combined social learning methods with nicotine replacement therapy, and the LHS group program was based, in part, on the intensive group program used in the MRFIT. Key features of the program were an intensive "quit week" with frequent contact, knowledge and skill acquisition, self-control activities, and attempts to increase participants' self-efficacy.[38] Support persons (spouse, relative, or friend) were encouraged to take part in the LHS group program to strengthen the participants' environment once abstinence was achieved. Nicotine gum served as an important adjunct to the behavioral program. Components of the comprehensive smoking intervention program are described briefly in the following paragraphs.

Physician Message

Delivered soon after randomization, the message was designed to influence the participants' decision to quit smoking early on and use the bronchodilator. The message accomplished the following:

1. It provided personalized health information about the presence of lung disease.
2. It stressed the concept of risk reduction.
3. It discussed how smoking relates to health problems.
4. It prescribed use of nicotine gum and inhaler.

Behavior Interview

Immediately following the physician message, an interventionist met with the participant to obtain an extensive smoking history and review the intervention program. A stop smoking date was scheduled.

Orientation

A group orientation session focused on preparation to stop smoking on quit day.

Group Intervention

Quit week consisted of a series of four group sessions on consecutive days, beginning with quit day. During session 1 (quit day), the aerosol inhaler and nicotine gum were explained and demonstrated, and their use was initiated among the participants. Cognitive and behavioral strategies for smoking cessation were introduced, and daily monitoring of adherence or usage problems of the aerosol inhaler and nicotine gum were addressed. Body weight and expired air carbon monoxide were measured at each session. Seven group sessions that included plans to prevent smoking relapse were scheduled between weeks 2 and 12. By week 5, the focus of the program shifted to topics on health behavior, stress management, and relapse prevention skills, including plans for tapering gum use. If participants did not cease gum use within 6 months, meetings were held with interventionists to discuss a reduction strategy.

Extended Intervention

Extended intervention was offered to participants who continued to smoke, who did not enter the group program, or

who stopped smoking but relapsed. Individual intervention, restart groups, stay-quit support groups, and LHS physician visits continued to be offered as options for smoking cessation.

Maintenance

The primary goals of maintenance were to prevent relapse, to maintain good rapport, and to facilitate compliance.[38] Special maintenance activities included at least three maintenance meetings annually, weight management programs offered twice each year, quarterly newsletters, and telephone or clinic contacts on a scheduled basis.

The quit rates for the SIA and SIP groups were virtually identical, so their smoking outcome data were combined.[37] Cotinine and expired air carbon monoxide served as objective measures of smoking status. Sustained quit rates refer to individuals who had stopped smoking at the time of the initial cessation program and maintained their abstinence through five annual visits. At year 1, the quit rate for SI was about 36 percent compared with about 9 percent for UC. The sustained quit rate declined each year to about 22 percent at year 5 for SI and about 5 percent for UC.[37]

Cross-sectional quit rates were based on the number of participants who were validated as not smoking at a given annual visit, irrespective of their previous status. Cross-sectional quit rates were about 36 percent for SI at year 1 and about 39 percent at year 5. For UC, the cross-sectional quit rates were about 9 percent at year 1 and 21 percent at year 5.

For participants who completed the fifth annual visit, the mean cumulative changes in postbronchodilator FEV_1, differed sharply between the two intervention groups and the UC group. Average decreases from baseline to annual visit 5 were UC; 267 mL; SIP, 209 mL; and SIA, 184 mL. All pairwise comparisons between groups were significant.[37] Moreover, when data from UC and SI participants were combined, it was strikingly apparent that continuing smokers experienced dramatically greater declines in FEV_1, than sustained quitters. Conclusions from the LHS were that an aggressive smoking intervention program significantly reduces the age-related decline in FEV_1 in middle-aged smokers with mild airway obstruction. Use of the bronchodilator did not influence the long-term decline of FEV_1.[37] Like the MRFIT, the LHS achieved high rates of sustained smoking cessation by use of a protocol which featured a strong medical component, group smoking intervention, and behavioral strategies for initial and long-term modification of smoking. The LHS also employed nicotine replacement therapy (see below). The combined use of medical, behavioral, and pharmacologic therapies will, no doubt, serve as an important model for future intervention on smoking.

VOLUNTARY HEALTH ORGANIZATIONS

A number of voluntary agencies have developed quit smoking programs. The most recent version of the American Cancer Society (ACS) program is called *Fresh Start*. The program consists of four 1-h, small-group sessions.[39] Reading assignments follow each meeting to help participants remember what was discussed. The first session provides an understanding of why people smoke and the effects of smoking. Approaches to quitting are described, with cold turkey recommended. The second session focuses on withdrawal symptoms: Participants are encouraged to drink a lot of water, suck cinnamon sticks, exercise daily, and engage in deep breathing. Stress management and assertiveness training also are stressed. The third session deals with barriers to quitting, such as weight gain. The fourth session deals with relapse prevention and nonsmoking maintenance.

The American Lung Association developed the *Freedom From Smoking* (FFS) *Guide* for clinic leaders.[39] The clinic program is based on the premise that smoking is a learned habit. Each clinic is conducted by a trained group leader and consists of seven 1½- to 2-h sessions held during a 6 week period.[39]

The initial clinic meeting provides information on the health effects of smoking. Session 2 deals primarily with the triggers for smoking and coping strategies. Quit night occurs at the third session to provide support and encouragement to participants over their initial period of nonsmoking. Maintenance is a key feature of the FFS program. Group process and support, insight, and various behavioral techniques, including methods of relaxation and coping with tension, are offered to help overcome nicotine dependence.[39]

Lando and coworkers[40] compared the effectiveness of the ACS' Fresh Start, the ALA's Freedom From Smoking, and Lando's laboratory-based clinic method. Lando's group program featured cognitive-behavioral techniques, including aversive smoking procedures, which were developed in his and others' laboratory over several years. The 1041 smokers were assigned randomly to one of the three group quit smoking methods. Quit rates for the three programs at 3, 6, and 12 months were as follows: ACS, 24.17, 23.56, and 22.36 percent; ALA, 28.93, 27.27, and 24.79; Lando, 37.18, 29.11, and 28.53 percent. Although the above point prevalence differences are no longer statistically significant after 3 months, sustained abstinence differences were significant at all follow-up points. ACS's Fresh-Start fared most poorly, and the Lando program achieved better outcome than the ALA's Freedom From Smoking program. Saliva thiocyanate served as an objective measure of smoking.

Rosenbaum and O'Shea[41] studied 494 smokers who attended 42 Freedom from Smoking Clinics in Western New York State. The reported quit rate at the end of the clinic was 52 percent; at one year, 29 percent. These outcome data are consistent with a prior study of outcome data for 590 smokers who attended the ACS or ALA clinics over a 6-year period.[41] The mean reported quit rate at the end of the group was 56 percent; at 12 months, the mean quit rate was 25 percent. When subjects were asked to identify the most helpful aspects of the Freedom From Smoking clinic, the two most important components were group support and being with others with the same problem.

The Kaiser-Permanente Stop Smoking Clinic is part of the Northern California region of the Kaiser-Permanente Medical Care Program, a health maintenance organization serving more than a million members.[42] The clinic covers an 8-week period with thirteen 90-min meetings. Groups meet twice weekly for the first nine meetings and once weekly for the remaining four meetings. Group reunions are held at 3, 6, and 12 months after quitting. Groups have an average of 10 members.

Prior to the group, the group leader interviews each potential participant. The confidential consultation is regarded as initial treatment as well as a process during which the most appropriate treatment mode is selected. Information gathered during the interview can be used by the group leader to motivate smokers during the group meetings.

During sessions 1 to 8, smokers monitor their behavior and identify situations which influence smoking. They also come into contact with the functional value of smoking. Other key features of the program are the emphasis on addiction, management of craving, and a quit date (session 5). During session 5, group members are instructed to leave the room and smoke their last cigarette together. A buddy system is then introduced, and care packages (sugarless gum, cinnamon sticks, and other items) are distributed. Four days after quitting, the group meets for breakfast (seventh meeting). Ex-smokers share experience and support each other. Meetings 9 to 13 are devoted to maintaining abstinence. Exercise, assertiveness training, and active coping are stressed. Group reunions are held at approximately 3, 6, and 12 months after cessation.

Harrup and colleagues[42] reported outcome data for 1128 smokers seen during 1973 to 1977. At the end of group, 90 percent of the participants reported not smoking. At 2 months, the quit rate was 78 percent; at 6 months, 57 percent; and at 12 months, 47 percent, with no difference between males and females.

Hypnosis

Schwartz[39] noted that the popularity of hypnosis as a smoking cessation method is suggested by a survey of the telephone yellow pages, which found that hypnosis was the most frequently advertised method. Scientific opinion regarding its effectiveness, however, is mixed. Schwartz[39] concluded that hypnosis produces only modest results when used alone, but when combined with other methods, success rates are enhanced. The skill and experience of the therapist are very important. While a single treatment of hypnosis may be cost-effective initially, multiple sessions appear to improve quit rates.

Whereas the initial reports of the effectiveness of hypnosis for smoking cessation specifically focused on hypnosis, later reports included studies in which hypnosis was combined with other treatment modalities. In addition, later studies included control groups and objective measures of smoking status. These improvements in methodology and design permitted less ambiguous assessment of the efficacy of hypnosis.

The APA Steering Committee on Practice Guidelines[17] noted that three metaanalyses reported that hypnosis was efficacious, whereas the Agency For Health Care Policy and Research (AHCP) clinical practice guideline[43] metaanalysis concluded that hypnosis was not efficacious. The APA steering committee noted that the discordance reflects the fact that most hypnosis trials have poor methodologies and were excluded from consideration in some metaanalyses or reviews. Given the conflicting evidence, the APA Steering Committee[17] rated hypnosis as a promising treatment.

Simon and Salzberg[44] described five approaches to hypnotic procedures for smoking cessation: (1) use of hypnosis to give smokers direct suggestions to change; (2) use of hypnosis to alter the smoker's perceptions with regard to addictive behavior; (3) use of hypnosis as an adjunct to verbal psychotherapy (hypnotherapy); (4) use of hypnosis to help the patient develop aversion to addictive behavior substances (hypnoaversion); and (5) self-hypnosis, used as an adjunct to supplement hypnotic treatment.

Spiegel[45] popularized a single-treatment method for stopping smoking using ancillary self-hypnosis. According to Spiegel, the primary strategy in this treatment is the three-point affirmation by the patient of a commitment to respect and protect his or her body. As a "facilitating technique, hypnosis aids in creating an expectant, receptive state of attention and aroused concentration that permits a new perspective on an old smoking habit. When the patient accepts the commitment to respect his or her body, it distracts attention from the urge to smoke. The patient now experiences two urges simultaneously—the urge to smoke and the urge to protect the body. By locking them together and emphasizing respect for the body, the patient concurrently ignores the urge to smoke."[45]

The technique consists of a brief clinical history and a test for hypnotizability. (Hypnotizability gives the treatment greater impact; however, sufficient motivation can compensate for a patient's inability to be hypnotized.) After being hypnotized, patients are asked to close their eyes and concentrate on three basic points:

1. For your body smoking is a poison. You are composed of a number of components, the most important of which is your body. Smoking is not so much a poison for you as it is for your body.
2. You cannot live without your body. Your body is a precious physical plant through which you experience life.
3. To the extent that you want to live, you owe your body respect and protection. . . . When you make this commitment to respect your body, you have within you the power to have smoked your last cigarette.

Once patients learn the physiologic and subjective sensations that distinguish the hypnotized state, they are immediately shown how to induce this state by themselves and how to bring themselves out of self-hypnosis. Patients then induce self-hypnosis several times under the therapist's supervision and repeat the three basic points of treatment each time. The therapist then teaches a "camouflage" technique so that reinforcement exercises can be carried out for 15 to 20 s any number of times daily without attracting attention. Finally, an abbreviated "secondary reinforcement" gesture, like stroking the side of the face, is demonstrated, concluding the 45-min session.[45]

Survey questionnaires were sent to 615 patients who were ready for a 6-month follow-up. Of those, 271 (44 percent) responded. Assuming, conservatively, that all those who did not respond had resumed smoking, 6 months or more after a single treatment, 20 percent reported that they were still not smoking.[45] Others reduced their daily smoking rate and/or stopped for a brief period of time.

Berkowitz and coworkers[46] attempted to replicate Spiegel's report. Spiegel's treatment protocol was applied in a private psychiatric setting to 40 consecutive patients, 20 males and 20 females. Follow-up was conducted via telephone. The 6-month reported quit rate was 25 percent, a finding consistent with Spiegel's earlier report.

More recent studies of single-session hypnosis, individual and group, included comparison groups, an important methodologic improvement. Javel[47] compared groups of 10 patients (not randomly assigned to conditions) receiving formal hypnotic induction plus suggestion, suggestion alone, and no treatment (waiting list control). Three-month telephone follow-up revealed reported quit rates of 60, 40, and 0 percent, for patients receiving the full treatment, suggestion only, and no treatment, respectively.

Sanders[48] applied mutual group hypnosis to the smoking problem. Mutual group hypnosis is a group hypnosis experience during which one hypnotized subject gives suggestions to another hypnotized subject. This method appears to have particular utility in providing social support and feedback to group members. Sander's basic assumption was that to change the habit of smoking, it is important to change smokers' view of themselves, expectations, and environmental supports.

Group hypnosis is induced by a combination of eye fixation and progressive relaxation.[48] Trance deepening is effected by imagery of a comfortable place. Additional techniques, carried out while subjects are in a relaxed state, include the following:

1. *Brainstorming:* The group brainstorms about reasons for wanting to be a nonsmoker.
2. *Time progression and imagery:* Imagery is the prototype of all thinking, and time progression permits liberation from the present and permits consideration of change in the future.
3. *Hypnotic dream:* Hypnotic dreams permit escape from the usual ways of thinking and reflect motivation for change or resistance to it.
4. *Rehearsal of imagery:* Rehearsing the role of being a nonsmoker and practicing new alternatives provides the opportunity to obtain group support for the new role by other group members.
5. *Self-hypnosis:* Self-hypnosis enables the group member to practice the technique and the role of being a nonsmoker independently of the group.

The smoking clinic study was carried out at the University of North Carolina.[48] Nineteen persons were seen in the smoking clinic over a period of 8 months. They were divided into four groups, each seen for four consecutive weeks. The same therapist worked with all four groups.

Questionnaires were sent to all members of the group 10 months after the group had terminated. After the fourth session, 84 percent, or 16 of 19 smokers, reported no smoking. At 10 months, 68 percent (13 of 19) reported that they still were nonsmokers. The results suggest that mutual group hypnosis is useful in providing a milieu which facilitates the change from being a smoker to becoming a nonsmoker.[48]

There are, of course, many variations on a theme and many different approaches to hypnotherapy. Hypnosis combined with individual counseling or psychotherapy may be more effective than hypnosis alone, and extended group hypnotherapy sessions may be even more effective.[49] It should also be noted that people differ in their susceptibility to be hypnotized. Hence, it might be predicted that highly susceptible subjects would benefit more from hypnotherapy for smoking cessation than less susceptible smokers. Although several reports consistent with this hypothesis are available, not all findings concur.[49,50]

Lambe and colleagues[51] conducted a randomized controlled trial of hypnotherapy for smoking cessation. The patient population at the Rochester Family Medicine Program received a screening questionnaire to determine eligibility for the study. Patients were eligible if they wished to quit smoking and were willing to undergo hypnosis. Recruitment continued until 180 eligible patients were identified. They were randomized to hypnosis or control groups.

All control patients received a letter notifying them that the physicians at the family medicine center hoped they would quit smoking. They also received a copy of the National Institutes of Health booklet *Calling It Quits*. Follow-up began with the date of this letter.

The hypnotherapy consisted of two 40-min sessions, 2 weeks apart.[51] At the first visit, the hypnotist followed a standard protocol. After the trance was terminated, the method of autohypnosis was explained and a list of instructions given. At the time of the second session, a trance was induced again and suggestions reinforced. During the trance, the subject was asked to choose a quit date. Follow-up began on the date of the second session.

In the hypnosis group, 45 patients underwent at least one hypnosis session, 6 quit before hypnosis, 18 declined hypnosis, and 21 were lost to follow-up. At the 3-month follow-up telephone contact, verbal report data indicated that hypnosis patients were significantly more successful in quitting smoking (21 versus 6 percent). However, at 6-month (18 versus 19 percent) and 12-month follow-up (22 versus 20 percent), the quit rates for the two conditions were virtually identical. The authors concluded that hypnosis accelerates the rate at which smokers quit but offers no long-term advantage beyond sympathetic contact with a health care professional.

Rabkin and coworkers[52] carried out a randomized trial comparing smoking cessation programs utilizing behavior modification, health education, or hypnosis. Serum thiocyanate served as an objective measure of smoking status. Participants were recruited by use of the media, included men and women between 20 and 65 years of age, and accepted random assignment to one of four treatment conditions: no treatment control (delayed treatment), hypnosis, health education, or behavior modification. Three weeks after completion of the program, participants were asked to return for a follow-up questionnaire and blood samples for serum thiocyanate, an objective measure of smoking. Six months later the participants were contacted by mail.

The behavior modification program consisted of four groups of 10 subjects conducted by a leader skilled in behavior modification. The program consisted of five evening meetings (45 to 90 min) over a 3-week period. The sessions followed a group format and focused on "stimulus control" techniques and other strategies for changing smoking behavior rather than on health hazards and scare tactics.

The health education program followed the format of cessation programs emphasizing the biologic effect of smoking and incorporated data on behavioral factors, such as perception of risk and efficacy. Most of the material was presented in a didactic format.

The hypnosis sessions were conducted on a one-to-one basis by a psychiatrist with special training and expertise in hypnosis. The technique used was that of Spiegel's single treatment method. Subjects were also given the following suggestions while in the trance. "Every hour or hour and a half over the next week and whenever necessary afterward you will sit down and induce a trance state through the use of the technique shown to you. You will repeat the statements regarding smoking three times with each self-induced trance state."[52]

The quit rates at the 3-week follow-up visit were as follows: for the hypnosis group, 29 percent (11 of 38) of those with follow-up data and 22.9 percent (11 of 48) of all those randomized to hypnosis; for health education, 32 percent (10 of 31) of those with follow-up data and 24 percent (10 of 41) of all participants; for the behavior modification, 37 percent (14 of 38) of those with follow-up data and 30 percent (14 of 46) of all those randomized to this intervention. No one in the control group quit. There were no significant differences between the three intervention groups with regard to the proportion that quit smoking, the number of cigarettes smoked, change in the number of cigarettes, or decrease in serum thiocyanate concentration.[52] The reported quit rates at the 6-month assessment (questionnaire) for intent-to-treat were 19, 22, and 17 percent for hypnosis, health education, and behavior modification, respectively. Between-group differences were not found.

Pederson and colleagues[53] studied the effects on smoking cessation of no treatment waiting list control, counseling, and hypnosis plus counseling. Subjects were 48 volunteers who were randomly assigned to one of three groups with each group containing equal numbers of men and women. The three groups were similar with respect to age, years smoked, and baseline smoking rate.

The subjects in the counseling groups underwent pulmonary function testing, had their medical history taken, and participated in six weekly group discussions about smoking and quitting (i.e., cold turkey versus gradual reduction, withdrawal symptoms, self-monitoring and self-regulatory techniques, alternative behaviors). The 16 subjects in the hypnosis-plus-counseling group participated in a single session of group hypnosis in addition to the counseling group. The 1½-h hypnosis session contained a description of the benefits of not smoking and instruction in simple relaxation techniques. Subsequent to the formal program, members of the latter two groups met once a month for 6 months and were then contacted by telephone at 10 months.

Zero percent of the waiting list control group was abstinent at 3 months (at least 3 months of no smoking) and 2 of 16 (12.5 percent) were abstinent at 10 months. At 3 months posttreatment, 56.25 percent (9 of 16) of the hypnosis-plus-counseling group and 12.50 percent (2 of 16) of the counseling group were successful. At 10 months, 50 percent of the hypnosis-plus-counseling group was abstinent compared with 0 percent of the counseling group.[53] Group differences at 3 and 10 months were highly significant.

Fifty additional people selected from the files were contacted by telephone 8 to 12 months following a single office visit for a group hypnosis session for quitting smoking. Only 8 percent (4 of 50) were successful. The investigators concluded that neither hypnosis alone nor group counseling alone yielded satisfactory long-term quit rates. However, the combination of techniques yielded a fairly high success rate.[53]

Frank and coworkers[54] examined the effects of hypnotic smoking cessation methods augmented with behavioral techniques. Subjects were 63 employees of the University of Missouri. They were randomly assigned to one of three experimental treatments: group 1, two 1-h sessions of hypnosis plus one booster session 3 weeks after the end of treatment; group 2, four 1-h sessions of hypnosis plus one booster session 3 weeks after the end of treatment; and group 3, two 1-h sessions of hypnosis and two 1-h sessions of behavioral self-management training, followed by a booster session 3 weeks after the end of treatment. All sessions were scheduled once every 2 weeks. A fourth group of subjects was later recruited and treated with four sessions of hypnosis and a booster session 3 weeks after the last treatment session. In group 4, subjects were seen twice per week for a total of 2 weeks with a booster session 3 weeks after the end of treatment.

The hypnotic treatment was drawn largely from Sanders'[48] mutual group hypnosis procedure. Several hypnotic procedures were used during different sessions including group problem-solving, self-hypnosis as a coping strategy, and personalized suggestion for motivation to quit and for maintenance. During the first hypnotic session, Sanders' procedure was augmented by suggestion similar to Spiegel's one-session treatment method.

The cognitive behavioral treatment included self-monitoring, learning of alternative behaviors, stimulus control, environmental management, self-reinforcement, target reduction with a gradual quitting date, and problem-solving strategies.

At the 3-month follow-up, a subset of 23 subjects was asked to provide a saliva sample to test for the presence of thiocyanate. All subjects who reported having quit were asked to provide a saliva sample. Six months after treatment subjects were interviewed by telephone and filled out a questionnaire to determine long-term smoking status.

At the end of treatment, no differences in the number of cigarettes smoked or quit rate (31 percent) between groups 1, 2, and 3 were found. Only 20 percent were still abstinent 6 months later. The performance of subjects in group 4 was the same as those in groups 1, 2, and 3.

Byrne and Whyte[55] also employed a randomized design to compare the effectiveness of hypnosis to other treatment modalities (behavioral self-management, behavior modification with a psychologist, and a more intensive behavior modification program—six consecutive daily sessions).

Complete data at baseline and at follow-up points were available for only 41.3 percent of the sample ($n = 131$; original sample size = 274). Analysis of reported smoking rates revealed similar declines in rate of smoking at the end of the group, with considerable relapse by the 3-month follow-up. Thereafter, smoking rates for each condition remained fairly stable through 12 months. Individual quit rate data for each condition were not reported although the overall quit rates for subjects on whom follow-up data were available (end of program, 59 percent; 3 months, 32 percent; 7 months, 30 percent; and 12 months, 31 percent) were said to be similar for each treatment modality. If the intent-to-treat analysis were used, quit rates would be much lower.

Acupuncture

Acupuncture is the most widely known treatment method in the field of Eastern medicine.[56] Acupuncture treatment may be applied to traditionally described points ("body points") and/or to loci defined in specialized, more recently developed systems, such as the ear points (auriculotherapy) or hand points (*Koryo Sooji Chim*). Most practitioners prefer to combine traditional and specialized points, particularly auricular points.[56]

Stimulation of the points may be accomplished by needle insertion, electrical current, laser beams, moxibustion (a form of heat treatment), application of magnets, or a combination of these methods.[56] Schwartz[39] describes two methods of treating smokers by means of acupuncture. Nasopuncture consists of selecting points on the surface of the nose in such a way as to decongest the respiratory tract and generate in the patient a feeling of disgust toward tobacco. The second method, auriculopuncture, is said to regulate the neurovegetative system.

Needles are usually left in place for 10 to 40 min, although most practitioners consider 20 min optimal.[56] In addition to treatment in the acupuncture clinic, it is common practice to provide means for ongoing stimulation of ear or hand points between treatments. This may be accomplished by taping down intradermal needles or, less frequently, magnets, metallic pellets, or herbal seeds at auricular or hand points.[56]

Review of a report by Choy, Lutzker, and Meltzer[57] may be instructive. In 1976, during use of acupuncture in the treatment of two obese nurses who smoked, an unexpected side effect was discovered: the treatment not only induced anorexia, it also induced aversion to tobacco smoke and a sharply diminished desire to smoke. This effect on smoking was unknown at the time.

During the following year, 33 patients were treated in the same manner. Of these, 55 percent stopped smoking, with a recurrence rate of 20 percent.[57] The "hunger" point was located in the center of the tragus of the ear. Before insertion of the needles, the patient was given a short lecture on the medical reasons for not smoking and shown slides of smokers' and nonsmokers' lungs. A detailed list of instructions also was provided. They included the following: use an empty cigarette-holder as a pacifier; for 4 weeks avoid social situations where smoking is part of the scene; enlist the support of friends, family, and colleagues; chew sugarless gum, celery, or carrot sticks as substitutes; drink at least four glasses of water per day; when experiencing a craving for a cigarette, count mentally up to and backward from 100, take a long hot shower, and rub the press needles with a gentle circular motion for 1 min; get rid of all cigarettes and do not buy any more; brush teeth after each meal with a strong tasting toothpaste; and return for booster treatments at the first sign of "backsliding."

From the inception of the program in May 1976 to December 14, 1982, a total of 514 patients were enrolled. Of these, 339 completed the minimal course of 4 weeks of treatment. Of the 339, 297 patients reported that they succeeded in stopping cigarette smoking, for a success rate of 88 percent. At 2 years, follow-up of 220 patients showed that the rate of relapse was 31 percent.[57] The investigators concluded that tragus acupuncture is an effective treatment.

Before accepting this conclusion, the careful reader may very well desire more information, as well as answers to important questions. Is the initial quit rate 88 percent (297 of 339 patients) or 58 percent (297 of 514 patients)? Why was follow-up data available for only 220 patients? A more conservative estimate of the 2-year quit rate would be 30 percent (152 of 514 patients). How much faith should be placed on verbal report data? Objective measures of smoking status, such as serum thiocyanate, saliva cotinine, or expired air carbon monoxide, would enhance the validity of the outcome data.

The exact nature of the quit rate aside, the question arises over the precise contribution to quitting of acupuncture. Indeed, the smokers carried out a variety of other stop smoking strategies, not to mention the motivating effect of the cost of treatment. Clearly, a randomized control or comparison group would aid interpretation. Such a group of patients might be exposed to the same educational and behavioral strategies. Instead of receiving actual acupuncture, they could receive a "sham" procedure, with needle placement at an "incorrect" site.

Olms[58] also reported an instance of serendipity in which self-acupuncture treatment for a persistent cough (not tobacco-related) not only resulted in cure of the cough, but also cessation of smoking. Subsequent work with the "Tim Mee" acupuncture point "confirmed" its positive effect on smoking cessation.

The smoking patient is given a brief paper to read concerning Olms' experience with stopping smoking by employing point Tim Mee. In addition to the Tim Mee point, located near the wrist, Olms also used Dr. Nogier's auricular aggression point on the patient's dominant ear, or on both ears if the patient is ambidextrous or has problems with directions. A "gallbladder" point on the nose is also utilized. After the needles have been in place for 15 min, Olms treats each one with a soft laser. When this is done, the treatment is completed.

Olms tells the patient that he will repeat the treatment at no charge if the first treatment does not work or if they inadvertently start smoking within 1 month. If Olms does not hear from the patient, he regards the treatment as a success! If they return, Olms tries to find out why the patient failed. If the patient states that the treatment worked, but "I started again because I thought I could play with cigarettes," or "I tried one for a lark and started again," Olms counts this as a success.[58]

Olms reported outcome data for 2282 cases seen in 1981, 1982, and 1983. Of these, 1571 were successful the first time around (69 percent). Another 696 (30 percent) were successful after repeat treatment. No information is given about duration of follow-up, nor does the author speculate about other reasons why patients who went through treatment did not call him again.

More recently, Clavel-Chapelon and colleagues[59] utilized a 2 × 2 factorial design to study the effects of acupuncture and nicotine gum (i.e., nicotine replacement therapy) on smoking cessation. Participants were assigned randomly to one of four groups: double active treatment (nicotine gum and acupuncture), double placebo (placebo gum and "sham" acupuncture points), and the combination of one active treatment and placebo.

Criteria for inclusion in the study were 18 years of age or more and smoking a minimum of 10 cigarettes per day. Treatments were administered blindly during three sessions with 10 to 15 people, at days 1, 7, and 28 by an acupuncturist. The needles were placed bilaterally at the "Bitong" and "Shuaigou" acupoints. The placebo points were 2 cm from the real points. Each piece of gum contained 2 mg of nicotine.

The placebo contained 1 mg of unbuffered nicotine to reduce its biologic availability.

Only ex-smokers on day 28 were considered successes and were followed up every 3 months during the first year and subsequently after 2 and 4 years. Nonsmoking status at year 4 was validated by measurement of expired air carbon monoxide.

The first 996 subjects who responded to the mail solicitation and who met inclusion criteria were randomly assigned to one of the four treatment conditions. The rates of success, defined as complete smoking cessation, did not differ significantly among the four groups at any follow-up point. Success rates for the group receiving active acupuncture and active gum, for example, were 26.5, 11.2, and 6.1 percent at 1 month, 1 year, and 4 years. For the group receiving placebo gum and placebo acupuncture, the corresponding quit rates were 20.6, 10.3, and 7.3 percent. No significant interactions between treatments were found.[59]

Schwartz[39] reviewed six randomized control studies which used "correct" and "incorrect" sites. In only one study did the correct site show a clear advantage over the placebo site. More recently, Riet and coworkers[60] conducted a metaanalysis of studies which met minimal methodologic criteria. The number of studies with negative outcomes exceeded by far the number with positive outcomes. Riet and coworkers concluded that claims that acupuncture is efficacious for smoking cessation (as well as other addictions) are not supported by results from sound clinical research. The APA guidelines steering committee[17] similarly concluded that acupuncture lacks sufficient evidence to be recommended for smoking cessation.

Suggestion under Anesthesia

Until recently, it had been assumed that general anesthesia renders a patient oblivious to sensory events. However, this may not always be the case. Even when there is no indication that the depth of anesthesia is inadequate, some processing of intraoperative events has been demonstrated.[61] Aldrete[62] met with 16 patients who smoke in a preanesthetic interview to talk about smoking. They talked about the physical consequences of smoking, as well as the added risk smoking represents to their immediate recovery from surgery and anesthesia. Smokers who expressed intentions and desires to quit smoking were asked if they wanted to have stop smoking suggestions made to them repeatedly before, during, and immediately after anesthesia. A control group included nine other patients with a similar tobacco history. The same initial interview was done and the same warnings were mentioned. However, the suggestions and warnings were not repeated again.

The study group was divided into highly motivated patients who expressed definite interest in quitting and moderately motivated patients who recognized the health hazards of smoking but were not certain if they wanted to quit.

Of the 16 patients in the study groups, nine did not smoke again for an entire year.[62] This included seven who were highly motivated to quit and two who were moderately motivated. Only one patient in the control group reported abstinence after 1 year. The differences in reported rates of quitting between highly motivated experimental group patients and control group patients at 6 and 12 months were highly significant.

Hughes and colleagues[63] specifically studied the effect of a recorded message designed to discourage tobacco consumption, delivered during general anesthesia, on the smoking habits of patients undergoing elective surgery. After obtaining informed consent, patients were randomly allocated, using a double-blind procedure, to either a control or experimental condition. In the anesthetic room following completion of venous cannulation, headphones from a portable tape player were placed over the patient's ears. As the induction agent was introduced, the tape was started at a preset valiance. Each tape had a 15-s delay before the message started, to allow a reasonable time for arm-brain circulation of the drug.

Two tapes were used. The message on the active tape was "You will stop smoking. You will want to stop smoking. Smoking will no longer be a pleasurable activity for you. You will want to stop smoking as of now." On the control tape the voice merely counted numbers to give the same number of syllables of the active tape. The tapes played continuously until the surgical procedure was complete and the anesthetic agent discontinued.

Approximately 4 weeks after surgery, patients were visited at home. Patients who could not be contacted in three visits were excluded from the study. Those contacted were asked about their smoking habit and whether they remember having had the earphones positioned and the content of the message.

Data were obtained for 122 female patients, of which 22 (10 from the active tape and 12 from the control tape conditions) were excluded from the data analysis because they could not be contacted at the postoperative visits. The two groups were similar in age and in tobacco consumption prior to surgery. Eight patients, all of whom had the active message, reported being abstinent at 1 month (16 percent quit rate, 8 of 50). Only 36 percent of patients ($n = 100$) could recall the headphones being positioned, and none could recall hearing the message or were aware of its content. Differences between the two groups in quit rates (16 versus 0 percent) and cigarettes smoked per day were statistically significant.

A more recent double-blind randomized trial of smoking cessation during anesthesia failed to replicate the above findings.[64] Three hundred sixty-three smokers who wanted to stop smoking were allocated randomly to hear a taped message encouraging them to stop smoking or to a blank tape, played during general anaesthesia. Overall, 56 patients (15.4 percent) claimed to have stopped smoking at 2 months and 29 patients (8.0 percent) remained abstinent through 6 months (confirmed by expired air carbon monoxide). However, there was no significant difference between the groups at either 2 or 6 months.[64] This study does not support the hypothesis that intraoperative tape suggestion can change smoking behavior.

Behavioral Techniques

Literally hundreds of well designed studies have been conducted on the efficacy of behavior modification techniques. The APA guidelines steering committee[17] reviewed many of these and rated them in terms of stop smoking efficacy (Table

TABLE 28-1 American Psychiatric Association Practice Guideline Recommendations

Behavioral Technique	Recommendation
Skill training/relapse prevention	Recommended
Stimulus control	Recommended
Aversive therapy	Recommended
Social support	Insufficient evidence (promising)
Contingency management	Insufficient evidence
Cue exposure	Insufficient evidence
Nicotine fading	Insufficient evidence
Relaxation	Insufficient evidence
Physiological feedback	Insufficient evidence

28-1). The effectiveness of these techniques may differ when they are used as a component of a multicomponent smoking cessation program from when they are used as a stand alone technique. Relaxation training, deep breathing, and stress management, for example, may not be efficacious for smoking cessation by themselves. However, they may be extremely important as components of a comprehensive "multicomponent" quit smoking program (see below).

Skill training and relapse prevention (e.g., problem solving, coping skills, stress management), stimulus control (e.g., self-monitoring, avoiding stimuli associated with smoking), and aversive therapy (rapid smoking) have been shown to be effective quit smoking strategies and are recommended, either as stand alone treatments or as components of a comprehensive quit smoking program. Social support, contingency management, cue exposure, nicotine fading, relaxation, and physiologic feedback, on the other hand, have had rather mixed findings, and there is insufficient evidence to recommend them as effective treatments for smoking cessation.[17]

AVERSIVE SMOKE THERAPY

The rationale for aversive therapy is to make smoking aversive and less reinforcing by inducing mild nicotine intoxication symptoms like nausea and dizziness when the patient smokes.[17] The original version of this type of treatment was rapid smoking in which patients inhale cigarette smoke every few seconds. Many well-controlled studies of rapid smoking have been conducted, and most reviews and metaanalyses have concluded that rapid smoking is efficacious.[17] Rapid smoking is considered safe in healthy patients. The APA guidelines steering committee[17] concluded that rapid smoking is a recommended component of behavior therapy for those smokers willing to comply. The steering committee left as "debatable" whether other aversive techniques are equally effective.

In addition to rapid smoking, other smoke aversion methods are the use of smoky air, smoke satiation, regular paced aversive smoking, and smoke holding.[39] Common to each of these procedures are the assumptions that (1) the reinforcing aspects of almost any stimulus are reduced and may actually become aversive if that stimulus is presented at sufficiently elevated frequency and intensity and (2) aversion based on stimuli intrinsic to the target response (smoking) is more salient and generalized than that stemming from artificial sources.[39]

Two other approaches to aversion therapy include covert sensitization and shock therapy. The objective of covert sensitization is to produce avoidance behavior through use of the subject's imagination. Both the behavior to be modified and the noxious stimulus are imagined.[39] In shock therapy, electric shock is used as a punishing stimulus to suppress smoking behavior.

Wilde[65] used cigarette smoke mixed with hot air as an aversive stimulus, the presentation of which was made contingent on smoking in a laboratory setting. In addition, the presentation of lightly mentholated room temperature air plus the opportunity to eat a peppermint was made contingent on the subject putting out the cigarette and saying "I want to give up smoking." Daily sessions lasted approximately 25 min, and the subjects received 6 to 20 trials, depending on their tolerance. Between the treatment sessions subjects were instructed to try to recall the laboratory situation whenever they wanted a cigarette and to eat a peppermint or other substitute instead of smoking. If smoking did occur, subjects were told to hold the cigarette between their lips as long as it was tolerable and then extinguish it. Treatment continued to the point when subjects reported that they were not smoking and that there was no longer a need to exercise self-control.

Three of seven subjects quit smoking after one or two sessions, one reduced his rate of smoking by 95 percent after one session, one switched to a pipe after 20 sessions, and two dropped out of treatment. Wilde[65] reported that all five smokers who underwent treatment ultimately reverted to their original smoking pattern, preferring a resumption of smoking to further "booster" sessions.

Franks and colleagues[66] made the presentation of hot air and cigarette smoke contingent on smoking in a similar, though better controlled, laboratory situation. All subjects received 12 individual treatment sessions, consisting of approximately 10 trials per session, over a period of 4 weeks. Of the 23 subjects who began treatment, only nine completed the program. A 6-month follow-up mail survey of the nine subjects who completed treatment indicated that four were not smoking, yielding a success rate of 44 percent (4 of 9) or 17 percent (4 of 23), depending on how it is calculated.

Resnick[67] studied the effects of stimulus satiation on the smoking behavior of college students. Eight undergraduate students were instructed to increase their smoking rate to four packs per day, with the goal usually being reached in 2 days. The treatment procedure lasted for 1 week, at which point they were instructed to stop smoking. Resnick reported that six of eight subjects stopped smoking and had not returned to smoking 4 months later.[67]

Resnick[68] extended his study of satiation therapy. All subjects met with the experimenters for one 10-min session, which consisted of a structured interview. At this point, subjects were assigned randomly to one of three experimental conditions: (1) a control group that was told to remain at its present rate of smoking, (2) an experimental group instructed to double its smoking rate, and (3) an experimental group told to triple its consumption rate. All subjects were told to smoke at their assigned rate for 1 week, after which they were instructed to quit smoking. Two weeks after treatment, the quit rates were 65, 50, and 25 percent for the group that tripled its consumption, doubled its consumption, and did not change its consumption, respectively. The differences in quit rates for experimental and control groups were highly significant. At 4 months follow-up, reported quit rates for the double (60 percent) and triple (65 percent) satiation groups were significantly greater than controls (20 percent abstinent), although the two experimental groups did not differ from each other.

Lublin and Joslyn[69] used an apparatus similar to Wilde's which blew warm, stale cigarette smoke at subjects while they smoked at an increased rate. At a 12-month follow-up, 40 percent (31 of 78) of the subjects who completed at least three sessions reported that they were abstinent or greatly improved (15 abstinent, 16 < 50 percent of baseline smoking).

Schmahl and coworkers[70] systematically replicated the study by Lublin and Joslyn. A 2 × 2 experimental design with seven smokers per cell was employed. The subjects were recruited via posters placed on the University of Oregon campus. They were randomly assigned to either a rapid smoking plus warm, smoky air group condition or to rapid smoking plus mentholated air, and the groups were further broken down into 2- or 4-week follow-up interval groups.

The procedure was identical for the two groups. The subjects were instructed to light up whenever they wished. As they did so, the blower was started. Every 6 s, the experimenter verbally commanded "smoke," and subjects inhaled normally. The experimenter monitored the subjects' behavior during the trial and provided additional lighted cigarettes if they could be tolerated. A trial was terminated when subjects could not tolerate another inhalation and signified this by repeating an autosuggested phrase, "I don't want to smoke anymore" and crushing out the cigarette. As soon as subjects felt they could tolerate another cigarette, the next trial was begun. The procedure continued until subjects could not tolerate another cigarette (i.e., another cigarette would possibly cause physical illness, throwing up, dizziness, or choking).

Subjects were instructed not to smoke until the next session. If the desire for a cigarette became overpowering, subjects were instructed to contact the experimenter for an impromptu session. Subjects were always seen initially for 3 consecutive days, then less frequently according to their ability to control their smoking. Booster sessions were available to help maintain abstinence. Follow-up telephone contact was implemented on a 2-week or 4-week schedule, depending on the subject's experimental assignment. To verify cessation, subjects submitted the name of an informant.

All subjects stopped smoking at the end of treatment and 16 were abstinent at 6 months (57 percent). The 4-week telephone contact proved superior to the 2-week contact, and there was no difference between the hot smoky air and mentholated air groups. The high sustained quit rate at 6 months underscores the robustness of the rapid smoking procedure.

In a follow-up study, Lichtenstein and colleagues[71] assigned habitual smokers to one of four experimental conditions: warm smoky air plus rapid smoking; warm, smoky air only; rapid smoking only; and an attention placebo control group. All but one subject was abstinent at the end of treatment, and 21 remained abstinent 6 months later. The three aversion groups were quite similar and, taken together, were smoking less at 6-month follow-up than the controls (60 percent abstinent for each experimental group versus 30 percent for the control group). The relatively high quit rate among the control group suggests that additional nonspecific factors were at play.

Lando[72] sought to replicate Lichtenstein's studies of rapid smoking and to compare its effectiveness to that of Resnick's[67] satiation procedure. Lando employed an appropriate control group, and he also used expired air carbon monoxide as an objective measure of cigarette smoking. Subjects were randomly assigned to rapid smoking, excessive smoking, or control conditions. In the rapid smoking procedure, subjects smoked each cigarette for a 3-min period, taking one puff every 6 s. In the excessive smoking condition, subjects were instructed to double their daily cigarette intake. In the control condition, subjects were paced at one puff every 30 s, rather than one puff every 6 s.

The quit rate at week 1 for subjects in the rapid smoking, excessive smoking, and control groups were 57, 46, and 29 percent, respectively, a marginal between-group difference. At week 2, quit rates of 64 and 54 percent for the rapid smoking and excessive smoking groups, although not different from one another, were superior to that of the control group (29 percent). However, the difference between groups diminished by month 1 (43, 38, and 29 percent for rapid smoking, excessive smoking, and control groups, respectively). Twelve-month follow-up revealed marked relapse, with no difference between conditions.

While Lando's study failed to provide unequivocal support for the efficacy of aversive smoke paradigms, there was a general sense of enthusiasm that aversive smokers techniques were more effective than other techniques and methods available at the time. Subsequent studies began to address the question of how to enhance the effectiveness of aversive smoking, ultimately leading to the inclusion of aversive smoking in comprehensive multicomponent interventions (see below). Danaher[73] investigated the efficacy of combining rapid smoking and training in self-control skills for maintaining nonsmoking. Fifty habitual smokers were assigned a 3-week treatment program emphasizing rapid smoking plus self-control, rapid smoking plus "filler" discussion, normal-paced placebo smoking plus self-control, or placebo smoking plus "filler" discussion.

Treatment was divided into two sequential phases focused on preparation and aversive smoking. During preparation, subjects were told to delay quitting during the first week and to concentrate instead on preparation for quitting. A 23-page manual of self-control maintenance skills was used during that time (as well as throughout the treatment) by subjects assigned to the self-control conditions. The self-control manual included sections on stimulus control of smoking, deep muscle relaxation, alternative behaviors, cognitive control, and self-reward. Subjects assigned to the discussion conditions gained insight into their smoking. The rapid smoking procedures followed those of Lichtenstein and colleagues.[71]

The reported quit rates at end of treatment were 63.6, 72.7, 78.6, and 57.1 percent for subjects assigned to placebo smoking plus discussion, placebo smoking plus self-control, rapid smoking plus discussion, and rapid smoking plus self-control, respectively. The high quit rates for the placebo groups suggest that nonspecific factors played a significant role. At 13 weeks follow-up, the quit rates for the above conditions were 27.3, 27.3, 35.7, and 21.4 percent, respec-

tively. Between group differences were not obtained at either time period, and the study failed to enhance the impact of rapid smoking on smoking cessation by adding a self-management component.

Best and coworkers[74] undertook a series of studies aimed at developing effective smoking cessation procedures for public health and preventive medical utilization. Best's group sought to combine aversive smoking techniques to generate high initial cessation rates with self-management procedures to sustain abstinence in a community sample.

Two aversive smoking procedures, satiation and rapid smoking, were compared in the context of a self-management training smoking cessation program developed for public health utilization. Sixty male and female smokers were assigned to satiation only, rapid smoking only, or satiation plus rapid smoking. They were seen individually for four sessions. The aversive smoking and self-management procedures were introduced first in the clinic, with set protocols for carrying out the activities at home.

Outcome data for the study showed similar rates of smoking cessation for each group at the end of treatment and during follow-up. The reported quit rates at the end of treatment were 75, 50, and 75 percent for satiation only, rapid smoking only, and satiation plus rapid smoking, respectively. At 6 months, the quit rates were 40.7, 55, and 45 percent (based on subjects who completed treatment and were available for follow-up). The high sustained 6-month quit rate in this community sample provided further impetus for combining aversive smoking procedures with self-management and other behavioral techniques.

Hall and coworkers[75] studied the efficacy and safety of rapid smoking therapy in patients with cardiac and pulmonary disease. In a previous study of healthy smokers,[76] this research group successfully replicated the earlier works by Lichtenstein and colleagues (i.e., 60 percent abstinent at 6 months) by adhering closely to their original protocol. In the 1984 study, 18 smokers with documented cardiopulmonary disease underwent rapid smoking with follow-up visits 12 and 24 months after treatment. Biochemical verified self-report data showed that 50 percent of all subjects had not smoked through the 2-year follow-up visit, whereas a waiting list control group had 0 percent abstinent subjects at the 2-year follow-up visit. Moreover, monitoring and cardiac testing during the rapid smoking procedure failed to reveal evidence of myocardial ischemia or significant cardiac arrythmia. These findings support the use of the "original" rapid smoking method and its safe and effective use in patients with mild to moderate cardiopulmonary disease and those who have had previous uncomplicated heart attacks.[75]

The emerging picture is that the rapid smoking technique, and, perhaps, satiation therapy as well, are among the most effective techniques for generating initial smoking cessation, and the long-term abstinence rates obtained with these procedures also are quite good. Of course, not everyone obtained results consistent with these observations.[77,78] Hall and colleagues[75] speculated that much of the variability in the literature may be due to modification of the rapid smoking procedure. Since the original reports by Lichtenstein and his colleagues in the early 1970s, researchers and clinicians restricted or controlled the number of sessions, conducted treatment in groups, added additional components and/or booster sessions, or had clients rapid smoke at home.

A robust intervention should allow for variation of procedure, and it is necessary to try different approaches to meet the needs of smokers in diverse clinical, medical, public health, worksite, and research settings. As can be seen below, the next generation of studies on rapid smoking and other aversive smoke techniques imbedded the procedure within a multicomponent treatment program, which now has emerged as a standard behavioral approach to modifying smoking. In addition, inclusion of pharmacologic regimens in the mix have added to the impact of the rapid smoking procedure.

Concern about potential adverse health effects of aversive smoking cannot and should not be easily dismissed.[79-81] Miller and coworkers[81] concluded their thoughtful discussion with the following: "The potential acute dangers of rapid smoking should be recognized. The well documented health hazards of chronic cigarette smoking seem to justify the use of these techniques if appropriate precautions are taken. The search for safer and more effective means of helping smokers break the habit needs to be continued."

Hackett and Horan[82] developed an alternative, "risk-free," aversive smoking procedure for use within multicomponent behavioral treatment programs. They asked college students while smoking to focus on the realistic aversive consequences of smoking (e.g., stains on the fingers and teeth, burning sensation in the mouth and throat), hence the name *focused smoking*.

Briefly, their comprehensive program consists of eight treatment sessions extended over a period of 5 weeks following 2 weeks of baseline.[82] The subjects met four times during week 1, twice during week 2, and once in the third and fifth weeks. The sessions lasted approximately 1½ h, with the first 30 to 40 min devoted to the following counseling strategies: peer and family contracting, thought stopping, cognitive restructuring, and cue-controlled relaxation. During the remainder of each session, the subjects underwent the focused smoking treatment. Subjects sat facing a blank wall while smoking at their normal rate and being cued by the experimenter to focus on the discomforts of smoking (at first, burning in throat, bad taste in mouth, light headaches, and feelings of nausea, and later a dull headache, shakiness, sweating, an uncomfortable heavy tired feeling, and difficulty breathing). Reminders to concentrate only on the effects of smoking also were included.

At the end of treatment, all nine subjects reported they had stopped smoking (100 percent). Quit rates at 1, 3, and 6 months were 77.8, 66.7, and 55.6 percent. The 55.6 percent success rate at 6 months compares quite favorably with the 50 percent success rates obtained in their previous work with rapid smoking.[83] Moreover, subjects reported the focused smoking treatment to be as aversive as rapid smoking. The authors concluded that focused smoking is an effective alternative to the rapid smoking procedures.

Taste satiation or smoke holding was first reported by Tori.[84] He instructed subjects to draw smoke directly into their mouths and hold it there for 30 s while breathing normally through their nose and concentrating on the unpleasant sensations evolved by the smoke. When inhalation occurred, subjects were instructed to hold the smoke in their mouths while they breathed through their nose and to concentrate their attention on their lungs. After 20 s, they were allowed to inhale burning vapors and then to exhale the smoke through their nose. Smoke holding continued until feelings of discomfort and nausea caused loss of desire for cigarettes. Treatment lasted five consecutive days.

Tori also provided five weekly sessions of hypnotherapy, so it was not possible to assess the independent effects of smoke holding. At a 6-month follow-up, 68 percent of the 25 smoke-holding subjects reported that they were abstinent. Tori also treated 10 smokers with rapid smoking and hypnotherapy. Sixty percent reported abstinence at 6 months.[84]

As noted by Schwartz,[39] three other investigative groups have reported results for smoke-holding studies. Kopel and colleagues[85] achieved a 33 percent quit rate at 6-month follow-up. Lando and McGovern,[86] combining smoke holding with nicotine fading, reported a 1-year quit rate of 44 percent. (Nicotine fading had a 19 percent quit rate.) Walker and Franzini[87] achieved a 50 percent quit rate at 6 months. Schwartz[39] noted that smoke holding appears to be a safe procedure, but not enough data are available to assess its efficacy.

MULTICOMPONENT BEHAVIORAL GROUP PROGRAMS

Lando[88] assessed the efficacy of a multifaceted maintenance program against a control condition that was limited to aversive conditioning. All subjects underwent 1 week of aversive conditioning (satiation). For experimental subjects, this procedure was supplemented by an additional 2 months of formal treatment sessions that included contractual management, booster sessions, and structured group contact and support. At a 6-month follow-up, 13 of 17 experimental subjects (76 percent) were abstinent compared to 6 of 17 controls (35 percent).

Elliott and Denney[89] designed a study to evaluate a broad-based treatment package for the reduction of smoking and to compare its effectiveness with a single treatment procedure (rapid smoking), which constituted a major component within the treatment package. The selection of components for the treatment package was based on research examining the effectiveness of each component as a single treatment procedure.

Male and female subjects were assigned to one of four conditions: "package" treatment, rapid-smoking, nonspecific treatment, and untreated control. Each of the three treatment conditions was administered to groups of six to nine subjects. Subjects attended three sessions per week for 3 weeks. A description of each treatment follows:

Package treatment: In addition to nonspecific treatments, subjects received eight specific components: rapid smoking, relaxation training, covert sensitization (aversive scenes and relief scenes), systematic desensitization (i.e., relax and imagine scenes that commonly "elicit" smoking), self-reward and punishment (for reaching or not reaching targeted goals), cognitive restructuring, behavioral rehearsal, and emotional role playing (participants prepare and enact scenes in which they learned that they had lung cancer and had to inform loved ones).

Rapid smoking: This treatment was patterned after the rapid-smoking treatments described by Lichtenstein and coworkers.[71] Subjects received two rapid smoking trials during each of nine treatment sessions.

Nonspecific treatment: Subjects received the standard nonspecific procedure, including lectures, educational material,
mild encouragement, and data collection. Subjects engaged
in nondirective discussion.
Untreated controls: These subjects received no treatment. They
were told that they could use anything on their own to
quit smoking.

Subjects in each of the three treatment conditions were
randomly divided into three booster session conditions: specific booster condition (three booster sessions, each of which
included a brief refresher lecture, mild encouragement, and
two additional rapid smoking trials), nonspecific booster condition (three sessions of refresher lectures and mild encouragement), and no booster sessions.

At the end of treatment, the package condition contained
a statistically significant larger proportion of abstainers (65
percent) than the control condition (0 percent), rapid smoking
(26 percent), or the nonspecific condition (33 percent). At
6-month follow-up, the same findings held (45, 0, 17, and 12
percent for the package, no treatment, rapid smoking, and
nonspecific conditions, respectively). Booster sessions had
no effect.

Powell and McCann[90] evaluated the efficacy of a multiple
treatment program and three maintenance strategies. Fifty-
one subjects attended an introductory meeting and four
consecutive treatment meetings that were held 1 week later.
At the end of the initial treatment phase, subjects were randomly assigned to one of three maintenance conditions: (1)
a 4-week support group which offered an opportunity to
discuss feelings and thoughts, (2) a telephone contact system
which allowed subjects to phone one another, or (3) a no-
contact control group.

At the first group meeting, participants were given an
introductory booklet, *Quitter's Countdown,* which describes
a series of homework assignments to be carried out for the
5 days prior to treatment. The intensive treatment program
involved lectures, demonstrations, practice exercises, the
teaching of self-control procedures, and a novel aversion
method. Topics covered at the sessions included attitudes
related to the quitting process, cognitive control of cravings,
health hazards of smoking and the benefits of quitting, the
use of covert sensitization, eating management skills, relaxation training, mental imagery exercises, behavioral rehearsal, stimulus control, use of positive reinforcement, and
the development of incompatible behaviors.

Two aversive smoke strategies were used. The aversive
conditioning apparatus consisted of a large ashtray filled
with cigarette litter placed in front of each subject, cigarette
filters that were dipped in a bitter tasting anti-nail-biting
solution, a tape recording of loud white noise, and a slide
show presentation of diseased organs interspersed with popular magazine advertisements. Subjects were instructed to
smoke the first of four cigarettes using a procedure called
pinky puffing, in which the cigarette is held between the last
two fingers of the subject's nonsmoking hand, brought to
the side of the mouth opposite that with which the subject
usually smokes, and is puffed rather than inhaled. Puffing
causes a build up of bitter nicotine residue on the tongue.
Two other cigarettes were puffed quickly without inhaling
(smoke signaling), causing a hot sensation around the lips

and an accumulation of smoke in the eyes. Participants could
terminate the aversive procedure any time they chose.

At the end of the treatment phase, all 51 subjects reported
that they were abstinent. Reported abstinence rates at 2, 4, 6,
and 12 months were 84, 82, 76.5, and 63 percent, respectively.
There were no differences in abstinence rates among the
three maintenance conditions, and males and females were
equally successful.

MULTICOMPONENT BEHAVIORAL TREATMENT PLUS NICOTINE REPLACEMENT

Killen and colleagues[91] employed a multicomponent, aversive, smoke-holding procedure during the first week of the
cessation phase of a treatment protocol. Subjects then were
randomly assigned to one of three maintenance phase conditions for 6 weeks: (1) nicotine polacrilex (2 mg, ad lib basis);
(2) skills training and relapse prevention only; (3) combined
nicotine polacrilex (2 mg, ad lib) plus skills training. Expired
air carbon monoxide and serum thiocyanate served as objective measures of smoking.

Eighty-three percent stopped smoking at the end of the
1-week induction phase.[91] Nine months after the end of treatment, abstinence rates were as follows: nicotine polacrilex
alone, 23 percent; skills training alone, 30 percent; nicotine
polacrilex plus skills training, 50 percent.

Hall and coworkers[92] assigned 122 subjects to either (1)
intensive behavioral treatment, (2) nicotine gum (2 mg) in a
low-contact treatment, or (3) intensive behavioral intervention plus nicotine gum treatment. Subjects met in groups of
five to six with one of two psychologists experienced in the
treatment of tobacco dependence.

The behavioral treatment condition included 30-s aversive
smoking of three cigarettes, relapse-prevention skill training,
relaxation training, and written exercises to increase commitment, provided in fourteen 75-min sessions in an 8-week
period. Sessions were massed early in treatment and gradually faded. Subjects in the combined condition participated
in the same behavioral treatment. In addition, they received
2 mg nicotine gum (Nicorette). In the low-contact nicotine
gum condition, subjects met four times over a 3-week period.
They completed paper and pencil exercises on reasons for
smoking, read educational materials, and participated in
group discussion. In the latter two groups, gum was available
for 6 months from treatment start.

Assessments were held at 0, 2, 12, 26, and 52 weeks. Abstinence was verified by expired air carbon monoxide (<10
ppm) at all assessments. Also, serum thiocyanate levels (<85
mg/mL) and reports of significant others verified abstinence
at weeks 26 and 52. Biochemical measures failed to match
self-report in only three instances.[92]

Differences between the combined condition and the other
two conditions were significant at weeks 3, 12, and 26, but
not at week 52. For the combined condition, abstinence rates
were 95, 73, 59, and 44 percent at weeks 3, 12, 26, and 52.
Corresponding abstinence rates for the low-contact condition
were 81, 58, 47, and 37 percent. For the behavioral condition,
the quit rates were 78, 47, 31, and 28 percent, for weeks 3,
12, 26, and 52, respectively. Smokers with high blood cotinine
levels (i.e., highly dependent smokers) were more likely to be
helped by nicotine gum than were less-dependent smokers.
The utility of adding nicotine replacement to comprehen-

sive multicomponent behavioral treatment was similarly demonstrated by Baddely and coworkers.[93] Subjects were recruited by means of advertisements in the local press. From 65 volunteers, 24 subjects were selected, 12 of whom expressed a desire for nicotine gum (experimental group). They were matched as closely as possible for sex, number of cigarettes per day, years smoked, and number of past attempts to stop smoking, with 12 subjects who desired psychological treatment only.

The six-session multicomponent program was based on behavior modification principles. The program included set homework assignments, self-monitoring of smoking behavior, stimulus control techniques, nicotine fading, alternative behaviors, and structuring a system of rewards. The quit date was set for 3 weeks after the start of the program. One group of subjects received Nicorette (2 mg), whereas the other received behavioral treatment only. Subjects in the experimental group used the gum from the date on which they stopped smoking until they decided they could cope without it.

Smoking status was established by means of blood carbon monoxide levels. Blood samples were drawn at baseline, 6 weeks, and 6 months. Abstinence rates at 2 weeks, 6 weeks, and 6 months after the quit date were 67, 50, and 50 percent for the experimental group and 55, 27, and 27 percent for the control group.

Buchkremer and colleagues[94] studied the combination of multicomponent behavioral intervention and transdermal nicotine substitution ("patch"). One hundred thirty-one smokers, recruited via announcements in the local press, were randomly assigned to three different conditions. Although all smokers received behavioral training in self-controlled cigarette reduction, one group of smokers was additionally treated with nicotine patches, one group was additionally treated with placebo patches, and a third group did not receive any patch treatment.

The behavioral treatment consisted of a multimodal approach to a self-controlled, step-by-step reduction of cigarette smoking.[94] Key features of the program included an increase in cognitive dissonance, systematic control of smoking situations, contract management, and relapse prevention. The program consisted of nine weekly sessions held within small training groups under the direction of skilled psychologists.

The self-adhesive patches were applied subsequent to the first week of behavioral training. A gradual increase in dosage was achieved by increasing the size of the patch. One week before termination of the behavioral cessation program, application of the patches was stopped for all subjects, with a gradual decrease in dosage. The patches were worn continuously (i.e., 24 h per day). Urine specimens for nicotine and cotinine content validated smoking status.

At the end of the treatment, the nicotine-treated subjects reached a total abstinence rate of 60 percent, compared with 51.2 percent for the placebo-treated subjects and 44.4 percent for the no-patch controls. The difference between nicotine-treated and placebo-treated smokers was not significant ($p < .10$). The nicotine group was significantly superior to the no-nicotine control group ($p < .05$). Follow-up data were not reported.[94]

The Johns Hopkins Smoking Cessation Program was a multicomponent program that combined cognitive behavioral techniques (self-monitoring, nicotine fading, stimulus control, health education, carbon monoxide monitoring, group support, talks by ex-smokers, and supervised use of nicotine chewing gum).[95] The program consisted of 10 sessions held over a 9-month period. Eight groups of 10 to 15 participants were conducted over a 3-year period.

After responding to print media announcements of a hospital-based smoking cessation program, participants completed a baseline questionnaire on smoking and medical history, underwent weight, blood pressure, CO, and respiration rate measurement, and filled out the Fagerstrom Tolerance Questionnaire. Smoking status of participants was determined after completion of the program through telephone interviews conducted over a 3-month period. Self-report of nonsmoking was confirmed with breath samples of carbon monoxide (CO). The average time to follow-up was 20 months from program initiation, with a range of 12 to 31 months. The response rate was 80 percent (89 of 111 eligible interviews).

Participants were considered to be nonsmokers if they reported having been abstinent from cigarettes 1 year after the program and also were not smoking at the time of the follow-up interview.[95] At follow-up, 28 smokers of 111 possible interviewees were nonsmokers (25 percent). Individuals who successfully quit smoking were less-dependent smokers, were more educated, had lower levels of stress, and had fewer friends who were smokers. Women were more than twice as likely to be smokers at 1-year follow-up than were men.[95] Of the 89 participants interviewed, 82 percent quit for at least 24 h after the designated quit date. The majority of the relapses occurred within the first 60 days after quitting. In 57 percent of the smokers who relapsed, the relapse occurred during periods of stress at home or at work.

Participants were asked to rate the helpfulness of each of the 10 program components on a scale of 1 to 10. The highest ratings were for self-monitoring, group support, cutting down the number of cigarettes, and CO monitoring. The lowest ratings were for information on health risks, nicotine gum, and information on diet and exercise. The rating of the overall program was higher than the rating of any individual component.[95]

Self-Help Techniques for Smoking Cessation

BIBLIOTHERAPY

One of the most popular forms of self-help smoking cessation therapy is bibliotherapy, and there are numerous self-help books, brochures, and "kits" available.[39,96] Audiotapes, videocassettes, and computer and CD-ROM programs also are available. Glasgow and colleagues[97] studied the effects of self-help books and amount of therapist contact on smoking cessation. Eighty adult cigarette smokers were recruited via advertisement in local media. A 3×2 factorial design was employed to evaluate three treatments (two self-help behavior therapy manuals and a minimal treatment control condition) under self-administered and therapist-administered conditions.

The manuals employed were developed by Danaher and Lichtenstein[98] and Pomerleau and Pomerleau.[99] The former is a 154-page manual which emphasizes the importance of recording and combating urges to smoke. Progressive muscle relaxation is also encouraged. In preparation for quitting, readers are given three options: setting a target date and quitting on their own, a monetary contract with a friend for nonsmoking, or normal paced aversive smoking (Danaher and Lichtenstein also used rapid smoking, but Glasgow's group did not offer that option in its study). Later chapters discuss managing thoughts about smoking, controlling weight, and planning ahead for difficult situations.

The Pomerleau and Pomerleau[99] book is a 90-page manual which stresses gradual smoking reduction by eliminating smoking in progressively more difficult situations. Readers are presented with a large number of stimulus control techniques (e.g., no more smoking in the car, do not linger at the table after a meal, post no-smoking signs) and alternative behaviors (try deep breathing instead of smoking, brush teeth immediately after drinking coffee, chew on a cinnamon stick instead of smoking). The latter part of the book is devoted to dealing with problems that may arise when quitting smoking.

Subjects in the control condition received an *I Quit Kit,* published by the American Cancer Society (ACS).[100] The multimedia kit consists primarily of motivational material (e.g., poster, buttons, and information on health hazards of smoking). A variety of tips are listed in a 20-page booklet. Tips include setting a target quit date and engaging in alternative behaviors (i.e., drinking water, taking deep breaths, or taking a walk instead of smoking).

Subjects assigned to each of the above conditions were randomly assigned to self-administered or therapist-administered conditions.[97] Subjects in the therapist-administered condition met with a therapist in groups of four to six subjects eight times throughout the treatment. During the weekly meetings, therapists checked on subjects' progress, helped solve problems, reviewed material, and led subjects in demonstrations of treatment procedures (e.g., progressive relaxation training, deep breathing, ex-smokers' imagery ritual). Expired air carbon monoxide served as an objective measure of cigarette smoking.

The treatment programs lasted 8 weeks. A follow-up was scheduled 6 months later. Eighty-five of the eighty-eight subjects beginning the program completed treatment and were available for the posttest. Eighty subjects participated in the 6-month follow-up. A 3×2 analysis of variance of the proportion of subjects reporting abstinence at posttest revealed a significant effect of condition of administration and a significant condition $\times$ type of treatment interaction. In the Danaher and Lichtenstein and the Pomerleau and Pomerleau conditions, therapist presence was associated with a large improvement in abstinence rates (47 versus 8 percent for self-administered conditions). In contrast, subjects in the *I Quit Kit* program reported doing slightly better under self-administered than therapist-administered conditions (27 versus 14 percent abstinence).

Quit rates for all conditions diminished at 6 months follow-up (overall quit rate of 11 versus 27 percent at posttest). Otherwise, the pattern of results was similar to that of the posttest. For the Danaher and Lichtenstein manual, the self-administered condition yielded a quit rate of 8 percent compared with 17 percent for the therapist-administered condition. For the Pomerleau and Pomerleau manual, the 6-month quit rates were 0 and 24 percent for the self-administered

and therapist conditions, respectively. For the ACS's *I Quit Kit,* abstinence rates at 6 months were 14 percent for the self-administered condition and 0 percent for the therapist-administered conditions, respectively.[97]

The overall pattern of results is somewhat perplexing. It is possible that the manuals prepared by Pomerleau and Pomerleau and Danaher and Lichtenstein, while comprehensive, were a bit *too* complex. Thus, smokers did better with therapist assistance than on their own. The ACS's *I Quit Kit,* on the other hand, was less comprehensive, and, perhaps, more easy to use on their own. Therapist contact for this condition added very little. Overall, the 6-month quit rates were quite modest, particularly for the more costly therapist-led conditions. The 6-month quit rates of 8 and 14 percent for Danaher and Lichtenstein's manual and the *I Quit Kit* are more in line with what is expected for public-health-oriented low-cost minimal-intervention self-help programs.

The American Lung Association developed two manuals for helping smokers quit and remain abstinent. They are the 64-page cessation manual entitled *Freedom from Smoking in 20 Days* and the 28-page maintenance manual, *A Lifetime of Freedom from Smoking.*[101] *Freedom from Smoking in 20 Days* contains the Horn test of why a person smokes, a method of keeping records of smoking behavior, information on identifying smoking triggers, and behavioral contracts for quitting smoking. It also includes information on weight control, deep breathing and muscle relaxation exercises, and preparation for smoking situations. *A Lifetime of Freedom from Smoking* also emphasizes techniques for coping with situations which trigger the urge to smoke.

Davis and colleagues[101] studied the effectiveness of the ALA materials under conditions which involved no-face-to-face contact with smokers. Five local lung associations participated. They recruited participants ($n = 1237$) through newspaper advertisements, flyers, and media announcements. All program materials were mailed to the participants, and follow-up data were collected via telephone interviews at 1, 3, 6, 9, and 12 months after the materials were mailed.

Participants were randomly assigned to one of four experimental groups: ALA leaflets only (eight existing ALA leaflets on how to stop smoking, smoking and health, smokers' rights, effects of parental smoking on children, etc.), leaflets plus maintenance manual; cessation manual; and cessation manual plus maintenance manual.

The initial quit rate (verbal report) was about 20 percent of the total sample. This was followed immediately by substantial recidivism, dropping to 10 percent at 1 month follow-up.[101] The group which received leaflets and the maintenance manual had the highest initial quit rate (25 percent) and the group which received leaflets only, the lowest (16 percent).

After the initial recidivism, nonsmoking prevalence was stable through the first 6 months but rose steadily thereafter, yielding a 1-year point prevalence quit rate of 16 percent. Only about 3 percent of the subjects were continuously abstinent from end of treatment to 12 months. Although the initial and long-term quit rates are modest, so too was the intensity of treatment. From a public health point of view, this study lends considerable support for the efficacy of self-help cessation approaches.

A study conducted in Australia examined the effects of a four-lesson smoking cessation correspondence course designed to provide small manageable amounts of information, a structured program sequence, and external prompts and reminders.[102] The impact of tailoring (personalizing) the intervention was also examined.

Participants were recruited via media. Three hundred twelve smokers responded. They were sent a course registration form and cover letter, which gave a brief description of the course and requested that they complete a registration form and return it with a $20 course fee. Of those who responded initially, 67 percent (218) entered the program.

Participants were assigned randomly to a "quit kit" control condition or to one of two intervention conditions. Those in the control condition had their course fee returned with a letter of apology, explaining that the course was oversubscribed. A quit kit was enclosed, and they were advised to try it. The kit included a five-day cessation plan, tips for cessation, instruction in progressive muscle relaxation, a cigarette pack wrapping sheet for self-monitoring, and a card for listing reasons for cessation and potential benefits.

The "standard correspondence course" consisted of four lessons mailed at weekly intervals. Lessons dealt with preparing for cessation, initial cessation, coping with urges to smoke, and maintenance. Course content included advice on progressive muscle relaxation, deep breathing, cognitive and behavioral coping skills, self-instruction goal setting and covert verbalization techniques, and advice on social support and contingency contracts. The cessation technique recommended was to halve daily smoking rates for 3 days prior to a time chosen in advance as the quit date.

The "personalized course" used the same content, sequence of lessons, and mailing schedule as the standard course. Rather than being photocopied, the lessons for the personalized course were generated for each individual using a computer. Personalized course segments were sets of extra paragraphs inserted into the text of the standard course. The contents of these were determined by information from the course registration form relating to motivation to attempt cessation, number of cigarettes smoked per day, subjective belief in addiction, concerns about weight gain, and self-efficacy. For example, one personalized course segment stated, "From what you have told us, you are not very confident about being able to resist the offer of a cigarette in social situations. You should practice ways to say no nicely and plan in advance what to say; you could be firm, but also make a joke of it to help the other person not to feel offended by your refusal."[102]

Participants were sent the first lesson of the course within 2 weeks of returning the registration form. The three subsequent lessons were sent out at 1-week intervals. Feedback forms requesting information on use of course components and on current smoking status with a prepaid return envelop were inserted in each of the four lessons. Up to $10 of the course fee was refundable contingent on the return of feedback forms: $2.50 per form returned. Follow-up telephone calls were made to assess smoking status 5 days after the last mailing and again at 3 and 9 months. Saliva and urine thiocyanate were collected from a random sample of nonsmokers at the 5-day and 9-month data collection points.

At the end of the course, the reported quit rates were 2.5, 19, and 22 percent for the quit kit control, standard course, and personalized course. At 9 months, the quit rates were 7.5, 18, and 10 percent. Based on a small sample of thiocyanate determinations, cessation rates should be adjusted downward by one-fifth.[102] These data show modest efficacy for the correspondence course, at least initially, and little support for the value of personalizing the course. Overall, the findings are consistent with the general literature on self-help interventions.

Prochaska and coworkers[103] recruited 756 volunteers who responded to newspaper advertisements seeking participants to test self-help materials developed for smokers in various "stages of change." All subjects were cigarette smokers at the time of enrollment and were in one of three stages of change: precontemplation ($n = 93$), contemplation ($n = 435$), and preparation ($n = 228$). Subjects in precontemplation were not seriously considering quitting smoking within the next 6 months; those in contemplation were seriously considering quitting within the next 6 months; subjects in preparation were planning to quit within the next 30 days and had made at least one 24-h quit attempt in the past year.

Four interventions were compared: (1) standardized manuals (ALA's *Freedom from Smoking in 20 Days* and *Lifetime of Freedom from Smoking* and the American Cancer Society's *50 Most Often Asked Questions*); (2) individualized manuals based on Prochaska and colleagues'[104] transtheoretical model of behavior change; (3) interactive reports (in addition to the stage-appropriate individualized manuals, participants were sent a series of three personalized computer reports at the start of treatment and at 1 and 6 months); and (4) personalized counselor calls, including both the transtheoretical model-based manuals and the interactive computer-generated progress reports as well as a series of short calls from counselors to provide personalized feedback.

Five manuals corresponded to each stage of change: (1) precontemplation, (2) contemplation, (3) action, (4) maintenance, and (5) relapse. Table 28–2 provides a brief description of each stage-related manual. On the basis of their pretest scores, participants were sent the manual matched to their individual stage of change and manuals for all the subsequent stages. Participants who took action and relapsed were sent the recycling manual following assessment at either the 1-month or 6-month follow-up, depending on when they relapsed.

At 6- and 12-month follow-up, the standardized manual and individualized manual conditions yielded similar reported quit rates (24-h abstinence) of about 7 percent. At 18 months, the individualized manual yielded significantly

TABLE 28-2 Stage-Related Self-Help Manuals

Stage	Content
Precontemplation	Consciousness raising self-reevaluation how to develop more balanced views about smoking
Contemplation	Analysis of smoking and quitting histories; consequences of continuing to smoke; benefits of quitting. Self-image as smoker and former smoker; decisional balance
Action	Traditional behavioral interventions
Maintenance	Traditional relapse prevention
Relapse	Encouragement of recycling through each stage

SOURCE: Prochaska et al.[103]

higher quit rates than the standardized manual condition (about 18 versus 10 percent). The interactive report condition yielded the highest quit rates (about 15, 21, and 25 percent at 6, 12, and 18 months, respectively). The personalized counselor condition yielded somewhat lower quit rates of 13, 17, and 18 percent on assessments at 6, 12, and 18 months. A comparable pattern of results held for prolonged abstinence (not smoking at two consecutive follow-ups).

Prochaska and coworkers[103] concluded that the results suggest that providing smokers intervention feedback about their stages of changes, decisional balance, processes of change, self-efficacy, and temptation levels in critical smoking situations can produce greater success than just providing the best self-help manuals currently available. Moreover, the superiority of the computer system over personalized telephone counseling suggests that a computer system can deliver expert help in a much more cost-effective manner than trained counselors.

BIBLIOTHERAPY PLUS NICOTINE GUM

Lando and colleagues[105] tested the effectiveness of behavioral self-help materials specifically written to accompany nicotine-containing chewing gum (Nicorette). Subjects included 187 women and 117 men. Their average age was 41.5 years, and they smoked about 31 cigarettes per day. The self-help materials were provided to patients who received prescriptions for Nicorette from 15 participating study physicians.

The experimental self-help materials consisted of a typewritten booklet in which a number of topics were discussed, including coping strategies, self-reward, relaxation, weight gain, proper use of Nicorette, stressful situations, negative affect, "want/should" ratios, and "positive addictions." Patients assigned to a control condition received the American Cancer Society pamphlet entitled *Danger: The Facts about Smoking.* This pamphlet was oriented more to providing information than to offering self-help quit strategies.

Patients were instructed by physicians to quit smoking immediately and were provided with prescriptions for Nicorette. All patients began with the 2-mg dose of gum but were given the option to switch to a 4-mg dose at a second visit 5 to 7 days later. Follow-up assessments were conducted at 1, 3, 6, and 12 months after the quit date. A proportion of patients who claimed abstinence at 6 and 12 months provided saliva thiocyanate samples to corroborate their self-reported abstinence.[105]

One week after the initial physician visit, only 217 of 304 subjects reported using the nicotine gum. By one month, gum use was down to 152 subjects (50 percent of sample). While gum use declined further to approximately 25 percent of patients at 6-month follow-up, 20.7 percent of patients continued to use gum at 12 months.

Abstinence data at each follow-up visit failed to reveal a significant difference between use of the specially prepared self-help materials and the ACS brochure. For the self-help material group, quit rates were 42, 34, 28, 24, and 19 percent at 1 week, 1 month, 3 months, 6 months, and 12 months. The corresponding quit rates for the comparison group were 45, 39, 34, 29, and 22 percent. Continuing gum users were far more likely than non-gum users to be abstinent through 6-month follow-up. Users maintained more than 2 to 1 abstinence advantage over nonusers. Saliva thiocyanate data revealed a false reporting incidence of just under 10 percent.

A similar pattern of results was reported by Killen and coworkers.[106] Twelve hundred eighteen smokers who were able to quit smoking for 48 h (confirmed by expired air carbon monoxide) were randomly assigned to one of 12 cells in a 4×3 factorial experiment. A pharmacologic factor contained four levels: nicotine gum, delivered ad lib or on a fixed regimen, placebo gum, and no gum. A self-guided behavioral treatment factor contained three levels: self-selected relapse prevention modules, randomly administered modules, and no modules.

Those receiving nicotine gum were more likely to be abstinent at the 2- and 6-month follow-ups. However, the main effect for gum was significant only for men at each assessment. The fixed regimen accounted for most of the gum effect, 25 percent quit rate at 6 and 12 months. However, there was no gum effect for the relapse prevention module factor. Although participants in the trial said they liked the relapse prevention strategies, they failed to put them into practice.

GRADUATED EXTERNAL FILTER SYSTEMS

One Step at a Time is a smoking withdrawal product marketed in the United States by Teledyne Water Pik. It is a four-step, 8-week stop smoking system consisting of four progressively stronger external plastic filters. According to the manufacturer, filter 1 filters approximately 25 percent of tars and nicotine and filter 4 filters approximately 90 percent. Smokers advance from one filter to the next in 2-week steps and attempt to quit smoking in 8 weeks. If they are not successful, they may elect to use filter 4 to achieve a safer level of smoking.[107]

To study the efficacy of *One Step at a Time* for smoking cessation, Hymowitz and coworkers[107] recruited 130 men and women, age 35 or above, with no prior history of using *One Step at a Time.* Subjects were assigned randomly to one of three experimental groups (group 1, quit smoking on own; group 2, placebo filter; and Group 3, *One Step at a Time*).

All participants were invited individually to the clinic six times in a 16-month period. Following an initial interview and explanation of the study, paper and pencil and a variety of other tests were administered, including measurement of expired air carbon monoxide, which served as an objective measure of smoking. All subjects were given a brief stop smoking message and "assigned" a quit date in 8 weeks. They were scheduled to return for visit 2 within 1 week following their quit date.[107]

At visit 2, the reported quit rates for groups 1, 2, and 3 were 21, 14, and 26 percent, respectively. These differences were not statistically significant.[107] Sixty percent of smokers who quit smoking at visit 2 remained abstinent at visits 3, 4, 5, and 6. These data include 7 of 9 initial quitters (78 percent) in group 1, 3 of 6 (50 percent) in group 2, and 7 of 12 (58 percent) in group 3.

Participants in groups 1 and 2 who did not quit smoking at visit 2 were given *One Step at a Time* to use, and group 3 smokers at visit 2 were given additional filter 4s. Nine more participants stopped smoking for the first time at visits 3, 4, and 5. Seven quit smoking following use of the filters, and two quit on their own.[107]

Overall, the data fail to document the utility of the filters for smoking cessation. Yet, there may be a place for the filters and other stop smoking devices in the antismoking arena. They may serve as a stimulus to stop smoking for people who neither stop on their own nor seek professional assistance. Successful quitters in group 3 attributed their success at visit 2 to the filters, as did several other quitters in the other groups who used the filters to quit smoking after failing to quit smoking on their own or with placebos. Hymowitz and colleagues[107] suggested that future efforts should be directed toward improving the impact of various self-help smoking devices by using them in combination or as adjuncts to more formal stop smoking procedures.

There are, of course, many other approaches to self-help and minimal intervention on smoking. Recent reviews[108-110] include programs offered via print and electronic media, physician and dental offices, and mail (correspondence course). While the quit rates obtained with self-help approaches are modest when compared with more labor-intensive approaches, they have the potential of reaching a large diverse population of smokers who do not wish to participate in group programs. Self-help programs have an important role to play in national and international antismoking arenas, and it is likely they will continue to proliferate in the future.

Nicotine Replacement Therapy

The effectiveness of medications for stopping smoking has been examined in several recent reviews.[17,39,111] Research findings on the efficacy of lobeline, clonidine, naltraxone, benzodiazepine anxiolytics, beta blockers, and antidepressants for smoking cessation have been either negative or inconsistent.[111] At best, these medications may prove effective when used by skilled clinicians with selected patients. The APA[17] has classified clonidine, buspirone, antidepressants, and anorectics as promising regimens, worthy of further study and clinical testing.* Data on the efficacy of nicotine replacement therapy, on the other hand, are much stronger.[17]

The goal of nicotine replacement therapy is to relieve withdrawal, which allows the smoker to focus on habit and conditioning factors when attempting to quit. After the acute withdrawal period, nicotine replacement therapy is gradually reduced so that few withdrawal symptoms should occur.

---

* Since this chapter was prepared, a double-blind, placebo-controlled trial of a sustained-release form of the antidepressant, bupropion, for smoking cessation was undertaken (Hurt RD, Sachs DPL, Glover ED, et al: A comparison of sustained-release bupropion and placebo for smoking cessation. *N Engl J Med* 337:1195, 1997). At the end of 7 weeks of treatment, the rates of smoking cessation ($n = 615$), confirmed by carbon monoxide measurement, were 19.0 percent in the placebo group, 28.8 percent in the 100-mg group, 38.6 percent in the 150-mg group, and 44.2 percent in the 300-mg group ($p < .001$). At 1 year, the respective rates were 14.4 percent, 19.6 percent, 22.9 percent, and 23.1 percent. The rates for the 150-mg group ($p = .02$) and the 300-mg group ($p = .01$)—but not the 100-mg group—were significantly better than those for placebo. An editorial by Neal L. Benowitz ("Treating Tobacco Addiction-Nicotine or No Nicotine?", published in the same issue of *The New England Journal of Medicine*) provides additional discussion of the role of antidepressants and other forms of medication in the management of nicotine addiction.

There are four types of nicotine replacement products currently available (Table 28–3). They are nicotine gum, nicotine patch, nicotine nasal spray, and nicotine inhalers. Nicotine gum may be used ad lib, one piece every 15 to 30 min as needed, or according to a set schedule (e.g., one piece per hour). The gum is used for about 3 to 6 months, although some smokers may use it even longer.

The nicotine patch releases nicotine which is absorbed through the skin. Some patches are worn for 24 h, whereas one is used for 16 h per day. Typically, the initial patch dose is 21 to 22 mg (24 h) or 15 mg (16-h patch). After 4 to 6 weeks, patients are usually tapered to a middle dose for 2 to 4 weeks, and then to a lower dose for several weeks. Usually, the course of therapy is completed by 12 weeks.

Nicotine nasal spray is a nicotine solution in a nasal spray bottle similar to those used with antihistamines. Smokers are to use the product ad lib up to 30 times a day for 12 weeks, including a tapering period.

Nicotine inhalers are plugs of nicotine placed inside hollow cigarette-like rods. The inhaler is to be used ad lib for about 12 weeks.

EFFICACY

Many studies have shown that nicotine replacement therapy decreases withdrawal symptoms in outpatient settings.[17] Anxiety, anger or irritability, depression, difficulty concentrating, and impatience are usually relieved by nicotine replacement. Insomnia and weight gain are not consistently reduced.

Eleven metaanalyses of more than 50 studies that included a psychosocial therapy (usually behavioral therapy) along with nicotine replacement all conclude that nicotine gum and nicotine patch increase long-term quit rates by a factor of 1.6 to 2.4.[17] The three studies of nicotine nasal spray reported increases in abstinence in the same range, whereas the one study of nicotine inhaler found a tripling of the quit rate.[17]

Often, physician interventions for smoking cessation consist of brief advice plus prescription for nicotine replacement.[17] Although early reviews indicate nicotine gum was not more effective than placebo in this setting, more recent metaanalyses indicated nicotine gum increases quit rates by a factor of 1.5. In addition, controlled studies have found that nicotine gum doubles quit rates even when given with no adjunctive therapy.[17] The nicotine patch is also effective when given with minimal or no therapy, and it doubles quit rates.

NICOTINE GUM

Nicotine gum is available in two strengths, 4 and 2 mg nicotine in each piece of gum. The nicotine is bound to an ion-exchange resin which allows it to be released slowly as the gum is chewed. About 90 percent of the nicotine is released after 30 min of chewing, the rate of release depending on the vigor and rate of chewing.[112] The nicotine is absorbed through the buccal mucosa and, since the rate of absorption is pH-dependent, the gum contains a buffer that keeps the pH in the mouth at about 8.5 as the gum is chewed. Nicotine that is swallowed is largely wasted.

Absorption of nicotine from the gum is slower than from a cigarette.[112] This is partly caused by the slow release of

TABLE 28-3 Nicotine Replacement Products

Product	Dose	Mode of Nicotine Delivery	Duration
Nicotine gum	2 mg (ad lib)	Nicotine released from resin by chewing (buccal)	3–6 months
Nicotine patch	21–22 mg (24-h patch) 15 mg (16-h patch) Tapering doses 14 mg (24 h) 10 mg (10 h) 7 mg (24 h) 5 mg (16 h)	Transdermal absorption	6–12 weeks
Nicotine nasal spray	1 mg droplet per administration (ad lib up to 30 times per day)	Nasal absorption	12 weeks
Nicotine inhaler		Buccal absorption	12 weeks

nicotine—30 min compared with 5 to 10 min for a cigarette—but mainly by the small surface area of the mouth compared with the lungs.

Despite the slower rate of absorption, with repeated use the gum soon builds up blood nicotine concentrations similar to those in cigarette smoking. Blood nicotine concentration builds up faster with 4-mg gum, but most smokers are satisfied with the 2-mg gum. In the early stages of use, the gum tastes slightly aversive. Dislike of the taste, irritation of the tongue, mouth, and throat, and occasional nausea are common complaints during the first week[112] and may deter smokers from continuing. This is partly caused by excessive chewing, which releases the nicotine too rapidly and causes excessive salivation and swallowing of nicotine. Less common side effects are ulceration of the tongue, aching of the jaw due to chewing, flatulence, hiccups, epigastric discomfort, and, rarely, a feeling of faintness or dizziness.[112]

Although about 10 percent of heavy smokers develop some degree of dependence on the gum during clinical use, this is not considered a serious problem. Most can be encouraged to withdraw gradually without relapse to smoking.[112] Russell and colleagues[112] recommend that subjects practice chewing two or three gums a day for a few days to get used to it before the target date for giving up smoking. On the target date, subjects should stop smoking abruptly rather than cut down gradually. The gum should be used as necessary whenever the urge to smoke is strong.

Treatment should start with the 2-mg gum. Most smokers manage on about eight pieces of 2-mg gum per day.[112] Only those who exceed 15 pieces per day need be offered the 4-mg gum. Smokers should be encouraged to use the gum for about 4 months, after which it should be reduced gradually. More recent studies suggest 6-month usage, and some smokers may use the gum for up to a year. Smokers should stop smoking as soon as they start using the gum. If they have not stopped completely by 4 weeks, there is little to be gained by continuing gum use.[112]

Jarvis and coworkers[113] studied the effects of 2-mg nicotine gum on smoking cessation in a randomized double-blind placebo-controlled trial with a 1-year follow-up and biochemical validation of reported abstinence. A total of 116 subjects were treated in groups of about 10, each group being allocated at random to receive either the active or placebo gum. Plasma nicotine and expired air carbon monoxide served as objective measures of smoking.

All subjects were given the same instructions about the gum. They were told that it contained nicotine which would be absorbed through the lining of the mouth as it was chewed and that it would reduce the craving for cigarettes and help relieve other withdrawal symptoms.[113] They were encouraged to stop smoking completely on the first day of treatment and told to chew a piece of gum whenever the desire to smoke was particularly strong. No restrictions were placed on the number of gums chewed each day, and it was recommended that they use the gum for at least 3 months before attempting to do without it.

At one year follow-up, the abstinence rate for the active gum group was significantly greater (47 percent) than the placebo control group (21 percent). The continuous abstinence rate (no smoking at all from first week of treatment to 1 year of follow-up) was 31 percent for the active group compared with 14 percent for the placebo group. Of those abstinent at 1 year, six in the active treatment group and two in the placebo group were still using the gum.

Another placebo-controlled, double-blind trial was carried out by Schneider and colleagues,[114] this time in a clinic-supported setting. In the clinic-supported study, 60 subjects, recruited via advertisement on a news radio station, were randomly assigned to nicotine and placebo groups.

All subjects came to the "laboratory" on a Friday (while still smoking) for baseline measures (including expired air carbon monoxide) and questionnaires. They were instructed to stop smoking when arising the following Monday morning. Subjects were given two or three pieces of gum to use that morning if they so desired.

During the first week, subjects came to the clinic at the same time on a daily basis. At that time, subjects took all tests and discussed their daily program and problems (sessions lasted 45 min and interaction with the experimenter was on an individual basis). At the end of the first week, all subjects returned to the laboratory once a week for four more weeks. Thereafter, subjects were required to return to the clinic for 3-month, 6-month, and 1-year follow-up checks with expired air carbon monoxide serving as verification of abstinence. The gum was chewed ad lib both in terms of amount per day and length of time on gum.

The active gum group yielded superior quit rates to the placebo group. At 6 months, 48 percent of the nicotine group was abstinent compared with 20 percent of the placebo controls, a highly significant difference. Between 6 months and 1 year, relapse in the nicotine group reduced the difference between groups to 10 percent, with the nicotine subjects showing a 30 percent success rate versus 20 percent for placebo controls. A second study involving a comparison of nicotine and placebo gum with minimal intervention and contact yielded lower success rates, with no difference between active gum and placebo.

More recently, Herrera and coworkers[115] undertook a double-blind placebo-controlled trial within a behavior modification support program. The behavioral supportive treatment consisted of 12 group sessions over approximately 6 weeks, two sessions per week, each lasting 60 to 80 min. The group sessions (10 to 15 participants) were divided into four phases. The first phase (2 weeks) included increased awareness of the habit by record keeping (self-monitoring). The subjects were instructed to increase the interval between cigarettes to decrease total intake of nicotine. This was aided by a wrist alarm that signaled smoking at longer and longer intervals. Measurement of expired air carbon monoxide and saliva cotinine, administration of the Fagerstrom Tolerance Questionnaire, and a medical evaluation were also accomplished during the first phase.

Phase 2 (2 to 4 weeks) included continued monitoring, reduction of smoking, and stimulus control strategies. Relaxation techniques, covert conditioning (associating smoking with negative consequences), and alternative behaviors were among the recommended behavioral strategies.

Thereafter, the quit phase began. During this period (4 to 6 weeks), most of the information and discussions were centered on nicotine replacement treatment. Use of the behavioral methods was also encouraged and relapse prevention training began with instructions in stress management and cognitive restructuring. A maintenance phase (7 to 12 weeks) offered additional support with one session per week. Eventually, individual follow-up sessions at 6, 12, and 24 months were made. In addition, participants could come and see the therapist at a set time each week for up to 24 months if they so wished. Sixty-eight patients dropped out in phase 1 and 10 patients in phase 2, prior to randomization.

Three doses of gum were used, a placebo and gum containing 2 and 4 mg of nicotine (Nicorette). High-dependent smokers ($n = 168$) were randomly assigned to either the 2-mg ($n = 81$) or 4-mg ($n = 87$) dose. The low-to-medium dependent subjects ($n = 154$) received randomly placebo ($n = 78$) or 2-mg ($n = 76$) gum.

Among the high-dependent smokers, the 4-mg dose produced significantly higher sustained success rates throughout the 2 years of follow-up. After 6 months, the 4-mg users experienced a doubling of success rates compared with those of the 2-mg users. At 6 weeks, 41 percent of the 2-mg users were abstinent, which diminished to 16 percent at 2 years. For 4 mg, the corresponding figures were 60 and 34 percent.[115]

Among the medium-to-low dependent smokers, the 2-mg dose produced a doubling of the effect of placebo. At 6 weeks, 70 percent of the 2-mg users were abstinent, compared with 34 percent of placebo subjects. The figures at year 2 were 40 and 17 percent.

TRANSDERMAL NICOTINE PATCH

The four nicotine patches, Habitrol (CIBA-GEIGY), Nicoderm (Marion Merrell Dow), PROSTEP (Lederle), and Nicotrol (Warner-Lambert), are distinctive systems with differing total nicotine content per delivery system, method, and pattern of release.[116] Each device has five layers: protective liner, contact adhesive, internal membrane, drug reservoir, and impermeable backing. The patches vary in size and shape and are designed to release the drug at a predetermined rate. The amount and rate of release of nicotine is controlled in two of the systems (Nicoderm and Nicotrol) by a diffusion-controlling element. The mechanism for release of nicotine from PROSTEP and Habitrol is through a concentration gradient between the drug reservoir in the system and the concentration gradient prevailing in the skin. The clinical implications of these differences among the four products is unknown.[116]

The absorption of nicotine from the transdermal system is relatively gradual. The mean time to achieve peak blood concentrations varies among the nicotine patches from 4 to 12 h. Total absorption is approximately 21, 21, 15, and 22 mg for Nicoderm, Habitrol, Nicotrol, and PROSTEP, respectively.

Nicotine patches are generally well tolerated, and they are now available as over-the-counter items (Nicoderm and Nicotrol). Many of the adverse effects expected after administration of nicotine (e.g., nausea) are minimized because of the tolerance seen with chronic smokers. Topical reactions (e.g., erythema, pruritus, burning at the application site) were the most frequently reported effects.[116] Because of the increased potential for adverse effects, transdermal nicotine should be used with caution in people with peptic ulcer disease, skin disorders, cardiovascular disease, hyperthyroidism, pregnancy, and insulin-dependent diabetes mellitus.

Abelen and colleagues[117] conducted one of the first studies of the efficacy of transdermal nicotine replacement for smoking cessation. The study was a randomized double-blind placebo-controlled trial for 3 months in 21 general medical practices. Over 4 months, 199 cigarette smokers, including both healthy subjects and patients, were followed. Patients with overt cardiovascular risks, pregnant women, and nursing mothers were excluded.

The transdermal nicotine patch system (TNS) was available for 3 months in 21.2, 13.8, and 7.7 mg nicotine per 24 h. The corresponding placebo patches contained a small, pharmacologically irrelevant amount of nicotine to give an identical color and appearance. A new patch was applied every morning dorsolateral above the hip. Subjects who smoked more than 20 cigarettes daily were treated with the 21.2-mg patch; those who smoked less received the 13.8-mg patch. Psychological counseling was not done, and the number of consultations was kept small. Participants who succeeded in abstaining switched to the next smallest patch for the next month. Participants who relapsed switched to the largest patch for the next month.[117]

Participants were urged to refrain completely from smoking after the beginning of therapy. At monthly consultations, the doctor assessed the patient's smoking status. Abstinence was verified by measurement of expired air carbon monoxide. Participants who smoked from zero to three cigarettes and had a CO of 0 to 11 ppm were deemed abstinent.

The abstinence rates for the TNS groups for months 1, 2, and 3 were 41.0, 36.0, and 36.0 percent. Corresponding abstinence rates for the placebo group were 19.4, 20.4, and 22.5 percent. The differences between the two groups were significant for all 3 months. The difference between groups was largely due to the greater efficacy of the TNS for highly dependent subjects, as measured by the Fagerstrom Nicotine Dependence Score. Smokers with lower scores responded similarly to TNS and placebo.[117]

Craving for tobacco was moderate in both groups, but diminished more over the course of treatment in the abstainers in the nicotine group than in the placebo group. Similarly, other withdrawal symptoms and weight gain were less in the TNS group.

Hurt and coworkers[118] recruited 70 subjects ages 20 to 65 years, who smoked at least 20 cigarettes per day. Each subject was expected to keep weekly appointments for 6 weeks, wear the patch as directed, and make a genuine effort to stop. Volunteers with active cardiac disease, pregnant women, nursing mothers, and subjects with dermatoses were excluded from the study.

The screening procedure for each participant included a comprehensive medical examination and laboratory testing. Questionnaires were completed, including the Fagerstrom Tolerance Questionnaire. After entering the study, participants were instructed in use of the patch, reminded that they agreed to stop smoking when the first patch was applied, and given the ALA manuals *Freedom from Smoking in 20 Days* and *A Lifetime of Freedom from Smoking.*[118]

Subjects were assigned randomly to an active nicotine patch that contained 30 mg of nicotine or a placebo patch (no nicotine). Subjects were instructed to wear one patch for 24 h during the entire 6 weeks. The patch was applied to the inside of forearms or arms, and the sites were rotated.

During the first phase (through week 6), each subject returned weekly for a 30-min assessment visit, which included expired air carbon monoxide testing. The nurse coordinator briefly reviewed parts of *A Lifetime of Freedom from Smoking.*

During the second phase (6 to 18 weeks), subjects assigned active patches who had stopped smoking could taper the nicotine dose by using 15- or 30-mg patches or could discontinue entirely. Those assigned placebo patches who had stopped smoking by week 6 were not offered the active patch. Subjects still smoking at 6 weeks continued with the original patch assignment and remained in the blinded portion of the trial. Those assigned placebo patches and still smoking at week 12 were offered 30-mg active patches and 15-mg patches for tapering during weeks 12 through 18. Return visits were scheduled at weeks 12, 18, 26, 40, and 56.[118]

Of the 62 subjects enrolled and randomized into the study, 62 completed phase 1, 31 in each condition. Abstinence from smoking was defined as no puffs on a cigarette in the preceding 7 days and a CO <8 ppm at the weekly visit. At the end of week 6, 24 subjects (77 percent) (or 71 percent, if those entering the study are counted) who received the active nicotine patch and 12 (39 percent) (or 34 percent) who had received the placebo patches were abstinent ($p = .002$).

For the active patch subjects, the abstinence rate declined from 77 percent at week 6, to 42, 32, 29, and 29 percent at weeks 18, 26, 40, and 56.[118] Eight (26 percent) has sustained abstinence from smoking though week 56. For subjects who had not stopped smoking at week 12 and used an active patch during weeks 12 to 18, 53 percent had stopped smoking at week 18. However, only one of these subjects was still abstinent at week 56.[118]

Comparable efficacy for patch use was demonstrated in two multicenter controlled clinical trials.[119] Two 6-week randomized, double-blind, placebo-controlled parallel group trials were conducted. Successful abstainers from both trials enrolled in a third trial for blinded downtitration from medications (6 weeks) and subsequent off-drug follow-up (12 weeks).

Patients were randomly assigned to a transdermal nicotine system delivering nicotine at rates of 21, 14, or 7 mg (trial 1 only) over 24 h or to a placebo. Group counseling sessions were provided to all participants (weekly during trials 1 and 2 and biweekly during phase 1 of trial 3). The groups consisted of 5 to 25 subjects, lasted from 45 to 60 min, and included a discussion of behavior modification techniques as well as smokers' progress. Abstinence at the end of weaning and after 6 months required verbal reports of no cigarette use and an expired air CO ≤ 8 ppm at all clinic visits during these periods.[119]

The centers enrolled 935 subjects. Cessation rates during the last 4 weeks of the two 6-week trials (pooled data) were 61, 48, and 27 percent for 21 mg, 14 mg, and placebo patches, respectively ($p < .001$ for each active treatment versus placebo). Six-month abstinence rates for 21-mg transdermal nicotine and placebo were 26 and 12 percent, respectively ($p \le .001$).

Nicotine transdermal patch therapy for smoking cessation confers a distinct advantage on the user. Questions concerning dose, use of the patch in combination with nicotine gum, and combinations of nicotine replacement plus other pharmacologic agents remain. Dale and colleagues[120] specifically addressed the issue of high-dose nicotine patch therapy. Volunteer subjects interested in stopping smoking were recruited by a press release and from a list of patients who had been seen at the Mayo Nicotine Dependence Center and were known to be smoking at the time of the last follow-up. Seventy-one cigarette smokers were recruited and were stratified according to light ($n = 23$), moderate ($n = 24$), and heavy ($n = 24$) smoking rates.

After baseline measures were obtained, subjects were randomly assigned to placebo or an 11-, 22-, or 44-mg dose of transdermal nicotine and admitted to a special hospital unit for intensive inpatient treatment of nicotine dependence. During the 6-day inpatient stay, daily nicotine and cotinine levels were determined from blood samples. While hospitalized, subjects received intensive nicotine dependence treatment, including individual counseling, group counseling, lectures, exercise sessions, and other activities.

Following the hospital stay, subjects continued to receive patch therapy for an additional 7 weeks, and subjects initially assigned to the placebo patch were randomly assigned to the 11- or 22-mg dose for the remainder of patch therapy. After 4 weeks of patch therapy, those initially assigned to the 44-mg dose were reduced to 22 mg, which they continued to receive for the remaining 4 weeks. For the 7 weeks following hospital discharge, subjects returned for seven weekly group counseling sessions and then for follow-up visits at 3, 6, 9, and 12 months. At each visit, self-reported smoking status was obtained, and expired air carbon monoxide was measured. Self-reported abstinence in the previous 7 days was considered biochemically confirmed if the expired air carbon monoxide level was 8 ppm or lower.[120]

Of the 71 subjects who completed the study, 70 percent were abstinent from smoking at 8 weeks, 62 percent at 6 months, and 45 percent at 1 year. All 18 of the subjects randomized to the 44-mg patch were abstinent at week 8. The 8-week point prevalence "stop" rates for subjects whose patch dose was 11, 22, or 44 mg for weeks 2 through 4 were 59, 62, and 100 percent. However, no significant association between dose and cessation was detected at 6 months or 1 year. Percentage of nicotine replacement (based on cotinine measurement at baseline and while on the different patch doses) was also positively associated with smoking cessation at 8 weeks. No significant association was detected at 6 or 12 months.

The concept of percentage of nicotine replacement is an important one. Dale and coworkers[120] not only showed that the higher the percent of nicotine replacement, the higher the initial cessation, but they also showed that the higher the percent of replacement, the lower the intensity and frequency of withdrawal symptoms. The investigators emphasized that one standard dose of nicotine replacement is probably not adequate for all smokers and highlight the need to extend the upper limits to higher levels of dosing than previously used.

In Dale and colleagues' study,[120] the 44-mg patch did not produce signs of nicotine toxicity, although one subject dropped out (a light smoker who received the 44-mg patch) because of nausea, vomiting, dizziness, visual disturbance, and weakness within 2 h of the initial application of the patches. The adverse effects resolved after removal of the patch. Jorenby and coworkers[121] also studied nicotine patch dose (22 and 44 mg). Four weeks of the 22- or 44-mg patch was followed by dosage reduction (2 weeks of 11 mg). Subjects ($n = 504$) also received minimal intervention, individual counseling, or group counseling. Abstinence from smoking was based on verbal report and CO $\leq$ 10 ppm.

Smoking cessation rates for the two nicotine patch doses and three levels of counseling did not differ significantly at either 8 or 26 weeks following the quit date.[121] Among those receiving minimal contact, the 44-mg dose produced greater abstinence at 4 weeks than did the 22-mg dose (68 versus 45 percent, $p < .01$). Participants receiving minimal contact adjuvant treatment were less likely to be abstinent at the end of 4 weeks than those receiving individual or group counseling (56 versus 67 percent, $p < .05$). Nicotine doses of 44 mg produced a significantly greater frequency of nausea (28 percent), vomiting (10 percent), and erythema and edema at the patch site (30 percent) than did a 22-mg dose (10, 2, and 13 percent, respectively; $p < .01$ for each adverse effect). Three serious adverse events occurred during use of the 44-mg patch dose. Jorenby and colleagues[121] concluded that there does not appear to be any general sustained benefit of initiating transdermal nicotine therapy with a 44-mg patch dose or of providing intense adjuvant smoking cessation treatment. Higher dose (44 mg) nicotine replacement does not appear to be indicated for general clinical populations,

although it may provide short-term benefit to some smokers attempting to quit with minimal adjuvant treatment.

Kornitzer and coworkers[122] investigated combined use of nicotine patch and gum for smoking cessation. They randomized 374 healthy subjects at their work setting into a 1-year double-blinded placebo-controlled trial, 149 subjects to the active nicotine patch and active gum (group 1), 150 to the active nicotine patch and placebo gum (group 2), and 75 to the placebo patch and placebo gum (group 3). Treatment duration was 12 weeks, with a 16-h patch of 15 mg, followed by a 6 + 6 weeks weaning period on, respectively, 10 and 5 mg patches. Gum use was not restricted during the first 6 months. Nonsmoking status was verified by CO < 10 ppm.

Abstinence rates in group 1 and group 2 were 34.2 and 22.7 ($p < .05$) at 12 weeks, and 27.5 and 15.3 percent ($p = .01$) at 52 weeks. In group 3, abstinence rates were 17.3, 14.7, and 13.3 percent, respectively, at 12, 24, and 52 weeks. No significant differences between the three groups in systemic and local adverse drug effects were observed.

NICOTINE NASAL SPRAY

One potentially important difference between means of giving nicotine is the rate of absorption. It is slowest with the transdermal route (patch), somewhat faster via buccal absorption (gum), and faster, second only to inhalation, with the nasal route.[123] Because satisfaction and other positive reinforcing effects of smoking may depend, at least in part, on the very rapid rate of nicotine absorption, the nasal and inhalation routes may provide an effective means of nicotine replacement treatment.[123]

Two hundred seventy-four patients referred to the Maudsley Hospital Smokers Clinic in London were assigned randomly to active or placebo nasal spray groups. Patients were treated in groups of 9 to 16 smokers, with equal numbers assigned to active and placebo sprays in each group. Subjects and therapists were blind to spray assignments.[123]

The nicotine nasal spray (NNS) device (Kabi Pharmacia Therapeutics, Helsingborg, Sweden) consisted of a pocket-sized multidose bottle with a pump mechanism fitted to a nozzle for insertion into the nostril. The active spray delivered 0.5 mg nicotine per 50 μL shot. A dose consisted of two shots (1 mg), one to each nostril.[123] Spray use was left to the individual, who was allowed up to a maximum of five doses (5 mg). Subjects were advised to use the NNS whenever they felt an urge to smoke and were told to stop using the spray if they resumed smoking. The recommended duration of NNS use was 3 months, but subjects could continue beyond this time. No formal dose reduction regimen to wean subjects off NNS was used.[123]

Supportive group treatment consisted of six sessions over a month, each lasting 60 to 75 min. Each group was run by two therapists using a group-orientated treatment approach. Subjects were urged to stop smoking at the first session but were not excluded from subsequent sessions if they failed to do so or if they chose not to use the spray. Individual follow-ups were scheduled for 2, 3, 6, 9, and 12 months after start of treatment. At these times, subjects were called by telephone, and those reporting abstinence for at least the past week were asked to attend a validation appointment (expired air carbon monoxide).[123]

Twenty six percent of the active treatment group were

validated as being completely abstinent throughout the 12-month follow-up, compared with 10 percent of placebo subjects, a highly significant difference. At 1 month, the abstinence rates for active and placebo nasal spray groups were 68 and 42 percent, respectively. Placebo subjects were less likely to achieve abstinence during group and more likely to relapse within 2 months. Most important, for the placebo group, the likelihood of abstinence declined sharply with higher pretreatment smoking plasma nicotine levels, whereas for those on active spray, the likelihood of abstinence was not affected by their nicotine intake from cigarettes.[123]

The active spray was more effective than the placebo in reducing withdrawal symptoms during the first week of abstinence, and it reduced weight gain more so than placebo over 12 months of follow-up. Nicotine nasal spray generally was well tolerated. The most common side effect was local transient nasal irritation; others included a sore area in the nostril, blocked nose, nasal blood spotting, minor epistaxis, nasal ulceration, and vomiting. Forty three percent of active spray successes (11 percent of all active spray users) used the spray for the whole year. The corresponding figures from the Maudsley Clinic for long-term gum use are 25 and 6.3 percent, respectively.[123]

A randomized, placebo-controlled, double-blind study ($n = 248$) which took place in Goteborg, Sweden,[124] yielded similar results. Significantly more subjects in the active NNS group were continuously abstinent (CO validation) at 12 months than in the placebo group (27 versus 15 percent). At the end of group treatment (6 weeks), 53 percent of subjects in the active NNS group and 27 percent in the placebo NNS group were abstinent. Relapse rates after group treatment and throughout the study period were similar in the two treatment groups.

Ten of the thirty-four abstinent subjects in the nicotine group used the spray for 1 year. Most important, subjects with high scores (>7) on the Fagerstrom Tolerance Questionnaire had a significantly lower success rate with the placebo than with the nicotine spray. For subjects with low scores, there was no difference.

NICOTINE INHALER

Another method of ad libitum administration of nicotine for smoking cessation is through an inhaler in which air is saturated with nicotine before inhalation. Such an inhaler could supplement nicotine and also replace some of the oral, handling, and sensory reinforcement of the smoking behavior, which may be of importance to smokers.[125]

Tonnesen and coworkers[125] examined the efficacy and safety of a nicotine inhaler in a double-blind smoking cessation trial incorporating minimal levels of advice and support. Volunteers were recruited through advertisement in a local newspaper. Two hundred eighty-six subjects were randomly assigned to either active nicotine inhaler or placebo inhaler treatment.

Subjects were advised to use between 2 and 10 nicotine inhalers per day ad lib. They were instructed to inhale deeply and to puff about 10 times more often compared with smoking a cigarette. One inhaler would be good for 300 puffs, and subjects were told to replace it with a new one when they felt the nicotine inhaler had no more effect. After 3 months, they were offered a tapering period during the next 3 months, with a monthly reduction of 25 percent of the number of inhalers per day used in the third month. After the 6-month visit, no more inhalers were available. The placebo inhaler contained only the additive and was identical in appearance with the active inhaler.[125]

The target quit date for smoking was the subject's first visit to the clinic. A total of eight visits during 52 weeks were scheduled (weeks 0, 1, 2, 3, 6, 12, 24, 52). Expired air carbon monoxide served as an objective measure of smoking.

The sustained abstinence rates for the active inhaler group at 6 weeks and 3, 6, and 12 months were 27.6, 20, 17.2, and 15.2 percent, respectively. Corresponding abstinence rates for the placebo group were 12.1, 9.2, 7.6, and 5.0 percent. All active-versus-placebo comparisons were significantly different.[125]

MECAMYLAMINE AND SKIN PATCH

Rose and colleagues[126] evaluated the concurrent use of nicotine replacement therapy (patch) plus mecamylamine, a nicotine antagonist. The investigators reasoned that both nicotine and mecamylamine occupy the receptors that would otherwise be acted on by nicotine from cigarettes. Thus, nicotine and mecamylamine may work in concert to attenuate the rewarding effects of cigarette smoking, thereby facilitating smoking abstinence. Moreover, the agonist and antagonist would be expected to offset each other's potential side effects resulting from overstimulation or understimulation of nicotine receptors. Rose and coworkers[126] tested the hypothesis that mecamylamine, administered orally in low doses (2.5 to 5.0 mg twice a day), would improve the efficacy of nicotine skin patch treatment in promoting smoking cessation and preventing relapse.

Twenty-nine women and nineteen men participated in the study. They averaged 34 years of age and smoked 28 cigarettes per day for 16 years. Their mean expired air carbon monoxide level at baseline was 31 ppm.

The study was a randomized, double-blind placebo-controlled study (with regard to mecamylamine). The performance of a group of subjects receiving mecamylamine capsules plus nicotine skin patch (Habitrol, 21 mg in 24 h, Ciba-Geigy) was compared to a group receiving placebo plus nicotine patch. Subjects also were provided with self-help booklets (*Quit Smart*) giving advice on smoking cessation strategies, including use of the nicotine patch, avoidance of smoking related cues, coping with withdrawal symptoms, enlisting social support, and using exercise and self-reward strategies.[126] Expired air carbon monoxide served as the objective measure of smoking.

Continuous abstinence throughout the first 7 weeks after cessation was 50 percent in the mecamylamine condition and 16.7 percent in the placebo condition. The quit rate at 7 weeks was 58 percent in the mecamylamine condition. The continuous abstinence rate for the mecamylamine group at weeks 26 and 52 were 37.5 and 37.5 percent, respectively, compared with 12.5 and 4.2 percent, respectively for the placebo group. (Differences were highly significant.)

Citric Acid Inhaler

The sensory aspects of nicotine and other components of cigarette smoke may play an important role in maintaining cigarette smoking. Nicotine is an irritant and together with elements of tar provides the "throat scratch" sensation that many smokers report enjoying during the act of inhaling cigarette smoke. These important peripheral cues may be conditioned stimuli producing many of the immediate effects of smoking, including smoking satisfaction and reduction of craving for cigarettes.[127,128] A comparable effect is also obtained with the administration of a citric acid aerosol which contains no nicotine.[127] Levin and coworkers[129] studied the efficacy of a cigarette substitute which uses an ascorbic acid aerosol to provide some of the critical sensory cues of smoking to promote smoking reduction and abstinence.

Sixty-three smokers (25 men and 38 women) were recruited through newspaper advertisements. Their average age was 42.3 years, and they smoked an average of 31.1 cigarettes per day. They had been smoking for an average of 24.3 years.[129]

Subjects were randomly assigned to two conditions: ascorbic acid and cigarette substitute and no substitute. All subjects received behavioral treatment consisting of four group counseling sessions (4 to 10 participants per group) conducted over a 3-week period. The *Quit Smart* smoking cessation program of counseling was used.[130] Subjects received general information at the first session, and they were asked to switch to a cigarette brand delivering about 40 percent less nicotine for the next week. At the second meeting (1 week later) subjects were given advice to help them prepare to quit smoking. Subjects were asked to quit smoking at midnight just prior to the day of the third meeting; cigarette substitutes were distributed at this quit day meeting for groups of subjects belonging to the experimental condition. Subjects returned for a fourth group treatment session 2 days after quitting and a final group treatment session 1 week after quitting. At these sessions, they were counseled on how to cope with withdrawal symptoms (e.g., cope with urges, relaxation training, and exercise). Subjects in the experimental group also were advised in the use of the cigarette substitute. Subjects were assessed for smoking status at this time and at follow-up points 3, 6, and 12 weeks after cessation. Subjects in the ascorbic acid condition were able to use their cigarette substitute during the first 6 weeks and relinquished the substitute at the 6-week follow-up visit. Expired air carbon monoxide served as the objective measure of smoking status.[129]

The subjects given the ascorbic acid replacement device had significantly greater rates of continuous abstinence than controls as evaluated by survival analysis. The controls averaged 14.3 days of continuous abstinence (CO < 8 ppm), whereas the ascorbic acid subjects averaged 23.7 days of continuous abstinence. On day 1 after cessation, both groups averaged about 70 percent abstinence. On day 3 (85 versus 60 percent) and day 22 (60 versus 20 percent), the ascorbic acid group revealed significantly greater rates of abstinence than the "control" group. By day 4, both groups had a quit rate of 20 percent.

Behm and coworkers[131] recruited 74 smokers (39 men and 35 women) through local newspaper advertisements. A portable citric acid delivery system delivered an aerosol that could be inhaled in a fashion similar to smoking. The volume of the puff, the draw resistance, and the size of the mouthpiece were all designed to match typical cigarette smoking. The device also yielded a tobacco smoke "flavor."

The participants were randomly assigned to citric acid and placebo conditions, and they attended a six-session group smoking cessation program. The first three meetings occurred on three consecutive days. The first two sessions prepared subjects for quit day (session 3). The fourth, fifth, and sixth meetings were scheduled 1 week apart, at days 5, 12, and 19 after cessation. Subjects started using the actual and placebo inhalers on the morning of their quit date. Subjects were told to puff on the device only when they felt a strong urge for a cigarette and not to take more than 10 inhalations every 30 min. At the end of sessions 4 and 5, subjects turned in their used canisters and received a sufficient supply to last until the next session. By the fifth session, the subjects would have used a total of 12 canisters. Session 6 was a follow-up meeting held 1 week after discontinuing inhaler use. Expired air carbon monoxide served as the objective measure of smoking cessation.

The active inhaler had a significant effect in promoting the reduction in the carbon monoxide levels after the quit day for the subjects with higher than average baseline CO (heavier smokers). For the high baseline CO subjects, a significantly higher proportion of the citric acid group was abstinent at the end of the study (day 19 after cessation). The log rank test of continuous abstinence duration also showed a strong trend for longer abstinence in the citric acid aerosol condition ($p = .06$). Neither analysis showed any effect of treatment on the low-baseline CO subjects. For high CO subjects, those who used the citric acid inhaler yielded a quit rate of 30 percent on day 1 (after cessation), about 28 percent on day 12, and about 22 percent on day 19. For controls, the continuous abstinence rates on days 1, 12, and 19 were about 8, 7, and 0 percent. Low CO participants yielded higher quit rates (50, 25, and 25 percent on days 1, 12, and 19 after cessation).

In view of the effectiveness of the ascorbic acid and citric acid inhalers, it seemed reasonable to test the efficacy of sensory replacement in combination with nicotine replacement.[132] Westman and colleagues[132] studied the efficacy of a citric acid inhaler combined with the nicotine patch compared with a placebo inhaler combined with the nicotine patch.

One hundred subjects were assigned randomly to either active (citric acid) or placebo (lactose) inhalers. All subjects also used the Habitrol transdermal nicotine patch for a 6-week period (21 mg for 4 weeks, 14 mg for 1 week, and 7 mg for 1 week). Subjects reported five times to the research clinic over the first 10-week period. They were provided a self-help manual and were instructed to begin wearing the nicotine patches on the morning of their quit date. Subjects also were advised to puff on the inhalers just like a cigarette to cope with urges to smoke. At each follow-up visit, subjects were given inhaler refills and nicotine patches.

Abstinence was assessed by self-report and exhaled carbon monoxide. Expired air carbon monoxide levels were measured at the end of weeks 1, 4, 6, 10, and 24. Abstinence was defined as zero cigarettes smoked since the quit date, verified by exhaled carbon monoxide levels <8 ppm at the return visits.[132]

The primary outcome of abstinence at 10 weeks for the citric acid group was 19.5 versus 6.8 percent for the lactose group. Secondary outcomes of continuous abstinence at 4 and 6 weeks for the citric acid and lactose groups were 36.6 versus 18.6 percent and 34.1 versus 11.9 percent, respectively.

Silver Acetate Deterrent Therapy

Silver acetate was first introduced in Europe as an over-the-counter smoking-deterrent lozenge, Respaton,[133] and later as a chewing gum, Tabmit.[134] The silver interacts with smoke from cigarettes to cause a noxious metallic taste. The aversive taste causes smokers to discard the cigarette, and repeated aversive conditioning encounters lessen the urge to smoke.[135]

Support for the efficacy of the silver acetate lozenge for smoking cessation has been modest, at best, and the APA[17] does not recommend silver acetate for smoking cessation. Yet, aversive conditioning procedures, such as rapid smoking, are among the most effective stop smoking interventions, and the use of an over-the-counter smoking deterrent medication has considerable intuitive appeal.

Malcolm and coworkers[136] reported that in a double-blind controlled study, subjects using silver acetate gum for 3 weeks had a smoking cessation rate of 11 percent, compared with only 4 percent for subjects using a placebo gum. The between-group difference was statistically significant.

Jensen and colleagues[137] followed 496 smokers for 1 year. Smokers were given 1 week to quit smoking on their own, after which the ex-smokers were assigned randomly to 12-week therapy with nicotine gum (2 mg), 6-mg silver acetate gum, or ordinary gum. In addition to gum use, the ex-smokers participated in weekly group meetings for the first 5 weeks and intermittently thereafter to obtain support and encouragement for long-term abstinence.

At 12 weeks, the abstinence rates fell from 100 percent to 59, 50, and 45 percent for subjects assigned to nicotine gum, silver acetate gum, or ordinary gum, respectively. At 1 year, abstinence rates fell to 23.4, 22.6, and 23.2 percent. None of the between-group differences achieved statistical significance at either time point.[137] Neither the nicotine gum nor the silver acetate gum proved superior to ordinary gum.

Jensen and coworkers' study may not have offered an appropriate test of the efficacy of the silver acetate gum. For the gum to serve as a deterrent to smoking, it is important for smokers to experience the aversive taste which occurs when the silver acetate mixes with cigarette smoke. In the Jensen group's study, smokers did not experience the aversive reaction until they "slipped" or "relapsed."

Hymowitz and Eckholdt[138] used a more appropriate procedure. Five hundred adult male and female smokers were recruited via print and electronic media advertisements. The active lozenge contained 2.5 mg silver acetate, sugar, corn syrup, artificial cherry flavor, and artificial color. The placebo was similarly flavored but did not contain silver acetate. A small amount of quinine was added to the placebo to give it a somewhat medicinal or bitter taste to match that of the silver acetate lozenge.

Subjects were seen individually. During visit 1, they received an orientation, informed consent, brief smoking cessation counseling, and instruction on lozenge use. They were assigned randomly to the silver acetate lozenge condition or the placebo lozenge condition, and the study was conducted double-blind. Expired air carbon monoxide and urine cotinine served as objective measures of smoking. Subjects were given seven "blister" packs of six lozenges each to last them until their next visit (visit 2) in 1 week. They were instructed to use one lozenge approximately every 2 to 3 h, whether or not they smoked, not to exceed six per day, and to monitor cigarette smoking and lozenge use on a record card.

Visit 2 provided an additional opportunity for data collection, brief behavioral counseling, monitoring of side effects, and enhancing adherence. Each subject was "assigned" a quit date in 1 week and asked to return to the clinic for visit 3 in 2 weeks. Subjects were given a 2-week supply of lozenges.

To be considered a quitter at visits 2 and 3 and during 1-year follow-up, subjects must report no smoking and have an expired air carbon monoxide reading of <10 ppm. If subjects missed a follow-up visit, they were interviewed by telephone and either sent a kit via mail for collecting urine cotinine or visited at work or home to measure carbon monoxide. Subjects who received the urine cotinine kit by mail sent the urine vial with a preservative in a special envelope directly to a laboratory for analysis. If the urine cotinine was ≤0.6 mg, and they reported not smoking any cigarettes, they were considered a nonsmoker. At visit 3, all subjects were asked to rate the aversiveness of the lozenge when combined with cigarette smoke on a scale of 1 to 10.

At visit 3, subjects who were not smoking were given additional lozenges (25 pieces) to use on an as-needed basis for relapse prevention. Subjects who did not quit smoking left the study. Those who quit smoking were given appointments to return to the clinic in 1 week (visit 3A) to be sure they were using the product for relapse prevention and then to return once every 3 months (visits 4, 5, 6, and 7) for long-term follow-up. If they were still not smoking at visits 4, 5, and 6, they were given additional lozenges (25 pieces for 3 months) to use on an as-needed basis. If they reported any smoking, they left the study. No more lozenges were distributed at visit 7.

About 90 percent of the subjects in each group reported that they used the lozenges, each reporting slightly fewer than five lozenges per day. Smokers assigned to the active lozenge condition considered the lozenge to be more useful as an aid to stopping smoking and more aversive tasting when mixed with smoke than subjects in the placebo lozenge condition. Males and females rated the lozenge as equally aversive, and African Americans on average rated lozenge significantly more aversive than whites.[138]

Objectively verified quit rates at visit 3 were modest, 17 and 11 percent for the active and placebo conditions, respectively ($p = .071$). When the comparison was limited to the 142 and 144 smokers in the silver acetate and placebo lozenge conditions, respectively, who reported using the lozenges at visit 3, 26 percent in the silver acetate lozenge group and 16 percent in the placebo group were abstinent, a statistically significant difference. Even though more than 70 percent of the quitters in each experimental condition reported using the lozenges on an as-needed basis to prevent relapse, few subjects remained abstinent over the 12-month period with an overall quit rate at visit 7 of 11 and 9 percent for the active and placebo groups, respectively. The between-group difference was not statistically significant.

Logistic regression analysis showed that the variables which were associated with smoking cessation at visit 3 were race, lozenge-aversiveness rating, number of cigarettes smoked per day, and number of self-help behavioral techniques (e.g., self-monitoring, relaxation, postpone each cigarette, smoke only in one place). African Americans, those who rated the lozenge most aversive, those who smoked the fewest cigarettes at baseline, and those who used the most behavioral techniques were most likely to quit smoking initially.

Physician Intervention

Physicians have a unique role to play in the antismoking arena,[139] and recent reviews,[140,141] monographs,[142] and guidelines[17] underscore the importance of physician intervention on smoking. The Agency for Health Care Policy and Research (AHCPR) recently convened the smoking cessation guidelines panel to identify effective, experimentally validated smoking cessation treatments and practices.[43] The major findings and recommendations may be summarized as follows:

1. Effective smoking cessation treatments are available, and every patient who smokes should be offered one or more of these treatments.
2. It is essential that clinicians determine and document the tobacco-use status of every patient treated in a health care setting.
3. Brief cessation treatments are effective, and at least a minimal intervention should be provided to every patient who uses tobacco.
4. A dose-response relation exists between the intensity and duration of treatment and its effectiveness. In general, the more intense the treatment, the more effective the treatment and the more effective it is in providing long-term abstinence from tobacco.
5. Three treatment elements in particular are effective, and one or more of these elements should be included in smoking cessation treatment:

   • Nicotine replacement therapy
   • Social support (clinician-provided encouragement and assistance)
   • Skills training and problem solving (techniques on achieving and maintaining abstinence)

6. Effective reduction of tobacco use requires that health care systems make institutional changes that result in systematic identification of, and intervention with, all tobacco users at every visit.

The AHCPR guidelines emphasize the importance of systematically identifying all smokers, strongly advising all smokers to quit, and determining each patient's willingness to make a quit attempt. The patient not willing to commit to quitting should receive a motivational intervention to promote subsequent quit attempts (e.g., personalize the health message, provide brochures on smoking and health, discuss with the patient the costs and benefits of smoking and quitting). When the patient is willing to make a quit attempt, primary care clinicians may assist by encouraging the patient to set a quit date, preparing the patient for the quit date, encouraging nicotine replacement therapy, providing self-help materials, and providing key advice. All patients attempting quitting should receive follow-up contact and support.

When smokers enroll in a quit smoking program, it may be reasonably assumed that they are at least motivated to try to quit smoking. This is not always true of patients seen in physician or dental offices. Indeed, at any given time, only about 10 to 20 percent of smokers are "ready" to try to quit.[143] Hence, physicians and other health professionals must assess the patient's readiness for stopping smoking and adjust their intervention accordingly.

Physicians should take advantage of "clinical opportunities" to address the smoking issue, and they should utilize "open-ended" questions and other features of "motivational" interviewing[144] to engage the patient in a discussion about smoking, with a eye toward assessing the patient's readiness to quit, success or lack of success in quitting in the past, potentially effective behavioral strategies, and likelihood of benefiting from nicotine replacement therapy. For patients in "precontemplation" and "contemplation" stages of change,[104] the physician might engage the patient in a discussion about the costs and benefits of quitting and continuing to smoke ("decision balance"), review personal health issues which make quitting smoking particularly important, provide brochures and related material on smoking and health, and enhance the patient's sense of self-efficacy (i.e., that patients can succeed when they decide to try to quit). At a subsequent office visit, the patient may be more ready to try to stop smoking ("preparation" or "action" stages), at which time the physician may provide assistance.

There is a large body of evidence which suggests that physician intervention for smoking cessation is efficacious and cost effective.[145] In a classic study of family practices in London, Russell and colleagues[146] showed that if general practitioners said nothing about smoking, the 1 year quit rate among patients who smoke was about 0.03 percent. If the doctors merely distributed a smoking questionnaire, the year-end quit rate among smoking patients increased from 0.3 to 1.6 percent. By adding physician advice, the quit rate increased to 3.3 percent. When the practitioners distributed a questionnaire, offered advice, gave the patient a leaflet, and provided follow-up, the 1-year quit rate increased to 5.1 percent. When systematic behavioral counseling, use of self-help quit smoking materials, and nicotine replacement therapy are used, 1-year quit rates as high as 15 to 20 percent are within reach.[147,148]

For patients with frank disease, the quit rates may be even higher. Rose and Hamilton[149] showed that patients at risk of cardiorespiratory disease normally quit at a rate of about 9 percent. When physicians systematically advised such patients to quit, the quit rate increased to 39 percent. For heart patients, standard advice yielded a 1-year quit rate of 24.5 percent. "Intensive" advice increased the quit rate to 63.2 percent.[150]

Guidelines for physician office intervention on smoking are available from the National Heart, Lung and Blood Institute,[151] the National Cancer Institute,[152] and the American Medical Association,[153] as well as many other medical associations and societies. The National Cancer Institute has undertaken a special effort to train primary care physicians to intervene on smoking.[154] The recently completed Community Intervention Trial for Smoking Cessation (COMMIT)[155] included a major continuing medical education (CME) initiative to train physicians, dentists, and their staffs to intervene on smoking. Physicians who attended the special training programs reported that they felt better prepared to counsel smokers than nonattenders, and they reported more activity in smoking intervention.[156] Since physicians see about 70 percent of the smokers each year, they have unique clinical opportunities to intervene on smoking, and their use of brief interventions and nicotine replacement therapies may yield substantial quit rates among patients who smoke. Therefore, efforts to mobilize physicians and their offices to play an active role in tobacco prevention and control are likely to increase in the future.

Community Intervention Trial for Smoking Cessation

Societal norms—shared rules and expectations for behavior—produce a complex system of formal and informal guidelines for the appropriateness of behaviors.[157] The most effective strategies for tobacco control, at least from a public health perspective, are those that strike at the heart of social norms and mores that support smoking.[157] In community intervention studies, the entire community serves as the focus of the intervention.

Experience with community intervention for health promotion derives largely from multifactor studies of heart disease prevention, such as the Stanford Three Community Study, the North Karelia Project in Finland, the Stanford Five-City Project, the Minnesota Heart Health Program, and the Pawtucket Heart Health Program.[157] COMMIT was a large-scale unifactor trial involving 11 matched pairs of communities in North America.[155] The matched pairs of communities were assigned randomly to intervention or no-treatment control conditions, and telephone survey data collected prior to and after the 4-year intervention permitted analyses of changes in smoking rates in the intervention and comparison communities.

Each of the 11 intervention communities followed a common intervention protocol, and the intervention activities in each community were carried out under the direction of a community board and its task forces.[157] Intervention activities were delivered through predetermined intervention channels. They were the health site channel, worksite channel, school site channel, public education and media channel, and the cessation resources channel.[157]

Among the activities carried out under the direction of the community board and its task forces were media advocacy for implementation of smoke-free policies, the training of physicians and dentists for office-based intervention on smoking, "quit and win" contests for the entire city, worksite awareness and cessation programs, and participation of churches, schools, and community organizations in a host of activities associated with the American Cancer Society's Great American Smokeout.[157]

Information on changes in smoking behavior in the Intervention and Comparison communities was obtained via random digit telephone surveys conducted at the start and end of the study, as well as by analysis of survey data from a cohort of smokers followed during the 4-year intervention in each community.[155] A statistically significant difference was found in the proportion of light to moderate smokers who quit smoking in the intervention (30.6 percent) and comparison (27.5 percent) communities. However, there was no difference in smoking cessation between intervention and comparison communities among heavy smokers.[155]

The COMMIT findings regarding heavy smokers and cessation are consistent with other community studies,[28,157] and the difference detected in light to moderate smokers in consistent with findings reported earlier in eight community studies in seven different countries.[157]

Analyses of quitting during COMMIT in the intervention and comparison communities showed that 67 percent of the smokers reported making at least one serious attempt to stop smoking between 1988 and 1993.[158] The most common reasons given for quitting smoking were concern over health (91 percent), expense (60 percent), concern about exposing others to secondhand smoke (56 percent), and wanting to set a good example for others (55 percent). Statistically significant predictors of smoking cessation in COMMIT were male gender, older age, higher income, less frequent alcohol use, lower levels of daily cigarette consumption, longer time to first cigarette in the morning, initiation of smoking after age 20, history of past quit attempts, the use of premium cigarettes, a strong desire to stop smoking, and the absence of other smokers in the household.[159] Among successful quitters in COMMIT, the most popular quit smoking strategies were nicotine replacement therapy (27 percent), use of a self-help booklet (17.7 percent), attendance at a stop smoking program (9.5 percent), hypnosis or acupuncture (6.5 percent), consultation with a psychiatrist or psychologist (1.0 percent), or use of other stop smoking devices (2.4 percent).[159] Among smokers who made an attempt to quit smoking, the likelihood of successful quitting was more than twice as high among nicotine patch users compared with nonusers.[159]

Summary and Conclusions

The literature on smoking cessation has grown by leaps and bounds since the early 1960s, and any review of the literature is bound to be incomplete. This chapter is no exception. Some issues which were not given sufficient attention include the literature on proprietary programs, residential cessation programs, worksite stop smoking programs, and smoking cessation programs targeted specifically for pregnant women, the psychiatrically impaired, and hard-core smokers with frank disease.

This chapter identifies several important themes in the smoking cessation literature which merit attention and thought. The issue of relapse was identified in the early 1970s as a key problem area,[160] and this issue is just as critical today. Although nicotine replacement therapy and behavioral approaches to relapse prevention[161,162] represent important advances, high rates of relapse among smokers who succeed in quitting still is the rule rather than the exception.

The addicted heavy smoker also remains a challenge. Public health approaches to cessation, such as self-help manuals and minimal intervention strategies, as well as efforts to mobilize entire communities, seem not to have enough "firepower" to meet the needs of this hard-core group. Nicotine replacement therapy is a step in the right direction, and it appears to be the only intervention which is as effective for heavy and light smokers. Multicomponent interventions, whether on an individual or group basis, which include aversive therapy, behavioral strategies, and nicotine replacement, seem to offer the most clout for hard-core addicted smokers.

Adolescent and teen smoking represents another area of concern. While adult smoking rates have declined, recent surveys show that smoking rates among young people are rising, with more than 3000 new smokers each day.[163] Very little is known about how to help adolescents and teens stop smoking,[164] and the prevention of smoking onset and intervention for smoking cessation in young people represent important health priorities for the nation.

In summary, this chapter highlights close to four decades of progress in smoking cessation. There has been a vast improvement in the quality of research on smoking cessation, and the emphasis has shifted from clinical to public health cessation strategies. Both clinical and public health interventions have an important place in the antismoking arena. Most smokers prefer to try to stop smoking on their own, and public health interventions are required to meet the needs of literally millions of smokers who simply cannot be accommodated in clinical settings. Labor-intensive clinical interventions also have an important role to play, particularly for the hard-core heavy smokers, as well as others who are not able to quit smoking on their own. For smokers requiring intensive assistance, multicomponent group interventions, which include diverse behavioral strategies, aversion therapy, nicotine replacement therapy, and group support, seem to hold the most promise for success.

References

1. Vogt TM: Cigarette smoking: History, risks, and behavior change. *Int J Mental Health* 11:6, 1982.
2. U.S. Department of Health and Human Services: *Reducing the Health Consequences of Smoking: 25 Years of Progress,* DHHS Publication no CDC 89-8411, Washington, DC, U.S. Government Printing Office, 1989.
3. Warner KE: *Selling Smoke: Cigarette Advertising and Public Health.* Washington, DC, American Public Health Association, 1986.
4. Centers for Disease Control and Prevention: *State Tobacco Control Highlights—1996,* CDC Publication no 099-4895. Atlanta, Centers for Disease Control and Prevention, 1996.
5. U.S. Public Health Service: *Smoking and Health.* Report of the Advisory Committee to the Surgeon General of the Public Health Service, PHS Publication no 1103. Washington, DC, U.S. Government Printing Office, 1964.
6. American Cancer Society: *Cancer Facts and Figures—1997.* Atlanta, Centers for Disease Control and Prevention, 1997.
7. Bartecchi CE, Mackenzie TD, Schrier RW: The human costs of tobacco use. *New Engl J Med* 330:907, 1994.
8. U.S. Department of Health and Human Services: *The Health Consequences of Smoking: Nicotine Addiction. A Report of the Surgeon* General, DHHS Publication no CDC 88-8406. Washington, DC, U.S. Government Printing Office, 1988.
9. Schachter S: Recidivism and self-cure of smoking and obesity. *American Psychologist* 37:436, 1982.
10. Fiore MC, Novotny TE, Pierce JP, et al: Methods used to quit smoking in the United States. Do cessation programs help? *JAMA* 263:2760, 1990.
11. Hymowitz N: Smoking modification: Research and clinical application, in Stout CE, Levitt JL, Ruben DH (eds): *Handbook for assessing and treating addictive disorders.* New York, Greenwood, 1992; chap 7, pp 145–164.
12. Lichtenstein E, Glasgow RE: Smoking cessation: What have we learned over the past decade? *J Consult Clin Psychol* 60:518, 1992.
13. Bernstein DA: Modification of smoking behavior: An evaluative review. *Psychol Bull* 71:418, 1969.
14. Keutzer CS, Lichtenstein E, Mees HL: Modification of smoking behavior. *Psychol Bull* 70:520, 1968.
15. Schwartz JL: A critical review and evaluation of smoking control methods. *Pub Health Rep* 84:483, 1969.
16. Hall LA: Timing-of-punishment and response mode in aversion therapy. Unpublished doctoral dissertation, University of Arkansas, 1971.
17. American Psychiatric Association (APA): Practice guidelines for the treatment of patients with nicotine dependence. *Am J Psychiatry* (Oct Suppl) 153:1, 1996.
18. Lawton MP: A group therapeutic approach to giving up smoking. *Appl Ther* 4:1025, 1962.
19. McFarland JW: Physical fitness and tobacco, in *Exercise and Fitness.* Urbana, University of Illinois College of Physical Education, 1960.
20. McFarland JW, Gimbel HW, Donald WA, et al: The five-day program to help individuals stop smoking. Connecticut Medicine 28:885, 1964.
21. Thompson DS, Wilson TR: Discontinuance of cigarette smoking: "Natural" and with "therapy." *JAMA* 196:96, 1966.
22. Schlegel RP, Kunetsky M: Immediate and delayed effects of the "five day plan to stop smoking" including factors affecting recidivism. *Prevent Med* 6:454, 1977.
23. Bachman DS: Group smoking deterrent therapy. *GP* 86:86, 1964.
24. Ross CA: Smoking withdrawal research clinics. *Am J Pub Health* 57:677, 1967.
25. Schwartz JL, Dubitzky M: Maximizing success in smoking cessation methods. *Am J Pub Health* 59:1392, 1969.
26. Lichtenstein E, Keutzer C: The implications of psychological research for smoking control clinics. *Health Serv Rep* 88:536, 1973.
27. Janis IL, Mann L: Effectiveness of emotional role-playing in modifying smoking habits and attitudes. *J Exper Res Personality* 1:84, 1965.
28. Hymowitz N: Community and clinical trials of disease prevention: Effects on cigarette smoking. *Pub Health Rev* 15:45, 1987.
29. Multiple Risk Factor Intervention Trial Group: The Multiple Risk Factor Intervention Trial (MRFIT). *JAMA* 235:825, 1976.
30. Benfari RC, Sherwin R: Forum: The Multiple Risk Factor Intervention Trial (MRFIT). The methods and impact of intervention over four years. *Prevent Med* 10:544, 1981.
31. Hymowitz N: The Multiple Risk Factor Intervention Trial: A four year evaluation. *Int J Mental Health* 11:44, 1982.
32. Hughes GH, Hymowitz N, Ockene JK, et al: The Multiple Risk Factor Intervention Trial (MRFIT): Intervention on smoking. *Prevent Med* 10:476, 1981.
33. Ockene JK, Hymowitz N, Sexton M, et al: Initial and long-term cessation of smoking after four years of the Multiple Risk Factor Intervention Trial (MRFIT). *Prevent Med* 20:564, 1982.
34. Ockene JK, Hymowitz N, Lagus J, et al: Comparison of smoking behavior change for SI and UC study groups. *Prevent Med* 20:564, 1991.
35. Multiple Risk Factor Intervention Trial Group: The Multiple Risk Factor Intervention Trial: Risk factor changes and mortality results. *JAMA* 248:1465, 1982.
36. Hymowitz N, Sexton M, Ockene J, et al: Baseline factors associated with smoking cessation and relapse. *Prevent Med* 20:590, 1991.
37. Anthonisen NR, Connett JE, Kiley JP, et al: Effects of smoking intervention and the use of an inhaled anticholinergic bronchodilator on the rate of decline of FEV_1: The Lung Health Study. *JAMA* 272:1497, 1994.
38. O'Hara P, Grill J, Rigdon MA, et al: Design and results of the initial intervention program for the Lung Health Study. *Prevent Med* 22:304, 1993.
39. Schwartz JL: Review and evaluation of smoking cessation methods: The United States and Canada, 1978–1985, NIH Publication no 87-2940. Washington, DC, U.S. Government Printing Office, 1987.

40. Lando HA, McGovern G, Barrios FX, et al: Comparative evaluation of American Cancer Society and American Lung Association smoking cessation clinics. *Am J Pub Health* 80:554, 1990.

41. Rosenbaum P, O'Shea R: *Large-Scale Study of Freedom from Smoking Clinics—Factors in Quitting. Pub Health Rep* 107:150, 1992.

42. Harrup T, Hansen BA, Soghikian K: Clinical methods in smoking cessation: Description and evaluation of a stop smoking clinic. *Am J Pub Health* 69:1226, 1979.

43. U.S. Department of Health and Human Services (DHHS): *Smoking Cessation,* Clinical Practice Guideline no 18, AHCPR Publication no 96-0692. Washington, D.C., U.S. Government Printing Office, 1996.

44. Simon MJ, Salzberg HC: Hypnosis and related behavioral approaches in the treatment of addictive behaviors, in Hersen Eisler RM, Miller PM (eds): *Progress in Behavior Modification,* vol 13. New York, Academic, 1982, pp 51–78.

45. Spiegel H: A single-treatment method to stop smoking using ancillary self-hypnosis. *Int J Clin Exper Hypnosis* 18:235, 1970.

46. Berkowitz B, Ross-Townsend A, Kohberger R: Hypnotic treatment of smoking: The single treatment method revisited. *Am J Psychiatry* 136:83, 1979.

47. Javel AF: One-session hypnotherapy for smoking: A controlled study. *Psychol Rep* 46:895, 1980.

48. Sanders S: Mutual group hypnosis and smoking. *Am J Clin Hypnosis* 20:131, 1977.

49. West LJ: Hypnosis in treatment of the tobacco smoking habit, in Jarvik ME, Cullen JW, Gritz ER, et al (eds): *Research in Smoking Behavior,* National Institute on Drug Abuse Research Monograph 17, DHEW Publication no [ADM] 78–581. Washington, DC, U.S. Government Printing Office, 1977, pp 364–371.

50. Holroyd J: The uncertain relationship between hypnotizability and smoking treatment outcome. *Int J Clin Exper Hypnosis* 39:93, 1991.

51. Lambe R, Osier C, Franks P: A randomized controlled trial of hypnotherapy for smoking cessation. *J Fam Pract* 22:61, 1986.

52. Rabkin SW, Boyko E, Shane F, et al: A randomized trial comparing smoking cessation programs utilizing behaviour modification, health education or hypnosis. *Addictive Behaviours* 9:157, 1984.

53. Pederson LL, Scrimgeour WG, Lefcoe NM: Comparison of hypnosis plus counseling, counseling alone, and hypnosis alone in a community service smoking withdrawal programme. *J Consult Clin Psychol* 43:920, 1975.

54. Frank RG, Umlauf RL, Wonderlich SA, et al: Hypnosis and behavioral treatment in a worksite smoking cessation program. *Addictive Behaviors* 11:59, 1986.

55. Byrne DG, Whyte HM: The efficacy of community-based smoking cessation strategies: A long-term follow-up study. *Int J Addictions* 22:791, 1987.

56. Kutchins S: The treatment of smoking and nicotine addiction with acupuncture, in Cocores JA (ed): *The Clinical Management of Nicotine Dependence.* New York, Springer-Verlag, 1991, chap 14, pp 169–180.

57. Choy DSJ, Lutzker L, Meltzer L: Effective treatment for smoking cessation. *Am J Med* 75:1033, 1983.

58. Olms JS: Increased success rate using new acupuncture point for stop-smoking program. *Am J Acupuncture* 12:339, 1984.

59. Clavel-Chapelon F, Paoletti C, Benhamou S: Smoking cessation rates 4 years after treatment by nicotine gum and acupuncture. *Prevent Med* 26:25, 1997.

60. Riet GT, Kleijnen J, Knipschild P: A meta-analysis of studies into the effect of acupuncture on addiction. *Br J Gen Pract* 40:379, 1990.

61. Pearson RE: Response to suggestions given under general anesthesia. *Am J Clin Hypnosis* 4:106, 1961.

62. Aldrete JA: Cessation of cigarette smoking by suggestion in the perianesthetic period. *Anesthes Rev* 14:22, 1987.

63. Hughes JA, Sanders LD, Dunne JA, et al: The effects of suggestion during general anaesthesia on postoperative smoking habits. *Anaesthesia* 49:126, 1994.

64. Myles PS, Hendrata M, Layher Y: Double-blind, randomized trial of cessation of smoking after audiotape suggestions during anaesthesia. *Br J Anaesthesia* 76:694, 1996.

65. Wilde GJS: Behaviour therapy for addicted cigarette smokers: A preliminary investigation. *Behav Res Ther* 2:107, 1964.

66. Franks, CM, Fried, R, Ashem B: An improved apparatus for aversive conditioning of cigarette smokers. *Behav Res Ther* 4:301, 1966.

67. Resnick JH: The control of smoking behaviour by stimulus satiation. *Behav Res Ther* 6:113, 1968.

68. Resnick JH: Effects of stimulus satiation on the overlearned maladaptive response of cigarette smoking. *J Consult Clin Psychol* 32:501, 1968.

69. Lublin I, Joslyn I: Aversive conditioning of cigarette addiction. Paper presented at the meeting of the American Psychological Association, San Francisco, 1968.

70. Schmahl DP, Lichtenstein E, Harris DE: Successful treatment of habitual smokers with warm, smoky air and rapid smoking. *J Consult Clin Psychol* 38:105, 1972.

71. Lichtenstein E, Harris DE, Birchler GR, et al: Comparison of rapid smoking, warm smoky air, and attention placebo in the modification of smoking behavior. *J Consult Clin Psychol* 40:92, 1973.

72. Lando HA: A comparison of excessive and rapid smoking in the modification of chronic smoking behavior. *J Consult Clin Psychol* 43:350, 1975.

73. Danaher BG: Rapid smoking and self-control in the modification of smoking behavior. *J Consult Clin Psychol* 45:1068, 1977.

74. Best JA, Owen LE, Trentadue L: Comparison of satiation and rapid smoking in self-managed smoking cessation. *Addictive Behaviors* 3:71, 1978.

75. Hall RG, Sachs DPL, Hall SM, et al: Two-year efficacy and safety of rapid smoking therapy in patients with cardiac and pulmonary disease. *J Consult Clin Psychol* 52:574, 1984.

76. Hall RG, Sachs DPL, Hall SM: Medical risk and therapeutic effectiveness of rapid smoking. *Behav Ther* 10:249, 1979.

77. Raw M, Russell MAH: Rapid smoking, cue exposure, and support in the modification of smoking. *Behav Res Ther* 18:363, 1980.

78. Poole AD, Sanson-Fisher RW, German GA: The rapid smoking technique: Therapeutic effectiveness. *Behav Res Ther* 19:389, 1981.

79. Hauser R: Rapid smoking as a technique of behavior modification: caution in selection of subjects. *J Consult Clin Psychol* 42:625, 1974.

80. Hynd GW, O'Neal M, Severson HH: Cardiovascular stress during the rapid smoking procedure. *Psychol Rep* 39:371, 1976.

81. Miller LG, Schilling AF, Logan DL, et al: Potential hazards of rapid smoking as a technique for the modification of smoking behavior. *New Engl J Med* 297:590, 1977.

82. Hackett G, Horan JJ: Focused smoking: An unequivocally safe alternative to rapid smoking. *J Drug Ed* 8:261, 1978.

83. Hackett G, Horan JJ: Behavioral control of cigarette smoking: A comprehensive program. *J Drug Ed* 7:71, 1977.

84. Tori CD: A smoking satiation procedure with reduced medical risk. *J Clin Psychol* 34:574, 1978.

85. Kopel SA, Suckerman KR, Baksht A: Smoke holding: An evaluation of physiological effects and treatment efficacy of a new nonhazardous aversive smoking procedure. Paper presented at the 13th Annual Meeting of the Association for Behavior Therapy. San Francisco, 1979.

86. Lando HA, McGovern PG: Three-year data on a behavioral treatment for smoking: A follow-up note. *Addictive Behaviors* 7:177, 1982.

87. Walker WB, Franzini LR: Low-risk aversive group treatments, physiological feedback, and booster sessions for smoking cessation. *Behav Ther* 16:263, 1985.

88. Lando HA: Aversive conditioning and contingency manage-

ment in the treatment of smoking. *J Consult Clin Psychol* 44: 312, 1976.

89. Elliott CH, Denney DR: A multiple-component treatment approach to smoking reduction. *J Consult Clin Psychol* 46:1330, 1978.

90. Powell DR, McCann BS: The effects of a multiple treatment program and maintenance procedures on smoking cessation. *Prevent Med* 10:94, 1981.

91. Killen JD, Maccoby N, Taylor CB: Nicotine gum and self-regulation training in smoking relapse prevention. *Behav Ther* 15: 234, 1984.

92. Hall SM, Tunstall C, Rugg D, et al: Nicotine gum and behavioral treatment in smoking cessation. *J Consult Clin Psychol* 53:256, 1985.

93. Baddely GM, Schomer HH, Albrecht CF: Nicotine gum and psychological support in smoking cessation. *South African Med J* 73:409, 1988.

94. Buchkremer G, Bents H, Horstmann KO, et al: Combination of behavioral smoking cessation with transdermal nicotine substitution. *Addictive Behaviors* 14:229, 1989.

95. Edmunds M, Conner H, Jones C, et al: Evaluation of a multicomponent group smoking cessation program. *Prevent Med* 20: 404, 1991.

96. Curry SJ: Self-help interventions for smoking cessation. *J Consult Clin Psychol* 61:790, 1993.

97. Glasgow RE, Schafer L, O'Neill HK: Self-help books and amount of therapist contact in smoking cessation programs. *J Consult Clin Psychol* 49:659, 1981.

98. Danaher BG, Lichtenstein E: *Become an Ex-Smoker*. Englewood Cliffs, NJ, Prentice-Hall, 1978.

99. Pomerleau OF, Pomerleau CS: *Break the Smoking Habit: A Behavioral Program for Giving Up Cigarettes*. Champaign, IL, Research Press, 1977.

100. American Cancer Society: *I Quit Kit*, Publication no 2028. New York, American Cancer Society, 1977.

101. Davis AL, Faust R, Ordentlich M: Self-help smoking cessation and maintenance programs: A comparison study with 12 month follow-up by the American Lung Association. *Am J Pub Health* 74:1212, 1984.

102. Owen N, Ewins AL, Lee C: Smoking cessation by mail: A comparison of standard and personalized correspondence course formats. *Addictive Behaviors* 14:355, 1989.

103. Prochaska JO, DiClemente CC, Velicer WF, et al: Standardized, individualized, interactive, and personalized self-help programs for smoking cessation. *Health Psychol* 12:399, 1993.

104. Prochaska JO, DiClemente CC: Stages and processes of self-change of smoking: Toward an integrative model of change. *J Consult Clin Psychol* 51:390, 1983.

105. Lando HA, Kalb EA, McGovern PG: Behavioral self-help materials as an adjunct to nicotine gum. *Addictive Behaviors* 13:181, 1988.

106. Killen JD, Fortmann SP, Newman B: Evaluation of a treatment approach combining nicotine gum with self-guided behavioral treatments for smoking relapse prevention. *J Consult Clin Psychol* 58:85, 1990.

107. Hymowitz N, Lasser NL, Safirstein BH: Effects of graduated external filters on smoking cessation. *Prevent Med* 11:85, 1982.

108. Flay BR: Mass media and smoking cessation: A critical review. *Am J Pub Health* 77:153, 1987.

109. Glynn TJ, Boyd GM, Gruman JC: Essential elements of self-help/minimal intervention strategies for smoking cessation. *Health Ed Quart* 17:329, 1990.

110. Orleans CT, Glynn TJ, Manley MC, et al: Minimal-contact quit smoking strategies for medical settings, in Orleans CT, Slade J (eds): *Nicotine Addiction: Principles and Management*. New York, Oxford University, 1993, chap 10, pp 181–220.

111. Hughes JR: Non-nicotine pharmacotherapies for smoking cessation. *J Drug Develop* 6:196, 1994.

112. Russell MAH, Raw M, Jarvis MJ: Clinical use of nicotine chewing gum. *Br Med J* 280:1599, 1980.

113. Jarvis MJ, Raw M, Russell MAH, et al: Randomized controlled trial of nicotine chewing gum. *Br Med J* 285:537, 1982.

114. Schneider NG, Jarvik ME, Forsythe AB, et al: Nicotine gum in smoking cessation: A placebo-controlled, double-blind trial. *Addictive Behaviors* 8:253, 1983.

115. Herrera N, Franco R, Herrera L, et al: Nicotine gum, 2 and 4 mg, for nicotine dependence. *Chest* 108:447, 1995.

116. Gora ML: Nicotine transdermal systems. *Ann Pharmacother* 27: 742, 1993.

117. Abelin T, Buehler A, Muller P, et al: Controlled trial of transdermal nicotine patch in tobacco withdrawal. *Lancet* 1:7, 1989.

118. Hurt RD, Lauger GG, Offord MS: Nicotine-replacement therapy with use of a transdermal nicotine patch—A randomized double-blind placebo-controlled trial. *Mayo Clin Proc* 65:1529, 1990.

119. Transdermal Nicotine Study Group: Transdermal nicotine for smoking cessation. *JAMA* 266:3133, 1991.

120. Dale LC, Hurt RD, Offord KP, et al: High-dose nicotine patch therapy. *JAMA* 274:1353, 1995.

121. Jorenby DE, Smith SS, Fiore MC, et al: Varying nicotine patch dose and type of smoking cessation counseling. *JAMA* 274: 1347, 1995.

122. Kornitzer M, Boutsen M, Dramaix M, et al: Combined use of nicotine patch and gum in smoking cessation: A placebo-controlled clinical trial. *Prevent Med* 24:41, 1995.

123. Sutherland G, Stapleton JA, Russell MA, et al: Randomized controlled trial of nasal nicotine spray in smoking cessation. *Lancet* 340:324, 1992.

124. Hjalmarson A, Franzon M, Westin A, et al: Effect of nicotine nasal spray on smoking cessation. *Arch Intern Med* 154:2567, 1994.

125. Tonnesen P, Norregaard J, Mikkelsen K: A double-blind trial of a nicotine inhaler for smoking cessation. *JAMA* 269:1268, 1993.

126. Rose JE, Behm FM, Westman EC, et al: Mecamylamine combined with nicotine skin patch facilitates smoking cessation beyond nicotine patch treatment alone. *Clin Pharmacol Ther* 56:86, 1994.

127. Rose JE, Hickman CS: Citric acid aerosol as a potential smoking cessation aid. *Chest* 92:1005, 1987.

128. Rose JE, Levin ED: Inter-relationships between conditioned and primary reinforcement in the maintenance of cigarette smoking. *Br J Addictions* 86:605, 1991.

129. Levin ED, Behm F, Carnahan E, et al: Clinical trials using ascorbic acid aerosol to aid smoking cessation. *Drug Alcohol Depend* 33:211, 1993.

130. Shipley RH: *Quit Smart: A Guide to Freedom from Cigarettes*. Durham, NC, JB Press, 1990.

131. Behm FM, Schur C, Levin ED, et al: Clinical evaluation of a citric acid inhaler for smoking cessation. *Drug Alcohol Depend* 31:131, 1993.

132. Westman EC, Behm FM, Rose JE: Airway sensory replacement combined with nicotine replacement for smoking cessation. *Chest* 107:1358, 1995.

133. Rosenberg A: An investigation into the effect on cigarette smoking of a new anti-smoking preparation. *J Int Med Res* 2:310, 1974.

134. Rosenberg A: An investigation into the effect on cigarette smoking of a new anti-smoking chewing gum. *J Int Med Res* 5:68, 1977).

135. Fey M, Hollander M, Hymowitz N: Silver-acetate deterrent therapy: A minimal-intervention self-help aid, in Cocores JA (ed): *The Clinical Management of Nicotine Dependence*. New York, Springer-Verlag, 1991; chap 11, pp 150–156.

136. Malcolm R, Curry HS, Mitchell MO, et al: Silver acetate gum as a deterrent to smoking. *Chest* 89:107, 1986.

137. Jensen EJ, Schmidt E, Pedersen B, Dahl R: Effect of nicotine, silver acetate, and ordinary chewing gum in combination with group counseling on smoking cessation. *Thorax* 45:831, 1990.

138. Hymowitz N, Eckholdt H: Effects of a 2.5-mg silver acetate lozenge on initial and long-term smoking cessation. *Prevent Med* 25:537, 1996.

139. Sullivan LW: To thwart the tobacco companies. *JAMA* 266: 2131, 1991.

140. Richmond R: General practitioner interventions for smoking cessation: Past and future initiatives, in Richmond R (ed): Baltimore, Williams & Wilkins, 1994; chap 10, pp 217–256.

141. Glynn TJ, Manley MW, Mecklenburg R: Involvement of physicians and dentists in smoking cessation: A public health perspective, in Richmond R (ed): *Interventions for Smokers: An International Perspective.* Baltimore, Williams & Wilkins, 1994; chap 9, pp 195–216.

142. Shopland DR, Burns DM (eds): Smoking and tobacco control, Monograph 5, *Tobacco and the Clinician,* NIH Publication no 94-3693. Washington, DC, U.S. Government Printing Office, 1994.

143. Prochaska JO, Goldstein MG: Process of smoking cessation: Implications for clinicians. *Chest Med* 12:727, 1991.

144. Botelho RJ, Skinner H: Motivating change in health behavior. *Primary Care* 22:565, 1995.

145. Goldstein MG, DePrue J, Niaura R: The role of primary care physicians in smoking cessation. *Rhode Island Med* 76:515, 1993.

146. Russell MAH, Wilson C, Taylor C, et al: Effect of general practitioners' advice against smoking. *Br Med J* 2:231, 1979.

147. Herbert JR, Kristeller J, Ockene JK, et al: Patient characteristics and the effect of three physician-delivered smoking interventions. *Prevent Med* 21:557, 1992.

148. Ockene JK, Kristeller J, Goldberg R: Increasing the efficacy of physician-delivered smoking interventions: A randomized clinical trial. *J Gen Intern Med* 6:1, 1991.

149. Rose G, Hamilton PJS: A randomized controlled trial of the effect on middle-aged men of advice to stop smoking. *J Epidemiol Commun Health* 32:275, 1978.

150. Burt A, Illingworth D, Shaw PRD, et al: Stopping smoking after myocardial infarction. *Lancet* 1:304, 1974.

151. U.S. Department of Health and Human Services: *Clinical Opportunities for Smoking Intervention: A Guide for the Busy Physician,* NIH Publication no 86-2178. Washington, DC, U.S. Government Printing Office, 1986.

152. Glynn TJ, Manley MW: *How To Help Your Patients Stop Smoking: A National Cancer Institute Manual for Physicians,* NIH Publication no 92-3064, Washington, DC, U.S. Government Printing Office, 1991.

153. American Medical Association: *How To Help Patients Stop Smoking.* Chicago, American Medical Association, 1994.

154. Manley M, Epps RP, Husten C, et al: Clinical interventions in tobacco control: A National Cancer Institute training program for physicians. *JAMA* 266:3172, 1991.

155. COMMIT Research Group: Community Intervention Trial for Smoking Cessation (COMMIT). II. Changes in adult cigarette smoking prevalence. *Am J Pub Health* 85:193, 1995.

156. Ockene JK, Lindsay EA, Hymowitz N, et al: Tobacco control activities of primary care physicians in the Community Intervention Trial for Smoking Cessation (COMMIT). *Tobacco Control* 6(Suppl2):549–556, 1997.

157. Hymowitz N, Mueller MD, Lynn WR, et al: Background for a comprehensive community-based trial for smoking control, in Shopland DR, Thompson B, Burns DM, Lynn WR (eds): *Smoking and Tobacco Control,* Monograph 6, Community Based Interventions for Smokers: The COMMIT Field Experience, NIH Publication no 95-4028). Washington, DC, U.S. Government Printing Office, 1995; chap 2, pp 15–25.

158. Hymowitz N, Cummings KM, Hyland, et al: Predictors of smoking cessation in a cohort of adult smokers followed for five years. *Tobacco Control,* 6(Suppl2):557, 1997.

159. Cummings KM, Hyland H, Ockene JK, Hymowitz N, et al: Use of the nicotine skin patch by smokers in 20 U.S. communities, 1992–1993. *Tobacco Control,* 6(Suppl2):563, 1997.

160. Hunt WA, Bespalec DA: An evaluation of current methods of modifying smoking behavior. *J Clin Psychol* 30:431, 1974

161. Shiffman S: Coping with temptations to smoke. *J Consult Clin Psychol* 50:71, 1984.

162. Curry SJ, McBride CM: Relapse prevention for smoking cessation: Review and evaluation of concepts and interventions. *Annu Rev Pub Health* 15:345, 1994.

163. Lynch BS, Bonnie RJ (eds): *Growing Up Tobacco Free.* Washington DC, National Academy Press, 1994.

164. Burton D: Tobacco cessation programs for adolescents, in Richmond R (ed): *Interventions for Smokers.* Baltimore, Williams & Wilkins, 1994; chap 5, pp 95–105.

Chapter 29

RESPIRATORY MUSCLE STRETCHING AND EXERCISE

IKUO HOMMA

Muscle Training

It is well known that weight training is one of the exercises which increases the force a muscle can exert. Physiologically, the force of muscle contraction is proportional to the size of the muscle which, in turn, depends on the level of muscle hypertrophy. Muscle strength can be increased by training not only in young people but also in the middle-aged and the elderly.

Reduction of Muscle Strength with Aging

Muscle strength fails with age.[1] There are two factors which cause this decline: one is intrinsic to the muscle itself, and the other is due to changes in the nervous system and the motor nerves that supply the muscle.

Skeletal muscles have fibers which are morphologically, functionally, and metabolically divided into three types. Type I muscle fibers, which have a small diameter and contain a large amount of mitochondria, are characterized by low activity of the glycolysis enzyme and high activity of the oxidative enzyme. This type I fiber is called a *red muscle* because of its red appearance caused by a large amount of myoglobin. In addition, the contraction velocity of the type I fiber is rather slow and is, therefore, called a slow twitch fiber.

There are two subtypes of the type II fiber, type IIA and type IIB. Type IIB is made up of thick muscle fibers and less mitochondria. Both glycolysis enzyme activity and oxidative enzyme activity are high. Comparatively, type IIB is called a *white muscle,* a result of an absence of myoglobin. It is also called a *fast twitch fiber.* Type IIA plays a role as an intermediation between type I and type IIB. With aging, type II characterized by the thick twitch fibers becomes atrophic; type I acts dominantly in contractions.[2,3] The percentage of lipid droplets in the muscle fibers increases according to ultrastructural findings. The excessive storage of lipids is caused by a combination of inactivity of the muscle fibers and low utilization of lipid energy.[4] Other research suggests that a decrease of mitochondrial percentage per fiber is induced by a decrease of metabolic demand.[3] The reason for the atrophy of type II fibers is considered from a factor in the muscle itself. However, a neurogenic factor also has a large effect on this phenomena. With aging, a decrease of motor units has been observed while the motoneuron in the spinal cord changed morphologically.[5,6] Cross-sectional research on the maximal voluntary strength has revealed

that maximal voluntary strength began to reduce around age 60 in more than 100 people ages 20 to 100[7] (Fig. 29-1). In a subject 75 years old, a large amount of maximum voluntary strength had decreased; he had 80 percent of the strength of a young adult. He was not a sedentary elderly man but a normal worker. This phenomenon indicates that decreases of the motor unit and/or of type II fibers may take place with age. In some subjects motor units decreased by two-thirds, but most of the subjects' motor units did not decrease before age 60.[8,9] Studies in old animals suggest that a decrease of neuromuscular junction effectiveness is another important effect of aging.[10] Decrease in twitch potentiation with age induced by applying electrical stimulation on the peripheral nerve and by prolonging the muscle twitch, is due to the atrophy of type II muscle fibers. The characteristic of the twitch contraction depends on tension developed in type I fibers.

Is it possible to prevent the decrease in motor units and the degeneration of the neuromuscular junction? Partial recovery in decreased muscle strength with resistive exercise has been reported.[11,12] It is known that resistive exercise in young people induces hypertrophy of the muscle fibers.[13] In an older age, exercise can induce hypertrophy as well.[14] A larger training effect is seen on type II fibers than type I fibers (Table 29-1). Charette and coworkers[14] have confirmed the possibilities of improvement in neuromuscular recruitment and of an increase in the size of individual myocytes in older men.

Endurance Training

Continuous muscle activity fatigues muscle so it becomes harder for it to maintain a constant force. Muscle fatigue is divided into *central fatigue,* caused by a decrease in central motor output, and *peripheral fatigue,* produced by a lessening of transmission of central motor through the neuromuscular junction or by diminution in the contractive ability of the muscle. When there is continuous muscle contraction with maximum effort for a short term, a peripheral factor is more dominant than a central factor in muscle fatigue.[15,16]

The energy sources and their availability for adenosine triphosphate (ATP) production change as the level of exercise increases. With increasing exercise, the energy source for ATP production changes from the oxidation of fat to the oxidation of carbohydrates. In general, there is no alinear relationship between ATP availability and exercise level. High levels of exercise induce production and storage of lactic acid as the supply of O_2 to muscles becomes insufficient to meet energy requirements. Since the dissociation constant (pK_a) of lactic is as high as 3.86, the lactic acid produced in the muscles is completely dissociated into lactate and hydrogen ion (H^+). Accumulation of H^+ reduces pH and causes metabolic acidosis. With strenuous exercise, pH decreases to 6.5.[17] This decrease in muscle pH slows ATP production. Through an inhibition of glycolysis, simultaneously, the decrease of pH in the muscles causes an efflux of K^+, which impedes membrane depolarization. A decrease of pH also interferes with Ca^{2+} release and uptake. These factors could cause muscle fatigue.[15] Increased effluxes of H^+ and K^+ stimulate the chemoreceptor and increase respiratory activity.

So as not to limit muscle activity, the production of lactate

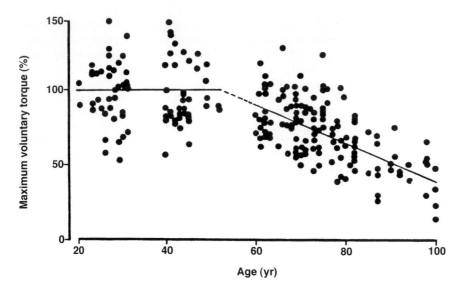

FIGURE 29-1 Maximum voluntary dorsiflexor and plantarflexor torques in 111 subjects, expressed as percentages of mean values for youngest groups (20 to 30 years) of men and women, respectively. Regression line for subjects 60 years and older was $y = -1.29x + 169.2$ ($r = -0.604$, $p < .001$). Horizontal line for subjects 52 years or younger reflects lack of significant influence of age ($r = 0.043$). (Reproduced with permission from Vandervoort AA, et al: *J Appl Physiol* 61:361–367, 1986.)

has to be restrained. Increasing the oxygen supply enhances the elimination of lactate. People with high V_{O_2}max have greater ability to oxidate and produce less lactate. The mean value of V_{O_2}max is usually 40 mL/kg per minute, and there is a correlation between V_{O_2}max and the amount of type I fiber.[18] V_{O_2}max reflects the ability of oxidative metabolism and is called the *aerobic work capacity*. Endurance training slows lactate production and hence increases the ability to eliminate lactate.[19,20]

Exercise in Patients with Respiratory Disease

There are two objectives of training respiratory muscles in patients with respiratory disease; one is to increase the strength of the respiratory muscle and the other is to improve its endurance of the respiratory muscle. In particular, training for patients with pulmonary disease is suitable for improving the endurance of the respiratory muscle. Usually PImax is used as an index to evaluate the strength of inspiratory muscles and PEmax for the expiratory muscles. Inspiratory resistive loading or inspiratory threshold loading, is routinely prescribed to increase PImax.

Exercise Prescription

GENERAL EXERCISE PRESCRIPTION

Detailed descriptions of exercise prescriptions are in the guidelines of the American College of Sports Medicine.[21]

In general, the prescription aims to avoid the possibility of developing disorders and to promote better health. However, increases in the frequency of exercise and time duration may aggravate some conditions. Thus, careful screening of patients before prescriptions are made decreases the risks and increases the effectiveness of the exercise. In general, both the effects and risk of exercise tend to be greater in previously inactive patients. The reverse is also true; in highly active people, both the effect and risk of exercise are low.

The effect of training depends on frequency, intensity, and time duration of the exercise which must exceed the usual level. According to the guidelines of American College of Sports Medicine, a dynamic exercise such as endurance training requires an activity level of 40 to 85 percent of V_{O_2}max and continuing for 15 to 60 min, three to five times a week. After 3 months of such training, V_{O_2}max is reported to increase 15 percent. In general, the level of exercise set according to the heart rate, which is proportional to V_{O_2}max. It is said that 40 to 85 percent of V_{O_2}max corresponds with 55 to 90 percent of the maximum heart rate. Research using the heart rate as an index of exercise level reported that training is ineffective if the heart rate does not reach 140 beats per minute.[22] A long period of exercise is more effective than a short period.[23] The actual duration of exercise depends on the individual's baseline physical strength. If exercise is being prescribed for a short period, it should be at least 5 to 10 min and at most 60 min.[24-27] A high-frequency exercise prescription is more effective according to a report by Pollock[28]; it said that exercise prescribed four times a week is more effective than two times a week. To promote good

TABLE 29-1 Initial and Final Muscle Fiber Areas

Group	n	TYPE I FIBER AREA, μm^2 Pre	TYPE I FIBER AREA, μm^2 Post	TYPE II FIBER AREA, μm^2 Pre	TYPE II FIBER AREA, μm^2 Post	PRE-POST FIBER AREA DIFFERENCE, μm^2 Type I	PRE-POST FIBER AREA DIFFERENCE, μm^2 Type II	% CHANGE IN FIBER AREA Type I	% CHANGE IN FIBER AREA Type II
Exercise	13	3967 ± 200	4205 ± 212	2532 ± 101	2988 ± 144*	238	456	7.3 ± 5.3	20.1 ± 6.8
Control	6	4631 ± 378	4427 ± 296	2941 ± 287	2273 ± 133	−204	−668	−6.1 ± 8.1	−18.3 ± 10.9

* Different from pre, p < .02.
NOTE: Values are means ± SE; *n*, no. of subjects.
SOURCE: Modified from Charette SL et al.[14]

health, it is enough that the exercise prescription should cause 1500 to 2000 kcal to be used each week.

EXERCISE PRESCRIPTION IN PATIENTS WITH RESPIRATORY DISEASE

Exercise plays an important role in respiratory rehabilitation for patients with respiratory disease. In an effective respiratory program, the exercise prescription is as important as a smoking cessation program, training of respiratory muscles, and O_2 therapy.[29] In general, both whole body exercise and respiratory muscle training or breathing maneuvers are useful and popular in patients with chronic respiratory disease. There has been a lot of discussion whether exercise for patients with chronic obstructive pulmonary disease (COPD) is effective. Exercise itself elicits dyspnea, and dyspnea is one of the symptoms that causes these patients to be sedentary. Many patients who are not very active physically feel dyspnea before exercise can be increased to a level that increases endurance. But decreased physical activity because of respiratory distress decreases respiratory muscle strength, which in turn results in increased dyspnea during movement. One of the early proponents of exercise in COPD, Alvan Barach stated, "Progressive improvement is the ability to walk without dyspnea."[30] Exercise training for COPD patients must first break the vicious cycle of dyspnea decreasing activity which leads to further dyspnea because of lower endurance. However, a satisfactory method has not yet been achieved.

Research studying a treadmill exercise for 10 to 60 min for 1 or 2 months was reported in the 1960s.[31–33] In the 1970s there were more studies of exercise employing an increased use of bicycles,[34–37] and walking has been popular as exercise since the 1980s.[38–41] A number of research studies showed that these exercises do not improve V_{O_2}max or spirometric measurements such as FEV_1, but did improve exercise endurance.

Since 1990, exercise has been the main method of rehabilitation for patients with COPD. However, the question whether exercise endurance really does alter COPD patients physiologically still remains unanswered, i.e., it is not clear whether patients are able to do heavy exercise with the same amount of ventilation and whether endurance is improved by suppressing dyspnea. Casaburi and coworkers[42] showed that endurance training using high exercise rates led to a decrease during exertion of ventilatory requirements by reducing lactic acidosis. They found that density of the capillaries in muscles increased with exercise; in addition, the number of mitochondria was greater, as were levels of aerobic enzymes. These effects increased aerobic work and delayed the development of lactic acidosis.[42]

Patients with COPD are usually capable of performing exercise for 15 to 60 min at a level of 40 to 85 percent of V_{O_2}max three to five times a week as recommended by *Guidelines for Exercise and Prescription*.[21] Leg fatigue is one of the symptoms which limits exercise in COPD patients.[43] The peripheral muscles are weak in COPD patients compared with normal individuals, and there is a correlation between the strength of major muscles and exercise tolerance.[44] Maltais and colleagues compared changes in oxidative enzymes in normal subjects with those in patients with COPD in a biopsy study. In both groups activity of oxidative enzymes de-

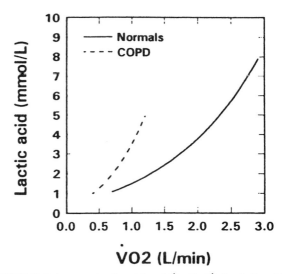

FIGURE 29-2 Average lactic acid and $\dot{V}_{O_2}$ ($La/\dot{V}_{O_2}$) relationships during exercise for control subjects (continuous line) and COPD patients (dashed line). These relationships were constructed from a group mean value of parameters *a* and *b*, and their ranges represent actual values observed in control subjects and COPD. For any given $\dot{V}_{O_2}$, the arterial lactic acid concentration was greater in COPD patients. (Reproduced with permission from Martais F, et al: *Am J Respir Crit Care Med* 153:288–293, 1996.)

creased significantly and lactic acid increased rapidly with exercise[45] (Fig. 29-2), but lactate levels increased more given V_{O_2} in COPD patients. The decrease in oxidative enzymes was greater in COPD. These changes in oxidative metabolism in skeletal muscle cells has also been confirmed by a noninvasive method, the nuclear magnetic resonance spectroscopy (^{31}P NMR).[46]

Casaburi and coworkers reported that the effect of an exercise program on normal subjects is the same as in patients with COPD.[42] Patients with COPD performed exercises for 45 min/day, 5 days/week for 8 weeks. The patients were divided into two groups, the COPD group who exercised at a high work rate (average, 71 W for a short period) and the COPD group at a low work rate (average, 30 W) for a long period of time each session. Both groups were tested on a cycle ergometer before and after the rehabilitation. In the group with a high work rate, both blood lactate and V_E increased significantly less with exercise after the rehabilitation compared to the baseline, whereas a significant change of lactate was not observed in the group on a low work rate; the decrease in V_E with rehabilitation was less than in the group on a high work rate. A correlation between the peak exercise lactate (average 8.5 mEq/L) and FEV_1 was not observed. Even though total work was the same in both groups, exercise endurance increased more in the high work rate group during a higher aerobic training.[47]

A number of other studies have reported that endurance improves even at a low work rate, but they did not find lactate and ventilation decreases. Continuation of exercise training often results in the improvement of symptoms of dyspnea in COPD patients.

No change in oxidative enzymes has been observed in biopsies of exercise muscle after training in COPD patients.[48] Crockoft and colleagues[49] observed that a 4-month continuation of a 6-week exercise training improved dyspnea and coughing, and Belman and Kendregan reported that with a 12-min walking distance, V_{O_2}max was also improved.[48]

A recent study using exercise on a treadmill has shown a decrease in symptoms in outpatients. Ten randomly assigned outpatients underwent 6 weeks of outpatient pulmonary rehabilitation (OPR), performing breathing training, relaxation techniques, and stress management together with upper extremity training, by light weightlifting, treadmill training, and inspiratory resistive training. In the OPR treatment group, the dyspnea, measured with a visual analog scale (VAS) decreased at the maximum workload, but the ratios of dyspnea to ventilation and dyspnea to V_{O_2}max were more than those in the control group.[50]

Unlike in normal subjects, a recent study of COPD patients found that improvement in exercise endurance was not associated with changes in enzyme activity in the exercised muscle but rather with increased motivation and tolerance toward exertional symptoms.[48] This study by Belman and Kendregan[48] focused only at certain levels of exercise.[48] Greater levels of exercise might also cause muscle enzyme changes in COPD.

Breathlessness is a common symptom which gives a limit to exercise in severe COPD.[43] During exercise, respiratory center drive increases together with other motor output and proprioceptive information from the peripheral muscles and joints. Accordingly, breathlessness during exercise arises from complex mechanisms. An increase of respiratory motor command caused by exercise is one of the factors causing an increased sense of effort or dyspnea. For example, when lifting weights, it is necessary to make a greater effort when the arm muscles are fatigued, even if the weight is the same as before the fatigue.[51] The perception of effort in exercise probably arises by sense rather than from increase in afferent information but by a corollary discharge of the central motor command to the muscle.[52] The sensations induced by elastic load or resistive respiratory loads probably arise from the increased motor output arised by adding load.[53]

A conscious awareness of the motor command may be the main sensation during muscular contraction. Normal subjects were tested on five levels of workload using a cycle ergometer, and their breathlessness was measured. There was a linear relationship between breathlessness and perception of respiratory muscle effort.[54] In respiratory patients, the effort demanded is considerably increased during exercise.

Patients with airflow obstruction are more dyspneic than normal subjects at comparable levels of ventilation. Airflow obstruction is associated with increased functional residual capacity (FRC). In COPD patients, inspiratory muscles at FRC are shorter so that increased effort is needed to move the chest wall, resulting in greater breathlessness. There is a linear relationship between oxygen uptake or CO_2 output and alveolar ventilation during low-intensity exercise. However, with increasing exercise intensity, ventilation increases more than for a given oxygen uptake because of lactic acid accumulation. This level is called the *anaerobic threshold* and is 50 percent of V_{O_2}max but lower in patients with pulmonary disease. Breathlessness is increased because of a combination of greater respiratory motor command to overcome airflow limitation because more ventilation is required as a result of lactic acid accumulation.

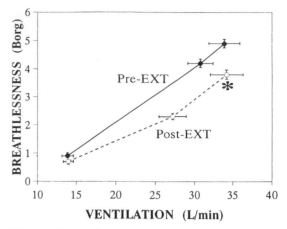

FIGURE 29-3 Slopes of Borg breathlessness ratings relative to ventilation fell significantly by 10 percent ($p < .025$ at asterisk) in response to EXT ($n = 30$). Values are mean ± SEM. (Reproduced with permission from O'Donnell DE, et al: *Am J Respir Crit Care Med* 152:2005–2013, 1995.)

One question is whether specific endurance exercise training (EXT) decreases the intensity of breathlessness. Physiotherapists define EXT as the following a training session that lasts 2.5 h and includes exercise of both the upper and lower limbs. It can include periods of walking, stair climbing, arm ergometry, cycle ergometry, treadmill exercise, and breathing exercises. The intensity of the training is limited by the level of symptom, and each subject performs at the highest attainable work rate and longest tolerable duration. Sessions are held three times a week for 6 weeks. Comparing the group on EXT with the control group, there was no difference in dyspnea at baseline between the two groups. Performing EXT for 6 weeks reduced breathlessness. Breathlessness per V_E and V_{O_2} and leg effort per V_{O_2} were also lessened (Fig. 29-3).[55] O'Donnell and Webb[56] suggest the factors responsible for the reduction of breathlessness are (1) lower ventilatory demand, (2) less impedance to ventilatory muscle action, (3) improved ventilatory muscle performance, and (4) psychological factors. The decrease of ventilatory demand may be caused by enhanced aerobic performance or mechanical efficiency. On the other hand, a decrease of breathlessness per V_E might be caused by a decrease of resistive or elastic forces opposing muscle contraction, inducing a concomitant decrease of central motor command.[53] The decrease of breathlessness might also be affected through another system since the pulmonary function was often not improved. There was no significant decrease of FRC after EXT.

Breathlessness could arise not only from the sense of effort but also by an increase in CO_2 or afferent traffic from intercostal muscle spindles. A recent study has suggested that conditioning the intercostal muscle spindles reduces breathlessness and improves pulmonary function.

Respiratory Muscle Stretch Gymnastics

MUSCLE STIFFNESS AND MUSCLE SPINDLE FIRING

Hagbarth and coworkers[57] have related muscle spindle firing to the stiffness of digit flexors in humans. Stiffness was evaluated by the change in the extension angle with the

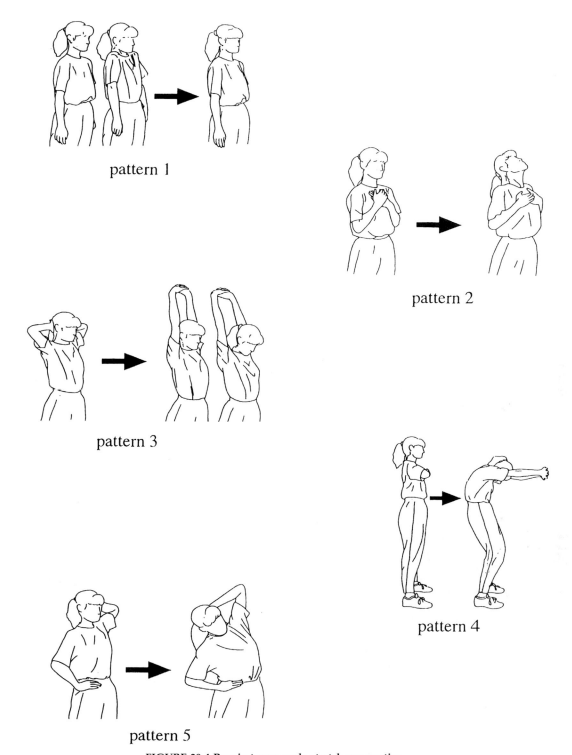

pattern 1

pattern 2

pattern 3

pattern 4

pattern 5

FIGURE 29-4 Respiratory muscle stretch gymnastics.

application of a fixed force (lengthening maneuver). Muscle spindle firing during such lengthening of the digit flexors was more frequent in stiffer muscles. The results indicate that there is a relatively parallel relationship in stiffness between the extrafusal and intrafusal muscles. It is possible that the stiffer chest wall in association with COPD[58] is caused by increased stiffness of the intercostal muscles. If this hypothesis stands, and the same feature is shared among digit flexors and intercostal muscles, intercostal muscle spindles could be firing more in the noncontracting lengthening phase (expiration) in patients with COPD compared with healthy subjects. Thus, in the stiffened chest wall, intercostal muscle spindles could be firing as if out-of-phase vibration were being applied, which could be partly responsible for dyspnea in these patients.[59] Muscle stretching of the intercostal muscles might reduce their stiffness.[57]

HOW TO PERFORM RESPIRATORY MUSCLE STRETCH GYMNASTICS

The object of the respiratory muscle stretch gymnastics (RMSG)[60] is to reduce the stiffness of the chest wall. It is easy to learn and can be performed at home on a daily basis (Fig. 29-4).

Patients are instructed in the following manner: (1) Perform the gymnastics in a sitting position. (2) Perform each pattern four or five times in sequential order, and then repeat pattern 1 again. This constitutes one session. Perform one session each in the morning, afternoon, and evening for a total of these three sessions per day. (3) If any pattern causes pain, simply bypass that pattern and perform only the patterns that feel comfortable.

Pattern 1: Elevate and lower the shoulders. While breathing slowly in through the nose, gradually elevate both shoulders. After taking a deep breath, slowly breathe out through the mouth, relax and lower the shoulders.

Pattern 2: Stretch the upper chest-wall inspiratory and neck muscles. Place both palms on the upper chest and stretch upward without leaning back. Then pull the elbows back and the chest down, inhaling deeply. Exhale slowly and relax.

Pattern 3: Stretch the lower chest wall expiratory muscles. Place both hands on back of the head. After taking a deep breath, turn both palms upward and stretch the arms, breathing out slowly.

Pattern 4: Stretch the upper chest wall inspiratory muscles and back muscles. Hold both hands in front of the chest. While slowly breathing out, move both hands forward and stretch the back. Keeping this position, take a deep inspiration.

Pattern 5: Twist the body and elevate the elbow. Hold one hand behind the head. While exhaling slowly, twist and stretch the torso to one side of the body, raising the elbow as high as possible.

Several studies indicate beneficial immediate and long-term effects of RMSG.[61] RMSG has an immediate effect in reducing dyspnea. Dyspnea at rest was measured by a 150-mm visual analog scale in 34 patients with COPD; it improved after RMSG as the VAS scores decreasing from 11.6 ± 3.4 to 6.2 ± 2.2 mm. After 4 weeks of RMSG, dyspnea after a 6-min walk test decreased. There were no significant differences between values measured before and after the RMSG session in blood pressure, pulse rate, and oxygen.

The circumference of the upper chest wall at maximal inspiration increased from 87.3 ± 1.0 to 88.1 ± 0.9 cm ($p < .01$) after 4 weeks of RMSG, but maximal inspiratory pressure did not increase.[62] There were few effects of RMSG on respiratory function tests for FRC. FRC significantly decreased 310 mL from 4.19 to 3.88 L after 4 weeks of RMSG.[61] In a randomized crossover study, the average FRC was 3.43 L before inspiratory muscle training (IMT) and 3.41 L after IMT, whereas a significant decrease was observed after 4 weeks of RMSG resulting in a decrease of 180 mL, from 3.46 to 3.28 L.[62]

Conclusion

Respiratory rehabilitation is an important technique in improving exercise tolerance and quality of life in patients with COPD.[63] Lacasse and colleagues,[64] using metaanalysis of studies from 1966 to 1995, emphasized that respiratory rehabilitation including exercise training is effective. Respiratory muscle stretch gymnastics seems to be a useful exercise and can be easily performed by every patient. RMSG not only reduces FRC but also decreases dyspnea.

Acknowledgment

The author thanks Suzanne Knowlton and Yuri Masaoka for their help in preparing this manuscript.

References

1. Larsson L, Grimby G, Karlsson J: Muscle strength and speed of movement in relation to age and muscle morphology. *J Appl Physiol* 46:451–456, 1979.
2. Larsson L, Sjodin B, Karlsson J: Histochemical and biochemical changes in human skeletal muscle with age in sedentary males, age 22–65 years. *Acta Physiol Scand* 103:31–39, 1978.
3. Poggi P, Marchetti C, Scelsi R: Automatic morphometric analysis of skeletal muscle fibers in the aging man. *Anat Rec* 217:30–34, 1987.
4. Scelsi R, Marchetti C, Poggi P: Histochemical and ultrastructural aspects of m. vastus lateralis in sedentary old people (age 65–89 years). *Acta Neuropathol Berl* 51:99–105, 1980.
5. Brown WF: A method for estimating the number of motor units in thenar muscles and the changes in motor unit count with aging. *J Neurol Neurosurg Psychiatry* 35:845–852, 1972.
6. Gutmann E, Hanzlikova V: *Age Changes in the Neuromuscular System.* Bristol, Scientechnica, 1972.
7. Vandervoort AA, McComas AJ: Contractile changes in opposing muscle of the human ankle joint with aging. *J Appl Physiol* 61(1):361–367, 1986.
8. Campbell MJ, McComas AJ, Petito F: Physiological changes in aging muscles. *J Neurol Neurosurg Psychiatry* 36:174–182, 1973.
9. McComas AJ, Fawcett PR, Campbell MJ, Sica REP: Electrophysiological estimation of the number of motor units within a human muscle. *J Neurol Neurosurg Psychiatry* 34:121–131, 1971.
10. Stebbins CL, Schultz E, Smith RT, Smith EL: Effect of chronic exercise during aging on muscle and end-plate morphology in rats. *J Appl Physiol* 58:45–51, 1985.
11. Fiatarone MA, Marks EC, Ryan ND, et al: High intensity strength training in nonagenarians. *JAMA* 263:3029–3034, 1990.
12. Fronterra WR, Meredith CN, O'Reilly KP, et al: Strength conditioning in older men: Skeletal muscle hypertrophy and improved function. *J Appl Physiol* 64:1038–1044, 1988.
13. MacDougall JD, Elder GCB, Sale DG, et al: Effects of strength training and immobilization on human muscle fibers. *Eur J Appl Physiol Occup Physiol* 43:25–34, 1980.
14. Charette SL, McEvoy L, Pyka G, et al: Muscle hypertrophy response to resistance training in older men. *J Appl Physiol* 70:1912–1916, 1991.
15. Sahlin K: Metabolic aspects of fatigue in human skeletal muscle, Marconnet P, Komi PV, Satin B, Sejersted OM (eds): *Muscle Fatigue Mechanisms in Exercise and Training. Med Sport Sci* 34:54–68, 1992.
16. Sejersted OM, Vollestad NK: Increased metabolic rate associated with muscle fatigue, Marconnet P, Komi PV, Satin B, Sejersted OM (eds): *Muscle Fatigue Mechanisms in Exercise and Training. Med Sport Sci* 34:115–130, 1992.
17. Hermansen L, Osnes J: Blood and muscle pH after maximal exercise in man. *J Appl Physiol* 32:304–308, 1972.
18. Karlsson J: OBLA: A new concept for exercise testing. *Int J Sports Med* (special issue), 1982.
19. Donovan CM, Brooks GA: Endurance training affects lactate clearance, not lactate production. *Am J Physiol* 244:E83–E92, 1983.

20. Favier RJ, Constable SH, Chen M, Holloszy JO: Endurance exercise training reduces lactate production. *J Appl Physiol* 61:885–889, 1986.

21. American College of Sports Medicine: *Guideline for Exercise and Prescription,* 4th ed. Philadelphia, Lea and Febiger, 1991.

22. Faria IE: Cardiovascular response to exercise as influenced by training of various intensities. *Res Quart* 41:44–50, 1970.

23. Shephard RJ: Intensity, duration and frequency of exercise as determinants of the response to training regime. *Int Z Angrew Physiol Einschl Arbeitsphysiol* 26:272–278, 1968.

24. Sharkey BJ, Holleman JP: Cardiorespiratory adaptation to training at specified intensities. *Res Quart* 38:698–704, 1967.

25. Jackson J, Sharkey B, Johnston L: Cardiorespiratory adaptations to training at specified frequencies. *Res Quart* 39:295–300, 1968.

26. Bryntenson P, Sinning WE: The effects of training frequencies on the retention of cardiovascular fitness. *Med Sci Sports* 5:29–33, 1973.

27. Kasch FW, Philips WH, Carter JEL, Boyer JL: Cardiovascular changes in middle-aged men during two years of training. *J Appl Physiol* 34:53–57, 1973.

28. Pollock ML, et al: Effects of training two days per week at different intensities on middle-aged men. *Med Sci Sports* 4:192–197, 1972.

29. Kida K, Koudoh S, the project team: Pulmonary rehabilitation program survey in North America and Europe. *Am J Respir Crit Care Med* 153:A781, 1996.

30. Barach AL, Bickerman HA, Beck G: Advances in the treatment of non-tuberculous pulmonary disease. *Bull NY Acad Med* 28:353–384, 1952.

31. Pierce AK, Paez PN, Miller WF: Exercise training with the aid of a portable oxygen supply in patients with emphysema. *Am Rev Respir Dis* 95:653–659, 1965.

32. Paez PN, Phillipson EA, Masangkay M, Sproule BJ: The physiologic basis of training patients with emphysema. *Am Rev Respir Dis* 95:944–953, 1967.

33. Woolf CR, Suero JT: Alterations in lung mechanics and gas exchange following training in chronic obstructive lung disease. *Dis Chest* 55:37–44, 1969.

34. Bass H, Whitcomb JF, Forman R: Exercise training: Therapy for patients with chronic obstructive pulmonary disease. *Chest* 57:116–121, 1970.

35. Vyas MN, Banister EW, Morton JW, Grzybowski S: Response to exercise in patients with chronic airway obstruction: 1. Effects of exercise training. *Am Rev Respir Dis* 103:390–400, 1971.

36. Degre S, Sergysels R, Messin R, et al: Hemodynamic responses to physical training in patients with chronic lung disease. *Am Rev Respir Dis* 110:395–402, 1974.

37. Alpert JS, Bass H, Szucs MM, et al: Effects of physical training on hemodynamics and pulmonary function at rest and during exercise in patients with chronic obstructive pulmonary disease. *Chest* 66:647–651, 1974.

38. Cockcroft AE, Saunders MJ, Berry G: Randomized controlled trials of rehabilitation in chronic respiratory disability. *Thorax* 36:200–203, 1981.

39. Tydeman DE, Chandler AR, Graveling BM, et al: An investigation into the effects of exercise tolerance training on patients with chronic airways obstruction. *Physiotherapy* 70:261–264, 1984.

40. Jones DT, Thomson RJ, Sears MR: Physical exercise and resistive breathing training in severe chronic airways obstruction: Are they effective? *Eur J Respir Dis* 67:159–165, 1985.

41. Ries AL, Moser KM: Comparison of isocapnic hyperventilation and walking exercise training at home in pulmonary rehabilitation. *Chest* 90:285–289, 1986.

42. Casaburi R, Storer TW, Ben-Dov I, Wasserman K: Effect of endurance training on possible determinants of VO_2 during heavy exercise. *J Appl Physiol* 62:199–207, 1987.

43. Killian KJ, P Leblanc, Martin DH, et al: Exercise capacity and ventilatory, circulatory, and symptom limitation in patients with airflow limitation. *Am Rev Respir Dis* 146:935–940, 1992.

44. Allard C, Jones NL, Killian KJ: Static peripheral skeletal muscle strength and exercise capacity in patients with chronic airflow obstruction. *Am Rev Respir Dis* 139:A90, 1989.

45. Maltais F, Simard AA, Simard C, et al: Oxidative capacity of the skeletal muscle and lactic acid kinetics during exercise in normal subjects and in patients with COPD. *Am J Respir Crit Care Med* 153:288–293, 1996.

46. Katsuzawa T, Shioya S, Kurita D, et al: P-NMR study of skeletal muscle metabolism in patients with chronic respiratory impairment. *Am Rev Respir Dis* 146:1019–1024, 1992.

47. Casaburi R, Patessio A, Loli F, et al: Reduction in exercise lactic acidosis and ventilation as a result of exercise training in patients with obstructive lung disease. *Am Rev Respir Dis* 143:9–18, 1991.

48. Belman MJ, Kendregan BA: Exercise training fails to increase skeletal muscle enzymes in patients with chronic obstructive pulmonary disease. *Am Rev Respir Dis* 123:256–261, 1981.

49. Cockcroft AE, Saunders MJ, Berry G: Randomized controlled trial of rehabilitation in chronic respiratory disability. *Thorax* 36:200–203, 1981.

50. Reardon J, Award E, Normandin E, et al: The effect of comprehensive outpatient pulmonary rehabilitation on dyspnea. *Chest* 105:1046–1052, 1994.

51. McCloskey DI: Kinesthetic sensibility. *Physiol Rev* 58:763–820, 1978.

52. Matthews PBC: Where does Sherrington's "muscle sense" originate? Muscles, joints, corollary discharge? *Annu Rev Neurosci* 5:189–218, 1982.

53. Killian KJ, Bucens DD, Campbell EJM: Effect of breathing patterns on the perceived magnitude of added loads to breathing. *J Appl Physiol* 52:578–584, 1982.

54. El-Manshawi A, Killian KJ, Summers E, Jones NL: Breathlessness during exercise with and without resistive loading. *J Appl Physiol* 61:896–905, 1986.

55. O'Donnell DE, McGuire M, Samis L, Webb KA: The impact of exercise recording on breathlessness in severe chronic airflow limitation. *Am J Respir Crit Care* 152:2005–2013, 1995.

56. O'Donnell DE, Webb KA: The efficacy of adjunct high dose anticholinergic therapy in relieving breathlessness in patients with severe chronic airflow limitation. *Am J Respir Crit Care Med* 149:A286, 1994.

57. Hagbarth KE, Hagglund JV, Nordin M, Wallin EU: Thixotropic behavior of human finger flexor muscles with accompanying changes in spindle and reflex responses to stretch. *J Physiol Lond* 368:323–342, 1985.

58. Cherniack RM, Hodson A: Compliance of the chest wall in chronic bronchitis and emphysema. *J Appl Physiol* 18:707–711, 1963.

59. Homma I, Obata T, Sibuya M, Uchida M: Gate mechanism in breathlessness caused by chest wall vibration in humans. *J Appl Physiol* 56(1):8–11, 1984.

60. Homma I, Kanamaru A, Sibuya M, et al: Respiratory muscle conditioning. Stretch gymnastics of the respiratory muscles. Tokyo, Respiratory Muscle Conditioning Group, 1993; pp 1–14.

61. Yamada M, Shibuya M, Kanamaru A, et al: Benefits of respiratory muscle stretch gymnastics in chronic respiratory disease. *Showa Univ J Med Sci* 8:63–71, 1996.

62. Fujinaga H, Miyagawa T, Kokubu F: Respiratory conditioning group: Randomized cross-over comparison between respiratory muscle stretch gymnastics and inspiratory muscle training. *Am J Respir Crit Care Med* 155:A451, 1997.

63. Feinlieb M, Rosenberg HM, Collins JG, et al: Trends in COPD morbidity and mortality in the United States. *Am Rev Respir Dis* 140:S9–18, 1989.

64. Lacasse Y, Wong E, Guyatt GH, et al: Meta-analysis of respiratory rehabilitation in chronic obstructive pulmonary disease. *Lancet* 348:1115–1119, 1996.

Chapter 30

FUNCTIONAL STIMULATION OF THE RESPIRATORY MUSCLES

IKUO HOMMA

Chest Wall Vibration

BACKGROUND OF VIBRATION STIMULI

Vibration stimuli have been used in audiometry to examine hearing using a tuning fork as in the Rinne or Weber tests. They have also been employed for the diagnosis of disturbances of the posterior column and the lateral column by testing *vibration sense,* that is, perception of vibration while touching the tuning fork to bones. The vibrator stimulates not only the touch receptor and pressure receptor in the pacinian corpuscle but also the muscle spindles. The effect of vibration on the muscle spindle has attracted interest.

Two kinds of intrafusal fibers make up the muscle spindles; one is the nuclear bag fiber, and the other is the nuclear chain fiber. The sensory nerve endings of group Ia afferent nerve endings (primary endings) are in the middle of both fiber types, whereas the group II afferent nerve endings (secondary endings) are located at both poles of the nuclear chain fiber. The center of the nuclear chain fiber is less viscous than other areas and more elastic.[1]

Accordingly, vibration stimuli such as rapid microstretches have greater effects on the central area. At either end of type Ia or II fibers are mechanical receptors which have the ability to respond to stretch, but there are reports that the primary sensory nerve endings have particularly high sensitivity.[2]

Afferent nerve activity from a primary sensory nerve ending causes a reflex known as the *classic stretch reflex,* which is brought about by monosynaptic activation of the motor neuron of the spinal cord. Early research by Granit in Sweden showed that vibration at the primary muscle spindle ending is quite effective as a stimulus and activates controlling mechanisms within the limb muscles.[3] In humans, Hagbarth and colleagues observed that vibration stimulation of limb muscle causes an autogenetic increasing muscle reflex contraction in the muscles which has become well known as the tonic vibration reflex (TVR).[4,5]

TVR is observed in all ages in normal persons, but the strength of TVR varies from individual to individual and depends on the vibratory frequency and amplitude. Frequencies around 100 Hz work well in producing TVR. A large-amplitude vibration produces a large effect; however, an uncomfortable sensation is induced when the amplitude is greater than 3 mm. Thus an amplitude of 1 mm seems to work best in humans in eliciting the reflex. TVR also depends on the precontraction muscle length; thus, TVR is greatest in stretched muscles. TVR is caused by afferent activity from the muscle spindle as shown by studies using microneurography in humans. Hagbarth and Vallbo recorded nervous activity with a percutaneously inserted tungsten electrode into the median nerve or the tibial nerve in humans.[6] The effects of vibration on the primary or secondary spindle endings on the afferent activities from Ia and II nerve fibers were examined. Both types of muscle spindle endings responded well to vibrations. Their activities ceased when the vibration stopped.[7] The time duration of this response corresponded to the TVR caused by stimulation of the primary endings. In general, the primary muscle spindle ending is more sensitive to vibration than the secondary muscle spindle. Furthermore, the responses of a voluntary contraction to vibration are much better at the primary than at the secondary ending.[8]

Breathing is an involuntary act controlled by a control system which employs the respiratory muscles to fulfill a metabolic requirement. The reflexes of the muscle spindles of respiratory muscles are an important part of this control system. Euler and coworkers studied the role of muscle spindles of the respiratory muscles. They found the disturbances to intercostal muscle contraction caused by airway occlusion cause the muscle spindle of the intercostal muscles to stretch through an alpha-gamma linkage. This results in increased activity of the intercostal muscles.[9] In particular, the motor neurons of synergistic muscles are excited by the activation of primary muscle spindle endings. Adding a load causes a greater contraction called the *load compensation reflex.*[10] It has been reported that respiratory activity decreases in patients after amputation of the dorsal root of the spinal cord for the treatment of intercostal neuralgia; this shows that impairment of the sensory afferent pathway decreases respiratory activity in humans.[11] The diaphragm, which is a major respiratory muscle, has tendon organs rather than muscle spindles.

METHOD OF CHEST WALL VIBRATION

In 1978, Homma and colleagues showed that in humans sustained vibration applied to the chest wall can elicit a reflex contraction in the intercostal muscle. Electromyograms recorded from the intercostal muscles with a needle electrode showed tonic and gradually augmenting activity when 100-Hz vibration was applied; this activity reverted to its initial level when the vibration was stopped.[12]

Muscles of limbs (when vibrated) showed the same features of TVR, that is, activity which gradually increased when vibration was applied. Vibration of the inspiratory muscles during the inspiratory phase and of the expiratory intercostal muscles during the expiratory phase causes TVR that produces the same effect as the load compensation reflex.

The inspiratory and expiratory intercostal muscles exist as a double layer in most parts of the chest wall so that both intercostal muscles respond simultaneously when given vibration. However, in humans, there are two places with a single layer of intercostal muscle; one is located in the upper chest wall at the second or third parasternal intercostal space, and the other is located in the lower chest wall from the seventh to tenth intercostals just anterior to the midaxillary line.[13] As shown in Fig. 30-1, activity can be recorded from the upper intercostal muscles during inspiration with a needle electrode. Activity from the lower muscles cannot always be recorded during quiet breathing, but the discharge from those muscles, when it is present, appears to be in the expiratory phase. Figure 30-1 shows the expiratory activity at

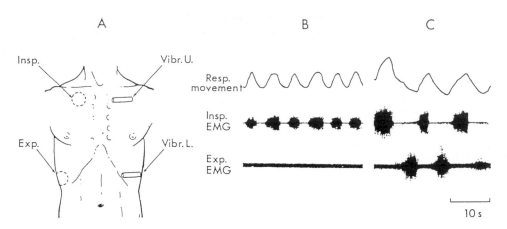

FIGURE 30-1 *A.* Diagram illustrating the upper and lower regions for EMG recording and application of vibratory stimulation. In (*B*) and (*C*) the upper trace indicates the respiratory movements as recorded by a strain gauge attached to a rubber band strapped around the thorax at the mamillary level. (In this as in succeeding figures inspiration gives upward deflection.) The middle trace shows inspiratory EMG and the lower expiratory EMG. Quiet breathing is shown in (*B*) and forced breathing (*C*). (From Homma et al.[14])

the expiratory phase during a large tidal volume.[12] Vibration applied to these two groups of intercostal muscles induces tonic activity. Applying vibration to the upper intercostal muscle during the inspiratory phase and to the lower intercostal muscle during the expiratory phase for short periods of time increases their activity, which assists inspiratory and expiratory contractions.[12] In patients with complete cervical spinal cord lesions at C6 or C7 who lack the ability to send a command from the central neural system, the intercostal muscle activity can be induced by applying vibration to the intercostal muscle (Fig. 30-2).[14] Vibrations of the upper chest wall during the inspiratory phase and of the lower chest wall during the expiratory phase are called in-phase vibration (IPV).[12] Vibration of the intercostal muscles stimulates spindles in the intercostal muscles. The vibration affects not only reflex effects through augmented afferent activity but also respiratory sensation. IPV decreases the sensation of dyspnea in normal subjects.[15] Out-of-phase vibration (OPV) refers to the application of vibration to the upper chest wall during the expiratory phase and to lower chest wall during the inspiratory phase.[12] In 1984, Homma's group suggested that the breathlessness may be induced by a mismatch between afferent activities and central respiratory commands.[16] In patients with chronic obstructive pulmonary disease (COPD), dyspnea decreases during IPV and increases during OPV (Fig. 30-3).[17] Cristiano and Schwartzstein also showed that IPV decreased dyspnea during hypercapnia in patients with COPD.[18] IPV also reduces breathlessness associated with

hypercapnia and resistive loading in normal subjects.[19] Homma's group developed the following vibrator system. The vibrator was installed inside a vest so that vibration could be applied to precise locations on the upper and lower chest on both sides. The apparatus for operating the vibrator and the triggering equipment to match stimulation to the appropriate phase of respiration were also installed in the vest (Fig. 30-4). Vibration of the chest wall causes not only TVR and affects the sensations related to respiration but may also produce a gas exchange increase referred to as high-frequency chest wall oscillation (HFCWO). This method is similar to the high-frequency ventilation (HFV) that increases gas exchange when vibration is applied to the airway directly at 2 to 20 Hz.[20]

SOMATOSENSORY EVOKED POTENTIALS FROM THE RESPIRATORY SYSTEM

Afferent information related to respiration from the intercostal muscles is relayed to centers in the medulla and to higher regions of the brain.[21] The relation between the output from the muscle spindle in the intercostal muscles and the sensory areas in the brain was examined in a study of somatosensory evoked potential (SEP). It is possible to record potentials (cortical SEP) induced by stimulation of sensory nerves in upper or lower extremities by means of electrodes applied to the skull. There is little research on respiration using the SEP. It has been reported that only signals from the sensory nerves with low-threshold receptors in the limb muscles project to the cortex.[22-24] In 1986, Davenport and coworkers reported that SEP is induced by airway occlusion, but the receptor involved was not specified.[25] The presence of evoked potentials from receptors in the chest wall was confirmed in a study in which there was electrical stimulation at the motor point of intercostal muscles and in another study by tapping of the chest wall. In 1989, Gandevia and Macefield[26] inserted a tungsten microelectrode percutaneously and applied electrical stimulation to the area where the efferent nerve contacts the muscles.

The tungsten microelectrode was inserted in the second intercostal space parasternally and the lateral part of the fifth intercostal space. The evoked potentials were observed 20 ms after stimulation.[26] In 1992, Kanamaru and colleagues produced evoked potentials by tapping the lower intercostal muscles. On one side, this study found that evoked potentials

FIGURE 30-2 Electromyogram (EMG) acrtivities from upper and lower intercostal muscles. Respiratory phase-locked vibrations were applied on both muscles alternatively. Vibration as indicated by bars. NOTE: Large spikes are electrocardiogram (ECG). (From Sibuya et al.[17])

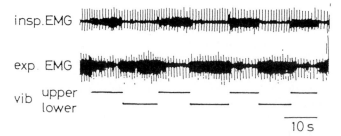

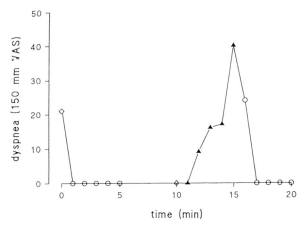

FIGURE 30-3 Typical time profile of the effect of chest wall vibration on dyspnea at rest in a patient with chronic respiratory disease. In-phase vibration (IPV; circles) eliminated dyspnea; out-of-phase vibration (OPV; triangles) increased dyspnea. Dyspnea intensity without vibration is shown by diamonds. In this particular case, IPV was repeated immediately after OPV. (From Homma et al.[14])

were observed in the contralateral parietal and occipital areas with a latency of 20 ms. Since evoked potentials could be induced even by tapping on a locally anesthetized area, the afferent activity which caused evoked potentials was considered to arise from muscle receptors.[27] That muscle receptors project to cortical areas has been confirmed in patients with brachial plexus injury after these patients underwent surgery in which the third or fourth intercostal nerve was sutured to the musculocutaneous nerve endings to restore function to the brachial biceps muscle after brachial plexus injury. A few months after surgery the patients were able to contract the brachial biceps muscle. Evoked potentials were observed on tapping the brachial biceps muscle which was controlled by the transferred intercostal nerve in these patients.[28] Reflex contractions were induced by tapping the reinnervated biceps muscle after reconstruction of the stretch receptors pathways.[29]

Electrical Stimulation

TEST OF DIAPHRAGM CONTRACTILITY

Electrical stimulation of the phrenic nerve can be used to examine the strength and contractility of the diaphragm in patients with respiratory problems. The force of a diaphragmatic twitch can be measured and induced by electrical stimulation of a phrenic nerve. Alternatively, the force produced by the diaphragm by maximal inspiratory efforts can be assessed.[30,31] Voluntary maximum inspiratory force is reduced by fatigue of the diaphragm as well as by respiratory muscle and other neuromuscular disorders.[32–34] The number of motor units activated by voluntary efforts, even maximal ones, is uncertain. Percutaneous tetanic electrical stimulation of the phrenic nerve, however, activates all motor units. Electrical stimulation at 10 Hz or more, however, causes subjects to feel pain.

Single twitch studies have been used to study the adductor pollicis muscle by Merton.[35] Bellemare and Bigland-Ritchie[36] and Aubier and coworkers[37] used the same technique to study fatigue of the diaphragm. In general, strength of the diaphragm is usually assessed from the transdiaphragmatic pressure achieved during maximal inspiratory efforts. Measurement during twitch contractions may be as useful as those produced by maximum inspiratory efforts in assessing diaphragm strength. Transdiaphragmatic pressure (Pdi) induced by inspiratory maximal sniffs and twitches induced by electrical stimulation have been compared in patients with diaphragm weakness and normal subjects.[38] There was a good relation between Pdi during a maximal sniff and electrically produced twitch Pdi. It is possible that the level of the twitch Pdi is potentiated by a voluntary contraction just before the electrical stimulation, as occurs in muscles of the extremities. This was confirmed in an experiment in which twitch Pdi increased to 5 to 10 s after a voluntary contraction of 50 to 100 percent of maximum.[39] Twitch Pdi is also utilized to test the effectiveness of therapy. Theophylline has been used extensively in the treatment of airway obstruction, not only because it relaxes bronchial smooth muscle, but also because it augments respiratory drive and improves the contractility of muscles.[40,41] Theophylline may improve diaphragm contractility in patients with chronic airflow limitation.[42] However, an analysis performed to examine the effect of aminophylline on the diaphragm in normal subjects using twitch Pdi demonstrated that there was no contractility effect.[43]

Maximal inspiratory and twitch Pdi decrease as lung volume increases because of shortening of precontraction muscle length.[23] In 1989 Hubmayr and colleagues[44] showed that an increase of 1 L of FRC in normal subjects reduced twitch Pdi by more than 7 cmH_2O. Thus, lung volume must be maintained at a fixed level to compare twitch Pdi during therapy.

DIAPHRAGM PACING

Electrical stimulation is useful not only for investigating the contractility of the diaphragm but also for supporting ventilation clinically. For example, electrical stimulation has been used for ventilator-dependent patients with high cervical cord lesion[45] and patients with central hypoventilation syndrome,[46] as well as for improving irregular breathing during sleep.[47]

The method for transcutaneous stimulation of the phrenic nerve is as follows: A moistened pad connected to the anode electrode is placed in contact with the skin on the back of the neck; the cathode electrode is placed on the operator's finger and is pressed against the skin overlying the anterior scalene muscle behind the lateral border of the sternocleidomastoid muscle. The stimulator is set to deliver impulses of 1-ms duration at a rate of one impulse per second at a current of 10 mA.[48]

Direct phrenic nerve stimulation is necessary for ventilatory support. The most common electrode used is the platinum ribbon type, which has an area of 0.17 to 0.20 cm^2.[49] The electrode is implanted against the perineum of the mediastinal surface of the phrenic nerve at a point between the base of the heart and the apex of the lung. The ribbon electrode and the wire are embedded in silicone to isolate them from tissues. The approach for implantation of the platinum ribbon electrode on the phrenic nerve in the chest is through the second interspace. The typical maximum strength re-

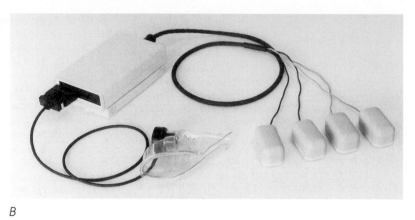

B

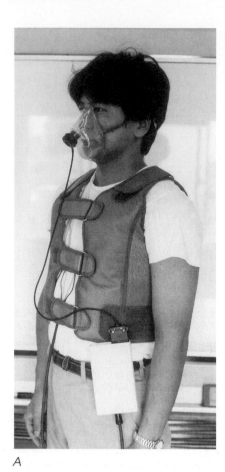

A

FIGURE 30-4 A vest installed with equipment, shown separately in (*B*), for giving vibration.

Magnetic Stimulation

quired to pace the diaphragm is 1.5 mA at a pulse width of 150 ms.[44] Ideal cases for diaphragm pacing are those with normal phrenic nerves, diaphragm, and lungs, and the technique has been used in central alveolar hypoventilation.[50]

Although improvements have been made, electrical stimulation of the diaphragm transcutaneously without causing pain remains a problem. Recently, magnetic stimulation has been used instead of the electrical stimulation. Magnetic stimulation does not need a high-density current as electrical stimulation does, so magnetic stimulation causes less discomfort since it does not stimulate skin receptor and the pain fibers.[51] Merton and Morton developed a way to examine the motor response of skeletal muscle by percutaneous electrical stimulation of cerebral motor area.[52] In the same way, diaphragm activity was induced by percutaneous electrical stimulation of motor area.[53] More recently, cortical magnetic stimulation has been used for the same purpose. This technique stimulates the agonists and antagonists simultaneously. Percutaneous stimulation of the motor area in the cortex activates the diaphragm only when the diaphragm is contracting and was not observed when the diaphragm was relaxed.[54,55] In magnetic stimulation, capacitors are charged from a high voltage source. When storage in the capacitor reaches a given voltage, then the stored energy is discharged through a coil. Structures in the discharge field are stimulated. Magnetic

transcranial stimulation has been combined with the stimulation of the cervical roots. In 1994, Lissens[56] demonstrated a technique which is useful in examining the function of central motor nerve pathways in respiratory muscles. Motor-evoked potentials (MEPs) were recorded with a 0.5-cm active cup electrode on the xiphoid process, with the reference electrode on the lower border of the rib cage at the midclavicular line and the ground electrode at the manubrium sterni. Magnetic transcranial stimulation was performed at 2 cm anterior to C3–C4 according to the 10–20 international system for placement of the EEG electrode. This place is close to the motor area of the right and left hemidiaphragm. The cervical root was stimulated at the C4 cervical level. Both transcortical stimulation and the cervical root stimulation were delivered by a circular magnetic coil (outer diameter 12.5 cm). The central motor conduction time was measured from the latency time of the MEP.

A technique for phrenic nerve trunk stimulation and phrenic nerve root stimulation was introduced by Chokroverty's group.[57] For nerve stimulation, a circular magnetic coil is held flat over the right or the left side of the neck with the handle of the coil pointing toward the acromion (Fig. 30-5). The midpoint of the outer edge of the coil faces the thyroid cartilage and is placed at the upper border of the thyroid cartilage posterior to the sternocleidomastoideus. For phrenic root stimulation, a circular magnetic coil is held flat on the upper cervical vertebrae with the handle pointing toward the feet. In 1996, Zifko and coworkers[58] compared of 9 cm was used. Transcortical stimulation was performed at 95 percent the maximal magnetic output; cervical stimulation, at 65 percent the maximal magnetic output. The latencies of the two different coils were similar; however, the amplitude was higher and the excitability thresholds were lower for the 9-cm circular coil. Accordingly, the result from stimulation with the 9-cm coil was preferable to the figure-of-eight coil. Magnetic stimulation seems to be a developing method for assessing the neurophysiology of respiration that may provide important diagnostic information.

References

1. Barker D: The innervation of the muscle spindle. *Quart J Microsc Sci* 89:143–186, 1948.
2. Bianconi R, Van der Meulen JP: The response to vibration of the end organs of mammalian muscle spindles. *J Neurophysiol* 26:117–190, 1962.
3. Granit R: Reflex self-regulation of the muscle contraction and autogenetic inhibition. *J Neurophysiol* 13:351–372, 1950.
4. Eklund G, Hagbarth K-E: Normal variability of tonic vibration reflexes in man. *Exp Neurol* 16:80–92, 1966.
5. Hagbarth K-E, Eklund G: Motor effects of vibration muscle stimuli in man, in Granit R (ed): *Proceedings of the First Nobel Symposium,* Stockholm, Almqvist and Wiksell, 1966; pp 177–186.
6. Hagbarth K-E, Vallbo AB: Discharge characteristics of human muscle afferents during muscle stretch and contraction. *Exp Neurol* 22:674–694, 1968.
7. Burke D, Hagbarth K-E, Löfstedt L, Wallin BG: The responses of human muscle spindle endings to vibration of non-contracting muscles. *J Physiol* 261:673–693, 1976.
8. Burke D, Hagbarth K-E, Löfstedt L, Wallin BG: The responses of human muscle spindle endings to vibration during isometric contraction. *J Physiol* 261:695–711, 1976.
9. Corda M, Eklund G, von Euler C: External intercostal and phrenic alpha motoneurons to changes in respiratory load. *Acta Physiol Scand* 63:391–400, 1965.
10. von Euler C: On the role of proprioceptors in perception and execution of motor acts with special references to breathing, in Campbell EJM (ed): *Loaded Breathing.* Canada, Hamilton Longman Ltd, 1973; pp 139–154.
11. Eccles JC, Eccles RM, Lundberg A: The convergence of monosynaptic excitatory afferents onto many different species of alpha motoneurones. *J Physiol* 137:22–50, 1957.
12. Homma I, Eklund G, Hagbarth K-E: Respiration in man affected by TVR contractions elicited in inspiratory and expiratory intercostal muscles. *Respir Physiol* 35:335–348, 1978.
13. Taylor A: The contribution of the intercostal muscles to effect of respiration in man. *J Physiol (Lond)* 151:390–401, 1960.
14. Homma I, Nagai T, Sakai T, et al: Effect of chest wall vibration on ventilation in patients with spinal cord lesion. *J Appl Physiol Respir Environ Exercise Physiol* 50(1):107–111, 1981.
15. Manning HL, Basner R, Ringler J, et al: Effect of chest wall vibration on breathlessness in normal subjects. *J Appl Physiol* 71(1):175–181, 1991.
16. Homma I, Obata T, Sibuya M, Uchida M: Gate mechanism in breathlessness caused by chest wall vibration in human. *J Appl Physiol Respir Environ Exercise Physiol* 56(1):8–11, 1984.
17. Sibuya M, Yamada M, Kanamaru A, et al: Effect of chest wall vibration on dyspnea in patients with chronic respiratory disease. *Am J Respir Crit Care Med* 149(5):1235–1240, 1994.
18. Cristiano LM, Schwartzstein M: Effect of chest wall vibration on dyspnea during hypercapnia and exercise in chronic obstructive pulmonary disease. *Am J Respir Crit Care Med* 155:1552–1559, 1997.
19. Edo H, Kimura H, Niijima M, et al: Effects of chest wall vibration

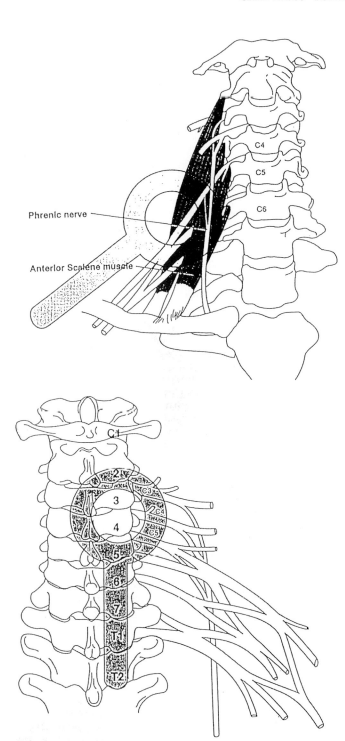

FIGURE 30-5 *Top*: **Schematic diagram showing position of the round magnetic coil (MC) stimulator on one side of the neck.** *Bottom*: **Schematic diagram showing position of the round magnetic coil (MC) stimulator over the upper cervical vertebral column. (Modified from Chokroverty et al.[57])**

two different kinds of devices for the magnetic stimulation; one is a circular stimulating coil, with a mean diameter of 9 cm and 2.0-T maximum magnetic density, and the other figure-of-eight circular stimulating coils, each with a mean diameter of 7 cm and 2.2-T maximal magnetic flux density. For cervical magnetic stimulation, the coil with a diameter on breathlessness during hypercapnic ventilatory response. *J Appl Physiol* 84(5):1487–1491, 1998.

20. Chang HK, Hart A: High-frequency ventilation: A review. *Respir Physiol* 57:135–152, 1984.

21. Shannon R, Bolser DC, Lindsey BG: Medullary expiration activity: Influence of intercostal tendon organs and muscle spindle endings. *J Appl Physiol* 62:1057–1062, 1987.

22. Burke D, Skuse NF, Lethlean AK: Cutaneous and muscle afferent components of the cerebral potential evoked by electrical stimulation of human peripheral nerves. *Electroencephalogr Clin Neurophysiol* 51:579–588, 1981.

23. Gandevia SC, Burke D, Mckeon B: The relationship between the size of a muscle afferent volley and the cerebral potential it produces. *J Neurol Neurosurg Psychiatry* 45:705–710, 1982.

24. Gandevia SC, Burke D, Mckeon B: The projection of muscle afferents from the hand to cerebral cortex in man. *Brain* 107:1–13, 1984.

25. Davenport PW, Friedman WA, Thompson FJ, Franzen O: Respiratory-related cortical potentials evoked by inspiratory occlusion in humans. *J Appl Physiol* 60:1843–1848, 1986.

26. Gandevia SC, Macefield G: Projection of low-thereshold afferents from human intercostal muscles to the cerebral cortex. *Respir Physiol* 77:203–214, 1989.

27. Kanamaru A, Sibuya M, Sai K, et al: Somatosensory evoked potentials induced by intercostal tapping. *Showa Univ J Med Sci* 4:59–66, 1992.

28. Kanamaru A, Suzuki S, Sibuya M, et al: Sensory reinnervation of muscle receptor in human. *Neurosci Lett* 161:27–29, 1993.

29. Sai K, Kanamaru A, Sibuya M, et al: Reconstruction of tonic vibration reflex in the biceps brachii reinnervated by transferred intercostal nerves in patients with brachial plexus injury. *Neurosci Lett* 206:1–4, 1996.

30. Agostoni E, Rahn H: Abdominal and thoracic pressures at different lung volumes. *J Appl Physiol* 15:1087–1092, 1960.

31. Milic-Emili J, Mead J, Turner JM, Glauser EM: Improved technique for estimating pleural pressure from esophageal balloons. *J Appl Physiol* 19:207–211, 1964.

32. Roussons C, Macklem PT: Diaphragmatic fatigue in man. *J Appl Physiol* 43:189–198, 1977.

33. Neusom DJ, Loh L: Alveolar hypoventilation and respiratory muscle weakness. *Bull Eur Physiopathol Respir* 15:45–51, 1979.

34. Bellemare F, Grassino A: Force reserve of the diaphragm in COPD patients. *J Appl Physiol* 55:8–15, 1983.

35. Merton PA: Voluntary strength and fatigue. *J Physiol* 123:553–564, 1954.

36. Bellemare F, Bigland-Ritchie B: Assessment of human diaphragm strength and activation using phrenic nerve stimulation. *Respiration Physiol* 58:263–277, 1984.

37. Aubier M, Farkas G, De Troyer A, et al: Detection of diaphragmatic fatigue in man by phrenic stimulation. *J Appl Physiol* 50:538–544, 1981.

38. Mier A, Brophy C, Moxham J, Green M: Twitch pressures in the assessment of diaphragm weakness. *Thorax* 44:990–996, 1989.

39. Wragg S, Aquilina R, Moran J, et al: Comparison of cervical magnetic stimulation and bilateral percutaneous electrical stimulation of the phrenic nerves in normal subjects. *Eur Respir J* 7:1788–1792, 1994.

40. Aubier M, De Troyer A, Sampson M, et al: Aminophylline improves diaphragmatic contractility. *N Engl J Med* 305:249–252, 1981.

41. Eldridge FL, Millhorn DE, Waldrop TG, Kiley JP: Mechanism of respiratory effects of methylxanthines. *Respir Physiol* 53:239–261, 1983.

42. Murciano D, Aubier M, Lecocguic Y, Pariente R: Effects of theophylline on diaphragmatic strength and fatigue in patients with chronic obstructive pulmonary disease. *N Engl J Med* 311:349–353, 1984.

43. Robert DL, Nava S, Gibbons L, Bellemare F: Aminophylline and human diaphragm strength in vivo. *J Appl Physiol* 68(6):2591–2596, 1990.

44. Hubmayr RD, Litchy WJ, Gay PC, Nelson SB: Transdiaphragmatic twitch pressure. *Am Rev Respir Dis* 139:647–652, 1989.

45. Glenn WWL: The treatment of respiratory paralysis by diaphragm pacing. *Ann Thorac Surg* 30:106–109, 1980.

46. Hyland RH, Jones NL, Powles ACP, et al: Primary alveolar hypoventilation treated with nocturnal electrophrenic respiration. *Am Rev Respir Dis* 117:165–172, 1978.

47. Bradley RD, Day A, Hyland RH, et al: Chronic ventilatory failure caused by abnormal respiratory pattern generation during sleep. *Am Rev Respir Dis* 130:678–680, 1984.

48. Shaw RK, Glenn WWL, Hogan JF, Phelps ML: Electrophysiological evaluation of phrenic nerve function in candidates for diaphragm pacing. *J Neurosurg* 53:345–354, 1980.

49. Glenn WWL, Hogan JF, Phelps ML: Ventilatory support of the quadriplegic patient with respiratory paralysis by diaphragm pacing. *Surg Clin North Am* 60:1055–1078, 1980.

50. William WL, Glenn MD, Mildred LP: Diaphragm pacing by electrical stimulation of the phrenic nerve. *Neurosurgery* 17:974–984, 1985.

51. Barker AT, Garnham CW, Freeston IL: Magnetic nerve stimulation—The effect of waveform on efficiency, determination of neural membrane time constants and the measurement of the stimulator output. *Electroencephalogr Clin Neurophysiol* 43:227–237, 1991.

52. Merton PA, Morton HB: Stimulation of cerebral cortex in intact human subjects. *Nature* 285:227, 1980.

53. Gandevia SC, Rothwell JC: Activation of the human diaphragm from the motor cortex. *J Physiol* 384:109–118, 1987.

54. Murphy K, Mier A, Adams L, Guz A: Putative cerebral cortical involvement in the ventilatory response to inhaled CO_2 in conscious man. *J Physiol* 420:1–18, 1990.

55. Maskill D, Murphy K, Mier A, et al: Motor cortical representation of the diaphragm in man. *J Physiol* 443:105–121, 1991.

56. Lissens MA: Motor evoked potentials of the human diaphragm elicited through magnetic transcranial brain stimulation. *Neurolog Sci* 124:204–207, 1994.

57. Chokroverty S, Shah S, Chokroverty M, et al: Percutaneous magnetic coil stimulation of the phrenic nerve roots and trunk. *Electroencephalogr Clin Neurophysiol* 97:369–374, 1995.

58. Zifko U, Remtulla H, Power K, et al: Transcortical and cervical magnetic stimulation with recording of the diaphragm. *Muscle Nerve* 19:614–620, 1996.

Chapter 31

MECHANICAL VENTILATION

RAJIV DHAND

MARTIN J. TOBIN

The development of acute or chronic respiratory insufficiency in a patient often necessitates the use of a mechanical device to replace or aid the work carried out by the ventilatory muscles. In the early part of this century, large tank-type negative pressure respirators ("iron lungs") were commonly employed to provide lifesaving ventilatory support. At midcentury, the benefits of positive-pressure ventilation were recognized, and this is now the usual method of providing ventilator assistance. The widespread popularity of positive-pressure ventilation has been dampened to some extent by the awareness that its use may worsen a patient's underlying lung injury. This awareness has led to a renewed search for alternative ventilatory strategies to support patients with respiratory insufficiency. In addition, the ability to provide long-term ventilation has resulted in several patients receiving mechanical ventilation outside the intensive care unit (ICU). Noninvasive means of providing positive pressure ventilation are being increasingly used to fulfill this role.

Mechanical Ventilation in the ICU

The objectives of mechanical ventilation are listed in Table 31–1.[1] In isolation, hypoxemia of mild to moderate severity can be managed by the administration of oxygen through a face mask. With more severe hypoxemia due to shunt and/or ventilation-perfusion ($\dot{V}/Q$) mismatching, it is difficult to guarantee the delivery of a high fractional inspired oxygen concentration ($F_{I_{O_2}}$) through a face mask. Moreover, these patients are also commonly in considerable distress, so that intubation helps by ensuring delivery of the required $F_{I_{O_2}}$ and positive-pressure ventilation helps by recruiting collapsed lung units leading to improved matching of ventilation and perfusion.

Acute progressive respiratory acidosis is a major indication for mechanical ventilation, although simpler measures can sometimes reverse the process.[2] If severe respiratory depression is expected to persist for some time (e.g., certain drug overdoses), intubation and mechanical ventilation should be instituted without delay.

A substantial proportion of patients who require (and benefit from) mechanical ventilation have relatively normal arterial blood gases but have clinical signs of increased work of breathing—nasal flaring; vigorous activity of the sternomastoid muscles; tracheal tug; retraction of the suprasternal, supraclavicular, and intercostal spaces; paradoxical motion of the abdomen; and pulsus paradoxus. These clinical signs of impending exhaustion, especially when they are coupled with the presence of hemodynamic instability (hypotension, tachycardia), are good indicators for initiating mechanical ventilation when the underlying clinical condition is not rapidly reversible. Depending on the nature of the underlying disease, work of breathing may be increased as a result of increased airway resistance, increased stiffness of the lungs or chest wall, or the presence of a threshold inspiratory load due to auto- or intrinsic positive end-expiratory pressure (PEEPi) (Fig. 31–1).[3,4] Increased respiratory work increases the O_2 cost of breathing to as much as 50 percent of total O_2 consumption.[5] In such circumstances, mechanical ventilation decreases the work of breathing and allows precious O_2 stores to be rerouted to other vulnerable tissue beds. In patients with atelectasis or acute lung injury, breathing occurs on the low flat portion of the pressure-volume curve. By shifting tidal ventilation to the steep compliant portion of the pressure-volume curve, mechanical ventilation can decrease the work of breathing (Fig. 31–2).[6]

POSITIVE-PRESSURE VENTILATION

INVASIVE POSITIVE-PRESSURE VENTILATION

Modes of Mechanical Ventilation

The term *mode* refers to the relationship between various possible breath types—mandatory, assisted, supported, spontaneous—and inspiratory phase variables.

CONTROLLED MECHANICAL VENTILATION   The ventilator delivers all breaths at a preset rate, and the patient cannot trigger the machine. In the volume-targeted mode, the breaths have a preset volume called *volume-controlled ventilation*. When the breaths are pressure limited and time cycled, it is termed *pressure-controlled ventilation*.[7] Use of volume-controlled ventilation is largely restricted to patients who are apneic as a result of brain damage, sedation, or paralysis.

ASSIST-CONTROL VENTILATION   In the assist control (AC) mode, the ventilator delivers a breath either when triggered by the patient's inspiratory effort (either pressure or flow triggered) or independently if such an effort does not occur within a preselected time period. All breaths are delivered under positive pressure by the machine, but unlike controlled mechanical ventilation the patient's triggering effort can exceed the preset rate. If the patient's spontaneous rate drops below the preset back-up rate, controlled ventilation is provided. The pressure to achieve the set tidal volume may be provided solely by the machine or in part by the patient. The amount of active work performed by a patient being ventilated in the AC mode is critically dependent on the trigger sensitivity and inspiratory flow settings. Even when these settings are selected appropriately, patients actively perform about one-third of the work performed by the ventilator during passive conditions.[8,9]

INTERMITTENT MANDATORY VENTILATION   With intermittent mandatory ventilation (IMV), the patient receives periodic positive-pressure breaths from the ventilator at a preset volume and rate, but the patient can also breathe spontaneously between these mandatory breaths.[10] Modifications of the ventilator to achieve synchronization of the delivery of machine breaths with the patient's own inspiratory rhythm led to the introduction of synchronized intermittent mandatory ventilation (SIMV). For this purpose, a patient-triggered demand valve, which functions essentially like assist control during windows of time set by the manu-

TABLE 31-1 Objectives of Mechanical Ventilation

Improve pulmonary gas exchange	Alter pressure-volume relationships
Reverse hypoxemia	Prevent and/or reverse atelectasis
Relieve acute respiratory acidosis	Improve compliance
Relieve respiratory distress	Prevent further injury
Decrease oxygen cost of breathing	Permit lung and airway healing
Reverse respiratory muscle fatigue	Avoid complications

SOURCE: From Tobin MJ: Mechanical ventilation. *N Engl J Med* 330:1056, 1994, with permission.

facturer (usually as a function of the set respiratory rate), is incorporated into the ventilator (Fig. 31–3). Any spontaneous inspiratory activity is sensed by the pressure sensor, the expiratory valve is closed, and the inspiratory valve is opened. The flow of gas through the inspiratory valve is matched to the patient's inspiratory flow rate; allowing the patient to breathe spontaneously through the ventilator.

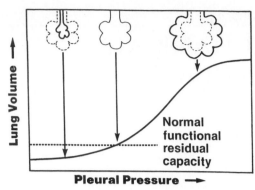

FIGURE 31-2 Normally a tidal breath begins at functional residual capacity (FRC), which is on the steep portion of the pressure-volume curve of the lung. A collapsed airway or alveolus results in a low FRC (on the low flat portion of the curve) where a large change in pleural pressure is required for even a small volume change. In this situation, PEEP shifts the end-expiratory lung volume to the steep portion of the curve; however, it may also cause a normal alveolus to move to the upper flat portion of the curve with consequent overdistention and risk of alveolar rupture. (From Tobin MJ: *Essentials of Critical Care Medicine.* New York, Churchill Livingstone, 1989; p 279, with permission.)

FIGURE 31-1 The inspiratory pressure-time product (PTP/min) can be partitioned into intrinsic positive end-expiratory pressure (PEEPi), non-PEEPi elastic, and resistive components. The contributions of each component to PTP/min are shown at the beginning and end of a weaning trial. Total PTP/min was higher at the beginning of the trial in patients who failed the weaning trial ($n = 17$) compared with those who were successfully extubated ($n = 14$). The difference was mainly due to higher contributions from PEEPi and resistive components in the failure group. By the end of the trial, PTP/min increased disproportionately in the patients who failed weaning compared to those who were successful. At the end of the trial, the increase in PTP/min in the failure group was due to increases in the PEEPi component by 111 percent ($p < .0001$ compared with values at the start of the trial), non-PEEPi elastic component by 33 percent ($p < .0001$) and resistive component by 42 percent ($p < .0001$). (From Jubran A, Tobin MJ: Pathophysiologic basis of acute respiratory distress in patients who fail a trial of weaning from mechanical ventilation. *Am J Respir Crit Care Med* 155:906–915, 1997, with permission.)

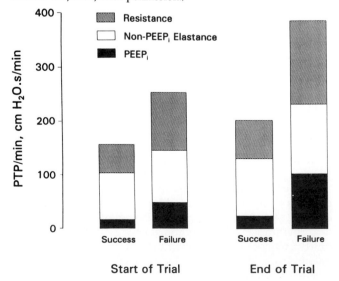

When a mandatory breath is due, the ventilator waits until the patient begins to inhale and then synchronizes the breath with the patient's inspiratory effort. If the patient makes an inspiratory effort while the window is open, a synchronized breath is delivered. If no effort occurs by the time the window closes, the ventilator delivers a controlled positive-pressure breath.

The occurrence of some complications, such as ventilator-induced barotrauma, is lower in patients receiving IMV compared with those receiving controlled mechanical ventilation.[11] Similarly, patients with normal left-ventricular function have a higher cardiac output with IMV than with controlled mechanical ventilation, but patients with poor left-ventricular function show lower cardiac output with IMV than with controlled ventilation.[12] The more negative intrathoracic pressure during IMV enhances venous return, which presumably accounts for the increased cardiac output in patients with normal left-ventricular function. However, negative intrathoracic pressure also increases left-ventricular afterload, and this effect dominates in patients with poor cardiac reserve, accounting for the reduction in cardiac output in this group.[13]

One of the main objectives of mechanical ventilation is to alleviate discomfort secondary to increased respiratory work. However, patients may have difficulty in adapting to the intermittent nature of ventilator assistance with IMV. In the past, it was assumed that the degree of respiratory muscle rest was proportional to the level of machine assistance during IMV. However, recent studies indicate that inspiratory effort is equivalent for spontaneous and assisted breaths during IMV[14–16] (Fig. 31–4). Indeed, the tension-time index for both the spontaneous and assisted breaths was above the threshold associated with respiratory muscle fatigue at IMV rates of 14 breaths per minute or less.[14] At a moderate level of machine assistance, that is, where the ventilator accounted for 20 to 50 percent of the total ventilation, electromyographic

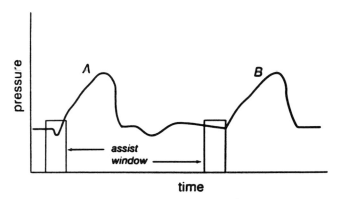

FIGURE 31-3 Synchronization of intermittent mandatory ventilation (IMV) through use of an assist window *A*. If the patient makes an effort during a window of time, the ventilator senses this effort and delivers a breath in synchrony with the patient's effort. *B*. If no effort is made while the window is open, a controlled breath is delivered. (From Kacmarek RM, Hess D, in Tobin MJ (ed): *Principles and Practice of Mechanical Ventilation*, New York, McGraw-Hill 1994; p 79, with permission.)

(EMG) activity of the diaphragm and sternomastoid muscles was equivalent for assisted and spontaneous breaths.[15] These findings suggest that respiratory center output is preprogrammed and that it does not adjust to breath-to-breath changes in load as occur during IMV. As a result, IMV may contribute to the development of respiratory muscle fatigue or prevent its recovery.

PRESSURE SUPPORT VENTILATION   Pressure support (PS) ventilation is patient triggered like AC and IMV, but differs in that it is pressure targeted and flow cycled.[17] The physician sets a level of pressure that augments every spontaneous effort, and the patient can alter respiratory frequency, inspiratory time, and tidal volume. A fall in airway pressure with the initiation of a breath by the patient triggers the ventilator, which then provides inspiratory airflow and raises the pressure to the preset value. Therefore, the energy to inflate the lungs and chest wall is provided partly by the patient and partly by the positive airway pressure generated by the ventilator. Tidal volume is determined by the pressure setting, the patient's effort, and pulmonary mechanics, in contrast to AC and IMV where a guaranteed volume is delivered. The lack of guaranteed ventilator assistance in the absence of patient effort can result in apnea in patients with unstable respiratory center output; some ventilators include safety features against this problem, but others (e.g., Siemens Servo 900C) do not. Cycling to exhalation is triggered by a decrease in inspiratory flow to a preset level, such as 5 L/min or 25 percent of the peak inspiratory flow, depending on the manufacturer's algorithm. Inspiratory assistance can also be terminated by a small increase in pressure (1 to 3 cmH₂O) above the preset level, resulting from expiratory effort.[17] If there is a leak in the system, neither of these mechanisms is effective and the patient is at risk of overinflation; inclusion of a time limit for inspiration prevents this hazard.

Several investigators have shown that PS is very effective in decreasing the work of inspiration. However, the degree of inspiratory muscle unloading is variable, with a coefficient of variation of up to 96 percent among patients.[18] PS does

not decrease PEEPi in patients with chronic obstructive pulmonary disease (COPD).[18,19] Thus, at a PS of 20 cmH₂O, PEEPi may account for approximately two-thirds of total inspiratory effort.[18] The algorithm used to terminate inspiratory assistance during PSV (a fall in inspiratory flow to a threshold value) can lead to excessive expiratory effort in patients with COPD. Patients with a prolonged time constant require more time for flow to fall to this threshold, and, consequently, mechanical inflation may persist into neural expiration. To counteract such neural-mechanical dysynchrony, patients may activate their expiratory muscles at a time when the ventilator is still inflating the thorax causing the patient to "fight the ventilator."[18]

There is no consensus as to the appropriate level of PS for an individual patient. In one study, the level of PS that minimized activity of the sternomastoid muscles was associated with reversal of EMG evidence of excessive diaphragmatic stress.[17] More commonly, PS is titrated to achieve a decrease in respiratory frequency and an increase in tidal volume. However, there is a considerable discrepancy among studies as to the preferred target or "optimal" level of PS. Titration of PS to achieve a low respiratory frequency will generally result in inspiratory muscle unloading, but activity of the expiratory muscles may increase *pari passu* and cause the patient to fight the ventilator. This makes selection of the optimal level of PS quite complex.[18]

Ventilator Settings
The settings on the ventilator are based on the patient's size and condition. This is a dynamic process that is based on

FIGURE 31-4 Electromyograms of the diaphragm (EMGdi) and the stenocleidomastoid muscles (EMGscm) in a patient receiving synchronized intermittent mandatory ventilation, showing similar intensity and duration of electrical activity during assisted (A) and spontaneous (S) cycles. Paw, airway pressure; Pes, esophageal pressure. (From Imsand C, Feihl F, Perret MD, Fitting JW: Regulation of inspiratory neuromuscular output during synchronized intermittent mechanical ventilation. *Anesthesiology* 80:13–22, 1994, with permission.)

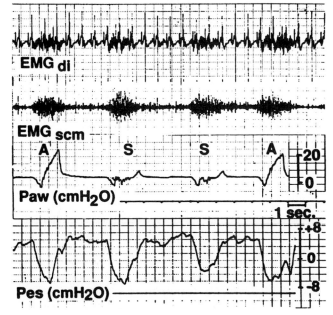

a patient's physiologic response rather than a fixed set of numbers. The settings require repeated readjustment over the period of dependency on the ventilator, and such iterative interaction requires careful respiratory monitoring.

TRIGGER SENSITIVITY Most mechanical ventilators employ pressure triggering, whereby a decrease in circuit pressure is required to initiate ventilator assistance. It is difficult to employ a trigger setting more sensitive than -1 to -2 cmH_2O without causing the ventilator to autocycle, but if the setting is less sensitive, the work of breathing increases significantly. The actual change in airway pressure with ventilator triggering is usually quite different from the set sensitivity.[20]

With flow triggering (sometimes termed *flow by*), a base flow of gas (usually set at 5 to 20 L/min) is delivered during both the expiratory and inspiratory phases of the respiratory cycle.[21] In the presence of patient effort, gas enters the lungs and is diverted from the exhalation port. The difference between inspiratory and expiratory base flow is sensed and causes the ventilator to switch phase; sensitivity is usually set at 2 L/min. A flow-triggered system is thought to be more responsive to a patient's ventilatory demand than a pressure-triggered system.[20] As a result, work of inspiration is less with flow triggering than with pressure triggering. However, ventilators using a flow-triggering mechanism are very susceptible to circuit leaks, condensation of water in the circuit, or movement caused by turbulence. These conditions may cause spurious triggering of the ventilator, thereby impairing patient-ventilator synchrony and increasing the work of breathing.

Triggering of the ventilator is more difficult in patients with airflow limitation and dynamic hyperinflation, where the end-expiratory lung volume exceeds the relaxation volume of the respiratory system. In this case, the patient must first generate sufficient pressure to offset the elastic recoil associated with hyperinflation and then overcome the sensitivity threshold. As a result, patients may make two or more efforts before successfully triggering the ventilator, and the patient's intrinsic rate exceeds that of the ventilator[16] (Fig. 31–5).

TIDAL VOLUME A tidal volume of 10 to 15 mL/kg of the patient's body weight has been the standard recommendation for several years. This recommendation has been challenged by convincing data in experimental animals indicating that alveolar overdistention can produce endothelial, epithelial, and basement-membrane injuries that are associated with increased microvascular permeability and lung rupture.[22] To minimize this risk, it would be ideal to monitor alveolar volume, but this is not feasible. A reasonable substitute is to monitor the peak alveolar pressure as estimated from the plateau pressure, which is measured in a relaxed patient by briefly occluding the ventilator circuit at end-inspiration.[23] The incidence of ventilator-induced lung injury increases markedly when the plateau pressure is high. Although data are incomplete, there is a growing tendency to decrease the delivered tidal volume from the 10 to 15 mL/kg recommended earlier to 5 to 7 mL/kg (or less). The objective is to achieve a plateau pressure no higher than 35 cmH_2O,[24] so as not to exceed total lung capacity. This ventilatory strategy is termed *permissive hypercapnia*, or *controlled hypoventilation*,[25] because it may lead to an increase in Pa$_{CO_2}$. It is impor-

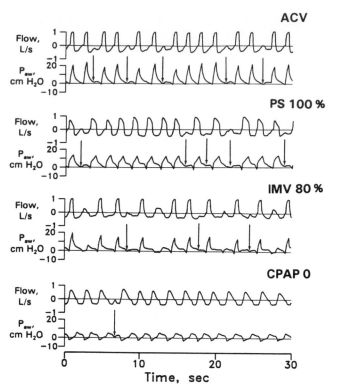

FIGURE 31-5 Recordings of flow and airway pressure in a patient receiving assist-control ventilation (ACV), pressure support of 100 percent (PS 100), intermittent mandatory ventilation of 80 percent (IMV 80), and unassisted breathing through the ventilator circuit (CPAP 0). PS 100 is the level of pressure support required to match the tidal volume on ACV, whereas IMV 80 represents an IMV ventilator rate setting at 80 percent of the patient's breathing frequency during ACV. Several inspiratory efforts by the patient failed to trigger opening of the ventilator valve (arrows). (From Leung P, Jubran A, Tobin MJ: Comparison of assisted ventilator modes on triggering, patient effort and dyspnea. *Am J Respir Crit Care Med* accepted for publication, with permission.)

tant to focus on the pH rather than the Pa$_{CO_2}$ when using this approach. If the pH falls below 7.20, some physicians recommend intravenous bicarbonate, but this is of unproven benefit.[25] In patients with severe asthma requiring mechanical ventilation, uncontrolled studies suggest that permissive hypercapnia results in lower mortality than conventional ventilation,[26,27] and the same may be true in patients with the acute respiratory distress syndrome (ARDS).[28]

RESPIRATORY RATE Setting the ventilator rate depends on the mode being employed. With AC ventilation, the ventilator supplies a breath in response to each patient effort. Two types of problems can occur if the machine rate is set much lower than the patient's spontaneous rate. One, if the patient has a sudden decrease in respiratory center output, a low machine rate will result in serious hypoventilation. Two, a large discrepancy between the patient's spontaneous rate and the backup rate results in a respiratory cycle with an inverse inspiratory-to-expiratory time (I:E) ratio.[21] Therefore, during AC the backup rate should be set at approximately four breaths fewer than the patient's spontaneous rate. With IMV, the ventilator or mandatory rate is set high

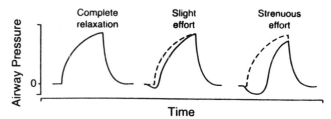

FIGURE 31-6 Airway-pressure waveforms recorded during assist-control ventilation. The tracings represent changes in airway pressure during inspiration in a completely relaxed patient and in patients making a slight effort and a strenuous effort to breathe. The distance between the dashed line (representing controlled ventilation) and the solid line (representing spontaneous breathing) is proportional to the patient's work of breathing. (From Tobin MJ: Mechanical ventilation. *N Engl J Med* 330:1056, 1994, with permission.)

at first and then gradually decreased according to patient tolerance. Unfortunately, titration is often based on arterial blood-gas data, and even a small number of ventilator breaths result in acceptable Pa_{O_2} and Pa_{CO_2} values but achieve little or no respiratory muscle rest in patients with an increased work of breathing. With pressure-support ventilation, the ventilator rate is not set.

INSPIRATORY FLOW RATE   In most patients receiving ACV or IMV, the initial (default) inspiratory flow rate is 60 L/min; with AC on certain ventilators (e.g., Siemens Servo 900C), however, such a flow cannot be attained without increasing V_T above desirable levels. In patients with COPD, increasing the flow rate to 100 L/min produces better gas exchange, as reflected by decreases of >20 percent in venous admixture ($\dot{Q}s/\dot{Q}T$) and V_D/V_T, probably because the resulting increase in expiratory time allows more complete emptying of gas-trapped regions.[29] A high inspiratory flow setting is also needed in patients with increased respiratory drive. An excessive flow setting should be avoided, and studies in healthy subjects demonstrate that increasing the inspiratory flow setting causes an immediate increase in respiratory frequency and respiratory drive.[30] When adjusting the flow rate and trigger sensitivity, it is helpful to examine the contour of the airway pressure waveform (Fig. 31–6). Ideally, the waveform should show a smooth rise and convex appearance during inspiration. In contrast, a prolonged negative phase with excessive scalloping of the tracing indicates unsatisfactory sensitivity and flow settings.

FRACTIONAL INSPIRED OXYGEN CONCENTRATION   Correction of hypoxemia and its prevention are major goals in ventilator-supported patients. Many predictive equations have been published to aid in the selection of an appropriate $F_{I_{O_2}}$, but none is sufficiently accurate to substitute for a trial-and-error approach. Initially, $F_{I_{O_2}}$ is set at a high value, often 1.0, to ensure adequate oxygenation. Thereafter, the lowest $F_{I_{O_2}}$ that achieves satisfactory arterial oxygenation should be selected. The usual target is a Pa_{O_2} of 60 mmHg or an arterial saturation (Sa_{O_2}) of 90 percent, since higher values do not substantially enhance tissue oxygenation. Although it is customary to wait 30 min to assess the response to a change in $F_{I_{O_2}}$, the effect is usually well defined within 10 min.[31] When using arterial blood samples to assess oxygenation, a Sa_{O_2}

target of 90 percent is appropriate, but if pulse oximetry is employed this target (Sp_{O_2} of >90 percent), while satisfactory in white patients, can be associated with Pa_{O_2} values as low as 41 mmHg in some African American patients.[32] Therefore, values of Sp_{O_2} may be useful in following trends in the patient's oxygenation, but changes in $F_{I_{O_2}}$ should always be guided by arterial blood-gas analysis.

Positive End-Expiratory Pressure

DEFINITION   The term PEEP signifies that pressure in the airway is elevated above that of the atmosphere at the completion of expiration; it provides no information on airway pressure during inspiration, and by convention it refers to patients receiving mechanical ventilation. A reduction in functional residual capacity (FRC) occurs in patients with ARDS or those who are anesthetized, comatose, or have recently undergone upper abdominal surgery. The reduction in FRC may be associated with airway closure in dependent regions of the lung before the end of expiration, leading to hypoventilation of these areas, $\dot{V}A/\dot{Q}$ mismatching, and hypoxemia. Application of PEEP maintains a constant positive pressure in the lungs which keeps them slightly inflated even at the end of expiration, thereby increasing FRC.[33]

EFFECTS OF PEEP   The beneficial effects of PEEP include improvement in arterial oxygenation, improvement in lung compliance, alleviation of the work of breathing due to PEEPi in patients with airflow limitation, and perhaps a decrease in lung injury resulting from repeated alveolar collapse and reopening. The principal beneficial effect of PEEP is an increase in Pa_{O_2}, which permits a decrease in $F_{I_{O_2}}$ and, thus, reduces the risk of O_2 toxicity. As stated above, the major mechanism for the increase in Pa_{O_2} with PEEP is by an increase in end-expiratory lung volume (EELV) (Table 31–2). PEEP increases EELV by distending already open lung units and preventing collapse of unstable alveoli at end-expiration, recruiting collapsed lung units, and by redistributing liquid within the lung.[34-38] The decrease in $\dot{Q}s/\dot{Q}T$ with PEEP is proportional to alveolar recruitment.[37] In pulmonary edema, the beneficial action of PEEP is due to the redistribution of edema fluid from the alveolar space into the perivascular cuffs.[38] An increase in Pa_{O_2} is the anticipated response with application of PEEP, but a paradoxical response can sometimes occur in patients with unilateral lung disease. PEEP may overdistend the good lung with consequent increase in pulmonary vascular resistance; as a result, blood flow is diverted to the diseased lung with worsening of $\dot{V}/\dot{Q}$ relationships, resulting in hypoxemia.[39]

The presence of PEEPi increases the effort required to trigger the ventilator (*vide supra*) (Fig. 31–5). The addition of exter-

TABLE 31-2 Mechanisms of Increased Pa_{O_2} with PEEP

Increase in end-expiratory lung volume	Redistribution of fluid within the lung
Distention of patent lung units	Decrease in shunt
Recruitment of collapsed lung units	Increase in end-expiratory lung volume
	Decrease in cardiac output

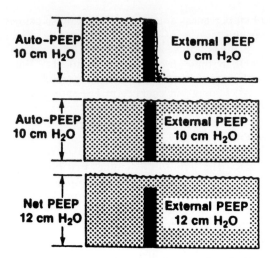

Auto-PEEP 10 cm H₂O — External PEEP 0 cm H₂O

Auto-PEEP 10 cm H₂O — External PEEP 10 cm H₂O

Net PEEP 12 cm H₂O — External PEEP 12 cm H₂O

FIGURE 31-7 The analogy of a waterfall over a dam (indicated by the solid block) is used to explain the effect of external PEEP ("downstream pressure") on PEEPi ("upstream pressure") during expiration. (From Tobin MJ, Lodato RF: PEEP, auto-PEEP, and waterfalls. *Chest* 96(3):613–616, 1993, with permission.)

airflow or the pressure upstream (PEEPi) from the site of critical closure (Fig. 31–7A). This situation exists until downstream pressure is elevated to a value equal to the critical closing pressure (Fig. 31–7B). However, once downstream pressure is elevated above the critical closing pressure (height of the waterfall), the pressure upstream increases immediately, and hyperinflation is exacerbated (Fig. 31–7C). This effect of external PEEP to decrease inspiratory work operates only in the setting of airflow limitation.

Ancillary Therapy

The plumbing of the ventilator circuit needs to be repeatedly evaluated by a knowledgeable person because several problems in the circuit, such as the characteristics or location of the humidifier or the type of expiratory valve, can increase the work of breathing and/or predispose patients to barotrauma. Adequate humidification and suctioning are required to prevent secretions from blocking the tracheal tube. In addition to other general aspects of care, bronchodilator therapy and the potential benefit of a change in body posture should be considered.

Bronchodilator aerosols are widely used in ventilator-dependent patients. The efficiency of aerosol delivery to the lower respiratory tract depends on several factors that are not a concern in ambulatory patients (Fig. 31–8). Until recently nebulizers were routinely employed, because metered-dose inhalers (MDIs) were considered ineffective owing to aerosol impaction in the ventilator circuit and endotracheal tube. Recent studies have established the efficacy of MDI-delivered bronchodilators in mechanically ventilated patients provided a proper technique of administration is employed.[43] A special adapter is required to connect the MDI canister to the ventilator circuit, and several different devices have become commercially available. Efficacy differs considerably between these devices, and aerosol delivery is much higher with an

nal PEEP can be helpful in this setting in patients with airflow limitation, because alveolar pressure needs to be decreased only below the level of external PEEP, rather than below zero, to trigger the ventilator.[40–42] This may seem paradoxical: external PEEP, which is commonly used to induce hyperinflation in patients with microatelectasis, is being used to decrease the work of breathing induced by hyperinflation consequent to PEEPi. This paradox can be explained by employing the analogy of a waterfall.[42] The height of the waterfall represents the critical closing pressure of airways in patients with PEEPi and COPD (Fig. 31–7). Thus, elevating downstream pressure, such as with external PEEP, has no influence on either expiratory

Ventilator Related
- Mode of ventilation
- Tidal volume
- Respiratory rate
- Duty cycle
- Inspiratory waveform
- Breath triggering mechanism

Device Related-MDI
- Type of spacer or adapter used
- Position of spacer in circuit
- Timing of MDI actuation

Drug Related
- Dose
- Aerosol particle size
- Duration of action

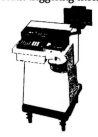

Device Related-Nebulizer
- Type of nebulizer used
- Continuous/intermittent operation
- Duration of nebulization
- Position in the circuit

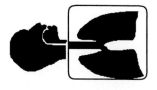

Circuit Related
- Endotracheal tube
- Inhaled gas humidity
- Inhaled gas density/viscosity

Patient Related
- Severity of airway obstruction
- Mechanism of airway obstruction
- Presence of dynamic hyperinflation
- Patient-ventilator synchrony

FIGURE 31-8 A multitude of factors influence lower respiratory tract deposition of aerosol delivered by a metered-dose inhaler (MDI) in mechanically ventilated patients. With dry air in the circuit, ≈30 percent of the dose is delivered to the major air ways if the MDI is actuated into a cylindrical spacer; whereas delivery decreases to ≈16 percent if inspired gas is humidified. (Modified from Dhand R, Tobin MJ: *Euro Respir J* 9:585–595, 1996, with permission.)

TABLE 31-3 Technique for Using Metered-Dose Inhalers in Mechanically Ventilated Patients

Ensure $V_T > 500$ mL (in adults) during assisted ventilation.
Aim for an inspiratory time (excluding the inspiratory pause) >0.3 of total breath duration.
Ensure that the ventilator breath is synchronized with the patient's inspiration.
Shake the MDI vigorously.
Place canister in actuator of a cylindrical spacer situated in inspiratory limb of ventilator circuit.[a]
Actuate MDI to synchronize with precise onset of inspiration by the ventilator.[b]
Allow a breath hold at end-inspiration for 3–5 s.[c]
Allow passive exhalation.
Repeat actuations after 20–30 s until total dose is delivered.[d]

[a] With MDIs, it is preferable to use a spacer that remains in the ventilator circuit, so that disconnection of the ventilator circuit can be avoided at the time of each bronchodilator treatment. Although bypassing the humidifier can increase aerosol delivery, it prolongs the time for each treatment and requires disconnection of the ventilator circuit.
[b] In ambulatory patients with a MDI placed inside the mouth, actuation is recommended briefly after initiation of inspiratory airflow. In mechanically ventilated patients when a MDI and spacer combination is used, actuation should be synchronized with onset of inspiration.
[c] The effect of a postinspiratory breath hold has not been evaluated in mechanically ventilated patients.
[d] The manufacturer recommends repeating the dose after 1 min. However, MDI actuation within 20 to 30 s after the prior dose does not compromise drug delivery.[120]
NOTE: MDI, metered-dose inhaler.

in-line chamber device than with an elbow adapter.[43] As in nonintubated patients, it is necessary to follow carefully several key steps to achieve maximal aerosol delivery, especially the synchronization of MDI actuation with the precise onset of inspiratory airflow by the ventilator. Because of concerns with aerosol deposition in the endotracheal tube and ventilator circuit, the dosage in mechanically ventilated patients is commonly increased much above the usual two to four puffs used in nonintubated patients. However, when the technique of administration is carefully controlled (Table 31–3), maximal bronchodilation is achieved in stable, ventilator-dependent patients with COPD with as little as four puffs of a sympathomimetic aerosol (Fig. 31–9).[44] MDIs offer several advantages over nebulizers, including ease of administration, decreased cost, reliability of dosing, and freedom from contamination.

In patients with ARDS, a substantial increase in Pa_{O_2} occurs in more than half of patients when turned from the supine to the prone position.[45,46] However, the degree of improvement and response among patients is variable, and some patients even develop a fall in Pa_{O_2}. The alteration in gas exchange on adopting the prone position appears to be related primarily to changes in regional ventilation. In the supine position, the gravitational gradient in pleural pressure is increased so that pleural pressure is positive in the dependent region.[47] Consequently, large areas of the lung are below closing volume, and there is little, if any, ventilation of the dependent dorsal regions. On turning to the prone position regional ventilation decreases from the dorsal to the ventral regions, but the gravitational gradient in pleural pressure is smaller, so that the rate of decrease in regional inflation is less than in the supine posture.[45,47] Thus, regional ventilation becomes more homogenous in the prone posture. Achieve-

ment of a more even distribution of ventilation appears to be a major factor in producing better oxygenation.

Monitoring
Several devices can be used to monitor pulmonary gas exchange, respiratory neuromuscular function, respiratory mechanics, and patient-ventilator interaction. Use of the derived information permits the physician to better tailor ventilator settings to an individual patient's requirements with the promise of enhancing patient comfort. Monitoring of key variables helps to minimize the risk of iatrogenic complications and also alerts the physician to the likelihood of an impending catastrophe and allows sufficient time for the institution of lifesaving measures.[48] A full discussion of monitoring modalities during mechanical ventilation is outside the scope of this chapter.

Complications
Patients receiving mechanical ventilation are at risk of numerous complications, including oxygen toxicity, volutrauma and air leaks, infection, endotracheal-tube complications, and decreased cardiac output. These problems occur frequently, and they can be life-threatening if they are not detected and treated promptly. Recently, there has been a growing awareness of more subtle injuries associated with mechanical ventilation. In addition, several adverse physiologic effects are attributed to mechanical ventilation. The interested reader is referred elsewhere for details.[22,49–52]

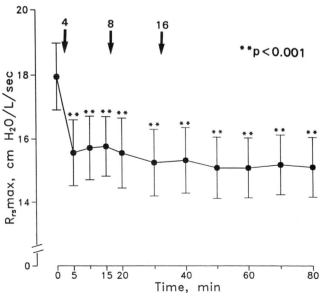

FIGURE 31-9 Effect of albuterol on minimal inspiratory airway resistance (Rrsmin) in 12 mechanically ventilated patients with COPD. Significant decreases in Rrsmin occurred within 5 min of administration of 4 puffs of albuterol with a MDI and chamber spacer, and were sustained following administration of 8 and 16 puffs (cumulative doses of 12 and 28 puffs, respectively). However, the effect of 12 and 28 puffs was not significantly greater than that with 4 puffs ($p > .05$). Bars represent SE. Double asterisks indicate $p < .001$. (From Dhand R, Duarte AG, Jubran A, et al: Dose response to bronchodilator delivered by metered-dose inhaler in ventilator-supported patients. *Am J Respir Crit Care Med* 154:388–393, 1996, with permission.)

OXYGEN TOXICITY Administration of a high F_{IO_2} causes a number of disturbances, including ciliary dysfunction, tracheobronchitis, impaired alveolar macrophage function, and parenchymal injury resembling ARDS.[53] Healthy human subjects who inhale 100% O_2 develop acute tracheobronchitis—which manifests as substernal discomfort and cough—sore throat, nasal congestion, eye and ear discomfort, paresthesia, and fatigue.[53] These symptoms begin within 4 h, and bronchoscopic features of tracheal inflammation are evident after 6 h of breathing 100% O_2.[54] Hyperoxia causes absorption atelectasis in lung units with low $\dot{V}A/Q$ ratios, because the rate of absorption of O_2 from the alveoli into the bloodstream is faster than the rate of replenishment from inspired gas.[53]

The possibility of O_2 toxicity should be considered in any patient receiving an F_{IO_2} of more than 0.50 to 0.60 for 24 to 48 h or longer. In the face of potential O_2 toxicity, all attempts should be made to reduce the F_{IO_2} to the lowest level that produces acceptable systemic oxygenation. To achieve these goals, meticulous attention is required to treat the underlying conditions that interfere with adequate oxygenation (e.g., pneumonia, pulmonary edema), use of PEEP, nursing in the prone posture, and inotropic agents. Simultaneously, the systemic transport of oxygen can be optimized by blood transfusions and fluid management and by providing cardiovascular and respiratory support. If these measures fail, inhaled nitric oxide and/or extracorporeal membrane oxygenation are sometimes employed. While unnecessary O_2 toxicity should be avoided, it is important to keep in mind that there is more to fear from severe hypoxemia than the potential damage that might result from hyperoxia.

BAROTRAUMA The presence of extraalveolar air due to pneumomediastinum, subpleural air cysts, subcutaneous emphysema, pneumothorax, or pneumoperitoneum is collectively termed *pulmonary barotrauma*. These findings have been described in 10 to 20 percent of patients receiving mechanical ventilation,[55,56] and they are associated with a high mortality.[55,57] Rupture of overdistended alveoli into the adjacent perivascular sheath appears to be the common underlying event in all forms of pulmonary barotrauma. Barotrauma usually occurs in the presence of underlying lung disease such as aspiration pneumonia,[58] ARDS,[55] or COPD.[59] An increased regional lung volume rather than airway pressure is the primary determinant of alveolar rupture. However, airway pressures are easier to measure, and they correlate with the presence of alveolar overdistention. Thus, peak inspiratory pressures >40 cmH$_2$O are associated with an increased risk of alveolar rupture during mechanical ventilation. The relationship of PEEP to the occurrence of barotrauma is not clear-cut, with some investigators showing an increase in barotrauma with PEEP levels higher than 8 cmH$_2$O, others reporting no demonstrable increase in barotrauma with increasing levels of PEEP,[56,58,59] and still others showing decreased incidence of barotrauma with application of PEEP.[60] In view of the concerns to limit alveolar distention during mechanical ventilation, a recent consensus conference on mechanical ventilation recommended that the peak alveolar pressures (plateau pressures) should not be allowed to exceed 35 cmH$_2$O.[24]

The occurrence of subcutaneous emphysema, pneumomediastinum, and pneumoperitoneum rarely produce major clinical problems, but the development of a pneumothorax

in a patient receiving mechanical ventilation can have devastating consequences. Progression to a tension pneumothorax can be rapid and occurs frequently (60 to 90 percent of pneumothoraces).[61] Therefore, prompt diagnosis of a pneumothorax is necessary, and drainage by tube thoracostomy is recommended. If air continues to leak from the chest for more than 24 h after the placement of a chest tube, the presence of a bronchopleural fistula is suspected.[50] The occurrence of a bronchopleural fistula can lead to failure of the lung to reexpand, loss of tidal volume and PEEP, unwanted cycling of the ventilator if negative suction applied to the chest tube is transmitted to the airway and triggers the ventilator, and pleural infection. Under these circumstances the fewest number of ventilator-delivered breaths compatible with adequate gas exchange should be used (low level of pressure support or SIMV with a low set rate). Reduction in delivered tidal volume, inspiratory time, and PEEP to the lowest acceptable level is advised. The level of chest tube suction should be reduced to the minimal level that can keep the lung inflated. Weaning from the ventilator should be attempted at the earliest opportunity. Generally, bronchopleural fistulas improve with the resolution of the underlying disease. Several measures have been suggested to try and reduce the size of the air leak from a bronchopleural fistula, but these are of questionable value and are rarely needed.[50]

INFECTION The development of pneumonia has been reported in 21 percent of patients receiving mechanical ventilation for longer than 48 h.[62] A number of factors related to the ventilator, other respiratory care equipment, and the host's defenses are responsible for the increased incidence of pneumonia among ventilator-dependent patients.[51]

The development of nosocomial pneumonia has a profoundly adverse effect on the outcome of ventilator-dependent patients,[63] with various investigators reporting mortality rates for nosocomial pneumonia in ventilator-dependent patients ranging from 30 to 76 percent.[62–65] Aerobic gram-negative bacilli are the most common etiologic agents for nosocomial pneumonia, but gram-positive pneumonias and polymicrobial infections occur frequently.[63,65] The difficulty in identifying the causative organism is a major stumbling block in treating nosocomial pneumonia effectively. Classic clinical criteria for diagnosing pneumonia are unreliable in mechanically ventilated patients,[66] and conventional bacteriologic methods usually provide misleading information because of the high rate of airway colonization.[67,68] Therefore, routine culture of secretions aspirated through an endotracheal tube inevitably result in recovery of a mixture of potential pathogens and are of no help in guiding appropriate antibiotic selection. Blood and pleural fluid cultures are helpful in identifying the causative organism(s) in fewer than 10 percent of nosocomial pneumonias.[64,69] Samples obtained from an involved area of the lung with a telescoping catheter brush passed through the flexible bronchoscope provide an accurate bacteriologic diagnosis in patients with ventilator-associated pneumonia.[70] Quantitative cultures of bronchoalveolar lavage (BAL) fluid have been attempted with conflicting results.[71–74] A plugged double-lumen catheter which is blindly wedged into the distal airways[72,75] or a protected balloon-tipped catheter can be used to lavage a distal segment of the lung.[76] The diagnosis of ventilator-associated pneumonia on the basis of results obtained by the blind mini-

TABLE 31-4 Complications Related to Endotracheal and Tracheostomy Tubes

Complications during endotracheal intubation	Complications associated with the cuff
Tooth avulsion	Tracheal mucosal ulceration
Perforation of retropharynx or hypopharynx	Tracheal dilatation
Vocal cord hematoma	Tracheoesophageal fistula
Pulmonary aspiration	Tracheal rupture
Dislodgement of tube	Complications associated with tracheostomy
Nasal bleeding	Hemorrhage
Arrhythmias	Stomal infection
Cardiac arrest	Subcutaneous or mediastinal emphysema
Complications occurring when endotracheal tube is in place	Pneumothorax
Laryngeal edema	Tracheo-innominate fistula
Laryngeal hematoma	Tracheoesophageal fistula
Posterior glottic ulceration	Tracheal stenosis
Subglottic stenosis	Tracheomalacia
Obstruction of lumen	
Paranasal sinusitis	

bronchoalveolar lavage agreed closely with results obtained by using the protected specimen brush.[75] Further studies are needed to determine the influence of quantitative cultures of fluid obtained by the protected specimen brush or BAL on the outcome of treatment. Accurate diagnosis of pneumonia is undoubtedly a key factor in determining the success of treatment.

COMPLICATIONS OF ENDOTRACHEAL AND TRACHEOSTOMY TUBES   Endotracheal intubation is associated with a variety of complications[77] (Table 31–4). The frequency of complications depends on the setting and urgency with which the procedure is performed. Thus, in the ICU some complication occurred in almost two-thirds of all patients during intubation or while the tube was in place.[52] The complications noted during insertion of the tube, while the tube is in place within the trachea, and following extubation are listed in Table 31–4. Some of the problems associated with endotracheal tubes have been reduced by the use of specialized plastic materials and by introduction of high-volume, low-pressure (high-compliance) cuffs. These cuffs require much less pressure to seal the airway compared with the hard, low-compliance cuffs used earlier, and they minimize tracheal mucosal damage associated with prolonged intubation. Other problems associated with endotracheal intubation include kinking or disconnection of the tube, herniation of the cuff over the tip of the tube, and self-extubation.

Tracheostomy is needed for patients requiring long-term positive-pressure ventilation. Complications associated with insertion of a tracheostomy tube are generally greater than those with endotracheal intubation[52] (Table 31–4).

Certain precautions can minimize the risk of complications associated with endotracheal intubation. The procedure should ideally be performed under controlled conditions by a skilled operator. Tubes with high-compliance cuffs should be used, and the lowest cuff pressure used to seal the airway. Higher cuff pressures may be needed if aspiration is suspected to occur through the wrinkles in the cuff and when PEEP is being applied. Maintenance of the cuff pressure below 25

cmH$_2$O at end-exhalation helps to reduce tracheal mucosal damage.[78] The previous policy of substituting a tracheostomy tube for an endotracheal tube after a certain period of mechanical ventilation has been revised. Management of the patient should be individualized based on the assessment of the likely duration of mechanical ventilation and the needs of the patient.[79] With improvements in the design of endotracheal tubes and cuffs, and with proper attention to preventing laryngeal injury, mechanical ventilation may be continued for longer periods with endotracheal tubes than was thought previously. On the other hand, if long-term ventilation is contemplated, it is preferable to perform a tracheostomy early in the course because of the ease of airway maintenance and nutritional support.

EFFECT ON CARDIAC OUTPUT   Reduction in cardiac output is a well recognized complication of mechanical ventilation, particularly with the use of PEEP or high tidal volumes.[13] Decreased venous return is thought to be the major mechanism responsible for this effect (Fig. 31–10). In addition, pul-

FIGURE 31-10 Factors decreasing cardiac output during positive-pressure mechanical ventilation. An increase in intrathoracic pressure compresses the vena cava and thus decreases venous return. Alveolar distention compresses the alveolar vessels, and the resulting increases in pulmonary vascular resistance and right-ventricular afterload produce a leftward shift in the interventricular septum. Left-ventricular compliance is decreased by both the bulging septum and the increased juxtacardiac pressure resulting from distended lungs. (From Tobin MJ: Mechanical ventilation. *N Engl J Med* 330:1056–1061, 1994, with permission.)

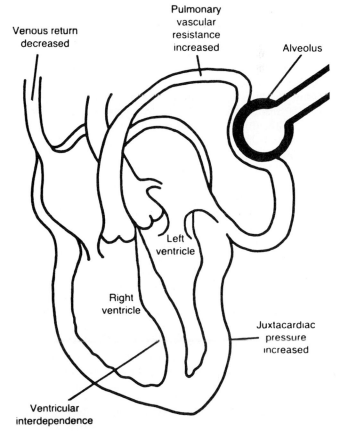

TABLE 31-5 Causes of Respiratory Muscle Pump Failure

Decreased neuromuscular capacity	Endocrinopathy
Decreased respiratory center output	Drug-induced abnormalities
Phrenic nerve dysfunction	Disuse muscle atrophy
Decreased respiratory muscle strength and/or	Respiratory muscle fatigue
endurance	Increased respiratory muscle pump load
Hyperinflation	Increased ventilatory requirements
Malnutrition	Increased CO_2 production
Decreased oxygen supply	Increased dead space ventilation
Respiratory acidosis	Inappropriately increased respiratory drive
Metabolic abnormalities	Increased work of breathing

SOURCE: From Tobin MJ (ed): *Principles and Practice of Mechanical Ventilation*. New York, McGraw-Hill, 1994; p 1178, with permission.

monary vascular resistance is elevated as the increase in alveolar volume by positive-pressure ventilation stretches the alveolar vessels, reduces their lumina, and increases resistance to flow. The increase in right ventricular afterload may shift the interventricular septum to the left with a reduction in left ventricular compliance. Increased juxtacardiac pressure as the distended lung comes into contact with the heart also decreases left ventricular distensibility. The hemodynamic response to mechanical ventilation depends on the patient's fluid status, and any reduction in cardiac output subsequent to an increase in pleural pressure can be corrected by increasing the intravascular fluid volume, but only at the expense of an increase in microvascular pressures.

Weaning

In most instances, patients receiving mechanical ventilation can resume spontaneous breathing with little or no difficulty. About 20 to 30 percent of patients fail initial attempts of discontinuing mechanical ventilation.[80] Overall, about 40 percent of the time that a patient receives mechanical ventilation is spent trying to wean the patient from the ventilator, and in patients with certain disease states, such as COPD, the weaning process accounts for ≈60 percent of ventilator time.[81]

CAUSES OF WEANING FAILURE Weaning failure is most commonly due to respiratory muscle dysfunction, and it may also result from problems with oxygenation and psychological difficulties.[82] Respiratory muscle dysfunction results from an imbalance between respiratory neuromuscular capacity and the load on the respiratory system (Table 31–5). Causes of decreased respiratory neuromuscular capacity that are important in the difficult-to-wean patient include dynamic hyperinflation (which decreases the contractile force), malnutrition, electrolyte abnormalities (hypokalemia, hypocalcemia, and hypophosphatemia decrease muscle contractility), respiratory acidosis, and the aftereffects of neuromuscular blocking agents. An increase in respiratory load may result from excessive ventilatory requirements, increased resistance, decreased compliance, and the presence of PEEPi (which poses an inspiratory threshold load). Hypoxemia is a less common primary cause of weaning failure, partly because weaning is not attempted in patients who appear to be susceptible to the development of hypoxemia. The factor that we know least about is psychological problems, which may significantly aggravate difficulties in weaning in a substantial number of patients.

TIMING OF THE WEANING PROCESS One of the major challenges in mechanical ventilation is deciding when is the best time to wean a patient from the ventilator. If a physician is too conservative and postpones weaning onset, the patient is placed at an increased risk of life-threatening, ventilator-induced complications. If weaning is commenced prematurely, the patient may suffer severe cardiopulmonary and/or psychological decompensation, which sets the patient back in his/her clinical course. Weaning is initiated when the disease process that precipitated the need for mechanical ventilation has resolved sufficiently that the patient has a reasonable chance of being able to sustain spontaneous ventilation. Although careful clinical assessment is necessary in deciding when to wean a patient, this alone is not sufficient.[83] Accordingly, functional tests are helpful in determining a patient's readiness for weaning (Table 31–6). In general, discontinuation of mechanical ventilation is not even contemplated in a patient with cardiopulmonary instability or persistent hypoxemia (e.g., Pa_{O_2} less than 55 mmHg with an $F_{I_{O_2}}$ of 0.40 or higher). However, many patients fail attempts at weaning despite satisfactory oxygenation. A minute ventilation of <10 L/min and maximum inspiratory pressure are both very inaccurate in predicting weaning outcome.[82] Instead, checking for the absence of rapid shallow breathing [respiratory frequency/tidal volume (f/V_T) ratio < 100 breaths per minute per liter] is more helpful in deciding when to attempt weaning (Fig. 31–11).[84]

WEANING TECHNIQUES A trial of spontaneous breathing through a T-tube circuit, performed several times a day, was the original method of weaning. Typically, this approach begins with brief trials (lasting about 5 min), which are gradually increased in accordance with a patient's performance as assessed by bedside clinical examination. The optimal period of rest between these trials has never been defined, but is commonly as little as 1 to 3 h. When the patient is able to sustain spontaneous ventilation for some fixed time, such as 1 to 2 h, extubation is performed.

IMV and PS were introduced in the early 1970s and early

TABLE 31-6 Variables Used to Predict Weaning Success

Gas exchange	Ventilatory pump
Pa_{O_2} of ≥60 mmHg with $F_{I_{O_2}}$ of ≤0.35	Maximum negative inspiratory pressure <−30 cmH$_2$O
Alveolar-arterial P_{O_2} gradient of <350 mmHg	Minute ventilation <10 L/min
$Pa_{O_2}/F_{I_{O_2}}$ ratio of >200	Frequency-to-tidal-volume ratio (f/V_T) < 100 breaths/min/L

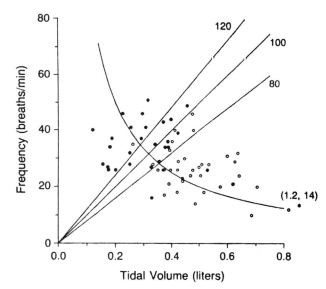

FIGURE 31-11 Isopleths for the ratio of frequency to tidal volume (f/V_T) representing different degrees of rapid shallow breathing. Patients who fell to the left of the isopleth at 100 breaths per minute per liter had a 95 percent likelihood of failing a weaning trial, whereas patients who fell to the right of this isopleth had an 80 percent likelihood of a successful weaning outcome. The hyperbola represents a minute ventilation of 10 L/min, a criterion commonly used to predict weaning outcome; it is apparent that this criterion was of little value in discriminating between weaning success (open circles) and weaning failure patients (solid circles). Values for one patient (V_T 1.2 L, f 14 breaths per minute) lay outside the graph. (From Yang KL, Tobin MJ: A prospective study of indexes predicting the outcome of trials of weaning from mechanical ventilation. *N Engl J Med* 324:1445–1450, 1991, with permission.)

1980s, respectively, and these are now the most popular approaches to weaning. When using IMV for weaning, the mandatory rate from the ventilator is reduced in steps of one to three breaths per minute, and an arterial blood gas is obtained after ≈30 min. Unfortunately, as little as two to three positive-pressure breaths per minute can achieve acceptable blood-gas values, but these values provide no information regarding the patient's work of breathing, which may be excessive. Consequently, use of IMV may actually contribute to the development of respiratory muscle fatigue or prevent its recovery. When PS is used for weaning, the level of pressure is reduced gradually in decrements of 3 to 6 cmH_2O, titrated on the basis of respiratory frequency. Several investigators have shown that PS can be used to counteract the work of breathing imposed by the endotracheal tube and ventilator circuit. This has led to the notion that a patient who can sustain spontaneous ventilation at this "compensatory level" of pressure support will tolerate extubation. The problem with this strategy is that a compensatory level of pressure support varies between 3 and 14 cmH_2O,[85] and there is no reliable method for accurately determining the level of PS required in an individual patient.[86]

The fourth possible method of weaning patients is to employ a single daily trial of spontaneous breathing through a T-tube circuit. The trial is conducted while a physician is in the ICU, and a patient who can sustain spontaneous ventilation for 30 to 60 min without undue distress is extubated. If the patient develops signs of distress on physical examination, the trial is stopped and mechanical ventilation is reinstituted. To allow the respiratory muscles to recover from excessive stress, the patient is rested for ≈24 h with a high level of ventilator assistance such as with assist-control ventilation,[87] and the trial of spontaneous breathing is repeated the following morning.

Two rigorously controlled, prospective studies were recently performed to compare the relative efficacy of different weaning strategies in the subgroup of patients who are difficult to wean.[80,88] In both studies, IMV was found to delay the weaning process. In one study, a single daily trial of spontaneous breathing was found to achieve a twofold increase in the rate of successful weaning and extubation compared with pressure support (Fig. 31–12),[80] whereas in the other study pressure support was found to result in faster weaning than T-tube trials.[88] The different outcome in the studies is probably due to the specific criteria employed at different stages of the weaning process.

A weaning strategy consisting of performing a trial of spontaneous breathing once a day was evaluated in a recent trial in adult patients receiving mechanical ventilation for acute respiratory failure from multiple causes.[89] When certain predetermined screening criteria for weaning were met, the patients underwent daily trials of spontaneous breathing. In the intervention group, if the patients were able to breathe spontaneously for 2 h, their physicians were notified that the patient had a high likelihood of breathing without mechanical ventilation. Patients who were unable to breathe spontaneously for 2 h underwent daily screening and trials of spontaneous breathing for 2 h until successful extubation or death. In contrast, patients in the control group were screened daily but did not undergo trials of spontaneous breathing, nor was any feedback provided to their physicians. The patients in the intervention group received mechanical ventilation for shorter duration (median 4.5 days) compared with those in the control group (6 days). The rate of complications was also lower in the intervention group.[89] Therefore, the technique of using single daily trials of spontaneous breathing is a simple and efficient method to wean patients from mechanical ventilation.

NONINVASIVE VENTILATION IN ACUTE RESPIRATORY FAILURE

Introduction of more comfortable nasal masks for continuous positive airway pressure (CPAP) in patients with obstructive sleep apnea led to a renewed interest in noninvasive positive-pressure ventilation (NIPPV). Substitution of a mask for an endotracheal tube has considerable appeal, in that (1) it is more comfortable; (2) there is less need for sedation, with enhanced alertness and ability to communicate; (3) it avoids the complications of endotracheal or tracheostomy tubes, such as airway trauma, sinusitis, and pneumonia; (4) it maintains airway defenses and permits speech and swallowing; and (5) the patient has a greater sense of control and independence than when intubated.[90,91] Reports on the use of NIPPV in patients with acute respiratory failure have mainly consisted of patients with COPD. The approach has also been employed in an uncontrolled fashion to treat acute respiratory failure in postoperative patients and in those with cardiac failure, pneumonia, cystic fibrosis, chest wall disorders, and obstructive sleep apnea.[90]

Three prospective controlled studies have recently been

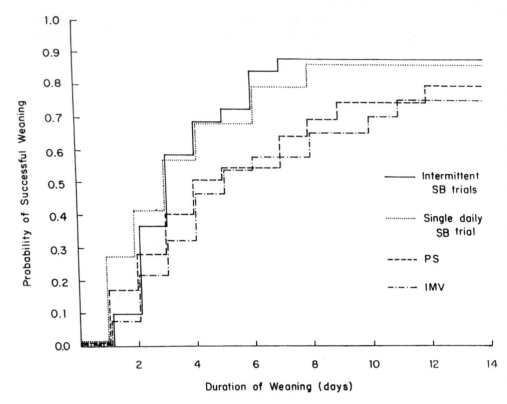

FIGURE 31-12 Kaplan-Meier curves of the probability of successful weaning with intermittent mandatory ventilation, pressure-support ventilation, intermittent trails of spontaneous breathing, and a once-daily trial of spontaneous breathing. After adjustment for baseline characteristics in a Cox proportional-hazards model, the rate of successsful weaning with a once-daily trial of spontaneous breathing was 2.83 times higher than that with intermittent mandatory ventilation ($p < .006$) and 2.05 times higher than that with pressure-support ventilation ($p < .04$) (From Esteban A, Frutos F, Tobin MJ: A comparison of four methods of weaning patients from mechanical ventilation. *N Engl J Med* 332:345–350, 1995, with permission.)

published describing a beneficial effect of NIPPV plus standard therapy versus standard therapy alone in patients with acute respiratory failure.[92-94] Patients in the NIPPV group required intubation less frequently, had a lower rate of complications, and a shorter hospital stay compared with the control group. The mortality rates in patients treated with NIPPV were lower than that in the control group in two of the three studies.[93,94]

Controlled and uncontrolled studies show that NIPPV is successful in ≈70 percent of patients with acute respiratory failure. There are still no firm indications for its use, but patients should have objective evidence of acute respiratory distress on physical examination and/or acute respiratory acidosis. Patients with exacerbations of COPD and cardiogenic pulmonary edema and those who are not suitable for intubation or refuse intubation can be supported by NIPPV. Patients need to be able to cooperate and follow instructions. NIPPV should be avoided in patients with a respiratory arrest, those who are unstable (hypotension, uncontrolled arrhythmias), those with a high risk of aspiration (obtunded, swallowing problems, gastrointestinal bleeding, or vomiting), and those who have excessive secretions.[95] Success appears more likely if NIPPV is used early rather than later in the progression of acute respiratory failure.[92,94] The optimal settings and duration of use have not been defined. NIPPV is generally used for ≈7 h/day,[92,94] although in one study it was used for 20 of the first 24 h.[93] Most patients are completely weaned from NIPPV after 3 to 6 days,[93] although some patients use it for as long as 23 days.[93] The decision to stop NIPPV is based on clinical judgment with the advantage that it is easy to reinstitute NIPPV if ventilatory failure recurs. Patients who do well with NIPPV typically show considerable improvement within the first hour of therapy, as indicated by a decrease in respiratory frequency,[94] a fall in Pa_{CO_2}, and an increase in pH.[92] If respiratory frequency is not significantly decreased after the first hour of therapy, intubation and conventional mechanical ventilation should be considered.

NIPPV has a number of limitations. About 20 to 25 percent of patients cannot adapt to its use, mainly because of discomfort from the mask.[91] The mask needs to be carefully selected and applied to minimize discomfort. The likelihood of skin ulceration (especially over the bridge of the nose) makes it difficult to use NIPPV continuously for more than 1 to 2 days.[90] With nasal masks, a better fit is generally achieved with smaller sizes, and the ideal mask fits closely to the lateral contour of the nose.[96] An excessive leak at the bridge of the nose causes intolerance as a result of air blowing into a patient's eyes. Excessive nasal dryness can be ameliorated by humidification, rhinorrhea can be helped by ipratropium bromide nasal drops, and nasal blockage may respond to ephedrine nasal drops.[90] A chin strap can be used when there is a large leak through the mouth. Other limitations with NIPPV include the lack of direct access to the patient's airway, so that, when secretions are copious, mucus plugging and atelectasis may develop. Aerophagia and gastric distention can occur, especially in patients who breathe out of synchrony with the ventilator,[90] and, if suspected, a nasogastric tube should be inserted.

NEGATIVE-PRESSURE VENTILATION

Negative-pressure ventilators work by intermittently creating a subatmospheric pressure around the patient's thorax and abdomen. The volume of air entering the lungs (tidal volume) depends on the surface area over which the negative pressure is applied and the compliance of the patient's lungs and chest wall. The respiratory rate and degree of negative pressure generated can be set, and these devices can be used in patients without the need for a tracheostomy, nasal mask, or mouthpiece. The iron lung is the most effective negative-pressure ventilator, and it can be synchronized with the patient's breathing. The negative pressure generated can be adjusted to achieve the target minute ventilation. To overcome the problems associated with the weight and bulkiness of the iron lung, a lighter version which can be fitted on a standard hospital bed has been developed (Portalung; Puritan Bennett, Boulder, CO). Patients who are being considered for negative-pressure ventilation must have adequate control of their upper airway. The disadvantages of using these negative-pressure ventilation devices is that they limit access to the patient and do not ensure patency of the upper airway. Furthermore, patients find negative-pressure ventilators to be cumbersome and uncomfortable, and they are often noncompliant with the use of these devices.

The "poncho wrap" and "cuirass" ventilators are designed to fit snugly over the patient's anterior chest and upper abdomen. Generation of a negative pressure within the device by a pump allows chest expansion to occur. However, the pressure required to achieve effective ventilation with these devices is more negative than that required with the iron lung. Although these devices are portable and easier to apply than the iron lung, they are less effective and often uncomfortable to wear, particularly in patients with chest wall deformities.

The "rocking bed" and the exsufflation belt, or "pneumobelt," function by displacing abdominal contents and affecting diaphragmatic motion. Upward displacement of the diaphragm produces exhalation, and gravity assists inhalation by returning the diaphragm to its original position. These devices can be helpful in patients with bilateral diaphragmatic paralysis. Both devices are relatively inefficient for providing ventilatory support. Furthermore, the pneumobelt cannot be used in the supine position. Thus, it may be used at night only if the patient can sleep in a semirecumbent position.

The use of negative-pressure ventilation (iron lung or poncho wrap) for providing ventilatory support in patients with COPD who develop acute respiratory failure has appeared in case reports and a few uncontrolled studies.[97,98] One group of investigators from Europe reported that patients with COPD and acute respiratory failure were ventilated successfully with negative-pressure ventilation, and 93 of 105 patients were weaned from the ventilator.[99] Similarly, 12 of 15 patients with neuromuscular disease who developed acute hypercapnic respiratory failure were managed successfully by ventilation with an iron lung.[100] Although negative-pressure ventilation could be considered an option for ventilating these patients, prospective, randomized, and controlled studies are needed to compare the efficacy of negative-pressure ventilation with positive-pressure ventilation with or without an endotracheal tube.[101]

Mechanical Ventilation outside the ICU

A variable proportion of patients remain ventilator dependent after an episode of acute respiratory failure. The fre-

quency of ventilator dependence has been shown to decrease as the duration of mechanical ventilation increases.[102] Estimates of the frequency of ventilator dependence in previous studies are unreliable because there is no uniformity of opinion about the duration for which patients should receive mechanical ventilation before being labeled ventilator dependent. The choices for providing long-term ventilation to these patients are similar to those for patients with acute respiratory failure admitted to the ICU, but several logistical and socioeconomic problems have to be overcome to make long-term ventilation feasible.

POSITIVE-PRESSURE VENTILATION

INVASIVE POSITIVE-PRESSURE VENTILATION
Ventilator-dependent patients who require full ventilator support need to have placement of a permanent tracheostomy. Patients who cannot protect their upper airway adequately, have excessive secretions, or who have failed a trial of NIPPV are also candidates for invasive mechanical ventilation. Fitting the ventilator on a specially designed device allows patients to be mobile while receiving mechanical ventilation.

NONINVASIVE POSITIVE-PRESSURE VENTILATION
NIPPV is gaining in popularity for long-term ventilation because it is more portable, convenient, and economical compared with intermittent positive-pressure ventilation (IPPV) or negative-pressure ventilation. In patients with chronic respiratory failure due to neuromuscular disease,[103–107] restrictive chest wall disorders,[108–111] or posttuberculosis complications,[110,111] several investigators have reported benefit from the use of NIPPV. Although these studies were not controlled and randomized, a few hours of nighttime ventilation was shown to improve nocturnal gas exchange and to decrease daytime symptoms of lethargy and somnolence.[103,104,106–111] Patients reported improvement in their quality of life[107,111] and had a prolonged survival.[111] In contrast, the benefits of NIPPV in chronically ventilator-dependent patients with COPD have not been as obvious.[112,113]

Many patients are unable to use NIPPV because of the discomfort caused by the mask or their inability to tolerate air pressure. Furthermore, some patients require several weeks to months of adaptation to the masks used for NIPPV before they are fully adjusted.

NEGATIVE-PRESSURE VENTILATION

A few investigators have concluded on the basis of uncontrolled studies that use of negative-pressure ventilation for 6 to 8 h every night lowered daytime Pa_{CO_2}, increased Pa_{O_2}, and eliminated symptoms of hypoventilation in patients with chronic respiratory failure due to neuromuscular disease,[114,115] restrictive chest wall disorders,[116,117] or hypoventilation syndromes.[118] However, in a controlled double-blind study that compared nocturnal ventilation by poncho wrap with sham ventilation in 184 patients with severe COPD,[119] approximately one-third could not complete treatment over the 12 weeks of the study. Since the patients were unable to tolerate the device at night, many used the device only during the day for a mean duration of 3.5 h. These workers were unable to demonstrate any improvement in 6-min walking distance, respiratory muscle strength, dyspnea, arterial blood gases, quality of life, or exercise endurance in the ventilated patients.[119] In general, negative-pressure ventilators are less reliable for providing ventilatory assistance compared with positive-pressure ventilators. They should be used only in selected patients with mild chronic respiratory failure who have good control of their upper airway.

In summary, patients with chronic respiratory failure who exhibit daytime somnolence and lethargy, hypoventilation, abnormal gas exchange, or inability to wean from the ventilator require long-term ventilation. If the patient needs mechanical ventilation most of the time, support has to be provided by invasive positive-pressure ventilation. On the other hand, when intermittent ventilation is needed, the airway is intact, and the airway function is normal, it is preferable to use NIPPV. If the patient cannot tolerate NIPPV or refuses to use it, a trial with negative-pressure ventilation may be given. Patients who do not benefit by either of these techniques may require IPPV through a tracheostomy.

Team Approach to Mechanical Ventilation

The complexity of modern ventilators and other monitoring systems necessitates their operation by specially trained personnel. The combined expertise of a multidisciplinary team is of great value in providing comprehensive care to the mechanically ventilated patient.

The role of the physician, as a team leader, is to assess the patient's medical status, to provide specific guidelines, and to coordinate the care given by various team members. The physician also interacts with the patient's family and makes decisions about the complex ethical issues often involved in the care of critically ill patients. Specially trained nurses provide bedside care for the patient, assess and record the patient's condition, administer drugs, and provide feedback to the physicians about the patient's condition. Respiratory therapists help the physicians in providing mechanical ventilation and other respiratory management. Their major role is to determine the need for ventilator changes, make the prescribed ventilator changes, regularly assess and evaluate the patient's response to ventilator changes, monitor and maintain the ventilator and associated equipment, and perform arterial blood-gas studies. At some centers, respiratory therapists can manage patients according to predetermined protocols which have been approved by the medical staff, such as those for initiation of, maintenance of, and weaning from mechanical ventilation. Nutritionists assess the daily caloric needs of the patient and recommend the appropriate method of providing the patient's nutritional requirements. At this center, the authors have found the input provided by a clinical pharmacist who accompanies the team on bedside rounds to be most valuable. The clinical pharmacist ensures that patients receive appropriate medications and monitors their efficacy, dosage, adverse effects, or drug interactions. Optimal management of mechanically ventilated patients requires the extensive support of laboratory and radiologic services. In addition, speech therapists are needed to devise methods to improve the patient's communication and to assess the ability to swallow effectively. Physical therapists suggest means to minimize or prevent pressure sores and contractures, assess any physical limitations, and devise plans to optimize the patient's muscle strength, endurance, and coordination. Later in their course, patients may need the help of occupational therapists to provide them with mechanical aids that help them overcome functional limitations. The psychologist, chaplain, social worker, and home care coordinator are needed to look after the complex emotional, social, and financial issues involved, particularly with long-term mechanical ventilation.

References

1. Tobin MJ: Mechanical ventilation. *N Engl J Med* 330:1056–1061, 1994.
2. Mountain RD, Sahn SA: Clinical features and outcome in patients with acute asthma presenting with hypercapnia. *Am Rev Respir Dis* 138:535–539, 1988.
3. Coussa ML, Guerin C, Eissa NT, et al: Partitioning of work of breathing in mechanically ventilated COPD patients. *J Appl Physiol* 75:1711–1719, 1993.
4. Jubran A, Tobin MJ: Pathophysiologic basis of acute respiratory distress in patients who fail a trial of weaning from mechanical ventilation. *Am J Respir Crit Care Med* 155:906–915, 1997.
5. Field S, Kelly SM, Macklem PT: The oxygen cost of breathing in patients with cardiorespiratory disease. *Am Rev Respir Dis* 126:9–13, 1982.
6. Katz JA, Marks JD: Inspiratory work with and without continuous positive airway pressure in patients with acute respiratory failure. *Anesthesiology* 63:598–607, 1985.
7. Marini JJ: Pressure-controlled ventilation, in Tobin MJ (ed): *Principles and Practice of Mechanical Ventilation.* New York, McGraw-Hill, 1994; pp 305–317.
8. Marini JJ, Capps JS, Culver BH: The inspiratory work of breathing during assisted mechanical ventilation. *Chest* 87:612–618, 1985.
9. Ward ME, Corbeil C, Gibbons W, et al: Optimization of respiratory muscle relaxation during mechanical ventilation. *Anesthesiology* 69:29–35, 1988.
10. Sassoon CSH: Intermittent mandatory ventilation, in Tobin MJ (ed): *Principles and Practice of Mechanical Ventilation.* New York, McGraw-Hill, 1994; pp 221–237.
11. Mathru M, Rao TLK, Venus B: Ventilator-induced barotrauma in controlled mechanical ventilation versus intermittent mandatory ventilation. *Crit Care Med* 11:359–361, 1983.
12. Mathru M, Rao TLK, El-Etr AA, Pifarre R: Hemodynamic response to changes in ventilatory patterns in patients with normal and poor left ventricular reserve. *Crit Care Med* 10:423–426, 1982.
13. Miro AM, Pinsky MR: Heart-lung interactions, in Tobin MJ (ed): *Principles and Practice of Mechanical Ventilation.* New York, McGraw-Hill, 1994; pp 647–671.
14. Marini JJ, Smith TC, Lamb VJ: External work output and force generation during synchronized intermittent mechanical ventilation. *Am Rev Respir Dis* 138:1169–1179, 1988.
15. Imsand C, Feihl F, Perret C, Fitting JW: Regulation of inspiratory neuromuscular output during synchronized intermittent mechanical ventilation. *Anesthesiology* 80:13–22, 1994.
16. Leung P, Jubran A, Tobin MJ: Comparison of assisted ventilator modes on triggering, patient effort and dyspnea. *Am J Respir Crit Care Med* 155: 1940–1948, 1997.
17. Brochard L: Pressure support ventilation, in Tobin MJ (ed): *Principles and Practice of Mechanical Ventilation.* New York, McGraw-Hill, 1994; pp 239–257.
18. Jubran A, Van de Graaff WB, Tobin MJ: Variability of patient-ventilator interaction with pressure support ventilation in patients with chronic obstructive pulmonary disease. *Am J Respir Crit Care Med* 152:129–136, 1995.
19. Appendini L, Patessio A, Zanaboni S, et al: Physiologic effects

of positive end-expiratory pressure and mask pressure support during exacerbations of chronic obstructive pulmonary disease. *Am J Respir Crit Care Med* 149:1069–1076, 1994.

20. Sassoon CSH, Gruer SE: Characteristics of the ventilator pressure and flow-trigger variables. *Intensive Care Med* 21:159–168, 1995.

21. Hubmayr RD: Setting the ventilator, in Tobin MJ (ed): *Principles and Practice of Mechanical Ventilation.* New York, McGraw-Hill, 1994; pp 191–206.

22. Dreyfuss D, Saumon G: Ventilator-induced injury, in Tobin MJ (ed): *Principles and Practice of Mechanical Ventilation.* New York, McGraw-Hill, 1994; pp 793–811.

23. Tobin MJ: State of the art: Respiratory monitoring in the intensive care units. *Am Rev Respir Dis* 138:1625–1642, 1988.

24. ACCP Consensus Conference: Mechanical ventilation. *Chest* 104:1833–1859, 1993.

25. Tuxen DV: Permissive hypercapnia, in Tobin MJ (ed): *Principles and Practice of Mechanical Ventilation.* New York, McGraw-Hill, 1994; pp 371–392.

26. Darioli R, Perret C: Mechanical controlled hypoventilation in status asthmaticus. *Am Rev Respir Dis* 129:385–387, 1984.

27. Tuxen DV, Williams TJ, Scheinkestel CD, et al: Use of a measurement of pulmonary hyperinflation to control the level of mechanical ventilation in patients with acute severe asthma. *Am Rev Respir Dis* 146:1136–1142, 1992.

28. Amato MBP, Barbas CSV, Medeiros DM, et al: Beneficial effects of the "open lung approach" with low distending pressures in acute respiratory distress syndrome: A prospective randomized study on mechanical ventilation. *Am J Respir Crit Care Med* 152:1835–1846, 1995.

29. Connors AF Jr, McCaffree DR, Gray BA: Effect of inspiratory flow rate on gas exchange during mechanical ventilation. *Am Rev Respir Dis* 124:537–543, 1981.

30. Puddy A, Younes M: Effect on inspiratory flow rate on respiratory output in normal subjects. *Am Rev Respir Dis* 146:787–789, 1992.

31. Sasse SA, Jaffe MB, Chen PA, et al: Arterial oxygenation time after an F_{IO_2} increase in mechanically ventilated patients. *Am J Respir Crit Care Med* 152:148–152, 1995.

32. Jubran A, Tobin MJ: Reliability of pulse oximetry in titrating supplemental oxygen therapy in ventilator-dependent patients. *Chest* 90:1420–1425, 1990.

33. Ashbaugh DG, Petty TL, Bigelow DB, Harris TM: Continuous positive-pressure breathing (CPPB) in adult respiratory distress syndrome. *J Thorac Cardiovasc Surg* 57:31–39, 1969.

34. Daly BDT, Edmonds CH, Norman JC: In vivo alveolar morphometries with positive end expiratory pressure. *Surgical Forum* 24:217–219, 1973.

35. Dueck R, Wagner PD, West JB: Effects of positive end-expiratory pressure on gas exchange in dogs with normal and edematous lungs. *Anesthesiology* 47:359–366, 1976.

36. Katz JA, Ozanne GM, Zinn SE, Fairley HB: Time course and mechanisms of lung-volume increase with PEEP in acute pulmonary failure. *Anesthesiology* 54:9–16, 1981.

37. Gattinoni L, Pesenti A, Bombino M, et al: Relationships between lung computed tomographic density, gas exchange, and PEEP in acute respiratory failure. *Anesthesiology* 69:824–832, 1988.

38. Malo J, Ali J, Wood LDH: How does positive end-expiratory pressure reduce intrapulmonary shunt in canine pulmonary edema? *J Appl Physiol* 57:1002–1010, 1984.

39. Kanarek DJ, Shannon DC: Adverse effect of positive end-expiratory pressure on pulmonary perfusion and arterial oxygenation. *Am Rev Resp Dis* 112:457–459, 1975.

40. Rossi A, Gottfried SB, Zocchi L, et al: Measurement of static compliance of the total respiratory system in patients with acute respiratory failure during mechanical ventilation: The effect of intrinsic positive end-expiratory pressure. *Am Rev Respir Dis* 131:672–677, 1985.

41. Smith TC, Marini JJ: Impact of PEEP on lung mechanics and work of breathing in severe airflow obstruction. *J Appl Physiol* 65:1488–1499, 1988.

42. Tobin MJ, Lodato RF: Editorial: PEEP, auto-PEEP, and waterfalls. *Chest* 96:449–451, 1989.

43. Dhand R, Tobin MJ: Bronchodilator delivery with metered-dose inhalers in mechanically-ventilated patients. *Eur Respir J* 9:585–595, 1996.

44. Dhand R, Duarte AG, Jubran A, et al: Dose response to bronchodilator delivered by metered-dose inhaler in ventilator-supported patients. *Am J Respir Crit Care Med* 154:388–393, 1996.

45. Gattinoni L, Pelosi P, Valenza F, Macheroni D: Patient positioning in acute respiratory failure, in Tobin MJ (ed): *Principles and Practice of Mechanical Ventilation.* New York, McGraw-Hill, 1994; pp 1067–1076.

46. Chatte G, Sab JM, Dubois JM, et al: Prone position in mechanically ventilated patients with severe acute respiratory failure. *Am J Respir Crit Care Med* 155:473–478, 1997.

47. Albert RK. Editorial: For every thing (turn. . . turn. . . turn. . . .). *Am J Respir Crit Care Med* 155:393–394, 1997.

48. Jubran A, Tobin MJ: Monitoring during mechanical ventilation. *Clin Chest Med* 17:453–473, 1996.

49. Pingleton SK: Complications associated with mechanical ventilation, in Tobin MJ (ed): *Principles and Practice of Mechanical Ventilation.* New York, McGraw-Hill, 1994; pp 775–792.

50. Pierson DJ: Barotrauma and bronchopleural fistula, in Tobin MJ (ed): *Principles and Practice of Mechanical Ventilation.* New York, McGraw-Hill, 1994; pp 813–836.

51. Chastre J, Fagon JY: Pneumonia in the ventilator-dependent patient, in Tobin MJ (ed): *Principles and Practice of Mechanical Ventilation.* New York, McGraw-Hill, 1994; pp 857–890.

52. Stauffer JL: Complications of translaryngeal intubation, in Tobin MJ (ed): *Principles and Practice of Mechanical Ventilation.* New York, McGraw-Hill, 1994; pp 711–747.

53. Lodato RF: Oxygen toxicity, in Tobin MJ (ed): *Principles and Practice of Mechanical Ventilation.* New York, McGraw-Hill, 1994; pp 837–855.

54. Sackner MA, Landa J, Hirsch J, Zapata A: Pulmonary effects of oxygen breathing: A 6-hour study in normal men. *Ann Intern Med* 82:40–43, 1975.

55. Petersen GW, Baier H: Incidence of pulmonary barotrauma in a medical ICU. *Crit Care Med* 11:67–69, 1983.

56. Gammon BR, Shin MS, Buchalter SE: Pulmonary barotrauma in mechanical ventilation: Patterns and risk factors. *Chest* 102:568–572, 1992.

57. Zwillich CW, Pierson DJ, Creagh CE, et al: Complications of assisted ventilation: A prospective study of 354 consecutive episodes. *Am J Med* 57:161–170, 1974.

58. deLatorre FJ, Tomasa A, Klamburg J, et al: Incidence of pneumothorax and pneumomediastinum in patients with aspiration pneumonia requiring ventilatory support. *Chest* 72:141–144, 1977.

59. Kumar A, Pontoppidan H, Falke KJ, et al: Pulmonary barotrauma during mechanical ventilation. *Crit Care Med* 1:181–186, 1973.

60. Webb H, Tierney D: Experimental pulmonary edema due to intermittent positive pressure ventilation with high inflation pressures: Protection by positive end-expiratory pressure. *Am Rev Respir Dis* 110:556–565, 1974.

61. Albelda SM, Gefter WB, Kelley MA, et al: Ventilator-induced subpleural air cysts: Clinical, radiographic, and pathologic significance. *Am Rev Respir Dis* 127:360–365, 1983.

62. Craven DE, Kunches LM, Kilinski V, et al: Risk factors for pneumonia and fatality in patients receiving continuous mechanical ventilation. *Am Rev Respir Dis* 133:792–796, 1986.

63. Fagon JY, Chastre J, Hance A, et al: Nosocomial pneumonia in ventilated patients: A cohort study evaluating attributable mortality and hospital stay. *Am J Med* 94:281–288, 1993.

64. Fagon JY, Chastre J, Domart Y, et al: Nosocomial pneumonia in patients receiving continuous mechanical ventilation: Prospective analysis of 52 episodes with use of a protective specimen brush and quantitative culture techniques. *Am Rev Respir Dis* 139:877–884, 1989.

65. Torres A, Aznar R, Gatell JM, Jimenez P, et al: Incidence, risk and prognosis factors of nosocomial pneumonia in mechanically ventilated patients. *Am Rev Respir Dis* 142:523–528, 1990.

66. Fagon JY, Chastre J, Hance A, et al: Evaluation of clinical judgement in the identification and treatment of nosocomial pneumonia in ventilated patients. *Chest* 103:547–553, 1993.

67. Johanson WG Jr, Pierce AK, Sanford JP, Thomas GD: Nosocomial respiratory infections with gram negative bacilli: The significance of colonization of the respiratory tract. *Ann Intern Med* 77:701–706, 1972.

68. Niederman MS, Mantovani R, Schoch P, et al: Patterns and routes of tracheobronchial colonization in mechanically ventilated patients: The role of nutrition status in colonization of the lower airway by *Pseudomonas* species. *Chest* 95:155–161, 1989.

69. Bryan CS, Reynolds KL: Bacteremic nosocomial pneumonia. *Am Rev Respir Dis* 129:668–671, 1984.

70. Chastre J, Viau F, Brun P, et al: Prospective evaluation of the protected specimen brush for the diagnosis of pulmonary infections in ventilated patients. *Am Rev Respir Dis* 130:924–929, 1984.

71. Chastre J, Fagon JY, Soler PR, et al: Diagnosis of nosocomial bacterial pneumonia in intubated patients undergoing ventilation: Comparison of the usefulness of bronchoalveolar lavage and the protected specimen brush technique. *Am J Med* 85:499–506, 1988.

72. Rouby JJ, Rossignon MD, Nicolas MH, et al: A prospective study of protected bronchoalveolar lavage in the diagnosis of nosocomial pneumonia. *Anesthesiology* 71:679–685, 1989.

73. Torres A, De La Bellacasa JP, Xaubet A, et al: Diagnostic values of quantitative cultures of bronchoalveolar lavage and telescoping plugged catheters in mechanically ventilated patients with bacterial pneumonia. *Am Rev Respir Dis* 140:306–310, 1989.

74. Jourdain B, Joly-Guillou ML, Dombret MC, et al: Usefulness of quantitative cultures of BAL fluid for diagnosing nosocomial pneumonia in ventilated patients. *Chest* 111:411–418, 1997.

75. Kolleff MH, Bock KR, Richards RD, Hearns ML: The safety and diagnostic accuracy of minibronchoalveolar lavage in patients with suspected ventilator-associated pneumonia. *Ann Intern Med* 122:743–748, 1995.

76. Meduri GU, Beals DH, Maijub AG, Baselski V: Protected bronchoalveolar lavage: A new bronchoscopic technique to retrieve uncontaminated distal airway secretions. *Am Rev Respir Dis* 143:855–864, 1991.

77. Stauffer JL, Olson DE, Petty TL: Complications and consequences of endotracheal intubation and tracheotomy. A prospective study of 150 critically ill patients. *Am J Med* 70:65–76, 1981.

78. Heffner JE: Tracheal intubation in mechanically-ventilated patients. *Clin Chest Med* 9:23–35, 1988.

79. Heffner JE: Timing of tracheotomy in mechanically ventilated patients. *Am Rev Respir Dis* 148:768–771, 1993.

80. Esteban A, Frutos F, Tobin MJ, et al: A comparison of four methods of weaning patients from mechanical ventilation. *N Engl J Med* 332:345–350, 1995.

81. Esteban A, Alfa I, Ibanez J, et al, Spanish Lung Failure Collaborative Group: Modes of mechanical ventilation and weaning: A national survey of Spanish hospitals. *Chest* 106:1188–1193, 1994.

82. Tobin MJ, Alex CG: Discontinuation of mechanical ventilation, in Tobin MJ (ed): *Principles and Practice of Mechanical Ventilation.* New York, McGraw-Hill, 1994; pp 1177–1206.

83. Stroetz RW, Hubmayr RD: Tidal volume maintenance during weaning with pressure support. *Am J Respir Crit Care Med* 152:1034–1040, 1995.

84. Yang KL, Tobin MJ: A prospective study of indexes predicting the outcome of trials of weaning from mechanical ventilation. *N Engl J Med* 324:1445–1450, 1991.

85. Brochard L, Rna F, Lorino H, et al: Inspiratory pressure support compensates for the additional work of breathing caused by the endotracheal tube. *Anesthesiology* 75:739–745, 1991.

86. Nathan SD, Ishaaya AM, Koerner SK, Belman MJ: Prediction of minimal pressure support during weaning from mechanical ventilation. *Chest* 103:1215–1219, 1993.

87. Laghi F, D'Alfonso N, Tobin MJ: Pattern of recovery from diaphragmatic fatigue over 24 hours. *J Appl Physiol* 79:539–546, 1995.

88. Brochard L, Rauss A, Benito S, et al: Comparison of three methods of gradual withdrawal from ventilatory support during weaning from mechanical ventilation. *Am J Respir Crit Care Med* 150:896–903, 1994.

89. Ely EW, Baker AM, Dunagan DP, et al: Effect on the duration of mechanical ventilation of identifying patients capable of breathing spontaneously. *N Engl J Med* 335:1864–1869, 1996.

90. Elliott M, Moxham J: Non-invasive mechanical ventilation by nasal or face mask, in Tobin MJ (ed): *Principles and Practice of Mechanical Ventilation.* New York, McGraw-Hill, 1994; pp 427–453.

91. Meyer TJ, Hill NS: Noninvasive positive pressure ventilation to treat respiratory failure. *Ann Intern Med* 20:760–770, 1994.

92. Bott J, Carroll MP, Conway JH, et al: Randomised controlled trial of nasal ventilation in acute ventilatory failure due to chronic obstructive airways disease. *Lancet* 341:1555–1557, 1993.

93. Kramer N, Meyer TJ, Meharg J, et al: Randomized, prospective trial of noninvasive positive pressure ventilation in acute respiratory failure. *Am J Respir Crit Care Med* 151:1799–1806, 1995.

94. Brochard L, Mancebo J, Wysocki M, et al: Noninvasive ventilation for acute exacerbations of chronic obstructive pulmonary disease. *N Engl J Med* 333:817–822, 1995.

95. Abou-Shala N, Meduri GU: Noninvasive mechanical ventilation in patients with acute respiratory failure. *Crit Care Med* 24:705–715, 1996.

96. Kacmarek RM, Hess D: Equipment required for home mechanical ventilation, in Tobin MJ (ed): *Principles and Practice of Mechanical Ventilation.* New York, McGraw-Hill, 1994; pp 111–154.

97. Marks A, Bocles J, Morganti L: A new ventilatory assister for patients with respiratory acidosis. *N Engl J Med* 268:61–67, 1963.

98. Sauret JM, Guitart AC, Frojan GR, Cornudella R: Intermittent short-term negative pressure ventilation and increased oxygenation in COPD patients with severe hypercapnic respiratory failure. *Chest* 100:455–459, 1991.

99. Corrado A, Bruscoli G, Messori A, et al: Iron lung treatment of subjects with COPD in acute respiratory failure: Evaluation of short and long-term prognosis. *Chest* 101:692–696, 1992.

100. Corrado A, Gorini M, De Paola E: Alternative techniques for managing acute neuromuscular respiratory failure. *Sem Neurol* 15:84–89, 1995.

101. Levine S, Henson D: Negative pressure ventilation, in Tobin MJ (ed): *Principles and Practice of Mechanical Ventilation.* New York, McGraw-Hill, 1994; pp 393–411.

102. Menzies R, Gibbons W, Goldberg P: Determinants of weaning and survival among patients with COPD who require mechanical ventilation for acute respiratory failure. *Chest* 95:398–405, 1989.

103. Ellis ER, Bye PTP, Bruderer JW, Sullivan CE: Treatment of respiratory failure during sleep in patients with neuromuscular disease: Positive-pressure ventilation through a nose mask. *Am Rev Respir Dis* 135:148–152, 1987.

104. Kerby GR, Mayer LS, Pingleton SK: Nocturnal positive pressure ventilation via nasal mask. *Am Rev Respir Dis* 135:738–740, 1987.

105. Bach JR, Alba AS: Management of chronic alveolar hypoventilation by nasal ventilation. *Chest* 97:52–57, 1990.

106. Heckmatt JZ, Loh L, Dubowitz V: Night-time nasal ventilation in neuromuscular disease. *Lancet* 2:579–582, 1990.

107. Gay PC, Patel AM, Viggiano RW, Hubmayr RD: Nocturnal nasal ventilation for treatment of patients with hypercapnic respiratory failure. *Mayo Clin Proc* 66:695–703, 1991.

108. Ellis ER, Grunstein RR, Chan S, et al: Noninvasive ventilatory support during sleep improves respiratory failure in kyphoscoliosis. *Chest* 94:811–815, 1988.

109. Carroll N, Branthwaite MA: Control of nocturnal hypoventilation by nasal intermittent positive pressure ventilation. *Thorax* 43:349–353, 1988.

110. Leger P, Jennequin J, Gerard M, et al: Home positive pressure ventilation via nasal mask for patients with neuromusculoskeletal disorders. *Eur Respir J* 7(suppl):640S–644S, 1989.

111. Leger P, Robert D, Langevin B, Guez A: Chest wall deformities due to idiopathic kyphoscoliosis or sequelae of tuberculosis. *Eur Respir Rev* 2:362–368, 1992.

112. Elliott MW, Mulvey DA, Moxham J, et al: Domiciliary nocturnal nasal intermittent positive pressure ventilation in COPD: Mechanisms underlying changes in arterial blood gas tensions. *Eur Respir J* 4:1044–1052, 1991.

113. Strumpf DA, Milman RP, Carlisle CC, et al: Nocturnal positive-pressure ventilation via nasal mask in patients with severe chronic obstructive pulmonary disease. *Am Rev Respir Dis* 144: 1234–1239, 1991.

114. Celli BR, Rassulo J, Corral R: Ventilatory muscle dysfunction in patients with bilateral idiopathic diaphragmatic paralysis: Reversal by intermittent external negative pressure ventilation. *Am Rev Respir Dis* 136:1276–1278, 1987.

115. Braun SR, Sufit RL, Giovannoni R, et al: Intermittent negative pressure ventilation in the treatment of respiratory failure in progressive neuromuscular disease. *Neurology* 37:1874–1875, 1987.

116. Goldstein RS, Molotiu N, Skrastins R, et al: Reversal of sleep-induced hypoventilation and chronic respiratory failure by nocturnal negative pressure ventilation in patients with restrictive ventilatory impairment. *Am Rev Respir Dis* 135:1049–1055, 1987.

117. Sawicka EH, Loh L, Branthwaite MA: Domiciliary ventilatory support: An analysis of outcome. *Thorax* 43:31–35, 1988.

118. Garay SM, Turino GM, Goldring RM: Sustained reversal of chronic hypercapnia in patients with alveolar hypoventilation syndromes: Long-term maintenance with noninvasive nocturnal mechanical ventilation. *Am J Med* 70:269–274, 1981.

119. Shapiro SH, Ernst P, Gray-Donald K, et al: Effect of negative pressure ventilation in severe chronic obstructive pulmonary disease. *Lancet* 340:1425–1429, 1992.

120. Shalansky KF, Htan EYF, Lyster DM, et al: In vitro evaluation of the effect of metered-dose inhaler administration technique on aerosolized drug delivery. *Pharmacotherapy* 13:233–238, 1993.

Chapter 32

NONINVASIVE MECHANICAL VENTILATION

ANTHONY F. DiMARCO

JEFFREY P. RENSTON

The aim of pulmonary rehabilitation is to alleviate symptoms, improve quality of life, and restore patients to their highest level of independent functioning.[1] Rehabilitation of the patient with respiratory disease often necessitates the application of complete or partial mechanical ventilation to overcome ventilatory failure and impairment of oxygenation. In the acute setting, nasal or orotracheal intubation or tracheostomy are often required. However, in chronic respiratory disease, tracheal intubation is not practical owing to its invasiveness and consequent association with complications, including infection, tracheal tube dislodgement, and potential for vascular erosion and serious hemorrhage. Noninvasive ventilatory support (NIVS) is an alternative means of providing long-term mechanical ventilation in the rehabilitation of patients with respiratory diseases. NIVS utilizes external body devices which apply negative (subatmospheric) pressure over the thorax (negative pressure ventilation) or positive pressure to the nose and/or mouth (positive pressure ventilation) to overcome chronic respiratory insufficiency. This chapter outlines selected elements of NIVS, including a brief description of available devices, methods of application, and efficacy of these devices in various patient groups; it includes an evaluation of published studies and provides recommendations for the use of NIVS in the rehabilitation of patients with chronic respiratory failure. A number of excellent recently published articles review the technical and financial aspects of NIVS devices; these aspects of NIVS, therefore, are not discussed here.[2-4]

Available Devices and Their Methods of Application

A variety of systems are available for the delivery of NIVS. These can be grouped into those providing (1) negative pressure to the chest wall, (2) positive pressure to the respiratory system via nasal or face masks, and (3) other miscellaneous systems. Negative-pressure devices include tank ventilators, cuirass (or chest shell), poncho, pneumosuit and pulmowrap systems, and the Hayek oscillator; positive-pressure devices include systems designed to deliver continuous positive airway pressure (CPAP), bilevel positive airway pressure (BiPAP), and conventional pressure or volume-cycled ventilation. There are also other types of systems, such as the rocking bed, which employs gravitational forces, and pneumobelt, which applies positive pressure to the abdominal wall. A brief description of each of these systems is provided below.

The mechanical mechanism, and advantages and disadvantages of each method are also summarized in Table 32-1.

Negative-Pressure Devices

TANK VENTILATOR

The tank ventilator, or iron lung, was developed in the 1920s and used almost exclusively in the management of respiratory failure associated with the polio epidemic for more than three decades.[3,5-13] This device consists of a large metal cylinder or tank with a flexible bellows or diaphragm operated by a motorized piston rod at the distal end. Outward and inward movement of the piston generates negative intratank pressure swings. The patient lays supine on a mattress-covered frame connected to movable rails on the inner sides of the tank. After being sealed inside the tank, only the head is exposed to the atmosphere.[4] The tank ventilator functions optimally at pressure settings of -10 to -35 cmH$_2$O and at respiratory rates of 14 to 24 cycles per minute.[3] Ongoing care to patients is usually provided via side portholes equipped with rubber gaskets to minimize pressure leaks.[14,15] The tank ventilator results in almost complete suppression of diaphragm electromyographic activity and significant reductions in accessory muscle activity[15] in patients with chronic hypercapnia indicating that this device significantly reduces inspiratory muscle work. Familiarization of the patient with the respirator appears to be necessary to achieve suppression of inspiratory muscle activation, however.[16]

Although this device is the most efficient and reliable method of negative-pressure ventilation (NPV), it is quite large, weighing approximately 300 kg, and requires a considerable amount of operational space. This device also presents difficulties with regard to ingress and egress, always requires an attendant, and imposes limitations on patient access.[5] The tank ventilator can also result in musculoskeletal pain and interfere with sleep.

CHEST CUIRASS

The success of the tank ventilator in the treatment of patients with paralytic polio led to the development of devices which were more portable and less confining and allowed easier access to patients by medical personnel. The chest cuirass and body suit ventilators are examples of such devices which are applied directly to the body surface.[3,5,10-14,17,18] The chest cuirass consists of a hard fiberglass or plastic shell, either of generic shape or custom fit, which is affixed using straps over the anterior thorax and abdomen. To function properly, the cuirass should encompass both the rib cage and at least the upper portion of the abdomen. The cuirass is in turn attached to a negative-pressure ventilator, via a flexible pressure hose. Negative pressure within the cavity of the cuirass shell acts to expand the rib cage and abdominal wall. The device is lightweight, portable, and relatively easy to apply independently and can be used in either the supine or upright position. Optimum inspiratory pressures range between -15 and -45 cmH$_2$O, at respiratory rates of 14 to 28 breaths per minute.[3,5]

A major disadvantage of this device is the difficulty in obtaining a proper fit. Too snug a fit and improper positioning of the device can actually impede inspiration and possibly

TABLE 32-1 Advantages and Disadvantages of Various Devices

Devices	Mechanism of Action	Advantages	Disadvantages
Negative-Pressure Devices			
Tank ventilator	Vacuum applied to body surface	Simple operation; reliable	Bulky; poor patient access; Requires assistance from others
Chest cuirass	Vacuum applied to body surface	Portable; easy to apply	Poor fit at neck, pelvis; inefficient in kyphotic or obese patients
Body suit	Vacuum applied to body surface	Portable; easy to apply	Musculoskeletal pain; temperature changes
Hayek oscillator	High-frequency ventilation	Portable	Poor fit; excessive noise
Positive-Pressure Devices			
CPAP	Continuous airway pressure	Easy to fit; Eliminates upper airway obstruction	Local discomfort from mask; gastric distension
BiPAP	Pressure-support	Higher inspiratory pressure	Local discomfort from mask; gastric distension; CO_2 rebreathing; no alarms
Volume-cycled	Fixed tidal volume	Can deliver higher airway pressure; safety alarms; more reliable	Bulky; lacks pressure-support mode
Miscellaneous Devices			
Rocking bed	Gravity	Simple; good patient mobility and access	Bulky; limited effectiveness in patients with kyphosis; decreased chest/abdominal compliance
Pneumobelt	Gravity	Well tolerated; easy to apply	Must be upright; limited effectiveness in obese

worsen respiratory failure. A loose fit and poor contact around the perimeter, on the other hand, can markedly reduce the ventilator's efficiency. Complications of the chest cuirass include skin abrasions and pressure sores which can develop in areas where the device is in contact with the body.

BODY-WRAP VENTILATORS

Body-wrap ventilators are modifications of the cuirass.[3,5,14,19] Several different types of similar basic design are available and include the poncho, pneumosuit, zip suit, pneumowrap, pulmowrap, and raincoat. These devices consist of a flat rigid plate, large plastic grid, and air-tight nylon parka- or windbreaker-like jackets or jumpsuits, which can be sealed at the neck, wrists, and legs using Velcro straps to prevent air leakage. Within the suit, the patient lies on the plate which extends the length of the thoracic spine. The grid arches anteriorly several inches over the chest. The suit is connected to a negative pressure ventilator via a flexible pressure hose in a fashion similar to the chest cuirass. Like the chest cuirass, optimum pressure settings range between −15 and −45 cmH₂O; optimum respiratory rates range between 14 and 28 breaths per minute.[3] Body suits are portable and fairly easy to use. Although they can be applied in the upright position, body suits are generally worn while supine.

An advantage of these devices compared with the cuirass is greater patient comfort since the device does not have direct contact with the chest wall. Complications of these devices include back, chest, and shoulder pain, a result of lying on the rigid back plate. It is therefore recommended that the plate be cushioned with some type of soft fabric. Other potential problems include inability to sleep, increases in temperature within tightly sealed suits, and the inconvenience of getting in and out of the device.[12]

HAYEK OSCILLATOR

The Hayek oscillator (HO) is a relatively new device for assisting ventilation.[20,21] Respiration is generated by a plastic chest cuirass which fits snugly over the anterior rib cage and upper abdomen. The cuirass is connected to a power unit by flexible tubing which, in turn, is connected to a pump which generates oscillating pressures at high frequency (8 to 999 cycles per minute). A separate pump allows the oscillating pressures to be superimposed on a negative baseline pressure.[20,21]

The short-term efficacy of the HO has been evaluated in a group of patients with chronic obstructive pulmonary disease (COPD).[20] The oscillator was employed at frequencies of 60 to 140 cycles per minute at pressures between −26 and +10 cmH₂O with an inspiratory/expiratory ratio of 1:1 over 3-min periods. This resulted in suppression of spontaneous ventilation and significant reductions in end-tidal P_{CO_2} (6 to 9 mmHg) in both eucapnic and hypercapnic patients and improvement in oxygen saturation. Disadvantages of this device include difficulty obtaining proper fitting, air leakage resulting in loss of oscillatory pressure, and excessive noise.[21,22] The Hayek oscillator therefore may be a potentially useful device in the management of respiratory failure. Its use as a mode of NIVS in the rehabilitation of patients with respiratory failure, however, requires further study.

Potential Complications of Negative-Pressure Ventilation

One of the more common and serious complications of all negative pressure devices is the development of upper airway obstruction. Negative pressure applied to the thorax is transmitted to the upper airway, where it induces a collapsing force. In the absence of synchronous activation of the upper airway musculature during inspiration to oppose this force, the applied pressure results in a reduction in caliber or complete collapse of the upper airway during inspiration.[23–25] Fortunately, the respiratory rhythm of most patients becomes entrained with that of the ventilator such that respiratory drive to the upper airway musculature occurs in synchrony with the negative pressure applied by the ventilator. However, this potential complication is not uncommon and occurs to some extent in many patients. Consequently, these devices are contraindicated in patients at risk for the development of obstructive apneas, weakness of the pharyngeal muscles, or significant defects in central ventilatory drive.

Gastroesophageal reflux disease can also be induced by NPV. These devices have been shown to reduce the pressure gradient between the lower esophageal sphincter and the stomach, leading to reflux of gastric material into the esophagus. This phenomenon has been demonstrated in both healthy individuals and in patients with COPD during negative-pressure ventilation.[26]

Finally, cyclical NPV can affect cardiac function. Decreased intrathoracic pressure may result in increases in venous return, right ventricular preload, and also increased left ventricular afterload. While these effects may be inconsequential in patients with normal cardiac function, they may result in adverse consequences in patients with underlying lung disease.[27] The overall effect of NPV on cardiac output, however, remains controversial.[14,27,28]

In summary, NPV can provide excellent ventilatory support in selected patients. Negative pressure devices, however, are generally more cumbersome to employ and are less well tolerated compared with some positive-pressure methods. Consequently, negative pressure devices are currently used less frequently. Nonetheless, NPV is the preferred method of NIVS for many patients owing to some of the disadvantages of positive-pressure devices. Clinicians, therefore, should be aware of these modalities as an alternative method of NIVS for certain patients.

Positive-Pressure Devices

CONTINUOUS POSITIVE AIRWAY PRESSURE

Use of this modality results in a constant preset pressure being maintained throughout the respiratory cycle. Theoretically, by expanding closed alveoli and increasing functional residual capacity, CPAP improves oxygenation and reduces the work of breathing. In patients with obstructive apnea, CPAP acts to splint open the upper airway, thereby reducing airway obstruction.[29,30,30a] In patients with COPD, CPAP has been shown to reduce inspiratory muscle effort.[31] CPAP can be delivered to the patient via a nasal or full-face mask or via a tracheostomy tube connected to a positive pressure source. CPAP pressures of 5 to 15 cmH$_2$O are generally utilized clinically.

The application of CPAP can be quite uncomfortable for many patients and, thus, poorly tolerated. Studies evaluating patient home use of nasal CPAP for the management of sleep apnea have, in fact, documented poor compliance.[32] Many patients complain of a variety of symptoms including nasal dryness and congestion, nosebleeds, or rhinorrhea. Some patients develop sinusitis. CPAP compressors can also be quite cumbersome and very noisy.

BI-LEVEL POSITIVE AIRWAY PRESSURE

The ability to separately adjust inspiratory positive airway pressure (IPAP) and expiratory positive airway pressure (EPAP) makes bilevel positive airway pressure (BiPAP) unique among the positive-pressure NIVS devices. BiPAP utilizes a flow-triggered system; that is, patient-generated inspiratory airflow of approximately 40 mL/s triggers onset of gas delivery at a high rate, until the preset IPAP is achieved. Flow continues at this pressure until inspiratory airflow falls to a minimal value at end-inspiration, at which time EPAP is initiated. Both IPAP and EPAP can be delivered at pressures ranging from +2 to +20 cmH$_2$O. Because BiPAP utilizes a continuous low-level (or "bias") airflow, it can sense and compensate for air leaks. BiPAP can be delivered via a nasal or full-face mask, utilizing four modes: spontaneous, timed, spontaneous and timed, and CPAP. In the spontaneous mode, patients trigger airflow with spontaneous breaths. The timed mode functions like conventional intermittent mandatory ventilation, while the spontaneous and timed mode allows for spontaneous patient breaths, which are augmented by a preset backup rate. Since BiPAP provides pressure support ventilation, patients maintain independent control of tidal volume, respiratory rate, inspiratory time, and inspiratory flow rate.[33,34] Unlike IPPB, flow continues when the preset IPAP is achieved using BiPAP. Increasing IPAP has the effect of increasing tidal volume. Increasing EPAP mimics delivery of positive end-expiratory pressure (PEEP), resulting in recruitment of closed alveoli and an increase in functional residual capacity (FRC), which may lead to improved oxygenation.

Because of its small size, portability, relatively low cost, and lower degree of discomfort, BiPAP offers significant advantages over other NIVS systems.[35] Disadvantages of BiPAP include mouth leaks, skin irritation from the nasal and face masks (especially over the bridge of the nose), dryness of the nasal mucosa, eye irritation, and interference with sleep.[36,37] In addition, BiPAP is poorly tolerated in patients who have increased airway secretions or nasal congestion. Since the BiPAP system lacks alarms, patients who have unstable ventilatory patterns, or who have the potential to become apneic, may be at risk for respiratory failure. Finally, CO$_2$ rebreathing may occur in the setting of minimal EPAP, elevated breathing frequency, or reduced expiratory time, resulting in increased work of breathing. This can be overcome, however, with the use of a non-rebreathing valve.[38]

CONVENTIONAL POSITIVE-PRESSURE VENTILATION

Standard volume or pressure-cycled ventilators, which deliver a preset tidal volume or pressure via nasal or full-face masks or mouthpiece, have been shown to effectively deliver NIVS to patients with various forms of chronic respiratory failure.[32,39–47,47a] There are a large number of different devices, most of which can function in either the assist-control or control mode. Positive-pressure ventilation

(PPV) is particularly useful in patients who require high airway pressures for ventilation, such as those with severe restrictive pulmonary abnormalities. A wide variety of models are available, and their technical aspects have been reviewed elsewhere.[4]

Potential Complications of Positive-Pressure Ventilation

Positive-pressure ventilation has the potential to impair cardiac function. Positive intrathoracic pressure may decrease venous return, resulting in significant reductions in preload and consequent reductions in cardiac output. Positive-pressure ventilation, however, can also have beneficial effects on cardiac output in patients with chronic congestive heart failure.[48] The reduction in preload and afterload associated with CPAP leads to improvement in cardiac function. In the setting of cardiogenic pulmonary edema, CPAP improves gas exchange, decreases respiratory work, and reduces circulatory stress.[49] Positive-pressure ventilation also carries the risk of barotrauma. The incidence of these complications is much less than that associated with PPV via endotracheal intubation, however, owing to the more modest pressures usually associated with NIVS. Rapid large changes in Pa_{CO_2} resulting from PPV can also cause acid-base disturbances. End-tidal P_{CO_2} or arterial blood gases should therefore be monitored during PPV.[35]

In summary, with the relatively recent development of noninvasive means of applying positive pressure to the respiratory system, these modalities have become the preferred method of NIVS. In addition to added convenience and greater degree of tolerability for most patients, there is also evidence that PPV may have greater efficacy when compared with portable negative-pressure devices.[50] The poncho-wrap ventilator (negative pressure) was compared with volume cycled positive-pressure ventilation via a nasal mask, in normal subjects and patients with COPD.[50] PPV was shown to be more effective in reducing diaphragmatic activity and Pa_{CO_2} values. Other studies have confirmed significant reductions in inspiratory muscle activation with use of nasal PPV in patients with chronic respiratory failure of diverse etiologies.[51,52] Despite these results however, PPV should not necessarily supplant the use of NPV, however, since these latter devices may provide sufficient ventilatory support in many patients with less discomfort or fewer side effects. Moreover, it is not yet clear that substantial respiratory muscle rest is necessary to reverse the clinical sequelae of chronic respiratory failure.

Miscellaneous Devices

ROCKING BED

The rocking bed, also developed in response to the poliomyelitis epidemic, has been in use for several decades. It consists of a hospital bed affixed to a mechanical frame capable of moving (or rocking) the bed through an arc from the head-down to the head-up position in continuous motion. The device relies on gravity to alter the position of the abdominal viscera, which in turn assists diaphragm movement. When the head is rocked downward, the abdominal contents push the diaphragm cephalad, resulting in positive intrathoracic pressure and exhalation; when the head rocks upward, abdominal contents fall, displacing the diaphragm downward, resulting in the generation of negative intrathoracic pressure, leading to inspiration.[2–4,53–55] Although tidal volumes of as much as 1.5 L can be achieved with this device, the head-down position contributes little to ventilation, whereas the greatest diaphragm movement, and hence inspiratory effect, occurs when rocking cycles from near horizontal to the 40-degree foot-down position.[54] At rates greater than about 20 cycles per minute, tidal volume falls, suggesting that the optimum rocking rate is 15 to 16 cycles per minute.[2]

Patients who have only diaphragm weakness or paralysis are particularly well suited for use of the rocking bed. However, those with severe kyphoscoliosis, poor abdominal wall or diaphragm compliance or short abdominal length are poor candidates, since use of this device in these patients is likely to be ineffective in achieving adequate ventilation.[2,56,57] Patients should be in stable condition, have some spontaneous respirations, and be capable of synchronizing their breathing with rocking.

An obvious advantage of this device compared with the cuirass and body suit is that it does not involve equipment attached to the chest wall, which some patients find too confining. Since the rocking bed does not require use of any masks or other attachments to the face, this device also has significant advantages when compared with positive-pressure devices, in some patients. Complications resulting from the use of the rocking bed are few. Motion sickness is rare, possibly due to the fact that the bed rocks only in one plane. As with negative-pressure ventilators, patients may develop upper airway obstruction during inspiration.

PNEUMOBELT

The pneumobelt (or intermittent abdominal pressure respirator) is a device which, like the rocking bed, utilizes gravity to alter intrathoracic pressure to effect ventilation. A corset-like abdominal binder containing an inflatable rubber bladder, is intermittently inflated and deflated in synchrony with the patient's spontaneous breathing.[58] Pressurization of the rubber bladder leads to compression of the abdominal contents, passive elevation of the diaphragm, positive intrathoracic pressure, and consequent exhalation of air. Depressurization results in a fall of the abdominal contents and of the diaphragm, generation of negative intrathoracic pressure and, hence, inhalation. Pressurization of the pneumobelt is accomplished using a positive-pressure ventilator. Optimal ventilation is achieved using pressures of 15 to 60 cmH$_2$O, at a cycle rate of 12 to 14 breaths per minute.[58] Since the mechanism of action of this device requires that the patient be in a vertical or near-vertical position (less than 60 degrees from vertical) for optimal function, its use is primarily restricted to the daytime, when patients are in an upright and seated position. This device therefore is often coupled with nocturnal use of alternative methods of NIVS. It is not surprising that the pneumobelt functions poorly in patients at the extremes of weight (either very thin, or obese) or who have significant kyphoscoliosis. Use of the pneumobelt is contraindicated in patients with acute respiratory failure, excessive secretions, or upper airway abnormalities.[2] Like the rocking bed, this device is well tolerated and associated

TABLE 32-2 Patient Groups Which May Benefit from the Application of Noninvasive Mechanical Ventilation

Neuromuscular diseases
    Muscular dystrophy
    Acid-maltase disease
    Multiple sclerosis
    Postpolio syndrome
    Amyotrophic lateral sclerosis
    Spinal cord injury
    Guillain-Barré syndrome
Chest wall diseases
    Kyphoscoliosis
    Ankylosing spondylitis
    Postthoracoplasty
Disorders affecting central control mechanisms
    Primary hypoventilation syndrome
    Sleep apnea syndrome with predominant central component
Parenchymal lung disease
    Chronic obstructive lung disease (COPD)
    Cystic fibrosis
Obstructive sleep apnea

with few complications, but also carries the risk of upper airway obstruction.

Efficacy of NIVS

With the onset of chronic respiratory failure, patients usually develop the insidious occurrence of a variety of symptoms including headaches (often worse in the morning), impaired cognition, daytime somnolence, fatigue, and overall reduction in life quality.[59,60] The common association of hypoxemia also results in deterioration in cognitive abilities. Moreover, hypoxemia causes reductions in the overall level of physical function and the development of cor pulmonale and cardiac arrhythmias. Further complicating matters, both hypoxemia and hypercapnia[61–63,61a] are known to have deleterious effects on respiratory muscle function, contributing to a vicious cycle of deterioration in respiratory muscle function followed by even further arterial blood-gas abnormalities. Consequently, the development of hypercapnic respiratory failure in these conditions is usually a harbinger of a rapid clinical deterioration leading to early death. The goal of NIVS is to prevent the development of, or ameliorate, these symptoms, improve life quality, and prolong life.

Previous studies have shown that patients in several disease categories, each with the propensity to develop chronic respiratory failure, may benefit from the application of NIVS (Table 32-2). These include patients with (1) neuromuscular disease who suffer primarily from severe reductions in respiratory muscle strength,[36,44,56,58–60,64–79] (2) chest wall disorders such as kyphoscoliosis,[37,39,40,59,63,80–84] (3) disorders primarily affecting central control mechanisms such as primary hypoventilation syndromes and certain forms of sleep-disordered breathing,[41,85–88] (4) parenchymal lung diseases such as COPD in which a high mechanical workload is coupled with reductions in muscle strength,[39,51,89–97] and (5) obstructive sleep apnea characterized primarily by upper airway obstruction. The use of NIVS in the management of sleep apnea is beyond the scope of this chapter, but several excellent reviews on this subject have been published recently.[32]

It should be noted that NIVS is generally provided at night during sleep because the application of ventilatory support (to a greater or lesser extent depending upon the specific device) is quite restrictive and requires prolonged periods of application (usually 4 to 8 h). In addition, the degree of hypoventilation and hypoxemia often worsens at night in many of these disorders. Consequently, the application of NIVS is best suited for nocturnal application allowing patients the freedom to pursue their usual daytime activities. The effectiveness of NIVS in the above-mentioned patient groups is reviewed below.

Neuromuscular and Chest Wall Disease

The largest clinical experience concerning the use of NIVS is in patients with various forms of neuromuscular and chest wall diseases and secondary respiratory failure. The efficacy of this modality in these patient groups was established by studies performed more than a decade ago. Garay and colleagues,[59] for example, evaluated the use of nocturnal NIVS, predominantly negative-pressure ventilation, in a diverse group of patients with neuromuscular disease including muscular dystrophy, kyphoscoliosis, and postpolio syndrome. These patients presented with carbon dioxide narcosis, and somnolence or coma. The application of NIVS resulted in a reduction in arterial carbon dioxide levels, increases in arterial oxygenation, reduction in the number of required hospitalizations, and significant reductions in the degree of pulmonary hypertension. NIVS did not significantly affect lung function. Since ventilation was provided only at night, these patients were able to resume their usual daytime activities. Moreover, the clinical benefit of this therapy was sustained for many years following the initiation of therapy. Goldstein and coworkers[71] also found that negative-pressure ventilation improved daytime arterial blood-gas tensions in patients with neuromuscular disease. In addition, they demonstrated that this modality prevents sleep-induced hypoventilation. In this study, the complication of upper airway obstruction was managed successfully with either a tricyclic medication or the addition of nasal CPAP. A number of subsequent studies utilizing positive pressure ventilation have assessed the effects of NIVS on respiratory muscle function and exercise tolerance in patients with neuromuscular and chest wall disease. Using a volume-cycled pressure-limited ventilator applied with a nasal mask, Goldstein's group[44] demonstrated improvements in both inspiratory muscle endurance and 6-min walking test after 3 months of therapy. Moreover, these improvements were sustained 14 months following initiation of therapy. Respiratory muscle strength, however, was not significantly affected. More recently, nasal BiPAP has also been shown to reverse nocturnal hypoventilation and symptoms associated with chronic respiratory failure in patients with various forms of restrictive disorders.[40,80,98] Further establishing the efficacy of NIVS, withdrawal of this modality resulted in worsening gas exchange during sleep and morning headaches,[79,79a] increased dyspnea at rest, daytime somnolence, and less energy— symptoms associated with chronic respiratory failure.[80]

The uniformly favorable results of studies evaluating the effectiveness of NIVS using both negative- and positive-pressure ventilation has made the performance of a randomized

TABLE 32-3 Neuromuscular and Chest Wall Diseases in Which NIVS May Be Efficacious

Neuromuscular disease
  Muscular dystrophy
  Spinal muscular atrophy
  Nemaline myopathy
  Minimal change myopathy
  Mitochondrial myopathy
  Postpolio syndrome
  Amyotrophic lateral sclerosis
Chest wall disease
  Kyphoscoliosis
  Thoracoplasty
  Rigid spine syndrome

controlled trial of this modality unethical.[99] A close approximation of such a study, however, was performed by Vianello and associates[75] by comparing the outcomes of five patients with Duchenne muscular dystrophy treated with nasal positive pressure ventilation with five similar patients who had refused ventilatory support. After 6 months of follow-up, mean loss of forced vital capacity (FVC) and maximum voluntary ventilation (MVV) was higher in the nonventilated patients. After 2 years of follow-up, all patients treated with nasal PPV were alive, whereas four of the five untreated patients had died. The striking results of this study confirmed previous clinical impressions that NIVS significantly prolongs survival in patients with neuromuscular and chest wall disease. Noninvasive ventilatory support, therefore, should be attempted in virtually all patients with hypercapnic respiratory failure secondary to neuromuscular and / or chest wall disease. Specific disease states in which NIVS has been shown to be of benefit are listed in Table 32-3.

It is important to note that although NIVS may attenuate the decline in pulmonary function in patients with neuromuscular disease, there is no evidence to suggest that this mode of therapy will prevent it.[60,76] This fact is well illustrated by the studies of Mohr and colleagues,[76] who followed patients with Duchenne muscular dystrophy for an average of 39 months. These patients experienced a gradual but progressive loss of pulmonary function over a 3-year period of follow-up. To compensate, patients gradually increased the duration of ventilatory support. Ultimately, patients had to resort to more effective forms of ventilatory assist devices including the iron lung and positive pressure via tracheostomy.

Previous uncontrolled investigations had suggested that early NIVS could limit the progression of restriction and possibly improve survival.[47,100] In a randomized controlled trial, NIVS was prophylactically applied to patients with muscular dystrophy who had not yet developed respiratory failure.[74] Surprisingly, and for unclear reasons, the application of NIVS in these patients resulted in a greater mortality compared with the control group. Consequently, the prophylactic administration of NIVS should be avoided in patients with neuromuscular disease.

Primary Hypoventilation Syndrome

Due to the rarity of these disorders, there is much less clinical data regarding the effects of NIVS in patients with primary

hypoventilation syndrome. In cases where NIVS has been applied, utilizing either negative-pressure ventilation (NPV) or nasal PPV, marked clinical improvement was noted. In one of the first applications of nasal PPV, nocturnal use of this modality resulted in increased mental alertness and improved exercise tolerance and arterial blood-gas values.[41] This patient had marked CO_2 retention which worsened during sleep. Application of NIVS resulted in marked improvement in arterial blood-gas values within a few days. Further decrements in Pa_{CO_2} values were noted after 2 weeks of therapy. The pattern of response is shown in Fig. 32-1. A 6-year-old patient with this disorder was also treated successfully with nasal PPV and 5 cmH_2O PEEP.[86] Of interest, treatment with NIVS also resulted in improvements in CO_2 responsiveness, suggesting a resetting of the central chemoreceptors.

CHRONIC OBSTRUCTIVE PULMONARY DISEASE

In contrast to patients with neuromuscular disease, the therapeutic benefit of NIVS in patients with obstructive lung disease is controversial.[43] Employing both negative- and positive-pressure systems, several studies have demonstrated

FIGURE 32-1 Adapted from Robert et al: *Eur Respir J* 6:599–606, 1993. Pattern of changes in oxygen saturation (upper panel) and arterial P_{CO_2} (lower panel) before and after institution of nasal positive pressure breathing in a patient with primary hypoventilation syndrome. (Adapted from DiMarco et al: Management of chronic alveolar hypoventilation with nasal positive pressure breathing. *Chest* 92:952–954, 1987.)

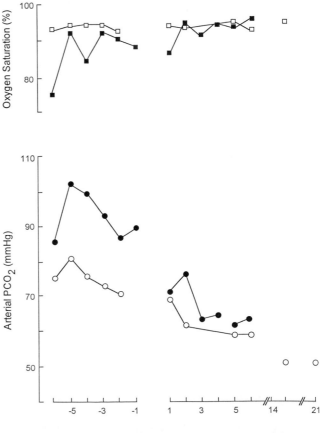

TABLE 32-4 Noninvasive Ventilation in Severe COPD and Chronic Respiratory Failure

Investigator	Year	Sample Size	Method	Control Group	Study Duration	Compliance	Decrease in Pa_{CO_2} (>5 mmHg)	Subjective Improvement	Improved RMS[g]	Improved RMF[h]	Improvement in Exercise Tolerance
						Positive Results					
Braun and Marino	1984	18	NPV[a]14, PPV[b]4	No	5 mo	Unknown	Yes	Yes	Yes	NM[f]	NM
Cropp and DiMarco	1987	15	NPV	Yes	3 days	Yes (s)[e]	Yes	Yes	Yes	Yes	NM
Gutierrez et al.	1988	5	NPV	No	4 mo	Yes (s)	Yes	Yes	Yes	NM	Yes
Caroll and Branthwaite	1988	4	NPPV[c]	No	3–9 mo	Yes	Yes	Yes	NM	NM	Yes
Scano et al.	1990	11	NPV	Yes	7 days	Yes	Yes	Yes	Yes	NM	NM
Fernandez et al.	1991	13	NPV	No	2 days	Yes (s)	Yes	Yes	Yes	NM	NM
Elliot et al.	1991	8	NPPV	No	6 mo	Yes	Yes	NM	No	NM	NM
Elliot et al.	1992	12	NPPV	No	12 mo	Yes	Yes	Yes	NM	NM	NM
Renston et al.	1994	17	NPPV	Yes	5 days	Yes (s)	No	Yes	No	NM	Yes
Meecham Jones et al.	1995	14	NPPV	Yes	3 mo	Yes	Yes	Yes	NM	NM	No
						Negative Results					
Zibrak et al.	1988	20	NPV	Yes	4–6 mo	Poor	No	Yes	No	No	No
Shapiro et al.	1992	184[d]	NPV	Yes	3 mo	Poor	No	No	No	NM	No
Gay et al.	1996	13	NPPV	Yes	3 mo	Poor	No	No	NM	NM	No

[a] NPV = negative pressure ventilation.
[b] PPV = positive pressure ventilation.
[c] NPPV = nasal positive pressure ventilation.
[d] 56 patients in this study were hypercapneic.
[e] (s) = supervised.
[f] NM = not measured.
[g] RMS = respiratory muscle strength.
[h] RME = respiratory muscle endurance.

significant improvements in ventilatory function, respiratory muscle strength and endurance, exercise tolerance, and sense of dyspnea following the application of NIVS in patients with severe COPD.[39,51,59,78,90–96] In contrast, other studies have failed to demonstrate any improvement in either subjective or objective parameters of respiratory system function in these patients.[101–106] One explanation for the varying results between studies may relate to the fact that NIVS may only be effective in certain subsets of patients with COPD. Close analysis of these studies provides some insight into factors which may distinguish the responders from nonresponders.

Celli and associates[102] found that the application of NPV to nine patients with predominantly eucapnic COPD (mean Pa_{CO_2} = 45 mmHg) did not result in increased benefit over that achieved by a pulmonary rehabilitation program. It is interesting that one patient in this group with the highest Pa_{CO_2} value did experience significant improvement with NIVS. Following 3 weeks of NPV, exercise tolerance improved markedly in association with a fall in Pa_{CO_2} from 56 to 46 mmHg. Previous studies that have demonstrated subjective and/or objective improvements in patients with COPD have almost uniformly been performed in hypercapnic patients. Moreover, other studies evaluating the effectiveness of NIVS in eucapnic COPD patients have generally found negative results.[105,107] The reasons NIVS may benefit only patients with hypercapnia are not clear. It is possible that the presence of hypercapnia reflects greater severity of illness. Also, these patients may suffer from greater degrees of respiratory muscle impairment since hypercapnia alone is known to adversely affect respiratory muscle function.[61]

Numerous studies have evaluated the use of NIVS in hypercapnic COPD patients. A brief description of these studies and outcome parameters are provided in Table 32-4. Those studies in which NIVS had some beneficial impact are listed in the upper panel, whereas those which found no benefit are listed below. Although the number of studies reflecting beneficial effects outnumber those that did not, this may merely be a reflection of reporting bias.

Marino and Braun[90] first reported that NIVS resulted in significant improvements in respiratory muscle strength, reductions in Pa_{CO_2} values (from 54 to 43 mmHg), and reduction in number of hospitalizations per year. This was an uncontrolled study, however, and since it was published only in abstract form, many of the specific details remain unknown. In a short-term prospective controlled trial, Cropp and DiMarco[89] reported improved respiratory muscle strength, endurance, and reduced hypercapnia when negative pressure was applied using a tank or cuirass ventilator for 3 to 6 h/day for three consecutive days. Other investigators utilizing NPV in short-term studies also demonstrated significant subjective improvement associated with increases in respiratory muscle strength and reductions in the level of hypercapnia.

Renston's group[51] performed a short-term controlled trial using a BiPAP ventilator for only 2 h/day for five consecutive days. Patients using BiPAP experienced symptomatic improvement as determined by a reduction in their Borg dyspnea score during spontaneous breathing and significant improvement in the distance they could walk in 6 min following BiPAP use.

Long-term studies lasting 3 to 12 months have also demonstrated beneficial effects of NIVS. In an uncontrolled study, Gutierrez and associates[91] showed that only weekly use of a cuirass ventilator was adequate to achieve improvements in respiratory muscle function, exercise tolerance, quality of life, and level of hypercapnia. Using nasal PPV, Caroll and Branthwaite[84] evaluated 10 patients with nocturnal hypoventilation, four of whom had COPD. Patients were reassessed 3 to 9 months after initiation of therapy. All patients reported an improvement in exercise tolerance. The level of hypercapnia fell in each patient, and the degree of nocturnal oxygen desaturation was reduced. Also using nasal PPV, Elliot and colleagues[97] found similar significant reductions in Pa_{CO_2} and an improved breathing pattern, but no change in respiratory muscle strength after 6 months of use. In a separate study, Elliot and coworkers[96] confirmed reductions in Pa_{CO_2} following use of nasal PPV for a 6-month period, with further reductions after 12 months of use. Most patients also realized symptomatic benefit which in some cases was marked. However, these studies were also uncontrolled.

Most recently, Meecham Jones and coworkers[108] performed a randomized crossover study of the effects of the combination of nasal BiPAP and home oxygen therapy, compared with home oxygen therapy alone in hypercapnic COPD patients over 3-month periods. Nasal BiPAP resulted in significant improvements in daytime Pa_{O_2} and Pa_{CO_2} values, sleep time, sleep efficacy, and quality of life.

In contrast to the previously described studies, other investigators have failed to demonstrate any improvement following use of NIVS in patients with COPD. Notable is the work of Shapiro's group,[105] who studied 184 patients, 56 of whom were hypercapnic. Negative-pressure ventilation was applied for 12 weeks after a 5-day inpatient trial period. Patients were instructed to use NPV for 5 h/day. Approximately one-third of the patients either stopped using the ventilator before the end of the trial or didn't use it at all. Moreover, mean time of ventilator use per patient was approximately 50 percent of that expected based on prior patient instruction. Despite this, all the study patients were included in the analysis, which failed to demonstrate any improvement in outcome parameters including exercise tolerance, respiratory muscle strength, arterial blood-gas tensions, dyspnea, and quality of life. As these investigators admit, NPV may not have been successful since patient compliance was poor. This study and others[101] demonstrate the difficulties in applying chronic NPV in patients with COPD. This modality is not well accepted, most likely owing to its inconvenience and discomfort. Nasal PPV ventilation is also poorly tolerated in some patients with severe COPD.[106] It is not suprising that these studies also failed to demonstrate any improvement in gas exchange, respiratory muscle strength, or exercise tolerance, because of high patient dropout rates and/or limited time of application. In summary, a major factor affecting the outcome of NIVS trials in patients with severe COPD is patient acceptance, motivation, and ability to tolerate the applied devices. Compared with neuromusclar and restrictive disorders, it appears that patients with COPD have greater difficulty tolerating NIVS. These devices often fit poorly, can be quite uncomfortable and are cumbersome to use. Nonetheless, there is increasing evidence that highly motivated patients capable of adapting to chronic use of NIVS, can derive significant clinical benefits.

It should be noted that NIVS does not significantly affect pulmonary function in COPD, since no study has found significant changes in spirometry or lung volumes. Elliot and colleagues,[97] however, found a correlation between the reduction in Pa_{CO_2} and both decreased gas trapping and reduction in residual volume. They speculated that the observed reduction in Pa_{CO_2} was secondary to reductions in small airway obstruction, that is, decreased load. However, they found no significant changes in the degree of gas trapping or residual volume for the group, nor did the study design include controls. Nevertheless, this is an interesting observation that warrants further study.

For NIVS to be successfully applied in patients with COPD, it is apparent that a period of patient education and acclimatization is particularly important. Frequent supervision and adjustments with the type of interface or mode of pressure application may be necessary. Although some patients may be unable to tolerate these devices or are not motivated to use them, NIVS appears to provide a striking benefit in selected patients with COPD and chronic hypercapnia.

CYSTIC FIBROSIS

Nasal PPV has also been applied in patients with end-stage cystic fibrosis and secondary chronic respiratory failure. In a study of four patients with hypercapnia and severe disease,[104,104a] nocturnal nasal PPV resulted in improved length and quality of sleep, reduction in the degree of hypercapnia and increases in both inspiratory and expiratory muscle strength. These patients also experienced a lessening of their level of dyspnea and improvement in their level of daily activities. Moreover, the observed improvements were maintained for up to 18 months.

MECHANISM OF ACTION

For the most part, each of the disorders in which NIVS has been shown to be of clinical benefit is characterized by marked reductions in respiratory muscle function.[60,109,110] Indeed, in many of these diseases, such as the muscular dystrophies, this represents the primary pathophysiology, since lung and chest wall mechanics are normal. A leading hypothesis to explain the beneficial effects of NIVS in these disorders, therefore, relates to the fact that NIVS unloads (i.e., rests) the respiratory muscles.[79,89,92,109] Although never completely proved, it has been suggested that the markedly weakened respiratory muscles develop a state of chronic fatigue leading to their reduced performance and chronic respiratory failure.[111] A period of rest, usually provided at night, is believed to improve their performance, leading to improvement in symptoms and in daytime blood-gas tensions. In support of this hypothesis is the fact that NIVS does reduce respiratory muscle work and leads to improvement in both respiratory muscle strength and endurance following NIVS.[44,52,89,91,92,112]

Another leading hypothesis is that chronic respiratory failure is associated with blunting of the centrol chemoreceptors, resulting in progressive alterations in blood-gas tensions.[79,80,113] This may occur as a protective mechanism to prevent weakened respiratory muscles from developing muscle fatigue and acute respiratory failure.[111,114] Reductions in central chemosensitivity would result in a reduced ventilatory requirement, thereby reducing the workload placed on the respiratory muscles. By reversing nocturnal hypoventilation, NIVS may reset the central chemoreceptors and thereby improve daytime gas tensions. In support of this theory are several studies which have shown clinical improvement, including reduction in the degree of hypercapnia and improved oxygenation but no changes in respiratory muscle function following use of NIVS.[84,97] The observation that tem-

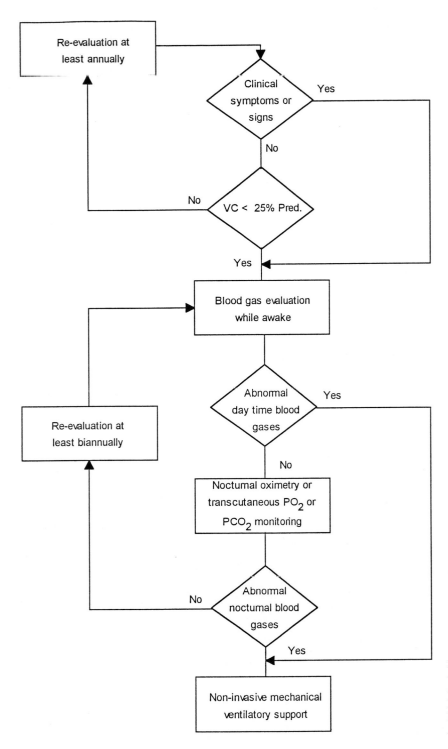

FIGURE 32-2 Management strategy of ventilatory support in patients with neuromuscular disease. (Adapted from Robert D, Willig TN, Leger P.: Long-term nasal ventilation in neuromuscular disorders: Report of a consensus conference. *Eur Respir J* 599–606, 1993.)

porary withdrawal of NIVS results in worsening of nocturnal gas exchange and symptomatology without changes in respiratory muscle strength or daytime gas exchange also favors this theory.[80]

As pointed out by previous authors,[79] these different theories are not mutually exclusive. It is quite likely that reversal of both respiratory muscle fatigue and depressed chemoreceptor sensitivity accounts for the clinical improvement observed following use of NIVS. The relative importance of these two factors may also vary significantly among various disease entities which result in chronic respiratory failure. For example, the observed improvement in daytime gas tensions following nocturnal use of NIVS in patients with primary hypoventilation syndrome,[41,86] who have normal respiratory muscle function, strongly suggests improved chemoreceptor sensitivity as the primary mechanism in this patient group. Further research directed at specific mechanisms by which NIVS exerts its beneficial effects in different patient groups is likely to lead to further refinements in this mode of therapy.

Recommendations

Unfortunately, there are no absolute criteria for the initiation of NIVS in patients with chronic respiratory failure. Useful general guidelines, however, have been proposed for the management of patients with neuromuscular and chest wall diseases[60,73] and obstructive lung disease.[115]

Clinical guidelines are best defined for patients with neuromuscular and chest wall disorders in whom the benefits of NIVS are universally accepted. Based on the results of a consensus conference on long-term nasal ventilation in neuromuscular disorders,[60] a simple algorithm was developed for patient evaluation and use of NIVS (Fig. 32-2). Although, developed for patients with Duchenne muscular dystrophy, these recommendations are applicable to most patients with other forms of progressive neuromuscular disease, as well. Some general guidelines concerning the point in the clinical course at which NIVS should be instituted include symptoms of fatigue, shortness of breath, daytime somnolence, or evidence of chronic respiratory failure by arterial blood gases (i.e., $Pa_{CO_2} > 45$ mmHg or $Pa_{O_2} < 60$ mmHg). Spirometric indexes are also useful in the evaluation of these patients. Previous work by Splaingard and coworkers[73] have shown that elective initiation of NIVS based on a vital capacity <25 percent predicted in addition to signs and/or symptoms of respiratory failure resulted in much shorter duration of hospitalization compared with those patients who were first treated much later in the course of their disease, when emergency lifesaving ventilatory support was required. With greater recognition of the natural history of these disorders, however, NIVS is now generally instituted on an outpatient basis prior to the onset of overt acute respiratory failure. In patients with normal daytime blood gases, with symptomatology suggestive of chronic respiratory failure, nocturnal sleep studies should be performed, since the first signs of blood-gas abnormalities usually occur during sleep.[60]

The indications for NIVS in patients with obstructive lung disease are much less clear, reflecting the controversial nature of this modality in this patient group. Despite the variability of results in clinical studies and lack of benefit found in a large randomized clinical trial,[105] it appears likely that certain subgroups of patients with obstructive disease may derive substantial benefit. Esau and associates[115] have suggested that NIVS be considered when one or more of the key variables listed in Table 32-5 fall below a certain threshold. Parameter values below these thresholds are generally considered harbingers for the subsequent development of acute respiratory

TABLE 32-5 Criteria for Use of Noninvasive Mechanical Ventilation in Patients with COPD

Variable	Value
Maximum inspiratory pressure	<40 cm H_2O
FEV_1	<30% predicted
MVV	<30% predicted
Tidal volume	<6 mL/kg
Pa_{CO_2}	>50 mmHg

failure. Based on the results of studies previously reviewed, it appears that hypercapnia and evidence of marked respiratory muscle weakness are important physiologic abnormalities that should be present prior to the institution of NIVS.

The presence of physiologic abnormalities alone, as described for these different patient groups, however, is not likely to identify those patients who will derive clinical benefit. It is also critically important that patients are highly motivated, are provided with an adequate acclimatization period (which may require an extensive trial-and-error period with various devices and levels of support), and have sufficient family and ancillary respiratory support services in the home. In all patients, subjective and objective parameters should be reassessed after institution of these devices to evaluate their clinical response.

References

1. Punzal PA, Ries AL, Kaplan RM, Prewitt LM: Maximum intensity exercise training in patients with chronic obstructive pulmonary disease. *Chest* 100:618–623, 1991.
2. Hill NS: Use of the rocking bed, pneumobelt, and other noninvasive aids to ventilation, in Tobin M, (ed): *Principles and Practice of Mechanical Ventilation.* New York, McGraw-Hill, 1994; pp 413–425.
3. Hill NS: Clinical applications of body ventilators. *Chest* 90:897–905, 1986.
4. Kacmarek R: Home mechanical ventilation equipment, in Branson R, Hess D, Chatburn R (eds): *Respiratory Care Equipment.* Philadelphia, Lippincott, 1995; pp 425–457.
5. DiMarco AF: Negative pressure ventilation, in Nochomovitz M, Montenegro H (eds): *Ventilatory Support in Respiratory Failure.* Mt. Kisco, NY, Futura, 1987; pp 27–49.
6. Emerson JH: *The Evaluation of Iron Lungs.* Cambridge, MA, J.H. Emerson, 1978.
7. Drinker P, Shaw LA: An apparatus for the prolonged administration of artificial respiration. *J Clin Invest* 7:229–247, 1929.
8. Drinker P, McKhann CF: The use of a new apparatus for artificial respiration. *JAMA* 92:1658–1660, 1929.
9. Drinker P: Prolonged administration of artificial respiration. *Lancet* 1:1186, 1931.
10. Wiers PW, LeCoultre R, Dallinga OT, et al: Cuirass respirator treatment of chronic respiratory failure in scoliotic patients. *Thorax* 32:221–228, 1977.
11. Newson Davis J, Goldman M, Loh L, Casson M: Diaphragm function and alveolar hypoventilation. *Quart J Med* 45:87–100, 1976.
12. Powner DJ, Hoffman LG: Bedside construction of a custom cuirass for respiratory failure in kyphoscoliosis *Chest* 74:469–471, 1978.
13. Plum F, Lukas DS: An Evaluation of the cuirass respirator in acute poliomyelitis with respiratory insufficiency. *Am J Med Sci* 221:417–424, 1951.
14. Levine S, Henson D: Negative pressure ventilation, in Tobin MJ (ed): *Principles and Practice of Mechanical Ventilation.* New York, McGraw-Hill, 1994; pp 393–411.
15. Rochester DF, Braun NMT, Laine S: Diaphragmatic energy expenditure in chronic respiratory failure. The effect of assisted ventilation with body respirators. *Am J Med* 63:223–232, 1977.
16. Rodenstein DO, Stanescu DC, Cuttita G, et al: Ventilatory and diaphragmatic EMG responses to negative-pressure ventilation in airflow obstruction. *J Appl Physiol* 65:1621–1626, 1988.
17. O'Leary J, King R, LeBlanc M, et al: Cuirass ventilation in childhood neuromuscular disease. *J Ped* 94:419–421, 1979.
18. Collier CR, Affeldt JJE: Ventilatory efficiency of the cuirass respi-

rator in totally paralyzed chronic poliomyelitis patients. *J Appl Physiol* 6:531–538, 1954.

19. Spalding JMK, Opie L: Artifical respiration with the Tunnicliffe Breathing-Jacket. *Lancet* 1:613–615, 1958.

20. Spitzer SA, Fink G, Mittelman M: External high-frequency ventilation in severe chronic obstructive pulmonary disease. *Chest* 104:1698–1701, 1993.

21. Hardinge FM, Davis RJ, Stradling JR: Effects of short term high frequency negative pressure ventilation on gas exchange using the Hayek oscillator in normal subjects. *Thorax* 50:44–49, 1995.

22. King M, Phillips DM, Gross D, et al: Enhanced tracheal mucus clearance with high frequency chest wall compression. *Am Rev Respir Dis* 128:511–515, 1983.

23. Sanna A, Veriter C, Stanescu D: Upper airway obstruction induced by negative-pressure ventilation in awake healthy subjects. *J Appl Physiol* 75:546–552, 1993.

24. Bach JR, Penek J: Obstructive sleep apnea complicating negative-pressure ventilatory support in patients with chronic paralytic/restrictive ventilatory dysfunction. *Chest* 99:1386–1393, 1991.

25. Scharf SM, Feldman NT, Goldman MD, et al: Vocal cord closure. A cause of upper airway obstruction during controlled ventilation. *Am Rev Respir Dis* 117:351–357, 1978.

26. Marino WD, Jain NK, Pitchumoni CS: Induction of lower esophageal sphincter (LES) dysfunction during use of the negative pressure body ventilator. *Am J Gastroenterol* 83:1376–1380, 1988.

27. Murray R, Criner G, Becker P, et al: Negative pressure ventilation impairs cardiac function in patients with severe COPD. *Am Rev Respir Dis* 139:A15, 1989.

28. Marks A, Bocles J, Morganti L: A new ventilatory assister for patients with respiratory acidosis. *New Engl J Med* 268:61–68, 1963.

29. Sullivan CE, Berthon-Jones M, Issa FG: Remission of severe obesity-hypoventilation syndrome after short-term treatment during sleep with nasal continous positive airway pressure. *Am Rev Respir Dis* 128:177–181, 1983.

30. Sullivan CE, Issa FG, Berthon-Jones M, Eves L: Reversal of obstructive sleep apnea by continuous positive airway pressure applied through the nares. *Lancet* 1:862–865, 1981.

30a. Piper A, Sullivan C: Effects of short-term IPPV in the treatment of patients with severe obstructive sleep apnea and hypercapnia. *Chest* 105:434–440, 1994.

31. Petrof BJ, Kimoff RJ, Levy RD, et al: Nasal continuous positive airway pressure facilitates respiratory muscle function during sleep in severe chronic obstructive pulmonary disease. *Am Rev Respir Dis* 143:928–935, 1991.

32. Hudgel DW: *Treatment of obstructive sleep apnea—A review. Chest* 109:1346–1358, 1996.

33. Sanders M, Black J, Stiller R, Donahoe M: Nocturnal ventilatory assistance with bilevel positive airway pressure. *Head Neck Surg* 2:56–62, 1991.

34. Elliott M, Moxham J: Noninvasive mechanical ventilation by nasal or face mask, in Tobin MJ (ed): *Principles and Practice of Mechanical ventilation.* New York, McGraw-Hill, 1994; pp 427–453.

35. Claman DM, Piper A, Sanders MH, et al: Nocturnal noninvasive positive pressure ventilatory assistance. *Chest* 110:1581–1588, 1996.

36. Gay PC, Patel AM, Viggiano RW, Hubmayr RD: Nocturnal nasal ventilation for treatment of patients with hypercapnic respiratory failure. *Mayo Clin Proc* 66:695–703, 1991.

37. Leger P, Jennequin J, Gerard M, et al: Home positive pressure ventilation via nasal mask for patients with neuromusculoskeletal disorders. *Eur Respir J* 2(suppl 7):640s–644s, 1989.

38. Lofaso F, Brochard L, Touchard D, et al: Evaluation of carbon dioxide rebreathing during pressure support ventilation with airway management system (BiPAP) devices. *Chest* 108:772–778, 1995.

39. Carroll N, Branthwaite MA: Control of nocturnal hypoventilation by nasal intermittent positive pressure ventilation. *Thorax* 43:349–353, 1988.

40. Ellis ER, Grunstein RR, Chan S, et al: Noninvasive ventilatory support during sleep improves respiratory failure in kyphoscoliosis. *Chest* 94:811–815, 1988.

41. DiMarco AF, Connors AF, Altose MD: Management of chronic alveolar hypoventilation with nasal positive pressure breathing. *Chest* 92:952–954, 1987.

42. Marino W: Intermittent volume cycled mechanical ventilation via nasal mask in patients with respiratory failure due to COPD. *Chest* 99:681–684, 1991.

43. Martin JG: Clinical intervention in respiratory failure. *Chest* 97(suppl):105s–109s, 1990.

44. Goldstein RS, DeRosie JA, Avendano MA, Dolmage TE: Influence of noninvasive positive pressure ventilation on inspiratory muscles. *Chest* 99:408–415, 1991.

45. Kerby GR, Mayer LS, Pingleton SK: Nocturnal positive pressure ventilation via nasal mask. *Am Rev Respir Dis* 135:738–740, 1987.

46. Bach JR, Alba A, Mosher R, Delaubier A: Intermittent positive pressure ventilation via nasal access in the management of respiratory insufficiency. *Chest* 92:168–170, 1987.

47. Delaubier A, Guillou C, Mordelet M, Rideau Y: Assistance ventilatoire precoce par voie nasale dans la dystrophie musculaire de Duchenne. *Aggressologie* 28:737–738, 1987.

47a. Rodenstein DO, Stanescu DC, Delguste P, et al: Adaptation to intermittent positive pressure ventilation applied through the nose during day and night. *Eur Respir J* 2:473–478, 1989.

48. Naughton MT, Liu PP, Benard DC, et al: Treatment of congestive heart failure and Cheyne-Stokes respiration during sleep by continuous positive airway pressure. *Am J Respir Crit Care Med* 151:92–97, 1995.

49. Rasanen J, Heikkila J, Downs J, et al: Continuous positive airway pressure by face mask in acute cardiogenic pulmonary edema. *Am J Cardiol* 55:296–300, 1985.

50. Belman MJ, SooHoo GW, Kuei JH, Shadmehr R: Efficacy of positive vs negative pressure ventilation in unloading the respiratory muscles. *Chest* 98:850–856, 1990.

51. Renston JP, DiMarco AF, Supinski GS: Respiratory muscle rest using nasal BiPAP ventilation in patients with stable severe COPD. *Chest* 105:1053–1060, 1994.

52. Carrey Z, Gottfried SB, Levy RD: Ventilatory muscle support in respiratory failure with nasal positive pressure ventilation. *Chest* 97:150–158, 1990.

53. Colville P, Shugg C, Ferris BG Jr: Effects of body tilting on respiratory mechanics. *J Appl Physiol* 9:19–24, 1956.

54. Plum F, Whedon GD: The rapid-rocking bed: Its effect on the ventilation of poliomyelitis patients with respiratory paralysis. *N Engl J Med* 245:235–241, 1951.

55. Joos TH, Dickinson DG, Tainer NS, Wilson JL: The rocking bed and head position. *N Engl J Med* 255:1089–1090, 1956.

56. Bach JR, Alba AS: Intermittent abdominal pressure ventilator in a regimen of noninvasive ventilatory support. *Chest* 99:630–636, 1991.

57. Goldstein RS, Molotiu N, Skrastins R, et al: Assisting ventilation in respiratory failure by negative pressure ventilation and by rocking bed. *Chest* 92:470–474, 1987.

58. Miller HJ, Thomas E, Wilmot CB: Pneumobelt use among high quadriplegic population. *Arch Phys Med Rehabil* 69:369–372, 1988.

59. Garay SM, Turino GM, Goldring RM: Sustained reversal of chronic hypercapnia in patients with alveolar hypoventilation syndromes. Long-term maintenance with noninvasive nocturnal mechanical ventilation. *Am J Med* 70:269–274, 1981.

60. Robert D, Willig TN, Leger P: Long-term nasal ventilation in neuromuscular disorders: Report of a consensus conference. *Eur Respir J* 6:599–606, 1993.

61. Juan G, Calverley P, Talamo C, et al: Effect of carbon dioxide

on diaphragmatic function in human beings. *N Engl J Med* 310:874–879, 1984.

61a. Supinski GS, Nethery D, Ciufo R, et al: Effect of varying inspired oxygen concentration on diaphragm glutathione metabolism during loaded breathing. *Am J Respir Crit Care Med* 152:1633–1640, 1995.

62. Arora NS, Rochester DF: Effect of hypoxia and resistive work on diaphragm muscle ATP and glycogen concentration in the dog (abstract). *Clin Res* 30:425, 1982.

63. Leger P, Robert D, Langevin B: Chest wall deformities due to idiopathic kyphoscoliosis or sequelae of tuberculosis. *Eur Respir Rev* 2:362–368, 1992.

64. Celli B, Rassulo J, Corral R: Ventilatory muscle dysfunction in patients with bilateral idiopathic diaphragmatic paralysis: Reversal by intermittent external negative pressure ventilation. *Am Rev Respir Dis* 136:1276–1278, 1987.

65. Bach JR, Alba AS, Bohatiuk G, et al: Mouth intermittent positive pressure ventilation in the management of postpolio respiratory insufficiency. *Chest* 91:859–864, 1987.

66. Heckmatt JZ, Loh L, Dubowitz V: Night-time nasal ventilation in neuromuscular disease. *Lancet* 335:579–582, 1990.

67. Bach JR, Alba AS: Management of chronic alveolar hypoventilation by nasal ventilation. *Chest* 97:52–57, 1990.

68. Bach JR, Alba AS, Saporito LR: Intermittent positive pressure ventilation via the mouth as an alternative to tracheostomy for 257 ventilator users. *Chest* 103:174–182, 1993.

69. Sherman MS, Paz HL: Review of respiratory care of the patient with amyotrophic lateral sclerosis. *Respiration* 61:61–67, 1994.

70. Ellis ER, Bye PT, Bruderer JW, Sullivan CE: Treatment of respiratory failure during sleep in patients with neuromuscular disease. Positive-pressure ventilation through a nose mask. *Am Rev Respir Dis* 135:148–152, 1987.

71. Goldstein RS, Molotiu N, Skrastins R, et al: Reversal of sleep-induced hypoventilation and chronic respiratory failure by nocturnal negative pressure ventilation in patients with restrictive ventilatory impairment. *Am Rev Respir Dis* 135:1049–1055, 1987.

72. Segall D: Noninvasive nasal mask-assisted ventilation is respiratory failure of Duchenne muscular dystrophy. *Chest* 93:1298–1300, 1988.

73. Splaingard ML, Frates RL Jr, Jefferson LS, et al: Home negative pressure ventilation: Report of 20 years of experience in patients with neuromuscular disease. *Arch Phys Med Rehabil* 66:239–242, 1985.

74. Raphael JC, Chevret S, Chastang L, Bauvet F: Randomised trial of preventive nasal ventilation in Duchenne muscular dystrophy. French Multicenter Cooperative Group on home mechanical ventilation assistance in Duchenne de Boulogne muscular dystrophy. *Lancet* 343:1600–1604, 1994.

75. Vianello A, Bevilacqua M, Salvador V, et al: Long-term nasal intermittent positive pressure ventilation in advanced Duchenne's muscular dystrophy. *Chest* 105:445–448, 1994.

76. Mohr CH, Hill NS: Long-term follow-up of nocturnal ventilatory assistance in patients with respiratory failure due to Duchenne-type muscular dystrophy. *Chest* 97:91–96, 1990.

77. Heckmatt JZ, Loh L, Dubowitz V: Night-time nasal ventilation in neuromuscular disease. *Lancet* 335:579–582, 1990.

78. Curran FJ: Night ventilation by body respirators for patients in chronic respiratory failure due to later stage Duchenne muscular dystrophy. *Arch Phys Med Rehabil* 62:270–274, 1981.

79. Hill NS: Noninvasive ventilation: does it work, for whom and how? *Am Rev Respir Dis* 147:1050–1055, 1993.

79a. Jimenez JFM, Escuin JS, Vicente CD, et al: Nasal intermittent positive pressure ventilation. Analysis of its withdrawal. *Chest* 107:382–388.

80. Hill NS, Eveloff SE, Carlisle CC, Goff SG: Efficacy of nocturnal nasal ventilation in patients with restrictive thoracic disease. *Am Rev Respir Dis* 145:365–371, 1992.

81. Hoeppner VH, Cockroft DW, Dosman JA, Cotton DJ: Nighttime

82. Kinnear W, Hockley S, Harvey J, Shneerson J: The effect of one year of nocturnal cuirass-assisted ventilation in chest wall disease. *Eur Resp J* 1:204–208, 1988.

83. Leger P, Bedicam JB, Cornette A, et al: Nasal intermittent positive pressure ventilation. Long term follow-up in patients with severe chronic respiratory insufficiency. *Chest* 105:100–105, 1994.

84. Carroll N, Branthwaite MA: Control of nocturnal hypoventilation by nasal intermittent positive pressure ventilation. *Thorax* 43:349–353, 1988.

85. Hill NS, Redline S, Carskadon MA, et al: Sleep-disordered breathing in patients with Duchenne muscular dystrophy using negative pressure ventilators. *Chest* 102:1656–1662, 1992.

86. Ellis ER, McCauley VB, Mellis C, Sullivan C: Treatment of alveolar hypoventilation in a six-year-old girl with intermittent positive pressure ventilation through a nose mask. *Am Rev Respir Dis* 136:188–191, 1987.

87. Barbé F, Quera-Salva MA, deLattre J, et al: Long term effects of nasal intermittent positive-pressure ventilation on pulmonary function and sleep architecture in patients with neuromuscular diseases. *Chest* 110:1179–1183, 1996.

88. Bach JR, Robert D, Leger P, Langevin B: Sleep fragmentation in kyphoscoliotic individuals with alveolar hypoventilation treated by NIPPV. *Chest* 107:1552–1558, 1995.

89. Cropp A, DiMarco AF: Effects of intermittent negative pressure ventilation on respiratory muscle function in patients with severe chronic obstructive pulmonary disease. *Am Rev Respir Dis* 135:1056–1061, 1987.

90. Marino W, Braun NMT: Reversal of the clinical sequelae of respiratory muscle fatigue by intermittent mechanical ventilation (abstract). *Am Rev Respir Dis* 125(pt2):85, 1982.

91. Gutierrez M, Beroiza T, Contreras G, et al: Weekly cuirass ventilation improves blood gases and inspiratory muscle strength in patients with chronic air-flow limitation and hypercarbia. *Am Rev Respir Dis* 138:617–623, 1988.

92. Scano G, Gigliotti F, Duranti R, et al: Changes in ventilatory muscle function with negative pressure ventilation in patients with severe COPD. *Chest* 97:322–327, 1990.

93. Ambrosino N, Nava S, Fracchia C, et al: Evaluation of bi-level positive pressure device to deliver nasal pressure support ventilation in COPD patients (abstract). *Am Rev Respir Dis* 143:A79, 1991.

94. Fernandez E, Weiner P, Meltzer E, et al: Sustained improvement in gas exchange after negative pressure ventilation for 8 hours per day on 2 successive days in chronic airflow limitation. *Am Rev Respir Dis* 144:390–394, 1991.

95. Meecham Jones DJ, Braid GM, Wedzicha JA: Nasal masks for domiciliary positive pressure ventilation: Patients usage and complications. *Thorax* 49:811–812, 1994.

96. Elliot MW, Simonds AK, Carroll MP, et al: Domiciliary nocturnal nasal intermettent positive pressure ventilation in hypercapnic respiratory failure due to chronic obstructive pulmonary disease: Effects on sleep and quality of life. *Thorax* 47:342–348, 1992.

97. Elliot MW, Mulvey DA, Moxham J, et al: Domiciliary nocturnal nasal intermettent positive pressure ventilation in COPD: Mechanisms underlying changes in arterial blood gas tensions. *Eur Respir J* 4:1044–1052, 1991.

98. Waldhorn RE: Noctural nasal intermittent positive pressure ventilation with bi-level positive airway pressure (BiPAP) in respiratory failure. *Chest* 101:516–521, 1992.

99. Hill NS. Noninvasive positive pressure ventilation in neuromuscular disease. Enough is enough. *Chest* 104:337, 1994.

100. Rideau Y, Delaubier A: Management of respiratory neuromuscular weakness. *Muscle Nerve* 11:407–408, 1988.

101. Zibrak JD, Hill NS, Federman EC, et al: Evaluation of intermittent long-term negative-pressure ventilation in patients with

severe chronic obstructive pulmonary disease. *Am Rev Respir Dis* 138:1515–1518, 1988.

102. Celli B, Lee H, Criner G, et al: Controlled trial of external negative pressure ventilation in patients with severe chronic airflow obstruction. *Am Rev Respir Dis* 140:1251–1256, 1989.

103. Zibrak JD, Hill NS, Federman EC, et al: Evaluation of intermittent long-term negative-pressure ventilation in patients with severe chronic obstructive pulmonary disease. *Am Rev Respir Dis* 138:1515–1518, 1988.

104. Gay PC, Hubmayr RD, Stroetz RW: Efficacy of nocturnal nasal ventilation in stable severe chronic obstructive pulmonary disease during a three months controlled trial. *Mayo Clin Proc* 71:533–542, 1996.

104a. Piper AJ, Parker S, Torzillo PJ, et al: Nocturnal nasal IPPV stabilizes patients with cystic fibrosis and hypercapnic respiratory failure. *Chest* 102:846 to 850, 1992.

105. Shapiro SH, Ernst P, Gray-Donald K, et al: Effect of negative pressure ventilation in severe chronic obstructive pulmonary disease. *Lancet* 340:1425–1429, 1992.

106. Strumpf DA, Millman RP, Carlisle CC, et al: Nocturnal positive-pressure ventilation via nasal mask in patients with severe chronic obstructive pulmonary disease. *Am Rev Respir Dis* 144:1234–1239, 1991.

107. Strumpf DA, Millman RP, Carlisle CC, et al: Nocturnal positive-pressure ventilation via nasal mask in patients with severe chronic obstructive pulmonary disease. *Am Rev Respir Dis* 144:1234–1239, 1991.

108. Meecham Jones DJ, Paul EA, Jones PW, Wedzicha JA: Nasal pressure support ventilation plus oxygen compared with oxygen therapy alone in hypercapnic COPD. *Am J Respir Crit Care Med* 152:538–544, 1995.

109. Levine S, Henson D, Levy S: Respiratory muscle rest therapy. *Clin Chest Med* 9:297–309, 1988.

110. Rochester DF: Respiratory muscle weakness, pattern of breathing, and CO_2 retention in chronic obstructive pulmonary disease. *Am Rev Respir Dis* 143:901–903, 1991.

111. Aldrich TK: Respiratory muscle fatigue. *Clin Chest Med* 9:225–236, 1988.

112. Nava S, Ambrosino N, Rubini F, et al: Effect of nasal pressure support ventilation and external PEEP on diaphragmatic activity in patients with severe stable COPD. *Chest* 103:143–150, 1993.

113. Roussos C: Function and fatigue of respiratory muscles. *Chest* 88:124s–132s, 1985.

114. Begin P, Grassino A: Inspiratory muscle dysfunction and chronic hypercapnia in chronic obstructive pulmonary disease. *Am Rev Respir Dis* 143:905–912, 1991.

115. Esau SA, Truwit JD, Rochester DF: Respiratory muscle rest, in Roussos T (ed): *The Thorax Part C: Disease.* New York, Marcel Dekker, 1995; pp 2261–2300.

Chapter 33

NUTRITIONAL SUPPORT IN THE PATIENT WITH CHRONIC OBSTRUCTIVE PULMONARY DISEASE

STEVEN G. KELSEN

FRANCIS C. CORDOVA

Background

Body wasting, that is, loss of lean body (i.e., fat-free) mass, is extremely common in patients with advanced chronic obstructive pulmonary disease (COPD). The mechanism of body wasting in subjects with COPD is not well understood although it appears that a sizable percentage of subjects are hypermetabolic, that is, their daily energy requirements are greater than normal. In most subjects with COPD nutritional intake appears to be normal. Strictly speaking, therefore, it seems to be more accurate to describe the wasting process which occurs in patients with COPD as a state of bodily depletion causing a relatively inadequate nutritional intake.

It has been suggested that the loss of fat mass and lean body mass may be an adaptive response serving to reduce body oxygen consumption and carbon dioxide production and hence the demand for ventilation. However, the fact that weight-losing subjects with COPD are hypermetabolic and that depleted subjects have a poorer survival rate suggests that the response is maladaptive and contributes to the morbidity and mortality of the disease. In fact, the loss of body cell mass impairs respiratory muscle strength and endurance and immune function and may even accelerate the rate of progression of emphysema. Furthermore, nutritional intervention may reverse these abnormalities.

DEFINITION

Bodily depletion may manifest itself in a number of ways as changes in (1) body dimension (e.g., body weight, fat-free mass, body cell mass, midarm muscle circumference); (2) serum protein levels (e.g., reductions in albumin, prealbumin, transferrin); (3) body electrolyte composition; and (4) impaired immune system function. Although no single parameter adequately defines body cell mass in all clinical situations, perhaps the most widely accepted and clinically useful parameter is body weight. It is generally agreed that body weight less than 90 percent of ideal represents significant depletion of lean body mass. However, it is important to note that the precise body weight at which clinically important depletion supervenes is not well understood. Measurements of body weight alone may underestimate the true incidence of body depletion in patients with COPD. Of interest, simultaneous measurement of body weight, fat mass, and fat-free mass (FFM) indicates that changes in respiratory muscle function correlate best with FFM. Moreover, depletion of FFM may occur in patients with normal weight, and conversely FFM may be preserved in underweight subjects with COPD.[1] These several observations suggest that FFM is a more discrimating parameter than body weight and likely to provide more clinically and physiologically meaningful information. Assessment of FFM can be made relatively easily from measurement of bioelectrical impedance (see below).

PREVALENCE

When body weight of < 90 percent of ideal is used to define an underweight state, approximately 20 to 50 percent of subjects with COPD are subnormal.[2-8] The incidence of significant weight loss in COPD varies considerably across studies and depends at least in part on the severity of airway obstruction and hypoxemia. The greater the severity of airway dysfunction and hypoxemia, the greater the incidence of weight loss. In the National Institutes of Health (NIH) Intermittant Positive Pressure Breathing Trial of 779 men, 24 percent had body weight of < 90 percent.[7] However, 55 percent of subjects in the group with the most severe airflow obstruction (FEV_1 < 35 percent predicted) had body weight of < 90 percent, compared with only 16 percent of subjects with FEV_1 > 47 percent. A separate study of 255 Dutch patients with stable COPD admitted to an inpatient rehabilitation unit, yielded similar results.[1,9] Hypoxemia may be a more important factor than airflow obstruction since, in the Dutch study, body weight was < 90 percent ideal in 94 percent of subjects in whom the Pa_{O_2} was < 55 mmHg but in only 29 percent of subjects when the FEV_1 was < 50 percent predicted. Emphysematous patients appear more likely to be nutritionally depleted than patients with chronic bronchitis for unclear reasons.[6]

Adverse Effects of Undernutrition in COPD

The importance of undernutrition in patients with COPD lies with its effects on the morbidity and mortality of the disease. For example, respiratory muscle function and the ability to wean from mechanical ventilation are impaired, and the risk of respiratory failure and the 5-year mortality rate are increased in depleted patients.

MORTALITY

Beginning in the 1950s and 1960s, it was recognized that mortality was increased in patients with COPD whose body weight was less than 85 to 90 percent of ideal.[7,10-13] Vanderburg and colleagues[12] reported that patients with COPD who had lost 20 percent or more of their body weight in 5 years had a significantly higher mortality than those who had not. Because the depleted state correlates closely with the severity of airway function, it was not clear whether the depleted state is an independent factor or merely a surrogate marker for airway disease. The NIH sponsored Intermittant Positive-Pressure Breathing (IPPB) trial, however, suggests that body weight is, in fact, an independent predictor of mortality in COPD.[7] This multicenter study examined body weight and lung function annually for 3 years in 779 males with COPD

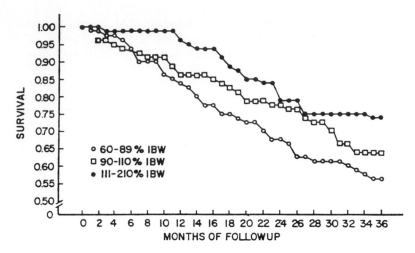

FIGURE 33-1 Survival of patients with COPD and FEV$_1$ = 35 percent of predicted versus months of follow-up. Data obtained in the National Institutes of Health Intermittant Positive Pressure Breathing Trial. Patients stratified by percent ideal body weight (%IBW). Note the lower survival in patients with lower body weight. (Data from Wilson et al.,[7] with permission.)

in whom FEV$_1$ was < 60 percent predicted total lung capacity (TLC) was > 80 percent predicted, and Pa$_{O_2}$ was > 55 mmHg.

Patients were classified on the basis of ideal body weight (IBW) (i.e., low < 90, normal > 90 and < 110, and high > 110 percent) and postbronchodilator FEV$_1$ (i.e., < 35, 35 to 46, and > 47 percent). Across the entire group, ideal body weight significantly correlated with FEV$_1$ (p < .0001 and r = 0.26), TLC, and DL$_{CO}$, indicating the importance of the severity of lung dysfunction on bodily weight. After adjusting for FEV$_1$, however, it was apparent that, subjects with low IBW had higher mortality rates than the normal and elevated ideal body weight (IBW) groups. For example, in subjects with FEV$_1$ < 35 percent, the survival rate over 3 years was 55 percent with IBW < 90 percent compared with a survival rate of 65 percent in the 90 to 110 percent IBW group and 75 percent in the > 110 percent IBW group (Fig. 33-1). It is interesting that the effect of body weight was most obvious in the subjects with the mildest airway obstruction (i.e., FEV$_1$ > 47 percent). In this group, the survival rate was 65 percent with < 90 percent IBW compared with a greater than 85 percent survival rate in the normal and greater than normal body weight groups (Fig. 33-2).

The NIH IPPB trial, the largest epidemiologic study performed to date, indicates that underweight patients with

COPD have more severe airway obstruction and emphysema (as reflected in a low DL$_{CO}$) than normal weight subjects. However, the mortality of underweight patients was greater when cohorts with equivalent FEV$_1$ were compared. Moreover, the greater effect of body weight on mortality in the cohort with the mildest airway obstruction strongly argues that body weight is, in fact, an independent variable affecting prognosis in COPD. The cause of death was not detailed in this study. Consequently, the mechanism(s) by which body depletion influences survival remains poorly understood.

RESPIRATORY MUSCLE STRUCTURE AND FUNCTION

The skeletal musculature of the body represents its primary reserve of proteins and calories. In chronic inflammatory and catabolic diseases, muscle tissue is mobilized for amino acids and calories.[14,15] For many years, it was believed that the striated muscles of the heart and respiratory system were spared the wasting effects of starvation and disease. However, it is now apparent that the respiratory skeletal muscles are not spared the effects of cachexia and wasting.[16,17]

Respiratory skeletal muscles, like skeletal muscles in other parts of the body are a mix of slow twitch (type I) and fast

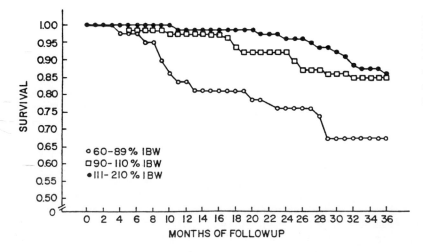

FIGURE 33-2 Survival of patients with COPD and FEV$_1$ > 47 percent of predicted versus months of follow-up. See legend for Fig. 33-1. Note that survival is much lower in subjects with lowest body weight, even in this group of patients with relatively mild airway obstruction (FEV$_1$ > 47 percent). (Data from Wilson et al.,[7] with permission.)

twitch (types IIA and IIB) fibers.[18,19] The mix of fiber types varies across the respiratory musculature. The metabolic and contractile properties of these three fiber populations varies. Type I fibers are highly oxidative and fatigue resistant but generate and dissipate force slowly. Types IIA and IIB fibers have both oxidative and glycolytic metabolism, are larger and generate greater force than type I fibers, but are more susceptible to fatigue. Moreover, the fiber types demonstrate a distinct pattern of motor unit recruitment in accordance with the size principle of Henneman.[20] In the diaphragm, motor units comprising type I fibers are active during eupneic breathing when the intensity of muscle contractions are low.[21] Types IIA and B fibers are recruited only with more strenuous efforts. Type IIA fibers are recruited next, followed by type IIB fibers when near maximal efforts are made.

ANIMAL STUDIES

Two to three days of starvation decreases the rate of protein synthesis in the isolated rat diaphragm and increases the rate of protein degradation.[19,22,23] Diaphragms from fasted rats oxidize branch-chain amino acids such as leucine, isoleucine, and valine at three times the control value and, at the same time, synthesize alanine and glutamine at increased rates. This process appears to be protective in nature in that oxidation of branched-chain amino acids provides energy for diaphragm muscle, spares glucose oxidation, and stimulates the synthesis of alanine and glutamine. Alanine and glutamine, in turn, are released into the circulation and become available for gluconeogenesis in the liver. In the isolated diaphragm from fasted animals, protein synthesis and degradation rates return to control values when the muscles are incubated with amino acids. Branched-chain amino acids produce greater effects than non-branch chain amino acids.

Chronic semistarvation produced over a 4-week period by limiting availability of feed to two-thirds the basal level causes a 25 to 30 percent reduction in body weight and atrophy of diaphragm muscle fibers and a reduction in maximum force output.[16,24] Kelsen and colleagues[16] found that the diaphragms from undernourished hamsters undergo atrophy of type II but not type I fibers. The magnitude of the reduction in cross-sectional area of types IIA and B fibers was proportional to the reduction in body weight. Diaphragm muscle bundles from undernourished hamsters have a normally shaped length-tension curve during electrically induced contractions (Fig. 33-3). However, maximal tetanic tension is reduced. Reductions in maximum muscle force are proportional to the reduction in diaphragm muscle cross-sectional area, suggesting that in the undernourished hamster, the cause of muscle weakness is a loss of contractile elements. Residual muscle contractile elements develop force normally.

In contrast, Lewis'[24] and Sieck's[17] groups found that 4 weeks of undernutrition in the rat, which reduces body weight by 50 percent, causes a reduction in the cross-sectional area of type I as well type II fibers. However, in agreement with Kelsen and coworkers,[16] greater atrophy was observed in the type II fiber population. Undernutrition in the rats caused a leftward shift of the force-frequency curve of the isolated diaphragm such that nutritionally depleted animals generated a greater proportion of maximal force at subtetanizing frequencies compared with control animals. Of interest, diaphragms from undernourished animals were less fa-

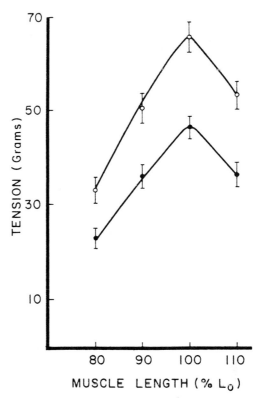

FIGURE 33-3 Effect of 4 weeks of undernutrition in the hamster induced by caloric restriction on the length-tension characteristic of isolated diaphragm muscle strips. Isometric tetanic tension (50 Hz electrical stimuli) is shown as a function of muscle fiber length expressed as a percentage of L_0, the length at which tension was maximum. Filled circles represent caloric-restricted groups; open circles represent ad lib fed control group. Note that tension was significantly less in calorie-restricted animals at any fiber length. (Data from Kelsen et al.,[16] with permission.)

tigued when stimulated subtetanically for a 2-min period. The greater endurance of the nutritionally depleted animals is misleading in the sense that electrically stimulated contractions do not replicate the pattern of activation of the muscle in vivo. During electrically stimulated contractions, all fibers are recruited simultaneously, but in vivo type II fibers are recruited only with strenuous efforts. It appears likely, therefore, that during eupneic breathing in vivo when only slow twitch fibers are activated there is no change in diaphragm endurance. Rather, preferential wasting of type II fibers in the diaphragm is likely to impair diaphragm endurance during the performance of strenuous efforts.

Acute fasting may also impair respiratory muscle function but by a different mechanism. Shindoh and colleagues[25] demonstrated that acute starvation for 36 h in the hamster had no effect on diaphragm muscle morphology but decreased force output and enhanced muscle fatigability in vitro. Impaired diaphragm function appeared to be a result of hypoglycemia since the changes in diaphragm strength and endurance could be reversed when the glucose level in the bath was raised to normal values. In contrast, Shindoh's and Lewis' groups[25,26] found that 90 h of starvation in the rat did not affect peak diaphragmatic twitch and tetanic tension, and diaphragm endurance was largely unaffected. However, Lewis and colleagues did not examine blood sugar in the

TABLE 33-1 Diaphragm Dimensions at Autopsy in COPD

	Weight	Thickness	Area
Steele and Heard, 1973[28] ($n = 14$)	Decrease	Decrease	Decrease
Ishikawa and Hayes, 1973[29] ($n = 9$)	Increase	Increase	Unaffected
Butler, 1976[30] ($n = 95$)	—	Unaffected	Decrease in proportion to the extent of the emphysema
Thurlbeck, 1978[31] ($n = 184$)	Decrease in proportion to severity of emphysema		
Arora and Rochester, 1987[32] ($n = 18$)	Decrease in proportion to body weight; no different from weight-height matched controls		

starved rats. Differences in the two studies may reflect differences in the blood sugar response to starvation in the two species.

HUMAN STUDIES

Respiratory Muscle Mass

In humans, diaphragm muscle mass correlates directly with body weight. Reductions in weight may be expected to decrease mass at the diaphragm (and probably other respiratory muscles). Diaphragm dimensions, heart weight, and body weight were measured at autopsy in 33 normal subjects and 33 patients with a variety of diseases excluding chronic lung disease, obesity, and overt edematous states.[27] The normal subjects died suddenly of trauma or poisoning. The patients died after a period of hospitalization ranging from one to several weeks. Both diaphragm muscle mass and heart weight were directly proportional to body weight. That is, diaphragm mass was less in underweight patients (< 91 percent of IBW) than those with normal weight (> 100 percent of IBW). Of interest, the diaphragm muscle mass–body weight relationship was unique, and data points of underweight and normal weight subjects fell along the same line. The area and the thickness of the diaphragm muscle changed in parallel with muscle mass. Reductions in diaphragm muscle mass in undernourished subjects were proportionally greater than reductions in heart mass. These data suggest that diaphragm muscle mass changes with nutritional state in the same way as other body muscles.

Although COPD per se is associated with reductions in diaphragm fiber length and deleterious changes in muscle shape which impair muscle contractility, it does not appear to have a consistent effect on muscle mass. Table 33-1 shows several studies which have compared the dimensions of the human diaphragm at autopsy in patients with COPD and in subjects who suddenly died of trauma.[18,28–32]

The disparate results on diaphragm morphology obtained to date in humans may relate to differences in the severity or duration of lung disease. Alternatively, they may be explained by differences in systemic factors which influence muscle structure and metabolism (e.g., corticosteroid, thyroid, or growth hormone levels, medication use, Pa_{O_2}).[15]

Respiratory Muscle Function

Respiratory muscle strength and endurance are impaired in subjects with body wasting. Arora and colleagues[33] have demonstrated that subjects with cachexia secondary to malignancy or poorly controlled infection but without disease manifest lower values for maximum inspiratory pressure (MIP) and maximum expiratory pressure (MEP) and maximum voluntary ventilation compared with a well nourished population (i.e., greater than 85 percent ideal body weight). The effects of undernutrition and muscle wasting on diaphragm endurance are less clear-cut.

Kelly and colleagues[34] studied the relationship between inspiratory muscle strength and body cell mass in 59 surgical patients requiring total parenteral alimentation. The patients studied by Kelly did not have chronic lung disease. Body cell mass was assessed from measurements of the radioactive potassium and sodium compartments. Maximal inspiratory pressure measured at functional residual capacity correlated directly with body cell mass. Neither inspiratory muscle function nor body cell mass correlated with total body weight in these subjects, probably because of edema. After 2 to 4 weeks of total parenteral hyperalimentation, maximal inspiratory pressure increased in 21 of 29 patients by an average of 37 percent. Body cell volume increased by 12 percent. The remaining eight patients had a 10 percent decrement in body cell mass and no significant change in maximal inspiratory pressure.

This study suggests that improvements in muscle function correlate with improvements in lean body mass but are proportionally greater in magnitude than the increase in body cell mass.

Nutrition and the Lung Parenchyma

In accordance with the protease-antiprotease theory of emphysema, reductions in the activity of serum antiproteases relative to serum proteases predispose to emphysema. Since the rates of protein synthesis and degradation are under nutritional control, it has been suggested that semistarvation could conceivably induce emphysema-like changes in the lungs of normal adults.[35]

ANIMAL STUDIES

Almost all the information available on the effects of weight loss on lung structure and function has been generated in animal models by food deprivation. Lung dry and wet weights are reduced by semistarvation and restored by refeeding.[14,35] DNA content is unchanged by fasting, indicating that cell number is unaffected. In starved animals, the volume of lamellar bodies and mitochondria and the content of dipalmitoyl lecithin is reduced in granular pneumocytes. Furthermore, in starved animals, the airspaces are enlarged and nonuniform, and elastin fibers in the interstitium are short, irregular, and fewer in number.

Semistarved animals manifest a rightward shift of the lung static pressure-volume (P-V) curve during air inflation but a leftward shift of the P-V curve when saline-filled. These findings suggest that semistarvation has a dual effect on lung mechanics. Semistarvation increases lung surface forces but decreases lung tissue elasticity.

Kerr and coworkers[36] deprived rats of both protein and calories for 6 weeks and compared results with controls and rats deprived only of calories. In the protein and calorie deprived rats the ratio of lung to body weight was increased and the alveoli were larger and demonstrated a reduced internal surface area. They concluded that depletion of proteins and calories was required to induce emphysema-like changes of the lungs of adult animals.

HUMAN STUDIES

Keys and associates[37] noted reductions in vital capacity in adult men semistarved for 24 weeks sufficient to lose 24 percent of initial body weight. After 12 weeks of rehabilitation and refeeding, the vital capacity returned to initial values. A separate study[38] observed that vital capacity was less and the RV/TLC (where RV is residual volume) ratio was higher than predicted in 10 females with anorexia nervosa.

In COPD, the extent of emphysema may correlate with the degree of weight loss. For example, Sukumalchantra and Williams[39] noted that reductions in maximum midexpiratory flow rate and increases in airway resistance occured only in those with COPD who lost more than 10 percent of their initial body weight during the 5-year period of observation. Reductions in the diffusing capacity for carbon monoxide were also more severe in patients who lost weight. Openbrier and colleagues[6] reported that declines in lung function were greater in undernourished (depleted) than normal weight patients.

Pathogenesis of Body Depletion in COPD

Weight loss generally occurs when daily energy expenditure exceeds energy intake in the diet. That is, weight loss occurs when subjects are in a condition of negative energy balance. In turn, daily energy expenditure has three main components: (1) the resting energy expenditure (REE), which accounts for ≈60 percent of total energy expenditure; (2) energy consumed during physical activity and the activities of daily living, which accounts for ≈30 percent of energy expenditure; and (3) diet-induced thermogenesis, the energy required to digest the nutrient intake, which accounts for < 10 percent.[15,40] In most normally active subjects, the largest fraction of total body energy requirements is the REE.

ENERGY EXPENDITURE

In subjects with advanced COPD, the REE is usually 10 to 20 percent greater than normal and is a greater fraction of the total energy expenditure (70 to 80 percent of total energy expenditure) than in normal subjects.[41-48] Approximately, two-thirds of subjects with advanced COPD have an REE > 110 percent of normal based on the Harris-Benedict equation or indirect calorimetry in age- and sex-matched controls. Resting energy expenditure is significantly correlated with

FEV_1 and is higher in weight-losing subjects with COPD than in weight-stable ones.

Increases in REE in patients with COPD have been attributed to the increased oxygen cost of breathing.[41,49] Greater work of breathing and lower efficiency and mechanical advantage of the respiratory muscles require a greater respiratory muscle oxygen consumption for a given level of minute ventilation.[50] Donahoe and coworkers[41] measured the oxygen cost of breathing in 19 patients with COPD (10 with body weight < 90 percent IBW; 9 with body weight > 95 percent IBW) and 7 control subjects. Of note, the nutritionally depleted subjects (< 90 percent IBW) were more hyperinflated and obstructed and had lower values of MIP and MEP than the normally nourished subjects. Respiratory muscle oxygen cost was assessed from the change in oxygen consumption induced by increasing minute ventilation by 6 to 10 L/min on a breathing circuit containing a large dead space. The oxygen cost of breathing for depleted subjects with COPD (4.28 mL O_2 per liter) was ≈1.7-fold greater than in normal-weight patients with COPD (> 95 percent IBW) (2.61 ml O_2 per liter) and ≈3.5-fold greater than in healthy controls (1.23 mL O_2 per liter). The oxygen cost of breathing was also a greater percentage of total oxygen consumption in the nutritionally depleted subjects, and the REE correlated directly with the oxygen cost of breathing. This study indicates that respiratory muscle oxygen consumption is greater in depleted than normal weight subjects with COPD, and it correlates with the severity of lung dysfunction.

However, the elevated REE alone is unlikely to explain the high prevalence of body wasting in COPD patients. First, if the work of breathing were the predominant factor determining the high REE, a close correlation would be expected between indexes of airway obstruction and REE. This is not the case. Second, nasal positive-pressure ventilation which reduces respiratory muscle activity (i.e., diaphragm and intercostal muscle EMG), does not reduce REE to the normal range in hypermetabolic COPD patients. Thus, although the increased work of breathing may contribute to the increased REE, it would not appear to be the sole factor. Other factors which stimulate metabolism may contribute. For example, beta$_2$ adrenergic bronchodilators increase resting energy expenditure in healthy subjects by approximately 8 to 10 percent.[51] An intriguing possibility is that inflammation within the lung and airways releases proinflammatory cytokines which stimulate muscle protein catabolism and alter the mobilization of amino acids (e.g., TNFα). Of interest, stimulated peripheral blood monocytes from weight-losing subjects with COPD (i.e., > 5 percent of body weight in the preceding year) produce significantly higher levels of TNFα protein than in weight-stable COPD patients and cells of healthy, age-matched controls.[52]

Regardless of mechanism, the increase in REE in subjects with advanced COPD is surprising since a decrease in REE in proportion to the reduction in lean body mass is the normal physiologic response.[15,40] The high REE in subjects with COPD contradicts the hypothesis that weight loss is an adaptive mechanism which acts to decrease oxygen consumption and CO_2 production in patients with COPD.

Exercise-induced energy expenditure is relatively small in patients with COPD, who are sedentary and largely inactive. Studies in a small number of patients with COPD demonstrate an average exercise-induced energy expenditure measured in the laboratory at 20 percent. Unfortunately, no data are available on daily energy expenditure in the free-living condition. Dietary induced thermogenesis is similar in normal subjects and those with COPD.[48]

DIETARY INTAKE

Gastrointestinal symptoms are frequent in patients with emphysema.[53] Those with COPD have reduced nutritional intake due to dyspnea because of gastric distention–induced reductions in functional residual capacity and/or early satiety because of compression of the stomach by the diaphragm. Suboptimal oral intake may also occur because chewing and swallowing require changes in the breathing pattern which may induce arterial oxygen desaturation.[53] Medications taken by the patient with COPD may contribute to suboptimal intake. For example, theophylline may produce anorexia by its effect on gastric acid production and gastric function. Also anxiety and depression, common psychological impairments in patients with COPD, may cause appetite supression. In fact, those patients with abnormally high scores for anxiety and depression have the subjectively reported poorest appetites.[54] In addition, dietary intake may be extremely low during acute exacerbations of disease when subjects are most intensely breathless. Finally, hypoxemia may impair intestinal absorption of nutrients.[55]

Contrary to popular belief, however, stable patients usually have normal caloric intake.[45,56] In a nutritional survey of 38 patients with COPD, total caloric and protein intake were 44 and 82 percent higher, respectively, than the recommended daily allowance.[56] However, weight-losing patients show a significantly lower dietary intake than weight-stable patients, both in absolute terms and in relation to the REE.[45]

The normal response to an increase in energy requirements induced by increases in physical activity (for example, the lumberjack) is a proportional increase in dietary intake sufficient to match the energy requirements. Under these conditions, body weight remains stable. The reason for the relatively inadequate energy intake in hypermetabolic patients with COPD is not well understood. The inadequate caloric intake indicates a state of "relative anorexia," perhaps because of cytokine-induced depression of appetite.[57] The contribution of cachexia-inducing cytokines, such as TNFα, to the depleted state in patients with COPD raises the possibility of novel forms of treatment for this disorder.[58]

Nutritional Assessment

The nutritional evaluation should assess the patient's tissue mass and function, identify the mechanisms causing the disturbance (e.g., malabsorption, inadequate intake), and develop an appropriate nutritional treatment plan. The nutritional assessment begins with the history and physical examination. Information should be obtained about body weight in the last 6 months, dietary habits, gastrointestinal symptoms, and functional capacity. Physical examination should include estimation of the subcutaneous fat stores by palpation of the skin fold in the triceps region and at the midaxillary level on the chest wall, determination of muscle bulk and tone by palpation of the quadriceps and deltoids, and identification of the presence of any edema, or ascites.

Detsky and colleagues[59] have used routine history and

TABLE 33-2 Features in the Clinical History and Physical Examination Used in the Subjective Global Assessment (SGA)

History	Weight change in last 6 mo and 2 wk
	Changes in dietary intake
	Presence of gastrointestinal symptoms for >2 wk (nausea, vomiting, diarrhea, anorexia)
	Functional capacity (working, ambulatory, bedridden)
	Presence of disease states and corresponding metabolic demands (low, moderate, high stress)
Physical examination	Loss of subcutaneous fat
	Presence of muscle wasting
	Ankle edema
	Sacral edema
	Ascites

SOURCE: Adapted from Detskey AS, McLaughlin JR, Baker JP, et al: *J Parenter Enter Nutr* 11:8–13, 1987, with permission.

physical examination to develop a subjective global nutritional assessment to classify surgical patients as well nourished, moderately malnourished, and severely malnourished. Important features included in the subjective global assessment are shown in Table 33-2. Clinical assessment using the subjective global nutritional assessment has high interobserver reproducibility (91 percent) and is highly correlated with objective nutritional measurements. The subjective global assessment has been advocated as a useful clinical tool applicable to medical as well as surgical patients. The major limitation of this clinical assessment is the lack of sensitivity in assessing change in nutritional status following nutritional support.

BODY WEIGHT

Body weight is usually normalized for differences in height, age, and body frame size and expressed as a percentage of ideal body weight according to the Metropolitan Life Insurance Height and Weight Tables (Table 33-3).[2] Frame size of the individual (i.e., small, medium, or large) is estimated by using elbow breadth or wrist circumference. The elbow breadth is measured as the distance between the two prominent bones on either side of the elbow with a tape measure while the forearm is flexed to a 90-degree angle to the arm. Frame size adjusted to height can then be estimated from Table 33-4. The height/wrist ratio can then be calculated and compared with standard reference values shown in Table 33-5. Body weight 10 to 20 percent above the reference value is considered overweight; weight > 20 percent above the reference is considered obesity. Body weight more than 10 percent below the reference weight is considered undernutrition. Without resorting to the tables, a quick estimate of ideal body weight can be obtained by using the following rule of thumb: for males, add 6 lb for every 1 in. above 5 ft, which has a value of 106 lb; for females, add 5 lb for every 1 in. above 5 ft which has a value of 100 lb. For large- or small-frame individuals, 10 percent of the reference weight is added or subtracted, respectively.

Alternatively, a body mass index (BMI) can be determined

TABLE 33-3 1983 Examples of Metropolitan Height and Weight Tables for Adults Age 25 to 29 Years

| MEN | | | | | | WOMEN | | | | |
| HEIGHT | | FRAME | | | HEIGHT | | FRAME | | |
Feet	Inches	Small	Medium	Large	Feet	Inches	Small	Medium	Large
5	2	128–134	131–141	138–150	4	10	102–111	109–121	118–131
5	3	130–136	133–143	140–153	4	11	103–113	111–123	120–134
5	4	132–138	135–145	142–156	5	0	104–115	113–126	122–137
5	5	134–140	137–148	144–160	5	1	106–118	115–129	125–140
5	6	136–142	139–151	146–164	5	2	108–121	118–132	128–143
5	7	138–145	142–154	149–168	5	3	111–124	121–135	131–147
5	8	140–148	145–157	152–172	5	4	114–127	124–138	134–151
5	9	142–151	148–160	155–176	5	5	117–130	127–141	137–155
5	10	144–154	151–163	158–180	5	6	120–133	130–144	140–159
5	11	146–157	154–166	161–184	5	7	123–136	133–147	143–163
6	0	149–160	157–170	164–188	5	8	126–139	136–150	146–167
6	1	152–164	160–174	168–192	5	9	129–142	139–153	149–170
6	2	155–168	164–178	172–197	5	10	132–145	142–156	152–173
6	3	158–172	167–182	176–202	5	11	135–148	145–159	155–176
6	4	162–176	171–187	181–207	6	0	138–151	148–162	158–179

SOURCE: From *Metropolitan Life Insurance Company Statistical Bulletin,* with permission.

from the measured body weight divided by the square of height as

$$BMI = \frac{weight\ (kg)}{height\ (m)^2}$$

BMI can be interpreted as shown in Table 33-6.

However, it is important to realize that the range of predicted normal is wide for both body weight and body mass index.[59] Accordingly, patients may still remain in the normal range despite significant weight loss. Thus, changes in body weight are important to note and may be clinically significant even when the weight is still within the predicted normal range. Furthermore body weight may be misleading in the presence of edema in COPD patients with cor pulmonale. Nonetheless, a number of studies have demonstrated the considerable usefulness of this simple, clinically applicable parameter.

ANTHROPOMORPHIC MEASUREMENTS

TRICEPS SKIN FOLD THICKNESS
Subcutaneous fat stores are assumed to be about 50 percent of total body fat. Accordingly, body fat can be assessed from

the triceps skin fold thickness, a simple, inexpensive, and noninvasive measurement. Triceps skin fold thickness (TSF) is measured using calipers applied at four sites: (1) triceps, (2) biceps, (3) subscapular area, and (4) suprailiac area.

Several studies have shown that body fat store is depleted in both stable patients and those with acute respiratory decompensation.[5,6,8,60,61] For example, triceps skin fold thickness was below the lower limit of normal in 68 percent of consecutive patients with COPD in acute respiratory failure.[8]

The major limitation of measurements of triceps skin fold thickness is that the proportion of subcutaneous fat to total body fat is not always constant. In fact, the triceps skin fold thickness has been shown to overestimate the fat-free mass in stable patients with COPD when compared with measurements obtained by bioelectrical impedance.[46] Moreover, interobserver variability is relatively high (coefficient of variation of 9 percent),[62] and the measurement can be misleading in edematous patients.

MIDARM MUSCLE CIRCUMFERENCE
Skeletal muscle bulk as reflected by lean body mass represents ≈ 60 percent of the total body protein store. Lean body muscle mass can be assessed from the midarm muscle

TABLE 33-4 Elbow Breadth Values[a]

| MEN | | WOMEN | |
Height in 1-inch Heels	Elbow Breadth	Height in 1-inch Heels	Elbow Breadth
5 ft 2 in to 5 ft 3 in	2½ to 2⅞ in	4 ft 10 in to 4 ft 11 in	2¼ to 2½ in
5 ft 4 in to 5 ft 7 in	2⅝ to 2⅞ in	5 ft 0 in to 5 ft 3 in	2¼ to 2½ in
5 ft 8 in to 5 ft 11 in	2¾ to 3 in	5 ft 4 in to 5 ft 7 in	2⅜ to 2⅝ in
6 ft 0 in to 6 ft 3 in	2¾ to 3⅛ in	5 ft 8 in to 5 ft 11 in	2⅜ to 2⅝ in
6 ft 4 in and over	2⅞ to 3¼ in	6 ft 0 in and over	2½ to 2¾ in

[a] Standard for elbow breadth measurement in men and women with medium body frame size of various heights. Elbow breadth size smaller than those listed indicates small frame size, and larger measurement indicates large frame size.
SOURCE: Adapted from Whitney EN, Cataldo CB, DeBruyne LK, et al: *Nutrition for Health and Health Care,* 1996, Metropolitan Life Insurance Company, with permission.

TABLE 33-5 Estimation of Frame Size Using Height-Wrist Circumference Ratios (r)[a]

Frame Size	Male r Values	Female r Values
Small	>10.4	>11.0
Medium	9.6–10.4	10.1–11.0
Large	<9.6	<10.1

[a] The wrist circumference is measured distal to the styloid process.
SOURCE: Whitney EN, Cataldo CB, DeBruyne LK, et al: *Nutrition for Health and Health Care*, 1996, and Metropolitan Life Insurance Company.

circumference (MAMC). The midarm muscle circumference is calculated as

$$MAMC \ (cm) = arm \ circumference \ (cm) - 3.14 \times triceps \ skin \ fold \ (cm)$$

The MAMC should be measured at the same location as the triceps skin fold thickness. Lean body mass assessed by midarm circumference is decreased in 42 percent of patients with COPD and acute respiratory failure.[8]

Like body weight, serial measurements of TSF and MAMC are more important than a single determination since the normal range is wide. Changes are likely to be meaningful even if values fall within the normal range.

MEASUREMENT OF BODY COMPOSITION

Measurement of FFM by bioelectrical impedance is a promising test.[46] Body resistance and its reciprocal, impedance, reflect body water volume since the electrical resistance of the fat-free mass (i.e., water and electrolyte component of lean tissue) is far lower than that of fat. Body resistance and impedance are calculated from the voltage drop between electrodes applied to the hand and foot in response to low-frequency alternating current (800 μA at 50 kHz). The higher the resistance, the lower the fat-free mass. The lean body mass is then estimated assuming a constant hydration fraction.

The technique is safe, and the equipment is portable and easy to use. The interobserver error is low, and the test can be performed repeatedly without risk. The technique, however, may be inaccurate in the presence of edema since the ratio of lean body mass to total body water is altered. The use of dual or multiple frequency bioelectrical impedance increases the accuracy of measurements of lean body mass and may circumvent this problem by discriminating intracellular from extracellular water. Low-frequency (< 1 kHz) current prefer-

entially passes through the extracellular fluid because it cannot easily pass through the cell membrane. Other techniques to measure lean body (e.g., deuterium dilution, total body potassium, dual-energy x-ray absorptiometry, in vivo neutron activation analysis) remain research tools.

Patients whose body weight is normal may have abnormally low FFM. Schols' group[9,46] measured fat-free mass using bioelectrical resistance in 255 patients with COPD undergoing outpatient pulmonary rehabilitation. Fat-free mass was reduced in a sizable minority of those with normal body weight (14 percent). These subjects also had abnormally low lean body mass measured by creatinine/height index and poorer exercise performance than patients with normal FFM.

SERUM PROTEINS

Serum protein levels are an index of visceral protein stores and, hence, nutritional status. However, decreases in serum proteins also reflect capillary permeability and the migration of proteins into the extravascular space.[63] For example, the daily exchange of albumin between the intravascular and extravascular space is 10 times greater than the rate of albumin synthesis. Accordingly, acute inflammation which causes albumin to leak from the capillaries to the extravascular space may cause severe hypoalbuminemia rapidly.

Serum albumin, which is synthesized in the liver, is decreased in 42 percent of patients in acute respiratory failure.[8] Unfortunately, the half-life of serum albumin (20 days) is long, making it an insensitive marker of acute nutritional deterioration.

Serum prealbumin is a better marker of changes in nutritional status because of its shorter half-life (2 days). Serum prealbumin is decreased in a greater percentage of patients with acute respiratory failure than is serum albumin (76 versus 42 percent, respectively).[8] Changes in serum prealbumin levels occur within 7 days after a change in nutritional intake. A rising prealbumin level correlates with positive nitrogen balance.

Serum transferrin level is also a useful marker of acute nutritional status because its plasma half-life is intermediate between that of prealbumin and albumin (i.e., $\approx$ 8 days). A rising transferrin level is a good indicator of positive nitrogen balance during nutritional therapy. However, iron deficiency states increase transferrin synthesis cofounding its use as a nutritional index.

MUSCLE PROTEIN STORES

CREATININE HEIGHT INDEX

Lean body mass can be estimated noninvasively from the amount of creatinine excreted in the urine normalized for body height (i.e., the creatinine/height index). Creatinine/height index (CHI) is the ratio of 24-h urinary creatinine to expected output for age-, gender-, and height-matched controls expressed as a percentage (Table 33-7). An index of 100 percent indicates normal muscle mass as long as urinary function is normal. Infection, injury, and a diet high in protein and creatinine may increase urinary creatinine and give a spuriously elevated CHI.

NITROGEN BALANCE

Nitrogen balance is the most common method of assessing protein turnover. A negative nitrogen balance indicates in-

TABLE 33-6 Interpretation of BMI for Both Men and Women

	Men	Women
Underweight	<20.7	<19.1
Acceptable weight	20.7 to 27.8	19.1 to 27.3
Overweight	≥27.8	≥27.3
Severe overweight	≥31.1	≥32.3
Morbid obesity	≥45.4	≥44.8

SOURCE: Adapted from Whitney EN, Cataldo CB, DeBruyne LK, Rayes SR: *Nutrition for Health Care*, Metropolitan Life Insurance Company, 1996, and *Journal of the American Dietetic Association*, 85:1117–1121, 1985.

TABLE 33-7 Creatinine-Height Index Standards

		MEN								
		SMALL FRAME			MEDIUM FRAME			LARGE FRAME		
HEIGHT		Ideal Weight, kg	CREATININE		Ideal Weight, kg	CREATININE		Ideal Weight, kg	CREATININE	
in	cm		(g/24 h)	(mmol/d)		(g/24 h)	(mmol/d)		(g/24 h)	(mmol/d)
61	154.9	52.7	1.21	10.7	56.1	1.29	11.4	60.7	1.40	12.4
62	157.5	54.1	1.24	11.0	57.7	1.33	11.8	62.0	1.43	12.6
63	160.0	55.4	1.27	11.2	59.1	1.36	12.0	63.6	1.46	12.9
64	162.5	56.8	1.31	11.6	60.4	1.39	12.3	65.2	1.50	13.3
65	165.1	58.4	1.34	11.8	62.0	1.43	12.6	66.8	1.54	13.6
66	167.6	60.2	1.39	12.3	63.9	1.47	13.0	68.9	1.59	14.1
67	170.2	62.0	1.43	12.6	65.9	1.52	13.4	71.1	1.64	14.5
68	172.7	63.9	1.47	13.0	67.7	1.56	13.8	72.9	1.68	14.9
69	175.3	65.9	1.52	13.4	69.5	1.60	14.1	74.8	1.72	15.2
70	177.8	67.7	1.56	13.8	71.6	1.65	14.6	76.8	1.77	15.6
71	180.3	69.5	1.60	14.1	73.6	1.69	14.9	79.1	1.82	16.1
72	182.9	71.4	1.64	14.5	75.7	1.74	15.4	81.1	1.87	16.5
73	185.4	73.4	1.69	14.9	77.7	1.79	15.8	83.4	1.92	17.0
74	187.9	75.2	1.73	15.3	80.0	1.85	16.4	85.7	1.97	17.4
75	190.5	77.0	1.77	15.6	82.3	1.89	16.7	87.7	2.02	17.9
		WOMEN								
56	142.2	43.2	0.79	7.0	46.1	0.83	7.3	50.7	0.91	8.0
57	144.8	44.5	0.80	7.1	47.3	0.85	7.5	51.8	0.93	8.2
58	147.3	45.4	0.82	7.2	48.6	0.88	7.8	53.2	0.96	8.5
59	149.8	46.8	0.84	7.4	50.0	0.90	8.0	54.5	0.98	8.7
60	152.4	48.2	0.87	7.7	51.4	0.93	8.2	55.9	1.01	8.9
61	154.9	49.5	0.89	7.9	52.7	0.95	8.4	57.3	1.03	9.1
62	157.5	50.9	0.92	8.1	54.3	0.98	8.7	58.9	1.06	9.4
63	160.0	52.3	0.94	8.3	55.9	1.01	8.9	60.6	1.09	9.6
64	162.5	53.9	0.97	8.6	57.9	1.04	9.2	62.5	1.13	10.0
65	165.1	55.7	1.00	8.8	59.8	1.08	9.5	64.3	1.16	10.3
66	167.6	57.5	1.04	9.2	61.6	1.11	9.8	66.1	1.19	10.5
67	170.2	59.3	1.07	9.5	63.4	1.14	10.1	67.9	1.22	10.8
68	172.7	61.4	1.11	9.8	65.2	1.17	10.3	70.0	1.26	11.1
69	175.2	63.2	1.14	10.1	67.0	1.21	10.7	72.0	1.30	11.5
70	177.8	65.0	1.17	10.3	68.9	1.24	11.0	74.1	1.33	11.8

NOTE: To convert urinary creatinine measure (g/24 h) to standard international units (mmol/d) multiply by 8.840.

SOURCE: Grant A, DeHoog S: *Nutritional Assessment and Support*, 3rd ed 1985 (available from Anne Grant and Susan DeHoog, P.O. Box 25057, Northgate Station, Seattle, WA 98125) and Metropolitan Life Insurance Company, Statistical Bulletin, with permission.

creased breakdown of tissue proteins and a catabolic state. Nitrogen balance is calculated by dividing 24-h protein intake by 6.25 and subtracting the sum of urinary nitrogen plus 2 to 4 g (the estimated gastrointestinal and cutaneous losses in the absence of malabsorption or protein-losing cutaneous diseases).

3-Methyhistidine is a constituent of actin and myosin in skeletal muscles. During catabolic states, 3-methyhistidine is released unchanged in the urine and is not reused for protein synthesis. Accordingly, measurement of 24-h urinary 3-methyhistidine estimates the extent of muscle breakdown.[64] The technique remains a research tool.

TESTS OF SKELETAL MUSCLE FUNCTION

The maximum voluntary grip strength is measured in the nondominant hand by dynamometry or bulb vigorometer. Muscle grip strength is highly correlated to total body protein stores and is an important indicator of postoperative complications. Electrical stimulation of the ulnar nerve can be used to assess the contraction-relaxation characteristics of the adductor pollicis muscle. In patients with energy malnutrition, force generation in response to low-frequency stimulation is increased, the maximum rate of relaxation is slower, and muscle fatigability is increased.[61]

Respiratory muscle function can also be measured easily from MIP and MEP.

TEST OF IMMUNOCOMPETENCE

Blood lymphocyte count and delayed skin testing, which have been used traditionally as markers of immunocompetence, provide some clues as to nutritional state. A lymphocyte count ≤ 1500 per square millimeter in the absence of chemotherapeutic agents is abnormal.

In delayed hypersensitivity skin testing, several antigens may be used (e.g., tuberculin, *Candida albicans*, *Trichophyton mentagrophytes*). A positive test is indicated by an induration > 5 mm after 48 h. The delayed skin test, however, may be affected by viral and bacterial infection, uremia, or drugs such as *corticosteroids* and cimetidine.

Delayed skin test reactions are depressed in about 33 percent of hospitalized patients with COPD.[5] The incidence of anergy may be even higher in those in acute respiratory failure.[65] Refeeding and weight gain increase the absolute lymphocyte count and skin reactivity.[66] Of interest, delayed skin test responses may be useful as prognostic indicators. In 282 seriously ill patients, 90 percent of those whose delayed skin test response improved or remained positive were discharged. In contrast, only 27 percent of patients whose delayed skin test response deteriorated or remained negative survived their hospital stay.[67]

Nutritional Intervention

TOTAL CALORIC REQUIREMENT

Development of a rational nutritional "prescription" requires both a knowledge of the total caloric needs of the patient and the mix of protein, carbohydrates, and fat required in the diet. Total caloric needs may be estimated using the Harris-Benedict equation or, better yet, measured by indirect calorimetry.[68,69]

INDIRECT CALORIMETRY

Indirect calorimetry is the preferred and the most accurate method of assessing resting energy expenditure. Using a metabolic chart, V_{O_2} and V_{CO_2} are continuously measured from the expired gases until a steady state is achieved ($\approx$20 min). Total energy is then calculated using the Weir equation, where

$$\text{Total calories} = (3.94 \times V_{O_2} + 1.11 \times V_{CO_2}) \times 1.44$$

Oxygen consumption is elevated by eating and physical activity. Accordingly, indirect calorimetry is performed in a quiet environment with the patient fasting and inactive. Measurements of V_{O_2} may be erroneous if subjects are breathing concentrations of oxygen > 50 percent. This is commonly a problem in patients receiving mechanical ventilation for acute respiratory failure, the precise group in which the measurement is so vital.

HARRIS–BENEDICT EQUATION

Resting energy expenditure can be estimated using the Harris-Benedict equation,[68] where

$$\text{REE males} = 66.5 + 13.8 \text{ (weight, kg)} + 5.0 \text{ (height, cm)} - 6.8 \text{ (age, years)}$$

$$\text{REE females} = 655.1 + 9.6 \text{ (weight)} + 1.8 \text{ (height)} - 4.7 \text{ (age)}$$

Stress factors related to the clinical condition (e.g., burns, fever) which increase the REE have been derived from indirect calorimetry measurements in critically ill surgical patients and can be used as modifiers with the Harris-Benedict equation. Stress factors in ventilated COPD patients increase the REE by 29 percent to 54 percent.[70]

Although the Harris-Benedict equation is simple to use, it suffers from a lack of precision. Values derived from the Harris-Benedict equation frequently differ considerably from the values obtained by indirect calorimetry. In addition, the Harris-Benedict equation does not provide a method of monitoring the metabolic response to refeeding. For example, Cortes and coworkers[71] performed simultaneous measurements of REE by indirect calorimetry and the Harris-Benedict equation with and without stress modifiers. Comparisons were made on 31 critically ill patients, 29 of whom were receiving mechanical ventilation. Resting energy expenditure determined by indirect calorimetry was significantly greater than that predicted from the Harris-Benedict equation without stress modifiers but less than that predicted using stress modifiers. Sources of error in the Harris-Benedict approach are unclear but may involve inaccurate weights due to fluid changes. Clinically, it would seem appropriate, therefore, to base initial caloric support on the Harris-Benedict equation multiplied by the appropriate stress factor. However, indirect calorimetry should be performed as soon as possible to derive a more accurate caloric prescription.

In general, depleted patients (i.e., < 80 to 85 percent IBW) require a total daily caloric intake amounting to 1.4 to 1.7 $\times$ REE to achieve a positive energy balance and gain weight.[69] Patients with normal body weight (i.e., > 95 percent IBW) require a total daily caloric intake amounting to 1.25 to 1.4 $\times$ REE to maintain weight.

PROTEIN REQUIREMENT

The amount of protein required for positive nitrogen balance depends on the severity of nutritional depletion, the amount of nonprotein calorie intake, and the desired rate of nutritional repletion. It is essential to provide sufficient total caloric intake to avoid burning protein for fuel. Restoration of lean body mass is not possible, even in the face of large amounts of protein if the total caloric intake is less than adequate. Accordingly, both carbohydrate and lipid are required in the diet in sufficient amount to have a "protein-sparing" effect.

In general, requirements range from 0.75 to 1.0 g protein per kilogram per day and should be administered as 15 to 30 percent of total calories. In depleted patients, protein intake as high as 1.5 to 2.0 mg/kg may be required.[69–71] Excessive protein intake should be avoided, however, since it increases minute ventilation and the ventilatory responses to hypoxia and hypercapnia, thus heightening the sense of dyspnea in patients with advanced COPD.[72,73]

CARBOHYDRATE AND FAT REQUIREMENT

The optimum proportions of dietary carbohydrate and fat as sources of nonprotein calories in patients with COPD is controversial. Carbohydrate has a respiratory quotient (RQ) of 1.0; fat has an RQ of 0.7. This means that for a given O_2 consumption, more CO_2 is produced by a gram of carbohydrate than a gram of fat. In theory, then, a diet high in carbohydrates may increase CO_2 production and ventilation more than an isocaloric diet high in fat. It has been suggested that large increases in CO_2 production with high carbohydrate intake may precipitate respiratory distress, hinder weaning, and impair exercise performance in patients with COPD.[74–76]

Supporting the above concerns, Brown and coworkers showed that marked carbohydrate loading (i.e., total calories more than two times REE and more than 60 percent of non-protein calories as carbohydrates) decreased exercise tolerance in COPD patients.[77] Moreover, COPD patients fed a single, 920-kcal carbohydrate meal increase oxygen consumption and CO_2 production by ≈ 10 and ≈ 20 percent, respectively.[78]

However, stable patients tolerate a moderate degree of carbohydrate loading without difficulty. Angelillo's group[79] showed that a low (28 percent of total calories) and moderate carbohydrate intake (53 percent total calories) with diet equal to $1.3 \times$ REE did not affect blood-gas tensions or ventilation in hypercapnic patients (mean $Pa_{CO_2} = 49$ mmHg). A high carbohydrate diet (74 percent total calories) raised CO_2 production and minute ventilation modestly. No patient developed symptoms.

Nonetheless, some authors have recommended a low-carbohydrate, high-fat diet (> 50 percent total calories) for patients with COPD. Enteral formulas with such a makeup high in fat content are commercially available (e.g., Pulmocare) and have been specifically marketed for COPD patients. The benefit of a high-fat regimen remains unproved. Total caloric intake is likely to be equally or even more important than a diet with a low carbohydrate-to-fat ratio as already discussed. Nonetheless, it would seem prudent to avoid high-caloric diets (i.e., > 1.7 to $1.8 \times$ REE) with a high carbohydrate composition (> 50 percent total calories) especially in hypercapnic patients with COPD.

In patients who require prolonged parenteral nutritional support, intravenous lipid emulsion prevents essential fatty acid deficiency in addition to providing a concentrated calorie source. The essential fatty acids in humans include linoleic acid, linolenic acid, and arachidonic acid.

Several investigators reported decreases in arterial Pa_{O_2} or diffusing capacity in patients with impaired baseline lung function following intravenous fat emulsions.[80–82] In normal subjects, 500 mL of 10% intralipid infused over 4 h transiently decreases diffusion capacity during submaximal exercise.[81] Infusion of 20 percent intralipid in mechanically ventilated patients did not affect gas exchange.[83] Lipid infusion increases prostaglandin synthesis, particularly PGE_2, which may alter pulmonary vasomotor tone and result in hypoxemia, which is blocked by pretreatment with indomethacin.[84]

The clinical significance of the decrease in arterial oxygenation and diffusion capacity following intravenous lipid emulsion is unclear since the magnitude of the changes are small. However, it would appear prudent to give intravenous lipid slowly (e.g., over 12 h) in patients with abnormalities in lung function.

Effectiveness of Nutritional Intervention in COPD

The repeated observations that depleted subjects with COPD are hypermetabolic and suffer from reductions of both fat and fat-free mass have led to investigations of the effects of nutritional intervention. Since 1986, at least eight studies have examined the effect of supplementary nutrition on body weight and respiratory and limb muscle function in patients with COPD. The results of these studies are summarized in Table 33-8.

Knowles and coworkers[85] performed a 16-week single-blind crossover study of 25 stable, ambulatory patients with COPD (body weight < 85 percent of ideal in 13 of the 25). Subjects were given an oral supplement to increase caloric intake by 50 percent over baseline for an 8-week period. The supplement was withdrawn for the subsequent 8-week period. Caloric intake assessed by a diet history increased significantly with the supplement ($+ 28$ percent) at 4 and 8 weeks. Body weight increased only 1 to 2 percent, however. Moreover, there was also no clear-cut effect on MIP, MEP, or sustainable inspiratory pressure at 10 min, an index of inspiratory muscle endurance.

Wilson and colleagues[86] studied six depleted subjects with emphysema (body weight < 85 percent ideal) during a 3-week stay in a clinical research center. During a 2-week period of nutritional intervention, caloric intake was increased to 110 to 170 percent above the REE assessed by indirect calorimetry. Three of the six subjects required oral supplements to achieve the nutritional target. Average body weight increased from 49.5 to 52.6 kg (from 75 to 81 percent of ideal). MIP, maximum voluntary transdiaphragmatic pressure (Pdi), hand grip strength, and serum transferrin all increased significantly. These investigators concluded that a vigorous, supervised nutritional supplementation program can increase caloric intake, body weight, respiratory muscle, and limb muscle function. Of interest, this study followed patients after 1 week of discharge and observed that some of the benefit was lost.

Lewis and associates[87] studied 21 outpatients with COPD over an 8-week period. Subjects were divided into control and dietary intervention groups. The intervention group received 500 to 1000 additional kilocalories a day as an enteral supplement. The control group continued its usual ad lib outpatient diet. Intake was assessed by a dietary history. The intervention group had a small increase in caloric intake (≈ 13 percent) but no change in body weight, MIP or MEP, albumin, or anthropomorphic indexes. These investigators concluded that it was not possible to provide enough calories to increase body weight when subjects were in an unsupervised outpatient setting.

Whitaker and coworkers[88] studied 10 depleted patients with COPD (body weight less than 85 percent ideal) who were fed nocturnally via nasoenteral tube in a hospital setting for an average of 16 days. Subjects were provided with 1000 kcal above their usual intake or a caloric intake 1.7 times the REE, whichever was greater. A control group was given an equal volume of enteral feed which contained fewer than 100 kcal. Initial body weight was 76 and 82 percent of IBW in the fed and the sham-fed groups, respectively. The caloric intake was increased in the fed group to $\approx 2.2 \times$ REE or approximately 175 percent of the caloric intake in the home setting. Average body weight increased by 2.4 kg, MIP by 20 percent, and MEP by 33 percent. Respiratory muscle endurance assessed from the sustainable inspiratory pressure increased approximately 100 percent. There was, however, no change in the contractile function of the adductor pollicis muscle during electrically stimulated contraction. The sham-fed subjects showed no change in any parameter. These authors concluded that a short period (≈ 2 weeks) of intensive

TABLE 33-8 Effect of Supplementary Nutrition on Respiratory Muscle Function

Weight	Population	Control	Duration Intervention	Route	Muscle Effect	Body
Wilson, 1986[86]	COPD (n = 6)	No	2 wk	Oral 1.5	↑ PImax, ↑ PDImax REE ↑ hand grip strength	Increased (+3.1 kg)
Whitaker, 1990[88]	COPD (n = 10)	Yes	16 ± 3 d	Eternally nocturnally +1000 kcal 1.7 REE	↑ PEmax, ↑ insp. thresh-old load No change adductor or pollicis strength	Increased (+2.4 kg)
Efthimiou, 1988[89]	COPD (n = 14)	Yes, crossover	12 wk	Oral to 2500 kcal	↑ Sternomast. strength and endurance ↑ PImax, PEmax ↑ Hand grip strength	Increased (+4.2 kg)
Lewis, 1987[87]	COPD (n = 21)	Yes	8 wk	Oral +500 1,000 kcal	NC PImax, PEmax, or MSVV	NC
Knowles, 1988[85]	COPD (n = 29)	Yes, crossover	8 wk	Oral 50% over-nor-mal calories	NC PImax, insp. com-pared to control group	±NC
Rogers, 1992[90]	COPD (n = 27)	Yes, ran-domized	3 wk inpt. and 4 mo outpt.	Oral 1.7 REE with 1.5 g/kg protein walking	↑ Hand grip and PI-max, PEmax and 12-min walking distance	Increased (+2.4 kg)
Shridar, 1994[91]	COPD (n = 12)	No	4 mo	Oral 1.3 REE with 1.5 g/kg protein	NC PImax and PEmax	Increased (+0.3 kg)
Schols, 1995[9]	COPD (n = 233)	Yes, ran-domized	8 wks	Oral, 420 kcal	NC PImax	Increased (+2.6 kg)

NOTE: MSVV, maximum sustained voluntary ventilation.

alimentation was sufficient to increase body weight and respiratory muscle function in depleted subjects with COPD.

Efthimiou's group[89] studied 14 depleted (< 90 percent IBW) subjects with COPD during a 9-month period as outpatients. During the initial 3 months, subjects consumed a normal diet. A high-calorie diet was provided during a subsequent 3-month period, and in the final 3 months a normal diet was resumed. An oral supplement was used to increase caloric intake to 2500 kcal/day with 90 g of protein in men and 2300 kcal containing 80 g of protein in women. Intake in the first 3 months of the study was 1429 kcal containing 53 g of protein. Caloric intake was significantly augmented during the 3 months of dietary supplementation to greater than 2100 kcal/day containing 82 g of protein. A well-nourished control group of subjects with COPD consumed 2200 calories and 90 g of protein. Efthimiou found that body weight, midarm muscle circumference, triceps skin fold thickness, MIP, sternomastoid muscle maximal voluntary contraction and fatigability during electrical stimulation, and hand grip strength all increased significantly and progressively during the 3-month period of supplementation but fell back toward original values with return to the baseline diet (Fig. 33-4). During the 3-month period of hyperalimentation, subjects noted an improved sense of well-being and 6-min walking distance.

These investigators concluded that malnourished subjects with COPD have decreased limb and respiratory muscle strength and evidence of heightened fatigability of the sterno-mastoid muscle. An increase in caloric intake tended to improve all the above parameters. Unfortunately, the benefit derived during the period of hyperalimentation tended to be lost when subjects were permitted to go back to an unsupervised, ad lib diet.

Rogers and coworkers[90] studied 27 depleted subjects with COPD (average body weight 79 percent ideal). The nutri-

tional intervention group received 3 weeks of oral supplementation as inpatients. Caloric intake was increased to 1.7 × REE with approximately 1.5 g/kg protein. Following the 3-week inpatient program, subjects were followed for a subsequent 4 months with the intervention continued on an outpatient basis. The control group received ad lib oral intake. The nutritional intervention group achieved significantly greater weight gain at 4 months after enrollment than the control population (+ 2.4 versus − 0.5 kg, respectively). Of importance, approximately three quarters of the weight gain was achieved during the 3-week inpatient stay. MEP, hand grip strength, and 12-min walk distance improved significantly, and MIP tended to increase in the nutritional intervention group. The indexes of respiratory muscle strength and exercise performance also showed greatest improvement following the period of hospitalization. However, the quality of life and dyspnea indexes were unaffected.

These authors concluded that significant improvements in body weight and limb and respiratory muscle strength could be achieved in depleted patients with COPD. However, improvements required a highly supervised inpatient environment and could be sustained but not enhanced during an outpatient period. Furthermore, important clinical parameters, such as the sense of breathlessness during exercise and the activities of daily living and the subjects' perception of the quality of life, were not made better.

Shridhar and colleagues[91] evaluated the effects of a 4-month outpatient nutritional intervention in 12 patients with COPD. Body weight was < 90 percent ideal. Subjects were instructed to increase caloric intake to 1.3 × REE and consume 1.5 g/kg protein. The study was not controlled. Nutritional supplementation was in the form of an oral supplement. Patients attended a monthly dietetic review at which adherence to the recommended diet was confirmed verbally. Body weight increased insignificantly (+ 0.3 kg). There was

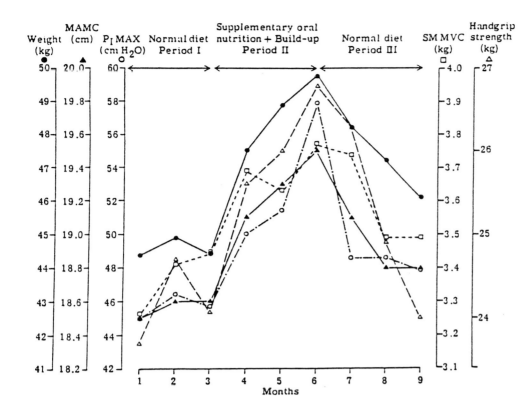

FIGURE 33-4 Effect a nutritionally supplemented diet in stable, outpatients with COPD. Subjects were studied over three 3-month periods (i.e., periods I to III). During period I, subjects consumed a normal diet. During period II, an oral supplement sufficient to raise caloric intake to 2500 kcal was consumed. During period III, subjects returned to their normal diet. Note the progressive increase in all parameters during the 3-month period of nutritional intervention followed by the gradual decline toward baseline values when the intervention was withdrawn. MAMC, midarm muscle circumference; PI-max, maximal static inspiratory pressure; SM MVC, sternomastoid muscle maximal voluntary contractile force. (From Efthimiou et al.,[89] with permission.)

no significant change in anthropomorphic measurements or PI and PEmax.

Schols and associates[9] studied the largest group of subjects with COPD investigated to date, 233 patients enrolled in an inpatient pulmonary rehabilitation program. Subjects with body weight less than 90 percent of ideal and/or fat-free mass less than 67 percent of ideal were defined as depleted. In contrast, subjects whose body weight exceeded 90 percent of ideal and/or fat-free mass greater than 67 percent of ideal body weight were considered to be nondepleted. In 63 percent of the subjects, the REE was greater than 110 percent of the Harris-Benedict reference values. Subjects were randomly allocated to receive (1) placebo alone, (2) supplemental nutrition sufficient to raise caloric intake by 420 kcal/day, or (3) nutritional supplement plus anabolic steroids every 2 weeks (nandrolone decanoate). Interventions were performed for an 8-week period. Subjects remained on their usual medications, and all subjects participated in an intensive regimen of exercise reconditioning in an inpatient setting.

Weight gain occured in both the nutritionally supplemented and nutritional plus anabolic steroid treated group. However, weight gain in the nutritional supplement group consisted primarily of an increase in fat mass, whereas both fat and FFM increased in the nutritional plus anabolic steroid group. Weight gain averaged 3 kg in the nutritional group and 2.6 kg in the nutritional plus anabolic steroid group. Of interest, some subjects in the nutritional group demonstrated increases in weight but decreases in fat-free mass. Conversely, some subjects showed no change in body weight, but significant improvements in fat-free mass. Changes in MIP were greatest in the group receiving the anabolic steroids plus supplementation. Subjects with the greatest increases in FFM demonstrated the greatest improvements in

MIP regardless of changes in body weight. In agreement with the study by Rogers and colleagues,[90] improvements in body composition and respiratory muscle function were not accompanied by improvements in the 12-min walking distance. These authors concluded that nutritional intervention achieved small but significant improvements in body composition and in respiratory muscle function. However, greater improvements could be achieved when the nutritional intervention was coupled with administration of an anabolic steroid.

Taken in aggregate, these studies demonstrate that the depleted state is reversible and that nutritional interventions can produce favorable changes in body composition and muscle function in patients with COPD. However, for most patients, nutritionally induced improvements in respiratory muscle performance are modest and correlate with increases in body weight and, more precisely, fat-free mass. Moreover, gains are made almost exclusively when dietary interventions are performed in a highly structured inpatient environment. It is somewhat disappointing that the gains achieved do not appear to be associated with improvements in exercise performance, the activities of daily living, or the quality of life. The effect of these modest changes in body composition on prognosis await further study. The prospect that greater changes can be accomplished when anabolic steroids are added to an intensive nutritional intervention suggests an additional therapeutic approach which also awaits further study.

At present it seems reasonable to consider nutritional intervention in patients with advanced COPD who are underweight, especially those subjects exhibiting rapid weight loss and/or profound impairment in inspiratory muscle function. The use of dietary supplements should ideally be provided in close consultation with a dietician and requires close supervision and much encouragement of the patient and family. Dietary therapy is essentially benign and may achieve impressive gains in selected, highly motivated patients.

References

1. Schols AMWJ, Soeters PB, Dingemans AMC, et al: Prevalence and characteristics of nutritional depletion in patients with stable COPD eligible for pulmonary rehabilitation. *Am Rev Respir Dis* 147:1151–1156, 1993.
2. Metropolitan Life Insurance Company: New weight standards for men and women. *Stat Bull Metro Insur Co* 64:14, 1983.
3. Stefee WP: Malnutrition in hospitalized patients. *JAMA* 244:2630–2635, 1980.
4. Kelly RM, Russle RM, Greenberg LB, et al: Nutritional status of adult patients in two acute care hospitals: A university hospital and an affiliated veterans administration medical center. *Nutr Res* 2:213–222, 1982.
5. Hunter AMB, Carey MA, Larsh HW: The nutritional status of patients with chronic obstructive pulmonary disease. *Am Rev Respir Dis* 124:376–381, 1981.
6. Openbrier DR, Irwin MM, Rogers RM, et al: Nutritional status and lung function in patients with emphysema and chronic bronchitis. *Chest* 83:17–22, 1983.
7. Wilson DO, Rogers RM, Wright EC, et al: Body weight in chronic obstructive pulmonary disease: The National Institutes of Health Intermittent Positive-Pressure Breathing Trial. *Am Rev Respir Dis* 139:1435–1438, 1989.
8. Laaban JP, Kouchakji B, Dore MF, et al: Nutritional status of patients with chronic obstructive pulmonary disease and acute respiratory failure. *Chest* 103:1362–1368, 1993.
9. Schols AMWJ, Soeters PB, Mostert R, et al: Physiologic effects of nutritional support and anabolic steroids in patients with chronic obstructive pulmonary disease. *Am J Respir Crit Care Med* 152:1268, 1995.
10. Dornhurst A: Respiratory insufficiency. *Lancet* 1:1185–1187, 1955.
11. Renzetti AD, McClement JG, Litt BD: The Veterans Administration Cooperative Study of Pulmonary Function. Mortality in relation to respiratory function in chronic obstructive pulmonary disease. *Am J Med* 41:115–129, 1966.
12. Vanderburg E, Van de Woestigne K, Gyselen A: Weight changes in the terminal stages of chronic obstructive lung disease. *Am Rev Respir Dis* 96:556–565, 1967.
13. Traverse GA, Cline MG, Burrows B: Predictors of mortality in chronic obstructive pulmonary disease. *Am Rev Respir Dis* 119:895–902, 1979.
14. Sahebjami H, Vassalo CL: Effects of starvation and refeeding on lung mechanics and morphometry. *Am Rev Respir Dis* 119:443–451, 1979.
15. Kinney JM, Weissman C: Forms of malnutrition in stressed and unstressed patients. *Clin Chest Med* 7:19–28, 1986.
16. Kelsen SG, Ference M, Kapoor S: Effects of prolonged undernutrition on structure and function of the diaphragm. *J Appl Physiol* 58:1354–1359, 1985.
17. Sieck GC, Lewis MI, Blanco CE: Effects of undernutrition on diaphragm fiber size, SDH activity, and fatigue resistance. *J Appl Physiol* 66:2196–2205, 1989.
18. Derenne J-P, Macklem PT, Roussos C: State of the art: The respiratory muscles: Mechanics, control, and pathophysiology. Parts I, II, III. *Am Rev Respir Dis* 118:119–133, 373–389, 581–601, 1978.
19. Kelsen SG: The effects of undernutrition on the respiratory muscles. *Clin Chest Med* 7(1):101–110, 1986.
20. Henneman E, Mendell LM: Functional organization of motorneuron pool and its inputs, in Brooks VB (ed): *Handbook of Physiology*, vol 2, *The Nervous System: Motor Control*. Bethesda, MD, American Physiological Society, 1981:423–508.
21. Fournier M, Sieck G: Mechanical properties of motor units in the cat diaphragm. *J Neurophysiol* 59:1055–1066, 1988.
22. Rannels DE, Pegg AE, Rannels SR, et al: Effect of starvation on initiation of protein synthesis in skeletal muscle and heart. *Am J Physiol* 235:E126–133, 1978.
23. Preedy VR, Smith DM, Sugden PH: A comparison of rates of protein turnover in rat diaphragm in vivo and in vitro. *Biochem* 233:279–282, 1986.
24. Lewis MI, Sieck GC, Fournier M, et al: Effect of nutritional deprivation on diaphragm contractility and muscle fiber size. *J Appl Physiol* 60:596–603, 1986.
25. Shindoh C, Dimarco A, Lust W, et al: Effect of acute fasting on diaphragm strength and endurance. *Am Rev Respir Dis* 144:488–493, 1991.
26. Lewis MI, Sieck GC, Fournier M: Effect of acute nutritional deprivation on diaphragm structure and function. *J Appl Physiol* 68:1938, 1990.
27. Donohoe M, Rogers RM: Nutritional assessment and support in chronic obstructive pulmonary disease. *Clin Chest Med* 11:487–504, 1990.
28. Steele RH, Heard BE: Size of the diaphragm in chronic bronchitis. *Thorax* 28:55–60, 1973.
29. Ishikawa S, Hayes JA: Functional morphometry of the diaphragm in patients with chronic obstructive lung disease. *Am Rev Respir Dis* 1208:135–138, 1973.
30. Butler C: Diaphragmatic change in emphysema. *Am Rev Respir Dis* 114:155–159, 1976.
31. Thurlbeck WM: Diaphragm and body weight in emphysema. *Thorax* 33:483–487, 1978.
32. Arora NS, Rochester DF: COPD and human diaphragm dimensions. *Chest* 91:719–724, 1987.
33. Arora NS, Rochester DF: Respiratory muscle strength and maximal voluntary ventilation in undernourished patients. *Am Rev Resp Dis* 126:5–8, 1982.
34. Kelley SM, Rose A, Field S, et al: Inspiratory muscle strength and body composition in patients receiving total parenteral nutrition therapy. *Am Rev Respir Dis* 130:33–37, 1984.
35. Sahebjami H: Nutritional and the pulmonary parenchyma. *Clin Chest Med* 7:111–130, 1986.
36. Kerr JS, Riley DJ, Lanza-Jacoby S, et al: Nutritional emphysema in the rat: Influence of protein depletion and impaired lung growth. *Am Rev Respir Dis* 131:644–650, 1985.
37. Keys A, Brozek J, Henschel A, et al: *Biology of Human Starvation*. Minneapolis, University of Minnesota Press, 1950:601–606.
38. Rochester DF, Esau SA: Malnutrition and the respiratory system. *Chest* 55:441–445, 1984.
39. Sukumalchantra Y, Williams MH: Serial studies on pulmonary function in patients with chronic obstructive pulmonary disease. *Am J Med* 39:941–945, 1965.
40. Swift RW, French CF: Energy metabolism and nutrition. Washington DC, Scarecrow Press, 1954:14–32.
41. Donahoe M, Rogers RM, Wilson DO, et al: Oxygen consumption of the respiratory muscle in normal and malnourished patients with chronic obstructive pulmonary disease. *Am Rev Respir Dis* 140:385–391, 1989.
42. Goldstein S, Askanazi J, Weissman C, et al: Energy expenditure in patients with chronic obstructive pulmonary disease. *Chest* 91:222–224, 1987.
43. Goldstein SA, Thomashow BW, Kvetan V, et al: Nitrogen and energy relationships in malnourished patients with emphysema. *Am Rev Respir Dis* 138:636–644, 1988.
44. Wilson DO, Donahoe M, Rogers RM, et al: Metabolic rate and weight loss in chronic obstructive lung disease. *J Parenter Enter Nutr* 14:7–11, 1990.
45. Schols AMWJ, Soeters PB, Mostert R, et al: Energy balance in chronic obstructive pulmonary disease. *Am Rev Respir Dis* 143:1248–1252, 1991.
46. Schols AMWJ, Fredrix EWHM, Soeters PB, et al: Resting energy

expenditure in patients with chronic obstructive pulmonary disease. *Am J Clin Nutr* 54:983, 1991.

47. Schols AMWJ, Schoffelen P, Ceulemans H, et al: Measurement of resting energy expenditure in patients with COPD in a clinical setting. *J Parenter Enter Nutr* 16:364–368, 1992.

48. Green JH: Comparisons between basal metabolic rate and diet-induced thermogenesis in different types of chronic obstructive pulmonary disease. *Clin Sci* 83:109, 1992.

49. Cherniack RM: The oxygen consumption and efficiency of the respiratory muscle in health and emphysema. *J Clin Invest* 38:494–498, 1959.

50. Sharp J, Danon TJ, Druz WS, et al: Respiratory muscle function in patients with chronic obstructive pulmonary disease. Its relationship to disability and to respiratory therapy. *Am Rev Respir Dis* 110:154–167, 1974.

51. Amoroso P, Wilson SR, Moxham J, et al: Acute effects of inhaled salbutamol on the metabolic rate of normal subjects. *Thorax* 43:882–885, 1993.

52. De Godoy I, Donahoe M, Calhoun WJ, et al: Elevated TNF-α production by peripheral blood monocytes of weight-losing COPD patients. *Am Rev Respir Dis* 153:33–37, 1996.

53. Browning RJ, Olsen AM: The functional gastrointestinal disorders of pulmonary emphysema. *Mayo Clin Proc* 36:537–543, 1961.

54. Schols A, Mostert R, Cobben N, et al: Transcutaneous oxygen saturation and carbon dioxide tension during meals in patients with chronic obstructive pulmonary disease. *Chest* 100:1287–1292, 1991.

55. Schols AMWJ, Schlosser MAG, Wouters EMF: The role of psychology in nutritional assessment of COPD. *Am Rev Respir Dis* 143:A806, 1991.

56. Milledge JS: Arterial oxygen desaturation and intestinal absorption of xylose. *Br Med J* 3:557–558, 1972.

57. Millward DJ, Waterlow JC: Effect of nutrition on protein turnover in skeletal muscle. *Fed Proc* 37:2283–2290, 1978.

58. Vaisman N, Hahn T: Tumor necrosis factor-α and anorexia—cause or effect? *Metabolism* 40:720–723, 1991.

59. Detsky AS, Baker JP, Mendelson RA, et al: Evaluating the accuracy of nutritional assessment techniques applied to hospitalized patients: Methodology and comparisons. *J Parenter Enter Nutr* 8:153–159, 1984.

60. Knapp TR: A methodological critique of the "ideal weight" concept. *JAMA* 250:506–510, 1983.

61. Braun SR, Keim NL, Dison RM, et al: The prevalence and determinants of nutritional changes in chronic obstructive pulmonary disease. *Chest* 86:558–563, 1984.

62. Fuller NJ, Jebb SA, Goldberg GR, et al: Inter-observer variability in the measurement of body composition. *Eur J Clin Nutr* 45:43, 1991.

63. Manning EMC: Nutritional assessment in the critically ill. *Crit Care Clin* 11:603, 1995.

64. Young VR, Munro HN: *N*-Methylhistidine (3-methylhistidine) and muscle protein turnover: An overview. *Fed Proc* 37:2291–2300, 1978.

65. Driver AG, McAlevy MT, Smith JL: Nutritional assessment of patients with chronic obstructive pulmonary disease and acute respiratory failure. *Chest* 82:568–571, 1982.

66. Fuenzalida CE, Petty TL, Jones ML, et al: The immune response to short-term nutritional intervention in advanced chronic obstruction pulmonary disease. *Am Rev Respir Dis* 142:49–56, 1990.

67. Harvey KB, Moldawer LL, Bistrian BR, et al: Biological measures for the formulation of a hospital prognostic index. *Am J Clin Nutr* 34:2013–2022, 1981.

68. Harris JA, Benedict FG: A biometric study of the basal metabolism in man. *Carnegie Institute* 279, 1919.

69. Head CA, McManus CB, Seitz S, et al: A simple and accurate indirect calorimetry system for assessment of resting energy expenditure. *J Parenter Enter Nutr* 8:45–48, 1984.

70. Harmon GS, Pingleton SK: Energy (calorie) requirements in mechanically ventilated COPD patients. *Am Rev Respir Dis* 131(A):203, 1986.

71. Cortes V, Nelson LD: Errors in estimating energy expenditure in critically ill surgical patients. *Arch Surg* 124:287–290, 1989.

72. Askanazi J, Weissman C, Rosenbaum H, et al: Nutrition and the respiratory system. *Crit Care Med* 10:163–172, 1982.

73. Wojnar MM, Hawkins WG, Lang CH: Nutritional support of the septic patient. *Crit Care Clin* 11:717–733, 1995.

74. Pingleton SK, Harmon GS: Nutritional management in acute respiratory failure. *JAMA* 257:3094–3099, 1987.

75. Askanazi J, Weissman C, LaSala PA, et al: Effect of protein intake on ventilatory drive. *Anesthesiology* 60:160, 1984.

76. Zwillich CW, Sahn SA, Weil JA: Effects of hypermetabolism on ventilation and chemosensitivity. *J Clin Invest* 60:900–906, 1977.

77. Brown SE, Wiener S, Brown RA, et al: Exercise performance following a carbohydrate load in chronic airflow obstruction. *J Appl Physiol* 58:1340–1346, 1985.

78. Gieseke T, Gurushanthaiah G, Glauser FL, et al: Effects of carbohydrates on carbon dioxide excretion in patients with airways disease. *Chest* 71:55–58, 1977.

79. Angelillo VA, Bedi S, Durfee D, et al: Effects of low and high carbohydrate feedings in ambulatory patients with chronic obstructive pulmonary disease and chronic hypercapnia. *Ann Intern Med* 103:883–885, 1985.

80. Talbot GD, Frayser R: Hyperlipidemia: A cause of decreased oxygen saturation. *Nature* 200:684, 1963.

81. Sundstrom G, Zauner CW, Mans A Jr: Decrease in pulmonary diffusing capacity during lipid infusion in healthy men. *J Appl Physiol* 34:816–820, 1973.

82. Greene HL, Hazlett D, Demaree R: Relationship between intralipid-induced hyperlipemia and pulmonary function. *Am J Clin Nutr* 29:127–135, 1976.

83. Jarnberg PO, Lindholm M, Eklund J: Lipid infusion in critically ill patients. Acute effects on hemodynamics and pulmonary gas exchange. *Crit Care Med* 9:27–31, 1981.

84. Mckeen CR, Brigham KL, Bowers RE, et al: Pulmonary vascular effects of fat emulsion infusion in unanesthetized sheep. *J Clin Invest* 61:1291–1297, 1978.

85. Knowles JB, Farbane MD, Wiggs DJ, et al: Dietary supplementation and respiratory muscle performance in patients with COPD. *Chest* 93:997–983, 1988.

86. Wilson DO, Rogers RM, Sanders MH, et al: Nutritional intervention in malnourished patients with emphysema. *Am Rev Respir Dis* 134:672–677, 1986.

87. Lewis MI, Belman MJ, Door-Uyemura L: Nutritional supplementation in ambulatory patients with chronic obstructive pulmonary disease. *Am Rev Respir Dis* 135:1062–1068, 1987.

88. Whitaker JS, Ryan CF, Buckley PA, et al: The effects of refeeding on peripheral and respiratory muscle function in malnourished chronic obstructive pulmonary disease patients. *Am Rev Respir Dis* 142:283–288, 1990.

89. Efthimiou J, Fleming J, Gomes C, et al: The effect of supplementary oral nutrition in poorly nourished patients with chronic obstructive pulmonary disease. *Am Rev Respir Dis* 137:1075–1082, 1988.

90. Rogers RM, Donahoe M, Constantino J: Physiologic effects of oral supplementation feeding in malnourished patients with chronic obstructive pulmonary disease. *Am Rev Respir Dis* 146:1511–1517, 1992.

91. Shridhar MD, Galloway A, Lean EMJ, et al: An out-patient nutritional programme in COPD patients. *Eur Respir* 7:720–724, 1994.

Chapter 34
EXERCISE RETRAINING

SANFORD LEVINE
BRUCE D. JOHNSON
TAITAN NGUYEN
KEVIN McCULLY

At present, exercise training is considered an essential component of a pulmonary rehabilitation program.[1-6] This chapter reviews the physiologic and biochemical bases of exercise training. Since most studies have concerned patients with chronic obstructive pulmonary disease (COPD), the focus is on this disease entity. However, the authors' comments are also germane to patients with interstitial lung disease.

Historical Background

Prior to the work of Barach and associates,[2,7] pulmonary physicians recommended that patients rest and avoid dyspnea. Indeed some of the pulmonary literature early in this century contains the assumption that dyspnea per se is harmful to patients with COPD. Viewing this approach retrospectively, Fig. 34-1 indicates that these physicians were converting patients who experienced dyspnea on mild to moderate exertion into deconditioned patients who experienced both dyspnea and fatigue while carrying out activities of daily living (ADL).

In 1952, Barach and coworkers[2,7] reported "an exercise program was instituted with subsequent marked improvement of capacity to exercise.... The progressive improvement in ability to walk without dyspnea suggested that a physiologic response similar to a training program in athletes may have been produced." As a result of this pioneering work and those of others,[8,9] virtually every current pulmonary rehabilitation program time contains an exercise component.

Evidence That an Exercise Program Is an Essential Component of a Pulmonary Rehabilitation Program

In the opinion of these authors, the strongest case for this concept is provided by the study of Toshima and Ries.[10] These investigators randomized 119 patients with COPD either to a comprehensive rehabilitation program including exercise reconditioning or to an educational control program. The exercise group received education, physical and respiratory therapy, psychosocial support, and supervised exercise training for 8 weeks, whereas the control group received twice-weekly classroom instruction in respiratory therapy, pharmacology, and diet, but did not exercise. Before and after the study, and for an additional 6 months, both groups underwent physiologic and psychosocial tests. The major finding of this study was that at 8 weeks the exercise group showed a mean increase in endurance walking time (on the treadmill) from 12.5 to 23 min compared with a nonstatistically signifi-

cant increase in the control group from 11 to 13 min. At 6 months, the exercise group maintained its advantage by exhibiting a treadmill endurance of approximately 21 min compared with 12 min in the control group. This study supports the notion that exercise therapy is an essential component of a successful pulmonary rehabilitation program.

The studies of O'Donnell's[11] and Reardon's[12] groups support the conclusions of Toshima and Ries.[10] However, these papers (or any other in the literature) do not demonstrate unequivocally that exercise training is an essential component of a pulmonary rehabilitation program. These authors believe that an adequate test of this hypothesis would require a control group which receives exactly the same treatment (i.e., same amounts of the following: contact with health care professionals, therapeutic expectation, education, number of diagnostic tests) as the experimental group. Additionally, to control for unexpected variation (e.g., air pollution indexes), the exercise group and the control group should be studied over the same period of time. Moreover, the outcome measurements of this proposed clinical trial must include ADL.

Philosophical Approach to Exercise Retraining

Figure 34-2 presents a model which indicates these authors' approach to exercise training. In this model, exercise tolerance or the lack of it is attributed to an interaction of the following four physiologic systems: musculoskeletal, respiratory, circulatory, and central nervous. The left panel shows that in healthy individuals, all systems are functioning at 100 percent of capacity, and therefore $\dot{V}_{O_2}$ max is 100 percent of predicted. The middle panel depicts the situation after the previously healthy individual develops an acute nonreversible lung disease which reduces respiratory system function to 45 percent of capacity. Simple linear control theory suggests that this "weak link" would limit the individual's $\dot{V}_{O_2}$ max to 45 percent of predicted.

Since the $\dot{V}_{O_2}$ max is markedly decreased, this individual will no longer be able to engage in strenuous physical activity. Therefore, even if it is assumed that the respiratory impairment remains constant, the right-hand panel indicates that the other three systems in this model will show adaptations of deconditioning. The stippled areas indicate that these deconditioning adaptations can cause the individual to have an even lower $\dot{V}_{O_2}$ max than that predicted by his or her lung disease. A major responsibility of the health care professional concerned with respiratory rehabilitation is to ensure that this scenario does not occur.

RELATIONSHIPS AMONG NORMAL, TRAINED, AND DECONDITIONED STATES

For the purpose of this chapter, maximal O_2 uptake ($\dot{V}_{O_2}$ max) expressed in milliliters per minute per kilogram is used to define these states. Since age and gender are major determinants of $\dot{V}_{O_2}$ max,[13-16] these terms are used to predict $\dot{V}_{O_2}$ max for specific individuals. A normal individual has a $\dot{V}_{O_2}$ max which falls within the range predicted by age and gender. A deconditioned individual has a lower than predicted $\dot{V}_{O_2}$ max, whereas a trained individual has a higher than predicted $\dot{V}_{O_2}$ max. A central concept of this chapter is

417

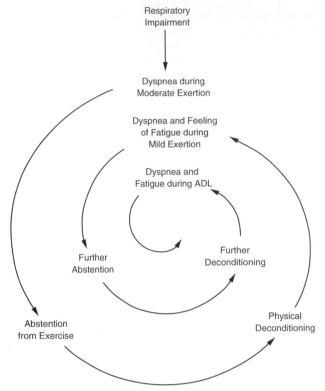

FIGURE 34-1 Dyspnea-deconditioning cycle. The schematic illustrates the progression from dyspnea during moderate exertion through progressive deconditioning; this progression leads to a deconditioned patient experiencing dyspnea during normal activities of daily living (ADL).

that these three states represent specific points on the following fitness continuum:

$$\text{deconditioned} \leftrightarrow \text{normal} \leftrightarrow \text{trained}$$

Therefore, a normal subject whose physical activity becomes markedly decreased (e.g., due to bed rest) will exhibit a decrease in $\dot{V}_{O_2}$ max; the term deconditioning is used to refer to this process. In contrast, a deconditioned subject who undergoes an endurance training program (see below) will increase $\dot{V}_{O_2}$ max to (or toward) the normal range; the term *training*, or *reconditioning*, is used to refer to this process.

Types of Exercise Training

In sports medicine, a distinction is made between two types of training, aerobic, or endurance, and strength. Endurance exercise seeks to improve an athlete's ability to perform sustained tasks, and this is the type of training utilized by long-distance runners, swimmers, rowers, bicyclists, and other athletes. In contrast, strength training seeks to improve an individual's ability to perform explosive tasks, and this type of training is used by jumpers, shot putters, weight lifters, and other athletes.[13,16] Whereas some pulmonary exercise programs have a strength component, all these programs utilize endurance exercise training, and this review focuses on this latter type of therapy. For the purpose of this chapter, endurance exercise training[17] is characterized by the following

triad: (1) it uses large muscle groups; (2) it can be maintained continuously in a rhythmic manner; and (3) the adenosine triphosphate (ATP) utilized for this type of exercise is largely provided by aerobic oxidative pathways (although a small anaerobic component may also be present).

Adaptations Elicited by Endurance Training

Table 34-1 presents the adaptations elicited in normal subjects by adequate endurance training, and this section assesses the evidence on whether endurance exercise training can elicit the same or similar adaptations in subjects with COPD.

GLOBAL EXERCISE PERFORMANCE

Casaburi and associates[18] studied global exercise performance (see Table 34-1) before and after their patients with COPD carried out a high-endurance bicycle ergometer training protocol for 8 weeks (5 days/week). The exercise intensity was approximately equal to 80 percent of $\dot{V}_{O_2}$ max. The closed circles in Fig. 34-3 represent pretraining values, and the open circles represent posttraining measurements.

The left set of panels depicts the results of an incremental test carried out on the bicycle ergometer; it shows that this type of endurance exercise training increases $\dot{V}_{O_2}$max [as well as maximum pulmonary carbon dioxide elimination ($\dot{V}_{CO_2}$ max)]. Additionally, it shows that the arterial blood lactate concentration ([art. lactate]) is less at any given work rate in the posttraining test. Lastly, the maximum ventilation (i.e., $\dot{V}_E$ max) is also increased posttraining.

The middle panels show the results of pre- and posttraining high constant work rate tests; this work rate was calculated from the preexercise incremental test, and it corresponded to the sum of (1) the lactate threshold (i.e., the $\dot{V}_{O_2}$ at which [art. lactate] begins to rapidly increase) and (2) 60 percent of the difference in $\dot{V}_{O_2}$ between the lactate threshold and $\dot{V}_{O_2}$ max. First, the panel shows that training prolonged the time that the patient with COPD was able to carry out this exercise (i.e., for the full 15-min time period). Additionally, [art. lactate] in the posttraining test is less than that measured pretraining.

The right-hand panels show the results of pre- and posttraining exercise tests carried out at a low constant work rate (i.e., a $\dot{V}_{O_2}$ corresponding to 90 percent of the pretraining lactate threshold). Both before and after training, the patient is able to carry out the work rate for the full 15 min. However, posttraining exercise is associated with a lower [art. lactate].

This study of Casaburi and colleagues[18] documents that endurance exercise training can produce the same global functional adaptations in COPD as those elicited in normal subjects.

MUSCULOSKELETAL SYSTEM

IMPORTANCE OF LEG EFFORT AS A SYMPTOM LIMITING EXERCISE

Killian and associates[19] recently analyzed the results of incremental exercise tests on the bicycle ergometer in 97 patients with COPD and 320 control subjects. At each work level, both control and COPD subjects rated both dyspnea and leg

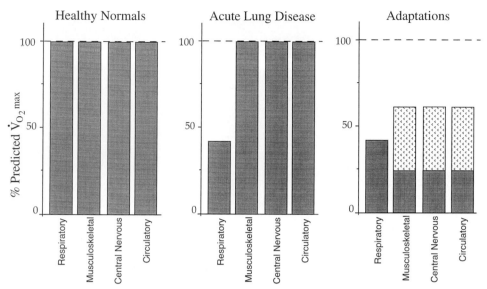

FIGURE 34-2 This simplified schematic indicates that four systems (i.e., respiratory, circulatory, musculoskeletal, central nervous) determine the magnitude of the exercise intolerance exhibited by the patient with chronic respiratory disease. The *left panel* illustrates the situation prior to the onset of respiratory disease; all these systems are functioning optimally and the patient's exercise tolerance is normal (i.e., 100 percent predicted $\dot{V}_{O_2}$ max). The *middle panel* indicates the onset of acute pulmonary disease which is severe enough to decrease the patient's predicted $\dot{V}_{O_2}$ max to 45 percent. This respiratory impair-

ment persists, and the other systems adapt to the increased sedentary nature of the patient dictated by his or her respiratory system disease (*right panel*). The *right panel* shows that these adaptations are of two types: an unavoidable component represented by the solid gray area and a component which can be prevented by exercise training depicted by the dotted area above the solid gray area. The figure indicates that even though the respiratory impairment causes the patient's $\dot{V}_{O_2}$max to decrease to 45 percent of predicted, failure to institute exercise training can result in $\dot{V}_{O_2}$max being limited to 25 percent of predicted.

effort on the 10-point Borg scale (see Fig. 34-4). As expected, patients with COPD stopped exercising at lower work rates, lower proportions of heart rate relative to maximum age-predicted heart rate, and higher fractions of $\dot{V}_E$ max relative to their estimate of $\dot{V}_E$ max. It is important that these investigators noted that at end-exercise, the median intensity of dyspnea (6, severe to very severe) and leg effort (7, very severe) was the same in both COPD and control groups. The rating of dyspnea exceeded that of leg effort in 26 percent of the COPD group and in 22 percent of the control group;

in contrast, the level of leg effort exceeded dyspnea in 43 percent of COPD subjects and 36 percent of control subjects. Lastly, both symptoms were rated equally in 31 percent of COPD subjects and 42 percent of controls. This report by Killian's group suggests that the sensation of leg effort may be as important in terminating incremental exercise in COPD patients as that of dyspnea.

OVERVIEW OF DECONDITIONING AND TRAINING IN LIMB MUSCLES

Human muscle is composed of one slow-twitch fiber type (i.e., type I) and three fast-twitch fiber types (i.e., types IIa, IIx, and IIb); Table 34-2 characterizes the different fiber types.[20] Four concepts are critical for the subsequent discussion. First, endurance training is associated with fast-to-slow fiber type transformations (i.e., IIb → IIx → IIa → I), whereas deconditioning is associated with slow-to-fast fiber type transformations (i.e., I → IIa → IIx → IIb). Second, some adaptations elicited by both training and deconditioning occur relatively quickly (e.g., mitochondrial oxidative enzyme activities which can show large changes within several weeks), whereas other adaptations [e.g., changes in myosin heavy chain (MHC) or capillarity] can take many months.[20,21] Third, different muscles as well as different regions of the same muscle have different fiber type proportions. Fourth and last, heredity is also a factor in determining fiber type proportions.[17,20,21]

EFFECT OF DECONDITIONING AND TRAINING ON MYOSIN AND FIBER TYPE ADAPTATIONS

Myosin is the ATPase in the muscle fiber which accounts for more than 80 percent of its ATP consumption during

TABLE 34-1 Adaptations Elicited by Endurance Training

Global exercise performance
  ↑ $\dot{V}_{O_2}$ max
  ↑ Duration of exercise at submaximal levels of work
  ↓ Blood lactate concentrations at submaximal exercise
Musculoskeletal system (trained limb muscle)
  ↑ Capacity for aerobic oxidation of fat and carbohydrate
  Fast-to-slow transformation of myosin heavy chains (MHC)
Respiratory system
  Functional: ↑ in "clinical tests of ventilatory muscle endurance"
  Structural: fast to slow transformation of myofibrillar proteins
Circulatory system
  Cardiac: ↑ maximum cardiac output due to ↑ stroke volume; additionally ↓ heart rate at rest and submaximal exercise
  Peripheral vasculature: ↑ capillarity of trained limb muscles
Central nervous system
  ↑ Sense of well-being

SOURCE: References 16, 59, and 60.

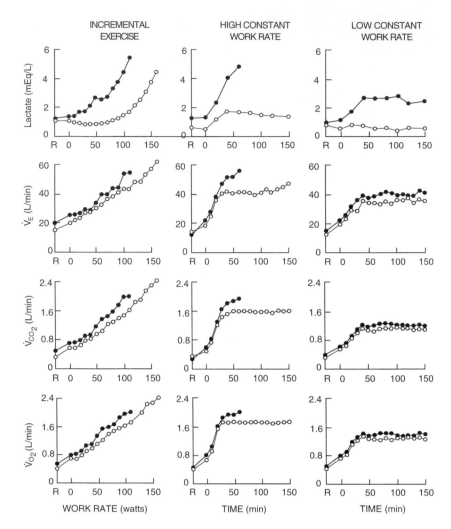

FIGURE 34-3 Relationships among $\dot{V}_E$, $\dot{V}_{O_2}$, carbon dioxide production ($\dot{V}_{CO_2}$) and arterial lactate concentration in patients with mild-to-moderate COPD. In all three panels, closed symbols represent pretraining data, whereas open symbols indicate posttraining data. The *left panel* shows responses to an incremental leg cycle ergometer test. The *middle panel* presents responses to a high-rate constant work test at a $\dot{V}_{O_2}$ between the lactate threshold (i.e., the $\dot{V}_{O_2}$ at which arterial blood lactate concentration begins to rapidly increase) and $\dot{V}_{O_2}$max. The *right panel* depicts responses to a low rate constant work test (i.e., at a $\dot{V}_{O_2}$ below the lactate threshold).

activity.[20,21] The MHC is the portion of the myosin molecule which determines the fiber type according to the most common method of classifying muscle fiber types.[22] Despite the classic studies of Saltin and Gollnick,[21] the literature does not contain any longitudinal data on the effect of deconditioning of the limb muscles of normal individuals on MHC or fiber type proportions. However, the observations of Larsson and Ansved[23] do provide longitudinal data on changes in fiber type proportions elicited by detraining 11 elite male athletes for a 1-year period and found that deconditioning elicited statistically significant decreases in the proportion of type I fibers in the quadriceps and deltoid muscles. Additionally, Jakobsson and associates[24] reported that patients with severe COPD contain a smaller proportion of type I fibers in the gastrocnemius muscle than do "normal subjects from the literature." Although one can fault this study because of the absence of longitudinal (i.e., pre- and post-) data, the conclusions of Jakobsson and associates are consistent with the observations of Larsson and Ansved as well as much animal data in the literature.[25–27] Accordingly, reasonable evidence exists to support the notion that deconditioning (i.e., relative or absolute) is accompanied by slow-to-fast transformations in limb muscle fiber types of both COPD and normal subjects.

In contrast to deconditioning, endurance exercise training elicits adaptations in MHCs characterized by fast-to-slow transformation. The data of Coggan's group[28] show that treadmill exercise training at 80 percent of maximum heart rate 4 days/week for 9 to 12 months decreases type IIb fibers, increases type IIa fibers, and causes no change in type I fibers. These observations indicate that endurance training can elicit fast-to-slow adaptations in human limb muscles. However, very few programs involving exercise training in patients with chronic respiratory disease (CRD) have been carried out for prolonged periods of time.[29–32] In those which have, fiber type or myosin heavy chain proportions were not assessed, so it is not known whether an exercise training program can cause these changes in the limb muscles of patients with COPD.

EFFECT OF DECONDITIONING AND TRAINING ON MITOCHONDRIAL OXIDATIVE ENZYME ACTIVITIES

Much work has demonstrated that muscles adapt to deconditioning by decreasing the activities of aerobic oxidative enzymes without changing the activities of the glycolytic enzymes. Recently, Maltais and associates[33] measured the enzymatic activities of three glycolytic enzymes [lactate dehydrogenase (LDH), hexokinase (HK), phosphofructoki-

0	Nothing at all
0.5	Very very slight (just noticeable)
1	Very slight
2	Slight
3	Moderate
4	Somewhat severe
5	Severe
6	
7	Very severe
8	
9	Very very severe (almost maximum)
10	Maximum

FIGURE 34-4 Borg scale. A perceived symptom scale which can be used to rate symptoms of breathlessness and limb muscle effort during exercise testing and activities of daily living (ADL). (Adapted from Borg GAV: Psychophysical bases of perceived exertion. *Med Sci Sports Exerc* 14:377–381, 1982, with permission.)

nase (PFK)] and two oxidative enzymes [citrate synthase (CS), beta-hydroxyacyl CoA dehydrogenase (HADH)] in biopsies of the vastus lateralis of nine patients with COPD (age 62 ± 2 years, $FEV_{1.0}$ 40 ± 3 percent predicted) and nine normal control patients of similar age. First, they noted that COPD and normal subjects did not differ with respect to LDH, HK, and PFK activities, but the activities of CS and HADH were less in the COPD patients than in the normal subjects. Once again, this study suggests that COPD patients are deconditioned but lacks longitudinal data.

In a subsequent study, Maltais and colleagues[34] studied 11 patients with COPD (age 65 ± 2 years; $FEV_{1.0}$ 36 ± 3 percent predicted; $\dot{V}_{O_2}$ max 54 ± 2 percent predicted) before and after bicycle ergometer exercise endurance training at a target work rate of 80 percent $\dot{V}_{O_2}$ max for 30-min sessions at a frequency of three times per week for 12 weeks. During the initial phases of the program, none of the subjects were able to maintain this exercise intensity; however, the exercise intensity that they could maintain progressively rose from 15 ± 3 to 69 ± 3 percent over the course of the program. By the end of the program, $\dot{V}_{O_2}$ max had increased by 14 percent and arterial lactate concentration fell from 3.4 ± 0.40 to 2.8 ± 0.27 mmol / L at the same (i.e., iso) workload. This type of training elicited no change in the glycolytic enzyme (i.e., LDH, HK, PFK) activities of the vastus lateralis, but the activities of CS and HADH increased by approximately 15 and

40 percent, respectively. Moreover, a statistically significant inverse relationship was found between the percent increases in each of these enzymes and the percent decrease in [art. lactate] at the same work rate. Thus, latter finding suggests that the increases in leg muscle oxidative enzyme activities attenuated the exercise-induced increase in [art. lactate]. Thus, endurance exercise training can elicit oxidative enzyme adaptations in the limb muscles of patients with COPD similar to those seen in normal subjects.

MAGNETIC RESONANCE SPECTROSCOPY—A NEW NONINVASIVE METHOD FOR EVALUATING THE EFFECTS OF ENDURANCE TRAINING

To examine the consequences of both endurance exercise and deconditioning on limb muscles, investigators[35-37] have begun to utilize magnetic resonance spectroscopy (MRS). Figure 34-5 shows some representative ^{31}P NMR spectra from the gastrocnemius muscle of a 35-year-old normal female at rest and during plantar flexion. As indicated, the lower spectrum shows resting measurements averaged over a 1-min time interval, whereas the middle and upper spectra represent submaximal and maximal exercise, respectively; each of these latter spectra represent 8-s averages. The resting spectra show five peaks of interest; i.e., from left to right, these peaks represent inorganic phosphate (Pi), phosphocreatine (PCr), and the gamma-, alpha-, and beta phosphate groups of ATP. A shift of the Pi peak to the right indicates a decrease in pH. Submaximal exercise is characterized by an increase in Pi, a decrease in PCr, and no appreciable change in pH.[35,37] Maximal exercise is characterized by further increases in Pi and decreases in PCr. However, in contrast to submaximal exercise, the Pi peak moves to the right (i.e., toward the PCr peak), reflecting a decrease in pH.[37]

In using magnetic resonance spectra to evaluate the effect of endurance training or deconditioning, the two key measurements are the changes in PCr concentration ([PCr]) and pH elicited by exercise of the relevant limb in the magnet. The change in [PCr] is used as a measure of the activity of the mitochondrial enzymes concerned with oxidative phosphorylation. [PCr] is used as a measure of oxidative enzyme activity because the "phosphocreatine shuttle"[38-40] serves as both a spatial and temporal buffer of the phosphate potential {i.e., [ATP]/ ([ADP] [Pi])} throughout the muscle fiber. A constant or a small decrease in [PCr] during exercise suggests that oxidative phosphorylation is adequate to maintain the phosphate potential, whereas appreciable reductions in [PCr] indicate that this mechanism is unable to maintain the phosphate potential. In this latter case, the muscle fibers will utilize a higher glycolytic flux to generate the necessary ATP, and the accompanying increase in the concentration of lactic

TABLE 34-2 Comparison of Muscle Fiber Types in Human Limb Muscles

Fiber Type	I	IIa	IIx	IIb
Predominant MHC isoform	I	IIa	IIx	IIb
Contractile speed	Slow	Fast	Fast	Fast
Myofibrillar ATPase activity	Low	Moderately high	High	High
Glycolytic enzyme activities	Low	Moderately high	High	High
Mitochondrial oxidative enzyme activities	High	High	Moderately high	Low

NOTE: MHC, myosin heavy chain.
SOURCE: References 20 and 21.

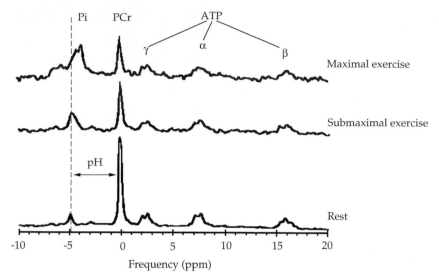

FIGURE 34-5 Magnetic resonance spectroscopy. ^{31}P NMR spectra from a 35-year-old normal subject at rest and during plantar flexion. As indicated, the lower spectrum shows rest measurements averaged over a 1-min time interval, whereas the middle and upper spectra represent submaximal and maximal exercise, respectively; each of these latter spectra represent 8-s averages. The resting spectra show five peaks of interest; that is, from left to right, these peaks represent inorganic phosphate (Pi), phos- phocreatine (PCr), and the gamma-, alpha-, and beta-phosphate groups of adenosine triphosphate (ATP). A shift of the Pi peak to the right indicates a decrease in pH. Submaximal exercise is characterized by an increase in Pi, a decrease in PCr, and no appreciable change in pH. Maximal exercise is characterized by further increases in Pi and decreases in PCr as well as the development of an appreciable decrease in pH manifest by a shift to the right in the Pi peak (i.e., toward the PCr peak).

acid will diminish muscle pH. Therefore, endurance-trained muscle will show less decrease in [PCr] and less decrease in pH than non-endurance-trained muscle.[41] Conversely, deconditioned muscle will show larger decrements in both [PCr] and pH than normal muscle.

Kutsuzawa and coworkers[42] used MRS to compare the extent of training or detraining in the forearm muscles of nine patients with COPD and nine age-matched normal controls. The exercise consisted of repetitive gripping of a lever attached to a 2-kg weight via a pulley system until the weight moved a specified distance; this was carried out at a rate of 20 per minute for 6 min. Figure 34-6 shows [PCr]/([PCr] + [Pi]) measurements on the ordinate for the two groups plotted against time on the abscissa. The figure shows that the two groups did not differ with respect to preexercise measurements. During exercise, the COPD group exhibited larger decreases in this ratio than controls; during recovery, this ratio returned to preexercise levels in both groups. Since the denominator of the fraction [PCr]/([PCr] + [Pi]) should be constant if the measurements are technically satisfactory (i.e., no loss of signal), the ordinate represents the magnitude of [PCr] depletion. The authors interpret this data as indicating that oxidative phosphorylation maintained [PCr] at a higher level in normal subjects.

Figure 34-7 compares the two groups with respect to pH measurements. The figure shows that the control group maintained a constant pH throughout the experiment, whereas subjects with COPD exhibited progressive decreases in pH during exercise. (It is interesting that both groups had a decrease in pH following the cessation of exercise which was due to resynthesis of PCr. The creatine kinase reaction liberates protons; i.e., $MgATP + Cr \rightleftharpoons PCr + MgADP + H^+$.) The decrease in muscle pH during exercise in the subjects with COPD is explainable by high rates of lactic acid

formation because of the enhanced glycolytic flux. Therefore, based on the data in Figs. 34-6 and 34-7, these authors conclude that the patients with COPD exhibited "impaired oxidative phosphorylation and the early activation of anaerobic glycolysis." This conclusion suggests that the forearm muscles of the subjects with COPD were deconditioned.

However, this conclusion is warranted only if Kutsuzawa and colleagues[42] had demonstrated that both groups of subjects were exercising at the same percent of maximum power. Indeed, tabular data in their paper indicate that the maximum handgrip strength was 28 to 40 percent greater in the normal group. Since both groups were carrying out exercise at the same absolute power, the percent of maximum power was greater in the COPD group. Indeed, above some percent of maximum power, normal subjects would exhibit MR features similar to those of the subjects with COPD.[38,41] Therefore, the possibility exists that the results of Kutsuzawa's group[42] can be attributed to the fact that the patients with COPD were working at a higher percentage of maximum power, and some data in their paper support this interpretation. More importantly, the fact that the above-noted indexes of MR spectra provide valid comparisons only in the special circumstances where power output is normalized to maximum power output has stimulated many researchers to develop more sophisticated MR indexes which are valid without this type of normalization (see below).

USE OF THE RECOVERY TIME CONSTANT TO CHARACTERIZE ACTIVITIES OF ENZYMES OF OXIDATIVE PHOSPHORYLATION

To control for differences in muscle strength, we measure the rate of PCr resynthesis after submaximal exercise, which depletes [PCr] to approximately 50 percent of control.[36,43] Figure 34-8 indicates that following the cessation of exercise,

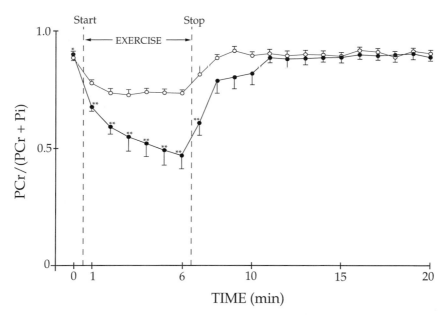

FIGURE 34-6 Magnetic resonance spectroscopy comparison of COPD and age-matched normal subjects with respect to exercise at the same work rate for the same amount of time; this work was carried out by the flexor digitorum superficialis and flexor digitorum profundus muscles. Open circles, normal subjects; filled circles, COPD patients. Values are expressed as mean $\pm$ SEM*, $p < .05$; **, $p < .01$ for group t test. Since the denominator of the ordinate should be constant if the measurements are technically satisfactory (i.e., no loss of signal), the ordinate represents the magnitude of [PCr] depletion. The authors interpret this data as indicating that oxidative phosphorylation maintained [PCr] at a higher level in the normal subjects. These results suggest clear metabolic differences between COPD patients and controls (see text for further explanation). (From Kutsuzawa T, et al: ^{31}P NMR study of skeletal muscle metabolism in patients with chronic respiratory impairment. *Am Rev Respir Dis* 146:1019–1024, 1992, with permission.)

[PCr] returns to its resting level in an exponential manner. This recovery of PCr to resting level can be described by the following equation: $PCr(t) = PCr_0 + \Delta PCr(1 - e^{-t/Tc})$, where PCr_0 represents the percent resting level of PCr at end-exercise, ΔPCR is the difference between PCr_0 and 100 percent PCr recovery, t is the number of seconds after cessation of exercise, and Tc represents the time constant of recovery. In theory, this recovery time constant should permit the formation of valid comparisons between muscle groups having different strengths, and this work is described in recent publications.[31,36] However, because Tc is also influenced by O_2 delivery to the muscle(s) under study, it is important to take this into account when interpreting Tc data in patient groups with impaired O_2 delivery to the muscles (i.e., anemia, congestive heart failure, and peripheral vascular disease). Therefore, these authors are currently developing methodologies which will differentiate the effects of O_2 delivery and mitochondrial oxidative capacity on the recovery time constant (i.e., Tc).

A final point concerns the relationship between in vitro

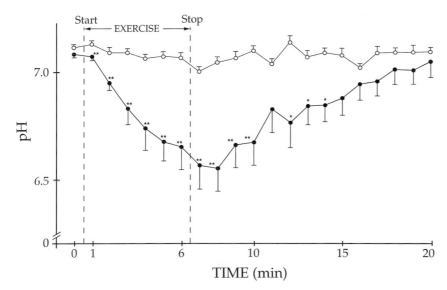

FIGURE 34-7 Magnetic resonance spectroscopy comparison of the same COPD and normal subjects with respect to muscle pH while carrying out the protocol described in Fig. 34-6. Symbols and abscissa are identical with those in Fig. 34-6. These data are consistent with the interpretation that oxidative phosphorylation cannot maintain the [PCr] at normal or near-normal levels in COPD subjects; therefore, these subjects activate glycolytic generation of ATP with the resultant formation of lactic acid. This high rate of lactic acid generation effects large decreases in pH. (Kutsuzawa T, et al: ^{31}P NMR study of skeletal muscle metabolism in patients with chronic respiratory impairment. *Am Rev Respir Dis* 146:1019–1024, 1992, with permission.)

(i.e., wet bench) measurements of the maximum rate of oxidative phosphorylation and MRS. The two are directly related by the following equation: Vmax oxidative phosphorylation = (1/Tc) × PCr end. When the Tc is stated in seconds and PCr end in millimoles per liter, this equation provides an estimate of Vmax in millimoles per second and this in vivo measurement can be compared with in vitro assessments of Vmax oxidative phosphorylation.[35,36,44]

RESPIRATORY SYSTEM

VENTILATORY MUSCLE ENDURANCE

The resistance of muscle to fatigue can be expressed as the endurance capacity, that is, the time that a particular work rate can be maintained. In 1976, Leith and Bradley[45] demonstrated that the endurance capacity of the ventilatory muscles of normal subjects can be increased by having the subjects carry out selective training of the ventilatory muscles on a daily basis for 5 weeks. Ventilatory muscle endurance was quantitated by the maximum sustainable ventilatory capacity (MSVC)—the maximum isocapnic $\dot{V}_E$ that a subject was able to maintain for a relatively long period of time (e.g., 10 to 15 min). These investigators also demonstrated that no change in MSVC was noted over a 5-week time interval in an age-matched normal control group who did not undergo ventilatory muscle endurance training (VMET).

Subsequently, Keens and associates[46] demonstrated that a 4-week course of VMET was associated with increases in MSVC in four teenage patients with cystic fibrosis as well as four normal teenage subjects. However, Belman and Mittman[47] were the first to use VMET therapy in adult patients with COPD. In each of their 10 subjects, they noted that a 5-week course of VMET was associated with increases in

MSVC. Coincident with these increases in MSVC, their subjects exhibited objective improvement in exercise tests. Therefore, following this seminal publication of Belman and Mittman, it appeared that MSVC constituted a clinically applicable test of ventilatory muscle endurance. However, subsequent work by Levine and colleagues[48] raised the possibility that the increases in MSVC elicited by VMET represented a "learning effect" as opposed to a "training effect."

In a subsequent study, Belman and Kendregan[49] examined the effect of arm and leg endurance exercise training on arm and leg muscle endurance as well as MSVC in 15 patients with symptomatic COPD (FEV$_{1.0}$ approximately 1.0 L). Although there was no statistically significant changes in spirometry, lung volumes, or MSVC, there were approximately 70 percent increases in the mean workload which could be performed for 20 min by either leg or arm exercise. This work by Belman and Kendregan raised the possibility that nonventilatory muscle exercise such as arm and leg cycling does not improve ventilatory muscle endurance. However, all the above-noted studies did not contain direct measurements of ventilatory muscle structure (i.e., MHC isoforms, fiber types, and activities of aerobic oxidative enzymes) or maximum activity of oxidative phosphorylation as assessed by MRS (see above-noted section on musculoskeletal adaptations to deconditioning and endurance exercise training). At the present time, it is not known if MSVC is an adequate test of ventilatory muscle endurance, and these authors believe that more direct assessments of ventilatory muscle histochemistry and biochemistry are needed.

STRUCTURAL ADAPTATIONS OF THE VENTILATORY MUSCLE

Because of increases in airway resistance and decreases in dynamic compliance, even at rest, the ventilatory muscles of patients with severe COPD can be thought of as undergoing constant moderate endurance-type exercise. To elucidate the adaptation of the diaphragm to this unusual situation, Levine and coworkers[50] compared the diaphragm of patients with COPD (FEV$_{1.0}$, 33 ± 4 percent predicted; RV, 256 ± 31 percent predicted) and age-matched control subjects who had normal or near-normal pulmonary function tests with respect to the proportions of MHCs and fiber types. These subjects with COPD had appreciably greater proportions of MHC I and lesser proportions of MHCs IIa and IIb. With respect to fiber type proportions, COPD diaphragms had higher percentages of slow fiber type I and lesser percentages of the fast fiber types (i.e., IIa and IIb). These results suggest that the diaphragm adapts to severe COPD by fast-to-slow transformation in MHCs and fiber types. Moreover, since these results suggest that the diaphragms of COPD patients are already maximally endurance trained, this may account for the failure of systemic endurance exercise to elicit increases in ventilatory muscle endurance. Lastly, since other workers[24] have demonstrated that the limb muscles of patients with severe COPD undergo slow-to-fast transformation, these results indicate that the diaphragm and the limb muscles adapt to severe COPD in a qualitatively different manner.

MECHANICAL CONSTRAINTS TO VENTILATION

During the past several years, Johnson and associates[51–53] have developed a method for determining whether a mechanical constraint (i.e., either in pulmonary mechanics or

FIGURE 34-8 Following the cessation of exercise, the concentration of creatine phosphate [PCr] returns to resting levels in an exponential manner characterized by the equation shown in the figure, where PCr$_0$ represents the percent resting level of PCr at end-exercise, ΔPCr is the difference between PCr$_0$ and 100 percent PCr recovery, t is the number of seconds after cessation of exercise, and Tc represents the time constant of recovery.

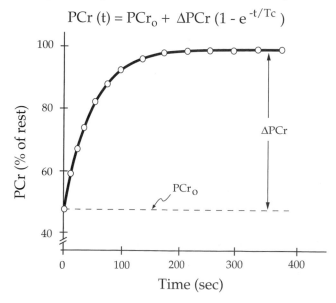

$$PCr\,(t) = PCr_0 + \Delta PCr\,(1 - e^{-t/Tc})$$

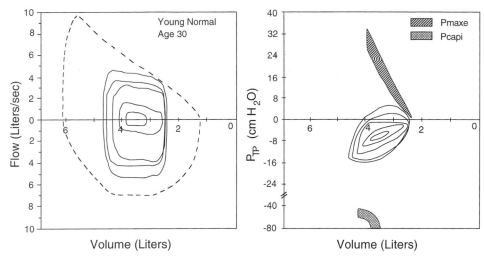

FIGURE 34-9 Flow- and pressure-volume responses to maximal exercise in a young normal untrained male (peak ventilation = 102 L/min and $\dot{V}_{O_2}$ max = 42 mL/min per kilogram). *Left panel:* maximal volitional expiratory and inspiratory flow-volume envelope (dashed line), exercise tidal flow-volume loops at increasing exercise intensities (solid lines). *Right panel:* tidal exercise pressure-volume loops (solid lines) plotted within the maximal effective pressure generation on expiration (Pmaxe) and the capacity for dynamic pressure generation on inspiration (Pcapi). The smallest solid flow- and pressure-volume loops represent resting breathing.

ventilatory muscle function) exists to $\dot{V}_E$ during incremental exercise testing. Since this type of analysis is useful in categorizing the cause of exercise limitation in patients with CRD undergoing exercise retraining, an overview of this approach is presented, which focuses on the flow-volume and pressure-volume relationships. Figure 34-9 shows the normal flow-volume relationships (*left panel*) and pressure-volume relationships (*right panel*) to incremental exercise in a young adult. These panels show the characteristic responses to exercise in a young healthy adult which include (1) decrease in end-expiratory lung volume (EELV); (2) equal encroachment on the inspiratory and expiratory reserve lung volumes; (3) minimal expiratory flow limitation (i.e., expiratory pressures produced during expiration do not meet or exceed the flow-limiting pressures over a significant portion of the tidal breath); and (4) inspiratory pressures during exercise, which reach <50 percent of the capacity of the inspiratory muscles for pressure generation. Thus, in this young average individual, a mechanical constraint to $\dot{V}_E$ does not exist at peak exercise.

In contrast, Fig. 34-10 presents an example of the flow- and pressure-volume responses to exercise in an older individual (age 70) with moderate COPD (maximal midexpiratory flow rate 35 percent predicted). Relative to the young adult, the following differences are noted in the ventilatory response to exercise: (1) EELV does not fall but instead stays close to resting functional residual capacity (FRC), with a subsequent increase at the highest level of exercise; (2) end-inspiratory lung volume (EILV) approaches total lung capacity (TLC); (3) tidal breathing exercise loops become flow-limited over the majority of expiration; and (4) peak inspiratory pressures equal the dynamic capacity of the inspiratory muscles for pressure generation. Therefore, in this older individual with COPD, a mechanical constraint to ventilation exists during peak exercise.

Pulmonary physiologists have long emphasized that aging per se results in loss of lung elastic recoil with its associated decreases in expiratory airflow.[51,53] The relative effects of age, training, and COPD on mechanical constraints to ventilation are indicated in Fig. 34-11, which shows the relationship between the percent of tidal volume that is flow-limited during expiration and the level of $\dot{V}_E$ in four individuals (i.e., young untrained, young trained, older trained, and older with moderate COPD). The young adults do not reach expiratory flow limitation (i.e., >20 percent of tidal breath) until a $\dot{V}_E$ of approximately 100 to 120 L/min is achieved. In contrast, the older normal adult reaches significant expiratory flow limitation at a $\dot{V}_E$ of 40 L/min, whereas the patient with COPD reaches a similar degree of flow limitation at a $\dot{V}_E$ of 25 to 30 L/min. [Older adults and patients with COPD attempt to avoid expiratory limitation at lower levels of $\dot{V}_E$ by increasing EELV and thereby moving the tidal breath away from the expiratory boundary of the maximum flow-volume loop (see Fig. 34-10).]

This method of Johnson and associates[51–53] allows the determination of whether an individual quits exercise because of a mechanical constraint. Although this is presumed to be the case with COPD and patients with other respiratory diseases, this is not necessarily true. Indeed, as indicated elsewhere, some of these patients quit because of pain or panic attacks.

PSYCHOLOGICAL EFFECTS

Exercise retraining elicits a host of positive psychological benefits in normal subjects which have been referred to as an "increased sense of well-being" (see Table 34-1). The specific studies in this area are summarized by the recent U.S. Surgeon General's report entitled *Physical Activity and Health.*[54]

These authors[48] have demonstrated that a pulmonary rehabilitation program containing an exercise component causes the following improvements on the Hopkins Psychological Check List 90 (SCL-90): (1) reductions in global psychological abnormalities manifest by decreases in both the positive symptom total and global severity index, and (2) decreases

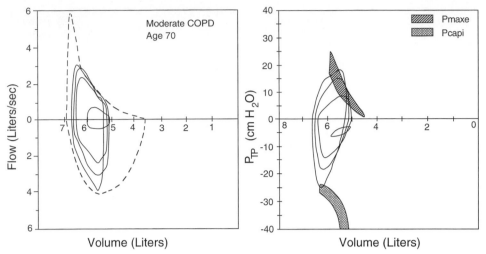

FIGURE 34-10 Flow (*left*) and pleural pressure (*right*) responses to exercise in a patient with moderate obstructive airway disease plotted within the maximal expiratory and inspiratory flow-volume envelope (*left*) and the maximal effective expiratory pressures and maximal available inspiratory pressure (*right*). Unlike the young healthy adult in Fig. 34-9, end-expiratory lung volume increases, end-inspiratory lung volume approaches TLC, tidal breathing exercise loops become flow-limited over the majority of expiration, and peak inspiratory pressures reach the dynamic capacity for inspiratory pressure generation. Little reserve exists to increase ventilation.

in the specific subscores for anxiety, somatization, and depression.[55] A fall in the depression subscale of the Minnesota Multiphasic Personality Index has also been demonstrated.[56] Other workers have reported similar improvements in psychological tests with pulmonary rehabilitation programs that have an exercise retraining component.[57] A major problem exists in determining the precise relationship of these improvements to exercise retraining versus other components of a comprehensive pulmonary rehabilitation program.

PERSONAL OBSERVATIONS

Some patients with moderate to severe COPD as well as patients with other types of CRD seem to be convinced that situations that cause high levels of dyspnea should be avoided because they can be fatal. This idea may trigger anxiety attacks in these patients which limit their usual activities and thereby causes further deconditioning.

Comprehensive pulmonary rehabilitation programs with an exercise retraining component are often successful in

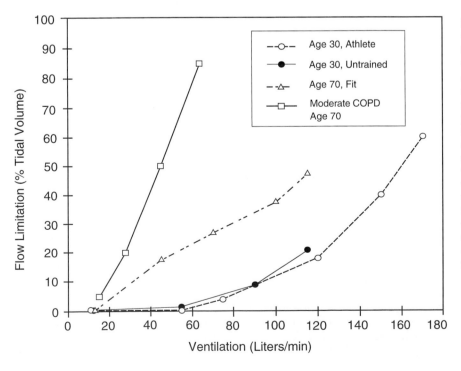

FIGURE 34-11 Expiratory flow limitation with progressive exercise in a young untrained adult (age 30), a trained athlete (age 30), a 70-year-old relatively fit subject, and a subject with obstructive airways disease. The young adults do not reach significant expiratory flow limitation (i.e., >20 percent of the tidal breath) until a ventilation of approximately 100 to 120 L is achieved. In contrast, the older adult reaches flow limitation over 20 percent of the tidal breath at 40 L/min, and the patient reaches a similar degree of flow limitation at a ventilation of 25 to 30 L/min. Some flow limitation is avoided early in exercise in the aging adult and patient by increasing EELV and moving the tidal breath away from the expiratory boundary of the maximum flow-volume loop.

breaking this cycle. However, in the experience of these authors, there is a subset of patients whose size depends on cultural, educational, and socioeconomic conditions—as well as the presence or absence of a support group—in whom exercise retraining does not reduce anxiety. This subset of patients can often be vastly improved by having them carry out incremental exercise protocols in a carefully monitored situation (i.e., ECG, pulse oximetry, end-tidal gas analysis, and rating of perceived dyspnea) under the supervision of a fully trained physician assisted by appropriate exercise physiologists and respiratory therapists. In this carefully controlled environment, the physician is able to reassure the patient that "everything is fine" and encourage the patient to reach higher exercise intensities. In the experience of these authors, confidence of the patient in the physician and a detailed explanation of the monitoring by the physician to the patient will usually be successful in convincing the patient that he or she can exercise to a higher level of dyspnea without dire consequences. Multiple iterations of this "anxiety desensitization" approach have been successful in the rehabilitation of the above-noted subset of CRD patients.[48,57,58]

CARDIOVASCULAR SYSTEM

CARDIAC

As shown in Table 34-1, endurance training in normal subjects increases maximum cardiac output by increasing stroke volume.[14,59,60] It is not clear if this occurs in COPD. Some older studies which directly measured cardiac output failed to demonstrate training-induced increases in cardiac output in patients with COPD.[61–64] Additionally, only one older study (i.e., that of Pierce and coworkers[9]) found a decrease in heart rate at the same work rate following training. However, since $\dot{V}_{O_2}$ was also decreased, their observation cannot be interpreted as a training-induced lessening of heart rate. A critical review of these studies does not provide any assurance that the training protocols used were adequate either in terms of work intensity or duration of training to elicit cardiac adaptations of endurance training. More measurements of cardiac function are needed (perhaps by state-of-the-art assessments such as echocardiography) over the course of endurance exercise training to see whether patients with COPD respond in the same ways as normals.

PERIPHERAL VASCULATURE

Until several years ago, some uncertainty existed as to whether exercise training elicited an increase in capillarity in the limb muscles of older individuals. However, the study of Coggan and associates[28] demonstrated that a high-intensity treadmill exercise program (i.e., 80 percent maximal heart rate for 45 min/day for 4 days/week) for 9 to 12 months elicited greater capillarity in the gastrocnemius muscles of 23 healthy older men and women (mean age 64 ± 3 years). Specifically, these investigators noted that this exercise program produced increases in the following measurements: (1) number of capillaries per unit area; (2) total number of capillaries per fiber (i.e., total number of capillaries per unit area divided by the number of fibers in that unit area); and (3) mean number of capillaries in contact with each muscle fiber. Despite the inherent difficulties in assessing capillarity, the combination of these three measurements demonstrates that capillarity was unequivocally increased in these older

normal subjects. Very few programs involving exercise training in patients with CRD have been carried out for this prolonged duration,[29–32] and in those which have, no assessment of capillarity of limb muscles was carried out. Therefore, at the present time, it is not known for certain if an exercise training program can elicit increased capillarity in the limb muscles of patients with COPD.

Exercise Retraining in Patients with Interstitial Lung Disease

Novich and Thomas have[65] recently reported on 23 patients with interstitial lung disease (ILD) who completed their 4-week pulmonary inpatient rehabilitation program. A major component of their program was at least one 45-min exercise session daily consisting of floor walking, treadmill walking, stationary bicycle riding, and work on an upper-body cycle ergometer. At the end of the 4 weeks, the amount of time that these patients could perform arm ergometry tripled, whereas the distance covered in 6 min of ambulation (i.e., 6-min walk) as well as the number of stairs climbed doubled; additionally, the amount of time they were able to carry out leg ergometry increased 47 percent. These observations of Novich and Thomas[65] suggest that exercise retraining elicits the increases in exercise performance in patients with ILD as have been observed in COPD.

Types of Exercise Retraining Which Should Be Included in a Comprehensive Rehabilitation Program

STATEMENT OF THE PROBLEM

At the present time, two different viewpoints exist with respect to exercise training, i.e., the physiologic approach versus the rehabilitation perspective. Cardiopulmonary and sports medicine physiologists and physicians believe that the purpose of exercise retraining is to elicit physiologic effects of endurance training manifested by increases in $\dot{V}_{O_2}$ max as well as the other items enumerated in Table 34-1. Surprisingly, some of the best publications of these authors[18] do not even mention the effect of an exercise retraining program on the patient's ability to carry out ADL.

In contrast, exercise retraining can be considered as a specific component of a comprehensive program which seeks to teach the patient how activities of daily living can be optimized. Therefore, this approach focuses on instructing the patient in the most efficient manner of carrying out such ADL as face washing, combing hair, surface-to-surface transfers, etc. This approach consists of constant practice of the correct methods for carrying out these ADL once the patient has mastered a technique which maximizes function and minimizes the sensation of dyspnea.

Both of these components should be included as part of exercise retraining.[66,67] For example, patients can start with one daily session of 45 to 60 min of general conditioning (i.e., the sports medicine approach) that includes floor walking, treadmill walking, stationary leg bicycle ergometer, and arm ergometer. Each of these should be performed repetitively to the patients' tolerance. Additionally, the patients should

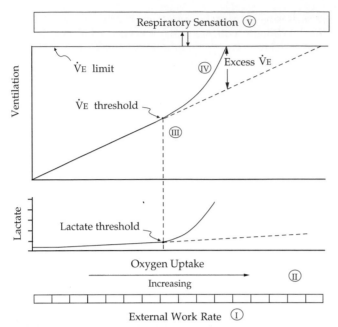

FIGURE 34-12 Mechanisms by which endurance exercise training can benefit patients with CRD. See text for complete description of this model. Roman numerals indicate the following mechanisms: I, increase external work rate; II, increase efficiency (i.e., work rate that can be achieved at a given $\dot{V}_{O_2}$); III and IV, increase $\dot{V}_{O_2}$ at which both lactate and $\dot{V}_E$ thresholds occur; IV, decrease excess $\dot{V}_E$ (e.g., correction of exercise-induced hypoxemia); and V, eliminate phobic anxiety and thereby increase the $\dot{V}_E$ limit.

also undergo daily sessions of 45 to 60 min which include surface-to-surface transfers, as well as repetitive practice of upper extremity tasks of ADL (e.g., face washing, hair combing). A combination of the sports medicine and occupational therapy approaches should be included in exercise retraining components of comprehensive pulmonary rehabilitation programs. Detailed protocols for exercise training must be customized for the type of patient to be treated and should use resources in a cost-efficient manner.

MECHANISMS BY WHICH EXERCISE TRAINING BENEFITS PATIENTS WITH CRD

Figure 34-12 provides a schematic of the mechanisms by which exercise training can benefit patients with CRD. The most important point is the concept that "sensations" produced by respiratory effort, and not the level of ventilation or $\dot{V}_{O_2}$ per se, is most important in terminating exercise. The following points are implicit in this schematic: (1) $\dot{V}_{O_2}$ increases as the external work-rate increases. (2) $\dot{V}_E$ is linearly related to $\dot{V}_{O_2}$ until the lactate threshold is reached, then $\dot{V}_E$ rises faster than $\dot{V}_{O_2}$. Alternatively stated, $\dot{V}_E$ at any point above the lactate threshold can be viewed as the sum of two components, that is the $\dot{V}_E$ dictated by the $\dot{V}_{O_2}$ and an additional component termed *excess $\dot{V}_E$* in the figure. (3) Incremental exercise is generally terminated at a more or less predictable level of $\dot{V}_E$ termed the *$\dot{V}_E$ limit*. (4) The perception that $\dot{V}_E$ cannot increase any more (or be continued at a given level) is affected by $\dot{V}_E$ as well as sensations from the extremities, anxiety, etc.

Exercise retraining can increase physical performance in the following ways (as indicated by the roman numerals in Fig. 34-12): (I) Limb muscle adaptations resulting from endurance exercise can increase the external work rate that the patient can carry on as well as $\dot{V}_{O_2}$ max. (II) The patient can carry on the same external work rate more efficiently, as many authors[15,19,48] have demonstrated. (III and IV) Endurance exercise training can increase both the lactate and $\dot{V}_E$ thresholds, and thereby excess $\dot{V}_E$ will begin at a higher $\dot{V}_{O_2}$. As a result of this perturbation, the $\dot{V}_E$ limit will be reached at a higher work rate and $\dot{V}_{O_2}$. (IV) Excess $\dot{V}_E$ can also be elicited by hypoxemia (both below and above the lactate threshold). Therefore, supplemental oxygen should be administered to avoid decreases in arterial P_{O_2}. (V) A decrease in inhibitory stimuli from brain areas primarily concerned with nonventilatory sensations (e.g., phobic anxiety) will prevent the cessation of exercise before the $\dot{V}_E$ limit is achieved.

Health Benefits of Physical Activity

The recent Surgeon General's report,[54] *Physical Activity and Health*, enumerates certain health benefits associated with increases in physical activity. Since the literature indicates that patients who have completed exercise retraining will have a greater activity level, these benefits are germane to patients with CRD who have undergone endurance exercise training. Accordingly, the beneficial effects of increases in physical activity are enumerated here: *Overall mortality:* Higher levels of regular physical activity are associated with lower mortality rates for both older and younger adults. Even those who are moderately active on a regular basis have lower mortality rates than those who are least active. *Cardiovascular disease:* Regular physical activity or cardiorespiratory fitness decreases the risk of cardiovascular disease mortality in general and of coronary heart disease (CHD) mortality in particular. It is interesting that the level of decreased risk of CHD attributable to regular physical activity is similar to that of other lifestyle factors, such as keeping free from cigarette smoking. Regular physical activity prevents or delays the development of high blood pressure, and exercise reduces blood pressure in people with hypertension. *Cancer:* Regular physical activity is associated with a decreased risk of colon cancer. *Non-insulin-dependent diabetes mellitus:* Regular physical activity lowers the risk of developing non-insulin-dependent diabetes mellitus. *Mental health:* Physical activity appears to relieve symptoms of depression and anxiety and improve mood.

Conclusions

The following conclusions are warranted: (1) Exercise retraining is an important component of a comprehensive pulmonary rehabilitation program. (2) Objective evidence exists that some patients with CRD are deconditioned. (3) Endurance exercise training in CRD patients can produce objective changes in global exercise performance as well as structural adaptations in the limb muscles. (4) Methodology exists to determine whether a mechanical constraint (i.e., either in pulmonary mechanics or ventilatory muscle function) exists at a given level of $\dot{V}_E$ in the patient with CRD. (5) Magnetic resonance spectroscopy is a new and powerful noninvasive method for evaluating the effects of both deconditioning and endurance training on limb muscles. (6) Endurance exercise training can decrease the phobic anxiety exhibited by many patients with CRD during exercise. (7) Although most of the data on the efficacy of exercise retraining relates to patients with COPD, exercise training also appears to be beneficial in the rehabilitation of patients with interstitial lung disease. (8) Rehabilitation of the patient with CRD is best accomplished by combining the endurance exercise approach of the physiologist with occupational therapy. (10) A recent Surgeon General's report[54] indicates that increased physical activity—a necessary accompaniment of exercise retraining—has beneficial effects on overall mortality, cardiovascular disease, some forms of cancer, non-insulin-dependent diabetes mellitus, and mental health.

References

1. Belman MJ: Therapeutic exercise in chronic lung disease, in Fishman AP (ed): *Pulmonary Rehabilitation*. New York, Marcel Dekker, 1996.
2. Casaburi R: Exercise training in chronic obstructive lung disease, in Casaburi R, Petty TL: *Principles and Practice of Pulmonary Rehabilitation*. Philadelphia, Saunders, 1993; p 204.
3. Reis AL: The importance of exercise in pulmonary rehabilitation. *Clin Chest Med* 15(2):327, 1994.
4. Casaburi R, Petty TL: *Principles and Practices of Pulmonary Rehabilitation*. Philadelphia, Saunders, 1993.
5. Fishman AP: *Pulmonary Rehabilitation*. New York, Marcel Dekker, 1996.
6. Bach JR: *Pulmonary Rehabilitation: The Obstructive and Paralytic Conditions*. Philadelphia, Hanley & Belfus, 1996.
7. Barach AL, Bickerman HA, Beck G: Advance in the treatment of nontuberculous pulmonary disease. *Bull NY Acad Med* 28:353, 1952.
8. Petty TL, Nett LM, Finigan MM, et al: A comprehensive care program for chronic obstructive airways: Methods and a pulmonary evaluation of symptomatic and functional improvement. *Ann Intern Med* 70:1109, 1069.
9. Pierce AK, Taylor HF, Archer RK, et al: Response to exercise training in patients with emphysema. *Arch Intern Med* 113:28, 1964.
10. Toshima MT, Ries AL: Experimental evaluation of rehabilitation in chronic obstructive pulmonary disease: Short-term effects on exercise endurance and health status. *Health Psychol* 9:237, 1990.
11. O'Donnell DE, Webb KA, McGuire MA: Older patients with COPD: Benefits of exercise training. *Geriatrics* 48:59, 1993.
12. Reardon J, Awad E, Normandin E, et al: The effect of comprehensive outpatient pulmonary rehabilitation on dyspnea. *Chest* 105:1046, 1994.
13. Astrand P, Rodahl K: *Text Book of Work Physiology: Physiological Bases of Exercise*. New York, McGraw-Hill, 1977.
14. Buskirk ER, Hodgson JL: Age and aerobic power: The rate of change in men and women. *Fed Proc* 46:1824, 1987.
15. Jones NL: *Clinical Exercise Testing*, 3d ed. Philadelphia, Saunders, 1988.
16. McArdle WD, Katche FI, Katch VL: *Exercise Physiology: Energy, Nutrition, and Human Performance*, 3d ed. Philadelphia, Lea & Febiger, 1991.
17. American College of Sports Medicine: The recommended quantity and quality of exercise for developing and maintaining cardiorespiratory and muscular fitness in healthy adults. *Med Sci Sports Exerc* 23:265, 1990.
18. Casaburi R, Patessio A, Ioli F, et al: Reductions in exercise lactic acidosis and ventilation as a result of exercise training in patients with obstructive lung disease. *Am Rev Respir Dis* 143:9, 1991.
19. Killian KJ, Leblanc P, Martin DH, et al: Exercise capacity and ventilatory, circulatory, and symptom limitation in patients with chronic airflow obstruction. *Am Rev Respir Dis* 146:935, 1992.
20. Booth FW, Baldwin KN: Muscle plasticity: Energy demand and supply processes, in Rowell LB, Shepherd JT: *Handbook of Physiology*, sec 12, *Exercise: Regulation and Integration of Multiple Systems*. New York, Oxford University, 1996; p 1075.
21. Saltin B, Gollnick PD: Skeletal muscle adaptability: Significance for metabolism and performance, in Peachy LD (ed): *Handbook of Physiology*, sec 10, *Skeletal Muscle*. Bethesda, MD, American Physiological Society, 1983; p 555.
22. Brooke M, Kaiser K: Three "myosin ATPase" systems. The nature of their pH lability and sulfhydryl dependence. *J Histochem Cytochem* 18:670, 1970.
23. Larsson L, Ansved T: Effects of long-term physical training and detraining on enzyme histochemical and functional skeletal muscle characteristics in man. *Muscle Nerve* 8:714, 1985.
24. Jakobsson P, Jorfeldt L, Brundin A: Skeletal muscle metabolites and fiber types in patients with advanced chronic obstructive pulmonary disease (COPD), with and without chronic respiratory failure. *Eur Respir J* 3:192, 1990.
25. Adams GR, Haddad F, Baldwin KM: Interaction of chronic creatine depletion and muscle unloading: Effects on postural and locomotor muscles. *J Appl Physiol* 77:1198, 1994.
26. Templeton GH, Sweeney HL, Timson BF, et al: Changes in fiber composition of soleus muscle during rat hindlimb suspension. *J Appl Physiol* 65:1191, 1988.
27. Thomason DB, Herrick RE, Surdyka D, Baldwin KM: Time course of soleus muscle myosin expression during hindlimb suspension and recovery. *J Appl Physiol* 63:130, 1987.
28. Coggan AR, Spina RJ, King DS, et al: Skeletal muscle adaptations to endurance training in 60- to 70-yr-old men and women. *J Appl Physiol* 72:1780, 1992.
29. Brudin A: Physical training in severe chronic obstructive lung disease: I. Clinical course, physical working capacity, and ventilation. *Scand J Respir Dis* 55:25, 1974.
30. Brudin A: Physical training in severe chronic obstructive pulmonary disease: II. Observations on gas exchange. *Scand J Respir Dis* 55:37, 1974.
31. Mertens DJ, Shepherd RS, Kavanagh T: Long-term exercise therapy for chronic obstructive lung disease. *Respiration* 35:96, 1978.
32. Sinclair DJM, Ingram CG: Controlled trial of supervised exercise training in chronic bronchitis. *Br J Med* 1:519, 1980.
33. Maltais F, Simard A-A, Simard C, et al: Oxidative capacity of the skeletal and lactic acid kinetics during exercise in normal subjects and in patients with COPD. *Am J Respir Crit Care Med* 153:228, 1996.
34. Maltais F, LeBlanc P, Simard C, et al: Skeletal muscle adaptation to endurance training in patients with chronic obstructive pulmonary disease. *Am J Respir Crit Care Med* 154:442, 1996.
35. Conley K: Cellular energetics during exercise. *Advan Vet Compar Med* 38A:1, 1994.
36. McCully K: Magnetic resonance spectroscopy as a tool to study sarcopenia. *Muscle Nerve* (suppl)5:S102, 1997.
37. Kent-Braun JA, Miller RG, Weiner MW: Human skeletal muscle metabolism in health and disease: Utility of magnetic resonance spectroscopy, in Holloszy JO (ed): *Exercise and Sports Science Reviews*. Baltimore, Williams & Wilkins, 1995; p 305.
38. Chance B, Leigh J, Kent J, et al: Multiple controls of oxidative metabolism of living tissues as studied by ^{31}P MRS. *Proc Natl Acad Sci USA* 83:9458, 1986.
39. Levine S, Tikunov B, Henson D, et al: Creatine depletion elicits structural, biochemical, and physiological adaptations in the rat costal diaphragm. *Am J Physiol* 271 (*Cell Physiol* 40): C1480, 1996.
40. Wallimann T, Wyss M, Brdiczka D, et al: Intracellular compartmentation, structure, and function of creatine kinase isoenzymes,

with high and fluctuating energy demands: The "phosphocreatine circuit" for cellular energy homeostasis. *Biochem J* 281:21, 1992.

41. Kent-Braun JA, McCully K, Chance B: Metabolic effects of training in man: A ^{31}P MRS study. *J Appl Physiol* 69:1165, 1990.

42. Kutsuzawa T, Shioya S, Kurita D, et al: ^{31}P NMR study of skeletal muscle metabolism in patients with chronic respiratory impairment. *Am Rev Respir Dis* 146:1019, 1992.

43. Walter G, Vandenborne K, McCully K, Leigh J: Noninvasive measurements of oxidative capacity in a single muscle. *Am J Physiol (Cell)* 272:C525, 1997.

44. Kemp G, Radda G: Quantitative interpretation of bioenergetic data from ^{31}P and ^{1}H magnetic resonance spectroscopic studies of skeletal muscle: An analytical review. *Mag Res Quart* 10:43, 1994.

45. Leith DE, Bradley M: Ventilatory muscle strength and endurance training. *J Appl Physiol* 41:508, 1976.

46. Keens TG, Krastins IRB, Wanamaker EM, et al: Ventilatory muscle endurance training in normal subjects and patients with cystic fibrosis. *Am Rev Respir Dis* 116:853, 1977.

47. Belman MJ, Mittman C: Ventilatory muscle training improves exercise capacity in chronic obstructive pulmonary disease patients. *Am Rev Respir Dis* 121:273, 1980.

48. Levine S, Weiser P, Gillen J: Evaluation of a ventilatory muscle endurance training program in the rehabilitation of patients with COPD. *Am Rev Respir Dis* 133:400, 1986.

49. Belman MJ, Kendregan BK: Physical training fails to improve ventilatory muscle endurance in patients with chronic obstructive pulmonary disease. *Chest* 81:440, 1982.

50. Levine S, Kaiser L, Leferovich J, et al: Cellular adaptations in the diaphragm in chronic obstructive pulmonary disease. *N Engl J Med* 337:1799, 1997.

51. Johnson BD, Badr MS, Dempsey JA: Impact of the aging pulmonary system on the response to exercise. *Clin Chest Med* 15(2):229, 1994.

52. Johnson BD, Reddan WG, Pegelow DF, et al: Flow limitation and regulation of functional residual capacity during exercise in a physically active aging population. *Am Rev Respir Dis* 143:960, 1991.

53. Johnson BD, Reddan WG, Seow KC, Dempsey JA: Mechanical constraints on exercise hyperapnea in a fit aging population. *Am Rev Respir Dis* 143:968, 1991.

54. U.S. Department of Health and Human Services: *Physical Activity and Health: A Report of the Surgeon General.* Atlanta, GA: U.S.
Department of Health and Human Services, Centers for Disease Control and Prevention, National Center for Chronic Disease Prevention and Health Promotion, 1996.

55. Derogatis LR: *SCL 90. Administration, Scoring, and Procedures Manual.* Baltimore, Derogatis, 1977.

56. Dahlstrom WG, Welch GS, Dahlstrom LE: *An MMPI Handbook,* vol 1, *Clinical Interpretation.* Minneapolis, University of Minnesota, 1982.

57. Agle DP, Baum GL, Chester EH, Wendt M: Multidiscipline treatment of chronic pulmonary insufficiency: 1. Psychological aspects of rehabilitation. *Psychosom Med* 35:41, 1973.

58. Carrieri-Kohiman V, Gormley JM, Stulbarg MS: Monitored exercise and coached exercise decrease dyspnea intensity. *Ann Behav Med* 15:S168, 1993.

59. American College of Sports Medicine: in Durstine JL, King AC, Painter PL, et al (eds): *Resource Manual for Guidelines for Exercise Testing and Prescription,* 2d ed. Philadelphia, Lea & Febiger, 1993.

60. Rowell LB, Shepherd JT: *Handbook of Physiology,* section 12, *Exercise: Regulation and Integration of Multiple Systems.* New York, Oxford University, 1996.

61. Alpert JS, Bass H, Szucs MM, et al: Effects of physical training on hemodynamics and pulmonary function at rest and during exercise in patients with chronic obstructive pulmonary disease. *Chest* 66:647, 1974.

62. Chester EH, Belman MJ, Bahler RC, et al: Multidisciplinary treatment of chronic pulmonary insufficiency: 3. The effect of physical training on cardiopulmonary performance in patients with chronic obstructive pulmonary disease. *Chest* 72:695, 1977.

63. Degre S, Sergysels R, Messin P, et al: Hemodynamic responses to physical training in patients with chronic lung disease. *Am Rev Respir Dis* 110:395, 1974.

64. Paez PN, Phillipson EA, Masangkay M, Sproule BJ: The physiologic basis of training patients with emphysema. *Am Rev Respir Dis* 95:944, 1967.

65. Novich RS, Thomas HM III: Pulmonary rehabilitation in chronic pulmonary interstitial disease, in Fishman AP (ed): *Pulmonary Rehabilitation.* New York, Marcel Dekker, 1996.

66. Hodgkin JE: Benefits of pulmonary rehabilitation, in Fishman AP (ed): *Pulmonary Rehabilitation.* New York, Marcel Dekker, 1996; p 33.

67. Rondinelli RD, Hill NS: Rehabilitation of the patient with pulmonary disease, in DeLisa JA (ed): *Rehabilitation Medicine: Principles and Practices.* Philadelphia, Lippincott, 1988; p 688.

Chapter 35

AIR TRAVEL IN PATIENTS WITH CHRONIC PULMONARY DISEASE

MORDECHAI R. KRAMER

Air travel is considered a safe and convenient mode of transportation for millions of people around the world. Thousands of takeoffs and landings occur daily without significant discomfort to the passengers. This is despite the fact that they are exposed to significant changes in their environment—in altitude, barometric pressure, and some decreases in inspired oxygen concentration. Indeed, the body's normal physiology can adapt quickly to such changes without any problem.

In fact, the incidence of medical emergencies during commercial flights is extremely low. Studies[1,2] have estimated the incidence of medical emergencies of any kind to be between 0.004 to 0.003 percent in series involving more than 80 million air travelers arriving at several airports. Most problems were cardiovascular (13 to 50 percent), neurologic (7 to 33 percent), gastrointestinal (12 to 26 percent), and respiratory (7.5 to 10 percent). In those series only 12 passengers died (out of 80 million passengers) during the flight, mostly from cardiac causes. In another large scale survey[2] involving 245 million passengers over a period of 7 years, 577 people died suddenly during flights (incidence of 0.0002 percent), 56 percent due to cardiac problems and 6 percent due to respiratory causes.

This low incidence of medical emergencies suggest that air travel is probably safer than car travel for healthy people. The situation may be different, however, for patients with respiratory disorders who may have been avoiding air travel because of their disease. Over the last decade major advances have been made in smoking cessation on aircraft, as well as providing an oxygen supply to hypoxemic patients during air travel, thus enabling almost any patient with lung disease with the proper preparation to travel almost anywhere.

Hypoxemia at Altitude

Oxygen levels remain approximately 21 percent of any barometric pressure. With increased altitude, barometric pressure decreases and the inspired partial pressure of oxygen falls proportionally. For example, at sea level barometric pressure is 760 Torr, inspired P_{O_2} is 159 mmHg. At a higher altitude of 10,000 feet (3049 m) atmospheric pressure is 523 Torr and inspired P_{O_2} is 110 mmHg while at 40,000 feet (12, 125 m) barometric pressure is about 230 Torr and inspired P_{O_2} is 36 mmHg[3-6] (Table 35-1).

By calculation of inspired P_{O_2} [inspired P_{O_2} = 0.21 × (barometric pressure − 47)] and by measuring arterial P_{O_2} one can see that for a normal person at 10,000 feet, alveolar P_{O_2} may reach as low as 61 mmHg and the arterial P_{O_2} at that level is about 53 mmHg, so that low oxygen saturation is between 80 to 90 percent.

Flight Hypoxemia

Most commercial aircraft cruise between 22,000 and 40,000 feet (6700 to 13,000 m) above sea level to improve their flight operation. Without pressurizing systems, flying above 10,000 feet will require oxygen supplementation to all passengers. Most aircraft have pressurizing systems that compress air into the cabin. The pressurization results in a cabin altitude equal to 5000 to 8000 feet during most cruising altitudes. When the aircraft is flying at 22,500 feet or less cabin pressure can reach sea level pressure but this rarely occurs (a point to remember in case of emergency). When actual measurement of cabin pressure was made, it was found that during air turbulence cabin pressure may temporarily reach levels of 9000 to 10,000 feet (levels that are allowed by the aviation authorities), although the 8000-foot level is the standard requirement. More modern aircraft maintain this same pressure even though they fly even higher than older models. Therefore, patients with hypoxemia are prone to additional hypoxia when flying.[4-6]

Other factors that may be important during flight are low cabin humidity, poor ventilation, and passive smoking around areas where smoking is permitted. All these factors may further impair ventilation and oxygenation of patients with underlying lung disease.

Normal Response to Hypoxemia

The physiologic response to hypoxemia has been investigated thoroughly for mountain climbers.[7,9] Hypoxemia causes reflex responses from carotid chemoreceptors that prevent a significant fall in arterial oxygen levels though the respiratory alkalosis may blunt the hypoxemic response. The increased ventilation causes a rise in arterial P_{O_2} and oxygen saturation increases towards 90% at altitudes of 10,000 feet. Beyond that level, hyperventilation does not keep saturation at a satisfactory level and oxygen supplementation is required. The normal hemodynamic response includes tachycardia and increase in cardiac output which is related to the degree of hypoxemia. Pulmonary vasoconstriction and mild pulmonary hypertension is a normal response to hypoxemia and is reversible when hypoxemia is corrected.[7-8] Hypoxemia may cause mild neuropsychological impairment with altered perception and judgment, fatigue and drowsiness. Severe hypoxemia may cause restlessness, altered behavior and altered level of consciousness.

Preflight Evaluation of Patients with Pulmonary Disease

The main factor that determines the safety of air travel for patients with pulmonary disease is their response to hypoxemia (Fig. 35-1). Some patients can fly without symptoms despite expected severe hypoxemia, but others may develop significant respiratory distress. Therefore, some investigators have proposed testing patients at hypoxemic conditions prior to flying.[9-11] Others, however, have suggested that the effects

TABLE 35-1 Effect of Cabin Altitude on Inspired Oxygen Levels in Normal Subjects

Cabin Altitude (Thousands Feet)	Barometric Pressure (mmHg)	PARTIAL OXYGEN PRESSURE (mmHg)			
		Cabin	Inspired	Alveolar	Arterial
0	760	159	149	103	98
2	707	148	138	94	90
4	656	137	128	85	80
6	609	127	117	77	64
8	565	118	108	69	60
10	523	109	100	61	53

of high altitude can be estimated from the lung function and blood gases obtained prior to the flight at low altitude.[12,13] The hypoxia-altitude stimulation test (HAST) can be performed at any pulmonary laboratory by having the patient breath 15% of oxygen with or without exercise. However, in my experience as well as that of others this is rarely needed and one may confidently rely on simple equations[13]:

1. Pa_{O_2} expected (8000 ft) = 0.41 Pa_{O_2} (sea level) + 17.65
   [for example, for Pa_{O_2} of 50 mmHg at sea level, expected Pa_{O_2} on flight will be 20.5 + 17.65 = 38.05 which requires supplemental oxygen]
   or based on FEV_1 and arterial Pa_{O_2} at sea level:
2. Pa_{O_2} (8000 feet) = 0.519 Pa_{O_2} (sea level) + 11.855 FEV_1 (liters) − 1.76
   For example, for patient with Pa_{O_2} of 60 mmHg and FEV_1 of 1.2 liters expected Pa_{O_2} will be 31.14 + 14.23 − 1.76 = 43.6 mmHg

In general, any patient with an arterial P_{O_2} at sea level lower than 60 mmHg on room air will require oxygen supplementation. Similarly, a patient who is on supplemental oxygen will require in-flight supplemental oxygen but at a higher level than used at home. Patients should be advised to bring their medication, particularly bronchodilators, and take them on schedule. Patients who are used to nebulized aerosols should arrange for battery charged devices. Patients with active bronchitis or other pulmonary or ear infections should be advised to delay their flight as it will further compromise their lung function and they may infect their flight cabin neighbors.

In-Flight Oxygen Supplement

Once the decision on oxygen supplement is made, several steps need to be taken.[14–17] As bringing along home oxygen is not allowed by most airline companies, the airline should be notified as to the amount of oxygen required. Most companies supply the oxygen as compressed gas tanks with two fixed options of oxygen flow rate (high/low) which equals 2 and 4 liters/min. In most cases this should be sufficient but if a higher flow is required special arrangements should be made. The airline company is responsible for the amount of oxygen required for the entire flight including delay time. A direct non-stop flight is always preferable to save time during the trip. Ground arrangements to and from the airplan, however, are the responsibility of the patient. Nasal canula are the more comfortable and therefore preferable way of oxygen administration during the flight[18] and patients are advised to bring another set with them with an adaptor, as a face mask is commonly supplied. Long tubing should also be brought along to facilitate going to the lavatory. Disconnecting the oxygen flow during use of the lavatory could be a very dangerous experience even for a short period of time. Additional small oxygen cylinders (20-min supply) are also available on board as an emergency back-up. In case of system malfunction or respiratory failure, the pilot should be informed so that the aircraft can be lowered to an altitude of 22,000 feet where cabin pressure is close to sea level.

Other Complications during Flight

INFECTION

Cabin air is renewed every several minutes. However, there are areas where air becomes stagnant and contaminants such as tobacco smoke or infective agents such as bacteria or viruses are circulated. Thus, the risk of acquiring infection

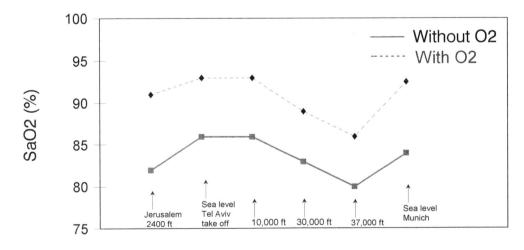

FIGURE 35-1 In flight oximetric arterial saturation in patient with severe emphysema flying to a transplant center. The patient was asked to remove the oxygen cannula for 5 min at different altitudes. Closed circles show saturation without oxygen and open circles, with oxygen.

TABLE 35-2 Management of Conditions That May Affect Flight Safety

Condition	Action
1. Active upper or lower tract infection	Delay flight till resolved
2. Bronchospasm	Bronchodilators/steroids, take on board inhalers or battery-charged nebulizer
3. Recent thromboembolism	Anticoagulation, avoid venous stasis
4. Pneumothorax or pneumomediastinum	Delay flight 3 months from event
5. Hypoxemia	Oxygen supplementation (see text)
6. Pulmonary hypertension	Oxygen supplementation
7. Myocardial infarction/ischemia	Delay flight 1 to 2 months
8. Congestive heart failure	Oxygen supplementation

from another passenger or adverse response to passive smoking is not negligible.[19,20] Epidemiologic studies on mini-epidemics of tuberculosis, meningococcal meningitis and bacterial pneumonia have been reported following crowded flights. It is advisable that any passenger with an active infection (fever, productive cough) should avoid flying. Obviously this cannot be enforced and the decision is left to the passenger.

BAROTRAUMA

According to Boyle's law, when pressure on gas decreases, the gas expands proportionally. Therefore patients with pneumothorax are advised not fly for at least 3 to 6 months following resolution of the problem.[21] Patients with emphysema or with large bulla may also be exposed to increased risk of pneumothorax although this has been rarely considered an absolute contraindication for air travel. Ear infection may account for pain or even ear drum perforation during flight descent and is considered a contraindication for high altitude flying.

THROMBOEMBOLISM

Sitting passively for many hours in a crowded cabin may lead to venous stasis or pooling and subsequent thromboembolism.[22] Patients with underlying coagulopathy, pregnancy, or history of deep vein thrombosis or other thromboembolism should be encouraged to move around the cabin and perform leg movements periodically to prevent stasis. Thromboembolism may occur later ("economy class syndrome") and the patient's problem may go unnoticed until 2 to 4 days later when symptoms develop.

Contraindications to Air Travel

Table 35-2 summarizes the contraindications to air travel for the pulmonary patient. Each condition can be dealt appropriately and many patients with similar conditions have been able to travel with the right preparation.[23] Once hypoxemia can be corrected and active infection or bronchospasm is treated the patient can travel by air.

Travel of High-Risk Patients

When severely ill patients need air transfer either to another facility or to a referral center for a specific treatment such as lung transplantation or thrombendarterctomy, special arrangements should be made.[24-25] In case the patient is intubated or hemodynamically unstable, an air ambulance with complete resuscitation facilities should be made available. In more stable cases such as patients waiting for lung transplantation a commercial flight may be adequate. The patient requires medical escort by a physician trained in intensive care medicine with continuous oximeteric monitoring equipment, intravenous access, intubation equipment and, of course, an appropriate oxygen supply. In our experience all patients with end-stage lung disease with severe hypoxemia (some with severe pulmonary hypertension and hypercarbia) needing lung transplantation can be transported safely by commercial aircraft for distances up to 10,000 miles.

In conclusion, air travel today is possible for almost any patient with lung disease. Preparation of the patient by evaluating the need for oxygen during the flight, oxygen supplement, and treating his bronchospasm and bronchial secretion prior to the flight will ensure that he will arrive safely at his destination.

References

1. Speizer C, Rennie LJ, Breton H: Prevalence of in flight medical emergencies in commercial airlines. *Ann Emerg Med* 18:26–29, 1989.
2. Cummins RO, Chapman PJC, Chamberlin DA, et al: In flight deaths during commercial air travel. How big is the problem? *JAMA* 259:1983–1988, 1988.
3. Gong H: Air travel in patients with pulmonary and allergic conditions. *J Allergy Immunol* 84:879–885, 1991.
4. Gong H: Air travel and oxygen therapy in cardiopulmonary patients. *Chest* 101:1104–1113, 1992.
5. Dillard TA, Beninati WA, Berg B: Air travel in patients with COPD. *Arch Intern Med* 151:1793–1795, 1991.
6. Schwartz JS, Bencowitz, Mosser KM: Air travel hypxemia with COPD. *Ann Intern Med* 100:473–477, 1984.
7. Lenfant C, Sullivan K: Adaptation to high altitude. *N Engl J Med* 284:1289–1309, 1971.
8. Finkelstein S, Tomashefski JF, Shillito FH: Pulmonary mechanics at altitude in normal and obstructive lung disease patients. *Aerospace Med* 36:880–884, 1965.
9. Gong H, Tashkin DP, Lee EY, Simmons MS: Hypoxia altitude simulation test: Evaluation of patients with chronic airway obstruction. *Am Rev Respir Dis* 130:980–986, 1984.
10. Gong H, Mark JA, Cowan MN: Preflight medical screening of patients. Analysis of health and flight characteristics. *Chest* 98:788–794, 1993.
11. Vohra KP, Klocke RA: Detection and correction of hypoxemia associated with air travel. *Am Rev Respir Dis* 148:1215–1219, 1993.
12. Berg B, Dillard TA, Dederian SS, Rajagopal KR: Hemodynamic effects of altitude exposure and oxygen administration in COPD. *Am J Med* 94:407–412, 1993.
13. Dillard TA, Berg B, Rajagopal KR, et al: Hypoxemia during air travel in patients with COPD. *Ann Intern Med* 111:362–367, 1989.
14. Gong H: Air travel and patients with COPD. *Ann Intern Med* 100:595–597, 1984.
15. Berg B, Dillard TA, Rajagopal KR, Mehm WJ: Oxygen supplemen-

tation during air travel in patients with COPD. *Chest* 101:638–641, 1992.

16. Gong H: Advising patients with pulmonary disease on air travel. *Ann Intern Med* 111:349–351, 1989.
17. Cottrel JJ: Altitude exposure during aircraft flight: Flying higher. *Chest* 92:81–84, 1988.
18. Dixon JP: Arterial oxygen saturation at altitude using a nasal cannula. *Aviat Space Environ Med* 53:1207–1210, 1982.
19. Henley JO: Risk of acquiring respiratory tract infection during air travel. *JAMA* 258:2764–2765, 1987.
20. Mattson ME, Boyd G, Byar D, et al: Passive smoking on commercial airline flights. *JAMA* 261:867–872, 1989.
21. Haid MM, Paladini P, Maccherini M, et al: Air transport and the fate of pneumothorax in pleural adhesion. *Thorax* 47:833–834, 1992.
22. Cruickshank JM, Gorlin R, Jennet B: Air travel and thrombotic episodes: "The economic class syndrome." *Lancet* 2:497–498, 1988.
23. Rodenberg H: Prevention of medical emergencies during air travel. *Am Fam Physician* 37:263–271, 1988.
24. Kramer MR, Jakobson DJ, Springer C, Donchin Y: The safety of air transportation of patients with advanced lung disease. *Chest* 108:1292–1296, 1995.
25. Bendrick GA, Nicollas DK, Krause BA, Castillo CY: Inflight oxygen saturation decrement in aeromedical evacuation patients. *Aviat Space Environ Med* 66:40–44, 1995.

Chapter 36

PHYSICAL MEDICINE PULMONARY AND HABILITATION INTERVENTIONS FOR PATIENTS WITH NEUROMUSCULAR DISORDERS

JOHN R. BACH

"Throughout the [amyotrophic lateral sclerosis] ALS process, I have learned many things. I have learned that having ALS does not necessarily mean a death sentence, that I am not living with a life-threatening disease, but rather with a life-enhancing condition."

—Spoken for The Honorable Justice Sam Filer, a ventilator user, by voice synthesizer at Beyond the ICU III, Perspectives on Ventilation, Committee for Independence in Living and Breathing, Toronto, Canada, April 19, 1991.[1]

Physical medicine interventions can be used for patients with neuromuscular or severe chest wall disorders to decrease the risk of pulmonary morbidity and mortality as well as to promote physical independence and enhance activities of daily living. Thus, physical medicine applications fall into two categories, those for maintaining pulmonary function and those for maximizing physical functioning. Patients with little or no respiratory muscle function can use noninvasive respiratory muscle aids as alternatives to tracheostomy on a long-term basis when they have sufficient bulbar muscle function to permit assisted peak cough flows (PCF) to exceed 160 L/m.[2] To benefit from physical medicine aids to enhance function and independence, patients need only have the volitional use of one muscle group such as the eyelids. Patients with the diagnoses listed in Table 36-1 are the most frequent beneficiaries of physical medicine aids. Both pulmonary and general physical medicine aid categories are considered in this chapter.

Physical Respiratory Muscle Aids

The inspiratory and expiratory muscles can be aided by applying forces manually or mechanically to the body or by applying intermittent pressure changes to the airway. Unfortunately, instead of using noninvasive respiratory aids, it continues to be common practice to use supplemental oxygen, bronchodilators, continuous positive airway pressure (CPAP), and other approaches that may be appropriate for patients with intrinsic lung disease but can only worsen the prognosis for these patients.[3] Oxygen therapy can exacerbate alveolar hypoventilation and decrease the effectiveness of noninvasive aids, bronchodilators can exacerbate tachycar-

dia for myopathic patients who commonly have cardiomyopathies, and although CPAP acts to maintain airway and alveolar patency, it does not assist respiratory muscle function. These approaches do not prevent acute respiratory failure.

INSPIRATORY MUSCLE AIDS

Cooperative patients who are not receiving sedation, narcotics, or high concentrations of supplemental oxygen, or who do not have seizure disorders and can attain assisted PCF over 160 L/m[2] are candidates to use noninvasive respiratory muscle aid alternatives to tracheostomy. Body ventilators and noninvasive intermittent positive pressure ventilation (IPPV) methods can be used. IPPV can be applied noninvasively via oral, nasal, or oral-nasal interfaces to assist inspiratory muscle function and support alveolar ventilation. Since the use of noninvasive IPPV methods is critical for long-term success, there must be no conditions that interfere with the use of IPPV interfaces such as facial fractures, inadequate bite for mouthpiece entry, presence of a nasogastric tube, or beards that hamper airtight seal.

The advantages of using noninvasive aids over tracheostomy include safety, convenience, comfort, and improved speech, swallowing, sleep, and appearance. In addition, patients receiving tracheostomy IPPV are generally hyperventilated. This can exacerbate respiratory muscle deconditioning,[4] and the resulting chronic hypocapnia may result in bone decalcification.[5]

BODY VENTILATORS

Negative-pressure body ventilators (NPBVs) act on the body by creating atmospheric pressure changes around the thorax and abdomen. Other body ventilators like the rocking bed ventilator and the intermittent abdominal pressure ventilator (IAPV) act directly on the body to move the diaphragm and thereby assist inspiratory muscle function.

The NPBVs, which include the iron lung, chest shell ventilator, and wrap-style ventilators, envelop the chest and abdomen. Iron lungs continue to be the mainstay of intensive care unit ventilatory support in some centers in Europe.[6] Currently, however, portable iron lungs (PortaLung, Lifecare International Inc., Westminster, CO) and the more portable chest shell and wrap-style devices are more commonly used for long-term nocturnal ventilatory support.

The chest shell ventilators consist of a firm shell that covers the chest and abdomen (Fig. 36-1). Negative pressure is cycled under the shell by a negative pressure generator. This ventilator can support ventilation with the patient sitting or supine, but it is only practical for the latter because the IAPV and noninvasive IPPV methods are more practical for patients when they are sitting.

The wrap-style ventilators, similar in principle and function to the chest shell ventilator, consist of a firm plastic grid that covers the thorax and abdomen. The grid and the body under it are covered by a windproof wrap or jacket that is sealed around the neck and extremities. Negative-pressure ventilators cycle subatmospheric pressure under the wrap and grid. Although more time consuming to don, they are more effective than chest shell ventilators because of more complete covering of the thorax and abdomen.

The NPBVs are suitable for overnight ventilatory support, but with time they become less effective because of the patients' decreasing pulmonary compliance with age. They also

TABLE 36-1 Patients with the Following Disorders Can Benefit from the Use of Physical Medicine Aids

Myopathies
  Muscular dystrophies including Duchenne and Becker
    Dystrophinopathies, limb-girdle, Emery-Dreifuss, facioscapu-
      lohumeral, congenital, childhood autosomal recessive, and
      myotonic dystrophies
  Inflammatory, congenital, and metabolic myopathies
  Myasthenia gravis
Neurological disorders
  Anterior horn cell disorders including the spinal muscular atro-
    phies, motor neuron diseases, and poliomyelitis
  Neuropathies including Charcot-Marie-Tooth disease
  Phrenic neuropathies
  Guillain-Barré syndrome
  Multiple sclerosis, Friedreich's ataxia, and familial dysauto-
    nomia
  Myelopathies including high-level traumatic tetraplegia
  Sleep-disordered breathing including obesity hypoventilation
  Restrictive lung or chest wall conditions such as lung resection
    and kyphoscoliosis
  Chronic obstructive pulmonary disease

cause obstructive sleep apneas which have been associated with systemic hypertension and indicate switching patients to noninvasive IPPV methods.[7,8]

The rocking bed ventilator (J.H. Emerson Company, Cambridge, MA) rocks the patient 15 to 30 degrees and allows gravity to cyclically displace the abdominal contents and thereby move the diaphragm. It is generally not as effective as other NPBVs and noninvasive IPPV.[9]

Largely because these body ventilators were only practical and effective with the user recumbent and the fact that an indwelling tracheostomy tube facilitated airway secretion management, tracheostomy and translaryngeal delivery of IPPV and suctioning have become the mainstay of conventional respiratory management since the late 1950s.[10] How-

ever, because of the many difficulties, complications, and the expense associated with this invasive approach when used in the long term,[10] and because of the recent advances in physical medicine respiratory muscle aids, tracheostomy is now as unnecessary[11] as it is undesirable[12] for the majority of patients with the diagnoses listed in Table 36-1.

NONINVASIVE IPPV AND THE INTERMITTENT ABDOMINAL PRESSURE VENTILATOR

The IAPV involves the intermittent inflation of an elastic bladder contained in a corset worn beneath a user's outer clothing by a positive pressure ventilator (Fig. 36-2) (Exsufflation Belt, Lifecare International Inc., Westminster, CO). Bladder action moves the diaphragm upward causing forced exsufflation and subsequently a passive insufflation. Since gravity is important for its action, it can be effective only with the patient sitting. The IAPV can augment tidal volumes by 300 to 700 mL, but volumes as high as 1200 mL have been reported.[13] Patients with more than 1 h of ventilator-free breathing ability usually prefer to use mouthpiece IPPV for daytime aid rather than the IAPV.[13] The IAPV is usually inadequate in the presence of scoliosis or obesity.

Noninvasive IPPV methods are more effective than body ventilators and are preferred over tracheostomy IPPV and NPBV use.[12] However, their use was not reported as alternatives to long-term invasive approaches until the 1980s. The recent availability of mechanical expiratory muscle (coughing) aids and newly described noninvasive IPPV methods now make it practical to prevent respiratory complications of neuromuscular diseases and manage long-term ventilatory insufficiency by strictly noninvasive approaches.

In the early 1950s many postpoliomyelitis body ventilator users with little or no ventilator-free breathing ability were advised to, but refused to, undergo tracheostomy. Many gradually discontinued body ventilator use in favor of up to 24-h mouthpiece IPPV. During daytime hours, some mouthpiece IPPV users hold the mouthpiece between their

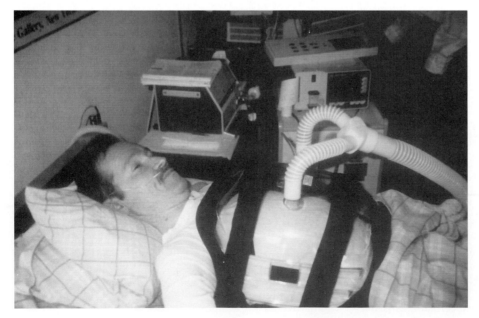

FIGURE 36-1 This patient with no measurable vital capacity since 1952 used a chest shell ventilator for nocturnal ventilatory support for 25 years before switching to nocturnal lipseal IPPV in 1980 and a regimen of 24-h mouthpiece IPPV.

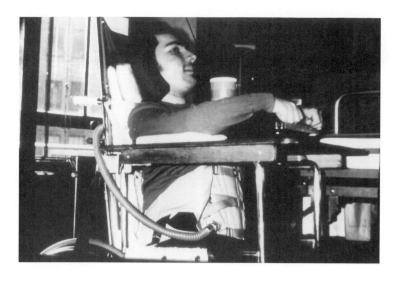

FIGURE 36-2 This 24-h ventilator-dependent individual with Duchenne muscular dystrophy used lipseal IPPV for nocturnal ventilatory support and an intermittent abdominal pressure ventilator (seen here) for daytime ventilatory support.

lips and teeth, but most prefer to have it held near the mouth by either a metal clamp attached to the wheelchair or fixed onto motorized wheelchair controls (Fig. 36-3) and receive assisted breaths as necessary to maintain normal alveolar ventilation.[14]

For effective mouthpiece IPPV, the patient must learn to

FIGURE 36-3 This 24-h noninvasive IPPV patient with Duchenne muscular dystrophy is using mouthpiece IPPV with the mouthpiece held adjacent to his mouth.

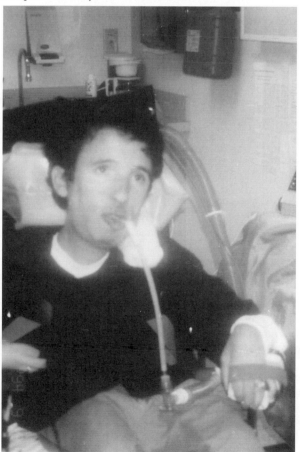

use the palate to prevent insufflation leakage out of the nose and to open the glottis with the initiation of each assisted breath. Adequate neck rotation and oral motor function are also necessary to grab the mouthpiece and receive IPPV without insufflation leakage out of the mouth.

Patients are also taught to air stack by consecutively taking and holding delivered ventilator volumes to approach the predicted inspiratory capacity. The maximum volume of air that can be held is the maximum insufflation capacity (MIC). Air stacking may help maintain static lung compliance and the higher volumes increase both unassisted and assisted PCF and permit the patient to raise voice volume as needed. Because of the importance of air stacking, volume-cycled ventilators rather than pressure-cycled ventilators or bilevel positive airway pressure machines are used. In addition, some patients benefit from the use of the low-pressure alarm on volume ventilators to maintain adequate alveolar ventilation by developing conditioned reflexes to accomplish this during sleep.

Although mouthpiece IPPV is delivered via a simple mouthpiece for daytime ventilatory support, patients occasionally nap and the mouthpiece is at risk of falling out of the mouth. This can be potentially hazardous. A mouthpiece IPPV should be used for sleep with lipseal retention (Fig. 36-4) (Puritan-Bennett Inc., Pickering, Ontario).[15] The lipseal seals the mouth and firmly retains the mouthpiece in the mouth. Orthodontic bite plates and custom fabricated acrylic lipseals can also increase comfort and efficacy and eliminate the risk of orthodontic deformity that can result from long-term use.

Aerophagia and abdominal distention often occur sporadically during sleep. The air passes as flatus once the patient gets up or is placed in a wheelchair in the morning. When severe, a rectal tube can decompress the colon.

Nasal IPPV was first described for 24-h ventilatory support for a patient with no ventilator-free breathing ability in 1984.[16] A nasal CPAP mask was used as the nasal interface. There are now many commercially available CPAP masks on the market that can be used for nasal IPPV. Each design applies pressure differently to the paranasal area. Patients must be offered various styles to determine the ones that are most comfortable and airtight. Many patients use different style

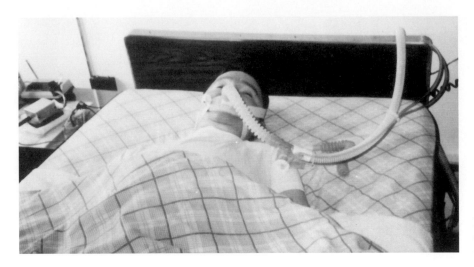

FIGURE 36-4 The same patient as in Fig. 36-1, who continues to use lipseal IPPV for nocturnal ventilatory support.

interfaces on alternate nights to vary skin contact pressure. Custom molded nasal interfaces[16–19] are also now both commercially (SEFAM company, distributed by Lifecare Inc., Westminster, CO) and individually available (Fig. 36-5).[19]

EXPIRATORY MUSCLE AIDS

A normal cough expels about 2.5 L of air[20] upon glottic opening after the glottis has been closed for about 0.2 s to permit the generation of high intrathoracic pressures. Peak transient expiratory flows or PCF normally exceed 6 L/s.[21,22]

The vital capacities (VCs), forced vital capacities (FVCs), and PCFs of patients with paralytic and/or restrictive pulmonary syndromes are further diminished during intercurrent respiratory tract infections and following general anesthesia because of fatigue, temporary weakening of both inspiratory

FIGURE 36-5 Custom molded acrylic low-profile nasal interface for nasal IPPV. (Available from the University of Medicine and Dentistry of New Jersey, Newark, NJ.)

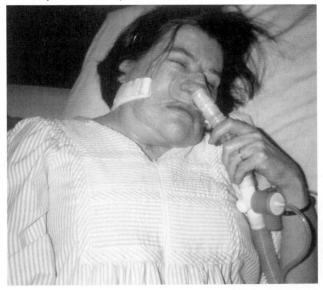

and expiratory muscles,[23] and bronchial mucus plugging. Concomitant weakness of oropharyngeal muscles exacerbates the problem. Nevertheless, because these patients have essentially normal airways, the use of expiratory muscle (abdominal muscle) aids can increase PCF and thereby prevent serious pulmonary complications.[24]

MANUALLY ASSISTED COUGHING

Both inspiratory and expiratory muscle function are important for effective coughing. If the VC is under 1.5 L, the MIC becomes an important parameter. Assisted PCF from insufflations over 1.5 L are always much greater than assisted PCF from patients with lower VCs who are not maximally insufflated before coughing. Following an optimally deep breath or insufflation, manually assisted coughing is performed by providing an abdominal thrust in conjunction with glottic opening. A manual resuscitator, intermittent positive-pressure breathing (IPPB) machine, or portable ventilator can be used to deliver the deep insufflations. Manually assisted coughing requires a cooperative patient, good coordination between the patient and caregiver, and adequate physical effort by the caregiver. When manually assisted coughing generates PCF greater than 160 L/min, safe tracheostomy tube removal and conversion to noninvasive ventilatory support is possible irrespective of the extent of respiratory muscle weakness,[11] and noninvasive ventilatory support methods can be used to prolong survival with minimal risk of complications.[25] Failure to achieve assisted PCF over 160 L/min despite good lung inflation usually indicates fixed upper airway obstruction or severe bulbar muscle weakness and upper airway collapse. Previous transtracheal intubation and subsequent tracheostomy has often caused granuloma formation and vocal cord adhesions or paralysis.[26] Since some lesions, especially the presence of obstructing granulation tissue, are amenable to surgical correction, laryngoscopic examination is warranted.

Neuromuscular patients with severe scoliosis may have poor assisted PCF because of a combination of limited insufflation capacity and inability of abdominal thrusts to capture the asymmetric diaphragm. Unlike patients with fixed upper airway obstruction, these patients are particularly good candidates to benefit from mechanical insufflation-exsufflation.

MECHANICAL INSUFFLATION-EXSUFFLATION

In February 1993, a mechanical insufflator-exsufflator (In-Exsufflator, J. H. Emerson Co., Cambridge, MA) came onto the market. This device can cycle instantaneously between positive and negative pressure. The addition of an abdominal thrust during the exsufflation cycle further increases PCF. One treatment consists of about five cycles of insufflation-exsufflation from about $+40$ to -40 cmH_2O. Treatments are continued until no further secretions are expulsed and VC and oxyhemoglobin saturation (Sa_{O_2}) return to pre-mucus plug baselines. Use can be required as often as every 10 min around the clock during intercurrent respiratory tract infections. Liquefaction of sputum using heated aerosol treatments with normal saline or mucolytic agents can facilitate exsufflation when secretions are inspissated.

Mechanical insufflation-exsufflation is also extremely effective via a tracheostomy tube. When used in this manner, the tube cuff should be inflated. A concomitant abdominal thrust is unnecessary. Since effective flows are created in both right and left airways without the discomfort or airway trauma of tracheal suctioning, patients invariably prefer it to suctioning, and airway suctioning can be discontinued entirely for many patients.

Besides being extremely effective for some patients, particularly those with functional bulbar musculature, in more than 650 patient-years and hundreds of applications by ventilator users at this institution as well as by patients in other studies,[27-29] there have been no episodes of pneumothorax, aspiration of gastric contents, or significant complications attributed to insufflation-exsufflation. The consistent increase in VC, forced expiratory flows, and Sa_{O_2} in the immediate post-exsufflation period indicates that no sustained airway collapse or obstruction results from its use.[30] Since the use of high insufflation pressures can cause intercostal muscle pulls for patients with low VCs who do not routinely receive maximal insufflations, insufflation pressures should be increased gradually for these patients.

The use of mechanical insufflation-exsufflation has permitted consistent extubation of ventilator-dependent neuromuscular patients immediately post-surgical anesthesia despite their having no ventilator-free breathing ability, and to convert them to the use of noninvasive IPPV. It has also permitted the avoidance of intubation or allowed quick extubation of neuromuscular patients in acute respiratory failure due to intercurrent infections with profuse airway secretions. It will not be very helpful if the patient cannot cooperate sufficiently to keep the airway open or if upper or lower airway collapse or obstruction is irreversible and not on the basis of bronchial mucous plugging.[31] This is most often the case for patients with advanced amyotrophic lateral sclerosis, spinal muscular atrophy type I, or chronic obstructive pulmonary disease.

OXIMETRY FEEDBACK AND
EVALUATION PARAMETERS

The evaluation of patients includes the measurement of VC (in sitting and recumbent positions), MIC, PCF, Sa_{O_2}, and end-tidal CO_2 (ET_{CO_2}). Since oxygen therapy is not used, the patient and care providers are instructed that Sa_{O_2} decreases below 95 percent are due to hypoventilation, bronchial mucous plugging, or intrinsic lung disease, usually pneumonia which is caused by inadequate attention to alveolar ventila-

tion and assisted coughing. Although Pa_{CO_2} levels can exceed 50 mmHg despite Sa_{O_2} levels of 95 percent or greater, provided that oxygen therapy is avoided, hypercapnia is usually minimal and asymptomatic when Sa_{O_2} levels are maintained within normal limits. Oximetry feedback guides the use of noninvasive IPPV during daytime hours. Patients are instructed to maintain Sa_{O_2} greater than 94 percent by autonomous breathing and to take mouthpiece-assisted breaths only when necessary to maintain normal Sa_{O_2}. An oximetry alarm set at 93 to 94 percent may be useful to remind the patient to take assisted breaths. The patient sees that by taking slightly deeper or assisted breaths the Sa_{O_2} will normalize within seconds. Usually, the patient uses noninvasive IPPV as needed when tiring. Eventually, once generalized weakness is severe, patients use noninvasive IPPV continuously. The use of oximetry in this manner can help to reset central ventilatory drive by reversing compensatory metabolic alkalosis and virtually guarantee the effectiveness of noninvasive IPPV during sleep as well as during waking hours. Oximetry feedback is also helpful when decanulating tracheostomized patients and switching them to noninvasive respiratory muscle aids.[2]

Whether or not totally ventilator dependent, these patients often require 24-h noninvasive IPPV to maintain alveolar ventilation and air stacking for assisted coughing during intercurrent respiratory infections. Since with ventilator use the lungs are rarely underventilated, desaturations are usually caused by bronchial mucus plugging for which both manually and mechanically assisted coughing are used until Sa_{O_2} returns to normal or to baseline levels. As respiratory tract infections clear, VC and Sa_{O_2}, which may decrease from normal baselines, return to normal and patients usually wean to their former regimen of ventilator use until the next respiratory tract infection. If the Sa_{O_2} baseline decreases below 93 percent despite aggressive mechanical insufflation-exsufflation and noninvasive ventilatory support, a chest radiograph and further work-up are warranted, since at this point patients usually have intrinsic lung disease. This is very uncommon, however, when patients use assisted ventilation, assisted coughing, and oximetry feedback as prescribed.

GLOSSOPHARYNGEAL BREATHING

In essence, any tracheostomized patient with sufficient bulbar muscle function to potentially master glossopharyngeal breathing (GPB) is a good candidate for tracheostomy tube decanulation and conversion to noninvasive aids. The mastery of GPB can provide individuals with no measurable VC otherwise to achieve normal alveolar ventilation for hours in perfect safety without using their ventilators or in the event of sudden ventilator failure day or night.[14,32] Approximately 60 percent of ventilator users with no ventilator-free breathing ability and good bulbar muscle function,[32,33] can use GPB for ventilator-free breathing.

Both inspiratory and, indirectly, expiratory muscle function can be assisted by GPB.[14] This technique involves the use of the tongue and pharyngeal muscles to project (gulp) boluses of air past the glottis. The glottis closes with each gulp. One breath usually consists of six to nine gulps of 60 to 200 mL each. During the training period the efficiency of GPB can be monitored by spirometrically measuring the milliliters of air per gulp, gulps per breath, and breaths per minute. An excellent training manual and video are available.[34,35]

DIFFICULTIES IN INITIATING THE USE OF NONINVASIVE AIDS

Despite patient and caregiver preferences for noninvasive approaches[12]; the ability of these methods to lower the cost of home mechanical ventilation[36]; the elimination of the need for hospitalization, intubation, and bronchoscopy for many patients; and their safety and efficacy for long-term ventilatory support and secretion management, they are not being widely used. Currently, invasive approaches are consistent with the general tendency to resort to the highest available and most costly technology. Physician and hospital reimbursement has been procedure based and directed toward inpatient management rather than preventive care. A physician is often remunerated for hospitalizing a patient for respiratory failure, intubating or placing a tracheostomy, and performing bronchoscopy, but outpatient preventive care has not been recognized and has often not been reimbursed by third-party payors even though it costs only a small fraction of the alternative. Further, the initial use of noninvasive aids requires a significant time commitment for evaluating the use of various IPPV interfaces to optimize comfort and effectiveness. Another difficulty is the low volume of these patients seen by pulmonologists and physiatrist pulmonary specialists. Neuromuscular patients are rarely referred before an episode of acute respiratory failure has led to their being intubated. This is in large part because the neurologists who run the Muscular Dystrophy Association clinics in the United States are not experienced in the use of noninvasive respiratory muscle aids.[37]

Habilitation Interventions

Prolonging the lives of patients with neuromuscular disorders by taking the humane measures described above would have little meaning if it were not possible to provide these patients with the means for self-actualization. The restoration or optimization of independent functioning is critical for the physically challenged individuals' self-esteem, personal interactions, and life satisfaction. It is now possible for all but those who have lost all voluntary muscle control, including the control of all facial muscles, to communicate and control all the appliances in their homes with the use of assistive technology. It is important that clinicians caring for these patients be aware of their patients' functional and vocational capacities despite severe disability and ventilator dependence.

The following principles maximize outcomes[38]:

1. Interventions are designed to facilitate home management and activities of daily living (ADL) and relieve care provider burdens;
2. Interventions are based on a realistic evaluation of the patient's needs, physical and cognitive capabilities, and resources.
3. Interventions are considered in the overall framework of cultural and social attitudes, timing, and patient and family acceptance.

ORTHOPEDIC AND PHYSICAL THERAPEUTIC INTERVENTIONS

Orthopedic and physical therapeutic interventions are important for optimizing quality of life and minimizing the risk of medical complications from immobility for ventilator users with neuromuscular conditions. Lower extremity musculotendinous contractures can be minimized by using a combination of orthopedic surgery and physical therapy.[39] Scoliosis prevention, which is only possible by surgical means,[40] is important to permit the patient to use convenient and cosmetic methods of noninvasive ventilatory assistance such as the IAPV and to prevent radicular low back pain, lumbar compression radiculopathy, ischial discomfort, and skin breakdown. Scoliosis can also hinder the use of mobile arm supports for self-feeding, and with severe scoliosis the patient's ribs impinge into the abdomen and prevent him or her from leaning forward to optimize upper extremity function and eventually from sitting at all. Determination of the plateau VC is of paramount importance for timing surgical intervention.[41]

RESPIRATORY MUSCLE EXERCISE

Although short daily sessions of inspiratory resistive exercise have not been reported to improve spirometric values or maximum inspiratory or expiratory pressures,[42–44] respiratory muscle endurance has been reported to have improved[42,43,45] as a function of the level of VC and maximum inspiratory pressure at the outset of training. No patient with less than 30 percent of predicted VC has been reported to have improved.[42] This, however, is the level of VC at which point patients often require ventilatory aid and have considerable difficulty eliminating airway secretions during respiratory tract infections.[17] There is also no evidence that beginning an exercise program earlier would preserve more muscle function to delay the time when the deteriorating patient requires ventilatory aid or experiences pulmonary complications.[42] There may also be a greater rate of loss of muscle strength in any temporarily strengthened muscles, and the training may be dangerous for advanced patients. Thus, for those most likely to have respiratory complications, the use of high resistance exercise is likely to be of little or no value. It is interesting, however, that the combination of interspersing respiratory muscle rest by ventilatory assistance and inspiratory muscle training has been reported to improve the respiratory muscle strength and endurance of neuromuscular patients during ventilator weaning.[46]

DEEP BREATHING AND INSUFFLATION

The use of range-of-motion exercises for hypomobile tissues is a basic rehabilitation principle. This may be an even more important principle to apply to the lungs and chest walls of patients with restrictive pulmonary conditions. This has already been discussed as the frequent application of deep insufflations.

Although short periods of mechanical hyperinflation can briefly increase the dynamic pulmonary compliance associated with airway changes and reverse acute atelectasis,[47–49] multiple daily periods of maximal mechanical hyperinflations of up to 30 cmH$_2$O pressure have not been shown to improve static compliance in adults.[50] It is not yet known whether more aggressive treatments or treatments introduced before lung compliance is greatly reduced would be of benefit.[51] At the very least, hyperinflation treatments, including training in and the use of GPB, may be indicated before the VC has declined to 50 to 60 percent of predicted.

MOBILITY

Some ventilator users, particularly those who require only nocturnal ventilator use, are not totally wheelchair dependent. Facilitation of safe ambulation with the use of one or two standard or wide-based canes, crutches, or walkers may be indicated. Except for postpoliomyelitis ventilator users with patchy and asymmetric muscular weakness who retain good triceps brachii, lower extremity bracing is rarely indicated for ventilator users with neuromuscular diseases. Either their conditions progress too rapidly to permit adaptation to bracing, or muscle weakness is primarily proximal. In this case bracing neither renders the gait safer nor permits getting up from a chair without assistance.

WHEELCHAIRS

When ambulation is no longer safe, strollers, wheelchairs, and scooters can be useful. Wheelchairs can be manual or powered (for patients with inadequate biceps or leg strength to self-propel them). Proper sizing allows room for wearing a coat and orthotics when applicable. Most wheelchairs have an overall width of 24 to 28 in. Wider, more heavily constructed chairs can be made for obese individuals. A seatbelt should be used for those with poor sitting balance or weak trunk musculature.

RIGID FRAME WHEELCHAIRS
Wheelchairs can have rigid or nonrigid frames. A rigid frame provides more stability, a smoother ride, and durability. These wheelchairs have solid wheelchair bases with immovable axles. Such chairs can carry more weight and accessories such as ventilators and robot arms and are particularly suited for very active users who navigate rough terrain. Rigid frame chairs cannot be simply folded and put into cars but "quick release" wheels can be used to accomplish this in many cases.

NONRIGID FRAME WHEELCHAIRS
Nonrigid frame wheelchairs have crossbars connecting one side of the wheelchair to the other. These chairs, though less durable, fold, decreasing their width in half, and can be placed on the back seats or in the trunks of cars.

OTHER OPTIONS
Most individuals with neuromuscular conditions require adjustable, removable leg rests with heel straps. Off-set foot plates and heel loops are used for individuals with severe ankle and foot deformities. The feet are maintained flat on the plates to discourage deformity. Elevating footrests often increases the turning radius of the wheelchair and are generally useful only in conjunction with a reclining back when lower extremity edema, postural hypotension, and skin pressure relief can not be medically managed. Individuals with poor endurance may also require a reclining seat. Neck rests with a forehead strap provide both lateral and anterior-posterior support.

The user has the option of having full-length wheelchair arms or desk arms. Desk arms are usually preferred because they permit the user to approach tables. Full-length arms may be useful to support a lap tray. A lap board can facilitate the performance of schoolwork, gainful employment, and recreational activities. Elevating arms are an option but are rarely required by users with neuromuscular weakness. However, the arms must be removable to facilitate transfers.

SEATING SYSTEMS
While sitting, posture and positioning are important for function and impeding the development of deformities. When bony prominences or pelvic obliquity are severe, a firm seat cushion is used to support the ischia and to keep the pelvis level. Many specialized cushions and padded inserts are available to relieve problem skin pressure areas. Each patient should be evaluated on several systems. Modular components can be added to the chair to support patients with poor sitting balance. Hip adductor or abductor wedges and thigh straps can help maintain pelvic and lower extremity alignment. Lateral trunk supports or full contouring of a seat are options.[52] Some seating systems permit users to vary their sitting positions independently or to come to a stand.

MOTORIZED WHEELCHAIRS AND SCOOTERS
Many of the prescription considerations for standard wheelchairs also apply to power wheelchairs. The operation system is an additional consideration, however. Power wheelchairs can be operated by joystick, tongue, chin, and sip-and-puff controls as well as by any muscle activity under the patient's control. Daytime ventilatory support is conveniently provided by the delivery of IPPV via a mouthpiece fixed onto wheelchair controls adjacent to the mouth (Fig. 36-3).

Motorized scooters have a maximum speed of 10 mi/h and a turning radius of about 20 in., and they can ascend a grade of 30 degrees and go about 20 mi on one battery charge. They have swivel seats and can have elevating seats when this is necessary for independent transfers. They are longer, however, and require more maneuvering space than wheelchairs. Trunk and upper extremity musculature must be functional to transfer to and from, and to operate a scooter. A wire basket is attached to the frame of the scooter for transporting objects.

BEDS AND MATTRESSES

Most ventilator users require hospital beds to assist care providers in positioning the patient at home. A major problem in caring for individuals with neuromuscular disease is the need for frequent overnight turning. Some individuals require repositioning in bed every hour.[53,54] Determining which mattresses provide the greatest comfort and reduce the nocturnal turning requirement is an empirical process. Available mattress surfaces include egg crate, water, alternating pressure pad, and other air mattresses. Each has advantages and disadvantages.[55] Some patients require frequent turning irrespective of mattress style. The Motion Bed (Emerson Co., Cambridge, MA), a bed that slowly rotates the user from side to side, can alleviate any need for turning. The movement, however, can at times loosen nasal or lipseal interfaces.

OTHER EQUIPMENT

Equipment and environment modifications must also be undertaken to facilitate toileting, bathing, hygiene, dressing,

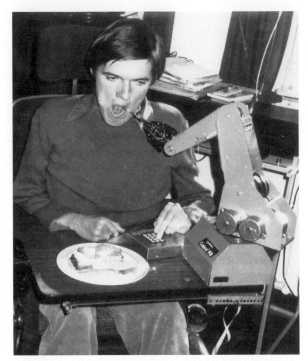

FIGURE 36-6 A Duchenne muscular dystrophy ventilator user using a programmable, wheelchair-mountable robot arm to feed himself.

eating, food preparation, environmental control,[55] and, at times, communication.[56] Splinting extremity articulations and service animals such as chimpanzees and dogs may be helpful.[55] Many patients can use joystick-controlled, programmable robot arms for self-feeding, opening doors, and manipulating smaller objects (Fig. 36-6).[57]

Periodicals that can provide valuable information about habilitation options for individuals with neuromuscular disease are published by the Jerry Lewis Muscular Dystrophy Association (Tuscon, AZ), Families of Children with Spinal Muscular Atrophy (Highland Park, IL), the National Easter Seal Society (Chicago, IL), the Polio Society (Washington, DC), the International Polio Network (St. Louis, MO), the ALS Association (Woodland Hills, CA), the Myasthenia Gravis Foundation (Chicago, IL), the Charcot-Marie-Tooth Association (Upland, PA), the National Ataxia Foundation (Wayzata, MN), the National Support Group for Myositis (Cooperstown, NY), the Guillain-Barré Syndrome Foundation International (Wynnewood, PA), the Malignant Hyperthermia Association of the United States (Westport, CN), New Mobility (North Hollywood, CA), and the National Association for Ventilator Dependent Individuals (New York, NY).

Psychosocial Issues

MARRIAGE

In a recent study of more than 600 community-based ventilator users with primarily neuromuscular conditions, of which 494 were supported by noninvasive means, there were 313 males with a mean age of 46.5 years and 306 females with a mean age of 52.2 years.[58] They had been dependent on ventilatory support for a mean of 21.1 years and, at the time of the survey, used aid a mean of 15.7 h/day. Two hundred seventy-seven (45 percent) ventilator users, 157 males and 120 females, had not married. However, 186, 97 males and 89 females, were married prior to requiring ventilatory support and remained married and living with their spouses. This included four individuals who were widowed prior to requiring ventilatory support and later remarried while using support and two males who were divorced prior to requiring support and remarried while on aid. Thirty-six individuals, 10 males and 26 females, were married prior to requiring ventilatory support and were divorced and have remained so while using ventilatory aids. An additional 60 individuals, 32 males and 28 females, who were single prior to requiring ventilator support, married as ventilator users. Thus, 20 percent of ventilator users who were single before requiring ventilator use, married for the first time after becoming ventilator users. The 16 percent divorce rate of the ventilator users who began using ventilators at the average age of 28 years is about one-half that of the general population for individuals married at age 28.[59]

EMPLOYMENT

Two hundred thirty-four ventilator users were gainfully employed. Seventeen other ventilator users reported being active daily as volunteers for various philanthropic causes, and 24 were students. In addition, 32 married women ventilator users reported being housewives.[58]

LIFE SATISFACTION

When asked to indicate how satisfied they were with their lives by circling a number from 1 to 7 where 1 is very dissatisfied and 7 is very satisfied, the 615 individuals who responded had a mean of 5.1. Two hundred forty-two health care professional controls with an average age of 33.0 ± 8 years (range 21 to 59 years) reported 5.33 ± 1.2 for satisfaction with their own lives. When asked how ADL-dependent, ventilator-dependent individuals would respond to this question, however, the health care professionals mean estimate of the ventilator users' responses was 2.42 ± 1.37. This was significantly worse than the ventilator users' actual responses ($p < .0001$). Differences between individuals using noninvasive ventilatory aids and those using tracheostomy IPPV were found. The noninvasive group was older than the tracheostomy group (50 versus 45.8 years, $p < .001$), had significantly less upper extremity function (1.13 versus 1.21, $p < .05$), used ventilatory support for fewer hours per day (15.5 versus 17.7, $p < .05$) but for more years (22 versus 17, $p < .005$). The tracheostomy IPPV group, however, had a mean satisfaction index of 4.68 as opposed to 5.04 for the noninvasive group ($p < .05$).

Thus, ventilator users, in general, are satisfied with their lives. Noninvasive ventilatory aid users are significantly more satisfied with their lives than tracheostomy IPPV users; and, as previously mentioned, they were also found to prefer noninvasive aid use over tracheostomy IPPV for safety, convenience, appearance, and comfort, and they reported that it hampered swallowing and speech less than did tracheostomy IPPV.[12] Thus, both physical medicine respiratory muscle aids and physical aids to function enhance quality of life and deserve wider application for this patient population.

References

1. Bach JR: Amyotrophic lateral sclerosis: Communication status and survival with ventilatory support. *Am J Phys Med Rehabil* 72:343, 1993.

2. Bach JR, Saporito LR: Criteria for extubation and tracheostomy tube removal for patients with ventilatory failure: A different approach to weaning. *Chest* 110:1566, 1996.

3. Bach JR, Rajaraman R, Ballanger F, et al: Neuromuscular ventilatory insufficiency: The effect of home mechanical ventilator use vs. oxygen therapy on pneumonia and hospitalization rates. *Am J Phys Med Rehabil* 77:8, 1998.

4. Bach JR: Case studies of respiratory management, in Bach JR (ed): *Pulmonary Rehabilitation: The Obstructive and Paralytic Conditions.* Philadelphia, Hanley & Belfus, 1996; chap 25, pp 331–346.

5. Bach JR, Haber II, Wang TG, Alba AS: Alveolar ventilation as a function of ventilatory support method. *Eur J Phys Med Rehabil* 5:80, 1995.

6. Corrado A, Gorini M, De Paola E: Alternative techniques for managing acute neuromuscular respiratory failure. *Semin Neurol* 15:84, 1995.

7. Bach JR: Inappropriate weaning and late onset ventilatory failure of individuals with traumatic quadriplegia. *Paraplegia* 31:430, 1993.

8. Bach JR, Alba AS, Bohatiuk G, et al: Mouth intermittent positive pressure ventilation in the management of postpolio respiratory insufficiency. *Chest* 91:859, 1987.

9. Goldstein RS, Molotiu N, Skrastins R, et al: Assisting ventilation in respiratory failure by negative pressure ventilation and by rocking bed. *Chest* 92:470, 1987.

10. Bach JR: Conventional approaches to managing neuromuscular ventilatory failure, in Bach JR (ed): *Pulmonary Rehabilitation: The Obstructive and Paralytic Conditions.* Philadelphia, Hanley & Belfus, 1996; chap 23, pp 285–301.

11. Bach JR, Saporito LS: Indications and criteria for decannulation and transition from invasive to noninvasive long-term ventilatory support. *Respir Care* 39:515, 1994.

12. Bach JR: A comparison of long-term ventilatory support alternatives from the perspective of the patient and care giver. *Chest* 104:1702, 1993.

13. Bach JR, Alba AS: Total ventilatory support by the intermittent abdominal pressure ventilator. *Chest* 99:630, 1991.

14. Bach JR, Alba AS, Bodofsky E, et al: Glossopharyngeal breathing and non-invasive aids in the management of post-polio respiratory insufficiency. *Birth Defects* 23:99, 1987.

15. Bach JR: Update and perspective on noninvasive respiratory muscle aids: Part 1—The inspiratory muscle aids. *Chest* 105:1230, 1994.

16. Bach JF, Alba A, Mosher R, Delaubier A: Intermittent positive pressure ventilation via nasal access in the management of respiratory insufficiency. *Chest* 92:168, 1987.

17. Bach JR, Alba AS: Management of chronic alveolar hypoventilation by nasal ventilation. *Chest* 97:52, 1990.

18. Leger P, Jennequin J, Gerard M, Robert D: Home positive pressure ventilation via nasal mask for patients with neuromuscular weakness or restrictive lung or chest-wall disease. *Respir Care* 34:73, 1989.

19. McDermott I, Bach JR, Parker C, Sortor S: Custom-fabricated interfaces for intermittent positive pressure ventilation. *Int J Prosthodont* 2:224, 1989.

20. Leith DE: Cough, in Brain JD, Proctor D, Reid L (eds): *Lung Biology in Health and Disease: Respiratory Defense Mechanisms,* part 2. New York, Marcel Dekker, 1977; pp 545–592.

21. Bach JR, Smith WH, Michaels J, et al: Airway secretion clearance by mechanical exsufflation for post-poliomyelitis ventilator assisted individuals. *Arch Phys Med Rehabil* 74:170, 1993.

22. Fugl-Meyer AR, Grimby G: Ventilatory function in tetraplegic patients. *Scand J Rehab Med* 3:151, 1971.

23. Mier-Jedrzejowicz A, Brophy C, Green M: Respiratory muscle weakness during upper respiratory tract infections. *Am Rev Respir Dis* 138:5, 1988.

24. King M, Brock G, Lundell C: Clearance of mucus by simulated cough. *J Appl Physiol* 58:1776, 1985.

25. Bach JR: Amyotrophic lateral sclerosis: Predictors for prolongation of life by noninvasive respiratory aids. *Arch Phys Med Rehabil* 76:828, 1995.

26. Richard I, Giraud M, Perrouin-Verbe B, et al: Laryngo-tracheal stenosis after intubation or tracheostomy in neurological patients. *Arch Phys Med Rehabil* 77:493, 1996.

27. Barach AL, Beck GJ: Exsufflation with negative pressure: Physiologic and clinical studies in poliomyelitis, bronchial asthma, pulmonary emphysema and bronchiectasis. *Arch Int Med* 93:825, 1954.

28. Colebatch HJH: Artificial coughing for patients with respiratory paralysis. *Australasian J Med* 10:201, 1961.

29. Barach AL: The application of pressure, including exsufflation, in pulmonary emphysema. *Am J Surg* 89:372, 1955.

30. Bach JR: Mechanical insufflation-exsufflation: Comparison of peak expiratory flows with manually assisted and unassisted coughing techniques. *Chest* 104:1553, 1993.

31. Kobavashi I, Perry A, Rhymer J, et al: Relationships between the electrical activity of genioglossus muscle and the upper airway patency: A study in laryngectomised subjects. *Respir Crit Care Med* 149:A148, 1994.

32. Bach JR: New approaches in the rehabilitation of the traumatic high level quadriplegic. *Am J Phys Med Rehabil* 70:13, 1991.

33. Bach JR, Alba AS: Noninvasive options for ventilatory support of the traumatic high level quadriplegic. *Chest* 98:613, 1990.

34. Dail CW, Affeldt JE: *Glossopharyngeal Breathing* [video]. Los Angeles, Department of Visual Education, College of Medical Evangelists, 1954.

35. Dayman HG: Mechanics of airflow in health and emphysema. *J Clin Invest* 30:1175, 1951.

36. Bach JR, Intintola P, Alba AS, Holland I: The ventilator individual: Cost analysis of institutionalization versus rehabilitation and in-home management. *Chest* 101:26, 1992.

37. Bach JR: Ventilator use by muscular dystrophy association patients: An update. *Arch Phys Med Rehabil* 73:179, 1992.

38. Mann W, Lane J: *Assistive Technology for Persons with Disabilities: The Role of Occupational Therapy.* Baltimore, American Occupational Therapy Association, 1991; p 11.

39. Rideau Y, Duport G, Delaubier A, et al: Early treatment to preserve quality of locomotion for children with Duchenne muscular dystrophy. *Semin Neurol* 15:9, 1995.

40. Duport G, Gayet E, Pries P, et al: Spinal deformities and wheelchair seating in Duchenne muscular dystrophy: Twenty years of research and clinical experience. *Semin Neurol* 15:29, 1995.

41. Rideau Y, Glorion B, Delaubier A, et al: Treatment of scoliosis in Duchenne muscular dystrophy. *Muscle Nerve* 7:281, 1984.

42. DiMarco AF, Kelling JS, DiMarco MS, et al: The effects of inspiratory resistive training on respiratory muscle function in patients with muscular dystrophy. *Muscle Nerve* 8:284, 1985.

43. Martin AJ, Stern L, Yeates J, et al: Respiratory muscle training in Duchenne muscular dystrophy. *Develop Med Child Neurol* 28:314, 1986.

44. Rodillo E, Noble-Jamieson CM, Aber V, et al: Respiratory muscle training in Duchenne muscular dystrophy. *Arch Dis Childhood* 64:736, 1989.

45. Smith PEM, Coakley JH, Edwards RHT: Respiratory muscle training in Duchenne muscular dystrophy (letter). *Muscle Nerve* 11:784, 1988.

46. Aldrich JK, Karpel JP, Uhrlass RM, et al: Weaning from mechanical ventilation: Adjunctive use of inspiratory muscle resistive training. *Crit Care Med* 17:143, 1989.

47. Egberg LD, Laver MB, Bendixen HH: Intermittent deep breaths

and compliance during anesthesia in man. *Anesthesiology* 24:57, 1963.

48. Mead J, Collier C: Relation of volume history of lungs to respiratory mechanics in anesthetized dogs. *J Appl Physiol* 14:669, 1959.

49. O'Donohue W: Maximum volume IPPB for the management of pulmonary atelectasis. *Chest* 76:683, 1976.

50. McCool FD, Mayewski RF, Shayne DS, et al: Intermittent positive pressure breathing in patients with respiratory muscle weakness: Alterations in total respiratory system compliance. *Chest* 90:546, 1986.

51. De Troyer A, Deisser P: The effects of intermittent positive pressure breathing on patients with respiratory muscle weakness. *Am Rev Respir Dis* 124:132, 1981.

52. Gibson DA, Albisser AM, Koreska J: Role of the wheelchair in the management of the muscular dystrophy patient. *Can Med Assoc J* 113:964, 1975.

53. Firth M, Gardner-Medwin D, Hosking G, Wilkinson E: Interviews with parents of boys suffering from Duchenne muscular dystrophy. *Dev Med Child Neurol* 25:466, 1983.

54. Redding GJ, Okamoto GA, Guthrie RD, et al: Sleep patterns in nonambulatory boys with Duchenne muscular dystrophy. *Arch Phys Med Rehabil* 66:818, 1985.

55. Valenza J, Guzzardo SL, Bach JR: Functional interventions for individuals with neuromuscular disease, in Bach JR (ed): *Pulmonary Rehabilitation: The Obstructive and Paralytic Conditions.* Philadelphia, Hanley & Belfus, 1996; chap 28, pp 371–394.

56. Kazandjian MS, Dikeman KJ, Bach JR: Assessment and management of communication impairment in neuromuscular disease. *Semin Neurol* 15:52, 1995.

57. Bach JR, Zeelenberg A, Winter C: Wheelchair mounted robot manipulators: Long term use by patients with Duchenne muscular dystrophy. *Am J Phys Med Rehabil* 69:59–69, 1990.

58. Bach JR, Barnett V: Psychosocial, vocational, quality of life and ethical issues, in Bach JR (ed): *Pulmonary Rehabilitation: The Obstructive and Paralytic Conditions.* Philadelphia, Hanley & Belfus, 1996; chap 29, pp 395–411.

59. National Center for Health Statistics: *Vital Statistics of the United States, 1985,* vol III, *Marriage and Divorce,* DHHS Publication no (PHS) 89-1103. Public Health Service, Washington. US Government Printing Office, 1989; pp 4-23, 4-24.

PART V
SPECIFIC DISEASE MANAGEMENT

Chapter 37
PULMONARY REHABILITATION IN THE ELDERLY

E. PAUL CHERNIACK

Among the elderly, chronic lung diseases, such as chronic obstructive pulmonary disease (COPD), are common, disabling diseases whose prevalence is increasing. The ability of the aged to survive these diseases and maintain their quality of life is dependent on many parameters including age, remaining pulmonary function (as documented by a variety of indexes), response to bronchodilators, nutrition, continued smoking, exercise tolerance, and self-perception of breathing. Pulmonary rehabilitation provides the means to make a multifactorial intervention to improve as many of the causes of morbidity and mortality as possible. This chapter outlines the methods used in this intervention and examines the evidence for their efficacy.

Effects of Aging on Respiratory Muscle Physiology

Changes that occur in respiratory muscle function with aging may impact on the ability of the elderly individual to undergo rehabilitation. A reduction in muscle strength as measured by maximal inspiratory pressure (MIP) and maximum expiratory pressure (MEP) was initially noted 30 years ago by Rinquist,[1] who noted a curvilinear decline in muscle strength in approximately 200 subjects between ages 20 and 80, with the steep linear part occurring between ages 60 and 80 in both men and women. Since then, several other studies, including a recent study of 4463 volunteers, have shown a linear, but not a steep decline in MIP and MEP in individuals between 60 and 90 as that observed by Rinquist.[2-6] The muscle strength of the diaphragm has been shown to decline in age in one small comparison of 10 young (ages 18 to 32) and nine old people (ages 65 to 74).[7]

Muscle endurance may be similar in young and elderly subjects. This has been assessed using a weighted "threshold" loading device, in which volunteers breathed at sufficient pressure to open an air valve against which increasing amounts of weight were added.[8] The results in aged individuals were similar to earlier studies in young subjects, although the method used in the study of the young did not control for variability of breathing pattern.[7,9]

Aging is characterized by a number of changes in pulmonary function, including declines in residual volume, forced expiratory volume in one second, maximum breathing capacity, forced vital capacity, elastic recoil, diffusing capacity, maximal oxygen uptake, and an increase in closing capacity.[10] Arterial P_{O_2} tension declines with age in part because of the increase in closing capacity, whereas arterial P_{CO_2} is nearly the same in the young and the old. The result of these changes is that there is a lessening of maximal airflow.[10] The ability to exercise at increased lung volumes during exercise is pressure dependent, and in one study healthy elderly appeared to generate excessive pressures to maintain their ventilation.[11]

Takishima and associates[12] demonstrated a decreasing oxygen consumption with age in normal subjects by using an expandable dead space connected to a spirometer filled with 100% O_2. Oxygen consumption was assessed from the reduction in volume of the spirometer. However, only one subject in the study was older than 70.

Pulmonary Rehabilitation Team

As the approach to solving multiple potential problems in successfully rehabilitating the patient involves more than one professional discipline, a team approach to pulmonary rehabilitation programs has been recommended.[13-16] Components of a rehabilitation program have included physical examinations, judicious use of medication, patient education, psychological, social, and nutritional assessment, exercise, respiratory therapy, and training in breathing and relaxation techniques. Some suggested team numbers include a pulmonary physician, physical therapist, occupational therapist, nurse, dietician, psychiatrist or psychologist, and chaplain, but the composition of team can be variable; smaller programs need fewer members, and appropriately trained and motivated individuals can perform multiple functions.[13,14]

There have been no systematic studies of the necessity of given team members. It is unknown if programs with a larger team are more successful than those who have fewer, or if the elderly benefit more readily from teams of different compositions than younger individuals.

Patient Selection Criteria

While the variability in severity of and response to illness, including exercise tolerance, hyperpnea, and motivation, can affect how successfully a person can be rehabilitated, it has been suggested that all elderly patients impaired by long-standing pulmonary disease should be considered.[13,17] The severity of the disease may alter motivation, as those patients with very mild or very severe degrees of impairment may not believe that they might realize noticeable improvement in their health. However, patients have been shown to benefit with both COPD of varying severity and respiratory illnesses other than COPD.[13,17,18]

Compliance is an important issue in pulmonary rehabilitation.[13,19] Individuals must be able to have the capacity to learn about the nature of their illness to properly cope with the problems they may confront, such as how to recognize symptoms and manage them. They need to learn how to use their medications and, in some cases, oxygen, learn breathing and exercise techniques, and receive retraining on how to perform activities of daily living. They must be able to attend sessions several times a week for one to several months. Elderly patients may have cognitive deficits and medical, psychiatric, and social problems that may make attendance difficult. For these reasons, and because the elderly have many undetected potential problems treatable by rehabilitation, initial patient assessment is important.

Patient Assessment

A comprehensive assessment for potential candidates has been advocated. This assessment should include history and physical, nursing assessment using questionnaires to evaluate, for example, activities of daily living, disease-specific quality of life, and psychologic function. Evaluations by physiotherapists, occupational therapists, nutritionists, and social workers can also be helpful. The role of the history and physical examination is to identify limitations and intercurrent illnesses that might influence what therapies might be offered or what other medical conditions might have to be evaluated and treated before further participation can take place.[13] Aged COPD patients may have cognitive impairment, and cognitive assessment may be significant.[13] Certain varieties of psychiatric disorders, such as depression and anxiety are more common in this population, and questioning should be directed to detect these disorders.[13] Nursing assessments as referred to above can be used to set feasible targets for gains in activities of daily living and quality of life, and provide background for referral to other team members, such as the psychologist or the social worker.[13] At least eight different quality-of-life questionnaires have been studied for use in COPD. Of these, the Sickness Impact Profile, a 30-min, 136-item questionnaire, has been most thoroughly investigated. Even though it is long, it has been found to be reproducible and valid. However, its responsiveness (the ability to detect small but significant changes over a long period of time) has not been examined in COPD.[20] Three shorter questionnaires, the Medical Outcome Study (20 items, 3 min to complete), Quality of Well Being Questionnaire (50 items, 12 min, requiring a trained interviewer), and the Nottingham Health Profile (45 items, 10 min) are other quality-of-life instruments that have been applied to COPD with many of the same advantages as the Sickness Impact Profile, but since they are shorter, they obtain less information.[20] There are three questionnaires that have been developed specifically for COPD whose responsiveness, validity, and reproducibility have been shown, the Chronic Respiratory Disease Questionnaire (20 items, 20 min, given by trained interviewer), the St. George's Respiratory Questionnaire (76 items), and the Baseline Dyspnea Index (assesses dyspnea only, less than 5 min, requiring trained interviewer).[20]

Initial laboratory investigations, which can include pulmonary function testing, exercise testing, electrocardiogram, and blood-gas measurements, identify what potential causes limit the patient's ability to tolerate exercise, such as hypoxia, hypercapnia, or deconditioning.[13,15,21] Pulmonary function testing can ascertain the severity of illness, and diffusing capacity can predict, although not with certainty, hypoxemia during exercise.[13,21]

Ries[21] uses FEV_1 to stratify COPD patients into different groups, which help to base exercise training goals. Exercise testing which can include an 8- or 12-min walk or treadmill walking, such as performed in the Bruce protocol, serves multiple functions: it can determine how much exercise a patient can tolerate and what symptoms, blood-gas abnormalities, and concomitant medical conditions, such as ischemia, might influence a subject's ability to train. However, older patients may have increased difficulty in performing certain maneuvers, such as those required for pulmonary function testing.[22] Aged individuals can have reduced strength or mental impairment which can decrease their ability to cooperate in tests which are contingent on patient effort, often involving breath holding or repeated maximal expirations.[22] Exercise therapy is a critical element in pulmonary rehabilitation, decreasing symptoms, attempting to improve ventilatory muscle strength and endurance, and reducing deconditioning, which may impair ability to perform activities of daily living. The severity of COPD will determine the means and goals of exercise therapy.[13,21,23]

There are many physiologic changes in COPD which influence capacity for exercise. Subjects can have circulatory impairment from right ventricular dysfunction or be limited from exercise only by maximal heart rate.[24,25] The latter group of individuals during exercise has elevations of blood lactate with reserve ventilatory capacity and a decrease in P_{CO_2} while training.[24,25] Mechanical factors can preclude successful training in patients with more advanced COPD, such as curtailed end-expiratory flow.[24,25] Individuals circumvent this barrier by utilizing greater end-expiratory lung volumes, which increase flow, but which create positive pleural pressures even at rest, increase work, and place the chest muscles and diaphragm at a mechanical disadvantage.[24,25] As subjects exercise, more work is done by the inspiratory muscles and muscle fatigue may possibly occur. As the ratio of the mean transdiaphragmatic pressure to the maximal transdiaphragmatic pressure created during inspiration increases, diaphragm endurance decreases.[24,25] Subjects with emphysema have weak inspiratory muscles which fatigue easily.[24,25] COPD patients have less lung surface for gas exchange, and severely decreased diffusion can limit oxygen consumption and impair exercise tolerance.[25]

Exercise Training in Pulmonary Rehabilitation

Exercise training regimens have been devised to increase muscle strength and endurance. Regimens can include maneuvers to enhance the ability of specific muscle groups to meet respiratory needs (e.g., breathing against loads) and others (e.g., stationary cycling) that are not specific to the respiratory muscles but create other changes, such as greater stroke volume, cardiac output, and blood volume, which can increase respiratory endurance.[23,26,27]

Decisions about the intensity of the exercise to be given are based on the supposition that there is a threshold value beyond which a training effect will be perceived and that, above this threshold, the amount of work done will determine the outcome.[26] Heart rate, serum lactate, and oxygen uptake have been used to ascertain this threshold, but the amount of exercise that different individuals use to achieve a given level of these potential criteria vary.[26] Casaburi recommends that training be given in sessions of at least 20 min, based on data showing those of 30 to 60 min have a greater effect than those of 10 to 15 min. Three to five sessions a week will confer gains which may be obtained only minimally from two sessions. More frequent exercise has not been shown to produce any greater training effect.[26] The majority of studies examining results of training have used 5 to 10 weeks to produce a significant training effect.[26]

Regimens to improve respiratory strength have included multiple maximal inspiratory or expiratory maneuvers and breathing against inspiratory loads. Efforts to improve endurance training have focused on isocapneic hyperpnea and inspiratory loading. In isocapneic hyperpnea, patients breathe at a given target level of inspiration for up to 15 min.[27]

Inspiratory resistive load training involves breathing against inspiratory loads for 5 to 15 min, but subjects have the ability to modify their breathing pattern by breathing slowly and deeply, which is easier but can decrease the effort needed below that which is necessary to achieve a training response.[27] This possibility can be circumvented by inspiratory threshold loading, in which weights of differing amounts are applied via a spring or plunger via the port of a one-way valve.[28] Even using this technique, the respiratory pattern may still need to be controlled, and neither of these inspiratory resistive methods replicates the changes in lung volumes of unloaded exercise.[27]

Although many studies have shown success in respiratory muscle training,[13,16,21,22,24–32] a meta-analysis[33] did not show benefits of training. The authors of the meta-analysis (Smith and colleagues) screened 73 articles from computerized databases to obtain 17 well-randomized trials.

They evaluated the methodologies of all of the articles and gave each article a score based on quality of methodology. In addition, the results or measurements of a given criterion in each study were pooled through measurement of an effect size (the difference between treatment and control groups divided by the pooled standard deviation of that measure). There was a significant effect size for respiratory muscle strength but not for respiratory muscle endurance, exercise capacity, or functional status. It was concluded that evidence for the benefit of respiratory training was lacking, although it could not be concluded that certain populations of patients might not benefit from individual regimens. In a review of the use of exercise in pulmonary rehabilitation, Ries concludes that a simple method to select patients who might benefit from such training has yet to be found.[21]

Since the meta-analysis, Kim and coworkers[34] performed a double-blind, randomized study, subjecting 67 patients with COPD, mean age approximately 64, to 6 months of muscle training with an inspiratory load, or a sham lighter inspiratory load. Both groups had similar insignificant increases in maximal inspiratory pressure, 12-min walking distance, respiratory muscle endurance, and dyspnea.

A number of studies have been performed using exercise not specific to the respiratory muscles to improve exercise tolerance and ameliorate dyspnea. The techniques used include walking, with or without a treadmill, stair climbing, stationary cycling, muscle flexibility exercises, and arm ergometry or elevation. Many of these investigations showing benefits, which have consisted of improved exercise tolerance,[13,16,35–37] psychological parameters,[13,16,37,38] quality of life,[13,16,36,37] and dyspnea[13,16,39] have been uncontrolled, and the programs contain other components such as education, mak-

ing it difficult to ascertain whether the exercise alone was related to the improvement.

However, at least several controlled, albeit not necessarily masked, randomized, or appropriately exercise-supervised studies do show increases in exercise tolerance. McCavin and coworkers[40] compared 12 "chronic bronchitis" (mean FEV_1 approximately 1 L, mean age approximately 59) who climbed up and down stairs at home in a fixed amount of time, keeping a diary, to those who did not. The intervention group had statistically significant increases in 12-min walking distance, workload, and reported subjective improvement in symptoms. Sinclair and Ingram[41] studied 30 chronic bronchitics (mean FEV_1 approximately 1 L, mean age approximately 65) who were admitted for acute exacerbation of illness. When they had recovered, they were divided into control and intervention groups both of which did a daily 12-min walk test and climbed up and down two 24-cm steps for 1.5 to 2 min supervised by a nurse until discharge. The intervention group continued to exercise and kept a diary after discharge for 12 months. The control group did no further exercise. The subjects who continued their exercise after discharge developed the ability to walk significantly greater distances, which the control group did not. Cockcroft's group[42] randomized patients with COPD, mean age ≈60, into a treatment group who exercised in a rehabilitation center for 6 weeks with bicycle ergometry, rowing, swimming, walking, and home stair climbing, and a control group who did not exercise. The treated group showed a significantly greater increase in walking distance after 2 months. Busch and McClements[43] randomized a physical therapist-supervised home exercise group and a control group which did not exercise. Both groups were visited by a physical therapist every 2 weeks for 18 weeks. The treatment group performed exercises to increase flexibility, strength, and endurance with the physical therapist, and then repeated up to 20 times in the therapist's absence. Subjects were tested every 6 weeks on their ability to perform bicycle ergometry and stair climbing and their reported perception of dyspnea. The intervention group did have a significantly increased mean work capacity. There was no change in dyspnea in either group.

Several investigations have examined the utility of arm exercise as part of a training regimen. Couser and associates[44] utilized arm and bicycle ergometry and unsupported shoulder abduction and extension of a wooden dowel for 2 min for one or two sessions five times a week for 3 weeks in nine patients with COPD and found increased oxygen consumption and decreased minute ventilation in participants. Martinez and colleagues[45] randomized and compared 18 subjects who performed arm ergometry with 17 who did unsupported shoulder flexion and extension and elbow exercises. All performed bicycle ergometry and respiratory muscle training using a threshold-resistive training device) for 10 weeks. Both groups had increases in respiratory muscle strength, treadmill, walking distance, bicycle ergometry power output, and bicycle endurance time.

Several other studies have contrasted regimens including both respiratory muscle training and nonspecific exercises to those with either alone. Weiner and coworkers[46] divided 36 individuals with COPD, mean age approximately 65, into those who received either threshold inspiratory muscle training and general exercise (rowing, cycle ergometry, and muscle strengthening), general exercise, and sham inspiratory muscle training, or no exercise. The subjects trained for 1 h three times a week, for 6 months under the guidance of a physical therapist. All who exercised had significant gains in 12-min walking distance and bicycle ergometry, but those who received both forms of exercise had the most gain. Other studies showing an advantage to a combined respiratory muscle and general conditioning program, such as that of Dekhuijezen and associates,[47] which reported exercise and psychological gains,[47,48] were considered as part of the meta-analysis by Smith's group.[33]

The Effect of Age on Exercise Training

Most studies of the effects of exercise training have been done on subjects whose average mean age is early sixties. Many studies have included some older than 70, but almost none have considered the potential effect of age on the ability to exercise or the outcome of pulmonary rehabilitation. There are good theoretical reasons to suspect aging may have an impact. There are age-related physiologic declines in lung function, as previously mentioned; older individuals have more illnesses which decrease mobility; and the elderly have a higher incidence of sensory and cognitive deficits which can make training more difficult. Of the relatively few studies considering exercise in the elderly, none have the number of subjects and the sophistication of methodology to define the effect of aging on the outcome of exercise in rehabilitation, but those that do exist imply that subjects in their 60s or 70s have no worse outcomes than younger subjects.

Corriveau and coworkers[49] examined 40 patients with COPD, dividing them into two groups, those older than 60 (mean age 64, range 61 to 74) and those younger than 60 (mean age 53, range 32 to 60). The authors do not list inclusion criteria for their subjects.

The individuals trained as inpatients for 6 weeks with bicycle ergometry to 75 percent of the maximal heart rate or the maximal short of that and received flexibility training, physical therapy, recreation therapy, smoking cessation, and stress management. Resting minute ventilation increased in both the younger and the older participants.

O'Donnell and associates[50] assessed dyspnea in an initial study of 46 elderly with COPD. The selection criteria for patients was not given. The training regimen consisted of "aerobic training," including walking with and without a treadmill, stair climbing, and cycle ergometry. The intensity of the exercise was varied according to measurement of dyspnea index, and training was provided for 2 to 3 h, three sessions a week, for 8 weeks. Individuals were evaluated using four self-rated scales of breathlessness, the Breathless Dyspnea Index, the Oxygen Cost Diagram, the Medical Research Council Scale, and the Borg Scale. Trainees improved in all scales, whereas controls did not. In a larger uncontrolled series by the same authors, 102 subjects (ages not given) improved in 12-min walking distance and dyspnea as measured on the Borg Scale.

Couser and coworkers[51] did a restrospective study of all 134 patients undergoing rehabilitation at their institution with diagnosis of COPD (FEV_1 less than 70 percent of predicted and FEV_1/FVC less than 70 percent). Twelve-minute walking distance was measured in these patients before they entered a program which entailed 2 months of 2-h sessions once or twice a week. Participants with "severe exercise limitation" or other functional impairment received inpatient treatment. The older subjects (over 75 years, mean 78) had a statistically higher FEV_1 percent predicted than the younger (below 75, mean age 64) but had similar maximal inspiratory pressures. The exercises consisted of walking with and without a treadmill, stationary bicycling, and upper extremity exercises with weights. Educational sessions were provided for all individuals. Outcome measures examined were distance walked in 10 min and the results of a questionnaire assessing retention of the education they had received. The results of 12-min walking distances were tabulated for patients of each decade of age who participated in the study, and all significantly improved walking distances by an average of approximately 600 ft. Inpatients and outpatients both benefited, and all improved similarly on the educational questionnaire.

Respiratory Therapy in Rehabilitation

OXYGEN

Oxygen therapy can be used as an adjunctive therapy in rehabilitation. Compliance is an important consideration in selecting which aged person should receive oxygen and had the method used to deliver oxygen: compressed gas cylinder or electrically powered oxygen generator.[13] Transtracheal oxygen can reduce the amount of oxygen necessary and decrease tracheopharyngeal irritation, but catheter care may be more difficult for the aged.[13,52]

Supplemental oxygen has been shown in several studies to prolong life in hypoxemic individuals. As with exercise, investigations showing the benefit of oxygen have included individuals in their sixties and seventies, but have not specifically considered whether the benefit of oxygen is related to the age of the recipient. One of the largest studies, the Nocturnal Oxygen Therapy Trail (NOTT),[53] compared continuous oxygen to nocturnal oxygen therapy (13 h or less of oxygen a day, assessed by patient log and timer) in 203 patients with a P_{O_2} less than 55 whose mean age was approximately 65. The group using continuous oxygen had a 20 percent lower mortality than the nocturnal oxygen group after 3 years. The British Medical Research Council[54] divided 87 subjects, all below age 70, mean age in the upper 50s, but including some in their 60s, into groups of those receiving oxygen for at least 15 h/day and those receiving no oxygen. All subjects had COPD and a P_{O_2} between 40 and 60. Males receiving oxygen had a 25 percent greater survival after 5 years, and females had a 65 percent greater survival after 3 years. Cooper's group[55] examined males with COPD and cor pulmonale, mean age 60, given at least 15 h of O_2. The participants had a 5-year survival of 62 percent [higher than in the Medical Research Council study of oxygen-receiving males whose 5-year survival was approximately 40 percent],[54] but their 10-year survival was only 10 percent.

Oxygen has resulted in gains in neuropsychiatric testing and, to a less quantified extent, exercise tolerance, which may be particularly relevant in the aged.[22] A follow-up neuropsychiatric trial of NOTT patients showed gains in alertness and motor testing.[56] In a small study of six patients, subjects of a mean age of 64 were able to perform leg ergometry for a longer time on 30% oxygen.[57]

The potential adverse consequences of oxygen should be considered when oxygen is a potential therapy for the elderly, including drying of mucous membranes, fire hazard, or tank explosion.[22] Atelectasis and CO_2 retention are possible, although they are not common in home therapy.[22] The incidence of side effects, specifically in the elderly, has not been published.

HOME MECHANICAL VENTILATION

Home mechanical ventilation has been used in COPD, restrictive lung disease, chest wall diseases, and neuromuscular disorders. Mechanical ventilation can be used after acute respiratory failure and in individuals who develop hypoxia at night, using intermittent positive-pressure breathing via a nasal mask, mouthpiece, or tracheostomy and intermittent positive-pressure ventilation via a respirator.[58,59] The nasal mask is the least invasive and therefore has been widely considered a first choice, although air leaks may happen, particularly at night, which disturb sleep.[60] Tracheostomy may more be more difficult to care for in elderly recipients.[13] The relative feasibilities of techniques of home mechanical ventilation in specifically elderly individuals has not been studied.

TRAINING IN BREATHING TECHNIQUES

Training in breathing techniques such as pursed-lip and diaphragmatic breathing has been used as part of pulmonary rehabilitation programs. Rehabilitation techniques including yoga have also been advocated to relieve fear and anxiety.[13,61,62] Although the effects of these techniques have been studied for more than 40 years,[13,19,63–70] the outcome of such techniques on respiration has not been conclusively determined. Pursed-lip breathing, which is performed "voluntarily and instinctively" by individuals with COPD,[67] was shown in a study of 13 dyspneic patients with COPD to heighten accessory muscle and rib cage muscle recruitment in preference to the diaphragmatic recruitment during inspiration. Increased oxygen saturation was also noted. This technique, in an earlier study,[65] improved symptoms and blood gases at rest, but the blood-gas changes were not associated with reduced symptoms and did not continue during exercise. Pursed-lip breathing creates an end-expiratory pressure that is similar to continuous positive end-expiratory pressure.[68] Positive end-expiratory pressure improved ventilation in one investigation, but it increased dyspnea in the subjects as well.[68] Other investigations have differed as to whether IPPB altered blood gases, and several studies have shown there was no improvement in hospitalization rate or mortality.[19,69,70]

It is unfortunate that another prospective and randomized study[71] in which a program was devised utilizing breathing training and relaxing techniques as part of a comprehensive patient education program did not improve patients' sensation of dyspnea or quality of life. Eighty-nine patients with COPD (mean age approximately 67, mean FEV_1 percent predicted 50 percent) were randomized into control and treatment groups. The treatment group went to six weekly sessions in which patients received education on diaphragmatic and pursed-lip breathing, including instructions and practice sessions during rest and exercise, and the subjects were told to practice daily. Subjects in this group were also given education about the physiology of the disease, relaxation techniques (including practice sessions in which subjects practiced tensing and relaxing certain muscles), methods of how to save energy and pace oneself during strenuous activities, and panic and stress management. There were "activity stations" in which subjects role-played independent activities of daily living (e.g., stair climbing, doing laundry, vacuuming). Controls attended lectures on general health and exercise for the same amount of time as the treatment group. All participants were measured at baseline and 6 months later by 6-min walking distance, six different dyspnea indexes, the quality of well-being scale, and anxiety and depression scale. There were no significant differences between the two groups in any of the parameters measured, leading the authors to conclude that use of breathing techniques, relaxation techniques, and education were not in and of themselves sufficient to achieve the desired improvements.

Chest Physiotherapy

Percussion and postural drainage are commonly used techniques to mobilize secretions. It has been difficult to establish which are the most appropriate criteria to measure the efficacy of these techniques, and it is not easy to separate the effect of such maneuvers from other adjunctive measures such as medicine, mucolytic agents, or humidification.[19] These have been shown to be helpful in the segment of patients who produce a large amount of secretions, but investigations have failed to show benefit in subjects who were not great sputum producers.[13,19]

Psychological and Social Intervention

Numerous psychological problems have been found to be more common in elderly with COPD, such as depression, anxiety, excessive body preoccupation, sexual dysfunction, alcoholism, and paranoia.[13,72] Psychiatric illness per se is not more common in individuals with lung disease, and patients often best benefit by multiple forms of intervention.[73] Psychotherapy can be used successfully in many cases, and psychoactive medications can safely treat elderly individuals with pulmonary disease.[13,74]

Smoking cessation is of great importance to patient health, and efforts to achieve this should be considered.[13,75] Nicotine gum has been successful in smoking cessation programs, but its utility in general practice has been questioned.[76–78] Transdermal nicotine alone[79–81] or combined with behavior modification[82] has yielded good results, even in double-blind and placebo-controlled trials.[79,80,82] A study done in elderly smokers yielded a 29 percent 6-month quit rate.[83] Cessation is more likely with a structured program[75] and when users do not concomitantly smoke,[82] but smoking can be curtailed even in users of the transdermal patch who continue to smoke.[80,81] There can be ample opportunity for social intervention. Aged individuals with pulmonary disease can lack supportive caregivers, lack adequate help in performing activities of daily living, have difficulty with employment and recreational activities, and develop isolation. Fishman states that lack of social support and stresses of life are the best predictors of hospitalizations, even considering severity of illness, and married COPD subjects tolerate exercise better than unmarried patients, when controlled for disease severity and age.[75] Many sources of payment for medical care do not cover pulmonary rehabilitation.[75]

Nutrition

Alterations of nutritional state and body weight and are common in patients with pulmonary disease. Between 27 and 47 percent of individuals with emphysema are nutritionally depleted,[84,85] and the more severe the disease as measured by FEV_1, the more likely they are to be underweight.[86,87] Patients with COPD can also be overweight, for which a regimen of diet and exercise has been advocated.[13,88,89] There is a negative correlation between morbidity and mortality and weight loss in COPD, but the mechanism for this weight loss has not been determined.[86,90]

There is some evidence that measures of nutrition are more closely correlated with 12-min walking distance than body weight. Fat-free mass can be calculated from measurements of skinfold thickness and arm circumferences, or bioelectric impedance measurements.[91-93] The creatinine height index can also be used to measure fat-free muscle mass, but many factors other than mass can alter creatinine such as diet, age, stress, and exercise, and there can be great variability in the measurement of urinary creatinine.[93]

At least three theories may explain nutritional depletion in COPD, including increased COPD-induced dietary thermogenesis,[86,88,94] a limited delivery of nutrients resulting from the cardiopulmonary vascular alterations that occur in COPD,[86,88] and a hypermetabolic condition induced by increased respiratory muscle energy demand.[86,88,94-96] The fact that at least one study[88] showed that supplementation of COPD patients with a standard nutritional regimen used in other conditions resulted in an appropriate increase in weight makes the first theory less likely.[88] The possibility of a hypermetabolic state is uncertain; two studies showed an increased resting energy expenditure in subjects with COPD,[95,96] but a more recent study did not,[97] claiming methodologic improvements in measuring energy expenditure from the two previous studies.

The appropriate method of treatment and efficacy of nutritional supplementation is not certain. Rogers and colleagues[88] randomized 28 patients with COPD of a mean age of 64 who were below 90 percent of ideal body weight into an intervention group that received 1 month of inpatient monitoring and nutritional support and a control group that received 1 week of hospitalization and testing before returning home. Each had anthropomorphic measuring, spirometry, handgrip and inspiratory muscle strength testing, 12-min walking distance assessment, and dyspnea and quality-of-life questionnaire assessment, and were followed 4 months after hospital discharge. The treatment group did gain weight, improve walking distance, and increase handgrip and expiratory muscle strength, but almost all the weight gain occurred during hospitalization, and dyspnea and quality-of-life index were not improved. The authors believed their intervention to be "costly, time-intensive, and of limited therapeutic magnitude." The substitution of high-calorie foods for processed nutritional supplements has been suggested,[13] which may prove less expensive, but this has not yet been formally studied for efficacy.

In a small treatment series,[98] seven underweight patients with COPD were given subcutaneous injections of methionyl human growth hormone (0.05 mg/kg per day) for 3 weeks. There was a significant weight gain within a few weeks after the onset of therapy, and, after 3 weeks, there was a significant increase in maximal inspiratory pressure.

Education

Education for both the patient and the family has been advocated to help these individuals understand possible warning signs of potential illness-related difficulties; use their medications, oxygen, and components of a rehabilitation program properly; and develop realistic expectations of the outcomes. Education may help patient and family best adapt to the situation and become involved in care.[13] Topics can include potential symptoms and signs of illness; the use of medications and their side effects, breathing, energy conservation, and relaxation techniques; sexual counseling; equipment and oxygen use and care; community resources; and advice on travel.[99] As mentioned in the section on breathing techniques, at least according to one study, patient education in and of itself was not sufficient to relieve dyspnea and improve quality of life.[71]

Medications

Special attention must be given to medications and delivery systems used in the treatment of pulmonary disease in the elderly. The elderly may frequently experience the side effects of tertiary ammonium agents, such as atropine, including urinary retention, confusion, thickened secretions and narrow-angle glaucoma.[22] Quaternary ammonium agents, such as ipratropium may be better tolerated.[22] Sympathomimetics have been used successfully, although their arrythmiogenic properties should be noted when medicating the older patient.[22] Limited dexterity may preclude the successful use of metered dose inhalers in the elderly, and one study of 30 individuals with a mean age of 80 showed only 60 percent could use them properly.[100]

Outcome of Pulmonary Rehabilitation

To assess the efficacy of a pulmonary rehabilitation program, appropriate criteria showing benefit must be established. In the case of the rehabilitation of the elderly, this is especially difficult to accomplish. As was the case previously when trying to assess the efficacy of exercise, most of the studies include elderly subjects, especially "younger" elderly, since the mean of age of most of the participants was low to middle sixties, but almost no one has addressed the issue of whether the benefits are age-specific. Age was not shown to predict improvement in 12-min walking distance in one program, in which 50 ambulatory outpatients (mean age 62.2 ± 10.9 years) completed a comprehensive 6-week rehabilitation program (including inspiratory muscle training, treadmill exercise, cycle ergometry, stair climbing, upper extremity exercise, education, breathing exercises, and relaxation techniques).[17] The elderly may also receive special unquantifiable but real benefits from increased contact with a team of caring health professionals working in concert (e.g., identification of previously unnoticed health problems with atypical presentations or relief from social isolation).

Organizing appropriate clinical trials showing the efficacy of pulmonary rehabilitation in general is difficult because there are relatively few quantitative measures for all the potential criteria to consider and little information on the identity of subgroups within the populations studied who might be helped by the intervention. This increases the possibility of undetected differences between treatment and control groups (type II error).[75]

Studies assessing pulmonary rehabilitation have cited gains in exercise capacity and tolerance, improvement in measures of psychosocial functioning, augmentation in quality-of-life indexes, and reductions in hospitalizations and length of stay. A more complete listing of these studies, many of which are either unrandomized, uncontrolled, or not prospective can be found in the reviews of the subject by Rodrigues and Ilowite[13] and Hodgkin,[16] among others. In the past 2 years, several prospective controlled trials have continued to confirm benefit, although not entirely resolving many issues.

Goldstein's group[101] randomized 89 nonsmoking patients with COPD (FEV_1 less than 40 percent predicted, and mean age 66) into groups receiving rehabilitation or conventional treatment. The rehabilitation consisted of 30 min of stretching, range-of-motion activity, and diaphragmatic and pursed-lip breathing exercises, followed by treadmill and leisure walking and upper-extremity training three times a week. The duration of the treadmill walking was gradually increased. Subjects were trained in a home exercise program with gradually decreasing supervision by a physical therapist for 4 months. At the end of 6 months, statistically significant differences were noted between the two groups in 6-min walking distance, submaximal cycle time on a cycle ergometer, and symptoms of illness as measured by the Chronic Respiratory Disease Questionnaire. The actual mean values for the end points examined by the study for each group were not included, only the mean values of differences between groups. The intervention was, by the authors' admission, expensive.

Wijkstra and colleagues[102,103] used stratified randomization to divide 36 patients with COPD (FEV_1 less than 44 percent predicted, mean age approximately 62) into three groups, one of which received intervention once a month for 18 months, one once a week, and one no intervention. The intervention was preceded by a 12-week period in which subjects saw a local physical therapist twice a week for 30 min and met with a physician and nurse once a month. The intervention consisted of target-flow inspiratory training, upper-limb and breathing exercises, such as pursed-lip breathing and synchronization of thorax and abdominal movement, and cycle ergometry exercises consisting of cycling at 60 percent of baseline maximal workload for 4 min, which was gradually increased to 12 min at 75 percent. A nurse provided education, and all patients kept an activities log.

Individuals who received rehabilitation had significantly higher quality-of-life scores at 3, 6, 12, and 18 months after the start of the study, but those who had therapy only once a month had higher scores than those who had therapy once a week. Six-minute walking distance and maximal workload as measured by bicycle ergometry declined in those who did not receive therapy, and did not change in those who did. A dyspnea index and the duration of holding one's breath at 70 percent of maximum inspiratory pressure was slightly higher after 18 months in those who exercised once a week.

Ries and coworkers[104] examined 119 patients with COPD (mean age approximately 62) who included smokers willing to quit, randomly separating them into pulmonary rehabilitation or education groups. The rehabilitation group included an initial component of 12-h sessions for 8 weeks including education, instruction in chest physiotherapy, psychiatric group therapy, relaxation techniques, and individualized physical therapy consisting of treadmill walking, accompanied by supplemental oxygen for those whose P_{O_2} was less than 55, and upper extremity exercise including arm weight-lifting. The second component was a once-monthly session of monitored exercise and discussion. The education group received four 2-h sessions twice a week for 8 weeks, during which videotapes of health topics were followed by discussion. Subjects in the rehabilitation group had significantly improved treadmill walking times and self-reported breathlessness and muscle fatigue which persisted up to a year after the program started. There was no significant improvement in mean hospital days used or self-reported quality of life, and no changes at all in the education group. There was not a significant difference between groups in overall survival. After 1 year, the significant changes returned to baseline.

In an era of great upheaval in medical economics, establishing the cost benefit of pulmonary rehabilitation for the elderly might promote the greater availability of these services. It is unfortunate that the impact of pulmonary rehabilitation has not clearly been established. More than 20 years ago, Lertzman and Cherniack[105] asserted in a chapter on the topic that "the provision of home care has resulted in an average decrease of 20 hospital days a year" without providing data. Agle and colleagues[106] followed 24 middle-age patients in a 4-week rehabilitation program and found that five hospitalizations occurred in the group in the year after rehabilitation, whereas 20 occurred in the year before.

Several other investigators in larger series of patients found decreases in hospitalizations when comparing the rate for their populations after completing their rehabilitation programs to that before they started therapy.[104] Petty and associates,[35] in 1969, cut the average hospital days spent per patient by four in 182 individuals from the previous year, which was statistically significant. Johnson's group[107] noted a decline of 55 percent in hospital admissions for 96 individuals with COPD up to 1 year following treatment, Hudson and colleagues[108] achieved a 47 to 61 percent decrease from baseline in each of 4 years among a group of 64 patients, and Hodgkin and coworkers[109] maintained a greater than 90 percent decrease in 80 patients for 8 years.

Prospective controlled studies have been fewer. Jensen[110] stratified 59 subjects with COPD (median age 64) into a low- or high-risk group for stress based on a questionnaire and provided them for 6 months with either a nurse who educated them (including information on their illness, breathing techniques, and medications), a self-help support group, or no intervention. The high-risk control group had a significantly higher hospitalization rate compared with the previous 2 years than the education or self-help groups. There was no difference between groups in emergency room or clinic visits. In a double-blind prospective trial in 30 middle-aged asthmatics, Weiner and coworkers[111] found a significant decrease in hospitalization, emergency room visits, and school absences in the last 3 months of a 6-month respiratory muscle training program. Ries' group,[104] as has been previously stated, did not find a significant difference between the groups they studied and suggest that this might be attributable to the fact that since their study was more recent, it may have been influenced by the economically imposed stricter criteria for hospitalization.

Three years ago, a National Institutes of Health conference was held on pulmonary rehabilitation. Numerous questions that were raised in discussion on the topic of measurement of the outcomes still remain to be fully answered:

Is the traditional full team of physicians and allied health professionals necessary or could a smaller team suffice? . . . Is exercise, education or psychologic intervention the most important factor in promoting functional improvement as the result of a program in pulmonary rehabilitation? How can we predict who will benefit from interdisciplinary care? Should cost analysis be an integral part of the study design? From whose perspective is the study or analysis be conducted: the patient/client, the payer, or society?[75]

One conclusion is also apt:

In general, participants in this workshop, drawing on personal experiences, shared the belief that pulmonary rehabilitation epitomizing medical "caring" is beneficial for certain patients with pulmonary disease. However, proof of this supposition can be challenged: much of the research in support of this view suffers from methodologic problems such as small sample size, the lack of adequate control populations, incompletely validated outcome measures, and the absence of prospective data collection. Moreover, long-term benefits have yet to be proved.[75]

The additional complexities of aging make this even more true, specifically for the elderly.

References

1. Rinquist T: The ventilatory capacity in healthy subjects: An analysis of causal factors with special references to the respiratory forces. *Scan J Clin Lab Invest* 18:1, 1966.
2. Enright PL, Kronmal RA, Manolio TA, et al: Respiratory muscle strength in the elderly. *Am J Resp Crit Care Med* 149:430, 1994.
3. Black LF, Hyatt RE: Maximal static respiratory pressures: Normal values and relationship to age and sex. *Am Rev Resp Dis* 99:696, 1969.
4. Wilson SH, Cooke NH, Edwards RHT, Spiro SG: Predicted normal values for respiratory pressures in caucasian adults and children. *Thorax* 39:535, 1984.
5. Vincken W, Ghezzo H, Cosio MG: Maximal static respiratory pressures in adults: Normal values and their relationship to determinants of respiratory function. *Bull Eur Physiopathol Respir* 23:435, 1987.
6. McElvaney G, Blackie S, Morrison NJ, Wilcox PC, Fairbarn MS, Pardy RL: Maximal static respiratory pressures in the normal elderly. *Am Rev Resp Dis* 139:277, 1989.
7. Tolep K, Criner G, Kelsen SC: Transdiaphragmatic pressure generation in elderly, healthy subjects. *Am Rev Resp Dis:* A366, 1991.
8. Morrison NJ, Richardson J, Dip PT, et al: Respiratory muscle performance in normal elderly subjects and patients with COPD. *Chest* 95:90, 1989.
9. Martyn JB, Moreno RH, Pare PD, Pardy RL: Measurement of inspiratory muscle performance with incremental threshold loading. *Am Rev Resp Dis* 135:919, 1987.
10. Grinton SF: Respiratory limitations in the aging population. *South Med J* 87(5): S47, 1994.
11. Johnson BD, Reddam WG, Seow KC, Dempsey JA: Mechanical constraints on exercise hyperpnea in a fit aging population. *Am Rev Resp Dis* 143:968, 1991.
12. Takishima T, Shindoh C, Kikuchi Y, et al: Aging effect on oxygen consumption of respiratory muscles in humans. *J Appl Physiol* 69(1):14, 1990.
13. Rodrigues JC, Ilowite JS: Pulmonary rehabilitation in the elderly patient. *Clin Chest Med* 14(3):429, 1993.
14. Petty TL: Pulmonary rehabilitation in perspective: Historical roots, present status, and future projections. *Thorax* 48:855, 1993.
15. Clark CJ: Setting up a pulmonary rehabilitation programme. *Thorax* 49:270, 1994.
16. Hodgkin JE: Pulmonary rehabilitation. *Clin Chest Med* 11(3):447, 1990.
17. Niederman MS, Clemente PH, Fein AM, et al: Benefits of a multidisciplinary pulmonary rehabilitation program. *Chest* 99(4):798, 1991.
18. Foster S, Thomas HM III: Pulmonary rehabilitation in lung disease other than chronic obstructive pulmonary disease. *Am Rev Resp Dis* 141:601, 1990.
19. Sutton PP, Pavia D, Bateman JRM, Clarke SW: Chest physiotherapy: A review. *Eur J Resp Dis* 63:188, 1982.
20. Curtis JR, Deyo RA, Hudson LD: Health-related quality of life among patients with chronic obstructive pulmonary disease. *Thorax* 49:162, 1994.
21. Ries AL: The importance of exercise in pulmonary rehabilitation. *Clin Chest Med* 15(2):327, 1994.
22. Chalker RB, Celli BR: Special considerations in the elderly patient. *Clin Chest Med* 14(3):437, 1993.
23. Goldstein RS: Ventilatory muscle training. *Thorax* 48:1025, 1993.
24. Olopade CO, Beck KC, Viggiano RW, Staats BA: Exercise limitation and pulmonary rehabilitation in chronic obstructive pulmonary disease. *Mayo Clin Proc* 67:144, 1992.
25. Dekhuijjzen PNR, van Herwaarden CLA, Cox NJM, Folgering HTM: Exercise training during pulmonary rehabilitation in chronic obstructive pulmonary disease. *Lung* suppl:481, 1990.
26. Casaburi R: Principles of exercise training. *Chest* 101(5)(suppl):2636, 1992.
27. Pardy RL, Reid WD, Belman MJ: Respiratory muscle training. *Clin Chest Med* 9(2):287, 1988.
28. Reid WD, Samrai B: Respiratory muscle training for patients with chronic obstructive pulmonary disease. *Phys Ther* 75(11):996, 1995.
29. Larson JL, Kim MJ, Sharp JT, Larson DA: Inspiratory muscle training with a pressure threshold breathing device in patients with chronic obstructive pulmonary disease. *Am Rev Resp Dis* 138:689, 1988.
30. Levine S, Weiser P, Gillen J: Evaluation of a ventilatory muscle endurance and training program in the rehabilitation of patients with chronic obstructive pulmonary disease. *Am Rev Resp Dis* 133:400, 1986.
31. Belman MJ, Shadmehr R: Targeted resistive ventilatory muscle training in chronic obstructive pulmonary disease. *J Appl Physiol* 65:2726, 1988.
32. Harver A, Mahler DA, Daubenspeck JA: Targeted inspiratory muscle training improves respiratory muscle function and re-

duces dyspnea in patients with chronic obstructive pulmonary disease. *Ann Int Med* 111:117, 1989.

33. Smith K, Cook D, Guyatt GH, et al: Respiratory muscle training in chronic airflow limitation: A metaanalysis. *Am Rev Resp Dis* 145:533, 1992.

34. Kim MJ, Larson JL, Covey MK, et al: Inspiratory muscle training in patients with chronic obstructive pulmonary disease. *Nurs Res* 42(6):356, 1993.

35. Petty TL, Nett LM, Finigan MM, et al: A comprehensive care program for chronic airway obstruction: Methods and preliminary evaluation of symptomatic and functional improvement. *Ann Intern Med* 70:1109, 1969.

36. Vale F, Reardon JZ, ZuWallack RL: The long-term benefits of outpatient pulmonary rehabilitation on exercise endurance and quality of life. *Chest* 103:42, 1993.

37. Guyatt GH, Berman LB, Townsend MT: Long-term outcome after respiratory rehabilitation. *Can Med Assoc J* 137:1089, 1987.

38. Emery CF, Leatherman NE, Burker EJ, MacIntyre NR: Psychological outcomes of a pulmonary rehabilitation program. *Chest* 100:613, 1991.

39. Reardon J, Awad E, Normandin E, et al: The effect of comprehensive outpatient pulmonary rehabilitation on dyspnea. *Chest* 105:1046, 1994.

40. McGavin CR, Gupta SP, Lloyd EL, McHardy GJR: Physical rehabilitation for the chronic bronchitic results of a controlled trial of exercises in the home. *Thorax* 32:307, 1977.

41. Sinclair DJM, Ingram CG: Controlled trial of supervised exercise training in chronic bronchitis. *Br J Med* 280:519, 1980.

42. Cockcroft AE, Saunders MJ, Berry G: Randomised controlled trial of rehabilitation in chronic respiratory disability. *Thorax* 36:200, 1981.

43. Busch AJ, McClements JD: Effects of a supervised home exercise program on patients with severe chronic obstructive pulmonary disease. *Phys Ther* 68:469, 1988.

44. Couser JI, Martinez FJ, Celli BR: Pulmonary rehabilitation that includes arm exercise reduces metabolic and ventilatory requirements for simple arm elevation. *Chest* 103:37, 1993.

45. Martinez FJ, Vogel PD, Dupont DN, et al: Supported arm exercise vs unsupported arm exercise in the rehabilitation of patients with severe chronic airflow obstruction. *Chest* 103(5):1397–1402, 1993.

46. Weiner P, Azgad Y, Ganam R: Inspiratory muscle training combined with general exercise reconditioning in patients with COPD. *Chest* 102(5):1351, 1992.

47. Dekhuijzen PNR, Folgering HTM, van Herwaarden CLA: Target-flow inspiratory muscle training during pulmonary rehabilitation in patients with COPD. *Chest* 99:128, 1991.

48. Dekhuijzen PNR, Beek MML, Folgering HTM, van Herwaarden CLA: Psychological changes during pulmonary rehabilitation and target-flow inspiratory muscle training in COPD patients with a ventilatory limitation during exercise. *Int J Rehab Res* 13:109, 1990.

49. Corriveau ML, Rosen BJ, Dolan GF: Exercise capacity following pulmonary rehabilitation. *Missouri Medicine* 86 (11):751, 1989.

50. O'Donnell DE, Webb KA, McGuire MA: Older patients with COPD: Benefits of exercise training. *Geriatrics* 48:59, 1993.

51. Couser JI, Guthmann R, Hamadeh MA, Kane CS: Pulmonary rehabilitation improves exercise capacity in older elderly patients with COPD. *Chest* 107:730, 1995.

52. Heimlich HJ: Respiratory rehabilitation with transtracheal oxygen system. *Ann Otol Rhinol Laryngol* 91:643, 1982.

53. Nocturnal Oxygen Therapy Trial Group: Continuous or nocturnal oxygen therapy in hypoxemic chronic obstructive lung disease. *Ann Intern Med* 99:612, 1980.

54. Report of the British Research Medical Council Working Party: Long-term domiciliary oxygen therapy in chronic hypoxic cor pulmonale complicating chronic bronchitis and emphysema. *Lancet* i:681, 1981.

55. Cooper CB, Waterhouse J, Howard P: Twelve year clinical study of patients with hypoxic cor pulmonale given long term domiciliary oxygen therapy. *Thorax* 42:105, 1987.

56. Heaton RK, Grant I, McSweeney AJ, et al: Psychologic effects of continuous and nocturnal oxygen therapy in hypoxemic chronic obstructive pulmonary disease. *Arch Intern Med* 143:1941, 1983.

57. Crier GJ, Celli BR: Ventilatory muscle recruitment in exercise with oxygen in obstructed patients with mild hypoxemia. *J Appl Physiol* 63:195, 1987.

58. Muir JF: Home mechanical ventilation. *Thorax* 48:1264, 1993.

59. Bach JR: Mechanical exsufflation, noninvasive ventilation, and new strategies for pulmonary rehabilitation and sleep disordered breathing. *Bull NY Acad Med* 68(2):321, 1992.

60. Make BJ: Mechanical ventilation in the home: Summary of the 3rd international conference on pulmonary rehabilitation and home mechanical ventilation. *Neuromuscular Disorders* 1(3):229, 1991.

61. Renfroe KL: Effect of progressive relaxation on dyspnea and anxiety state in patients with chronic obstructive pulmonary disease. *Heart Lung* 17:408, 1988.

62. Tandon MK: Adjunct treatment with chronic severe airway obstruction. *Thorax* 33:514, 1978.

63. Miller WF: A physiologic evaluation of the effects of diaphragmatic breathing training in patients with chronic pulmonary emphysema. *Am J Med* 17:471, 1954.

64. Motley HL: The effects of slow deep breathing on the blood exchange in emphysema. *Am Rev Resp Dis* 88:484, 1963.

65. Mueller RE, Petty TL, Filley GE: Ventilation and arterial blood gas exchange in emphysema. *J Appl Physiol* 28:784, 1970.

66. Sinclair JD: The effect of breathing exercises in pulmonary emphysema. *Thorax* 10:246, 1955.

67. Breslin EH: The pattern of respiratory muscle recruitment during pursed-lip breathing. *Chest* 101:75, 1992.

68. van der Schans CP, de Jone W, de Vries G, et al: Effect of positive expiratory pressure on breathing during exercise in patients with COPD. *Chest* 105:789, 1984.

69. Curtis JK, Liska AP, Rasmussen HK, Cree EM: IPPB therapy in chronic obstructive pulmonary disease. *JAMA* 206:1037, 1968.

70. Cherniack RM, Svanhill E: Long-term use of intermittent positive pressure breathing (IPPB) in chronic obstructive pulmonary disease. *Am Rev Resp Dis* 113:721, 1976.

71. Sassi-Dambron DE, Eakin EG, Ries AL, Kaplan RM: Treatment of dyspnea in COPD. *Chest* 107:724, 1995.

72. Agle DP, Baum GL: Psychological aspects of chronic obstructive pulmonary disease. *Med Clin North Am* 61 (4):749, 1977.

73. Dudley DL, Glaser EM, Jorgenson BN, Logan DL: Psychosocial concomitant to rehabilitation in chronic obstructive pulmonary disease. *Chest* 77 (3):677, 1980.

74. Glaser EM, Dudley DL: Psychosocial rehabilitation and psychopharmacology, in Hodgkin JE, Petty TL (eds): *Chronic Obstructive Pulmonary Disease: Current Concepts*. Philadelphia, Saunders, 1987; pp 128–153.

75. Fishman AP: Pulmonary rehabilitation research. *Am J Resp Crit Care Med* 149:425, 1994.

76. Lam W, Sze PC, Sachs HS, Chalmers TC: Meta-analysis of randomized controlled trials of nicotine chewing gum. *Lancet* 2:27, 1987.

77. Hughes JR, Gust SW, Keenan RM, et al: Nicotine vs placebo gum in general practice. *JAMA* 261:1300, 1989.

78. Jarvis MJ, Russell MAH: Treatment for the cigarette smoker. *Int Rev Psychiat* 1:149, 1989.

79. Hurt RD, Langer GE, Offord KP, et al: Nicotine replacement therapy with the use of a transdermal nicotine patch: A randomized double-blind placebo-controlled trial. *Mayo Clin Proc* 65:1529, 1990.

80. Russell MA, Stapleton JA, Feyerabend C, et al: Targeting heavy smokers in general practice: Randomised controlled trial of transdermal nicotine patches. *Br Med J* 306:1308–1312, 1993.

81. Pickworth WB, Bunker EB, Henningfield JE: Transdermal nicotine: Reduction of smoking with minimal abuse liability. *Psychopharmacol* 115:9, 1994.

82. Daughton DM, Heatley SA, Prendergast JJ, et al: Effect of transdermal nicotine delivery as an adjunct to low-intervention smoking cessation therapy. *Arch Intern Med* 151:749, 1991.

83. Orleans CT, Resch N, Noll E, et al: Use of transdermal nicotine in a state-level prescription plan for the elderly. *JAMA* 271 (8):601, 1994.

84. Braun SR, Kein NL, Dixon RM, et al: The prevalence and determinants of nutritional changes in chronic obstructive pulmonary disease.

85. Hunter AMB, Carey MA, Larsh HW: The nutritional status of patients with chronic obstructive pulmonary disease. *Am Rev Resp Dis* 124:276, 1981.

86. Wilson DO, Rogers RM, Openbrier D: Nutritional aspects of chronic obstructive pulmonary disease. *Clin Chest Med* 7 (4):643, 1986.

87. Renzetti AD, McClement JH, Litt BD: The Veterans Administration cooperative study of pulmonary function-mortality in relation to respiratory function. *Am J Med* 41:115, 1966.

88. Rogers RM, Donahoe M, Constantino J: Physiologic effects of oral supplemental feeding in malnourished patients with chronic obstructive pulmonary disease. *Am Rev Resp Dis* 146:1511, 1992.

89. Hodgkin JE: Nonexercise aspects of pulmonary rehabilitation. *Semin Resp Med* 2:148, 1993.

90. Vandenburg E, Van De Wostigne K, Gyselen A: Weight changes in the terminal stages of chronic obstructive lung disease. *Am Rev Resp Dis* 96:556, 1967.

91. Schols AMWJ, Mostert R, Soeters PB, Wouters EFM: Body composition and exercise performance in patients with chronic obstructive pulmonary disease. *Thorax* 46:695, 1991.

92. Schols AMWJ, Soeters PB, Dingemans AMC, et al: Prevalence and characteristics of nutritional depletion in patients with stable COPD eligible for pulmonary rehabilitator.

93. Donahoe M, Rogers RM: Nutritional assessment and support in chronic obstructive pulmonary disease. *Clin Chest Med* 11 (3):487, 1990.

94. Goldstein SA, Askanazi J, Weissman C, et al: Energy expenditure in patients with chronic obstructive pulmonary disease. *Chest* 91:222, 1987.

95. Goldstein SA, Thomashow BM, Kvetan V, et al: Nitrogen and energy relationships in malnourished patients with emphysema. *Am Rev Resp Dis* 138:636, 1988.

96. Wilson DO, Donahoe M, Rogers RM, Pennock BE: Metabolic rate and wight loss in chronic obstructive lung disease. *J Parenter Enter Nutr* 14:7, 1990.

97. Ryan CF, Road JD, Buckley PA, et al: Energy balance with stable malnourished patients with chronic obstructive pulmonary disease. *Chest* 103 (4):1038, 1993.

98. Pape GS, Friedmann JM, Underwood LE, Clemmons DR: The effect of growth hormone on weight gain and pulmonary function in patients with chronic obstructive lung disease. *Chest* 99 (6):1495, 1991.

99. Gilmartin ME: Patient and family education. *Clin Chest Med* 7 (4):619, 1986.

100. Allen SC, Prior A: What determines whether an elderly patient can use a metered dose inhaler. *Br J Dis Chest* 80:45, 1986.

101. Goldstein RS, Gort EH, Stubbing D, et al: Randomised controlled trial of respiratory rehabilitation. *Lancet* 344:1394, 1994.

102. Wijkstra PJ, TenVergert EM, van Altena R, et al: Long term benefits of rehabilitation at home on quality of life and exercise tolerance in patients with chronic obstructive pulmonary disease. *Thorax* 50:824, 1995.

103. Wijkstra PJ, van der Mark TW, Kraan J, et al: Long-term effects of home rehabilitation on physical performance in chronic obstructive pulmonary disease. *Am J Resp Crit Care Med* 153:1234, 1996.

104. Ries AL, Kaplan RM, Limberg TM, Prewitt LM: Effects of pulmonary rehabilitation on physiologic and psychosocial outcomes in patients with chronic obstructive pulmonary disease. *Ann Intern Med* 122:823, 1995.

105. Lertzman MM, Cherniack RM: Rehabilitation of patients with chronic obstructive pulmonary disease. *Am Rev Resp Dis* 114:1145, 1976.

106. Agle DP, Baum GL, Chester EH, Wendt M: Multidiscipline treatment of chronic pulmonary insufficiency. *Psychosom Med* 25:41, 1973.

107. Johnson HR, Tanzi F, Balchum OJ, et al: Inpatient comprehensive rehabilitation program in severe COPD. *Resp Ther* May/June:15, 1980.

108. Hudson LD, Tyler ML, Petty TL: Hospitalization needs during an outpatient rehabilitation program for severe chronic airway obstruction. *Chest* 70:606, 1976.

109. Hodgkin JE, Connors GL, Bell CW (eds): *Pulmonary Rehabilitation Guidelines to Success*, 2d ed. Philadelphia, Lippincott, 1993.

110. Jensen PS: Risk, protective factors, and supportive interventions in chronic airway obstruction. *Arch Gen Psychiat* 40:1203, 1983.

111. Weiner P, Azgad Y, Ganam R, Weiner M: Inspiratory muscle treatment in patients with bronchial asthma. *Chest* 102 (5):1357, 1992.

Chapter 38

REHABILITATION IN THE ASTHMA POPULATION

KATHLEEN ELLSTROM
ERIC C. KLEERUP
DONALD P. TASHKIN

Asthma affects 14 to 15 million Americans and results in over 100 million days of restricted activity each year.[1] Despite the availability of newer drugs for the treatment of asthma, morbidity and mortality due to asthma have increased in the United States and other countries.[2] This increase is notable in minority populations, especially African Americans. It is uncertain if this increase in asthma morbidity and mortality has been caused by changes in the disease, environment, or population; long-term exposure to triggers and allergens; lack of access to health care; unappreciated effects of the drugs used to treat asthma; or a failure to widely adopt optimal treatment (based on expert opinion).

Asthma is difficult to define as a disease and may represent a mixture of etiologies and mechanisms. The following is an operational definition:

"Asthma is a chronic inflammatory disorder of the airways in which many cells and cellular elements play a role, in particular mast cells, eosinophils, T lymphocytes, macrophages, neutrophils and epithelial cells. In susceptible individuals, this inflammation causes recurrent episodes of wheezing, breathlessness, chest tightness and coughing, particularly at night or in the early morning. These episodes are usually associated with widespread but variable airflow obstruction that is often reversible either spontaneously or with treatment. The inflammation also causes an associated increase in the existing bronchial hyperresponsiveness to a variety of stimuli."[3]

National panels in the United States,[3,4] Great Britain,[5-7] Canada,[8] and Australia and New Zealand[9] and an international consensus panel[10] have proposed guidelines for the management of asthma. Based on a combination of facts and the best guesses of experts, they all emphasize the importance of education, self-management, use of inhaled anti-inflammatory agents, and self-monitoring using peak expiratory flow measurements. However, the guidelines differ somewhat in the definitions of severity and permissiveness of the formulary recommended. The degree to which the guidelines have been implemented in the general care of asthmatics remains speculative.

Little has been studied regarding rehabilitation in the asthma population. Most studies mix patients with both asthma and chronic obstructive pulmonary disease (COPD) in traditional rehabilitation programs. Even studies reported to involve patients with asthma combine them with COPD, so that the results of the program on the asthma population are difficult to determine.[11,12] A pilot study recently examined the effect of a 12-day inpatient rehabilitation program on patients recruited from a mill who had respiratory symptoms, but had not been previously diagnosed with asthma.[13] More of those who participated in the rehabilitation program maintained their lung function and reversibility compared with a control group. According to the American College of Chest Physicians, pulmonary rehabilitation is defined as

"An art of medical practice wherein an individually tailored, multidisciplinary program is formulated which through accurate diagnosis, therapy, emotional support, and education, stabilizes or reverses both the physiopathology and psychopathology of pulmonary diseases and attempts to return the patient to the highest possible functional capacity allowed by his pulmonary handicap and overall life situation."

An integral part of rehabilitation for the asthma population is active participation of the patient in managing the disease and maintaining an active lifestyle while going to school or working. The discussion of asthma management and rehabilitation is preceded by a brief review of the pathobiology and pathophysiology of asthma.

Cellular Biology of Asthma

The exact mechanism(s) that cause the clinical syndrome of asthma are unclear. The underlying abnormality is inflammation of the airways (cellular infiltration, edema, nerve irritation, vasodilatation) resulting in bronchoconstriction (airway smooth muscle constriction), increased mucous secretions (submucosal gland and goblet cell hyperplasia and stimulation), and nonspecific airways hyperresponsiveness. A number of triggers or mediators produce asthma-like responses in susceptible individuals at much lower concentrations than in "normal" subjects. These stimuli may act by igniting cascades of cell activation with subsequent cytokine release and/or neurogenic excitation with neuropeptide and/or neurotransmitter release (Table 38-1). Other elements act to limit the responses triggered. Medications may act to inhibit, arrest, augment, or counteract one or more elements in the cascades.

Mast cells[14] and eosinophils[15] play a central role in asthma (Table 38-2). Helper T cells[15] orchestrate the activation and recruitment of eosinophils and mast cells through cytokines [interleukins-3, -4, -5 and granulocyte-macrophage colony stimulating factor (GM-CSF)]. Important end effectors include neuropeptides,[16,17] cysteinyl leukotriene (C_4, D_4, E_4) products of the 5-lipoxygenase pathway,[18] prostaglandin (PGD_2, PGE_2, PGI_2, PGF_{2a}) and thromboxane A_2 products of the cyclooxygenase pathway,[19] and platelet activating factor (PAF).[19] The neuropeptides are regulated by selective degradation by neutral endopeptidase,[20] chymase, and tryptase.[21,22]

In experimental antigen challenge, the immediate reaction is initiated by nerves and inflammatory cells already present in the airways with release of preformed or newly synthesized chemical mediators, such as histamine and the cysteinyl leukotrienes. The late-phase reaction (3 to 8 h) is the result of new cellular infiltration and activation. These cells then release mediators, resulting in a second bronchospastic response. The activation of cells, particularly T-helper and mast cells, may persist long after the antigenic challenge has ended. The late-phase reaction results in an increase in airway hyperresponsiveness, which may persist in a self-perpet-

TABLE 38-1 Mediators of Inflammation and Bronchospasm in Asthma

Effect	Mediator	Source
Airway Diameter		
Decreased	Leukotriene C_4, D_4, E_4	Mast cells and eosinophils
	Histamine	Mast cell degranulation
	Potentiated by chymase	Mast cell degranulation
	C3a	
	Activation of C3 by tryptase	Mast cell degranulation
	Prostaglandin D_2	Mast cells
	Release augmented by neuropeptide Y	Adrenergic nerves
	Substance P	C-fiber sensory nerves
	Degraded by chymase	Mast cell degranulation
	Degraded by neutral endopeptidase	Type II epithelial cells, submucosal glands, nerves, and airway smooth muscle
	Augmented by inhibition or down-regulation of neutral endopeptidase	Viral or mycoplasmal infections, hypertonic saline inhalation, toluene di-isocyanate (TDI)?
	Release augmented by neuropeptide Y	Adrenergic nerves
(Proximal)	Acetylcholine	Cholinergic nerves
(Peripheral)	Neurokinin A (tachykinin)	C-fiber sensory nerves
	Degraded by neutral endopeptidase	Type II epithelial cells, submucosal glands, nerves, and airway smooth muscle
	Augmented by inhibition or down-regulation of neutral endopeptidase	Viral or mycoplasmal infections, hypertonic saline inhalation, TDI?
Increased	Augmented by platelet activating factor (PAF)	Mast cells and eosinophils
(Peripheral)	Neurokinin B (tachykinin)	C-fiber sensory nerves
	Vasoactive intestinal peptide (VIP)	Cholinergic nerves
	Degraded by tryptase	Mast cell degranulation
(Proximal)	Nitric oxide	Nonadrenergic noncholinergic nerves
Mucous Secretion		
Increased	Substance P[a]	C-fiber sensory nerves
	Platelet activating factor (PAF)	Eosinophils
	Leukotriene C_4, D_4, E_4	Eosinophils
	Gastrin releasing peptide (GRP)	Neuroendocrine cells in the lower airways
	Degraded by chymase	Mast cell degranulation
	VIP[a]	Cholinergic nerves
Vascular Diameter		
Increased	VIP[a]	Cholinergic nerves
	Nitric oxide	Cholinergic nerves
	Substance P	C-fiber sensory nerves
	PAF	Eosinophils
	Leukotriene C_4, D_4, E_4	Eosinophils
	Prostaglandin D_2[a]	Mast cells
	Histamine[a]	Mast cell degranulation
	Angiotensin II	
	Activation of angiotensin I by chymase	Mast cell degranulation
	Bradykinin (kallidin I)	
	Degraded by chymase	Mast cell degranulation
(Arteriolar)	Calcitonin gene-related peptide (CGRP)	C-fiber sensory nerves
	Degraded by chymase	Mast cell degranulation
Decreased	GRP[a]	Neuroendocrine cells in the lower airways
(Arteriolar)	Norepinephrine	Adrenergic nerves
	Neuropeptide Y	Adrenergic nerves
Vascular Permeability		
Increased with	Substance P[a]	C-fiber sensory nerves
edema	PAF	Eosinophils
	Leukotriene C_4, D_4, E_4	Eosinophils
	Histamine[a]	Mast cell degranulation

[a] See previous entry for factors affecting level or action of mediator.

TABLE 38-2 Cellular Chemotaxis and Activation in Asthma

Cell	Mediator	Source
Mast cell	Proliferation and differentiation	
	Interleukin 3	T cells (equivalent to murine Th2 cells)
	Chemotaxis	
	Leukotriene E_4	Eosinophils
	Degranulation	
	IgE cross-linking	Specific antigens
	Substance P[a]	C-fiber sensory nerves
	Inhibited by VIP[a]	Cholinergic nerves
Eosinophil	Chemotaxis and priming	
	GM-CSF, IL-3, IL-5	T cells (equivalent to murine Th2 cells)
	PAF,[a] leukotriene E_4	Eosinophils
	Activation	
	IL-5	T cells (equivalent to murine Th2 cells)
	C3b	
	IgG, IgA	
	PAF[a]	Eosinophils
	Epidermal growth factor	
	IgE production	
	Interleukin-4	T cells (equivalent to murine Th2 cells)
	Degranulation	
	IgE cross-linking	Specific antigens

[a] See Table 38-1 entry for factors affecting level or action of mediator.

uating manner or be reinforced with continual reexposure to antigen triggers.[23]

Pathophysiology of Asthma

Asthma is characterized by reversible airway obstruction and airway hyperresponsiveness. Spirometry reveals low forced expiratory flow rates [forced expiratory volume in 1 s (FEV_1), forced expiratory flow between 25 and 75 percent of forced vital capacity ($FEF_{25-75\%}$), and peak expiratory flow (PEF)] with normal or increased lung volumes [functional residual capacity (FRC), residual volume (RV), and total lung capacity (TLC)]. The airway obstruction is partially or completely reversible spontaneously or with bronchodilators (improvement ≥ 13 percent in FEV_1, ≥ 23 percent in $FEF_{25-75\%}$, ≥ 20 percent in PEF[24]). The degree of obstruction varies with exacerbations, with therapy, and with time of day. Nonspecific triggers of bronchospasm (methacholine, histamine) induce bronchospasm at much lower concentrations in asthmatics than in nonasthmatics. For example, the provocative concentration (PC) of methacholine necessary to produce a 20 percent drop (PC_{20}) in FEV_1 is generally ≤ 8 mg/mL in asthmatic patients and may range from 20 to >200 mg/mL in nonasthmatic patients. Patients with allergic rhinitis have intermediate airway reactivity with some overlap to both sides (PC_{20} 5 to 50 mg/mL). Other nonspecific triggers, such as exercise and cold air, can also produce an immediate bronchospastic reaction in asthmatic patients. Antigen challenge is followed by a late-phase influx and activation of inflammatory cells. This results in an increase in nonspecific hyperresponsiveness and predisposes the patient to subsequent episodes of bronchospasm. Circadian variation in cortisol, epinephrine, vagal tone,

and inflammatory mediators results in a peak of bronchial reactivity and a nadir of PEF between 4 and 8 A.M. and may account for episodes of nocturnal bronchospasm.[25]

Exposure of asthma patients to irritants or allergens to which they are sensitive has been shown to increase asthma symptoms and precipitate asthma exacerbations. For at least those patients with persistent asthma despite daily medications, the clinician should identify allergen exposures, use the patient's history to assess sensitivity to seasonal allergens, use skin testing or in vitro testing to assess sensitivity to perennial indoor allergens, and assess the significance of positive tests in context of the patient's medical history.

Skin testing or in vitro testing is now specifically recommended for at least those patients with persistent asthma exposed to perennial indoor allergens.[3] Skin testing or in vitro testing should be used to determine the presence of specific IgE antibodies to the indoor allergens to which the patient is exposed year-round. Allergy testing is the only reliable way to determine sensitivity to perennial indoor allergens. For selected patients with asthma at any level of severity, detection of specific IgE sensitivity to seasonal or perennial allergens may be indicated as a basis for avoidance, for immunotherapy, or to characterize the patient's atopic status.

Determination of sensitivity to a perennial indoor allergen is usually not possible with a patient's medical history alone.[26] Increased symptoms during vacuuming or bed making and decreased symptoms when away from home on a business trip or vacation are suggestive but not sufficient. Allergy skin or in vitro tests are reliable in determining the presence of specific IgE,[27] but these tests do not determine whether the specific IgE is responsible for the patient's symptoms. That is why patients should be tested only for sensitivity to the allergens to which they are exposed and why the third step in evaluating patients for allergen sensitivity calls for assessing the clinical relevance of the sensitivity.

The recommendation to perform skin or in vitro tests for patients with persistent asthma exposed to perennial indoor allergens will result in a limited number of allergy tests for about half of all asthma patients. This is based on the prevalence of persistent asthma and the level of exposure to indoor allergens. It is estimated that about half of all asthma patients have persistent asthma based on data on children in the United States[28] and on adults in Australia.[29] About 80 percent of the U.S. population is exposed to house-dust mites,[30] 60 percent to a cat or dog, and a much smaller percentage to both animals.[31] Cockroaches are a consideration only in the inner city and southern parts of the United States.

Skin or in vitro tests for patients exposed to perennial allergens are essential to justify the expense and effort involved in implementing environmental controls. In addition, patient adherence to maintaining environmental controls (e.g., with regard to pets) is likely to be poor without proof of the patient's sensitivity.

Natural History of Asthma

HISTORY

Asthma is the most frequent chronic disease of childhood, affecting an estimated 7.2 percent of children.[32] The diagnosis of asthma in children may be missed, attributed to the child's having "weak lungs" or merely increased susceptibility to colds. During puberty, changes in allergic responses may cause a remission of asthma symptoms. These symptoms may recur with varying severity at any time thereafter, often after a bout of influenza and sometimes not until later years in the elderly. Thus, the diagnosis of asthma in later years may be met with disbelief or denial. Asthma severity not only varies widely from one patient to another but also, characteristically, fluctuates within the same patient. Mild asthma may escalate to more severe, persistent illness following exposure to allergens and/or nonspecific irritants or a viral respiratory tract infection; this requires a "step-up" in therapy (see below). With appropriate treatment, asthma severity is reduced, which permits a "step-down" in therapy. The major goal of asthma management is to control the disease with a minimum of medication.

Patients with mild, intermittent asthma have only infrequent symptoms (such as after exercise or allergen exposure) that are readily relieved or prevented by medication as needed. Although progression to more severe illness is certainly possible in the latter patients (for example, following a viral lower respiratory tract infection or as a result of heavy, ongoing allergen exposure), they generally do not require maintenance medication. On the other hand, patients with more persistent asthma (more frequent symptoms and/or lung function abnormality between attacks) appear to be at some risk for progression from mild to moderate disease to more severe disease unless the underlying inflammation is suppressed by maintenance anti-inflammatory medication.

CHRONIC PERSISTENT AIRFLOW LIMITATION AND AIRWAY WALL REMODELING

Some patients with asthma may have a fixed component of airflow obstruction that is not reversible with bronchodilator therapy, in addition to a responsive, reversible component. The fixed component may be due to structural alterations in airway wall histopathology, including the deposition of collagen beneath the epithelial basement membrane.[33,34] These changes in the extracellular matrix of the airway wall may be the consequence of long-standing, severe airway inflammation that is not adequately treated with anti-inflammatory therapy. The result is a fixed component of airflow obstruction that is not responsive to therapy. The potential for developing fixed airflow obstruction due to airway wall remodeling underscores the importance of early intervention in persistent asthma with therapy directed at long-term control of inflammation.

Differentiation of Asthma from COPD

The most common obstructive diseases are asthma and chronic obstructive pulmonary disease, which consists of varying combinations of emphysema and/or cigarette-related small airways disease ("chronic obstructive bronchitis"). Emphysema and small airways disease are generally lumped together under the single designation of COPD because of their common etiology (i.e., cigarette smoking) and their frequent coexistence, whereas asthma is usually distinguishable clinically and physiologically from COPD. Both disorders, asthma and COPD, are fairly common, with a prevalence in the United States of approximately 4 to 5 percent. Consequently, some patients with COPD (approximately 5 to 7 percent) also have asthma. In addition to this overlap, asthma and COPD share some clinical, physiologic, and pathologic features in common, sometimes making the distinction between these two types of disorders difficult. Characteristically, asthma and COPD are distinguished by a number of clinical features (Table 38-3).

These characteristic clinical differences between asthma and COPD are sometimes blurred, however. For example, asthma may occur later in life, whereas emphysema in patients with alpha$_1$-antitrypsin deficiency may occur relatively early in life. Moreover, occasional patients with asthma have a history of smoking, whereas a small proportion of patients with COPD are lifelong nonsmokers. Furthermore, some patients with COPD have a pronounced response to bronchodilator therapy and occasional patients with COPD respond favorably to anti-inflammatory therapy, whereas patients with asthma sometimes respond poorly to bronchodilators and occasionally asthma is refractory to anti-inflammatory treatment. Other "crossover" features, in addition to airflow obstruction, are characteristic of both asthma and COPD, such as air trapping and hyperinflation and nonspecific airways hyperresponsiveness, although the last is usually less pronounced in COPD. In addition, a familial predisposition may be present in both disorders.

Physiologically, asthma and COPD exhibit both similarities and differences.[35] In asthma, the FEV_1 usually improves >15 to 20 percent in response to a bronchodilator. Although a significant response may be absent in severe, refractory asthma, the response to a beta agonist is usually greater than that to an anticholinergic and the flow response is usually greater than the volume response. In COPD, the response to a bronchodilator is usually less than in asthma and absent in approximately a third of patients; moreover, the response

TABLE 38-3 Clinical Features of Asthma and COPD: Differences

	Asthma	COPD
Onset	Often early in life	Usually not until middle age
Cigarette smoking	Infrequent	Most often a long history
Nature of symptoms	Intermittent	Often chronic cough and/or exertional dyspnea
Bronchodilator response	Often dramatic	Relatively modest
Response to anti-inflammatory therapy	Very favorable, as a rule	Only a small minority appears to respond

to an anticholinergic is usually greater than to a beta agonist and the volume response is sometimes greater than the flow response. Nonspecific bronchial hyperresponsiveness (BHR) is the physiologic hallmark of asthma, correlates with asthma severity (but not well with baseline FEV_1), and is characterized by a steeper dose-response slope than in COPD and the absence, usually, of a maximal response plateau. In COPD, on the other hand, nonspecific bronchial hyperresponsiveness, while often present, is less prevalent and of lesser degree than the BHR of asthma, is strongly related to baseline FEV_1, and is associated with a shallower dose-response curve than in asthma. Moreover, a maximal response plateau is usually present in mild COPD. In asthma, the diffusing capacity is usually normal or increased, whereas in COPD it is decreased in emphysema to an extent that correlates well with scores for emphysema derived from high-resolution computer tomography (HRCT) and morphologic assessment of lungs obtained at surgery or autopsy. On the other hand, diffusing capacity is normal in COPD characterized mainly by intrinsic small airways disease without significant emphysema. In asthma chronic hypoxemia is generally absent and acute hypoxemia varies with the severity of the acute attack, whereas in COPD chronic hypoxemia is often present, frequently worsening with exercise, as well as with acute exacerbations. Hypocapnia is common in asthma during attacks, except when airflow obstruction is severe, whereas hypocapnia is uncommon in COPD and hypercapnia is generally present when FEV_1 is <0.75 L. In COPD, the age-related annual rate of decline in FEV_1 is accelerated (>120 mL in some patients), and smoking cessation typically slows this increased rate of decline toward normal. In asthma, the rate of decline in FEV_1 with age is increased on the average (50 mL/year versus 35 mL/year in normal controls) but is normal in some patients and has no consistent relationship with smoking.

A number of other features tend to distinguish asthma from COPD.[36] For example, asthmatic sputum typically contains Curschmann's spirals, creola bodies, Charcot-Leyden crystals, and eosinophils, whereas during exacerbations sputum in patients with COPD is generally purulent with increased numbers of neutrophils. Bronchoalveolar lavage (BAL) fluid from asthmatic patients contains sloughed epithelial cells, eosinophils and eosinophilic cationic protein, and major basic protein and increased levels of a variety of cytokines (IL-4 and IL-5 in stable asthma and IL-1, IL-2, IL-6, TNFα, and GM-CSF in symptomatic asthma). BAL fluid from COPD patients, on the other hand, exhibits a predominance of pigmented alveolar macrophages and variable numbers of neutrophils, whereas the cytokine profile has been poorly studied. Autopsy features of asthma include tenacious plugs of mucus containing desquamated epithelial cells, eosinophils, and lymphocytes occluding small bronchi without

morphologic evidence of emphysema or right ventricular hypertrophy, whereas postmortem changes in COPD are characterized by excess mucus (generally without plugs or the cellular changes noted in asthma), the frequent presence of moderate to severe anatomic emphysema, and right ventricular hypertrophy.

The clinical importance of distinguishing asthma from COPD is that in asthma an emphasis is placed on long-term control with anti-inflammatory agents, whereas in COPD bronchodilators, particularly anticholinergic aerosols, play a more important role as maintenance therapy. When the distinction is difficult, it is wise to treat the condition as asthma with reliance on anti-inflammatory as well as both maintenance and quick-relief bronchodilator therapy.

Medical Management of Asthma

GOALS OF THERAPY

Therapy for asthma is directed at treating the underlying causes and mechanisms of the disease. At present, most forms of asthma are not "curable" but can be treated with great success. For most patients asthma is a continual process with periodic exacerbations. Treatment must address both the underlying chronic inflammatory process as well as the overt symptoms apparent to the patient (Table 38-4).

For the patient, asthma is manifested by the symptoms perceived. Most commonly, cough, wheezing, dyspnea, and chest tightness may be present episodically or continuously. Nocturnal symptoms or symptoms on awakening in the morning are common due to the diurnal variation of endogenous catecholamines, vagal tone, and adrenocorticosteroids.[25] For any given patient, a particular symptom may be most prevalent or bothersome. Because of the often gradual onset of asthma and its chronic nature, it is not unusual for patients to ignore even marked symptoms as "normal" for them. Isolated cough is not uncommon. Rapid relief of symptoms reduces the impact of asthma on the patient and may be life-saving. Preferable is the prevention of symptoms and

TABLE 38-4 The Goals of Asthma Therapy

Prevent chronic and troublesome symptoms.

Maintain near-normal pulmonary function.

Maintain normal activities of daily living including work (school) and exercise.

Prevent recurrent exacerbations of asthma and minimize the need for emergency department visits and hospitalizations.

Provide optimal pharmacotherapy with minimal or no adverse effects.

Meet patients' and families' expectations of and satisfaction with asthma care.

particularly exacerbations manifested by more severe symptoms.

Relief and prevention of symptoms allows the asthmatic patient to participate fully in all physical and social activities. Patients with well-controlled asthma should not be restricted in their physical activity. With proper treatment, asthma should not result in excess loss of time from work or school or indeed from any activity. Clearly, poorly controlled asthma limits exercise capacity. Adequate therapy should relieve ventilatory limitation to exercise and prevent exercise-induced asthma. Some cases of occupational asthma may not be controllable without complete avoidance of inciting triggers in the workplace.

Perception of asthma varies greatly from patient to patient. On the one hand, symptoms may sometimes be present without measurable physiologic changes, or conversely, marked declines in lung function may not cause the patient any duress. A reversible obstructive ventilatory defect is the hallmark of asthma. With aggressive therapy most patients' lung function will return to normal or near-normal. A proportion of patients with severe asthma appears to have a component of fixed or permanent obstruction. However, patients generally also have a large component that is responsive to therapy.

All medications are associated with possible adverse reactions. Some side effects are an extension of the drug's intended pharmacologic actions and are at times unavoidable if doses are to be adequate to control the disease. It is fortunate that most of the medications used have relatively few side effects and a high degree of safety.

Inconvenience and lack of immediate benefit are the greatest impediments to any chronic therapy. Unfortunately, moderate and severe asthma requires some interventions that have no immediate effect. Daily medication regimens should be as simple as possible. Avoidance and environmental manipulations should also be designed with convenience and expedience in mind. Cost to the patient and third-party payors must be a consideration. The patient who cannot afford the treatment in terms of time or dollars will not take it. The cost of intervention must be weighed against the cost of poorly treated asthma.

EDUCATION

Outpatient asthma is ultimately managed by the patient. The physician must develop a partnership with the patient to guide this self-management.[37] The physician, with the patient's input, must develop a flexible management plan. Contingencies for acute and chronic worsening and improvement must be addressed proactively. The plan may change over time. A large degree of autonomy may be given to the patient, but the limitations of patients' ability to manage their asthma must also be clearly recognized. The latitude allowed a patient is influenced by the patient's knowledge, experience, confidence, and motivation. Patient autonomy does not absolve the doctor from being responsive and available. Training in self-management of asthma may require more initial time than the traditional paternalistic approach. Nurse educators and other health care professionals can provide a valuable extension to the physician's educational efforts. Education is central to asthma self-management and includes both transmission of information and training in skills (Table

TABLE 38-5 Principles of Asthma Management

Educate the patient.
Assess and monitor asthma severity with objective measures of lung function.
Avoid or control asthma triggers and factors contributing to severity.
Establish medication plans for long-term self-management.
Proactively establish action plans for self-management of acute exacerbations in partnership with the health care provider.
Provide regular follow-up care.

38-5). Elements must be repeatedly reviewed and reinforced. Time must also be allotted for questions and the expression of expectations and concerns by the patient.

Education of the patient is a team effort. Other providers of education may include nurses, advanced practice nurses, and pharmacists (Table 38-6). Unfortunately, many opportunities for education are missed owing to lack of information by the physician, lack of time, or assumptions that the patient already knows the information, especially if the patient has had a diagnosis of asthma for a long time. Teaching moments occur throughout the health care continuum, and each moment must be utilized to the utmost since time is limited for education and poorly reimbursed.

Educational programs are valuable sources of education and support for the patient with asthma (Table 38-7). However, many patients who work find weekly sessions inconvenient. One-on-one sessions with frequent reinforcements may be a reasonable alternative.

To understand the elements of self-management, patients require a fundamental understanding of the characteristics and causes of asthma. Explaining the inflammatory nature of asthma is important to understanding the basis for the pharmacologic and nonpharmacologic interventions. The patient must understand the role of different medications in the reduction of inflammation and relief of bronchospasm. Patients need skill in the use of metered-dose inhalers (MDIs) and peak expiratory flow (PEF) meters to effectively self-manage their asthma. Fears regarding medications and, in particular, corticosteroids must be addressed.

Patients do not have asthma in isolation. The understanding and support of the patient's family and supervisors or teachers at work or school must be facilitated. This process may entail discussions with parents, spouses, supervisors, teachers, athletic coaches, and school or work health professionals. It also includes liaison with other health professionals (specialists, primary care physicians, ancillary services) caring for the patient. Patients may also benefit from community support groups which can be identified through local branches of the American Lung Association or Asthma and Allergy Foundation.

Control of asthma is a long-term endeavor for both the patient and caregivers. Feedback and measurements of progress help retain interest and enthusiasm and facilitate adjustments to management. Symptoms are most important to the patient, but the importance of any particular symptom varies from patient to patient. It is useful to identify symptoms or asthma-provoking activities which are important to a particular patient and review the response to therapy in terms of improvement in those specific symptoms and activities.

TABLE 38-6 Education

Physician	Nurse or Advanced Practice Nurse	Pharmacist
Joint development of treatment goals Medication management Development and management of the action plan Encourage adherence	Asthma pathology and pathophysiology Inhaler and spacer or holding chamber techniques Ongoing assessment and self-monitoring Triggers avoidance and home and environmental controls Liaison with physician Monitoring adherence to plan	Inhaler and spacer or holding chamber techniques Drug interactions Side effects Dosages Monitor usage

TABLE 38-7 Sample Plan for Patient Education

Knowledge	Skills	Health Care Professional Interventions
Disease process		
Inflammation		Diagnosis
Bronchospasm		Assessment of severity
Hypersensitivity		Goals of therapy
Controlling asthma triggers		
Infections	Dust-proofing	Identification of triggers
Miscellaneous aeroallergens	Environmental controls	Instruction in avoidance
Weather	Dietary limitations	Home or environmental controls
Drugs		
Overexertion		
Occupational		
Nighttime		
Lung irritants		
Extreme emotion (laughing, anger, etc.)		
Foods		
Food additives		
Drug therapy		
Understanding medications	Inhaler technique	Stepped therapy
Inhaled anti-inflammatory agents	Use of spacers/holding chambers	Instruction in use of aerosol delivery devices and auxiliary devices
β_2 agonists	Nebulizers	Immunotherapy
Antileukotrienes	Special delivery devices	
Oral corticosteroids	Cleaning of devices	
Other medications		
Long-term-control and quick-relief medications		
Guidelines to taking medications		
Monitoring		
Peak flow monitoring	Symptom monitoring with diary	Personal best or predicted PEF
Warning signs and symptoms	Recognition of early signs of deterioration	Green, yellow, red zones
When to go to school or work	Peak expiratory flow (PEF) meters	
When to call MD	PEF diary	
Management		
Rx of exacerbations		Exacerbation treatment protocol
Action plan		
Complicating factors		
Allergic rhinitis, sinus disease		Identification and treatment
Gastroesophageal reflux		
Allergic bronchopulmonary aspergillosis (ABPA)		
Nasal polyps		
Psychological/stress		
Exercise and fitness	Panic control	Identification and treatment
Breathing techniques	Stress reduction	
Relaxation methods	Coping skills	
Intimacy issues		

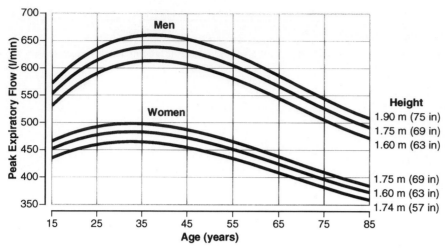

FIGURE 38-1 Predicted peak expiratory flow.[38]

Ultimately, symptoms are an imprecise assessment and subject to many confounding factors. Objective measurements of response are critical to assessment of asthma control. Peak expiratory flow monitoring is the most useful. It can be performed by the patient at frequent intervals to detect asymptomatic declines or improvements in lung function. It is inexpensive and reliable. Results can be compared with the patient's historical best or to sex-, age-, and height-adjusted normal subjects[38] (Fig. 38-1). Use of a peak flow meter or asthma diary helps the patient document changes over time and allows the health care professional (HCP) to review the changes to make adjustments in the action plan.

ASSESSMENT OF SEVERITY

The first step in developing a plan for management of asthma is assessment of the severity of the disease. Severity can be classified by clinical pattern, symptoms, need for medications and medical interventions, and severity of airflow obstruction (Table 38-8). These indicators of severity (or worsening of control) may not vary in concert with one another. A particular patient may be moderate in one category and mild in another. Patients with a previous near-fatal episode of

asthma have a marked decrease in perception of airway resistance (an altered sense of dyspnea). Less severe asthmatics also have reduced perception of dyspnea but overlap considerably with normal subjects.[39] There is little information regarding the comparative sensitivity of these measures for detecting exacerbations, but typically for any individual patient an exacerbation will occur in a reproducible pattern (e.g., increased frequency of nocturnal awakenings, followed by a fall in PEF; increased cough, wheeze, chest tightness, and/or shortness of breath, followed by increased inhaled albuterol use). Unfortunately, patients and physicians often underestimate the degree of severity of asthma. This may lead to undertreatment and increased morbidity and mortality.

In general, previously severe asthma portends future severe asthma and increased morbidity and mortality. Recognition of risk factors for morbidity and mortality should prompt close and aggressive management. Previous life-threatening exacerbations of acute asthma resulting in respiratory failure as evidenced by respiratory acidosis and/or intubation are most significant.[40] Any hospitalization for asthma within the past year, particularly while the patient is receiving chronic (long-term) oral corticosteroids, is a significant risk factor. A number of demographic risk factors have been identified, including age (late teens to early twen-

TABLE 38-8 Assessment of Asthma Severity at Presentation

Clinical Features before Treatment[a]	Intermittent	Mild, Persistent	Moderate, Persistent	Severe, Persistent
Symptoms	Intermittent and brief, ≤2 times/wk Asymptomatic and normal PEF between exacerbations	>2 time per week, <1 time per day	Daily Daily use of inhaled short-acting β_2 agonists	Continuous
Nocturnal asthma Physical activity	≤2 times/mo	>2 times/mo Exacerbations may affect activity	>Once per week Exacerbations affect activity	Frequent Limited by symptoms
Exacerbations	Brief (from a few hours to a few days) Intensity may vary	May affect sleep and activity	Affect sleep and activity ≥2 times/wk, may last days	Frequent
PEF or FEV$_1$	≥80% predicted Variability <20%	≥80% predicted Variability 20 to 30%	>60–≤80% predicted Variability >30%	≈60% predicted Variability >30%

[a] The presence of one of the features of severity is sufficient to place the patient in that category.
SOURCE: Reprinted, with permission, from Murphy.[3]

TABLE 38-9 Assessment of Asthma Severity after Initiation of Therapy

Treatment Necessary to Maintain Control[a]	Intermittent	Mild, Persistent	Moderate, Persistent	Severe, Persistent
Relievers	Intermittent use of inhaled β_2 agonists	Intermittent use of inhaled β_2 agonists	Intermittent use of inhaled β_2 agonists	Intermittent use of inhaled β_2 agonists
Controllers		Daily inhaled antiinflammatory (low dose), oral antileukotriene or, possibly, add a long-acting bronchodilator for nocturnal symptoms	Daily inhaled anti-inflammatory (low to moderate dose), *and* possibly long-acting bronchodilator for nocturnal symptoms	Anti-inflammatory medications (high-dose inhaled corticosteroids, and possibly an oral corticosteroid) plus long-acting bronchodilator

[a] The presence of one of the features of severity is sufficient to place the patient in that category.

SOURCE: Reprinted, with permission, from Murphy.[3]

ties), race (African American), and socioeconomic status (inner city, low income). Although asthma is not caused by emotion, the following psychological factors may affect its severity and treatment: depression, alcohol abuse, recent family loss and disruption, recent unemployment, and personality disorders.[41] Barriers or lack of access to medical care, whether due to economic, social, cultural, or psychological factors, affect control of asthma. Other risk factors that need to be assessed include noncompliance with maintenance antiinflammatory therapy and avoidance measures, dependence on high doses or frequent use of β_2 agonists, and recent reductions in or withdrawal from corticosteroids or other anti-inflammatory medications.

The nature and severity of symptoms reflect the severity of asthma in general. An increase in symptoms and acute exacerbations represent episodic worsening of asthma in response to exogenous stimuli (irritants, allergens, exercise, infection) or without identifiable provocation. Cough, chest tightness, wheezing, and breathlessness (with or without exercise) are common complaints. The frequency and duration range from rare to continuous. It is important to elicit a history regarding *nocturnal* symptoms, awakenings from sleep and early morning wheezing or chest tightness. Increased diurnal variability in peak expiratory flow rate implies increased susceptibility in the early morning. Symptoms may be induced by or present with or following exercise and result in dramatic exercise intolerance and avoidance. A significant measure of asthma severity is time lost from, or diminished effectiveness at, work or school. Patients with more than rare absences have inadequately controlled asthma or more severe disease than otherwise appreciated.

The level of treatment necessary to maintain good control is another index of asthma severity (Table 38-9). Patients with more severe asthma require more therapy to gain and retain control. Assessment of past therapies must include medications (dose, duration, and compliance), as well as effectiveness (symptoms and objective measures). Although patients may report that β_2 agonists provide short-term relief of symptoms, their asthma may remain poorly controlled in terms of objective measures (PEF, PEF variability, FEV_1/FVC ratio, and PC_{20}).

Monitoring of peak expiratory flow rate should be seriously considered in patients who take medications daily (moderate to severe asthmatics). In patients with mild asthma, it is less likely that PEF monitoring will result in a significant reduction in morbidity or mortality.[42,43] During adjustment of medications patients should record the best of three PEFs in the morning and evening at consistent times. If bronchodilators are used, PEFs should be recorded at least before and optimally after (10 to 15 min) inhaled bronchodilators. After good control has been established, it may be more convenient to record the best daily morning PEF alone. This strategy allows continued early detection of asymptomatic declines in lung function which may indicate impending exacerbation or decline in the degree of control. As evidence of good control, PEFs should be near the patient's personal best and near population normals. The zone system (Table 38-10), analogous to the traffic light, has been developed to grade changes in PEF.[44] Decline into the yellow zone may indicate the beginning of an acute exacerbation or chronic deterioration. Therapy may be changed to increase the dose of anti-inflammatory inhalers or initiate a short "burst" of oral corticosteroids (see below). Descent into the red zone indicates a severe deterioration and may require emergency intervention from the physician or in the hospital emergency department. The zones are approximations and need to be tailored to the individual patient based on his or her prior history and past response to therapy. Ideally, personal best peak expiratory flows are near population normals[38] [see Fig. 38-1 and Eq. (1)].

TABLE 38-10 Zone System of Peak Expiratory Flow Monitoring

Zone	Interpretation	% Personal Best PEF	A.M./P.M. PEF Variability, %
Green	All clear	>80	<20
Yellow	Caution	50–80	20–30
Red	Alert	<50	>30

Eq. (1): Predicted Peak Expiratory Flow for Men and Women[38]

Men:
$$\log_e \text{PEF (L/min)} = 0.544 \log_e \text{age} - 0.0151 \text{ age}$$
$$- 74.7/\text{height (cm)} + 5.48$$

Women:
$$\log_e \text{PEF (L/min)} = 0.376 \log_e \text{age} - 0.0120 \text{ age}$$
$$- 58.8/\text{height (cm)} + 5.63$$

Peak expiratory flow varies with time of day with the lowest values generally in the morning (8 to 10 A.M.) and the highest in the afternoon (3 to 5 P.M.) [see Eq. (2)]. Normal variability is probably less than 10 percent (4 to 18 percent) but may be greater than 25 percent (6 to 27 percent) in stable asthma. Following an asthma exacerbation PEF variability may be >50 percent.[45] The degree of PEF variability correlates with FEV_1 variability, severity of asthma, and airway hypersensitivity.

Eq. (2): Predicted Peak Expiratory Flow Variability

$$\text{PEF variability} = \left| \frac{\text{A.M. PEF} - \text{P.M. PEF}}{(\text{A.M. PEF} + \text{P.M. PEF})/2} \right|$$

CONTROL OF ASTHMA TRIGGERS

Nonpharmacologic interventions, particularly avoidance of asthma triggers, should be considered in all patients being treated for asthma. In some patients, specific environmental triggers of asthma can be identified and avoided (Table 38-11). The extent to which this is possible varies from patient to patient. The simplest approach is a careful history. Patients often associate worsening symptoms with certain activities, locations, or seasons. The ability to avoid triggers varies, depending on the nature and prevalence of the trigger. Avoidance of triggers such as dust mites for 2 to 9 months may result in a decrease in symptoms, medication use, and specific and nonspecific bronchial hyperresponsiveness.[46–48] Inhalation challenge with specific antigens is possible in some cases, but should be performed only by a specialist and usually is relevant only in a research setting.

Measures to control or limit exposure to triggers of inflammation and/or bronchospasm may require major lifestyle changes, which the patient or family may not be willing or able to make. Expensive changes such as removing carpeting may not be possible, and removing a beloved pet from an elderly patient's home may not be an option.

Pharmacologic Therapy

Pharmacologic therapy of asthma can be divided into two broad categories: long-term-control medications used routinely to continually prevent or relieve symptoms and quick-relief medications taken intermittently for short-term relief of symptoms (Table 38-12). The distinction quickly blurs in a patient whose asthma is poorly controlled. Ideally, patients unperturbed by an exacerbation of their asthma would have all their signs and symptoms of asthma continually prevented and/or relieved by their anti-inflammatory long-term-control medications, for example, either inhaled cortico-

steroids, cromolyn, nedocromil, or leukotriene modifiers. Symptoms or signs resulting from exposure to a trigger (e.g., cat dander, smoke, viral infection) ideally would resolve a short time after the use of their quick-relief medication like an inhaled short-acting β_2 agonist. Quick-relief medications may also be used to prevent symptoms before exposure to a known trigger (e.g., exercise). Patients with mild, intermittent asthma require only quick-relief medications for relief of infrequent symptoms. Patients with the most severe, persistent asthma often receive multiple anti-inflammatory medications and long-term bronchodilators. Despite this, they may continue to have frequent symptoms requiring more frequent quick-relief medication.

LONG-TERM-CONTROL MEDICATIONS

Anti-inflammatory agents, administered on a regularly scheduled basis, treat the underlying inflammation of asthma, resulting in reduced airway hyperreactivity and decreasing the frequency of acute bronchospasm and symptoms. The addition of long-acting bronchodilators to anti-inflammatory regimens may provide further relief from bronchospastic symptoms—wheezing, chest tightness, dyspnea. Optimal long-term-control medication regimens should result in a minimization of the signs and symptoms of asthma and of adverse effects and cost of medication.

INHALED CORTICOSTEROIDS
Airway inflammation is present even in asymptomatic asthmatics and correlates with disease severity. Inhaled corticosteroids are nonspecific suppressors of inflammation.[3] They inhibit arachidonic acid metabolism resulting in decreased production of leukotrienes and prostaglandins. They also reduce migration, activation, and survival of inflammatory cells through inhibition of cytokine production. In addition, inhaled corticosteroids increase the responsiveness of the β receptors on airway smooth muscle. The result is decreased frequency of acute exacerbations, symptoms, and need for concurrent medications. Diurnal variability in PEF and airway responsiveness to methacholine also decrease. Five inhaled corticosteroid preparations are currently available in the United States: beclomethasone dipropionate (Beclovent, Vanceril 42 μg per puff, and Vanceril DS, 84 μg per puff); budesonide (Pulmocort 200 μg per inhalation); triamcinolone acetonide (Azmacort, 100 μg per puff); flunisolide (AeroBid, 250 μg per puff); and fluticasone (FloVent, 44 μg per puff, 110 μg per puff, 220 μg per puff). Additional formulations of inhaled corticosteroids, including MDIs which deliver higher doses per puff and dry powder delivery devices, are available outside the United States. The relative strength of each preparation in the treatment of asthma is poorly defined. As a surrogate measure of topical anti-inflammatory activity, topical skin blanching efficacy has been used in the National Asthma Education and Prevention Program, Expert Panel Report II, guidelines for the diagnosis and management of asthma (NAEPP2), although this measure of efficacy does not take into account variable delivery of aerosol to the lung with different devices and different inhaler techniques. As a rough approximation, however, estimated relative skin-blanching potency has been converted to puffs in Fig. 38-2.

Detectable hypothalamic-pituitary-adrenal (HPA) axis suppression is uncommon at doses below 1000 to 1500 μg (24 to 30 puffs per day, 50 μg per puff) beclomethasone

TABLE 38-11 Asthma Triggers and Controls

Inducers of Inflammation and/or Bronchospasm	Alternatives for Home and Environmental Controls
Respiratory Viruses	Yearly influenza vaccination is recommended.
Occupational Sensitizers Toluene di-isocyanate (TDI), western red cedar sawdust, grain dust, cotton bract, resins, solvents, chemical or organic dusts, hardeners, latex, and many others	Alternative materials, ventilation/respirator protection may be inadequate, and a change of occupation may be necessary if exposure cannot be avoided.
Aeroallergens Indoors House dust, dust mite, cockroach, animal dander (cat, dog, feathers, down)	House dust and house-dust mite control: wash bedding in hot water [>55°C (131°F)]; remove stuffed toys or wash in hot water or deep freeze weekly; cover mattresses and pillows; replace upholstered furniture and drapes; adjust humidity to <50%; wear a mask when vacuuming; filter air with a high-efficiency particulate air (HEPA) filter; limit dust catchers. Pets: must be kept out of bedroom, consider washing pet weekly × 3 then every 2 to 3 weeks; give away the pet; a denaturant that is wiped on the pet (Allerpet C, D, and B) may be of benefit.

Molds
      Potted indoor plants, fish aquarium, leaks in bathrooms, Christmas trees
Outdoors
   Pollens (grasses, trees, molds)
	Molds: provide adequate ventilation; clean bathrooms carefully and frequently; limit houseplants; reduce humidity to <35%; clean walls and add mold inhibitor to paint; avoid humidifiers.
	
	Reduce exposure by closing windows and doors, using air conditioning and remaining indoors when pollen counts are high; filter air with HEPA air filters.

Medications Aspirin (10–30% of asthmatics), other nonsteroidal anti-inflammatory drugs β blockers (including eyedrops)	
Weather Changes in seasons Ozone, sulfur dioxide, smog Excessive humidity Cold air	Avoid unnecessary physical activity during episodes of high ozone or smog. Cold air or exercise may induce bronchospasm. Avoidance is not necessary, but pretreatment with bronchodilators may be useful.
Extreme Emotions Mood: sad, worried, angry Expressions of mood: laughing too hard, crying, hyperventilating	Avoid situations that may produce symptoms.
Overexertion Running fast, walking up stairs too fast, exercising too hard Coughing	
Nighttime Tiredness, lying down, accumulating mucus	
Lung Irritants Combustion products: cigar, cigarette smoke (including secondhand smoke), wood-burning fireplaces, barbecues Chemical irritants: cleaning fluids (bleach, sprays, strong odors), spray starch, newspaper print Volatile organic compounds: cooking fumes, paint and paint thinners, hair spray, perfume, furniture polish, potpourri and room deodorizers, fabric softener sheets	Avoid cigarette smoke (active or passive), fine aerosols from household sprays, and volatile organic compounds (polishes and cooking oils).
Foods Contaminating molds, nuts, peanut butter, soybean products Food additives: tartrazine, metabisulfite, monosodium glutamate (MSG) Other: chocolate, eggs, milk, orange juice, seafood (i.e. fish, shellfish)	If metabisulfite-sensitive, avoid beer, wine, dried fruits, processed potatoes, seafood, and meats; previously used on lettuce on salad bars but is no longer approved for such use.

TABLE 38-12 Available Preparations of Selected Asthma Medications in the United States

Drug	Metered-Dose Inhaler (MDI)	Breath-Activated MDI	Dry Powder Inhaler	Inhalation Solution	Oral	Oral Controlled Release	Subcutaneous	Intravenous
Anti-Inflammatory Agents								
Beclomethasone	•							
Budesonide	•							
Flunisolide	•							
Fluticasone	•							
Triamcinolone	•							
Cromolyn	•		•	•				
Nedocromil	•							
Zafirlukast					•			
Zileuton					•			
Bronchodilators								
Albuterol	•		•	•	•	•		
Bitolterol	•			•				
Epinephrine	•						•	
Metaproterenol	•			•	•			
Pirbuterol	•	•						
Terbutaline	•							
Salmeterol	•				•		•	•
Ipratropium	•			•				
Theophylline/ Aminophylline					•	•		•

(relative potency of 24 to 30 in Fig. 38-2). In mild, persistent asthma, relatively low doses of inhaled corticosteroids (e.g., eight puffs beclomethasone per day or equivalent) are usually sufficient for satisfactory asthma control. In severe asthma, however, higher doses are required and manufacturers' recommended doses are often exceeded.[49] The optimal dose of inhaled corticosteroids is that which effectively controls asthma. Even if HPA axis suppression is present, the degree of suppression is less than that caused by daily oral prednisone producing a comparable control of asthma.[50] Localized infections with *Candida albicans* may occur in the mouth, pharynx, or occasionally larynx. Clinically significant infection may be treated with topical antifungal agents and reduction in dose or discontinuation of the inhaled corticosteroid. The incidence of local oral effects may be reduced by using a spacer or holding chamber and rinsing the mouth

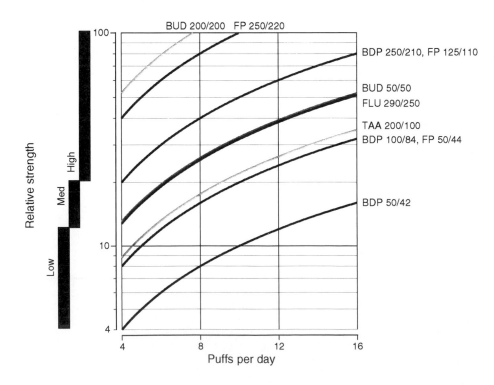

FIGURE 38-2 Relative strength of inhaled corticosteroids. Drug ex-valve dose/ex-mouthpiece dose are indicated in parenthesis (in the United States, the labeled dose is the ex-mouthpiece dose; outside the United States, it is generally the ex-valve dose). BDP, beclomethasone dipropionate (Becloforte, Beclovent, Vanceril); FP, fluticasone propionate (Flo Vent); TAA, triamcinolone acetonide (Azmacort response assumed to be proportional to the ex-valve dose); FLU, flunisolide (Aerobid); BUD, budesonide (Pulmocort in the Turbuhaler dry powder inhaler, which is assumed to have twice the lung delivery of a metered-dose inhaler).

following use. Cough due to the additive oleic acid may infrequently occur with beclomethasone preparations but is minimized by the use of spacers. Reversible dysphonia can occur as a result of deposition of the drugs on the vocal cords. Dermal thinning and purpura may occur, particularly in the elderly.[51,52] Laboratory studies indicate that inhaled corticosteroids in high doses ($\geq$1500 μg beclomethasone or equivalent) may decrease bone density, but the implications of these small-scale findings with respect to the risk of fractures are unclear. Recent reports link inhaled corticosteroid use, mainly in high doses administered over long periods of time, to an increased risk for cataracts[53] and glaucoma.[54] Therefore, regular eye examinations are recommended for patients on high-dose inhaled corticosteroids. Inhaled corticosteroids may also cause nausea, vomiting, diarrhea, headache, and sore throat.

Patients with unstable or severe asthma may benefit from tid or qid dosing. Stable patients with mild or moderate persistent asthma, however, achieve equivalent effectiveness with bid dosing with the same total number of puffs per day and are likely to be more compliant with the bid dosing regimen.[55] Frequent exacerbations indicate a failure of the chronic regimen and are an indication to intensify chronic therapy. Before increasing inhaled corticosteroid doses, it is important to review inhaler technique and compliance. In one study, 45 percent of subjects were estimated to be taking less than 51 percent of the prescribed doses of inhaled corticosteroids.[56] After asthma control is achieved, a stepwise decrease in anti-inflammatory therapy may be possible and is advisable. In a recent Finnish study, 74 percent of mild asthmatic subjects remained stable after a two-thirds reduction in dose of inhaled corticosteroids after 2 years at the higher dose.[57] The ideal dose of inhaled corticosteroids is the minimum dose necessary to attain and maintain the goals of therapy.

CHRONIC ORAL CORTICOSTEROIDS

Every effort should be made to minimize the use of chronic oral corticosteroids. For an equivalent degree of asthma control, daily oral corticosteroids cause significantly more systemic side effects than inhaled corticosteroids. Continual efforts should be made to reduce oral corticosteroid doses by increasing the dose of inhaled corticosteroids. Any patient without satisfactory control of his or her asthma on more than 10 mg of prednisone daily or 20 mg every other day should be referred to a specialist with this explicit goal. In patients previously on chronic maintenance therapy with oral corticosteroids, withdrawal of oral corticosteroids may result in adrenal insufficiency for up to 1 year. This complication is not prevented by inhaled corticosteroids. During adrenocortical stress, including surgery, oral corticosteroids may be necessary to prevent symptomatic hypoadrenalism.

INHALED NONSTEROIDAL ANTI-INFLAMMATORIES

Cromolyn sodium and nedocromil sodium are nonsteroidal, but less potent anti-inflammatory agents. Cromolyn inhibits mediator (histamine) release and degranulation from mast cells. Cromolyn also may possess tachykinin [substance P and neurokinin B(A)] antagonist properties.[58] Nedocromil inhibits release of histamine and PGD$_2$ from mast cells[59] and mobilization of neutrophils and eosinophils.[60] Nedocromil also inhibits

neural impulse propagation in the sensory C fibers of the airway wall, resulting in decreased neuropeptide release.[61] It has a greater protective efficacy than cromolyn sodium against bronchospasm induced by nonallergic stimuli (e.g., cold air, SO$_2$, metabisulfite, and hypertonic saline).[62] Cromolyn sodium (Intal) is available as an MDI inhaler, 800 μg per puff (as well as a dry powder inhaler and a solution for use with a powered nebulizer). Nedocromil sodium (Tilade) is available as an MDI inhaler delivering 1.75 mg per puff. Nedocromil may be slightly more effective than cromolyn.[63] Nedocromil (two puffs qid) is approximately equivalent to beclomethasone (two puffs qid). Because both nedocromil and cromolyn have very favorable side-effect profiles and no HPA axis suppression, they should be considered for patients with mild to moderate persistent asthma. No studies of the effectiveness of higher doses are available. If asthma control has been achieved, a reduction in the frequency of dosing from qid to tid or bid may be attempted several weeks after initiation of therapy. Prophylactic dosing with cromolyn or nedocromil is also useful for prevention of symptoms induced by exercise or trigger exposure; inhaled β_2 agonists, however, are more effective for the prevention of exercise-induced bronchospasm. Concomitant therapy with nedocromil and inhaled corticosteroids may permit reduction in the dose of inhaled corticosteroids in patients requiring high doses of the latter.[64] Nedocromil and cromolyn are generally well tolerated but occasionally associated with gastrointestinal symptoms (nausea, vomiting, dyspepsia, or abdominal pain) more often than placebo. Unpleasant taste, throat irritation, or dryness may also result in discontinuation or poor compliance. Intal (cromolyn) infrequently causes reflex bronchospasm, nasal congestion, cough, or laryngeal edema.

LONG-ACTING INHALED AND ORAL BRONCHODILATORS

Ultra-long-acting bronchodilators, such as salmeterol xinafoate (Serevent) (an ultra-long-acting inhaled β_2 agonist with a 12-h duration of bronchodilation), controlled-release oral albuterol (Proventil Repetabs, Volmax), and sustained-release theophylline all relieve bronchospasm for extended periods of time. Their role in the chronic therapy of asthma is unclear. In mild disease they may mask increasing symptoms that would be more appropriately treated with inhaled anti-inflammatory agents. In poorly controlled moderate or severe disease, they may lull the patient and physician into acceptance of less than optimal anti-inflammatory therapy. Nonetheless, around-the-clock bronchodilator therapy may be required in addition to relatively high or maximal doses of inhaled corticosteroids (with or without nedocromil) for adequate control of symptoms in moderate to severe asthmatics. Ultra-long-acting bronchodilators (sustained release theophylline or twice-daily salmeterol inhaler) provide more consistent around-the-clock bronchodilation than regularly scheduled (qid or q4 h) short-acting β_2 agonists, such as albuterol, and may be more effective in preventing nocturnal asthma symptoms.[65,66] Salmeterol also possesses a long duration ($\geq$8 h) of protective efficacy against exercise-induced bronchospasm (EIB). In some physically active young patients with mild asthma who frequently experience EIB, salmeterol taken in the morning may provide superior EIB prophylaxis than repeated doses of a short-acting β_2 agonist prior to each period of exercise.

TABLE 38-13 Comparison of Response to Doubling of Inhaled Steroid Dose versus Addition of Salmeterol[67]

	420 μg bid	420 μg bid	840 μg bid
Beclomethasone	420 μg bid	420 μg bid	840 μg bid
Salmeterol	42 μg bid	84 μg bid	None
Morning PEF Mean change % predicted	10	10	3
Evening PEF Mean change % predicted	7	6	1
FEV$_1$ Mean change % predicted	7	7	3
PC$_{20}$ or PD$_{20}$ (histamine) Change in doubling dose	0.75	0.58	0.43

NOTE: PC$_{20}$ and PD$_{20}$ represent provocative concentration or dose resulting in a 20 percent drop in FEV$_1$.

Salmeterol, 42 μg bid, has also been shown to improve control of asthma when added to a regimen of high-dose inhaled steroids (beclomethasone 840 μg bid) in patients not controlled in the latter regimen[67] (Table 38-13). Similarly, twice-daily salmeterol, when added to lower doses of beclomethasone (200 μg bid) in patients still symptomatic on the latter inhaled steroid regimen, led to better control of asthma than doubling the dose of inhaled steroids.[68]

METHYLXANTHINES AND PHOSPHODIESTERASE INHIBITORS

With the emphasis on anti-inflammatory drugs for chronic asthma therapy and fast-acting inhaled β_2 agonists for acute treatment, theophylline has been relegated to a minor role in the treatment of asthma. Theophylline does not appear to provide significant anti-inflammatory effects in tolerable pharmacologic doses. Superior bronchodilation is provided by β_2 agonists or anticholinergics without the attendant side effects. In acute asthma exacerbations, the addition of intravenous aminophylline to treatment with an inhaled β_2 agonist and intravenous corticosteroids increases the risk of side effects but does not provide improvement in objective measures of airflow. Adverse effects from theophylline may be seen at *therapeutic* levels (8 to 15 μg/mL), and severe side effects are common at higher levels. Adverse effects include nausea, vomiting, dyspepsia and gastroesophageal reflux, diarrhea, intestinal bleeding, aspiration, tachycardia, insomnia, headaches, irritability, life-threatening arrhythmias, seizures, cardiac arrest, and death. Inter- and intraindividual variations in metabolism and absorption of theophylline are complicated by interactions with common drugs. Clearance is increased by phenobarbital, phenytoin, intravenous β agonists (albuterol, isoproterenol), furosemide, and tobacco cigarette or marijuana smoking, thus requiring higher doses of theophylline for efficacy. Clearance is reduced with erythromycin, quinolones, isoniazid, cimetidine, calcium channel blockers, allopurinol, oral contraceptives, caffeine, influenza vaccine, liver disease, congestive heart failure, fever, and pregnancy, thereby increasing the risk of theophylline toxicity. The narrow therapeutic window necessitates careful monitoring, including serum theophylline levels. If used at all, theophylline must result in objective evidence of benefit beyond that achieved with primary lines of treatment in an individual patient.

Increases in intracellular cyclic adenosine monophosphate (cAMP) result in airways smooth muscle relaxation and bron-

chodilation. Stimulation of β_2 receptors results in increased synthesis of cAMP by stimulating adenylyl cyclase. Higher levels can also be maintained by preventing breakdown of cAMP by inhibition of cyclic nucleotide phosphodiesterases (PDE). PDE III and PDE IV inhibitors provide the greatest airway smooth muscle relaxation in humans.[69] Relaxation is also seen with nonselective PDE inhibitors, such as theophylline. The clinical efficacy of theophylline is disproportionately greater than the relatively small bronchodilator effect alone.

Phosphodiesterases are also present in immune-effector cells.[70] The combination of PDE III and PDE IV inhibition in vitro results in decreased lymphocyte proliferation and decreased release of TNF α from macrophages. The combination of a PDE IV inhibitor (decreased breakdown of cAMP) and a β_2 agonist (increased production) in vitro results in inhibition of PAF-induced chemotaxis for eosinophils and inhibition of C5a-stimulated degranulation of eosinophils. PDE III inhibition may result in unwanted cardiovascular side effects. Selective PDE IV inhibitors may provide both bronchodilation and anti-inflammatory properties that are desirable for the treatment of asthma. As a relatively weak nonselective PDE inhibitor, theophylline also provides bronchodilation and anti-inflammatory properties but is limited by cardiovascular and other side effects. A number of selective PDE IV or semiselective PDE III/IV inhibitors are under investigation in oral and inhaled form.

LEUKOTRIENE ANTAGONISTS

Leukotriene modifiers may be considered as alternative therapy to low doses of inhaled anti-inflammatory medications in mild persistent asthma in patients $\geq$ 12 years of age. Further clinical experience and research are needed to help establish their role in asthma therapy.

Zafirlukast is a leukotriene (LTD$_4$) receptor antagonist that is a selective competitive inhibitor of LTD$_4$ and LTE$_4$. It blocks the effects of sulfidopeptide leukotrienes, thereby inhibiting airway constriction, vascular permeability, vasodilation, mucous hypersecretion, mucosal edema, and reduced mucociliary clearance. No specific adverse effects have been noted to date, although there is a possibility of rare hypersensitivity or idiosyncratic reactions. High plasma concentrations may develop in patients with impaired metabolism due to liver disease. Zafirlukast is taken twice a day at least 1 h before or 2 h after meals, as food decreases bioavailability. It inhibits metabolism of warfarin and increases prothrombin time. It

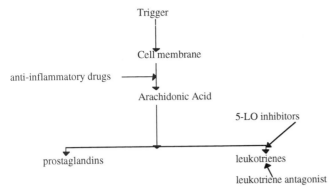

FIGURE 38-3 Inflammatory targets for asthma anti-inflammatory agents.

is a competitive inhibitor of the CYP2CP hepatic microsomal isozymes, although it does not affect elimination of drugs metabolized by these enzymes.

In the lipoxygenase pathway, leukotrienes are released into the tissues through the action of 5-lipoxygenase (5-LO) (Fig. 38-3). Blocking 5-LO prevents metabolism of arachidonic acid to leukotrienes. Zileuton is administered four times a day. Recent studies have shown that the dosage can be adjusted after 2 to 3 weeks of therapy and may be effective in twice-a-day dosage with selected patients. Elevation of liver enzymes has been reported, as has reversible hepatitis and hyperbilirubinemia. Zileuton can inhibit the metabolism of terfenadine, warfarin, and theophylline. Hepatic enzymes (ALT) should be monitored.

5-Lipoxygenase activating protein (FLAP) antagonists are currently in clinical development. FLAP antagonists inhibit leukotriene formation by binding tightly to FLAP.

IMMUNOTHERAPY

In contrast to its efficacy in allergic rhinitis, the role of immunotherapy in asthma is unclear. In carefully selected cases, a few very specific, well-defined antigens (grass pollen, housedust mite, *Alternaria*) may provide antigen-specific reduction in sensitivity. This mild benefit must be weighed against the potential for systemic reactions (5 to 30 percent), including anaphylaxis, and the cost and inconvenience of weekly physician visits.[71,72]

QUICK RELIEVERS

INHALED SHORT-ACTING β AGONISTS

The major role of bronchodilators is for the temporary relief of symptoms, primarily due to bronchoconstriction. Regularly scheduled, around-the-clock use of short-acting or long-acting bronchodilators may mask the severity of asthma resulting in undertreatment of the underlying inflammation.

Short-acting selective β_2 agonists are ideal for acute control of bronchospasm and prevention of EIB. Such agents include albuterol sulfate (Proventil, Ventolin), terbutaline sulfate (Brethaire), metaproterenol sulfate (Alupent), bitolterol mesylate (Tornalate), and pirbuterol acetate (Maxair), all available as MDIs. For mild symptoms, two puffs prn should be sufficient. Frequent use indicates a more significant exacerbation or poor chronic control. When used in higher doses, all "selective" β_2 agonists exhibit some β_1-agonist effects, most

often manifested by tachycardia, in addition to tremor and/or anxiety (both β_2-agonist effects). Less selective β agonists [epinephrine bitartrate (Primatene), isoproterenol hydrochloride (Isuprel), isoetharine mesylate (Bronkometer)] may cause a greater degree of cardiac side effects. In large doses, inhaled β_2 agonists may result in a slight lowering of serum potassium.

INHALED ANTICHOLINERGICS

Inhaled ipratropium bromide (Atrovent) is a second-line choice for acute bronchodilator therapy in asthmatics who are intolerant of side effects associated with β_2 agonists. The onset of action is somewhat slower than that of β_2 agonists, with a peak response in 20 to 30 min and 50 percent of maximal response in 3 to 4 min. The quaternary ammonium structure results in poor absorption and almost no systemic atropine-like effects. It is unclear if the maximal response achieved after a high dose of either a β_2 agonist or ipratropium or conventional doses of the combination of the two is greater. In general, however, two puffs of either a β_2 agonist or ipratropium gives a submaximal response, and further improvement may be seen with an additional dose of either the same drug or the other drug. Ipratropium may produce dry mouth and a bad taste. A closed-mouth technique is recommended for the MDI to prevent the spray from contacting the eyes, causing temporary blurring of vision.

INTERMITTENT ORAL CORTICOSTEROIDS

Oral corticosteroid therapy can be divided into two types, "burst" and chronic. Bursts of 7 to 14 days are appropriate for treatment of acute exacerbations and poorly controlled chronic asthma either at the initiation of therapy or when response to maintenance inhaled anti-inflammatory therapy is inadequate. Little residual effect on the HPA axis occurs after bursts, and tapering is not necessary to prevent adrenal insufficiency. During a burst, however, it may be useful to taper the corticosteroid dose to evaluate the effect of withdrawal on the patient's asthma. Gradual withdrawal allows early detection of relapse of asthma symptoms or objective declines in airflow without catastrophic exacerbations. An example of a burst is: prednisone in the morning 60 mg on days 1 to 3, 50 mg on day 4, 40 mg on day 5, 30 mg on day 6, 20 mg on day 7, 10 mg on day 8, and stop (dispense 33 tablets, 10 mg each). Divided doses (two-thirds in the morning and one-third in the afternoon) may also be used with daily doses greater than 30 mg. Prepackaged tapering doses of methylprednisolone decreasing by 4 mg/day from 24 mg are also available (Medrol Dosepak). In general, the requirement for a prednisone burst necessitates a temporary or long-standing increase of the patient's inhaled anti-inflammatory regimen.

BURSTS OF INHALED CORTICOSTEROIDS

Theoretically, delivering larger dose of inhaled corticosteroids directly to the lung during an exacerbation would be a useful adjunct to the more immediately acting bronchodilators and preferable to oral corticosteroids. There are no studies available to support this approach and no information on the dose which might be effective. Certainly worsening general control of asthma is often treated with an increase of inhaled corticosteroids in addition to a temporary increase in bronchodilators and a review for causes of worsening.

At present, inhaled corticosteroids cannot be considered a replacement for oral corticosteroids in severe exacerbations. However, inhaled corticosteroids should be resumed or begun before completion of an oral corticosteroid taper.

MEDICATIONS TO REDUCE ORAL CORTICOSTEROID DEPENDENCE

Combinations of long-term-control medications are used frequently in patients with severe persistent asthma. The first step to reduce oral corticosteroid dependence is to increase doses of inhaled corticosteroids. This may be accomplished by more puffs per day, more potent preparations, or both. Compliance and inhaler technique are also critical factors. The addition of long-acting inhaled bronchodilators to inhaled corticosteroids has been shown to improve symptom control. By extension, this combination may also allow a decrease in oral corticosteroid dose. The addition of inhaled nonsteroidal anti-inflammatory medication (cromolyn, nedocromil) is frequently tried but not proved to reduce oral steroid dose. In a subset of individuals, the addition of antileukotriene drugs may be beneficial in a failing regimen of high-dose inhaled steroids.

The goal of most experimental anti-inflammatory agents is to reduce dependence on oral corticosteroids, particularly in patients requiring treatment with high doses of oral prednisone (greater than 10 mg/day or 20 mg every other day) and maximal doses of inhaled corticosteroids. Troleandomycin (TAO), methotrexate, gold salts, and cyclosporin A have all been studied.[73] Frequent monitoring and intensive intervention, especially with inhaled corticosteroids, are often effective in reducing the dose of oral corticosteroids as evidenced by the marked response to placebo in studies of alternative anti-inflammatory agents. Experimental anti-inflammatory agents currently can be recommended only in rare cases after exhaustive attempts at reduction of oral corticosteroids using inhaled corticosteroids in maximal doses and other conventional therapies.

TROLEANDOMYCIN

TAO, a macrolide antibiotic, prolongs methylprednisolone elimination. Although the dose of methylprednisolone may be reduced, the corticosteroid-associated side effects are not attenuated.[74] A few open-label studies, however, have shown that some TAO-responsive patients subsequently may achieve acceptable control of asthma symptoms with relatively low doses of alternate-day methylprednisolone and resolution of cushingoid features,[75] although a recent double-blind placebo-controlled study failed to show any benefit.[74]

METHOTREXATE

Methotrexate, a folic acid analog, inhibits thymidylate synthesis resulting in an antiproliferative effect. It appears to inhibit interleukin-1 production, histamine release from basophils, and neutrophil chemotaxis by C5a and leukotriene B_4. Recent studies have demonstrated no significant difference between methotrexate and placebo in reducing oral corticosteroid dose.[76,77] It is possible, however, that a very small subset of patients respond to methotrexate.[75] Mild side effects include nausea, diarrhea, headache, rash, and elevated liver enzymes (up to 40 percent of patients). Severe side effects include liver fibrosis (up to 5 percent), methotrexate

pneumonitis, or fibrosis (3 to 5 percent) and opportunistic infections.

GOLD SALTS

Gold salts appear to inhibit release of histamine and leukotriene C_4 from mast cells and basophils, as well as having a range of other immunosuppressive effects. Studies are plagued by withdrawals due to side effects, but the remaining patients often show a slight reduction in corticosteroid use.[78-80] Side effects are common (20 to 37 percent) and include proteinuria, dermatitis, stomatitis, nausea, and diarrhea.

CYCLOSPORIN A

Cyclosporin A prevents mast cell degranulation and inhibits transcription of interleukins-2, -3, -4, and -5 and T-cell activation. The addition of cyclosporin A to the regimen of steroid-dependent asthma appears to improve PEF and FEV_1 and reduce exacerbations compared with placebo.[81] It has not been well studied in terms of steroid-sparing effect, however. Side effects include nephrotoxicity, hypertrichosis, paresthesias, headaches, hypertension, and herpes zoster.

ALTERNATIVE TREATMENT

Alternative medications are often sought by patients with side effects or concerns about side effects from pharmacologic therapy or those whose pharmacologic therapy is failing to control their asthma. Many of the current pharmacologic drugs are distant derivatives of herbal remedies. Albuterol is chemically related to ephedrine derived from ephedra bush (ma huang). Ipratropium has cholinergic properties similar to *Datura stramonium* (d'hatura). Cromolyn is related to a derivative of *Ammi visnga* (khella). Theophylline is closely related to caffeine. The active ingredient in marijuana, tetrahydrocannabinol (THC), is also a bronchodilator.[82] Corticosteroids are easily prepared from animal sources. Perhaps the greatest difficulties with "herbal" medications are the uncontrolled dose, poor delivery systems, and frequent addition of other unknown materials. Delivered orally, high doses are required for pulmonary effects, and this often results in undesirable systemic side effects. Smoked preparations deliver the medication directly to the lungs but also deliver the products of combustion which, similar to tobacco, may increase inflammation in the airways. Acupuncture, while providing beneficial relaxation effects and some "placebo effect," is not better than needles placed at control sites.[83]

Stepped Therapy

Initiation of therapy must be individualized depending on severity (Table 38-14). After treatment has begun at a level appropriate for the patient's severity, stepwise increases or decreases in therapy may be indicated. The presence of signs, symptoms, or abnormalities of objective measures of lung function (PEF, PEF variability, or spirometry) may signal a need to initiate or increase anti-inflammatory therapy. Good clinical response and normal or near-normal objective measurements of lung function may allow reductions in anti-inflammatory therapy. In patients with moderate to severe asthma, treatment appropriate for an acute exacerbation followed by aggressive initial maintenance therapy and gradual

TABLE 38-14 Stepped Therapy of Asthma[a]

	Severity	Controller	Reliever
4c	Severe Persistent	Experimental anti-inflammatory agents	Short-acting inhaled β_2 agonists as needed for symptoms[c]
4b	Severe Persistent	Addition of daily or alternate-day oral corticosteroids	Short-acting inhaled β_2 agonists as needed for symptoms[c]
4a	Severe Persistent	Inhaled corticosteroids 6–10 puffs[b] qid or more ("high" dose) and long-acting bronchodilator (long-acting inhaled or oral β_2 agonists or sustained-release theophylline)	Short-acting inhaled β_2 agonists as needed for symptoms[c]
Consider Referral to a Specialist			
3	Moderate Persistent	Inhaled corticosteroids 8–20 puffs[b] bid or 4–10 puffs[b] qid ("intermediate" to "high" dose) and long-acting bronchodilator (long-acting inhaled or oral β_2 agonists or sustained-release theophylline)	Short-acting inhaled β_2 agonists as needed for symptoms but fewer than 3–4 times in one day
2b	Mild Persistent	Inhaled corticosteroids 5–8 puffs[b] bid or inhaled corticosteroids 5 puffs[b] bid and long-acting bronchodilator (long-acting inhaled or oral β_2 agonists or sustained-release theophylline)	Short-acting inhaled β_2 agonists as needed for symptoms but fewer than 3–4 times in one day
2a	Mild Persistent	Inhaled corticosteroids 2–5 puffs[b] bid ("low" dose) or cromolyn/nedocromil 2 puffs qid or sustained-release theophylline	Short-acting inhaled β_2 agonists as needed for symptoms but fewer than 3–4 times in one day.
1	Intermittent	None needed	Short-acting inhaled β_2 agonists as needed for symptoms but less than once a week; inhaled β_2 agonists or cromolyn before exercise or anticipated exposure to triggers.

[a] As asthma increases in severity, patients proceed up the above steps from 1 to 4. With improvement, decreases in therapy may be possible and should be attempted on a regular basis (3 months).

[b] Doses of inhaled corticosteroids are in terms of puffs of beclomethasone, 42 μg per puff. Equivalent doses for other corticosteroid preparations can be found in Fig. 38-2.

[c] Patients with severe asthma may require around-the-clock maintenance bronchodilators to control symptoms, preferably either a sustained-release oral bronchodilator (theophylline or albuterol) or an ultra-long-acting inhaled bronchodilator (salmeterol).

increments or reductions in therapy as tolerated are appropriate. In milder cases, initial low-dose maintenance therapy may be instituted initially, followed by gradual stepwise increases or decrements as appropriate. Each patient should have rescue medication (short-acting selective β_2 agonist) available at all times for treatment of acute symptoms or exacerbations. Patients may also use a short-acting β_2 agonist (or cromolyn or nedocromil) as prophylaxis prior to exercise or anticipated exposure to asthma triggers. In selected cases of severe asthma, around-the-clock bronchodilators (short- or preferably long-acting oral or inhaled β_2 agonists, or sustained-release theophylline) may be necessary to control frequently recurrent symptoms, especially nocturnal symptoms, that persist in spite of high-dose or maximal anti-inflammatory therapy. Patients should always have available medications for treatment of acute exacerbations, usually a short-acting β_2 agonist (which may be used at frequent intervals, if necessary, during the exacerbation) and oral prednisone. Asthma in adults will often continue to be present to a greater or lesser extent for life. Constant vigilance is required for both recognition of deterioration in the level of control of asthma and opportunities for reducing pharmacologic therapy when asthma is well controlled.

Development of an Asthma Action Plan

PATIENT UNDERSTANDING

When developing the asthma action plan, the physician should consider the patient's level of understanding and capability of adjusting medication therapy according to symptoms or PEF monitoring. Additional relevant factors that need to be considered include knowledge level, belief in the chronic nature of asthma and in the ability of medications to control it, and economic, intellectual, and emotional ability to cope with asthma plus a plan of care.

CHRONIC THERAPY

Management of chronic asthma ideally is by the patient. However, if the patient does not understand or have an action plan, or cannot follow it, the physician must work with the patient to find out what the obstacles are. Patients should know (1) their symptoms, (2) what each medication does, (3) how to take it, and (4) what to do in an acute attack or with changes in symptoms. Some patients know their symptoms very well and are able to manage their asthma with medication therapy alone. Others may benefit from peak flow monitoring to identify changes that may necessitate alterations in therapy. Education is the key, but also knowing what the patient is able to learn and do is essential.

Compliance is an issue to identify problems with self-management. Patients who do not follow the prescribed medication therapy, use inhalers incorrectly, or fail to implement environmental controls may have various issues that need to be addressed. Young adults may not want friends and coworkers to know that they have asthma, since it may be viewed as a weakness, and therefore will not take the medications consistently, nor have rescue medication available. Pa-

TABLE 38-15 Goals for Evaluation and Treatment of Acute Exacerbations

Assess severity of exacerbation.
Relieve symptoms.
Restore lung function.
Prevent recurrence.

TABLE 38-16 Patient Criteria for Emergency Department Evaluation and Treatment

Rapid onset with poor response to initial therapy (see Table 38-18)
Previous history of severe attacks
Peak expiratory flow < 50%
Lack of response to initial therapy

tients who are working may not want coworkers and especially employers to know, since it may impact their jobs or health insurance. Socially, asthma is sometimes viewed as an excuse, and patients are treated in a negative manner. Pointing out that Olympic athletes have asthma and that it is against the law to discriminate against someone for health reasons may reduce their concerns. Support groups may also be useful in these situations, but patients need to be matched to support groups that are similar to their needs. Some groups are for working adults, others for adults with children with asthma, and still others are primarily made up of older adults who have retired.

Patients may not understand what is being taught if it is not at their comprehension level. Asking them to repeat the concepts discussed will help to determine if they truly understand. Patients with physical handicaps such as blindness, deafness, or arthritis present special challenges in teaching. Blind patients can be taught using marked inhalers to identify rescue versus controlling medication. Marking can be done by etching into the inhaler container or placing raised letters on the inhalers. Deaf patients should be provided with written literature, and may need to have a sign language interpreter to help discuss physiologic concepts. Patients who are unable to activate the inhaler owing to incoordination or arthritis may benefit from the Autohaler developed by 3M Pharmaceuticals for their rescue medication. Nebulized medications may be an alternative as well, though cleanliness of the nebulizer is then important.

It is common to provide written materials to patients for education, yet few patients are tested for ability to read. It is a sensitive area and may be difficult to determine, but in cases of continuing noncompliance, illiteracy may be the key. Asking the patient to read portions or find particular information in the educational materials may help to identify whether someone is unable to read. Excuses such as left reading glasses at home or need bifocals may alert the physician that the patient cannot read.

If physical and emotional issues have been eliminated as a cause for noncompliance, other alternatives may help patients to adhere to the medication regimen. Several devices have been developed that help to monitor patient use of inhalers. These include simple devices that measure date, time, and number of activations with one inhaler (e.g., Doser) to more complicated devices that also measure peak flow measurements before and after, measure proper inhaler technique, and can monitor more than one device (e.g., SmartMist by Aradigm). The devices range in price but are expensive and are not currently paid for by insurance. However, if use of the devices improves compliance, thereby decreasing exacerbations and use of medical resources, they may be a cost-effective benefit.

TREATMENT OF ACUTE EXACERBATIONS

Acute exacerbations represent either failure of chronic therapy, the impact of intercurrent viral upper respiratory tract infections, or unexpected exposure to patient-specific triggers of asthma (Table 38-15). Patients must be given clear guidelines (preferably in writing) for both assessment and treatment of acute exacerbations and, in particular, when to seek a higher level of care such as a hospital emergency department (Table 38-16).

ASSESS SEVERITY OF EXACERBATION

Patient guidelines for assessing the severity of exacerbation must be individualized (Table 38-17). The first indication of an exacerbation is usually either an increase in symptoms or a decline in PEF below the patient's normal range. The zone system (see Table 38-10) uses PEF to provide objective measurement of exacerbation severity. Exacerbations identified earlier, in the yellow range, are more easily treated. Many exacerbations may be treated at home by the well-instructed patient alone or in consultation with a physician.

TABLE 38-17 Assess the Severity of the Exacerbation

Severe exacerbations
  Characterized by rapid onset, lack of response to initial therapy and previous history of severe attacks
  Breathlessness at rest, hunching forward, speaking only words, agitation or confusion
  Respiratory rate > 30, pulse > 120 or bradycardia, loud wheezes or absent breath sounds due to severely reduced flow rates insufficient to generate wheezing sounds, accessory muscle use, respiratory muscle fatigue, paradoxical thoracoabdominal movement, pulsus paradoxus > 25 mmHg, cyanosis, hypoxemia (Sa_{O_2} < 90%), PEF after initial bronchodilators < 60% predicted or personal best, or < 100 L/min
Moderate exacerbations
  Breathless while talking, prefers sitting, speaking in phrases, agitated
  Respiratory rate increased, pulse 100–120, loud wheezes, accessory muscle use, pulsus paradoxus 10–25 mmHg, mild hypoxemia (Sa_{O_2} 90–95%), PEF 60–80% predicted or personal best after initial bronchodilators
Mild exacerbations
  Breathless while walking, can lie down, speaking in sentences, may be agitated
  Respiratory rate increased, pulse < 100, mild to moderate wheezes or wheezes present only on forced expiration, no accessory muscle use, no abnormal pulsus paradoxus (< 10 mmHg), no hypoxemia (Sa_{O_2} > 95%), PEF > 80% predicted or personal best after initial bronchodilators

TABLE 38-18 Response to Therapy and Appropriate Action

Response	Action
Good response, mild episode	
PEF > 80% of predicted or of personal best	Continue β_2 agonists every 3–4 h for 24 to 48 h
Response sustained for 4 h	
Incomplete response, moderate episode	
PEF 60–80% of predicted or of personal best	Continue β_2 agonists
	Add oral corticosteroid burst
Poor response, severe episode	
PEF < 60% of predicted or of personal best	Immediately repeat β_2 agonists
	Add oral corticosteroid
	Go to emergency department (consider ambulance)

RELIEVE SYMPTOMS (BRONCHOSPASM) AND RESTORE LUNG FUNCTION

Pharmacologic therapy of acute exacerbations is an intensification of chronic bronchodilator and anti-inflammatory therapy. Initial therapy with a short-acting β_2 agonist such as albuterol is directed at rapid relief of bronchospasm. An example is two to four puffs of albuterol every 20 min for three doses. This is followed by regular, around-the-clock use of β_2 agonists every 3 to 6 h for 1 to 2 days or until the episode resolves. The response is inadequate if (1) the initial response is not prompt and sustained for at least 3 h, (2) there is further deterioration in symptoms or PEF, or (3) frequent β_2 agonists are required for longer than 48 h (Table 38-18). The key to resolution of exacerbations is reduction of inflammation. For relatively mild and transient insults, removal of the trigger and the lapse of time may be sufficient if the acute bronchospasm is relieved by β_2 agonists. For mild to moderate attacks or gradual loss of chronic control, a temporary or long-term increase in inhaled corticosteroids may be adequate. However, many moderate to severe exacerbations are best treated initially with a short course ("burst") of oral prednisone. Failure of symptoms and PEF to show further improvement 3 to 6 h after oral corticosteroids indicates an inadequate response and consideration should be given to emergency department evaluation.

Early use of oral or parenteral corticosteroids may limit severity and shorten duration of symptoms. Antibiotics are indicated only when bacterial infection is suggested. Avoid theophylline and aminophylline in patients with unknown blood levels. Avoid sedation. Relieve hypoxemia if present.

PREVENT RECURRENCE

Identify the cause of the exacerbation and develop early intervention or avoidance strategies, if possible. Critical to the evaluation and treatment of exacerbations is the prevention of recurrence. It may be possible to avoid newly identified triggers or at least recognize the effects earlier. A review of compliance and inhaler technique is important before increasing anti-inflammatory therapy. Exacerbations without a defined trigger or in which the trigger is mild or unavoidable indicate a need for an increase in (or initiation of) chronic anti-inflammatory therapy.

MONITORING (PEF, SYMPTOMS, BRONCHODILATOR USE)

Peak flow monitoring is used as a tool for ongoing monitoring, not for diagnosing asthma. The measurement is very dependent on effort and technique, and patients need to be instructed on its use. If continuing monitoring is done, review of technique at each office visit should be done. Peak flow monitoring can be used for ongoing monitoring, short-term management, and management of exacerbations though an action plan.

Peak flow monitoring can be very useful to identify changes in lung pathology prior to occurrence of symptoms. However, the response is variable. All patients should be given a peak flow meter and taught how to use it and how to monitor their symptoms and measurements for several weeks to determine fluctuations in symptoms, response to therapy, and their personal best measurement. Some patients have very sensitive changes in peak flow monitoring with minimal changes in symptoms, then develop sudden severe symptoms. These patients may benefit from daily monitoring. Others have severe symptoms with minimal changes in peak flow measurements. These patients may not find peak flow monitoring useful. Without monitoring for a period of time, however, each patient's response is unknown.

The NAEPP2 guidelines suggest that peak flow monitoring should be used in patients with moderate-to-severe asthma. It can be used for monitoring during exacerbations to determine the severity and guide therapy. It is also recommended for long-term daily monitoring to detect early changes that may need therapy and to evaluate the response to those changes, assess the severity of air flow obstruction in those patients who are unable to detect changes readily, and provide an objective measurement of impairment for the clinician.

Most patients are amenable to measuring peak flows twice a day, in the morning and afternoon, preferably before medications. The measurements can be either before or after medication, but should be consistently done one way. Peak flow monitoring can also be used to identify responsiveness to environmental or occupational irritants or allergens. This may necessitate measuring several times throughout the day. Measurement of peak flows both before and after bronchodilator (quick-relief) use may help to identify responsiveness of the airways to relief from exposure to allergens. Patients who are stable with moderate asthma may need only to measure peak flows once a day in the morning before taking a bronchodilator to detect changes.

The first goal of peak flow monitoring is to identify the personal best measurement for each patient. This is measured against the predicted measurement to determine the degree of difference and helps identify how severe the airflow obstruction is. A course of oral steroids may be necessary to determine the personal best, especially if optimal treatment has not been in effect or if the patient has been noncompliant. The personal best measurement needs to be reevaluated periodically to monitor the progress of the disease and whether changes in the action plan should be made. Extremely high measurements that do not fit the clinical picture, or an outlier measurement, may be due to incorrect techniques such as spitting or coughing into the meter. Predicted values are based on height, age, and sex. African Americans usually have smaller thoracic diameters and shorter trunks for a given height and, therefore, have lower predicted values. The normal ranges for other minorities such as Hispanics, Asians, and Native Americans have been poorly studied but tend to lie between Caucasian and African-American values. Therefore, the best method of determining the goal for peak flow monitoring is to determine the patient's personal best value.

A three-color system has been developed to help patients self-manage an action plan. The system is based on the stoplight color scheme: green, yellow, and red. Green is 80 percent or greater of the predicted peak flow (or personal best if that is significantly different); yellow is 50 to 80 percent; and red is less than 50 percent of predicted. The green zone indicates that airflow is within normal and the patient should continue taking medications as usual (good control). The yellow zone indicates that airflow has diminished, either from infectious sources, exposure to irritants or allergens, or lack of compliance (caution). Short-acting bronchodilators should be used to increase the peak flow measurement. If the use of the bronchodilators does not improve the measurement and bring it back to the green zone, communication with the physician should occur to determine if additional medications or dosages should be provided. The red zone indicates a medical emergency (medical alert). Quick-relief bronchodilators should be taken immediately, and the physician should be called or the patient should go directly to the emergency room.

There are a variety of devices available that range from very small and simple to large and more cumbersome. Meters should meet the American Thoracic Society recommendations for monitoring devices.[84] Devices should be as small as possible to encourage use and portability. Peak flow meters which electronically record the date, time, and value of each maneuver are also available [AirWatch, which is downloaded over the telephone (Enact 800-267-9452), and SmartMist, which combines a PEF meter and breath-activated delivery system (Aradigm 510-783-0100)]. Newer devices also have the three-color system incorporated into the scale, which is important for identifying when the action plan should be used. Patients should use the same peak flow meter consistently and bring it with them to the office visit. There may be some variability between peak flow meters of different brands, but measurements should be consistent with the same meter and between meters of the different brands. If patients are given a new brand of peak flow meter, they should reestablish their personal best measurement with the new meter. The action plan may also need to be modified.

TABLE 38-19 Disorders Mimicking Asthma

Laryngeal dysfunction (vocal cord adductor dystonia)
Mechanical upper airway obstruction
Congestive heart failure ("cardiac" asthma)
Pulmonary embolism
Cigarette-related COPD with hyperreactive airways
Pulmonary infiltrates with eosinophilia (PIE)
Viral bronchiolitis or *Mycoplasma* infection

Complicating Factors

Many complicating factors may make asthma difficult or impossible to control. Compliance with the patient's asthma management plan and MDI technique must be reviewed meticulously in any patient with suboptimally controlled asthma or exacerbation. Inhaler technique greatly affects the delivery of drug to the lung and, therefore, the efficacy of therapy. Simply asking the patient to demonstrate use of the inhaler provides reinforcement of the importance of technique to the patient and an opportunity to correct any deficiencies. Compliance is a complex interaction between the patient's perceptions of the risks, benefits, and cost (time, convenience, and dollars) of therapy. Understanding the patients' perceptions of risk, benefit, and cost can help improve compliance with the current regimen, guide modifications to improve compliance, or direct educational interventions. Of particular concern are patients whose decrement in lung function greatly exceeds their perceived symptoms.

DIFFERENTIAL DIAGNOSIS

The signs and symptoms of asthma are nonspecific and may be mimicked by a variety of diseases not necessarily responsive to antiasthma medications (Table 38-19).

COEXISTING DISEASE

A number of coexistent diseases including gastroesophageal reflux, rhinitis and sinusitis, allergic bronchopulmonary aspergillosis, and anxiety and panic disorders make asthma more difficult to control. Each patient, at evaluation and at reevaluation following exacerbation, should have consideration given to these possibly complicating factors.

Gastroesophageal reflux may trigger severe bronchospasm and increase airway hyperresponsiveness. Reflux of acidic fluid into the upper esophagus or with microaspiration into the trachea is a common cause of refractory asthma. Patients with significant reflux proved by 24-h esophageal pH probe may not complain of heartburn or other reflux symptoms. Neutralization of the stomach contents by treatment with a histamine H_2 blocker (cimetidine, ranitidine, etc.) or a proton pump inhibitor (omeprazole), with or without a prokinetic agent (cisapride, metoclopramide), removes the insult, but reductions in hyperresponsiveness and improvements in asthma may take up to 6 months.

Rhinitis and particularly sinusitis may also make asthma difficult to control. Recurrent postnasal drip irritates the larynx and trachea and increases airway hyperresponsiveness. Treatment of sinusitis and/or rhinitis may result in dramatic improvements in control of asthma, but seldom eliminates asthma.

Allergic bronchopulmonary aspergillosis is caused by an aggressive immune response to noninvasive growth of *Aspergillus* in the airways. The intense local inflammatory response may result in very severe asthma which requires high doses of oral corticosteroids for even marginal control. Patients typically present with episodes of fever, wheezing, productive cough, minimal hemoptysis, shortness of breath, leukocytosis, and sputum and blood eosinophilia, particularly during the winter months. Patients may expectorate brownish plugs or flecks (56 percent) and, occasionally, bronchial casts. The syndrome is characterized by asthma with (1) proximal bronchiectasis, (2) peripheral blood eosinophilia (>1000/mm^3), (3) markedly elevated serum IgE (>1000 U/mL), (4) transient or fixed pulmonary infiltrates, (5) immediate and intermediate skin reactivity to *Aspergillus* antigen on prick or intradermal testing, and (6) serum precipitating antibodies against *Aspergillus* antigen.

Panic attacks are associated with the subjective sensation of breathlessness—dyspnea.[85] Unfortunately, bronchospasm from asthma may produce emotional distress—anxiety. Many patients with panic disorder will initially present to medical attention for evaluation of dyspnea, and certainly the asthma and panic disorder may coexist. Panic attacks are a discrete period of intense fear or discomfort in which four or more of the following symptoms develop abruptly and reach a peak within 10 min: (1) palpitations, pounding heart or accelerated heart rate; (2) sweating; (3) trembling or shaking; (4) sensation of shortness of breath or smothering; (5) feelings of choking; (6) chest pain or discomfort; (7) nausea or abdominal distress; (8) feeling dizzy, unsteady, lightheaded, or faint; (9) derealization or depersonalization; (10) fear of losing control or going crazy; (11) fear of dying; (12) paresthesias; (13) chills or hot flushes. Patients who meet these criteria should be referred for psychiatric evaluation in addition to continuing treatment of asthma if appropriate. Patients who do not meet the criteria for panic attacks often benefit from breathing relaxation techniques, and some require pharmacologic intervention for anxiety.

SURGERY

It is preferable to optimize asthma management prior to surgery and general anesthesia. Patients with poor asthma control or experiencing an exacerbation should receive a burst of corticosteroids in an effort to optimize asthma control prior to surgery, if possible. Intubation, anesthesia, and mechanical ventilation may trigger asthma exacerbations. Prophylactic intervention may avoid or minimize complications. Patients with mild asthma may require only routine β_2 agonists prior to, during, and immediately following surgery. Moderate or severe asthmatics may benefit from a very brief oral (or parenteral when NPO) course of corticosteroids, in addition to around-the-clock β_2 agonists. The patient's usual regimen of inhaled corticosteroids should be resumed as the systemic corticosteroids are tapered or discontinued. For patients treated with daily corticosteroids continuously for more than 3 weeks within the past year or with long-term inhaled corticosteroids in high doses (e.g., beclomethasone

≥1500 μg/day or equivalent), stress-dose corticosteroids for possible adrenal suppression are indicated regardless of need for control of asthma.

WOMEN'S ISSUES

Many women report fluctuations in symptoms throughout their menstrual cycle. Little research has been done in this area, although more research findings are beginning to emerge. Action plans should take these fluctuations into account and adjust medications accordingly to prevent exacerbations.

Preparation for pregnancy in patients with asthma should begin well in advance with achievement of good asthma control. In approximately equal proportions of patients, asthma will improve, worsen, or remain unchanged during pregnancy. The same stepped approach used for general asthma care is appropriate for care during pregnancy.[86,87] No therapy has been proved absolutely safe for use during pregnancy. For mild asthma treated with prn β_2 agonists, reassuring clinical experience exists with terbutaline, albuterol, and metaproterenol. For patients requiring anti-inflammatory therapy, use of inhaled beclomethasone or cromolyn is supported by human studies and long experience. Bursts of oral corticosteroids are appropriate as for routine care, and treatment of exacerbations with corticosteroids is preferable to the deleterious physiologic effects of withholding treatment.

Postmenopausal women may need supplements of calcium and vitamin D. Estrogen replacement therapy may be considered for patients on doses of >1000 μg inhaled corticosteroid a day.

GERIATRIC POPULATION

Older patients may have coexisting chronic diseases such as liver disease, diabetes, or congestive heart failure. These chronic diseases may affect drug metabolism, necessitating adjustment in the dosage. Medications taken for these chronic conditions may have interactions with asthma medications or with the disease itself (e.g., propranolol). Asthma medications may aggravate coexisting diseases (e.g., cardiac disease, osteoporosis), and adjustments in the plan may have to be made. At every visit it is imperative that *all* medications are known, not just those taken for asthma. Chronic bronchitis or emphysema may coexist with asthma. A trial of systemic corticosteroids could help determine the extent of benefit and reversibility.

Older patients may have difficulty actuating the metered-dose inhaler; in such patients, use of an automated device (Autohaler) or spacer may facilitate effective delivery of medications to the lung.[88] The elderly frequently find a nebulizer easier to use, although care must be taken that they clean the nebulizer adequately to prevent infection. Review of inhaler technique and correction should be done at each visit. Elderly patients also forget timing of medications and dosage. Compliance is enhanced if therapy is as simple as possible, for example, twice-a-day medication as opposed to three or four times a day, taking medications at the same time instead of spread out through the day, using a schematic to remind when to take the medication, and writing out the prescription for the patient in lay terms.

Older patients are generally more comfortable following

directions than self-managing and therefore may require more support. Giving them a phone number of the nurse or HCP to call for questions may prevent exacerbations since problems can be corrected early. Support groups may be of additional help to provide encouragement and ideas on how to cope with asthma. Family support is essential, and at least one primary member should be educated regarding asthma, symptoms, warning signs, monitoring, and the action plan to support the patient and help prevent exacerbations.

Patient Selection for Rehabilitation

ESTABLISHING A PARTNERSHIP WITH HEALTH CARE PROFESSIONAL

Success in living with and controlling asthma is dependent on an active partnership between patient and the health care provider delivering the asthma care. From the first visit when the diagnosis of asthma is made, goals should be mutually agreed on and worked toward. Understanding asthma, including recognizing that asthma is an inflammatory disease of the airway, expectations of therapy, recognition of the worsening control of asthma, and recognition of the need for seeking urgent help, is of primary importance. Asthma self-management should be taught to each patient who is able to comprehend a self-management program and work with the provider. Cultural beliefs and practices must be incorporated into action plans. The action plan should be provided from the first visit and incorporate a plan of daily management of chronic asthma, as well as providing a written action plan for exacerbations. This is especially important for those patients with moderate to severe asthma or those who have a history of frequent exacerbations. Aspects of a partnership that encourage adherence include: (1) open communication during and between visits, (2) developing individualized learning, (3) individualizing the action plan, (4) reviewing the plan on an ongoing basis and adjusting it as needed, (5) establishing mutual goals, (6) emphasizing outcomes as a measure of success, and (7) encouraging family support and involvement. Successful self-control of asthma is evidenced by control of symptoms, decreased use of quick-relief medications, and improvement in peak expiratory flow monitoring.

ASSESSING READINESS TO LEARN

Prior to instituting an action plan, patients have to be able and willing to manage their asthma in partnership with the health care provider. This ability and willingness can be determined at the first visit during goal setting. Clark and associates proposed a framework for assessing ability for self-regulation.[89] Patients are able to participate in self-management according to the phase of asthma self-regulation in which they are found. Each phase is mutually exclusive, but hierarchical. Patients move from a lower to higher phase with knowledge and confidence in their ability to self-manage (Table 38-20).

PHASE 1

Asthma Unawareness
The patient or family may have some knowledge of asthma as a disease (including symptoms), but they do not accept the conclusion that they have it as a chronic (recurrent) condition. They may perceive that they wheeze or cough periodically (or their child does), but they do not attribute such symptoms to an inherent physiologic vulnerability with serious health-threatening outcomes if untreated.

Health Beliefs
The patient and/or family does not know about asthma as a serious disease, nor do they see the patient as susceptible to it.

Implications for Teaching
Patients and families are reluctant to return for follow-up visits. They tend not to follow instructions. Teaching should focus on what is immediate and necessary: proper inhaler use, appropriate medications to take, whom to call in an emergency.

PHASE 2

Asthma Acceptance
The patient or family personally accepts asthma as a chronic and serious health-threatening disease but responds to it reactively rather than proactively. They are aware of the patient's wheezing and sleep disturbances, and they keep the patient at home when symptoms become worse. They worry about the health consequences of asthma and restrict the patient's activities to avoid serious outcomes. They seek information about asthma, but they are not aware or convinced of the importance of the preventive treatment of the disease through continuing care by a physician.

TABLE 38-20 Asthma Self-Regulation

	1	2	3	4
Asthma Phase	Unawareness	Acceptance	Compliance	Self-Regulation
Health beliefs	Not serious Not susceptible	Increased costs React to symptoms	Compliant with instructions	Value prevention Self-efficacious
Implications for teaching	Medications Inhaler technique Whom to call	Pathophysiology Medications Technique When to go to school or work	Simple action plan Rescue medications When to call Triggers Home and environmental controls Peak flow monitoring	Peak flow monitoring Asthma peak flow monitoring diary Action plan Manage on own

Health Beliefs

The family accepts that asthma can have serious health consequences and that the patient has this chronic disease, but they see the costs and barriers to obtaining continuing care as high.

Implications for Teaching

Patients and families accept the diagnosis and symptoms. They respond reactively, yet seek information. They are not convinced of the benefits of prevention through a continuing relationship with the physician and may not keep appointments. Teaching should focus on the pathophysiology of asthma, use of medications in addressing pathology, inhaler technique, and when to go to work or school.

PHASE 3

Asthma Compliance

The patient or family seeks to prevent and better control asthma symptoms by following the physician's treatment recommendations. They highly regard the personal attention and concern that the physician devotes to them. Enjoying a compliant relationship with the physician, they are not as likely to seek emergency room treatment for asthma exacerbations, but they are not confident about managing asthma on their own.

Health Beliefs

The benefits of continuing care by a physician are perceived as high, but self-efficacy to self-regulate an asthma care plan is low.

Implications for Teaching

Patients and families are able to follow physician direction for treatment and prevention. Teaching should focus on a simplified action plan that relates use of rescue medications to symptoms, when to call the physician, how to do peak flow monitoring, triggers or allergies, immunotherapy, and allergy-proofing the home.

PHASE 4

Asthma Self-Regulation

The patient or family seeks to develop the underlying skills to implement a flexible medical plan to prevent and manage asthma symptoms. To accomplish this goal, they learn how to observe, evaluate, and react to the asthma symptoms on a daily basis. The physician and the patient (or parent) consult together to work out an adaptable treatment plan that is tailored to the unique living conditions and personal reactions that occur. Patient or family may discuss how to evaluate asthma triggers, make decisions about medicine use, and manage or prevent breathing problems. The patient or parent will gradually acquire a sense of self-efficacy in implementing the plan and will feel open to contacting the physician when modifications are required.

Health Beliefs

The benefits of preventive and managed asthma care are viewed as high, and self-efficacy to follow systematic personal plan is high. These plans cue the enactment of self-regulatory activities.

Implications for Teaching

Patients and families are able to manage their asthma and self-regulate their treatments. Teaching should focus on using the three-color system (see Table 38-10) and asthma diary with peak flow monitoring and medications to prevent and manage asthma symptoms (Fig. 38-4).

Some cultures and elderly patients prefer to allow the physician to make decisions regarding management of their disease. These patients may do well at stage 3, but are not able to perform the critical thinking necessary to progress to stage 4. Each patient and family is different and should be taught at their own level.

LEARNING THEORIES

Education needs to be tailored to each patient. Specific issues to be assessed include cultural or ethnic beliefs or practices

FIGURE 38-4 Sample patient asthma diary.

Asthma Diary for:

		Date	11/7		11/8		11/9	
		Time	7A	9P	8A	8P	7A	11P
100%	500							
	450							
80%	400							
	350							
	300							
50%	250							
	200							
Quick relief *albuterol*			II	III	III I	II	I	I
Long-term control *beclomethasone*			4	4	4	4	0	4
Other								
Wheezing			2	5	5	1	1	0
Coughing			0	5	4	1	0	0
Short of breath			0	3	3	1	1	1
Nocturnal awake			-		+		1	
Other								
Triggers			Fred's cat!					
Comments			*itchy eyes*		*doing better at Noon*			
Activities			*Running in AM*				*Running in AM*	

that may interfere with the treatment goals, action plan, or self-management activities. For example, during the Muslim holy days of Ramadan, nothing can be taken by mouth from sunup to sundown. Thus, inhaled medications or other medications are not to be taken. Use of stronger and long-lasting medications that can be taken twice a day before and after sundown would be appropriate. In extreme cases, discussion with the religious leader may allow the patient to obtain dispensation for medication use during the day.

Patients should be queried as to their possible use of alternative therapies that are not considered conventional therapies for asthma. Otherwise, practices by the patient may not be known. Various teas have been promoted as "curing" asthma or other diseases; acupuncture, marijuana, and other herbal remedies are sometimes used. If the alternative therapy is not harmful, it may be incorporated into the daily management. By openly discussing alternative therapies and tolerating them, the clinician promotes open dialogue and the partnership becomes stronger. If the remedy is harmful, validating reasons should be given as to why it should not be used and what an alternative might be.

Whenever possible, the patient's native language should be used to discuss goals and treatment plans. Miscommunication frequently occurs if the patient does not fully understand the language being spoken. Interpreters should be fluent in the languages of both the clinician and patient and preferably in medical terminology as well. Family and friends may not always be appropriate interpreters since the patient may not be willing to discuss sensitive issues in their presence. Thus important information may be missed.

The special needs of the handicapped and elderly need to be recognized. Patients who are blind may not be able to perform peak flow monitoring. Those who have physical limitations from arthritis or neuromuscular disease may not be able to depress the inhaler canister for actuation. Women have smaller hands, and the elderly become weaker and thus may also have more difficulty in actuating the inhaler canister. Nebulized medication or a breath-actuated inhaler may be useful in this group. The elderly may not be able to remember dosage times; thus twice-a-day dosing that is tied to a routine activity such as brushing their teeth may be useful.

PROCESS OF EDUCATION

Patient education should begin at the time of diagnosis and continue throughout every visit with each health care provider. The plan of care established at the first visit must be communicated with all members of the team so that a coordinated and consistent approach is maintained. A partnership requires that open communication is promoted between the patient and providers and that treatment goals for both short- and long-term plans are mutually agreed on (Table 38-21). Open discussion of the plans encourages active participation by the patient, thus enhancing participation and promoting adherence. The patients' personal goals for treatment should be determined by asking how asthma affects lifestyle, what experiences they have had with others with asthma, and what life without asthma would be like for them. These responses help to direct the individual treatment goals. These goals should then be shared with other members of the team, as well as with the family.

TABLE 38-21 General Goals of Therapy

Freedom from severe symptoms day and night, including sleeping through the night
Having the best possible lung function
Ability to participate fully in any activities of choice
Not missing any work or school because of asthma symptoms
Need for fewer or no urgent care visits or hospitalizations for asthma
Use of medications to control asthma with as few side effects as possible
Satisfaction with asthma care

Adherence to a recommended treatment plan is increased when the treatment goals are mutually established and are individualized and when patients feel that the clinician is truly interested in their care and is invested in the outcome. Effective communication is essential to understand the goals of the patient and recognize when changes need to be made. Several techniques promote open communication: reflective listening, showing attentiveness, using open-ended questions to elicit concerns about treatment or goals, and reinforcing effective management skills. Use of open-ended questions is valuable to elicit concerns and issues that may not be expressed in response to "yes" or "no" questions. Sensitive issues such as personal experiences, beliefs, or cultural concerns may not be readily shared without probing questioning and may be a barrier to adherence. Asking about such concerns builds trust and facilitates development of the partnership.

Eliciting information about the perception of disease severity can alert the clinician to barriers that are anxiety-provoking. Patient experiences with asthma can be incapacitating, and the diagnosis may be perceived as a death sentence. Providing factual information such as pulmonary function results, peak flow monitor readings, or other objective measurements may help to alleviate anxiety. The action plan may also provide reassurance that the disease is manageable and is open to revision as the need arises. Involvement of family, close friends, or significant others may be key to effective use of the action plan and adherence with the treatment goals. The patient should be encouraged to share the diagnosis and treatment plan with family and close friends for support and help with actions they are able to help with. Asthma is not caused by stress, but stress may exacerbate symptoms and precipitate an acute attack. Stress, either emotional or social, may interfere with adherence to the treatment plan. Support groups may be useful to provide an outlet for concerns regarding anxiety and stressful situations. Referral to a professional counselor may also be necessary, although patients may resist.

Other issues of adherence to treatment goals include assessing the reasons a patient is not adhering to the plan. A patient who is using over-the-counter medications as the quick-relief medication instead of a prescription medication may not understand the side effects of the over-the-counter preparation (education), insurance will not pay for all the medications and the patient cannot afford them all (free samples, low-cost or free medication program with pharmaceutical company), or the patient finishes the prescription drugs before the next scheduled visit to the clinician (review medication treatment to adjust long-term therapy and thus reduce

TABLE 38-22 Breathing Exercise

Relax. Let shoulders and neck droop.
Breathe slowly in through nose.
Purse lips in whistling position and blow out slowly and evenly.
 Try to prolong expiration as much as possible.
Relax. Repeat the maneuver until shortness of breath resolves. If
 dizziness results, rest for a few breaths.

TABLE 38-23 Relaxation Breathing

Sit. Lean forward with a straight back and rest arms on knees.
Breathe slowly in through the nose.
Blow the air out slowly through the mouth. Keep chest still.

need for quick-relief medication). The action plan should be simple, flexible, and fit into the patient's daily lifestyle.

Many educational tools are available. These include (1) web pages on the Internet; (2) videotapes on asthma, triggers, medications, and inhaler technique; (3) brochures from various sources; (4) books targeted to lay persons; and (5) interactive computer games. It is best to have a variety of products available since patients learn in different ways—auditory, visual, and tactile. Pharmaceutical and medical device companies provide educational materials, although these may be useful primarily for the company's own particular product. Skills such as inhaler technique and peak flow monitoring should be demonstrated by the HCP and time then allowed for return demonstration until the technique is performed correctly.

Components of Rehabilitation

Most patients with asthma fall into the mild classification of severity. These patients go to school or work and maintain active lives between exacerbations. The focus of rehabilitation for this population is education with an emphasis on the disease, medications, and symptom management and when to contact the physician or go to the emergency department. This can be accomplished in a few visits. Patients with moderate to severe asthma may benefit, in addition, from exercise training, environmental control measures and avoidance of triggers, peak flow monitoring, and management of exacerbations by using an action plan. This type of program may require 4 to 6 weeks. The difference in time for education between the two groups is also related to the importance patients place on education and their willingness to participate in a program. Those who feel better are less likely to keep appointments or attend classes over several weeks and therefore need the education to be limited to the most essential information provided in the shortest amount of time. Follow-up with these patients may be necessary in short time frames to reinforce information. Studies have shown that it can take up to 6 months for adequate learning to take place. Families are integral to the educational process, since family dynamics play a role in emotional stressors that can exacerbate symptoms. Rehabilitation of the patient with asthma comprises exercise training, patient education, and addressing the psychosocial needs of the patient, as well as aspects of the disease.

EXERCISE TRAINING

The majority of patients with asthma are able to go to work or school and are not thought to be physically deconditioned. However, patients adjust their activity level to avoid shortness of breath and may indeed be deconditioned. Although asthma programs focus primarily on education rather than exercise, patients who are short of breath with minimal exertion should be evaluated by the rehabilitation physical therapist. Exercise prescriptions should be for home equipment or gymnasium centers since most patients are unable to attend a rehabilitation exercise program during the daytime. Older patients with asthma may benefit from participation in a traditional rehabilitation program. Studies on pulmonary rehabilitation programs with asthma patients often mix both chronic obstructive pulmonary disease and asthma patients together and find, at least in the aggregate group, improvement in both objective and subjective assessments. These programs also provide social support that may be missing in the patient's home life.

Exercise is often avoided by patients to prevent exercise-induced bronchospasm. Patients need to be instructed in effective preventive strategies that will permit them to exercise without inducing bronchospasm: do warm-up, take two puffs of quick-relief bronchodilator (e.g., albuterol), wait 10 min, then exercise.

Breathing exercises to "strengthen" respiratory muscles have not been shown to improve breathing. According to subjective reports, however, some exercises help decrease shortness of breath. Pursed-lip breathing has been found to be useful in emphysema and also seems to be useful anecdotally for asthma patients. It is easy to teach and can be included in simple breathing exercises (Table 38-22). Most patients tend to use pursed-lip breathing when dyspnea occurs, but it is also useful for preventing shortness of breath when climbing stairs or doing some other strenuous activity. The technique should be performed for several breaths prior to starting the activity.

Another exercise that may be useful for relieving shortness of breath or anxiety is relaxation breathing (Table 38-23). Breathing in this manner slows respirations and facilitates relaxation to avoid anxiety attacks.

Coughing attacks can be panic-provoking as well as embarrassing. When a patient feels a coughing spasm developing, a controlled coughing technique may be helpful to break the cycle (Table 38-24).

Other exercises that are helpful for controlling breathing and promoting relaxation while providing conditioning exercise are tai chi and yoga. These are especially useful for older

TABLE 38-24 Controlled Coughing[a]

Breathe in by sniffing gently.
Hold breath for a few seconds.
Cough twice, first to loosen the mucus, then to bring it up.
The cough should not be vigorous.
Multiple small coughs also can be used (huffing).
Rest.
Repeat as necessary.

[a] This technique facilitates mucous removal but also slows breathing and breaks the cough cycle.

TABLE 38-25 Sex and Asthma

Plan a date so that the patient is relaxed and not under stress.

Avoid perfumes, lotions, candles, or potpourri that may precipitate an attack.

Take two puffs of the rescue (short-acting) bronchodilator 10 to 15 min prior to initiating foreplay for prevention of symptoms.

Avoid positions that require vigorous activity if the patient has not been physically active.

Avoid areas that are dusty or may place the patient in contact with allergens or triggers (e.g., floor, garden).

---

patients who may not be able to keep up with younger, more vigorous patients or do aerobic activity.

Issues of intimacy or sexual performance may be difficult to elicit. A calm, relaxed, unhurried, and comfortable manner may put the patient at ease to discuss concerns. Some medications may affect desire or performance and possibly could be changed to another product. A common concern is fear of shortness of breath or an asthma attack during foreplay or intercourse (Table 38-25).

EDUCATIONAL COMPONENT

Education is the most important aspect of rehabilitation since all patients need the information, and the goal of asthma management is self-management. Studies of educational programs show such benefits as increased compliance with the plan of care, decreased use of health care resources, decreased frequency of exacerbations, and improved quality of life.[90] However, since these educational programs are of short duration and high intensity, they may not be feasible in a general clinical practice. It is unknown how long these benefits persist after completion of the program. Despite the documented benefits of education, education is generally not reimbursed or is reimbursed poorly by insurance companies. Many health maintenance organizations require asthma education as part of the contract for care but do not pay for it specifically.

Education must be provided at any available opportunity. As previously described, the education will be received by the patient depending on the patient's stage of learning.

Focusing on the patient's needs helps increase relevance and thereby compliance (Table 38-26). At every opportunity, questions should be asked such as: how are things going, what concerns does the patient have, what is the biggest problem the patient has dealing with asthma, what would the patient most like to improve, and what is the aspect of asthma that most impacts the patient's quality of life—

TABLE 38-26 Educational Topics to be Covered

Normal lung anatomy and physiology and alterations caused by asthma

Medications—side effects, interactions

Inhaler technique

Warning signs and symptoms

Triggers and troublemakers, home and environmental controls

Peak flow monitoring

Action plan

When to seek medical help

Stress reduction and relaxation techniques

Prevention

---

sleeping, social life, working, or something else? Awareness of these concerns should guide consideration of possible changes in therapy or the need for further education.

Education can be provided in many settings and formats. Any opportunity for education should be taken, such as checking inhaler technique, reinforcing adherence to the action plan, and ascertaining the appropriateness and accuracy of the patient's knowledge and understanding of asthma and its management.

Group classes are the most cost-effective and efficient but are frequently difficult to arrange at a convenient time for working patients. Groups also facilitate interaction between patients that allows a useful and reassuring exchange of information on how to manage living with asthma. Not all patients like groups or participation in support groups, however.

One-on-one education allows for intensive education and eliciting of problem areas of living with asthma or of implementing the action plan. It is not as cost-effective as group sessions but provides a greater opportunity to correct misunderstandings or incorrect information. Some patients are also more open and confiding in a one-on-one setting.

LUNG ANATOMY AND PHYSIOLOGY, ASTHMA PATHOPHYSIOLOGY

Basic anatomy and physiology of the lungs should be reviewed with the patient and family. Information regarding changes in the lung with asthma should then be discussed. This knowledge underscores the need for medication therapy and the necessity of continuous therapy, regardless of how the patient feels. Pictures and diagrams are the simplest teaching tools, but lung models and videotapes are very effective methods of demonstrating changes in lung pathology. Various teaching tools are available from pharmaceutical companies, although some products are thinly veiled promotional aids. Additional discussion of the causes of asthma is also appropriate at this point to elicit a history of possible coexisting diseases that may make asthma worse. Special situations in asthma may also be addressed, such as seasonal asthma secondary to allergies or other triggers, cough-variant asthma, and exercise-induced asthma.

MEDICATIONS

Education should focus on the reason for each medication and what aspect of asthma it addresses. The importance of the medication in reducing the pathophysiology and symptoms is emphasized. Differentiating between long-term control and quick-relief medications should also be stressed. Suggestions such as leaving long-term bronchodilator therapy (e.g., salmeterol) in the bathroom with the toothbrush may prevent its being available during an exacerbation, leading to inappropriate use. Instructions on frequency of medications, numbers of puffs (activations), and timing of medications should be reviewed verbally and given to the patient in written form. The patient should repeat the instructions since such simple directions as two puffs can be interpreted by patients as two puffs at the same time with the same breath, rather than two separate inhalations.

Inhaler technique is one of the essential teaching aspects. Patients cannot be expected to be able to perform the technique after one demonstration by the health care provider. Elderly patients and those with vision or other physical disability may need repeated demonstrations and return demonstrations over time to correct bad habits. Ideally, inhaler technique should be assessed at each visit with the health care provider. Use of a spacer device helps to reduce the need for precise breath-hand coordination.

Additional teaching items include side effects of medication and how to prevent them, identifying when the inhaler is empty, guidelines for taking medications, use of over-the-counter medications, and cleaning of the MDI nozzle and spacer. The best way to check whether the inhaler is empty is to count doses. Since rescue medications may be difficult to count, dropping the container in water to see if it floats (empty) may be helpful. Shaking the cannister is not sufficient. The patient should be discouraged from using a "priming" puff since it wastes medication.

Information about the patient's use of over-the-counter medications should be elicited, especially use of bronchodilators. Inquiry should also be made as to use of herbal teas or therapies for colds or acute attacks. Since patients will usually not volunteer the information, specific questions should be asked.

At the first visit with the clinician, a written, individualized, daily self-management plan should be developed in collaboration with the patient. The recommended doses and frequencies of daily medications as well as other activities such as trigger avoidance should be included. Linking the recommendations of therapy with treatment goals helps to reinforce previous education and encourage adherence. Reinforcement of the goals at each visit also helps elicit when goals have changed or if treatments are no longer working. Some patients may be more adherent if focused on long-term goals rather than short-term therapy.

INHALER TECHNIQUE

Inhaler techniques include open-mouth, closed-mouth, and spacer. Use of a spacer eliminates the need for precise hand-breath coordination and is the preferred method. Because many patients will not carry a spacer with them for use with rescue medications, open-mouth technique should be taught (except with ipratropium). Closed-mouth technique is the least preferred since most of the dose remains in the mouth, resulting in hoarseness, bad taste, and sore throat. The spacer should be as large as the patient will tolerate.[91] Small, short spacers are ineffective and give a false sense of security. Some pharmaceutical companies provide spacers free of charge, and some insurance companies pay for them. Spacers are recommended by the NAEPP2 guidelines.

WARNING SIGNS AND SYMPTOMS

Symptom identification is a first step in management. Patients experience various symptoms that are precursors to an exacerbation, and many patients do not know their symptoms well enough to manage them. An assignment can be made to have the patient keep track of symptoms for 1 to 2 weeks, as well as tracking severity, to identify those symptoms that may augur an exacerbation. Use of an asthma diary can facilitate the assignment. Once the specific symptoms applicable to the patient are identified, warning signs are then discussed and the patient instructed on when to seek medical care. Symptoms such as difficulty breathing, being unable to walk or talk, hunching over, chest and neck being pulled or sucked in with each breath, or cyanosis are empha-

sized as being dangerous. An action plan can be developed and reviewed periodically that addresses what to do in the event of an exacerbation. Specific danger signs need to be emphasized and written down and their knowledge reinforced at intervals. Many patients will ignore warning signs or try to treat themselves rather than to obtain professional help. Discussion with the patient may help elicit why this occurs, whether cost, or embarrassment, or fear of hospitals are issues. Educational interventions then should be utilized to address each. For example, if cost is an issue, calling the physician or primary care provider for help may prevent an emergency department visit. If fear is an issue, an educational visit to the hospital or emergency department may help—or attending a support group to discuss these issues may alleviate the concern.

Patients should be questioned regarding what they actually do during an acute exacerbation prior to being taught what should be done. This strategy will elicit information on use of over-the-counter medications.

Patients should be encouraged to identify what symptoms are warning signs that asthma is worsening. Some patients are in tune with their bodies and know when changes occur, but others may not identify a change and describe the attack as "coming out of nowhere" or occurring suddenly. Use of an asthma diary listing symptoms may help the patient identify symptoms that are warning signs.

TRIGGERS AND TROUBLEMAKERS, HOME AND ENVIRONMENTAL CONTROLS

Triggers, allergies, and troublemakers also need to be reviewed. If the patient has never had skin testing and the symptoms indicate an allergic source, skin testing with the common environmental allergens should be done. Before instituting expensive changes in the home or removing a beloved pet, a patient must be convinced that there is a need for the change. It is helpful to go through a list of possible troublemakers with the patient since there may be triggers that are not noticed or apparent until brought to the patient's attention.

Home and environmental controls that are inexpensive and easy to implement are the most successful. Items such as covering of mattress and pillows, washing linens in hot water, removing the pet from the bedroom, eliminating cockroaches, and investing in a HEPA filter are usually easy to implement and fairly inexpensive. Removing carpeting involves a big expense and may not be possible if the patient is renting a home or apartment. Several companies have products available for allergy-proofing and provide free books for ordering (Allergy Asthma Technology, Ltd., 1-800-621-5545; Allergy Control Products, 1-800-422-DUST; Allergy Free Inc., 1-800-ALLERGY; National Allergy Supply, Inc., 1-800-522-1448; Veterinary Products Laboratory, 1-602-285-1660). Some products, such as HEPA filters, are available more cheaply at local stores. *Asthma Resources Directory* from the American Allergy Association ($29.95) and the National Asthma and Allergy Network ($31.95) provides information on asthma triggers with products to control irritants and allergens, patient support, medical care with information on devices that help inhale medications more effectively, and information sources.

Occupational exposures also should be considered and symptoms discussed in relation to work hours. Work environments should be smoke-free and dust-free. Peak flow monitoring at the beginning and end of the workday and workweek is a useful means of evaluating the relationship between asthma and exposure in the workplace. In some cases, relocation within the workplace or changes in occupation may be necessary. Patient confidentiality may be an issue, since patients may be concerned with losing their job if it is known they have a problem with the work environment.

Nutritional consultations may be useful to discuss food allergies and ways to prepare foods to avoid the offending items.

PEAK FLOW MONITORING

Peak flow meters provide a guide to objective functioning of the lungs. There are various models of peak flow meters available. The patient should be taught how to measure and read peak flow and how to document the measurement on a peak flow monitoring diary. Having the patient complete the diary in front of the HCP assures that learning has taken place. The three-color system is the easiest to understand, and patients should know their personal best as well as what measurements should prompt a call for help or adjustment of their medications.

ACTION PLAN

Another essential step is to jointly develop an action plan for management of acute exacerbations of asthma. An effective plan includes monitoring of symptoms, peak flow measurements, frequency and doses of quick-relief medications, and restriction of physical activity. Patients should be taught how to identify symptoms of worsening asthma, either through use of a peak flow meter diary or asthma symptom diary. Action plans must be individualized to the patient's lifestyle, educational level, and ability to adjust medications and activities. Many action plans have been published and can be adapted to the needs of the patient and clinician. The action plan should also identify what peak flow measurements or asthma symptoms indicate the need to call the physician or seek emergency help. The plan for peak flow monitoring utilizing a three-color system is easy for patients to understand. Preprinted forms with the colors are available for purchase from PediPress (Amherst, MA).

WHEN TO SEEK MEDICAL HELP

Patients should always know when to seek medical help. Various reasons may inhibit the patient from seeking help: delays in getting an appointment, lack of funding for medications or clinic visits, denial of disease, underestimation of severity of disease, or fear. Despite the overwhelming evidence that early intervention saves money and prevents complications, education has not been successful in convincing many poor or uneducated patients to seek help earlier. An integral part of the patient-physician partnership is establishing a comfort level to call for help or questions. This helps prevent complications.

STRESS REDUCTION AND RELAXATION TECHNIQUES

Stress can exacerbate asthma symptoms and can result from physical changes (weight change, menopause) and various stressors: mental (school, work), emotional (negative attitude), relational (social isolation, divorce), or spiritual (feeling of worthlessness). Techniques to reduce stress are many

TABLE 38-27 Stress Reduction Techniques

Head and neck: Pull chin toward chest tightly and push back head, then let go. Turn head from side to side in a relaxed manner. Let it stop when it comes to a comfortable position.

Face: Tighten all the facial muscles. Hold, then let go.

Eyes: Focus eyes on something. While watching it, slowly let eyelids grow heavy. Open eyes as widely as possible and let close gradually until comfortable.

Shoulders: Shrug shoulders and tighten shoulder muscles as much as possible, then let go.

Arms: Do one hand and one arm at a time. Bend elbow and make a fist out of hand. Tighten as much as possible, then let go. Straighten arm and fingers. Tighten as much as possible, then let go.

Back: Arch back slowly and easily. Do not lift hips. Tighten as much as possible, then let go.

Buttocks: Squeeze muscles tightly, then let go.

Legs: Do one leg at a time. Pull toes toward nose and push heel and back of leg into bed. Tighten as much as possible, then let go.

and may have varied acceptance depending on the time and effort involved.

Progressive relaxation is the most commonly utilized technique for control of stress (Table 38-27). However, it must be practiced prior to need, and it requires a quiet, peaceful surrounding. The patient should lie down on a comfortable surface with a pillow under head and knees. Maximal relaxation follows maximal muscle contraction. Tighten muscles and relax them gradually. A tape recording can be made of the directions using a calm, low voice.

Guided imagery is a process of releasing tension by creating a mental image of an enjoyable setting. The image may be real or imagined and should elicit feelings of comfort and relaxation. The mental image is used to relax and reduce tension.

Self-hypnosis focuses on the mind's awareness and control over the body. Affirmations and biofeedback work in the same manner to tell the body to relax. Tapes are available from bookstores. Meditation consists of concentrating on a word and repeating it over and over. The word is repeated on exhalation, letting go of distracting thoughts and concentrating on the word. Yoga uses this technique for deep relaxation. Hobbies, television, movies, music, or reading can also be used for relaxation. Any method for stress reduction is useful as long as it produces results.

Acupuncture, when compared with simulated acupuncture, has not been shown to consistently improve asthma symptoms. The relaxation associated with an acupuncture treatment may be of some benefit, however. Marijuana, although providing modest short-term bronchodilation, can worsen asthma in the long-term because of chronic airway irritation form the many noxious ingredients in the smoke. Ephedra, an over-the-counter herbal remedy, does improve asthma symptoms as a result of its sympathomimetic properties, but patients should be counseled to avoid it because of its cardiac and central nervous system side effects. The FDA is currently evaluating whether to remove ephedrine-containing products from availability because of the deaths associated with their use.

PREVENTIVE MEASURES

Preventive measures should also be reviewed sometime during the educational process. Smoking history (for tobacco cigarettes, cigars, pipe, marijuana etc.), as well as exposure to second-hand smoke, should be elicited early. Smoking cessation options should be discussed. Programs are available through the American Lung Association and the American Cancer Society. Nicotine replacement products help to combat nicotine withdrawal. Products are available as gum, transdermal patches, and nasal sprays. Research has shown that the best outcomes result from combining a smoking cessation program with a replacement product. Many companies that market nicotine replacement products also provide education in the form of cassettes or videotapes, reading materials, and a telephone number to call for help or information. A new product available in oral form, bupropion (Zyban), holds promise as a pharmacologic method of reducing desire to smoke. The most enduring drive to smoke, however, is habit, and unless the habituation aspect is addressed and behavioral changes made, cessation will ultimately be unsuccessful.

Flu shots should be made available each fall and all patients encouraged to take advantage of this preventive measure. Postcards for reminders or a telephone call, especially to those mild asthmatics who are not seen frequently, may be all the encouragement needed. Patients who have episodes of pneumonia should also consider taking the pneumonia vaccine.

Severe asthmatics and those with life-threatening allergies should consider obtaining an identification (Medic Alert) bracelet. This will alert passersby or health care providers of any medications, conditions, or allergies that are important to know. Patients with life-threatening allergies should also be given an auto-injecting epinephrine dose (Epi-Pen) to carry and instructed on how to use it.

PSYCHOSOCIAL SUPPORT

Relaxation techniques are easy to teach and learn. Some patients, however, are not helped by those techniques and may need to be referred for psychological counseling. These include patients who have irrational fears and phobias, and panic and anxiety episodes unrelieved by breathing and relaxation techniques.

Support groups can be of help for some patients, especially those who have no family support or are socially isolated. Support groups for asthma are available through the Asthma and Allergy Foundation and the American Lung Association. It is important that the patient find a support group that is closely matched, that is, a working adult with other working adults, a parent with an asthmatic child with other parents, or older adults with other older adults.

Family support is essential since family members can sometimes undermine efforts to control symptoms consciously or unconsciously. Having the spouse or significant other in the room during education provides an opportunity to elicit family concerns and can be a valuable source of information on symptoms. Discussion of home and environmental controls helps elicit support from the family, for example, avoiding smoking or heavy perfumes and keeping pets out of the bedroom or home. Family members may also be sources of stress, which can be identified and dealt with in a neutral environment.

In addition chat rooms are available on the Internet for support and information. Patients must be cautioned that sources on the Internet are not necessarily professionals and they should discuss any advice they receive from these sources with their physician or other health care provider.

Resources

A wide variety of resources, many free of charge, are available for the patient with asthma. These range from expert sources, such as government entities and professional organizations, to pharmaceutical companies and the Internet. Printed educational materials should be available in the health care provider's office to help patients learn more about their disease and reinforce important information. Both patients and providers should know how to obtain these resources. Some of the most commonly available resources are listed in Table 38-28.

GOVERNMENTAL AGENCIES

Both educational materials and programs are available. The programs are directed primarily toward children with asthma. Resource materials are also available for health care providers. State health departments may also have educational resources and programs for asthma, frequently focused on children. States may also have initiatives focused on asthma programs as well.

PROFESSIONAL ORGANIZATIONS AND GROUPS

Many professional organizations have educational materials, as well as providing support groups. The National Jewish Center for Immunology and Respiratory Medicine (Denver, CO) has a telephone listing for patients with questions about lung disease (the Lung Line 800-222-LUNG). Nurses are available by telephone to answer questions, and educational information can be sent to the requester.

PHARMACEUTICAL COMPANIES

Most pharmaceutical companies have patient education materials available for the health care professional to use in teaching patients with asthma, and some have patient information as well. Educational materials available include slides, videotapes, cassette tapes, computer interactive programs, brochures, flip charts, models, and demonstration kits. Careful scrutiny of the materials usually can weed out products that are purely advertisement and select those items that can be used in an educational program.

INTERNET

Many home pages are available for information by using asthma as a search word. Care must be taken when reviewing information: sponsors are frequently not readily identifiable. Many pharmaceutical companies have home pages, as do many independent physicians and educational institutions. The National Jewish Institute for Immunology and Respiratory Medicine, for instance, has an excellent home page with several educational offerings. Patients should be cautioned to carefully scrutinize claims made on the Internet and identify the sponsor to evaluate claims and information available.

A chat room is also available on the Internet for patients

TABLE 38-28 Sources of Patient Educational Materials

Government resources
  NHLBI Asthma Reading Resource List
  National Asthma Education Program
  Resource List for Asthma Education in the Schools
    NHLBI Information Center, P.O. Box 30105, Bethesda, MD
      20824-0105
    Phone: 301-951-3260
  Global Initiative for Asthma (GINA)
  NHLBI and WHO
  U.S. Department of Health and Human Services
  Public Health Services, NIH, NHLBI
    NHLBI Information Center, P.O. Box 30105, Bethesda, MA
      20824-0105
    Phone: 301-951-3260
  British Lung Foundation
    8 Peterborough Mews, London SW6 3BL, England
  British Society of Allergy and Immunology
    Level D, South Academic Block, Southampton General Hospital
    Tremona Road, Southampton, England
  British Thoracic Society
    1 Andrews Place, London NW1 4LB, England
  Royal College of General Practitioners
    7 Prince's Gate, London SW7, England
Professional organizations and groups
  Asthma Resources Directory
    American Allergy Association, P.O. Box 640, Menlo Park, CA
      94026
    Phone: 415-322-1663
  American Academy of Allergy, Asthma and Immunology (education)
    611 E. Wells Street, Milwaukee, WI 53202
    Phone: 414-272-6071
  Allergy and Asthma Network and Mothers of Asthmatics, Inc.
    (newsletter)
    3554 Chain Bridge Road, Suite 200, Fairfax, VA 22030
    Phone: 703-385-4403
  The American College of Allergy, Asthma and Immunology
    85 West Algonquin, Suite 550, Arlington Heights, IL 60005
    Phone: 800-842-7777
  American Academy of Dermatology
    930 N. Meacham Road, Schaumburg, IL 60173-6016
    Phone: 708-330-0230
  American Lung Association (education and support groups)
    Phone: 800-LUNG USA
    Also, one should contact local chapter listings in the telephone book.
  Asthma and Allergy Foundation of America (education and
    support groups)
    1125 Fifteenth Street, Suite 502, Washington, DC 20005
    Phone: 800-7-ASTHMA or 202-466-7643
  Asthma Management Centre
    232 Tower Street, Brunswick Business Park, Liverpool L3 4BJ,
      England
  Asthma Training Centre
    Winton House, Church Road, Stratford Upon Avon,
      Warwickshire, England
  National Asthma Campaign
    Providence House, Providence Place, London NI ONT
  The Food Allergy Network
    10400 Eaton Place, Suite 107, Fairfax, VA 22030-2208
    Phone: 800-929-4040
  Allergy and Asthma Newsletter (subscription)
    Healthline Publishing, Inc.
    830 Menlo Avenue, Suite 100, Menlo Park, CA 94025

with asthma (http://www.alt.med.allergy and http://www.alt.support.asthma). An address that may also be of interest to obtain the most current pollen forecasts, information, and tips for allergy sufferers is http://www.allerdays.com. Again, patients should be cautioned to discuss any medication side effects and changes with the health care provider. Those who use the chat room are not professionals with expertise in asthma—only experience in living with the disease. The chat room can be a valuable resource for sharing experiences on how to deal with a chronic disease, but it is also used by hucksters to promote products that have little or no value.

READING MATERIALS IN THE LAY PRESS

Many publications are available in bookstores regarding asthma. Patients should be cautioned to obtain books that have a recent publication date (1996 and later) to obtain current recommendations for therapy and interventions. The most common publications available in bookstores are dated in the mid- to late 1980s. Examples of some good ones are: *Conquering Asthma,* 3d ed., by Michael T. Newhouse, MD, and Peter J. Barnes, DM, Empowering Press, 1998 (good introductory book written in lay terms); *The Asthma Self-Help Book,* 2d ed., by Paul J. Hannaway, MD, Prima Publishing, 1992 (good for more in-depth information, presents research basis for therapy); *Asthma and Exercise,* by Nancy Hogshead and Gerald S. Couzens, Henry Holt and Company, 1989 (good for patients who are athletes or primarily have exercise-induced asthma); *Asthma: Stop Suffering, Start Living,* 2d ed., by M. Eric Gershwin, MD, and E.L. Klingelhofer, PhD, Addison-Wesley Publishing Company, 1992 (this source is thorough, covering pregnancy, summer camps, traveling, and other issues, as well as alternative and home remedies).

Outcomes

Quality improvement must always be considered as part of program evaluation. The components of evaluating a health care program encompass structure, process, and outcome. Structure refers to factors in the institutional environment that impact on the success of the program (facilities, equipment, personnel). Process refers to the way the program is set up and administered, and includes guidelines, policies, and protocols. Most quality improvement programs have focused on these two aspects of program evaluation, but increasing emphasis is being made on evaluating outcomes. According to some schools of thought, the structure and process need not be evaluated unless the desired outcomes are not being achieved.

Although pulmonary rehabilitation programs are reasonably standardized, these focus primarily on the patient with COPD rather than the patient with asthma who is working or going to school. The success of any rehabilitation program is measured by assessing outcomes. These can be measured by looking at the more commonly assessed outcomes of mortality, complications, days lost from work or school, medication side effects, or utilization of medical resources, such as provider visits, emergency department visits, hospitalizations, and intubations.

Additional outcomes should be measured in the asthma population. For instance, compliance with a therapeutic regi-

TABLE 38-29 Instruments to Measure Quality of Life

Author	Instrument	Dimensions Measured	Validity	Reliability
Ware	SR-36 health survey	Physical functioning Role—physical Bodily pain General health Vitality Social functioning Role—emotional Mental health	$r = \geq 0.40$	0.68–0.93
Nelson, Wasson, Johnson, Hays	COOP charts	Physical Emotional Daily activities Social activities Social support Pain Overall health	$r = 0.62$ with SF-36	0.73–0.98
Damiano	Sickness Impact Profile	Physical category: ambulation, mobility, body care and movement Psychosocial category: communication, alertness behavior, emotional behavior, social interaction Independent categories: sleep and rest, eating, work, home management, recreation, and pastimes	$r = >0.49$	0.96
Jones	St. George's Respiratory Questionnaire	Symptoms Activity Impacts on daily life	$r = -0.35$ with 6-min walk $r = 0.50$ with MRC dyspnea grade	0.91
American Thoracic Society	Standardized Respiratory Disease Questionnaire	Demographic data Pulmonary symptomatology: cough, mucous production, wheezing		
Juniper	Asthma Quality of Life Questionnaire	Symptoms Emotions Exposure to environmental stimuli Activity limitation	$r > 0.5$ with changes in clinical control $r = 0.35$–0.5 with PEF and medication use	0.89–0.94

men is directly related to its ease of fitting into the patient's lifestyle and ability to be compliant. A medication prescribed to be taken four times a day is less likely to be taken consistently by patients who are working or in school than a medication that can be taken twice a day. Outcomes can also be measured by assessing health-related quality of life (physical, emotional, etc.) from both the clinician's and patient's point of view and bioeconomics.

Health-related quality of life (HRQL) has been defined and measured as purely objective (observed functional status, social economic status) or subjective (patient perceptions, attitudes). Both components provide important information on the success of a rehabilitation program. Most researchers in the area of quality of life (QOL) measure both subjective and objective components. Patients with chronic diseases frequently rate themselves as having a relatively high QOL, although observers may think they have a relatively low QOL. Since health is considered a dimension, or component, of QOL, a multidimensional tool must be used to adequately measure QOL. Quality of life can also be measured globally (e.g., how satisfied are you with your health at this time) or specifically (e.g., how much has your shortness of breath affected your ability to do activities of daily living this week).

SELECTING AN INSTRUMENT

Most researchers in QOL assessment recommend using both global and disease-specific measures of QOL, as well as a combination of patient-administered questionnaires and objective assessment. Global measures allow for comparison with other disease states, whereas disease-specific measures facilitate comparison with other samples of patients with the same disease.

Another concern is whether to use a single instrument or several instruments to measure the domains of quality of life. Factors to be considered when using multiple instruments include feasibility of completion by patients, time required to complete them, and costs related to duplication, follow-up, and analyzing the instruments. Three of the most common generic and disease-specific tools are discussed (Table 38-29).

The most frequently used measure of global QOL outcome measure in health care is the Medical Outcomes Study Short Form 36-item questionnaire (SF-36).[92] It evaluates five domains of quality of life: disease, personal functioning, psychological distress and well-being, general health perceptions, and social role functioning divided into eight subscales. It has also been validated in Denmark, Germany, Sweden, Canada, and the United Kingdom. Studies are in process for validation in Australia, France, Italy, and The Netherlands to develop norms. It has been used in many patient populations and settings, including asthma in which different treatments (drugs, monitoring, or provider) were compared.[93-96] Reliability for the eight subscales ranges from 0.68 (social functioning) to 0.93 (physical functioning), reliability for all but the social functioning scale being over 0.80. The SF-12 is a shorter version that is currently being used and validated in different populations.

Another commonly used global measure of QOL consists of the Dartmouth COOP Functional Health Assessment Charts.[97] Each chart asks a question referring to the patient's status over the past 2 to 4 weeks and is measured on a five-point ordinal scale. The dimensions measured include physical well-being, emotional well-being, daily activities, social activities, social support, pain, and overall health. It has been compared to the SF-36 and Sickness Impact Profile for validity and reliability. It is very simple to use and easy to administer in an outpatient setting.

The Sickness Impact Profile measures different levels of health and is sensitive to changes over time.[98] It consists of 136 items that describe activities associated with daily living. These items can be aggregated into 12 categories, and then into three dimensions: physical (three categories), psychosocial (four categories), and independent (five categories). Each item is checked if it applies and can be self-administered or be administered by interview. Validity and reliability have been measured against many other instruments, and reliability ranges from 0.41 to 0.96.

Asthma disease-specific QOL instruments are few, and none has been widely tested. These include the Asthma Quality of Life Questionnaire[99] by Marks, Living with Asthma Questionnaire[100] by Hyland, Life Activities Questionnaire for Adult Asthma[101] by Creer, Respiratory Illness Quality of Life Questionnaire[102] by Maille, and the Asthma Bother Profile[103] by Hyland. The most frequently used instrument in the United States is the Asthma Quality of Life Questionnaire[104] by Juniper. It is a 32-item questionnaire for adults and evaluates four domains: symptoms, emotions, exposure to environmental stimuli, and activity limitation. A seven-point Likert scale is used, and it can be completed in a short amount of time. Good reliability has been reported, with intraclass correlations ranging from 0.89 to 0.94.

The St. George's Respiratory Questionnaire[105] was developed in England and contains a few terms that may be confusing to Americans. It is widely used with COPD and less frequently in asthma. It evaluates the domains of symptoms, activity, and impacts on daily life. It is self-administered and consists of 76 items. Varying validity results have been found comparing it with other measures such as the Sickness Impact Profile ($r = 0.39$) and 6-min walk test ($r = 0.35$). The reliability has been reported to be 0.91.

The Standardized Respiratory Disease Questionnaire[106] was developed by the American Thoracic Society in 1978 and is currently under revision. It contains demographic data and information on pulmonary symptomatology such as dyspnea, wheezing, cough, and mucous production. Other information elicited includes historical information on pulmonary disease, occupational exposures, medication usage, and smoking. This instrument aids in evaluating the behavioral manifestations of dyspnea and can be used with both children and adults.

Other outcomes that can be assessed include the economics associated with asthma care. The latter outcome includes cost of medications and equipment, time lost from work or school, utilization of health care resources such as HCP appointments, phone calls, visits to the emergency department, hospitalizations, ambulance transportation, and costs associated with home and environmental controls.

Any program for asthma rehabilitation should include exercise training, education, and psychosocial support, as well as measurements of outcomes. Which outcomes to measure depends on the type of program, time available for collection of data, and what questions need to be answered.

References

1. Healthy People 2000, National Health Promotion and Disease Prevention Objectives. Washington, D.C.: US Department of Health and Human Services, 1990.
2. Centers for Disease Control and Prevention: Asthma—United States 1989–1992. *MMWR* 43:952–955, 1995.
3. Murphy S: National Asthma Education and Prevention Program, Expert Panel Report II: Guidelines for the Diagnosis and Management of Asthma. Washington, DC, National Heart, Lung and Blood Institute, 1997.
4. Sheffer AL: National Heart, Lung and Blood Institute, Asthma Education Program Expert Panel Report: Guidelines for the diagnosis and management of asthma. *Ped Asthma Allergy Immunol* 5:57–188, 1991.
5. British Thoracic Society, The National Asthma Campaign, Royal College of Physicians of London, et al: Guidelines for the management of asthma, 1995 review and position statement. *Thorax* 52:S1–S21, 1995.
6. British Thoracic Society, British Paediatric Association, Research Unit of the Royal College of Physicians of London, et al: Guidelines for the management of asthma. *Thorax* 48:S1–S24, 1993.
7. British Thoracic Society, British Paediatric Association, Research Unit of the Royal College of Physicians of London, Centre KsF, Campaign NA. Guidelines for the management of asthma in adults: II. Acute severe asthma. *Br Med J* 301:797–800, 1990.
8. Hargreave FE, Dolovich J, Newhouse MT: The assessment and treatment of asthma: A conference report. *J Allergy Clin Immunol* 85:1098–1111, 1990.
9. Woolcock AJ, Rubinfeld AR, Seale JP: Asthma Management Plan, 1989. *Med J Australia* 151:650–653, 1989.
10. International consensus report on diagnosis and treatment of asthma. *Clin Exp Allergy* 22:1–72, 1992.
11. van der Schoot TAW, Kaptein AA: Pulmonary rehabilitation in an asthma clinic. *Lung* 168(Suppl):495–501, 1990.
12. Cox NJM, Hendricks JC, van Herwaarden CLA: A pulmonary rehabilitation program for patients with asthma and mild chronic obstructive pulmonary disease (COPD). *Lung* 171:235–244, 1993.
13. Andersson L, Osterman M, Lundbäck B, Nygren A: Effects on lung function of a rehabilitation program for persons with asthma—a two year follow-up. *Am J Respir Crit Care Med* 155:A889, 1997.

14. Galli SJ: New concepts about the mast cell. *N Engl J Med* 328:257–265, 1993.

15. Kay AB: "Helper" (CD4+) T cells and eosinophils in allergy and asthma. *Am Rev Respir Dis* 145:S22–S26, 1992.

16. Barnes PJ, Baraniuk JN, Belvisi MG: Neuropeptides in the respiratory tract part 1. *Am Rev Respir Dis* 144.1107–1198, 1991.

17. Barnes PJ, Baraniuk JN, Belvisi MG: Neuropeptides in the respiratory tract part 2. *Am Rev Respir Dis* 144:1391–1399, 1991.

18. Smith LJ: Bioactive mediators in asthma. *Chest* 101:381S–384S, 1992.

19. Page CP: Mechanisms of hyperresponsiveness: Platelet-activating factor. *Am Rev Respir Dis* 145:S31–S33, 1992.

20. Nadel JA: Regulation of neurogenic inflammation by neutral endopeptidase. *Am Rev Respir Dis* 145:S48–S52, 1992.

21. Nadel JA: Biologic effects of mast cell enzymes. *Am Rev Respir Dis* 145:S37–S41, 1992.

22. Schwartz LB: Cellular inflammation in asthma: Neutral proteases of mast cells. *Am Rev Respir Dis* 145:S18–S21, 1992.

23. Lemanske RF: Mechanisms of airway inflammation. *Chest* 101:372S–377S, 1992.

24. Pennock BE, Rogers RM, Mc Caffree DR: Changes in spirometric indices. What is significant? *Chest* 80:97–99, 1981.

25. Martin RJ: Nocturnal asthma: Circadian rhythms and therapeutic interventions. *Am Rev Respir Dis* 147:S23–S28, 1993.

26. Murray AB, Milner RA: The accuracy of features in the clinical history for predicting atopic sensitization to airborne allergens in children. *J Allergy Clin Immunol* 96:588–596, 1995.

27. Adinoff AD, Rosloniec DM, Mc Call LL, Nelson HS: Immediate skin test reactivity to Food and Drug Administration-approved standardized extracts. *J Allergy Clin Immunol* 86:766–774, 1990.

28. Taylor WR, Newacheck PW: Impact of childhood asthma on health. *Pediatrics* 90:657–662, 1992.

29. Boston Consulting Group: Report on the cost of asthma in Australia: New South Wales, Australia, National Asthma Campaign, 1992.

30. Nelson HS, Fernandez-Caldas E: Prevelence of house-dust mites in the Rocky Mountain States. *Ann Allergy Asthma Immunol* 75:337–339, 1995.

31. Ingram JM, Sporik R, Rose G, et al: Quantitative assessment of exposure to dog (Can f 1) and cat (Fel d 1) allergens: Relation to sensitization and asthma among children living in Los Alamos, New Mexico. *J Allergy Clin Immunol* 96:449–456, 1995.

32. National Heart LaBI. Data fact sheet, October 1995, asthma. Bethesda, MD, National Heart, Lung and Blood Institute, 1995.

33. Laitinen A, Laitinen LA: Airway morphology: Endothelium/basement membrane. *Am J Respir Crit Care Med* 150:S14–S17, 1994.

34. Djukanovic R, Roche WR, Wilson JW: Mucosal inflammation in asthma. *Am Rev Respir Dis* 142:434–457, 1990.

35. Tashkin DP, Altose MD, Connett JE, et al: Airway hyperresponsiveness in "irreversible" chronic obstructive pulmonary disease, in Spector SL (ed): *Provocation Testing in Clinical Practice*, vol 5. New York, Marcel Dekker, 1995; pp 575–598.

36. Jeffrey PK, Wardlaw AJ, Nelson FC, et al: Bronchial biopsies in asthma. An ultrastructural, qualitative study and correlation with hyperreactivity. *Am J Respir Dis* 140:1745–1753, 1989.

37. Mayo PH, Richman J, Harris HW: Results of a program to reduce admissions for adult asthma. *Ann Intern Med* 112:864–871, 1990.

38. Nunn AJ, Gregg I: New regression equations for predicting peak expiratory flow in adults. *Br Med J* 298:1068–1070, 1989.

39. Kikughi Y, Okabe S, Tamura G: Chemosensitivity and perception of dyspnea in patients with a history of near fatal asthma. *N Engl J Med* 330:1329–1334, 1994.

40. Ruffin RE, Latimer KM, Schembri DA: Longitudinal study of near fatal asthma. *Chest* 99:77–83, 1991.

41. Strunk RC: Identification of the fatality-prone subject with asthma. *J Allergy Clin Immunol* 83:477–485, 1989.

42. Clark NM, Evans D, Mellins RB: Patient use of peak flow monitoring. *Am Rev Respir Dis* 145:722–725, 1992.

43. Drummond N, Abdalla M, Beattie JAG: Effectiveness of routine self-monitoring of peak flow in patients with asthma. *Br Med J* 308:564–567, 1994.

44. Lewis CE, Racheletsky G, Lewis MA, et al: A randomized trial of A.C.T. (asthma care training) for kids. *Pediatrics* 74:478–486, 1984.

45. Troyanov S, Ghezzo H, Cartier A, Malo J: Comparison of circadian variations using FEV_1 and peak expiratory flow rates among normal and asthmatic subjects. *Thorax* 49:775–780, 1994.

46. Murray AB, Ferguson AC: Dust-free bedrooms in the treatment of asthmatic children with house dust mite allergy: A controlled trial. *Pediatrics* 71:418–422, 1983.

47. Platts-Mills TAE, Tovey ER, Mitchell EB, et al: Reduction of bronchial hyperreactivity during prolonged allergen avoidance. *Lancet* 2(8300):675–678, 1982.

48. Boner AL, Peroni D, Sette L, et al: Effects of allergen exposure-avoidence on inflammation in asthmatic children. *Allergy* 48:119–124, 1993.

49. Toogood JH: High-dose inhaled steroid therapy for asthma. *J Allergy Clin Immunol* 83:528–536, 1989.

50. Bosman HG, van Uffelen R, Tamminga JJ, Paanakker LR: Comparison of inhaled beclomethasone dipropionate 1000 micrograms twice daily and oral prednisone 10 mg once daily in asthmatic patients. *Thorax* 49:37–40, 1994.

51. Roy A, Leblanc C, Paquette L, et al: Skin bruising in asthmatic subjects treated with high doses of inhaled steroids: Frequency and association with adrenal function. *Eur Respir J* 9:226–231, 1996.

52. Capewell S, Reynolds S, Shuttleworth D, et al: Purpura and dermal thinning associated with high dose inhaled corticosteroids. *Br Med J* 300:1548–1551, 1990.

53. Cumming RG, Mitchell P, Leeder SR: Use of inhaled corticosteroids and the risk of cataracts. *N Engl J Med* 337:8–14, 1997.

54. Gasarbe E, LeLorier J, Boivin J, Suissa S: Inhaled and nasal glucocorticoids and the risk of occular hypertension or open-angle glaucoma. *JAMA* 277:722–727, 1997.

55. Tashkin DP: Multiple dose regimens. Impact on compliance. *Chest* 107:176S–182S, 1995.

56. Yeung M, O'Conner SA, Parry DT, Cochraine GM: Compliance with prescribed drug therapy in asthma. *Respir Med* 88:31–35, 1994.

57. Haahtela T, Järvinen M, Kava T: Effects of discontinuing inhaled budesonide in patients with mild asthma. *N Engl J Med* 331:700–705, 1994.

58. Crossman DC, Dashwood MR, Taylor GW, et al: Sodium cromoglycate: Evidence of tachykinin antagonist activity in human skin. *J Appl Physiol* 75:167–172, 1993.

59. Pearce FL: Effects of nedocromil sodium on mediator release from mast cells. *J Allergy Clin Immunol* 92:155–158, 1993.

60. Bruijnzeel PLB, Warringa RAJ, Kok PTM, et al: Effects of nedocromil sodium on in vitro induced migration, activation and mediator release from human granulocytes. *J Allergy Clin Immunol* 92:159–164, 1993.

61. Verleden GM, Belvisi MG, Stretton CD, Barnes PJ: Nedocromil sodium modulates nonadrenergic, noncholinergic bronchoconstrictor nerves in guinea pig airways in vitro. *Am Rev Respir Dis* 143:114–118, 1991.

62. Barnes PJ: Effect of nedocromil sodium on airway sensory nerves. *J Allergy Clin Immunol* 92:182–186, 1993.

63. Lal S, Dorow PD, Venho KK, Chatterjee SS: Nedocromil sodium is more effective than cromolyn sodium for the treatment of chronic reversible obstructive airways disease. *Chest* 104:438–447, 1993.

64. Bone MF, Kubik MM, Keaney NP: Nedocromil sodium in adults with asthma dependent on inhaled corticosteroids: A double blind, placebo controlled study. *Thorax* 44:654–659, 1989.

65. Joad JP, Ahrens RC, Lindgren SD, Weinberger MM: Relative efficacy of maintenance therapy with theophylline, inhaled albuterol and the combination for chronic asthma. *J Allergy Clin Immunol* 79:78–85, 1987.

66. D'Alonzo GE, Nathan RA, Henochowicz S, et al: Salmeterol xinafoate as maintenance therapy compared with albuterol in patients with asthma. *JAMA* 271:1412–1416, 1994.

67. Woolcock A, Lundback B, Ringdal N, Jacques LA: Comparison of addition of salmeterol to inhaled steroids with doubling of the dose of inhaled steroids. *Am J Respir Crit Care Med* 153:1481–1488, 1996.

68. Greenin AP, Ind PW, Northfield M, Shaw G: Added salmeterol versus higher-dose corticosteroid in asthma patients with symptoms on existing inhaled corticosteroids. *Lancet* 344:219–224, 1994.

69. Raeburn D, Advenier C: Isoenzyme-selective cyclic nucleotide phosphodiesterase inhibitors: Effects on airways smooth muscle. *Int J Biochem Cell Biol* 27:29–37, 1995.

70. Schudt C, Tenor H, Hatzelmann A: PDE isoenzymes as targets for anti-asthma drugs. *Eur Respir J* 8:1179–1183, 1995.

71. Frew AJ: Conventional and alternative allergy immunotherapy: Do they work? Are they safe? *Clin Exp Allergy* 24:416–422, 1994.

72. Bousquet J, Michel FB: Specific immunotherapy in asthma: Is it effective? *J Allergy Clin Immunol* 94:1–11, 1994.

73. Kane GC, Peters SP, Fish JE: Alternative anti-inflammatory drugs in the treatment of bronchial asthma. *Clin Pulm Med* 1:69–77, 1994.

74. Nelson HS: Beta-adrenergic bronchodilators. *N Engl J Med* 333:499–506, 1995.

75. Wald JA, Friedman BF, Farr RS: An improved protocol for the use of troleandomycin (TAO) in the treatment of steroid-requiring asthma. *J Allergy Clin Immunol* 78:36–43, 1986.

76. Coffey MJ, Sanders G, Eschenbacher WL: The role of methotrexate in the management of steroid-dependent asthma. *Chest* 105:117–121, 1994.

77. Erzurum SC, Leff JA, Cochran JE: Lack of benefit of methotrexate in severe, steroid-dependent asthma, a double-blinded, placebo-caontrolled study. *Ann Intern Med* 114:353–360, 1991.

78. Nierop G, Gijzel WP, Bel EH: Auranofin in the treatment of steroid dependent asthma: A double blind study. *Thorax* 47:349–354, 1992.

79. Klaustermeyer WB, Noritake DT, Kwong FK: Chrysotherapy in the treatment of corticosteroid-dependent asthma. *J Allergy Clin Immunol* 79:720–725, 1987.

80. Muranaka M, Miyamoto T, Shinda T: Gold salts in the treatment of bronchial asthma—A double-blind study. *Ann Allergy* 40:132–137, 1978.

81. Alexander AG, Barnes NC, Kay AB: Trial of cyclosporin in corticosteroid-dependent chronic severe asthma. *Lancet* 339:324–328, 1992.

82. Tashkin DP, Shapiro BJ, Frank IM: Acute effects of smoked marijuana and oral delta₉-tetrahydrocannabinol specific airway conductance in asthmatic subjects. *Am Rev Respir Dis* 109:420–428, 1974.

83. Tashkin DP, Bresler DE, Kroening RJ, et al: Comparison of real and simulated acupuncture and isoproterenol in methacholine-induced asthma. *Ann Allergy* 39:379–387, 1977.

84. American Thoracic Society: Standardization of spirometry. 1994 update. *Am J Respir Crit Care Med* 152:1107–1136, 1995.

85. Smoller JW, Pollack MH, Otto MW, et al: Panic, anxiety, dyspnea and respiratory disease, theoretical and clinical considerations. *Am J Respir Crit Care Med* 154:6–17, 1996.

86. Luskin AL: Program WgoAaPotNAE. Report of the working group on asthma and pregnancy, Management of asthma during pregnancy. Bethesda, MD, National Institutes of Health, Heart, Lung, and Blood Institute, National Asthma Education Program, 1993.

87. Clark SL: National Asthma Education Program working group on Asthma and Pregnancy. Asthma in pregnancy. *Obstet Gynecol* 82:1036–1040, 1993.

88. Chapman KR, Love L, Brubaker H: A comparison of breath-actuated and conventional metered-dose inhaler inhalation techniques in elderly subjects. *Chest* 104:1332–1337, 1993.

89. Clark NM, Evans D, Zimmerman BJ, et al: Patient and family management of asthma: Theory-based techniques for the clinician. *J Asthma* 31:427–35, 1994.

90. Boulet LP, Boutin H, Cote J, et al: Evaluation of an asthma self-management education program. *J Asthma* 32:199–206, 1995.

91. Mukai DS, Wilson AF: Aerosol movement and pressures in spacer. *Am J Respir Crit Care Med* 155:A670, 1997.

92. Stewart AL, Hays RD, Ware JEJ: The MOS short-form general health survey. Reliability and validity in a patient population. *Med Care* 26:724–735, 1988.

93. Skaer TL, Wilson CB, Sclar DA, et al: Metered-dose inhaler technique and quality of life with airways disease: Assessing the value of the Vitalograph in educational intervention. *J Int Med Res* 24:369–375, 1996.

94. Vollmer WM, O'Hollaren M, Ettinger KM, et al: Specialty differences in the management of asthma. A cross-sectional assessment of allergists' patients and generalists' patients in a large HMO. *Arch Intern Med* 157:1201–1208, 1997.

95. Mahajan P, Okamoto LJ, Schaberg A, et al: Impact of fluticasone propionate powder on health-related quality of life in patients with moderate asthma. *J Asthma* 34:227–234, 1997.

96. Okamoto LJ, Noonan M, DeBoisblanc BP, Kellerman DJ: Fluticasone propionate improves quality of life in patients with asthma requiring oral corticosteroids. *Ann Allergy Asthma Immunol* 76:455–461, 1996.

97. Jenkinson C, Lawrence K, McWhinnie D, Gordon J: Sensitivity to change of health status measures in a randomized controlled trial: Comparison of the COOP charts and the SF-36. *Quality of Life Res* 4:47–52, 1995.

98. Bergner M, Bobbit RA, Carter WB, Gilson BS: The Sickness Impact Profile: Development and final revision of a health status measure. *Med Care* 19:787–805, 1981.

99. Marks GB, Dunn SM, Woolcock AJ: An evaluation of an asthma quality of life questionnaire as a measure of change in adults with asthma. *J Clin Epidemiol* 46:1103–1111, 1993.

100. Hyland ME, Finnis S, Irvine SH: A scale for assessing quality of life in adult asthma sufferers. *J Phychosom Res* 35:99–110, 1991.

101. Wigal JK, Stout C, Brandon M, et al: The knowledge, attitude, and self-efficacy asthma questionnaire. *Chest* 104:1144–1148, 1993.

102. Maille AR, Koning CJ, Zwinderman AH, et al: The development of the "Quality-of-Life for Respiratory Illness Questionnaire (QOL-RIQ)": A disease-specific quality-of-life questionnaire for patients with mild to moderate chronic non-specific lung disease. *Respir Med* 1997:5, 1997.

103. Hyland ME, Ley A, Fisher DW, Woodward V: Measurement of psychological distress in asthma and asthma management programmes. *Br J Clin Psych* 34(pt 4):601–611, 1995.

104. Juniper EF, Guyatt GH, Ferrie PJ, Griffith LE: Measuring quality of life in asthma. *Am Rev Respir Dis* 147:832–838, 1993.

105. Jones PW, Quirk FH, Baveystock CM: The St George's Respiratory Questionnaire. *Respir Med* 85(suppl B):25–31; discussion 33–37, 1991.

106. Ferris BG, Speizer F, Gaensler E, Greene R: Epidemiology standardization project. *Am Rev Resp Dis* 118:1–120, 1978.

Chapter 39

MANAGEMENT OF CHRONIC OBSTRUCTIVE PULMONARY DISEASE

MURRAY ALTOSE

NEIL S. CHERNIACK

Chronic obstructive pulmonary disease (COPD) is a group of diseases that result in progressive reductions in expiratory flow rates and ultimately, in reduced blood oxygenation and respiratory acidosis. Unlike asthma, which produces episodes of airways narrowing that may resolve completely or nearly completely, a significant portion of the obstruction in COPD cannot be reversed even by intensive treatment.[1]

Rehabilitation programs for patients with COPD are increasingly recognized as enhancing therapeutic outcomes. While a variety of drugs help alleviate the symptoms of acute exacerbations of COPD, there is still no treatment that will restore normal lung function. Thus, many patients are left to cope with a chronic largely irreversible process. Rehabilitation attempts to improve the patients' disability from the disease through a comprehensive approach that includes medication but, in addition, involves physical and behavioral techniques.

At one end the spectrum of COPD are patients in whom the disease primarily affects the airways, causing chronic bronchitis with increased cough and sputum production. At the other end of the spectrum are patients with emphysema, where the disease leads to dilatation and destruction of the alveolar walls and enlargement of air spaces. In most patients with COPD, the disease affects both the airways and the lung parenchyma in varying degrees. The loss of lung tissues diminishes the elastic traction of the lung tissues on the airways, allowing the airways to collapse during expiration.[2]

Cigarette smoking is the chief cause of COPD, but other injurious agents in the inhaled air can contribute to the inflammatory process to which leukocytes and macrophage are attracted and oxidants and proteases are released, causing further damage. Abnormalities in the mechanisms that protect the lung and airways against injury (the immune system, the mucociliary escalator, and antiproteases) all increase susceptibility to COPD.[3,4]

Pathophysiologic Basis

COPD is characterized by increased airway resistance which causes a reduction of the FEV_1 (forced expiratory volume in 1 s) with little change in the forced vital capacity (FVC). In normal individuals, the FEV_1 is at least 80 percent of the FVC, but in COPD it is reduced.[1,2]

Airway obstruction usually leads to overinflation of the lungs and thereby shortens the resting length of the inspiratory muscles so that the force they generate when they contract is reduced. Overinflation also flattens the diaphragm and changes the direction of the forces produced by dia-phragmatic contraction, decreasing the ability of the diaphragm to lift and expand the rib cage. As a result, the accessory respiratory muscles must be used even during quiet breathing. Both the greater airway resistance and the diminished capacity of the respiratory muscles increase the O_2 cost of breathing. Dyspnea, often an incapacitating symptom in COPD, arises from the lessening of the ability of the respiratory muscles to satisfy breathing demands despite increased efforts.[3,4]

Neither bronchitis nor emphysema affects all parts of the lungs uniformly. As COPD becomes more severe, the mechanisms that help maintain the balanced distribution of ventilation to perfusion in the lung fail. A greater fraction of the inspired air is wasted, filling the dead space instead of gas-exchanging alveoli. More of the pulmonary arterial blood traverses the lung without being exposed to freshly inspired air. As a consequence, hypoxia and hypercapnia develop. Hypoxia causes pressures in the pulmonary circulation to rise, leading eventually to right-sided heart failure and malfunctions in multiple organ systems.[1,2]

Assessment of the Patient with COPD

Comprehensive rehabilitation programs are not needed by every patient with COPD. As in other comprehensive programs, patients require careful assessment by a multidisciplinary team of experts as well as consultation with the patients' primary care physician and family.[5] Treatment is often long term. The total program includes exercise and muscle training, as well as psychosocial support and is suited for the patient who is stable after maximal therapy with drugs, pulmonary hygiene, and O_2 if necessary.[6–8] However, the development of lung reduction and lung transplantation surgery has demonstrated that even brief courses of muscle reconditioning can be beneficial pre- and postoperatively.[9] Also, even with inpatients who have mild disease, careful health maintenance programs which include smoking cessation and immunizations and exercise help prevent further deterioration in breathing function.

METHODS OF ASSESSMENT

Assessment starts with a careful history and physical examination. Measurement of lung function and exercise tolerance is essential. The patients' medical record should be reviewed to help identify other medical problems that might preclude or delay portions of the comprehensive program.[8]

Patients with COPD are usually over 40 and are predominantly male. Almost every patient with COPD has smoked cigarettes, and if there is no history of cigarette smoking, conditions other than COPD should be considered. Shortness of breath is the most common symptom in patients with COPD, correlating roughly with the degree of airways obstruction. Dyspnea may occur only during exertion, but unlike shortness of breath associated with exercise-induced asthma it will improve rather than worsen in the postexercise recovery period. COPD-associated dyspnea rarely awakens the patient from sleep, as does the dyspnea caused by obstructive sleep apnea or the breathlessness occasioned by nocturnal asthma. The patient with COPD may adopt certain characteristic positions to relieve dyspnea, such as leaning forward with arms supported, a posture that improves the force that the accessory respiratory muscles of the neck can produce.[1,2,8]

Cough, often productive, is a common symptom in COPD. Wheezing may be present in COPD patients and may be particularly prominent during exposure to cold air and during intercurrent upper respiratory infections. Other signs of airway obstruction, hyperinflation, ineffectual respiratory muscle function, and right-sided heart failure can all be present in patients with COPD. Some COPD patients may breathe through pursed lips which slows their usual tachypneic breathing and seems to relieve dyspnea.[1,2,7,8] Weight loss is not uncommon in severe, end-stage COPD.

Because of hyperinflation, the diaphragm may move less than the usual 5 to 6 cm during maximal inspiration and expiration. In addition, because the flattened diaphragm is less able to expand the rib cage, the lower ribs may move inward rather than outward during inspiration (Hoover's sign). The greater negative pleural pressure required to expand the overinflated lungs in patients with COPD may lead to pulsus paradoxus, a decrease in systolic blood pressure by 10 mmHg or more during inspiration. When the thorax is overexpanded, the inspiratory muscles are shortened and cannot generate as much force as usual, which changes the pattern of chest wall movement during breathing. To compensate for ineffectual diaphragm contractions, intercostal muscle contraction may move the abdomen toward rather than away from the spine during inspiration. Also, because the inspiratory muscles are more likely to fatigue, the muscles of respiration in the neck tend to become prominent, particularly when the FEV_1 falls below 1 liter.[1,2,8]

PULMONARY FUNCTION EVALUATION

The severity of COPD is assessed by measurements of airflow made during maximal expiratory efforts. The $FEV_{1.0}$, the volume of air that can be expired from total lung capacity (TLC) in one second by maximal effort is the test most frequently used. Patients with COPD will have an $FEV_{1.0}$ less than 80 percent of predicted normal values; an FEV_1 below 35 percent of the predicted normal value indicates severe obstructive disease.

Unlike patients with asthma, COPD patients will not respond to acute treatment with a bronchodilator; the improvement in $FEV_{1.0}$ is usually less than 10 to 15 percent.[10]

If airflow is directly measured during a forced vital capacity maneuver, both inspiratory and expiratory flow can be plotted against volume (flow-volume curve), and upper airway obstruction can be detected by decreases in inspiratory flow.

Characteristically, patients with COPD have an increased residual volume and an enlarged functional residual capacity. Total lung capacity is also enlarged. Lung compliance is increased, and diffusing capacity is either normal or mildly reduced. Arterial blood gas measurements show hypoxemia and a widened alveolar-arterial O_2 gradient; and with severe disease there may be hypercapnia.[1,2,10]

Malnutrition contributes to the reduction of the maximal force that can be generated by the inspiratory muscles. Patients with decreased sensitivity to changes in O_2 and CO_2 levels may not be able to compensate well for the increased load on the respiratory muscles caused by the heightened airway resistance. Ventilation is a poor index of respiratory output in COPD because respiratory mechanics are impaired. Thus, tests of respiratory regulation in COPD patients frequently use occlusion pressure or even the electrical activity of the respiratory muscles as a measure of respiratory chemoreceptor responses.[11,12]

OTHER ASSESSMENT TECHNIQUES

Typically the chest radiograph in COPD patients shows some or all of the following signs: a low, flattened diaphragm, an increased retrosternal airspace (greater than 4.5 cm), and a vertical heart. Bullae may be present and vascular markings are decreased; but in centrilobular emphysema, vascular markings may be more prominent than normal.

When there is significant bronchitis, bronchial markings may be enhanced. If fibrosis complicates COPD, cystic changes are found on radiographs. As pulmonary vascular pressure increases, blood vessels become prominent in the hila and these changes may need to be distinguished from tumor masses. Computed tomography (CT) or magnetic resonance imaging (MRI) may be useful in this regard. CT also is useful in delineating bullae.[13]

Erythrocytosis can be a result of hypoxemia and occasionally requires treatment. Leukocytosis suggests infection, and eosinophilia, the presence of allergies. Microscopic examination and culture of the sputum is useful. The most frequently encountered bacterial organisms in COPD are hemophilus, streptococcus pneumoniae, klebsiella, staphylococcus, and moraxella; but many respiratory infections in COPD are viral.

Determinations of serum alpha-1 antitrypsin levels can assist in the diagnosis and treatment of nonsmoking patients who develop COPD. Low concentrations of prealbumin may confirm the presence of malnutrition.[14,15]

The electrocardiogram in COPD typically shows exaggerated P waves in leads 2, 3, and AVF; prominent T waves in the same leads; and a vertical heart with counterclockwise rotation. Increased pulmonary vascular pressures may cause electrocardiographic signs of right ventricular hypertrophy and necessitate a more extensive evaluation with catheterization of the heart to assess the pulmonary circulation.[16]

EXERCISE TESTING

Exercise capacity depends considerably on the patient's perception and tolerance of dyspnea. Exercise tests help evaluate the current level of functioning. The exercise evaluation is best done using the same exercise mode as is planned during rehabilitation (e.g., treadmill for a walking training program). Ventilation, the heart rate, electrocardiogram, arterial oxygenation, and symptoms should be measured during the test. Expired gas analysis can be made to calculate oxygen uptake ($\dot{V}_{O_2}$). Noninvasive techniques such as transcutaneous oximetry to estimate arterial oxygen saturation can be used for continuous monitoring. In some patients it may be useful to measure blood lactate levels.[6–8,17]

NUTRITIONAL EVALUATION

Malnutrition is now recognized as common among patients with advanced emphysema and has been shown to adversely influence defense mechanisms as well as the function of the respiratory muscles.[11] Correction of anemia and electrolyte imbalances helps improve cardiopulmonary performance. To reduce dyspnea after meals the patient should take small amounts of food at more frequent intervals to lessen abdominal distention. Supplemental oxygen can be used at meal time if significant desaturation occurs. Finally, food high in carbohydrates may increase carbon dioxide production increasing minute ventilation thereby worsening dyspnea and decreasing exercise tolerance.

PSYCHOSOCIAL ASSESSMENT

Successful rehabilitation requires attention to psychological, emotional, and social problems.[6] Neuropsychological impairment is common in patients with COPD and cannot be explained just by physical disease. Commonly, patients become depressed, frightened, anxious, and more dependent on others to care for their needs.[6,18] Progressive dyspnea is frightening and may lead to a "fear-dyspnea" cycle, which can severely affect functional capacity and life quality. High stress and poor social support in one study of COPD patients were better predictors of subsequent hospitalizations than severity of illness.

Evaluation should include an assessment of the patient's psychological state and close attention should be given to the degree of family and social support, living arrangements, ability to perform activities of daily living, hobbies, and employment potential.[19,20] Nonverbal signals of the patient produced by changes in posture and facial expression may be informative. Cognitive impairment that may limit the ability to participate in the rehabilitation program is important to detect. Interviews with spouses, family members, and close friends may provide valuable insights.

Elements of a Comprehensive Treatment and Rehabilitation Program in COPD: General Approach

The complex difficulties that COPD patients encounter requires a multidisciplinary team approach to rehabilitation.[6-8,17] A physician who may be a pulmonologist or physiatrist usually directs the pulmonary rehabilitation team. This level of specialization and expertise is needed because of the many complicated problems which frequently arise during the rehabilitation process. The physician acts as team leader, educator, counselor, and motivator. Depending on the patients' needs, and the resources available, therapy may be administered by skilled professionals such as nurses, respiratory, physical or occupational therapists. The goal of the programs is to raise the patient to the highest possible level of physiologic and psychological function.

Comprehensive rehabilitation programs in COPD include the elements listed in Table 39-1. Not all patients require all program elements. Programs must be customized for each patient and carefully explained to both the patient and the patients' family. Objectives need to be clear. Every patient should be educated about COPD individually or in groups.

Patience is needed because patient compliance may be poor to demanding programs in which improvements occur slowly. Behavioral modification and support groups frequently help.

Smoking Cessation

Smoking cessation programs have met with only limited success, but can be effective even in the long time smoker

TABLE 39-1 Comprehensive Program of Treatment in COPD

1. Patient Evaluation
   History, physical, review of medical records
2. Laboratory Testing
   Pulmonary function tests, exercise testing, psychosocial assessment
3. Consultation with primary health care givers
   Patient and family to establish goals and set and explain treatment programs
4. Prevention of further lung injury
   Education, smoking cessation, immunization
5. Drug therapy
   Bronchodilators
   Anti-inflammatory agents
   Mucolytics
   Antibiotics
6. Oxygen
   During exercise, sleep, and continuously
7. Bronchial hygiene
8. Exercise
   Leg, arm
9. Training
   Ventilatory muscle exercise for strength and/or endurance
   Breathing (pursed lip, diaphragm use)
10. Psychosocial support
    Occupational therapy
    Group therapy
    Control of anxiety and depression
    Improve ability to carry on activities of daily living
11. Surgical
    Lung reduction therapy
    Lung transplantation

and in the elderly. The use of nicotine replacement therapy and the more recent use of antidepressants have considerably improved results of smoking cessation programs.

Medications

BRONCHODILATORS

Laboratory testing is of limited use in predicting the clinical efficacy of bronchodilator therapy in COPD. Hence it seems reasonable to suggest that there should be a clinical trial in all patients. Regular therapy should be continued if dyspnea, exercise tolerance, and cough is improved.[21,22]

Three classes of bronchodilator are available and appropriate for therapeutic trial: inhaled sympathomimetics (beta$_2$-agonists), inhaled anticholinergics, and oral sustained-release theophyllines. Combinations of two drugs are probably better than monotherapy.

SYMPATHOMIMETICS

Beta$_2$-agonists are commonly used for bronchodilatation in patients with COPD. Because of their selective beta$_2$ activity, effects on heart rate and rhythm resulting from the stimulation of beta$_1$-adrenergic receptors on the heart are minimized. Beta$_2$-agonists are preferentially administered by inhalation to further minimize circulatory side-effects and tremor that commonly accompany oral administration. Inhaled beta$_2$-agonists are usually given in a dosage of two puffs from a metered-dose inhaler every 6 h. During acute exacerbations it may be necessary to increase this dosage. Spacer devices improve aerosol deposition on intrathoracic airways.[21-23]

ANTICHOLINERGICS

Bronchial smooth muscles which regulate airway caliber are under cholinergic control, and anticholinergic therapy is useful in COPD.[24] Quaternary ammonium congeners of atropine, such as ipratropium bromide, have local anticholinergic actions and are not significantly absorbed and so do not produce significant systemic side effects. Ipratropium is selective for muscarinic receptor subtypes.[24,25] However, ipratropium, and possibly other quaternary agents, have less effect on inhibiting respiratory tract secretions than on relaxing airway smooth muscle. Anticholinergic agents have a slower onset of action and longer time to peak effect than do adrenergic agents. Typically, the peak effect following inhalation of an anticholinergic agent occurs at 60 to 120 min, compared with 15 min following an adrenergic agent. Its effect at peak bronchodilatation tends to persist longer and decline more slowly, particularly following larger doses of a quaternary agent. Anticholinergic agents which are usually administered by inhalation have their predominant effect on large airways. This contrasts with the action of adrenergic agents that dilate both central and peripheral airways.[24,26]

A very large number of trials have compared anticholinergic drugs to other bronchodilators in stable COPD. Trials that have employed conventional doses of each agent almost universally show that an anticholinergic agent results in more bronchodilatation than an adrenergic agent in this patient population. This finding contrast with studies in asthmatic patients which show that adrenergic agents are more effective bronchodilators. Some patients with COPD are resistant to adrenergic agents but respond well to anticholinergic agents. When recommended doses are used, a combination of anticholinergics and beta agonists may provide the speed of onset of the adrenergic with the prolonged duration of action of the anticholinergic together with the additive potency of the two agents at intermediate times.[24,26-28]

METHYLXANTHINES

They are available in oral and intravenous forms; the intravenous form is used for acute exacerbations and the oral form, in sustained-release formulation, for maintenance therapy.[29] The benefits of theophyllines are to an extent offset by their narrow therapeutic-toxic range and serum levels must be measured to guide management.

Theophyllines have useful effects aside from bronchodilatation. These include augmentation of cardiac and diaphragmatic contractility, lowering pulmonary vascular resistance, and enhancement of mucociliary clearance.

CORTICOSTEROIDS

Numerous studies have evaluated the efficacy of steroids in stable COPD, but less than 10 percent of patients show a significant increase in FEV_1 after 2 weeks of 40 mg of prednisone daily. On the other hand, some believe that a significant response to steroids can be predicted from responsiveness to inhaled bronchodilator and from the presence of eosinophils in sputum. Inhaled steroids are less effective in COPD than they are in asthma and they are associated with oropharyngeal candidiasis and dysphonia.[30] When symptoms of COPD are poorly controlled by standard medications with theophylline, anticholinergic agents, and beta$_2$-agonists, a trial of corticosteroid therapy seems justified and is warranted.

MUCOLYTICS AND ANTIBIOTICS

Iodide compounds are frequently used as mucolytics but hydration may work equally well. Overhydration should be avoided.

Even if there is no obvious bacterial etiology, many physicians use antibiotics (e.g., ampicillin) when the sputum in patients with COPD becomes purulent. Certainly respiratory infections need to be treated early. Recently, a number of new macrolide agents and quinolones became available for use in acute infectious exacerbations of COPD.[23,31,32]

Bronchial Hygiene

As part of a comprehensive program, each patient's needs for chest physiotherapy to enhance mucociliary clearance and removal of secretions should be assessed and instruction provided in best techniques. These are especially important for patients with heavy sputum production (more than 30 ml/day) during acute exacerbations and as a prevention measure.

Several studies have reported benefits from these techniques which include controlled coughing, postural drainage, vibration and/or percussion.[33] Available evidence suggests that postural drainage and controlled coughing (or the forced expiration technique) may be the most effective components. Inhalation of nebulized saline or bronchodilator, may increase secretion clearance. IPPB alone is not effective.[34]

Oxygen Therapy

Hypoxemia in COPD patients is caused by ventilation-perfusion mismatching and can be corrected by low-flow oxygen administration. Hypoxemia has been shown to induce pulmonary vasoconstriction and secondary polycythemia. The increased blood viscosity resulting from an elevated hematocrit level increases vascular resistance, worsens heart failure, and decreases cerebrovascular perfusion.

Neff and Petty first showed that long-term home oxygen therapy could improve survival in patients with severe hypoxemia.[35] Two controlled clinical trials have demonstrated conclusively that long-term oxygen therapy prolongs life in COPD. These two studies reported data on patients who had fixed airways obstruction and chronic hypoxemia ($P_{O_2} < 55$ mmHg, when breathing air when awake). Many had CO_2 retention, and modest pulmonary hypertension. The results indicated that without oxygen, only about 30 percent of patients survive for 3 years, that oxygen for 12 to 15 h per day produces a significant improvement in survival, and that the best survival is obtained when oxygen is given for more than 19 h per day.[36,37]

Expectations that oxygen therapy would reverse pulmonary hypertension and polycythemia have been partially fulfilled. Neuropsychiatric assessments (e.g., intelligence quotient, brain age quotient, and average impairment rating), have shown improvement after 6 months of oxygen therapy. These encouraging results suggest that any patient with advanced lung disease should be assessed for oxygen therapy.[36,37]

Any patient who, after optimal medical therapy, has an arterial Pa_{O_2} equal to or less than 55 mmHg, should receive continuous (24-h) supplemental oxygen. If the Pa_{O_2} is between 55 and 59 mmHg but the patient has polycythemia, heart failure, or "p" pulmonale on electrocardiogram, supplemental oxygen should be administered to raise the Pa_O to above 60 mmHg. Because an elevated Pa_{O_2} occasionally induces CO_2 retention, arterial blood gases should be measured after oxygen administration. If there is no rise in arterial partial pressure of carbon dioxide (Pa_{CO_2}), the patient can be followed with simple determinations of transcutaneous oxygen saturation. Because COPD patients with adequate resting Pa_{O_2} may develop significant hypoxemia during exercise or sleep, they may require long-term supplemental oxygen for those activities.[36,37]

Nasal cannula is the usual method of supplying O_2. Transtracheal oxygen with a small catheter has gained popularity because it is cosmetically more appealing and, often, more comfortable. Oxygen-conserving devices may be used such as devices with a reservoir and devices that deliver oxygen only during inspiration.

Oxygen may be supplied in the form of cylinders of compressed gas, liquid oxygen, or by an electric powered concentrator. The long-term goals of oxygen therapy should be thoroughly understood by the patient because the benefits may not be noticeable in the short-term.

Exercise Conditioning

Exercise conditioning is based on the principle that training will occur only when exercise intensity reaches a critical level that stresses the peripheral muscles. In general, training effects are specific, so that improvement is limited to the particular form of exercise that is practiced. A number of controlled trials show that exercise conditioning significantly reduces the sense of dyspnea in COPD patients. The improvement seen has been attributed to a desensitization to dyspnea. In addition, a significant increase in muscle enzymes involved in oxidative metabolism has been demonstrated after exercise conditioning. A reduction in lactic acidosis with training has also been reported.[6-8,10]

Patients may increase their maximum capacity and/or endurance for physical activity even though lung function does not usually change. Patients may also benefit from learning to perform physical tasks more efficiently. Exercise training also provides an ideal opportunity for patients to learn their limits for work and to use methods for controlling dyspnea (e.g., breathing and relaxation techniques).[3,8,39-41]

To be successful, the program should be tailored to the individual patient and be based on the results of initial exercise testing. Training should use methods easily adapted to the home setting such as walking which is particularly useful for older and physically limited patients. Other types of exercise such as cycling and swimming are also effective. But it is best that techniques used be simple and inexpensive. Patients should try to incorporate exercise into the daily activities they enjoy. Because many patients with COPD have limited

exercise tolerance, increasing endurance should be emphasized. Changes in exercise endurance are often greater than changes in maximal exercise levels attained.[6-8]

EXERCISE PRESCRIPTION

The selection of training targets is usually based on achieving certain percentages of maximum heart rate or $\dot{V}_{O_2}$. In healthy people targets are often 50 to 60 percent of maximum. In patients with chronic lung diseases, however, the best method of choosing an appropriate training prescription is not clearly defined. Exercise tolerance in patients with advanced lung disease is often limited by the reduced ventilatory capacity and breathlessness, rather than by cardiac or peripheral muscle performance. On the other hand, Wasserman and coworkers reported that about two thirds of patients with moderate to severe COPD will have a significant metabolic acidosis develop during exercise.[42] For these patients exercise training may increase the capacity for aerobic work and reduce the rate of lactate production.

Many patients, even with advanced COPD, can be trained at exercise levels approaching their maximum exercise tolerance and achieve levels of ventilation during exercise training that approach their maximum voluntary ventilation. In one study, patients achieved a sustained exercise workload of 86 percent of the baseline maximum workload after 8 weeks of training.[43] In another study, after 3 months of training, patients were able to reach a peak exercise ventilation of nearly 100 percent of their maximum voluntary ventilation.[44]

Some pulmonary rehabilitation programs define exercise targets by symptom tolerance rather than by heart rate, work level or other physiologic measurements. Ratings of perceived symptoms such as breathlessness, help patients to exercise to "target" levels of breathing discomfort. Therefore, after the initial exercise test to assess a patient's maximal exercise tolerance, the patient begins training at a level sustainable with reasonable comfort for several minutes. Increases in time or level of exercise are then made according to the patient's symptom tolerance. Patients can be encouraged to exercise daily and to increase exercise time up to 15 to 30 min of continuous activity to improve their tolerance for the sustained activity required for tasks of daily living.[6,8,9]

UPPER-EXTREMITY EXERCISE

Exercise conditioning in COPD patients has emphasized lower extremity use as in walking or riding a bicycle.[7,8] But some patients with COPD report severe dyspnea during daily activities that require the use of their arms. Ventilation is greater at a given work level with arm than leg exercise. Arm muscles can serve both respiratory and postural functions. The muscles of the shoulder girdle support the upper rib cage and in patients with severe COPD, they provide important assistance with breathing. When the arms are used for lifting, reaching, or carrying, they are unable to assist with breathing. If the arms are trained to perform more work or if the ventilatory requirement for the same work is decreased, the capacity to carry out usual daily activities is improved. Reis and colleagues found that training programs that involved the upper extremities specifically improved the function of only those arm muscles trained.[45]

Arm exercise can be performed by using an arm ergometer or by gravity resistive methods. In the first method, the arms are supported but not in the second. Unsupported arm exercise seems to be more effective. Unsupported arm training has been shown to reduce oxygen uptake at the same workload compared with arm cranking training.[46]

Celli and coworkers randomized 26 patients with COPD to either unsupported arm training (11 patients) or resistance breathing training (14 patients).[47] After 24 sessions, arm endurance increased only for the unsupported arm training group and not for the group who practiced resistance breathing. Maximal inspiratory pressure increased significantly for both groups. Although this suggests a possible effect of arm training on respiratory muscle function, other studies with similar objectives have found no change in ventilatory muscle performance.[47]

Breathing Retraining

Breathing retraining tries to teach patients a breathing pattern that will decrease dyspnea and the work of breathing by improving the position and function of the respiratory muscles. One maneuver is pursed lip breathing. Patients inhale through the nose and exhale for 4 to 6 seconds through lips pursed in a whistling position. Because the levator palatini is elevated, the nasopharynx is occluded and the air exits through the mouth. The exact mechanism by which pursed lip breathing decreases dyspnea is unknown.[6–8,10,48,49] Pursed lip breathing prolongs exhalation, slows breathing frequency, and may decrease the end-expiratory lung volume and thereby improve the mechanical advantage of the inspiratory muscles.

Breathing while leaning forward with the arms supported decreases dyspnea in some patients with severe COPD, both at rest and during exercise. This posture may lengthen the accessory muscles of the neck so that they can contract more effectively.[6–8]

Abdominal compression increases gastric pressure and this may serve to lengthen the diaphragm and place it in a better position to generate force. With improved diaphragmatic contraction, the use of accessory muscles is diminished and dyspnea may be ameliorated. With abdominal strapping or weights on the abdomen, breathing often becomes slower and deeper and overall ventilation decreases.[48]

Diaphragmatic breathing aims at changing the breathing pattern from one in which the rib cage muscles predominate to a more normal pattern, in which the diaphragm predominates. The patient starts the training in the supine position and then trains upright two or three times a day for about 20 min. The patient tries to inspire while displacing a hand on the abdomen. The patient then exhales with pursed lips while using the abdominal muscles to return the diaphragm to a more lengthened resting position. Although many patients report improvement in dyspnea, diaphragmatic breathing results in minimal, if any, improvement in gas exchange. Some reports actually indicate that diaphragmatic breathing increases the work of breathing.

Ventilatory Muscle Training

Leigh and Bradley first demonstrated that respiratory muscle like skeletal muscle could be trained to increase strength and endurance.[50] Training has generally focused on the inspira-

tory muscles. High-tension, low-repetition tasks such as breathing against very large resistive or threshold ventilatory loads increases respiratory muscle strength, while low-tension, high-repetition training by voluntary isocapnic hyperventilation increases respiratory muscle endurance.[51,52] These maneuvers often improve strength as well. Although ventilatory muscle training may result in improved ventilatory muscle function or symptoms for some patients with COPD, it is not yet clear that training helps everyone.[17] It is likely that more research is needed to identify patients who will benefit from this type of training.[17]

Respiratory Muscle Rest

Patients with severe COPD are predisposed to develop respiratory muscle fatigue. A critical factor in the development of fatigue is the percentage of maximal muscle tension (P/Pmax) generated in a required task and the length of inspiration as a fraction of the total respiratory cycle time.[53,54] Their product TTI (tension time index) determines if fatigue will occur. Recent studies indicate that respiratory muscle endurance at a given TTI also depends on the velocity of muscle shortening. Increases in the velocity of airflow during inspiration and increases in lung volume diminish inspiratory muscle endurance.

The force reserve of the diaphragm in COPD patients is markedly reduced because hyperinflation alters the length and shape of the diaphragm and reduces maximal transdiaphragmatic pressure. In addition, hypoxemia, hypercapnia, and/or malnutrition further impair function, both by increasing the demand for ventilation and by diminishing maximal force. Patients with COPD, therefore are predisposed to develop respiratory muscle fatigue with increases in ventilation or changes in breathing pattern.

Therapy in COPD aims at reducing the load on the muscles in addition to improving respiratory muscle contractility by alleviating airway obstruction, by controlling secretions and by correcting derangements in Pa_{O_2} and Pa_{CO_2}. Theoretically, respiratory muscle contractility can be enhanced pharmacologically (e.g., by methylxanthines, beta-agonists), by oxygen, and by proper nutritional support. Ventilatory muscle training as described may be beneficial. However, once a respiratory muscle fatigues, rest is the preferred form of treatment.

Studies of intermittent ventilatory support in patients with severe COPD have yielded conflicting results. Braun and Marino provided 4 to 10 h of daily ventilatory support (uncontrolled) to 18 patients, 13 of whom suffered from hypercapnia and severe COPD.[55] Results following mechanical ventilation were compared to data obtained during the baseline period. Following 5 months of daily intermittent ventilation, increases were noted in vital capacity and maximum inspired pressures. Pa_{CO_2} fell while the number of days of hospitalization were also reduced by ventilation support. However, other studies have failed to show any increase in respiratory muscle strength or exercise endurance with intermittent mechanical ventilation in patients with COPD.[56]

Most studies using intermittent mechanical ventilation to rest the respiratory muscles in patients with severe COPD are difficult to evaluate because they included only small numbers of patients and lacked proper controls or were not conducted in a prospective fashion. Furthermore, most studies did not satisfactorily document that respiratory muscle rest actually occurred during mechanical ventilation.

Psychosocial Support

An essential component of a comprehensive pulmonary rehabilitation program is psychosocial support to combat feelings of hopelessness and inability to cope with the disease.[57-60] Patients may show symptoms of anxiety and isolation and are often forced to rely on family, friends, and medical services to provide for their needs. Overconcern with physical problems is common. Fear of sexual activities is frequent in patients with COPD but this can be alleviated by advice from physicians. COPD patients may have neuropsychological dysfunction that may be related to arterial oxygen desaturation.

Psychosocial support is provided best by a caring well-motivated staff who have good communication skills. Key family members should be included in educational programs so that they help provide support. Group therapy may be effective as may be innovative approaches such as art and music therapy.

Jensen measured stress and social support in 59 patients with COPD and randomly assigned 30 "high-risk" patients to a pulmonary rehabilitation, self-help support, or a control group. She found that the "high-risk" control subjects were hospitalized significantly more frequently than either "low-risk" or "high-risk" patients in the rehabilitation or self-help groups.[61]

Relaxation Training

Because dyspnea in COPD is made worse by fear and anxiety, relaxation training techniques have been used in some pulmonary rehabilitation programs. Progressive muscle relaxation training, which involved sequentially tensing and then relaxing 16 different muscle groups, was evaluated in 10 patients with COPD and compared with a control group that was advised to relax but not given specific instructions.[62] After the relaxation sessions, the experimental group demonstrated significantly greater reduction in dyspnea and anxiety than the control group. Changes in dyspnea were significantly correlated with change in anxiety.

Quality of Life

With rehabilitation, quality of life may improve because of decreased respiratory symptoms, better exercise tolerance and physical activity, more independence and ability to perform activities of daily living and increased feelings of hope and self-esteem. Several "quality of life" instruments that incorporate aspects of physical, emotional, and psychological function into a small number of measures are used in the evaluation of patients with COPD.[17,20,63]

A disease-specific measure that has been used frequently is the chronic respiratory questionnaire (CRQ) developed by Guyatt and colleagues.[64] In a long-term study of multidisciplinary pulmonary rehabilitation in 31 consecutive patients, Guyatt and coworkers, using the CRQ, found that 24 demonstrated improvement in all four measured dimensions of quality of life (dyspnea, fatigue, emotional function, mastery) after rehabilitation.

The quality of well-being scale is a comprehensive measure of health-related quality of life. The quality of well-being scale is considered to be valid for evaluating interventions that affect general health status. Atkins and coworkers reported greater changes in the quality of well-being in three experimental exercise and behavioral groups compared with a no-treatment control group.[65] The investigators concluded that even a modest treatment program resulted in significant cost-benefits for these patients. However, in a subsequent randomized clinical trial of pulmonary rehabilitation in 119 patients with COPD, no significant changes were observed in well-being in either treatment or control groups despite marked changes in exercise tolerance and breathlessness after rehabilitation.

Treatment Compliance

A number of studies have reported high levels of noncompliance with prescribed medical regimens by COPD patients. Only half the patients in the multicenter Intermittent Positive Pressure Breathing (IPPB) Trial sponsored by the National Heart, Lung, and Blood Institute, used their IPPB machines as instructed.[66] Another study showed that despite improvements in inspiratory force and walking ability, many patients failed to continue exercise after a program of exercise with O_2 and inspiratory muscle training concluded.[67] There are several possible explanations for noncompliance with treatment regimens. Patients and caregivers can have different opinions as to the efficacy of treatment. If a physician recommends a treatment that the patient does not perceive to be effective, the patient may be noncompliant. Better patient education may improve compliance and health outcomes in COPD.

Behavioral Modification

Various strategies have been shown to be effective in promoting voluntary changes in behavior. The strategies used are all loosely based on the principles of social learning theory.[68]

According to social learning theory, individuals are motivated to perform in a particular way if they believe that the behavior leads to a desirable consequence and because the behavior can actually be performed well enough to produce a desired outcome.

There are four major ways that personal expectations of efficacy can be altered:

Practicing the behavior
Seeing others perform it
Encouragement and positive reinforcement
Techniques to overcome fear of the behavior

Kaplan and colleagues have applied behavior modification techniques to the management of COPD.[69] To increase compliance with an exercise program in COPD, they randomly assigned patients to one of five groups: behavior modification, cognitive modification, behavior-cognitive modification, attention only, or no treatment. Patients who received some form of intervention directed at behavior modification

TABLE 39-2 Potential Effects of Rehabilitation

1. Reduction of hospitalization, emergency room
2. Less dyspnea, depression fear
3. Improved quality of life, information about disease and independence
4. Little change in pulmonary function
5. Longer survival with O_2 therapy

exercised more and achieved better results from exercise (well-being and exercise tolerance) than did patients who received attention only or no treatment.

Lung Reduction Surgery

Much of the pathophysiology of COPD is related to over-distention of the lungs and over-expansion of the thorax.[12] If the over-distended regions could be removed, one might expect changes in lung volume, thoracic size and considerable improvement in the actions of both inspiratory and expiratory muscle. For example, in some patients, COPD takes the form of bullous emphysema in which there are a few giant air sacs (bullae) while the intervening lung is normal.[13] In this case resection of the bullae may dramatically improve lung function and blood gases.[70] Best results are obtained in patients with giant bullae which occupy more than one third of a lung and when $FEV_{1.0}$ is less that 50 percent of predicted value. The technique has been improved by the use of lasers through a thoracoscope to destroy bullae.[71,72]

In 1995, Cooper and colleagues reported their experience with volume reduction surgery in patients with severe emphysema in whom 25 to 30 percent of each lung had been removed through a median sternotomy.[9] In the relatively small group of patients thus far studied, lung function, arterial blood gases, exercise tolerance, and quality of life measures have improved.

All patients who are being considered for lung volume reduction surgery should first be enrolled in an exercise rehabilitation program for 6 to 8 weeks before being finally accepted for surgery. Experience has shown that exercise tolerance reaches a plateau at about 2 months. Preoperatively, even after maximal therapy, the average $FEV_{1.0}$ has been less than 750 ml. Over 90 percent of the patients used O_2 at rest or during exercise. The mortality rate of the operative procedure is 5 percent.

Lung transplantation is a final resort when lung reduction surgery is not possible and is used in patients whose age is less than 60 and whose life expectancy is less than 2 years. Those patients should be nonsmokers with no complicating disease. Single lung transplants are now generally used instead of combined heart-lung transplantation.

Efficacy of Rehabilitation Programs in COPD

Table 39-2 lists the potential benefits of a comprehensive treatment program. In a recent special report, a committee composed of members of the American Association of Cardiovascular and Pulmonary Rehabilitation and the American College of Chest Physicians reviewed studies on pulmonary rehabilitation and suggested some guidelines for treatment.[17] They recommended that a rehabilitation program for patients with COPD include a program of lower extremity and upper extremity exercises with ventilatory muscle training in selected patients. They felt that while the evidence is not conclusive, education and psychosocial interventions should be a part of the comprehensive rehabilitation program for patients with COPD. Besides these opinions the report is an excellent review of many of the studies of pulmonary rehabilitation in patients with COPD.

References

1. American Thoracic Society: Standards for the diagnosis and care of patients with chronic obstructive pulmonary disease (COPD) and asthma. *Am Rev Respir Dis* 136:225, 1987.
2. Fletcher C, Pride N: Definitions of emphysema, chronic bronchitis, asthma, and airflow obstruction; 25 years GBA symposium. *Thorax* 89:81, 1984.
3. Huchon G: Risk factors for chronic bronchitis and obstructive lung disease. *Respiration* 58 (Suppl):10, 1991.
4. Burrows B: Airways obstructive diseases: Pathogenetic mechanisms and natural histories of the disorders. *Med Clin North Am* 74:547, 1990.
5. Novitch RS: Pulmonary rehabilitation: An overview with evidence for its utility in chronic obstructive pulmonary disease. *Am J Managed Care* 3:1735–1741, 1997.
6. Reis AL: Pulmonary rehabilitation. *Curr Pulmonol* 15:441–463, 1994.
7. Celli BR: Pulmonary rehabilitation for patients with advanced lung disease. *Clin Chest Med* 18:521–534, 1997.
8. Tiep BL: Disease management of COPD with pulmonary rehabilitation. *Chest* 112:1630–1656, 1997.
9. Cooper JD, Trulock EP, Triantafillou AN, et al: Bilateral pneumonectomy (volume reduction) for chronic obstructive pulmonary disease. *J Thorac Cardiovasc Surg* 109:106–119, 1995.
10. Pride NB: The assessment of airflow obstruction: role of measurement of airway resistance and tests of forced expiration. *Br J Dis Chest* 65:135, 1971.
11. Edelman NH, Rucker RB, Pear HH: NIH workshop summary: Nutrition and the respiratory system. Chronic Obstructive pulmonary disease. *Am Rev Respir Dis* 134:347, 1986.
12. Zackon H, Despas I, Anthonisen NR: Occlusion pressure responses in asthma and chronic obstructive pulmonary disease. *Am Rev Respir Dis* 114:417, 1979.
13. Hayhorst MD, MacNee W, Flenely DC, et al: The diagnosis of emphysema. A computer tomographic pathologic correlation. *Am Rev Respir Dis* 133:541, 1986.
14. Larrson C: Natural history and life expectancy in severe alpha1-antitrypsin deficiency. *Acta Med Scand* 204:345, 1978.
15. Janoff A: Elastases and emphysema. Current assessment of protease-antiprotease hypothesis. *Am Rev Respir Dis* 134:147, 1985.
16. Millard FTC: The electrocardiogram in chronic lung disease. *Br Heart J* 29:43, 1967.
17. ACCP/AACVPR Pulmonary Rehabilitation Guidelines Panel: Pulmonary rehabilitation: Joint ACCP/AACVPR Evidence-Based Guidelines. *Chest* 112:1363–1396, 1997.
18. Sandhu HS: Psychosocial issued in chronic obstructive pulmonary disease. *Clin Chest Med* 7:629–642, 1986.
19. Jensen PS: Risk, protective factors, and supportive interventions in chronic airway obstruction. *Arch Gen Psychiatry* 40:1203–1207, 1983.
20. Dudley DL, Sitzman J: Psychobiological evaluation and treatment of COPD, in McSweeney AJ, Grant I (eds): *Chronic Obstructive*

Pulmonary Disease: A Behavioral Perspective, New York, Marcel Dekker, 1988:39–57.

21. Anthonisen NR, Wright EC, IPPB Group: Response to inhaled bronchodilators in COPD. *Chest* 19(Suppl 5):365, 1987.

22. Rebuck AS, Chapman KR, Abbood R, et al: Nebulized anticholinergic and sympathomimetic treatment of asthma and chronic obstructive airways disease in the emergency room. *Am J Med* 82:59, 1987.

23. Ferguson GT, Cherniack RM: Management of chronic obstructive pulmonary disease. *N Engl J Med* 328:1017–1022, 1993.

24. Anthonisen NR, Connett JE, Kiley JP, et al: Effects of smoking cessation and inhaled anticholinergic bronchodilators on the rate of decline of FEV1: The Lung Health Study. *JAMA* 272:1497–1505, 1994.

25. Mann JS, George CF: Anticholinergic drugs in the treatment of airways disease. *Br J Dis Chest* 79:209–228, 1985.

26. Tashkin DP, Ashutosh K, Bleecker ER, et al: Comparison of the anticholinergic bronchodilator ipratropium bromide with meta proterenol in chronic obstructive pulmonary disease: A 90-day multicenter study. *Am J Med* 81(Suppl 5A):81–89, 1986.

27. Rennard SI, Serby CW, Ghafoori M, et al: Extended therapy with ipratropium is associated with improved lung function in patients with COPD: A retrospective analysis of data from seven clinical trials. *Chest* 110:62–70, 1996.

28. Georgopoulos D, Wang D, Anthonisen NR: Tolerance to beta$_2$ agonists in patients with chronic obstructive pulmonary disease. *Chest* 97:280–289, 1990.

29. Dull WL, Alexander MR, Kasik JR: Isoproterenol challenge during placebo and oral theophylline therapy in chronic obstructive pulmonary disease. *Am Rev Respir Dis* 123:340, 1987.

30. Renkema TE, Schooten JP, Koeter GH et al: Effects of long-term treatment with corticosteroids in COPD. *Chest* 109:1156–1162, 1996.

31. Saint S, Bent S, Vittinghoff E, et al: Antibiotics in chronic obstructive pulmonary disease exacerbations. *JAMA* 273:957–960, 1995.

32. Jacoby GA: Prevalence and resistance mechanisms of common bacterial respiratory pathogens. *Clin Infect Dis* 18:951–957, 1994.

33. Kirilloff LH, Owens GR, Rogers RM, et al: Does chest physical therapy work? *Chest* 88:436–444, 1985.

34. Sutton PP: Chest physiotherapy a time for a reappraisal. *Br J Dis Chest* 82:127–137, 1988.

35. Neff RA, Petty TL: Long-term continuous oxygen therapy with chronic airways obstruction. *Ann Intern Med* 72:621–626, 1970.

36. Nocturnal Oxygen Trial Group: Continuous or nocturnal oxygen therapy in hypoxemic chronic obstructive pulmonary disease. *Ann Intern Med* 93:391–398, 1980.

37. Medical Research Council Working Group: Long term domicillary oxygen therapy in chronic hypoxic corpulmonale complicating chronic bronchitis and emphysema. *Lancet* 1:681–686, 1981.

38. Foster S, Lopez D, Thomas HM: Pulmonary rehabilitation in COPD patients with an elevated P_{CO_2}. *Am Rev Respir Dis* 138:1519–1523, 1988.

39. Vale F, Reardon JZ, SuWallack RL: The long-term benefits of outpatient pulmonary rehabilitation on exercise endurance and quality of life. *Chest* 103:42–45, 1993.

40. Casaburi R, Patessio A, Ioli F, et al: Reductions in exercise lactic acidosis and ventilation as a result of exercise training in patients with obstructive lung disease. *Am Rev Respir Dis* 143:9–18, 1991.

41. Maltais F, LeBlanc P, Simard C, et al: Skeletal muscle adaptation to endurance training in patients with chronic obstructive pulmonary disease. *Am J Respir Crit Care Med* 154:442–447, 1996.

42. Wasserman K, Sue DY, Casaburi R, et al: Selection criteria for exercise training in pulmonary rehabilitation. *Eur Respir J* 2(Suppl 2):604S–610S, 1989.

43. Punzal PA, Reis AL, Kaplan RM, et al: Maximum intensity exercise in patients with chronic obstructive pulmonary disease. *Chest* 100:618–623, 1991.

44. Carter R, Nicotra B, Clark L, et al: Exercise reconditioning in the rehabilitation of patients with chronic obstructive pulmonary disease. *Arch Phys Med Rehabil* 69:118–122, 1988.

45. Reis AL, Ellis B, Hawkins RW: Upper extremity exercise training in chronic obstructive pulmonary disease. *Chest* 93:688–692, 1988.

46. Martinez FJ, Vogel PD, Dupont DN, et al: Supported arm exercise vs. unsupported arm exercise in the rehabilitation of patients with chronic airflow obstruction. *Chest* 103:1397, 1993.

47. Celli BR: The clinical use of upper extremity exercise. *Clin Chest Med* 15:339, 1994.

48. Rochester DF, Goldberg SK: Techniques of respiratory physical therapy. *Am Rev Respir Dis* 122(Suppl):133–146, 1980.

49. Paul G, Elridge F, Mitchell J, et al: Some effects of slowing respiration rate in chronic emphysema and bronchitis. *J Appl Physiol* 21:877–882, 1966.

50. Leith DE, Bradley M: Ventilatory muscle strength and endurance training. *J Appl Physiol* 4:508, 1976.

51. Levine S, Weiser P, Gillen J: Evaluation of a ventilatory muscle endurance training program in the rehabilitation of patients with chronic obstructive pulmonary disease. *Am Rev Respir Dis* 33:400, 1986.

52. Lisboa C, Munoz V, Berioza T, et al: Inspiratory muscle training in chronic airflow limitation: Comparison of two different training loads with a threshold device. *Eur Respir J* 7:1266, 1994.

53. MacKlem PT, Roussos CS: Respiratory muscle fatigue: A cause of respiratory failure? *Clin Sci Mol Med* 53:419–422, 1977.

54. Clanton TL, Dixon GF, Drake J, Gadek JE: Effects of breathing on inspiratory muscle endurance in humans. *J Appl Physiol* 60:299–320, 1986.

55. Braun NMT, Marino W: Effect of daily intermittent rest of respiratory muscles in patients with severe airflow limitation (CAO). *Chest* 85(Suppl):59–60, 1984.

56. Lee H, Criner G, Rassulo J, et al: A controlled study of rehabilitation vs. rehabilitation and respiratory muscle resting with negative external ventilation in patients with severe COPD. *Am Rev Respir Dis* 133:A168, 1985.

57. McSweeny AJ, Grant I, Heaton RK, et al: Life quality of patients with chronic obstructive pulmonary disease. *Arch Intern Med* 142:473–478, 1982.

58. Porzelius J, Vest M, Nochomovitz M: Respiratory function, cognitions, and panic in chronic obstructive pulmonary patients. *Behav Res Ther* 301:75–77, 1992.

59. Keele-Card G, Foxall MJ, Barron CR: Loneliness, depression and social support of patients with COPD and their spouses. *Public Health Nurs* 10:245–251, 1993.

60. Inculzi RA, Gemma A, Marra C, et al: Chronic obstructive pulmonary disease: An original model of cognitive decline. *Am Rev Respir Dis* 148:418–424, 1993.

61. Jensen PS: Risk, protective factors, and supportive interventions in chronic airways obstruction. *Arch Gen Psychiatry* 40:1203–1207, 1983.

62. Renfroe KL: Effect of progressive relaxation on dyspnea and state of anxiety in patients with chronic obstructive pulmonary disease. *Heart Lung* 17:408–413, 1988.

63. Cox JM, Hendricks JC, Binkhorst RA, et al: A pulmonary rehabilitation program for patients with asthma and mild chronic obstructive lung disease. *Lung* 171:235–244, 1993.

64. Guyatt GH, Berman LB, Townsend M, et al: A measure of quality of life for clinical trials in chronic lung disease. *Thorax* 42:773–778, 1987.

65. Atkins CJ, Kaplan RM, Timms RL, et al: Behavioral exercise programs in the management of chronic obstructive pulmonary disease. *J Consul Clin Psychol* 52:591–603, 1944.

66. Intermittent Positive Pressure Breathing Trial Group: Intermittent positive pressure breathing therapy of chronic obstructive pulmonary disease: A clinical trial. *Ann Intern Med* 99:612–620, 1983.

67. Zack MB, Palange AV: Oxygen-supplemented exercise of ventilatory and non-ventilatory muscles in pulmonary rehabilitation. *Chest* 88:669–675, 1988.

68. Bandura A: Self-efficacy: Toward a unified theory of behavioral change. *Psychol Rev* 84:191–215, 1977.

69. Kaplan RM, Atkins CJ, Timms R: Validity of a quality of well being scale as an outcome measure in chronic obstructive pulmonary disease. *Chest* 64:317–322, 1973.

70. Rogers RM, Dubois AB, Blakemore WS: Effect of removal of bullae on airway conductance and conductance-volume ratios. *J Clin Invest* 47:2569–2579.

71. Brenner M, Kayaleh RA, Milne EN, et al: Thorascopic laser ablation of pulmonary bullae: Radiographic selection and treatment response. *J Thorac Carciovasc Surg* 107:883–900, 1994.

72. Cooper JD: Lung transplantation: A new era. *Ann Thorac Surg* 44:447, 1987.

Chapter 40

MANAGEMENT OF NEUROMUSCULAR DISEASES

PEGGY M. SIMON

Many of the same principles of pulmonary rehabilitation that operate for patients with chronic obstructive pulmonary disease (COPD) can be applied to patients with neuromuscular disorders. The goal to restore patients to an independent, productive, and quality life may not always be obtainable, particularly during the latter stages of disease. However, even in those patients who spend the majority of their life on ventilatory assistance through pulmonary rehabilitation, certain interventions can decrease the risk of complications, such as pneumonia, and can improve certain aspects of health-related quality of life. Patients may be better able to assume responsibility for their management decisions and for directing those who provide rehabilitative care. Unlike patients with COPD, patients with neuromuscular disease frequently have nonpulmonary impairments that need to be addressed as part of a rehabilitation program.

The first two sections of this chapter provide a brief overview of the pathophysiology of respiratory muscle weakness and of specific features of the more common neuromuscular disorders. The remainder of the chapter is devoted to a discussion of the management of patients with neuromuscular disorders.

Pathophysiology of Neuromuscular Weakness

Ventilatory failure may appear at the onset of the disease (e.g., Guillain-Barré syndrome and myasthenia gravis) or may develop slowly over years (e.g., muscular dystrophy and amyotrophic lateral sclerosis). The acute syndrome is frequently characterized by involvement of inspiratory and expiratory muscles, a rapid decline in vital capacity, and a rapid progression of alveolar hypoventilation. The mechanisms responsible for the development of chronic respiratory failure in patients with chronic neuromuscular disorders are usually multiple and include not only the direct effect of respiratory muscle weakness but also altered mechanical properties of the lungs and of the chest wall and "(mal)adaptive" changes in the respiratory center.

PULMONARY MECHANICS

A number of studies have confirmed that vital capacity (VC) is reduced as a consequence of respiratory muscle weakness and continues to decrease as the disease progresses.[1,2] VC is frequently used to follow the disease process. Although VC is highly correlated with respiratory muscle strength, the reductions in VC are usually greater than expected for the degree of respiratory muscle weakness[3,4] (Fig. 40-1). The disproportionate loss of VC is related to alterations in the mechanical properties of the lung and chest wall. Whether consistent changes occur in functional residual capacity (FRC) and residual volume (RV) is debated.[5-7] Differences in patient populations, extent of involvement of muscle groups, and the position in which patients were studied may explain these conflicting observations.

Many patients with long-standing severe respiratory muscle weakness have reduced lung distensibility,[4,8] an important determinant of volume loss in these patients. Several mechanisms have been proposed. One mechanism is an overall increase in the surface tension of the alveolar lining due to breathing at a low lung volume.[9,10] The second mechanism is an alteration in lung tissue elasticity[8,11-13] related to a chronic limited range of movement of the lung. Both mechanisms are plausible; however, direct evidence is lacking for either of these mechanisms. Patients with long-standing neuromuscular disorders also have been shown to have a decrease in chest wall compliance to approximately two-thirds of normal values[14,15] resulting from an increase in the stiffness of the rib cage.

The effectiveness of cough is significantly reduced in patients with neuromuscular diseases secondary to weak expiratory muscles. Normally, cough produces vigorous contractions of expiratory muscles that lead to large positive-pressure swings. These pressure swings cause dynamic compression of the intrathoracic airways, resulting in high flow velocities that cause suspension and propulsion of secretions toward the mouth. In patients with expiratory muscle weakness, pleural pressures generated with coughing are decreased and, therefore, so are flow velocities. This impairment in the clearance of secretions is a significant contributor to the high incidence of bronchopulmonary infections in these patients.

CONTROL OF BREATHING

Patients with respiratory muscle weakness develop a breathing pattern similar to that of patients with interstitial lung disease, i.e., a faster breathing rate and smaller tidal volumes.[11,16,17] Several potential mechanisms have been proposed for this altered breathing pattern. Vagal-mediated reflexes related to pulmonary stretch receptors are one potential mechanism for the tachypnea seen in patients with respiratory muscle weakness whose pulmonary compliance is reduced. An alternative mechanism for the tachypnea may be related to altered afferent feedback from the weakened respiratory muscles themselves.[16]

Hypoventilation and blunted responses to carbon dioxide and/or hypoxia have been reported in patients with neuromuscular disorders.[18,19] However, interpretation of these studies is difficult. A decrease in ventilatory responsiveness can be a specific indicator of an abnormal medullary respiratory center only if respiratory mechanisms are normal. Otherwise, whether a decrease in ventilatory responsiveness is related to an abnormal medullary respiratory center in patients with lower motoneuron disease, respiratory muscle weakness, and/or abnormal lung mechanics is difficult to determine. Several studies have reported normal mouth occlusion pressures, an index of respiratory drive, during CO_2 rebreathing in patients with various chronic neuromuscular disorders who had a normal or slightly elevated arterial P_{CO_2}.[11,12,16]

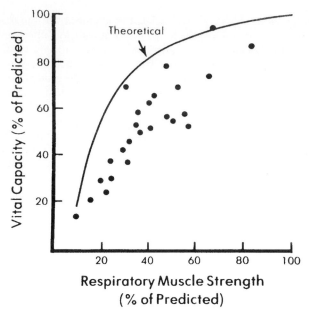

FIGURE 40-1 Relationship between respiratory muscle strength and vital capacity in 25 patients with long-standing neuromuscular disorders. The solid curve indicates the theoretical effect of respiratory muscle weakness (with proportionate effects on inspiratory and expiratory muscles) on vital capacity. This relationship is calculated from the standard maximal pressure-volume curve, assuming that respiratory system recoil in such patients is the same as that measured in normal subjects. Note that the reductions in vital capacity are disproportionate to the degree of muscle weakness. (Reproduced from De Troyer et al.,[4] with permission.)

SLEEP-RELATED CHANGES IN VENTILATION AND DEVELOPMENT OF RESPIRATORY FAILURE

Patients with chronic neuromuscular disorders are more predisposed to nocturnal desaturation and alveolar hypoventilation for several reasons. The fall in alveolar ventilation observed during sleep is a normal physiologic response related to the removal of the wakefulness stimulus on respiratory drive. Alveolar ventilation is further reduced because of inhibition of the intercostal and accessory muscles during rapid eye movement (REM) sleep (Fig. 40-2); the magnitude of this reduction in ventilation is greater in patients with weakened diaphragms. A decrease in tone of the upper airway, that is, an increase in upper airway resistance that occurs during sleep, is more profound in patients whose disease process involves the pharyngeal muscles. Coexisting processes, such as chest wall deformities or obesity, also can accentuate the degree of nocturnal desaturation by affecting mechanics and ventilation-perfusion mismatching.

Recent insights into the spectrum and mechanisms of respiratory abnormalities during sleep in neuromuscular diseases are provided primarily by descriptions of small series of patients with differing neuromuscular disorders. White and colleagues[20] performed sleep studies on four patients with generalized muscle weakness due to various myopathies and contrasted them with the results of four patients with isolated bilateral diaphragm weakness. Mean and nadir oxyhemoglobin saturations were significantly lower during REM sleep.

Desaturations were due chiefly to central hypopneas involving intercostal and expiratory abdominal muscle suppression during periods of phasic eye movements in REM sleep. Two of the eight subjects also had obstructive apneas. The severity of desaturation in all patients correlated inversely with diaphragmatic strength.[20] Generally, chronic respiratory failure is not observed routinely in patients with isolated diaphragmatic weakness unless other disorders, for example, other respiratory muscle involvement, are present.[21]

Sleep-related breathing changes may be an important determinant of daytime Pa_{CO_2} and subjective well-being in individuals with neuromuscular disorders. There are several observations that support this. Hypoventilation during sleep usually is present well before the development of daytime hypoventilation.[22,23] Hypercapnia is uncommon in patients who have normal gas exchange during sleep. The severity of the desaturation during REM sleep correlates with the severity of the daytime CO_2 retention.[22] Further supportive evidence is the observation that daytime blood gases improve with the use of noninvasive positive-pressure ventilation during sleep in patients with various neuromuscular disorders.[24–26] The significance of sleep-related breathing changes on daytime gas exchange may explain the failure of several investigators to find a simple association between respiratory muscle strength in patients with neuromuscular disease and daytime Pa_{CO_2} levels.[27,28]

How sleep-disordered breathing leads to daytime CO_2 retention and worsening symptoms of hypoventilation is not entirely clear. Alveolar hypoventilation and hypoxemia are frequently worse in the setting of abnormal respiratory mechanics, especially during REM sleep. Hypercapnia and hypoxemia can lead to frequent arousals, resulting in sleep fragmentation. Sleep fragmentation further depresses chemosensitivity[29] and upper airway dilatory muscle activity.[30] Concurrent obstructive sleep apnea (OSA), to which these patients may be predisposed by virtue of their illness and/or sleep deprivation, can further worsen gas exchange and sleep fragmentation. If the Pa_{O_2} falls on the steeper portion of the oxyhemoglobin dissociation curve, sleep-disordered breathing leads to proportionally greater reductions in oxyhemoglobin desaturation. Conceivably, the alterations in gas exchange during sleep progressively decrease the sensitivity of central and peripheral chemoreceptors. Prolonged periods at higher levels of Pa_{CO_2} during sleep may lead to an upward readjustment of the CO_2 setpoint. The development of metabolic alkalosis (bicarbonate retention) in response to hypoventilation can continue during the day because of slow HCO_3^- elimination. Alternatively, the respiratory center may set a lower level of ventilation to avoid overt muscle fatigue. Regardless of which mechanisms are operative, failure to detect and treat sleep-disordered breathing in patients with an underlying neuromuscular disorder ultimately may lead to respiratory failure.

Features of Specific Neuromuscular Disorders

An in-depth discussion of all neuromuscular disorders is well beyond the scope of this chapter. This section will focus on the more common disorders most likely to cause respiratory dysfunction.

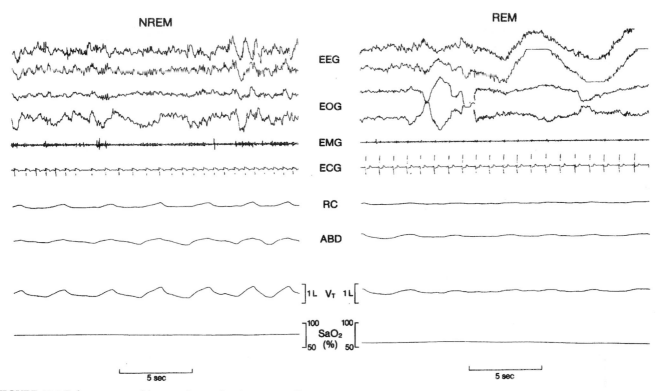

FIGURE 40-2 Polysomnographic recorder tracing in a postpolio patient. The channels show (from top to bottom) electroencephalogram (EEG), electrooculogram (EOG), submental electromyogram (EMG), electrocardiogram (ECG), excursion of the rib cage (RC) and the abdomen (ABD), and their sum (V_T), and arterial saturation (Sa_{O_2}). The pattern of breathing is rapid and shallow, and during REM sleep, the baseline saturation falls. This is accompanied by decreased excursion of both the rib cage and abdomen. (Reproduced from Goldstein et al.,[23] with permission.)

LOWER MOTONEURON DISORDER

Paralytic poliomyelitis was at one time the most common cause of lower motoneuron disease. With the polio epidemic came the advent of assisted ventilatory devices such as the iron lung. Respiratory motor function was affected in several ways. Involvement of the respiratory motor nuclei led to diaphragm and other respiratory muscle dysfunction. Disease involvement of the lower cranial nerves caused problems with upper airway obstruction, pooling of secretions, and aspiration. Direct involvement of the medullary cardiorespiratory center resulted in an irregular respiratory pattern and apnea. Overall mortality was considerably higher in patients with bulbar involvement. Nevertheless, many patients demonstrated significant muscle recovery over time. Approximately 25 percent of patients with a prior history of either paralytic or nonparalytic poliomyelitis can present later with postpoliomyelitis muscular atrophy, a syndrome of recurrent muscle weakness and fatigue as well as muscle and joint pain occurring 20 to 40 years after the initial infection. Fortunately, the decline in overall muscle strength progresses slowly. The most life-threatening complications of postpoliomyelitis occur when respiratory muscles are involved. Over time, patients can develop progressive respiratory failure. Additional respiratory compromise can occur from aspiration with new bulbar involvement and restriction from thoracic cage deformities that develop from asymmetric muscle weakness.

Amyotrophic lateral sclerosis (ALS) involves the anterior horn cells of the spinal cord and brain stem; however, upper motoneurons also can be involved. Initially, there is distal weakness, with respiratory and bulbar involvement occurring later in the disease. Abdominal muscles are usually the first to become involved, with sparing of intercostals and diaphragm muscles. Serial pulmonary function testing reveals a progressive decline in VC and TLC and an increase in RV.[31] Progression to respiratory failure is faster than in other patients with chronic neuromuscular disorders. Over half of patients with ALS die within 3 years of their diagnosis from respiratory failure associated with aspiration and pneumonia.

ABNORMALITIES OF NEUROMUSCULAR TRANSMISSION

The most common disorder involving the neuromuscular junction is myasthenia gravis. The initial onset of symptoms is usually insidious but can be rapid. Significant respiratory muscle dysfunction can occur despite minimal involvement of peripheral muscles. Respiratory failure is not uncommon and develops most often with an acute crisis. Although less common, long-standing respiratory muscle weakness may lead to chronic respiratory failure. The major causes of death in these patients are pulmonary infections and complications associated with respiratory failure and mechanical ventilation.

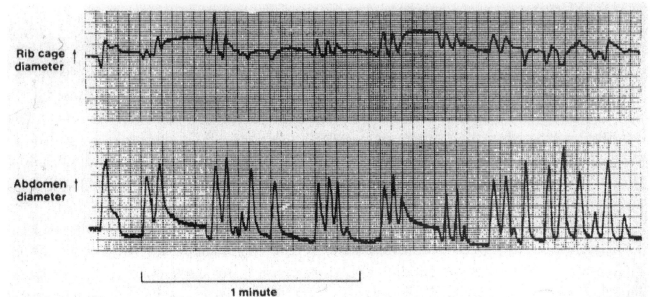

FIGURE 40-3 Patterns of breathing in a patient with myotonic dystrophy. The patient was awake and breathing at rest in the supine posture, and the respiratory changes in rib cage (*upper trace*) and abdomen (*lower trace*) anteroposterior diameter were measured with pairs of magnetometers (increase upward). The pattern was grossly disorganized ("chaotic") in both the rate and depth of breathing. (Reproduced from Serisier et al.,[36] with permission.)

PERIPHERAL NEUROPATHIES

Guillain-Barré syndrome is the most common peripheral neuropathy causing respiratory failure. The disease progresses rapidly, with approximately 15 to 30 percent of patients requiring ventilatory support.[32] The average duration of ventilatory support is 8 weeks, but patients requiring up to 30 months of support have been reported.[33] Most patients recover without sequelae. However, rehabilitation is usually necessary in those patients with prolonged mechanical ventilation and a long hospital course. Approximately 5 percent of patients will have relapsing demyelination, that is, chronic relapsing dysimmune polyneuropathy, which usually affects the limbs, but occasionally respiratory failure does occur.

Polyneuropathy of the critically ill is an acquired polyneuropathy occurring after sepsis and multiple organ system failure. It is characterized by muscle atrophy, profound weakness, diminished reflexes, and failure to wean from mechanical ventilation. Recovery is generally good, but patients usually require a long period of rehabilitation.

MUSCLE DISORDERS

Seventy-five percent of patients with Duchenne's muscular dystrophy die of respiratory failure, often in association with pneumonia.[6,34] Respiratory muscle weakness develops at an early stage of the disease. Chronic hypercapnic respiratory failure usually develops late in the disease process[6] and generally is considered a poor prognostic sign. The preservation of gas exchange is felt to be related to sparing of the diaphragm until late in the illness.[35]

Respiratory muscle weakness is commonplace in myotonic dystrophy and can be severe, even in those with only mild limb muscle weakness. Chronic hypercapnia is found more commonly with myotonic dystrophy.[18,36] Previous reports have documented irregular breathing patterns during wakefulness and sleep (including REM-related hypoventilation, central apneas, and obstructive apneas) in patients with myotonic dystrophy[37] (Fig. 40-3). The irregular breathing patterns found in 11 myotonic dystrophy patients could not be attributed to muscle weakness alone because they were not found in a control group of nonmyotonic patients with similar weakness.[37] The mechanisms underlying the increased incidence of irregular breathing patterns during both wakefulness and sleep in myotonic dystrophy patients is unclear, but alterations in central control mechanisms have been proposed by Veale and coworkers,[38] who noted that the disordered respiratory rhythm of wakefulness and during stage I-II sleep disappeared during stage III-IV non-REM sleep. An alternative explanation is that the chaotic breathing pattern is related to disordered afferent information from muscle spindles.[28] Mechanosensory feedback would have more of an effect on breathing pattern during wakefulness and the lighter stages of sleep than it would have on breathing during stage III-IV sleep, when ventilation is more dependent on chemoreceptor feedback.

Patients with limb-girdle dystrophy are also more likely to develop chronic hypercapnia than those patients with Duchenne dystrophy.[39,40] Gas-exchange involvement is felt to be related to early and severe impairment of the diaphragm. However, many patients have only moderate respiratory muscle weakness and maintain normal arterial blood gases.[18]

Management Principles: Respiratory Interventions

Many physicians have taken a pessimistic "nontreatment" approach to the management of patients with neuromuscular disease and respiratory failure because of the lack of specific treatment of the primary neuromuscular disease and the

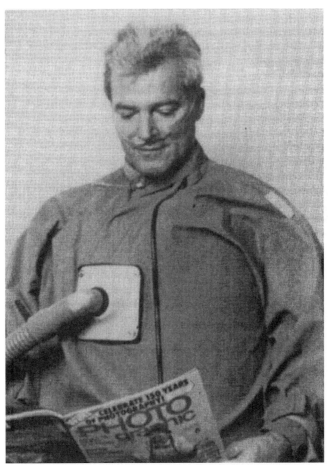

FIGURE 40-4 Subject seated in a body suit NPV applicator (cuirass). (Reproduced from Levine S, Levy S, Henson D: Negative pressure ventilation. *Crit Care Clin* 3:505–531, 1990, with permission.)

frequently predictable course of worsening respiratory muscle function followed by ventilatory failure and recurrent pulmonary infections. Although the disease is incurable, an aggressive approach to this population of patients can lead not only to a longer life but also to a better quality of life. Noninvasive modalities are available to facilitate airway clearance, which can help to avoid intubation and mechanical ventilation during respiratory infections. There are now numerous reports that the use of noninvasive mechanical ventilation at night in patients with neuromuscular disease and chronic respiratory failure can result in improvements in daytime gas exchange and a decrease in symptoms.[24-26] Tracheostomy sometimes can be avoided or delayed with application of respiratory muscle aids, implementation of noninvasive assisted ventilation (NAV) following onset of CO_2 retention, and use of NAV on a more continuous basis as the disease progresses. Furthermore, in those patients who eventually require tracheostomy and continuous mechanical ventilation, quality of life has been shown to be greatly underestimated.[41,42]

RESPIRATORY MUSCLE EXERCISE

The role of inspiratory muscle training remains controversial in patients with neuromuscular diseases. There have been a

few studies in patients with muscular dystrophy with stable or slowly progressive disease that suggest that short daily sessions of exercise training with increased inspiratory resistance can increase the endurance of the respiratory muscles.[43,44] However, improvements in lung volumes or maximum inspiratory or expiratory pressures were not always observed. The degree of improvement in endurance correlates directly with the VC and maximum inspiratory pressure at the initiation of respiratory muscle exercise.[43,44] Patients with severely impaired ventilatory function, i.e., VC values less than 25 to 30 percent of predicted and $Pa_{CO_2} > 45$ mmHg, showed no rise in respiratory muscle forces.[45-47] In general, caution should be practiced in instituting a respiratory muscle "training" program in this patient population. Adding an inspiratory resistance can be particularly hazardous to patients with more advanced disease, with the possibility of precipitating respiratory failure.[48]

NONINVASIVE ASSISTED VENTILATION: VENTILATORS

The negative-pressure ventilators were the first widely used devices to assist ventilation at night. Associated with the use of negative-pressure ventilators (e.g., the curaiss or poncho wrap) are some inherent problems (Fig. 40-4). These devices are cumbersome to apply and usually need an additional person to assist the patient. They are limited in their portability. Not all patients, particularly those who have developed chest wall deformities, can be properly fitted with one of the negative-pressure devices. In addition, negative-pressure ventilation is frequently associated with upper airway obstruction, particularly during REM sleep, when tone to the dilating muscles of the upper airway is significantly reduced. Because of the inefficiency of the negative-pressure ventilators, adequate ventilation cannot be achieved in all neuromuscular patients. Despite these limitations, there are still some patients who prefer negative-pressure devices, such as those who are claustrophobic with a mask or head gear or those who suffer from painful gastric distention with positive-pressure devices.

The rocking bed (Fig. 40-5) and pneumobelt (Fig. 40-6) are two other noninvasive ventilators that were developed and used during the latter years of the polio epidemic. Both work by a similar mechanism to cause diaphragmatic movement producing displacements of the abdominal viscera within the thoracic cavity. The major difference between these devices is that the pneumobelt assists expiration by applying positive pressure rather than just allowing gravitational force to act, as with the rocking bed. Any volume-limited positive-pressure ventilator will operate the pneumobelt successfully. A few postpolio survivors continue to use the rocking bed. Most of the other postpolio survivors with chronic respiratory failure have switched to a positive-pressure device or have died. The pneumobelt is still used sometimes as a daytime supplement in combination with positive-pressure ventilation administered noninvasively or with a tracheostomy. It provides time off the ventilator, frees the face of encumbrances, and improves speech and mobility. Efficacy of the rocking bed and pneumobelt is marginal at best and depends on a relatively normal body habitus.

With the recognition that positive-pressure ventilation could be used with a nasal mask, the use of positive-pressure

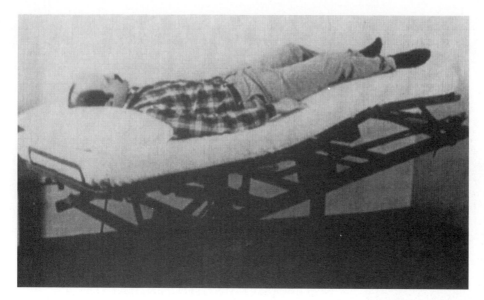

FIGURE 40-5 Rocking bed in head-down position. Sliding of the viscera and diaphragm cephalad assists exhalation. (Reproduced from Hill NS: Use of the rocking bed, pneumobelt, and other noninvasive aids to ventilation, in Tobin MJ (ed): *Principles and Practice of Mechanical Ventilation*. New York, McGraw-Hill, 1994, chap 18, pp 413–425, with permission.)

FIGURE 40-6 Pneumobelt is shown attached via a connecting hose to a Bantam positive-pressure ventilator (Puritan-Bennett Corp., Lenexa, KS). (Reproduced from Rondinelli RD, Hill NS: in Delisa JA (ed): *Rehabilitation Medicine: Principles and Practice*. Philadelphia: Lippincott, 1988, with permission.)

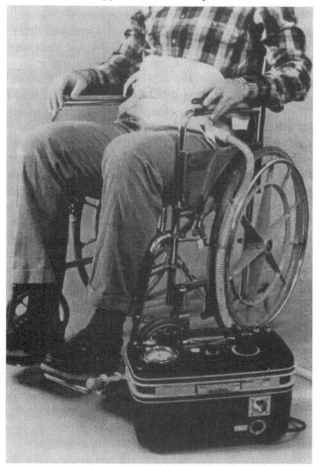

ventilators in the home has increased dramatically. There have been several studies, predominantly in patients with neuromuscular disorders,[26,49] that have noted resolution of symptoms of chronic alveolar hypoventilation and improvement in daytime gas exchange when patients have transferred from intermittent negative-pressure ventilation to intermittent positive-pressure ventilation at night. Positive-pressure ventilation can be delivered via a mouthpiece or an oral, nasal, or oral-nasal interface (Figs. 40-7 and 40-8).

NONINVASIVE ASSISTED VENTILATION: RATIONALE IN CHRONIC RESPIRATORY FAILURE

The efficacy of noninvasive assisted ventilation (NAV) in patients with chronic respiratory failure secondary to neuromuscular disease has been shown in multiple studies.[24–26,49–52] Although the majority of these studies were small and uncontrolled,[24–26,49–52] their results were overwhelmingly positive. NAV restored daytime CO_2 tension and in some patients improved respiratory muscle strength.[24–26,49–52]

There are several reasons that NAV may help. In neuromuscular diseases, substantial stress is placed on weak and/or inefficient muscles, which leads to respiratory muscle fatigue. Resting these muscles with mechanical ventilation may relieve this fatigue. Diaphragm and accessory muscle use have been shown to decrease when awake patients are ventilated with either negative- or positive-pressure ventilation.[53,54] Whether or not respiratory muscles are actually rested during mechanical ventilation is still debated. The apparent improvement in daytime arterial blood gases following nocturnal mechanical ventilation reported in some studies may be a result of factors other than the relief of respiratory muscle fatigue.[25,55] One possibility is that the reduction or removal of nocturnal hypercapnia leads to chemoreceptor "resetting" and relief of daytime CO_2 retention. It is conceivable that prolonged periodic mechanical input also could lead to changes in respiratory pattern generation. All the mechanisms responsible for the improvement in daytime symptoms and gas exchange associated with nocturnal ventilation have not been elucidated, but it is likely that more

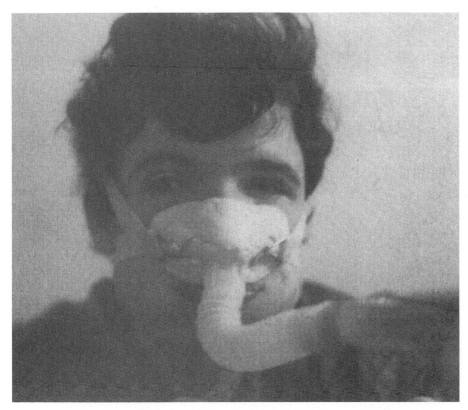

FIGURE 40-7 Duchenne muscular dystrophy patient who has required 24-h ventilatory support for 7 years and currently has less than 2 min of ventilator-free breathing time. Since his lips are too weak to grab a simple mouthpiece, he uses 24-h nasal IPPV alternating with use of various nasal interfaces. Here he is using one of three nasal interface styles custom-molded to his nose (available from Lifecare International, Inc., Westminster, CO). He also has a custom-made, molded mouthpiece, which he uses about 2 h each morning. (Reproduced from Bach JR: Pulmonary rehabilitation in musculoskeletal disorders, in Fishman AP (ed): *Lung Biology in Health and Disease,* vol 91: *Pulmonary Rehabilitation.* New York, Marcel Dekker, 1996; chap 30, pp 701–723, with permission.)

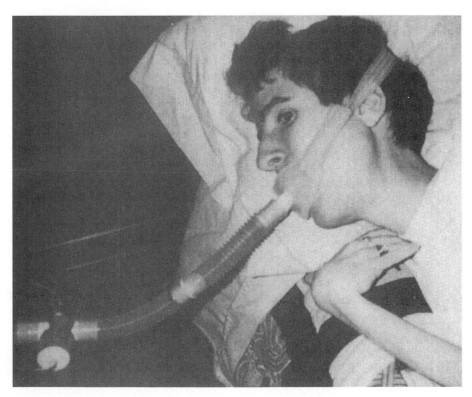

FIGURE 40-8 Duchenne muscular dystrophy patient using lipseal (Puritan-Bennett, Inc., Pickering, Ontario) IPPV for nocturnal ventilatory support prior to switching to nocturnal nasal IPPV. (Reproduced from Bach JR: Pulmonary rehabilitation in musculoskeletal disorders, in Fishman AP (ed): *Lung Biology in Health and Disease,* vol 91: *Pulmonary Rehabilitation.* New York, Marcel Dekker, 1996; chap 30, pp 701–723, with permission.)

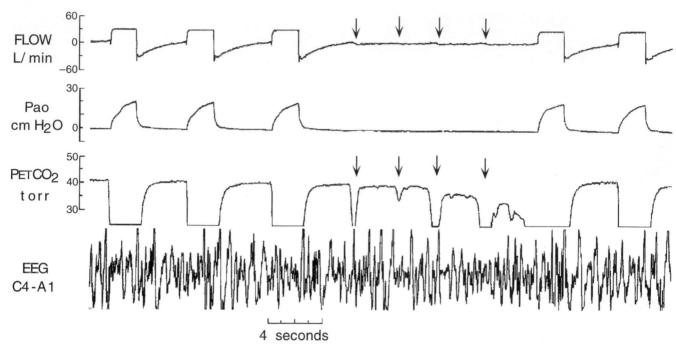

4 seconds

FIGURE 40-9 A strip-chart recording of flow, mouth pressure (Pao), $P_{ET_{CO_2}}$, and EEG in a sleeping subject with tidal volume set at 800 cc and inspiratory flow at 24 L/min in the absence of CO_2 supplementation. Shown is a long machine pause with periodic perturbations in the flow tracing, Pao tracing, and gas flow reversal in the $P_{ET_{CO_2}}$ waveform indicative of feeble respiratory efforts that fail to trigger the ventilator, i.e., "wasted efforts." (Reproduced from Tobert DG, Simon PM, Stroetz RW, Hubmayr RD: The determinants of respiratory rate during mechanical ventilation. *Am J Respir Crit Care Med* 155:485–492, 1997, with permission.)

than one mechanism may be operative. In general, the goal is to prevent hypoventilation during sleep.

NONINVASIVE ASSISTED VENTILATION: IMPLEMENTATION

Questions remain concerning the optimal time to implement NAV. The lack of consensus on indications for nocturnal NAV prompted a conference on the subject.[56] It was proposed that NAV be instituted in symptomatic patients with alveolar hypoventilation. Those patients with a $Pa_{CO_2} > 45$ mmHg and/or $Pa_{O_2} < 60$ mmHg obtained from blood-gas samples early in the morning or late in day were considered candidates. Realistically, patient are usually reluctant to start NAV unless they are symptomatic. The use of NAV does not appear to benefit patients with hypoxia alone. Evidence is also lacking to support the "prophylactic" use of NAV to prevent the onset of alveolar hypoventilation.

How to set the ventilator cannot be easily answered from prior studies in patients receiving NAV because of vast differences in study design, underlying disease, equipment used, modes of ventilation, and ventilator settings. Despite these differences, clinicians and researchers from many different medical centers and countries have reported success using NAV in patients with neuromuscular disorders. Therefore, it is reasonable to conclude that perfect application of NAV is not necessary to achieve benefit and that improvement is likely if nocturnal hypoventilation can be prevented.

There have been few studies to indicate whether patients are best ventilated with a pressure-limited or a volume-cycle ventilator. Pressure- or volume-preset breaths can be delivered via several different interfaces. Since the impedance of the respiratory system is determined by its resistive and elastic properties, higher pressures are required to overcome the impedance of the respiratory system in patients with high upper airway resistance, for example, when the state of arousal changes from wakefulness to non-REM sleep, in patients with noncompliant lungs or a stiff chest wall, or when machine breaths are delivered during the exhalation phase. This is less of a problem in a mechanically ventilated patient whose upper airway is bypassed with an endotracheal tube or a tracheostomy. During wakefulness, cortical influences can adjust breathing pattern to avoid discomfort, for example, alter timing to facilitate a machine breath. However, in sleeping patients receiving NAV, there is a limit to the amount of pressure or volume delivered. Too much of either can lead to an air leak around the mask or cause a startle response with arousal. In patients in whom the impedance to inflation is high or changing, pressure-limited ventilators may not be suitable because an adequate tidal volume may not be achieved.

It is not clear whether alveolar hypoventilation can be prevented during sleep when the ventilator is set such that the patient has to trigger each breath, that is, without a timed backup rate. When the Pa_{CO_2} of a sleeping normal volunteer is lowered by mechanically augmenting tidal volume, inspiratory motor output declines.[57] A reduction in the intensity of inspiratory effort during volume-assist ventilation can cause uncoupling of machine breaths and inspiratory efforts[58] (Fig. 40-9). Similar degrees of erratic, periodic breathing have been observed in normal sleeping subjects during pressure-support ventilation[59] (Fig. 40-10). During sleep, patients with neuromuscular disease may be more prone to "wasted ef-

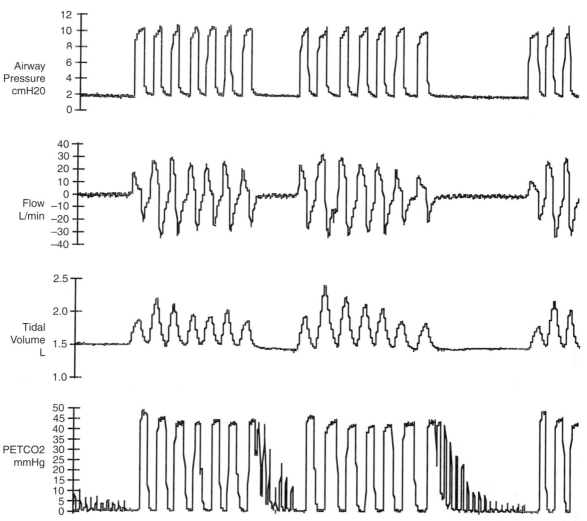

FIGURE 40-10 Example of ventilator-induced periodic breathing in a sleeping normal volunteer. Mechanical ventrilation was provided through a nasal mask using a bilevel pressure device (BiPAP; Respironics, Inc.) set to deliver an inspiratory pressure of 10 cmH$_2$O. The panel labeled PET$_{CO_2}$ shows the CO$_2$ tension in one of the nares. (Reproduced from Simon PM: Ventilatory control in the critical care setting, in Dantzker D, Scharf S (eds): *Cardiopulmonary Critical Care*, in press, with permission.)

forts," that is, inspiratory efforts not detected by the mechanical ventilator because of their underlying weakness. Generally, backup rates have been used in both volume-cycled ventilation and with bilevel positive airway pressure (BiPAP) [e.g., the spontaneous-timed (S/T) mode] to prevent apnea in patients with neuromuscular weakness (Fig. 40-11). Synchronization between the ventilator and the patient appears to be less of a problem in patients with neuromuscular disease compared with patients with COPD, who are more prone to developing autoPEEP (positive end-expiratory pressure).

In summary, there is no ideal method of NAV. Selection for an individual patient has to be based on efficiency, patient comfort, and the physician's expertise with a particular device. Generally, patients are started with ventilator settings that are most easily tolerated; this frequently includes initially setting a spontaneous mode, allowing the patient to determine his or her own rate. A timed backup rate can be added after the patient is comfortable with the mask and the device. Overnight oximetry studies are helpful before and after introduction of NAV to titrate fractionated inspired oxygen requirements. Repetitive oxygen desaturations also may indicate problems with synchronization with the device. Arterial blood gases initially can help to adjust settings, particularly to avoid overventilation. Improvements in CO$_2$ retention can take week(s) to month(s); specific studies addressing this issue are lacking. Therefore, attempts to adjust ventilator settings when introducing NAV with the purpose of documenting significant improvements in CO$_2$ retention will likely lead to patient intolerance and poor compliance. Furthermore, patients may feel distressed after NAV is removed because of changes in acid-base status over a short period of time or possibly because of a disparity between breathing patterns on versus off NAV, which can lead to dyspnea. Additional changes in ventilator settings are sometimes necessary with follow-up visits.

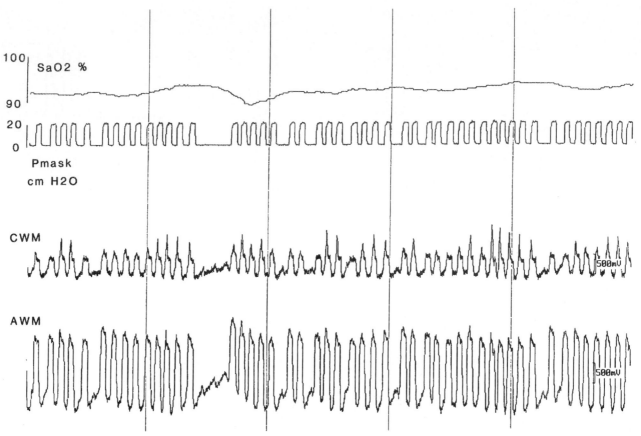

FIGURE 40-11 A 5-min epoch showing percent of oxygen saturation, mask pressure (Pmask), and chest wall (CWM) and abdominal wall (AWM) movements. The BiPAP was used in the spontaneous (S) mode, and episodes of apnea are seen, with associated desaturation. These occurred because the patient failed to initiate breaths and there was no timed backup to maintain ventilation. (Reproduced from Elliott M, Moxham J: Noninvasive mechanical ventilation by nasal or face mask, in Tobin MJ (ed): *Principles and Practice of Mechanical Ventilation*. New York: McGraw-Hill, 1994; chap 19, pp 427–453, with permission.)

GLOSSOPHARYNGEAL BREATHING

Glossopharyngeal breathing (GPB), sometimes called "frog breathing," is a technique used by some ventilator-dependent patients with neuromuscular disease to increase breathing time off the ventilator, to increase maximal inspiration, to assist coughing, and to increase the volume of the voice.[60] The technique consists of gulping boluses of air past the vocal cords using the tongue and pharyngeal muscles. Six to eight gulps of 60 to 100 mL constitute one breath. Utilizing this method, patients with no measurable VC can maintain adequate minute ventilation for several hours off ventilatory support.

ASSISTED COUGHING

In normal adults, an inspiration of 1000 to 1500 mL can generate 5 to 12 L/s of peak cough expiratory flow (PCEF) driven by pressure generated from the thoracic and abdominal walls during expiratory muscle contraction.[61] Cough flows will be diminished (1) when in an adult the inspiratory muscles cannot provide volumes of at least 1.5 L or when the lungs cannot accomodate this volume, (2) when an adequate volume of air and glottic control of the expiratory muscles cannot generate the required thoracoabdominal pressures, or (3) when neuromuscular impairment of bulbar-innervated

muscles precludes firm glottic closure or upper airway stability during the expiratory phase of the cough. Effective mobilization of loose airway secretions requires a minimum PCEF of 5 to 6 L/s.[62] Ventilator-assisted individuals with progressive neuromuscular disease rarely can generate effective PCEFs because of one or more of the problems outlined earlier. In such patients, unassisted PCEFs are often very brief and under 2 L/s. Mobilizing airway secretions during intercurrent respiratory tract infections or other periods of profuse airway secretion can be very difficult in patients receiving NAV.

Many patients can benefit from manually assisted coughing techniques such as anterior chest compression and abdominal thrust. When these maneuvers are delivered during the expiratory phase of the coughing effort, significant increases in peak expiratory flow rates have been shown.[63] The maximum insufflation capacity (MIC), a function of the strength of the oropharyngeal muscles, is the maximum volume of air that can be delivered to the patient and held with a closed glottis. The MIC is achieved by stacking air during ventilator-delivered insufflations, without exhaling, followed by GPB when possible. Either air stacking or GPB alone can sometimes achieve optimal volumes for coughing. However, the MIC is greater if air stacking precedes GPB. The PCEF can approach 5 L/s when this combination is used prior to initiating the expiratory phase of an attempted cough and the MIC exceeds 1.0 L. Significant augmentation of PCEFs can occur when anterior chest compression and/or abdominal thrust are delivered simultaneously with the expiratory phase of the cough after the insufflation maneuver.[63] PCEFs almost invariably exceed 5 L/s. This technique also can be used successfully on patients with indwelling tracheostomy tubes, provided they are capped. Manually assisted coughing requires that a caregiver has sufficient upper extremity strength and endurance to effectively apply the thrusts to the patient. It also requires cooperation and coordination between the caregiver and the patient.

Manually assisted coughing techniques may be inadequate in some patients, such as those with chest wall deformities and/or an MIC of less than 1.0 L. The most effective way to clear airway secretions in this group of patients is with the use of mechanical exsufflation.[62,64,65] A mechanical exsufflator delivers a deep, adjustable insufflation via a mask or tracheostomy tube followed by a sudden drop in pressure of about 80 cmH$_2$O in less than 0.2 s. This negative pressure is usually sustained for 1.5 to 2 s and is capable of generating PCEFs of 6 to 11 L/s.[62]

Long-term noninvasive ventilation has been successful in part because of the ability to provide adequate airway secretion clearance by using the technique of maximum insufflations followed by manually assisted coughing or a mechanical exsufflator. In many cases, use of these techniques has eliminated the need for intubation for airway suctioning even where there is intercurrent respiratory tract infections.

TRACHEOSTOMY

NAV is greatly preferred to tracheostomy by both patients and caregivers because of convenience, appearance, comfort, speech facilitation, swallowing, and overall acceptability. However, in some patients with neuromuscular disease, it cannot be avoided. Tracheostomies should be considered in patients who have oropharyngeal muscle dysfunction leading to problems with swallowing and saliva control (which places them at risk for aspiration) and in patients who can no longer effectively cough and clear secretions (which is usually when the assisted or unassisted peak cough expiratory flows drop below 3 L/s). Furthermore, when patients require mechanical ventilation for long periods of time, a tracheostomy is sometimes preferred. However, good results with NAV using an oral interface for up to 24 h per day have been reported.[66] Other indications for tracheostomy include inability of the patient to cooperate; impediments, because of orthopedic reasons, to IPPV interface use; significant use of narcotics; or uncontrolled seizures.

Management Principles: Nutrition

The limited range of physical activity can predispose patients with neuromuscular disorders to obesity. Excessive weight has a deleterious effect in patients who are already weak. Obesity is associated with a reduction in chest wall compliance and an increase in the mechanical work of breathing.[67] It is important that patients' weights are followed and that those patients who are overweight be placed on a weight-reducing diet. In general, heavy meals should be avoided, and calories should be restricted to about one-half of normal levels in wheelchair-dependent patients.

Malnutrition can become a problem in the advanced stages of the disease. Dysphagia and fear of choking can limit oral intake to thick liquids and high-calorie dietary supplements. Malnutrition can have significant effects on locomotion, respiratory muscle function, and other body systems. Specific nutritional deficiencies also can have deleterious effects on respiratory function. Placement of a gastrostomy tube may become necessary when full nutrition and hydration can no longer be taken by oral feedings. Eating difficulties also can be due to shortness of breath and overall fatigue associated with chronic hypoventilation.[49] Sometimes these difficulties resolve with NAV.

Management Principles: Orthopedic Interventions

Patients experience a significant reduction in overall functional status leading to physical discomfort and loss of emotional well-being with the development of extremity contractures. Premature loss of ambulation can occur with lower extremity contractures. Early intervention may prolong ambulation and slow the loss of function.[68] Surgical intervention such as musculotendinous releases can be done once the patient is wheelchair-dependent.[69]

Kyphoscoliosis is a common occurrence in patients with neuromuscular disease and can affect diaphragm function and chest wall mechanics. Whether surgical correction of the spinal deformity slows the rate of decline in VC is argued. However, correction of the spinal deformity allows the use of a wider variety of assisted devices to improve ventilation. Because surgery can prevent or impede the development of scoliosis in these patients, it should be done in a timely manner for all pediatric patients with neuromuscular disease who develop it.[70] Adult patients with spinal deformities have more rigid and less reversible curves, tend not to fare as well, and have a predisposition to surgical complications.

References

1. Hapke EJ, Meek JC, Jacobs J: Pulmonary function in progressive muscular dystrophy. *Chest* 61:41–47, 1972.
2. Keltz H: The effect of respiratory muscle dysfunction on pulmonary function: Studies in patients with neuromuscular disease. *Am Rev Respir Dis* 91:934–938, 1965.
3. Braun NMT, Rochester DF: Muscular weakness and respiratory failure. *Am Rev Respir Dis* 119:123–125, 1979.
4. De Troyer A, Borenstein S, Cordier R: Analysis of lung volume restriction in patients with respiratory muscle weakness. *Thorax* 35:603–610, 1980.
5. Ferris BG, Whittenberger JL, Affeldt JE: Pulmonary function in convalescent poliomyelitic patients: I. Pulmonary subdivisions and maximum breathing capacity. *N Engl J Med* 246:919–923, 1952.
6. Inkley SR, Oldenburg FC, Vignos PJ: Pulmonary function in Duchenne muscular dystrophy related to stage of disease. *Am J Med* 56:297–306, 1974.
7. Kreitzer SM, Saunders NA, Tyler HR, Ingram RH: Respiratory muscle function in amyotrophic lateral sclerosis. *Am Rev Respir Dis* 117:437–447, 1978.
8. De Troyer A, Deisser P: The effects of intermittent positive pres-

sure breathing on patients with respiratory muscle weakness. *Am Rev Respir Dis* 124:132–137, 1981.

9. Mead J, Collier C: Relation of volume history of lungs to respiratory mechanics in anesthetized dogs. *J Appl Physiol* 14:669–678, 1959.

10. Ferris BG, Pollard DS: Effect of deep and quiet breathing on pulmonary compliance in man. *J Clin Invest* 39:143–149, 1960.

11. Baydur A: Respiratory muscle strength and control of ventilation in patients with neuromuscular disease. *Chest* 99:330–338, 1991.

12. Bégin R, Bureau MA, Lupien L, et al: Pathogenesis of respiratory insufficiency in myotonic dystrophy. *Am Rev Respir Dis* 125:312–318, 1982.

13. Braun NMT, Arora NS, Rochester DF: Respiratory muscle and pulmonary function in polymyositis and other proximal myopathies. *Thorax* 38:616–623, 1983.

14. McCool FD, Mayewski RF, Shayne DS, et al: Intermittent positive pressure breathing in patients with respiratory muscle weakness: Alterations in total respiratory system compliance. *Chest* 90:546–552, 1986.

15. Estenne M, Heilporn A, Delhez L, et al: Chest wall stiffness in patients with chronic respiratory muscle weakness. *Am Rev Respir Dis* 128:1002–1007, 1983.

16. Bégin R, Bureau MA, Lupien L, Lemieux B: Control and modulation of respiration in Steinert's myotonic dystrophy. *Am Rev Respir Dis* 121:281–289, 1980.

17. Newsom Davis J, Stagg D, Loh L, Casson M: The effects of respiratory muscle weakness on some features of the breathing pattern. *Clin Sci* 10:10P–11P, 1976.

18. Kilburn KH, Eagan JT, Sieker HO, Heyman A: Cardiopulmonary insufficiency in myotonic and progressive muscular dystrophy. *N Engl J Med* 261:1089–1096, 1959.

19. Riley DJ, Santiago TV, Daniele RP, et al: Blunted respiratory drive in congenital myopathy. *Am J Med* 63:459–466, 1977.

20. White JES, Drinnan MJ, Smithson AJ, et al: Respiratory muscle activity and oxygenation during sleep in patients with muscle weakness. *Eur Respir J* 8:807–814, 1995.

21. Laroche CM, Carroll N, Moxham J, Green M: Clinical significance of severe isolated diaphragm weakness. *Am Rev Respir Dis* 138:862–866, 1988.

22. Bye PTP, Ellis ER, Issa FG, et al: Respiratory failure and sleep in neuromuscular disease. *Thorax* 45:241–247, 1990.

23. Goldstein RS, Molotiu N, Skrastins R, et al: Reversal of sleep-induced hypoventilation and chronic respiratory failure by nocturnal negative pressure ventilation in patients with restrictive ventilatory impairment. *Am Rev Respir Dis* 135:1049–1055, 1987.

24. Ellis ER, Bye PTB, Bruderer JW, Sullivan CE: Treatment of respiratory failure during sleep in patients with neuromuscular disease. *Am Rev Respir Dis* 135:148–152, 1987.

25. Gay PC, Patel AM, Viggiano RW, Hubmayr RD: Nocturnal nasal ventilation for treatment of patients with hypercapnic respiratory failure. *Mayo Clin Proc* 66:695–703, 1991.

26. Heckmatt JZ, Loh L, Dubowitz V: Night-time nasal ventilation in neuromuscular disease. *Lancet* 2:579–582, 1990.

27. Newsom Davis J, Goldman M, Loh L, Casson M: Diaphragm function and alveolar hypoventilation. *Q J Med* 45:87–100, 1976.

28. Gibson GJ, Gilmartin JJ, Veale D, et al: Respiratory muscle function in neuromuscular disease, in Jones NL, Killian KJ (eds): *Breathlessness.* The Campbell Symposium, Hamilton, Canada, Boehringer Ingelheim (Canada), Inc., 1992; pp 66–73.

29. White DP, Douglas NJ, Pickett CK, et al: Sleep deprivation and the control of ventilation. *Am Rev Respir Dis* 128:984–986, 1983.

30. Leiter JC, Knuth SL, Barlett D: The effect of sleep deprivation on activity of the genioglossus muscle. *Am Rev Respir Dis* 128:984–986, 1983.

31. Nakano KK, Bass H, Tyler RH, Carmel RJ: Amyotrophic lateral sclerosis: A study of pulmonary function. *Dis Nerv Syst* 37:32–35, 1976.

32. Gracey DR, McMichan JC, Divertie MB, Howard FM: Respiratory failure in Guillain-Barré syndrome: A 6-year experience. *Mayo Clin Proc* 57:742–746, 1982.

33. Knoedler JP: Delayed recovery from respiratory paralysis due to the Guillain-Barré syndrome. *Chest* 80:119–120, 1981.

34. Smith PEM, Calverley PMA, Edwards RHT, et al: Practical problems in the respiratory care of patients with muscular dystrophy. *N Engl J Med* 316:1197–1205, 1987.

35. Newsom Davis J: The respiratory system in muscular dystrophy. *Br Med Bull* 36:135–138, 1980.

36. Serisier DE, Mastaglia FL, Gibson GJ: Respiratory muscle function and ventilatory control: I. In patients with motor neuron disease. II. In patients with myotonic dystrophy. *Q J Med* 51:205–226, 1982.

37. Ververs CCM, Van der Mech FGA, Verbraak AFM, et al: Breathing pattern awake and asleep in myotonic dystrophy. *Respiration* 63:1–7, 1996.

38. Veale D, Cooper BG, Gilmartin JJ, et al: Breathing pattern awake and asleep in patients with myotonic dystrophy. *Eur Respir J* 8:815–818, 1995.

39. Skatrud J, Iber C, McHugh W, et al: Determinants of hypoventilation during wakefulness and sleep in diaphragmatic paralysis. *Am Rev Respir Dis* 121:587–593, 1980.

40. Neustadt JE, Levy RC, Spiegel IJ: Carbon dioxide narcosis in association with muscular dystrophy. *JAMA* 187:616–617, 1964.

41. Bach JR, Campagnolo D, Hoeman S: Life satisfaction of individuals with Duchenne muscular dystrophy using long-term mechanical ventilatory support. *Am J Phys Med Rehabil* 70:129–135, 1991.

42. Bach JR, Campagnolo D: Psychosocial adjustment of post-poliomyelitis ventilator-assisted individuals. *Arch Phys Med Rehabil* 73:934–939, 1992.

43. DiMarco AF, Kelling JS, DiMarco MS, et al: The effects of inspiratory resistive training on respiratory muscle function in patients with muscular dystrophy. *Muscle Nerve* 8:284–290, 1985.

44. Martin AJ, Stern L, Yeates J, et al: Respiratory muscle training in Duchenne dystrophy. *Dev Med Child Neurol* 28:314–318, 1986.

45. Smith PEM, Coakley JM, Edwards RHT: Respiratory muscle training in Duchenne muscular dystrophy. *Muscle Nerve* 11:784–785, 1988.

46. Rodillo E, Noble-Jamieson CM, Aber V, et al: Respiratory muscle training in Duchenne muscular dystrophy. *Arch Dis Child* 64:736–738, 1989.

47. Stern LM, Martin AJ, Jones N, et al: Training inspiratory resistance in Duchenne dystrophy using adapted computer games. *Dev Med Child Neurol* 31:494–500, 1989.

48. Schiffman PL, Belsh JM: Effect of inspiratory resistance and theophylline on respiratory muscle strength in patients with amyotrophic lateral sclerosis. *Am Rev Respir Dis* 139:1418–1423, 1989.

49. Bach JR, Alba AS: Management of chronic alveolar hypoventilation by nasal ventilation. *Chest* 97:52–57, 1990.

50. Kerby GR, Mayer LS, Pingleton SK: Nocturnal positive pressure ventilation via nasal mask. *Am Rev Respir Dis* 135:738–740, 1987.

51. Leger P, Jennequin J, Gerard M, et al: Home positive pressure ventilation via nasal mask for patients with neuromusculoskeletal disorders. *Eur Respir J* 7:640s–644s, 1989.

52. Hill NS, Eveloff SE, Carlisle CC, Goff SG: Efficacy of nocturnal nasal ventilation in patients with restrictive thoracic disease. *Am Rev Respir Dis* 145:365–371, 1992.

53. Carrey Z, Gottfried SB, Levy RD: Ventilatory muscle support in respiratory failure with nasal positive pressure ventilation. *Chest* 97:150–158, 1990.

54. Elliott MW, Mulvey DA, Moxham J, et al: Inspiratory muscle effort during nasal intermittent positive pressure ventilation in patients with chronic obstructive airways disease. *Anaesthesia* 48:8–13, 1993.

55. Mohr CH, Hill NS: Long-term follow-up of nocturnal ventilatory assistance in patients with respiratory failure due to Duchenne-type muscular dystrophy. *Chest* 97:91–96, 1990.

56. Robert D, Willig TN, Paulus J, Leger P: Long-term nasal ventila-

tion in neuromuscular disorders: Report of a consensus conference. *Eur Respir J* 6:599–606, 1993.

57. Henke HG, Arias A, Skatrud JB, Dempsey JA: Inhibition of inspiratory muscle activity during sleep. *Am Rev Respir Dis* 138:8–15, 1988.

58. Tobert DG, Simon PM, Stroetz RW, Hubmayr RD: The determinants of respiratory rate during mechanical ventilation. *Am J Respir Crit Care Med* 155:485–492, 1997.

59. Rajagopalan N, Simon PM, Gay PC, et al: Effects of nasal BiPAP on breathing in normal sleeping humans. *Am J Respir Crit Care Med* 153:A371, 1996 (abstr).

60. Bach JR, Alba AS, Bodofsky E, et al: Glossopharyngeal breathing and noninvasive aids in the management of postpolio respiratory insufficiency. *Birth Defects* 23:99–113, 1987.

61. Leith DE: Cough, in Brain JD, Proctor D, Reid L (eds): *Lung Biology in Health and Disease: Respiratory Defense Mechanisms*, part 2. New York, Marcel Dekker 1977; pp 545–592.

62. Barach AL, Beck GJ, Smith RH: Mechanical production of expiratory flow rates surpassing the capacity of human coughing. *Am J Med Sci* 226:241–248, 1953.

63. Massery M, Frownfelter D: Assisted cough techniques: There's more than one way to cough. *Phys Ther Forum* 9:1–4, 1990.

64. The OEM Cof-flator Portable Cough Machine, Shampaine Industries, Inc., St. Louis, MO.

65. Barach AL, Beck GJ, Bickerman HA, Seanor HE: Physical methods simulating cough mechanisms. *JAMA* 150.1380–1385, 1952.

66. Bach JR, Sortor SM, Saporito LR: Interfaces for non-invasive intermittent positive pressure ventilatory support in North America. *Eur Respir Rev* 3:254–259, 1993.

67. Naimark A, Cherniack RM: Compliance of the respiratory system and its components in health and obesity. *J Appl Physiol* 15:377–382, 1960.

68. Bach JR, McKeon J: Orthopedic surgery and rehabilitation for the prolongation of brace-free ambulation of patients with Duchenne muscular dystrophy. *Am J Phys Med Rehabil* 70:323–331, 1991.

69. Spencer GE: Orthopaedic care of progressive muscular dystrophy. *J Bone Joint Surg [Am]* 49:1201–1204, 1967.

70. Rideau Y, Glorion B, Delaubier A, et al: Treatment of scoliosis in Duchenne muscular dystrophy. *Muscle Nerve* 7:281–286, 1984.

Chapter 41

REHABILITATION OF PATIENTS WITH PULMONARY VASCULAR DISEASE

JONATHAN B. ORENS
LEWIS J. RUBIN

Disorders of the pulmonary circulation comprise a heterogeneous group of conditions which deleteriously affect cardiopulmonary function. Because of the anatomy of the chest, virtually every disease affecting the lung will have effects on the lung vasculature. As opposed to other lung diseases, such as COPD, information related to rehabilitation for the pulmonary vascular diseases is quite limited; patients with these disorders are infrequently placed into aggressive rehabilitation programs involving exercise because of potential harmful effects on cardiovascular function. This chapter will focus on primary pulmonary hypertension (PPH) as a model for pulmonary vascular disease, with a discussion of the physiologic consequences of pulmonary hypertension on gas exchange and pulmonary function both at rest and during exercise. Current therapy and the implications of these treatments relative to rehabilitation potential for PPH will also be reviewed.

Primary Pulmonary Hypertension

The National Heart, Lung, and Blood Institute Registry for Primary Pulmonary Hypertension defined pulmonary hypertension (PH) as a mean pulmonary artery pressure greater than 25 mmHg at rest and 30 mmHg during exercise.[1] An increased pulmonary artery pressure appears with a variety of clinical entities including parenchymal lung diseases, pulmonary thromboembolic disease, congestive heart failure, valvular heart disease, congenital heart disease, liver disease, certain medications, HIV infection, connective tissue disease, and hypoxemia.[2] Pulmonary vascular disease which occurs in the setting of one of these disorders is termed secondary pulmonary hypertension.[2-6] A diagnosis of primary pulmonary hypertension (PPH) can be established only by excluding a definable cause of pulmonary vascular disease.[2]

Primary pulmonary hypertension is a rare disease with an estimated incidence between 1 to 2 per 1 million.[7] Symptoms are nonspecific and often develop insidiously. By the time symptoms occur, pulmonary artery pressure is usually at least twice the normal level. In the NIH Registry the average time from the initial development of symptoms until the recognition of pulmonary hypertension was 2 to 5 years[1] (Fig. 41-1). The most common symptom of PPH is exertional dyspnea, which occurs in 60 percent of all patients at presentation, and nearly 98 percent over the course of the disease.[1] The etiology of dyspnea in PPH has not been elucidated: Suggested mechanisms include stimulation of pulmonary stretch receptors and an inability to augment cardiac output to meet metabolic demands.[8,9] Other symptoms include fatigue, chest pain, and syncope.[1] The chest pain is similar in character to the discomfort associated with ischemic heart disease and occurs in up to 47 percent of patients by the time of diagnosis.[1] The pain is believed to be due to overdistention of the right ventricle which leads to poor perfusion of the right ventricular wall. Syncope may occur with exertion or, in severe cases, at rest,[1] and has been attributed to inadequate cerebral perfusion resulting from an impaired cardiac output due to the extremely high right ventricular afterload.[2]

Pulmonary function testing is useful to exclude significant pulmonary parenchymal disease. Patients with PPH may have a mild restrictive ventilatory defect associated with a reduced diffusing capacity (DLCO).[1,10] The cause of the reduced lung volumes is thought to be due to overdistention of the pulmonary vessels with surrounding adventitial fibrosis and a decrease in lung compliance.[10] Reduction in DLCO is likely due to overall loss of capillary volume and possibly increased red blood cell transit time through the limited capillary bed. Arterial blood gases usually reveal a mildly reduced P_{CO_2} with an elevated pH compatible with a chronic respiratory alkalosis.[1] Although the findings from blood gas analysis are not specific for PPH, the study should be performed to exclude hypoventilation or significant hypoxemia.

Despite its invasive nature, right heart catheterization is the most suitable method to assess the hemodynamic profile of patients with PPH. Accurate measurements of pulmonary artery pressure, cardiac output, and right atrial pressure are essential for therapeutic decisions and assessing prognosis.[11] Ventilation/perfusion lung scanning and pulmonary angiography may be useful to exclude chronic pulmonary thromboembolic disease.[12] Pulmonary angiography is a safe procedure when properly performed in patients with PPH.[13,14] Open lung biopsy is rarely required to establish the diagnosis of PPH, but may be necessary to exclude parenchymal lung disease, pulmonary venoocclusive disease and vasculitis.[15]

Exercise Responses in Pulmonary Vascular Disease

It is reasonable to speculate that supervised cardiopulmonary rehabilitation programs may be beneficial by improving conditioning in patients with pulmonary vascular disease. However, it is important to recognize that strenuous exercise may raise pulmonary artery pressures acutely in patients with pulmonary hypertension.[16,17] An abrupt rise in pulmonary artery pressure may be associated with a sudden fall in cardiac output which could lead to syncope or sudden death. Because of the theoretical dangers associated with strenuous exercise, large cohorts of patients have not been studied to accurately define the utility or safety of pulmonary rehabilitation in this condition.

D'Alonzo and colleagues[18] examined the cardiopulmonary exercise responses in 11 patients with PPH during incremental cardiopulmonary exercise testing (CPET). Maximal oxygen consumption (V_{O_2}) was reduced and was associated with an early anaerobic threshold and low oxygen-pulse. Minute ventilation was elevated relative to V_{O_2}, and dead space to tidal volume (Vd/Vt) did not fall with exercise. These find-

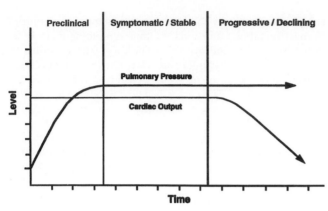

FIGURE 41-1 Hemodynamic and symptomatic progression of primary pulmonary hypertension.

ings are consistent with the expected cardiovascular consequences of pulmonary hypertension, since high pulmonary artery pressures adversely affect cardiac output and, as a result, O_2 delivery. We recently studied six untreated patients with severe PPH (New York Heart Association class III and IV) using symptom-limited maximal incremental CPET.[19] Arterial blood gases and lactate levels were obtained every minute of exercise to accurately assess anaerobic threshold and Vd/Vt. Right heart catheterization was performed on the same day to document the hemodynamic profile. These studies revealed a significant variability in the responses to exercise compared to the studies of D'Alonzo and coworkers. In particular, the "classic" findings of a low V_{O_2}, early anaerobic threshold and low O_2 pulse were not consistently present. There was no significant difference in the hemodynamic profile of these patients compared to those who displayed the findings of D'Alonzo and associates (Table 41-1). In a study of 51 patients with pulmonary hypertension resulting from various causes, Janicki and coworkers found a linear relationship between mean pulmonary artery pressure and cardiac

TABLE 41-1 Cardiopulmonary Exercise Responses in 6 Patients with Severe PPH

Hemodynamics at Rest	Mean $\pm$ SE	Range
PA systolic (mmHg)	83 $\pm$ 7.6	59–99
PA diastolic (mmHg)	31 $\pm$ 3.6	20–38
PA mean (mmHg)	49 $\pm$ 4.9	33–58
CO (mmHg)	4 $\pm$ 0.58	2.8–6
PVR (mmHg/L/min)	12 $\pm$ 2.2	9–16

Exercise Variable	Mean $\pm$ SE	Range
V_{O_2}max (% pred)	55 $\pm$ 4.8	40–69
Watts max (% pred)	68 $\pm$ 14.2	29–110
AT (% pred V_{O_2}max)	37 $\pm$ 4.5	24–52
O_2 pulse max (% pred)	67 $\pm$ 7.7	40–86
Ventilatory reserve (%)	26 $\pm$ 8.3	7–57
Vd/Vt max	0.3 $\pm$ 0.03	0.22–0.41
P(A–a)$_{O_2}$max (mmHg)	67 $\pm$ 15.6	14–95

NOTE: Data from maximal symptom limited incremental exercise performed on a cycle ergometer following a resting right heart catheterization. A significant correlation exists between Vd/Vt max and resting PA mean pressure ($r = 0.99$, $p = .002$) and between maximal work rate (watts) and resting PA systolic pressure ($r = 0.82$, $p = .03$).

output.[17] Similar to the findings of D'Alonzo and colleagues, anaerobic threshold occurred early, V_{O_2}max was reduced and ventilation was abnormal with an elevated VE for any given level of V_{O_2}.[20]

In normal subjects, there are three phases of V_{O_2} kinetics during the dynamic response to steady state exercise beginning from rest[21]: Phase 1, or the immediate increase in V_{O_2}, lasts for about 15 s followed by phase 2, which is represented by a more gradual rise in V_{O_2} until a steady state is achieved in phase 3 which begins around 3 min.[21] The V_{O_2} rise during phase 1 is predominantly due to the sudden rise in pulmonary blood flow, while the V_{O_2} rise in phase 2 is due to a further increase in pulmonary blood flow and a progressive fall in central venous O_2 saturation.[21] Sietsema[22] studied the kinetics of oxygen uptake during exercise in patients with pulmonary hypertension of various etiologies, including PPH, sarcoidosis, chronic thromboembolic disease, and congenital heart disease. The V_{O_2} kinetics in patients with pulmonary hypertension was abnormal, with a small rise in V_{O_2} during phase 1, and a long-time constant for the phase 2 increase and a prolongation of the time to reach a steady state. The V_{O_2} kinetics improved in two patients whose pulmonary hypertension was successfully treated surgically. These findings are consistent with an impairment in O_2 delivery due to a diminished right ventricular output resulting from an increased afterload.

Treatment

The past 15 years has witnessed significant advances in the therapy of patients with PPH. Treatment of PPH requires a comprehensive plan including medications, avoiding circumstances that may increase pulmonary artery pressure and, in selected patients, lung transplantation. Several measures should be instituted to prevent further worsening of pulmonary artery pressure or cardiac output. Hypoxic vasoconstriction must be avoided by preventing or correcting hypoxemia, particularly during physical activity. Sympathomimetic drugs and nonsteroidal anti-inflammatory agents should be avoided because of their vasoconstrictive properties. Agents which depress cardiac output should also be avoided. Aggressive exercise should be discouraged because of the acute increase in pulmonary artery pressure associated with this activity. Wood's description of the vasospastic component of PPH established both a fundamental pathologic mechanism for the disease, as well as the possibility that vasodilators could be utilized therapeutically.[23–25] Vasodilators coupled with anticoagulation prolong life and are the mainstay of therapy for PPH.[26–29] Acute responsiveness to vasodilators established by right heart catheterization with a decrease in pulmonary artery pressure and an increase in cardiac output portends the best outcome in this disease.[27,30] The calcium channel blockers nifedipine and diltiazem are the most widely used vasodilators, and dose requirements to produce a beneficial pulmonary vascular effect may be quite high.[30] Recently the United States Food and Drug Administration approved prostaglandin I2 (prostacyclin, epoprostenol) for the treatment of PPH which is refractory to other therapies.

Anticoagulation with oral warfarin is used by most centers as part of the therapy for PPH. Two arguments justify anticoagulation, including: (1) pulmonary artery pathology which has revealed in situ thrombosis, and (2) potential increased risk for pulmonary embolism because of inactivity coupled with poor cardiac output. Indeed, a retrospective study from the Mayo Clinic[26] and a more recent small, prospective study[27] suggest that chronic anticoagulation may provide a lengthened survival in patients with PPH.

Lung transplantation should be considered for patients who fail therapy with vasodilators. Successful combined heart and lung transplantation have been performed since the early 1980s with reasonable improvement in quality of life, exercise tolerance, and survival.[31-33] As experience with thoracic transplantation has grown, most centers in the United States now recommend lung transplantation alone rather than combined heart-lung transplantation for PPH. There are several reasons for this recommendation: (1) there is a significant scarcity of donor organs (two or three patients may benefit from one donor); (2) the right ventricle has a tremendous capability to recover after reduction of the markedly elevated afterload following lung transplantation; (3) a high rate of chronic lung allograft rejection (bronchiolitis obliterans) was reported in heart-lung transplantation recipients.[34] There is still controversy whether single lung or sequential double lung transplantation is the best approach. Advocates for single lung transplantation argue that a reasonable benefit from both a functional and survival standpoint can be achieved, while preserving a limited supply of donor organs. Sequential double lung transplantation is a longer operation with potentially higher immediate perioperative morbidity. However, double lung transplantation may provide a better long-term benefit, as it has been recognized that patients with PPH who undergo single lung transplantation may have more difficulties tolerating bouts of acute allograft rejection. The reason for this is that following single lung transplantation blood preferentially perfuses the low-resistance vascular bed of the allograft compared to the native lung. Thus, during a rejection episode, when ventilation of the allograft is disrupted, there may be severe shunting creating profound hypoxemia. Sequential double lung transplantation may also provide a small functional benefit over the long term when compared to single lung transplantation.[35] The timing of lung transplantation for patients with PPH is also not clearly defined. Because of the long waiting period for lung transplantation at most centers (12 to 18 months), and the unpredictable rate of decline for some patients, many centers advocate listing patients for transplantation as soon as the diagnosis of PPH is established. Data from the NIH Registry for PPH have been used to develop an equation to predict survival based upon hemodynamic measurements made from right heart catheterization.[11]

$$A\,(x, y, z) = e\,(0.007325x) + (0.0526y) - (0.3275z)$$

where x = mean pulmonary artery pressure
y = mean right atrial pressure
z = cardiac index
The probability of surviving 1, 2, and 3 years would be:
$p\,(1) = 0.75^A$
$p\,(2) = 0.65^A$
$p\,(3) = 0.55^A$
In general, most centers recommend that patients be listed for transplantation when 2-year survival is limited. Although

this formula is applicable to large groups of patients with PPH, individuals may decline at an unpredictable rate. Accordingly, the overall clinical picture must be assessed for each patient in order to allow an ample waiting time for this potential life-saving therapy. Many transplant centers advocate a program of cardiopulmonary rehabilitation for patients awaiting lung transplantation in order to minimize the consequences of deconditioning postoperatively.

IMPACT OF THERAPY ON EXERCISE TOLERANCE

Treatment with continuous intravenous PGI_2 has been shown to improve exercise tolerance as assessed by 6-min walk studies.[28,29,36] In a 12-week prospective multicenter study by the PPH Study Group, 6-min walk distance increased by a mean of 31 m in the group treated with prostacyclin combined with conventional therapy, while the group treated with conventional therapy alone experienced a mean decrease of 29 m in 6-min walk distance over the course of the study.[36] Interestingly, there was a significant inverse correlation between the changes in 6-min walk distance and pulmonary artery pressure, right atrial pressure, mean systemic-artery pressure, pulmonary vascular resistance, and systemic vascular resistance. Most importantly, performance in the baseline 6-min walk study was an independent predictor of survival. These data support the notion that exercise limitation in PPH is due to an inability of the heart to augment cardiac output due to the high pressures in the pulmonary vascular bed, and that exercise tolerance may be a useful indicator of progression and severity of the disease.

While the effects of exercise on pulmonary artery pressure and cardiac responses have not been studied in PPH, these responses have been assessed in patients with exercise-induced pulmonary hypertension in severe COPD.[37-39] Pulmonary vascular resistance and pulmonary artery pressure increase during exercise in some patients with severe COPD.[37] Exercise-induced pulmonary hypertension in COPD is due to both reactive and fixed vascular changes. Hypoxemia is responsible for the reactive component, while fixed changes are due to such factors as destruction of the vascular bed, increased alveolar pressure, increased hematocrit and blood volume, and combined respiratory and metabolic acidosis.[37]

Alpert and coworkers[38] studied the effects of exercise training in five subjects with moderately severe COPD and exercise-induced pulmonary hypertension. The training consisted of exercise on a bicycle ergometer for 20 min, 3 times per day. At the end of the training period, there was a significant fall in V_{O_2} and heart rate for the same work rate during submaximal exercise studies.

However, there was no significant difference in cardiac index, pulmonary vascular resistance, mean resting or exercising pulmonary artery pressure. These findings suggest improvement in efficiency or coordination of skeletal and/or respiratory muscles, without any pulmonary hemodynamic states. Two additional studies by Degre and coworkers[39] and Chester and colleagues[40] failed to show any significant changes in pulmonary hemodynamics as a consequence of exercise training in patients with COPD and pulmonary hypertension.

The effects of acute exercise on pulmonary hemodynamics have been examined in PPH. Laskey and coworkers[41] compared the hemodynamic responses during acute exercise be-

TABLE 41-2 Hemodynamic Data Obtained by Right Heart Catheterization during Rest and Steady State Exercise in a 60-Year-Old Male Patient with Mild PPH

Work Rate (watts)	PA Pressure, Systolic/Diastolic (mean)	Cardiac Output (liters/m)	Total Pulmonary Resistance (units)
0 (rest)	32/15 (22)	3.7	5.9
10	42/18 (29)	5.5	5.3
20	46/17 (25)	5.6	4.5
30	41/18 (21)	6.5	3.2
40	43/19 (30)	6.2	4.8
50	51/17 (27)	6.3	4.3

NOTE: The patient presented with dyspnea on exertion. Resting pulmonary hemodynamics were normal while a significant rise in pulmonary artery pressure occurred during exercise.

tween normal individuals and patients with PPH. Mean resting pulmonary artery pressure was 14 mmHg in the normal individuals and 50 mmHg in those with PPH. The mean pulmonary artery pressure rose insignificantly during exercise in the normal subjects. PPH patients demonstrated a significant rise in mean pulmonary artery pressure to 71 mmHg during exercise. We have also observed similar abnormal increases in pulmonary artery pressure in patients with less severe PPH. A subset of patients with early PPH may present with significant exercise-induced pulmonary hypertension while resting hemodynamics remain normal to mildly abnormal (Table 41-2). Taken together, these data suggest that significant exercise may affect already altered pulmonary hemodynamics.

Summary

Pulmonary vascular disease is associated with significant long-term morbidity and mortality. Studies assessing responses to acute exercise reveal significant increases in pulmonary artery pressure suggesting that this activity may be deleterious over the long term. This observation has led us to advise our patients with pulmonary vascular disease to perform activities with which they feel comfortable, while limiting strenuous exercise.

At the present time, several therapeutic options exist which may lead to improved exercise tolerance and survival. These include vasodilators, anticoagulation, continuous intravenous prostacyclin, and, in certain cases, surgery (lung transplantation and pulmonary thromboendarterectomy). These interventions provide the best hope for improvement in quality of life and long-term survival.

References

1. Rich S, Dantzker D, Ayres S, et al: Primary pulmonary hypertension. A national prospective study. *Ann Intern Med* 107:216–223, 1987.
2. Rubin L: Pulmonary vasculitis and primary pulmonary hypertension, in Murray J, Nadel J (eds): *Textbook of Respiratory Medicine*, 2d ed. Philadelphia, W.B. Saunders, 1994; pp 1683–1709.
3. McDonnell P, Toye P, Hutchins G: Primary pulmonary hypertension and cirrhosis: Are they related? *Am Rev Respir Dis* 127:437–441, 1983.
4. Chapman P, Bateman E, Benatar S: Primary pulmonary hypertension and thromboembolic pulmonary hypertension-similarities and differences. *Respir Med* 84:485–488, 1990.
5. Polos P, Wolfe D, Harley R, et al: Pulmonary hypertension and human immunodeficiency virus infection: Two reports and a review of the literature. *Chest* 101:474–478, 1992.
6. D'Alonzo G, Bower J, Dantzker D: Differentiation of patients with primary and thromboembolic pulmonary hypertension. *Chest* 85:457–462, 1984.
7. The International Primary Pulmonary Hypertension Study Group: The international primary pulmonary hypertension study (IPPHS). *Chest* 105 (suppl):37S–41S, 1994.
8. Levine S, Huckabee W: Ventilatory response to drug-induced hypermetobolism. *J Appl Physiol* 38:827–833, 1975.
9. Reeves J, Groves B: Approach to the patient with pulmonary hypertension, in Weir E (ed): *Pulmonary Hypertension*. Mt Kisco, NY, Futura Publishing, 1984; pp 1–44.
10. Scharf S, Feldman N, Graboys T, Wellman J: Restrictive ventilatory defect in a patient with primary pulmonary hypertension. *Am Rev Respir Dis* 118:409–413, 1978.
11. D'Alonzo G, Barst R, Ayres S, et al: Survival in patients with primary pulmonary hypertension. Results from a national prospective registry. *Ann Intern Med* 115:343–349, 1991.
12. Moser K, Page G, Ashburn W, et al: Perfusion lung scans provide a guide to which patients with apparent primary pulmonary hypertension merit angiography. *West J Med* 148:167–170, 1988.
13. Nicod P, Peterson K, Levine M, et al: Pulmonary angiography in severe chronic pulmonary hypertension. *Ann Intern Med* 107:565–568, 1987.
14. Perlmutt L, Braun S, Newman G, et al: Pulmonary arteriography in the high-risk patient. *Radiology* 162:187–189, 1987.
15. Wagenvoort C: Lung biopsy specimens in the evaluation of pulmonary vascular disease. *Chest* 77:614–625, 1980.
16. Reeves J, Dempsey J, Grover R: Pulmonary circulation during exercise, in Weir E, Reeves J (eds): *Pulmonary Vascular Physiology and Pathophysiology*. Mount Kisco, NY, Futura Publishing, 1989; pp 107–133.
17. Janicki J, Weber K, Likoff M, et al: The pressure-flow response of the pulmonary circulation in patients with heart failure and pulmonary vascular disease. *Circulation* 72:1270, 1985.
18. D'Alonzo G, Gianotti L, Pohil R, et al: Comparison of progressive exercise performance of normal subjects and patients with primary pulmonary hypertension. *Chest* 92(1):57–62, 1987.
19. Orens J, Moore W, Martinez F, Rubin L: Variability in the responses to cardiopulmonary exercise in primary pulmonary hypertension (abstr). *Chest* 108(supp)(3):181S, 1995.
20. Janicki J, Weber K, Likoff M, et al: Exercise testing to evaluate patients with pulmonary vascular disease. *Am Rev Respir Dis* 129(suppl):S93–S95, 1984.
21. Wasserman K, Hansen J, Sue D, et al: *Principles of Exercise Testing and Interpretation*, 2d ed. Philadelphia, Lea & Febiger, 1994.
22. Sietsema K: Oxygen uptake kinetics in response to exercise in patients with pulmonary vascular disease. *Am Rev Respir Dis* 145:1052–1057, 1992.
23. Wood P: Pulmonary hypertension. *Br Med Bull* 8:348–353, 1952.
24. Wood P, Besterman E, Towers M, McIlroy M: The effect of acetylcholine on pulmonary vascular resistance and left atrial pressure in mitral stenosis. *Br Heart J* 19:279–286, 1957.
25. Wood P: Pulmonary hypertension with special reference to the vasoconstrictive factor. *Br Heart J* 28:557–570, 1958.
26. Fuster V, Steele P, Edwards W: Primary pulmonary hypertension: Natural history and the importance of thrombosis. *Circulation* 70:580–587, 1984.
27. Rich S, Kaufmann R, Levy P: The effect of high doses of calcium-channel blockers on survival in primary pulmonary hypertension. *N Engl J Med* 327:76–81, 1992.
28. Barst R, Rubin L, McGoon M, et al: Survival in primary pulmo-

nary hypertension with long-term continuous intravenous prostacyclin. *Ann Intern Med* 121:409–415, 1994.

29. Rubin L, Mendoza J, Hood M: Treatment of primary pulmonary hypertension with continuous intravenous prostacyclin (Epoprostenol): Results of a randomized trial. *Ann Intern Med* 112:485–491, 1990.

30. Rich S, Brundage B: High dose calcium channel blocking therapy for primary pulmonary hypertension: Evidence for long-term reduction in pulmonary arterial pressure and regression of right ventricular hypertrophy. *Circulation* 76:135–141, 1987.

31. Reitz B, Wallwork J, Hunt S, et al: Heart-lung transplantation: Successful therapy for patients with pulmonary vascular disease. *N Engl J Med* 306:557–564, 1982.

32. Cooper J, Patterson G, Trulock E: Results of single and bilateral lung transplantation in 131 consecutive recipients. Washington University Lung Transplantation Group. *J Thorac Cardiovasc Surg* 107:460–470, 1994.

33. Pasque M, Trulock E, Cooper J, et al: Single lung transplantation for pulmonary hypertension: Single institution experience in 34 patients. *Circulation* 92:2252–2258, 1995.

34. Theodore J, Jamieson S, Burke C, et al: Physiologic aspects of human heart-lung transplantation: Pulmonary function status of the post-transplanted lung. *Chest* 86:349–357, 1984.

35. Orens J, Martinez F, Becker F, et al: Cardiopulmonary exercise testing following lung transplantation for different underlying diseases. *Chest* 107(1):144–149, 1995.

36. Barst R, Rubin L, Long W, et al: A comparison of continuous intravenous epoprostenol (prostacyclin) with conventional therapy for primary pulmonary hypertension. *N Engl J Med* 334:296–301, 1996.

37. Rogers T, Howard D: Pulmonary hemodynamics and physical training in patients with chronic obstructive pulmonary disease. *Chest* 101(suppl 5):289S–292S, 1992.

38. Alpert J, Bass H, Szucs M, et al: Effects of physical training on hemodynamics and pulmonary function at rest and during exercise in patients with chronic obstructive pulmonary disease. *Chest* 66:647–651, 1974.

39. Degre S, Sergysels R, Messin R, et al: Hemodynamic responses to physical training in patients with chronic lung disease. *Am Rev Respir Dis* 110:395–402, 1974.

40. Chester E, Belman M, Bahler R, et al: Multidiscipline treatment of chronic pulmonary insufficiency, III: the effect of physical training on cardiopulmonary performance in patients with chronic obstructive disease. *Chest* 72:695–702, 1977.

41. Laskey W, Ferrari V, Palevsky H, Kussmaul W: Pulmonary artery hemodynamics in primary pulmonary hypertension. *J Am Coll Cardiol* 21(2):406–412, 1993.

Chapter 42
VENTILATORY MUSCLE TRAINING

CARMEN LISBOA
GISELLA BORZONE

Since Leith and Bradley[1] demonstrated that it was possible to improve inspiratory muscle function in normal subjects by specific training, there has been increasing research in this area.[2-4]

Although several studies have shown better strength and endurance of respiratory muscles with training, the clinical significance of the improvement of certain indices of respiratory muscle function remains controversial. Most studies have centered on the changes in respiratory muscle function, without assessing their clinical effects in terms of improvements in dyspnea, exercise capacity, and quality of life. We are not aware of any reports on the effects of ventilatory muscle training (VMT) on morbidity or mortality.

Moreover the indications and best methods for VMT is another important area which will be better defined and more likely vary among patients.

General Aspects of VMT

Training modifies the structure and function of skeletal muscles. However, to obtain a training response it is necessary to apply a sufficiently large stimulus. According to Faulkner[5] three basic principles must be taken into consideration in devising training regimes:

1. *Intensity:* For a skeletal fiber to alter its structure and functional capacity, the stimulus must exceed a threshold or a critical intensity level.
2. *Specificity:* The type of stimulus applied determines the nature of the changes. Thus, strength training results in increased strength, while endurance training improves endurance.
3. *Reversibility:* The effects of training decline after training stops.

With regard to specificity, different stimuli have been used for VMT in normal subjects and in patients. For strength training, low repetitive, high-intensity inspiratory or expiratory near maximal maneuvers are recommended. Endurance training is generally achieved by performing highly repetitive, low-tension contractions such as occurs with maximal voluntary ventilation (MVV) maneuvers. It has been shown that by repetitively using intermediate levels of contraction it is possible to increase both strength and endurance.[6,7]

The author's research in this article was supported by FONDECYT. Grants: 90/715, 92/96, 195/1149.

Methods of VMT

The most frequently employed methods for training the respiratory muscles are:

1. *Voluntary isocapnic hyperpnea:* This consists in sustaining the highest possible level of minute ventilation for 10 to 15 min. A rebreathing circuit is required to maintain normocapnia. Since this circuit can be rather complex, there are few clinical studies using this method. The outcome of this type of training is generally measured by evaluating the changes in MVV or in maximal sustainable voluntary capacity (MSVC).
2. *Inspiratory resistive breathing:* Subjects inspire by mouth through devices (resistive loads) with orifices of progressively decreasing diameter. With resistive loads like this, the level of the load varies with the inspiratory flow and, therefore, is highly dependent on the pattern of breathing adopted by the subject during the training maneuvers. In order to assure the maintenance of a constant load, it is necessary to control both the breathing pattern and the target pressure. The response to resistive breathing training is generally evaluated by assessing changes in PImax and in endurance time during loaded breathing.
3. *Threshold inspiratory training:* The training stimulus is a combination of pressure and flow loads, applied through devices in which the subject must first develop a given pressure to open a valve and thereby initiate inspiratory flow. Once the valve is opened, by the subject's effort, inspiration is unhindered. Thus, the inspiratory muscles must overcome first a pressure load and then a low flow load. The training responses are evaluated in terms of changes in both strength and endurance.

Belman and associates[8] examined the characteristics of the load imposed on the inspiratory muscles (IM) by each of the three training methods described in COPD patients. They showed that important qualitative differences in ventilatory muscle loading are determined by the type of training device and the breathing strategy used. Therefore, to properly assess the outcome of a VMT protocol, particular attention should be given to the type of load that the respiratory muscles must overcome while training.

Ventilatory Muscle Training in Normal Subjects

In the study of Leith and Bradley[1] in normal subjects, the specificity of training was clearly shown. High intensity, low repetitive stimulus (maximal inspiratory and expiratory maneuvers) were able to induce a 55 percent increase in maximal respiratory pressures, but no changes in endurance were found. On the other hand, highly repetitive active like isocapnic hyperpnea produced a 19 percent increase in endurance with no changes in strength. This study also showed that the effects of training were reversible since strength and endurance returned to pretraining levels 15 weeks after training ceased.

Clanton and coworkers[9] using a threshold device with a load high enough to elicit respiratory muscle fatigue, also observed an increase in strength and endurance of respiratory muscles. A positive effect on endurance was also obtained by Belman and colleagues[10] using isocapnic hyperventilation in normal elderly subjects.

Recently, Tzelepis and coworkers[11] assessed the effects of different training protocols on inspiratory muscle function in normal subjects and confirmed that the effects of VMT are determined by the load and the method used (specificity). Their data suggest that ideally respiratory muscle training would use devices which would allow both flow and pressure experience, since in this way, it would be possible to improve both and thereby increase power output.

All these studies so far described were conducted in a laboratory setting with close supervision of training protocols so that their applicability could be questioned to clinical settings.

Ventilatory Muscle Training in Disease

Ventilatory muscle training has been used in patients with several disease states, with variable results. This may be due to differences in protocols, poor control of the training stimulus, and the use of different and at times inappropriate indices for the assessment of outcome.[2,12,13]

We will concentrate on the effects of training in COPD and neuromuscular diseases, in which the most research has been done. We will also describe the effects of VMT in patients with chronic congestive heart failure, since this group of patients has been reported to benefit from VMT.

Chronic Obstructive Pulmonary Diseases

RATIONALE FOR TRAINING RESPIRATORY MUSCLES IN COPD

In obstructive pulmonary disease maximal inspiratory pressures are reduced.[14,15] The rationale for VMT in this condition rests on the possibility of increasing inspiratory muscle reserve, and augmenting PImax during breathing. It is known that airways obstruction increases resistive work of breathing and contributes to dynamic hyperinflation with a consequent increase in elastic work. Therefore, for a given tidal volume patients with COPD must generate higher pressures (PI) as has demonstrated in studies using esophageal balloon catheters. On the other hand, hyperinflation places the inspiratory muscles, particularly the diaphragm, at a mechanical disadvantage, reducing their capability to generate tension (PImax). In addition to inspiratory muscle dysfunction derived from hyperinflation, COPD patients often have malnutrition which contributes to muscle weakness.[15,16]

The situation observed at rest (a high ratio of PI:PImax) is worsened when ventilatory requirements increase, such as occurs even during ordinary daily activities. With exercise increased, the ventilation demanded not only requires development of higher tensions by the inspiratory muscles, but also an increase in the velocity of muscle shortening. In patients with COPD, MSVC is also reduced, indicating impaired endurance, which crucially affects exercise tolerance. In addition, the discoordinated contraction of the breathing muscles, the inability to maintain adequate contraction of abdominal muscles, and the progressive hyperinflation all contribute to increasing the mechanical disadvantage of the inspiratory muscles, particularly the diaphragm during exercise.[17,18]

It is reasonable to expect that a ventilatory muscle training protocol which increases strength, endurance, and velocity of shortening of respiratory muscles would help in improving exercise capacity and, consequently, quality of life in these patients.

In COPD patients, dyspnea, although multifactorial, has been shown to be related to the proportion of maximum inspiratory muscle force used by the subject while breathing.[19,20] Muscle weakness and the increase in the work of breathing diminish inspiratory reserve. The reduction in inspiratory reserve and hyperinflation have been shown to correlate with hypercapnia in COPD patients.[21] Theoretically, at least, VMT by increasing strength, could improve inspiratory muscle reserve and thus, reduce dyspnea and hypercarbia.

VENTILATORY MUSCLE TRAINING IN COPD

Respiratory muscle training in COPD has been studied for more than 20 years, but its clinical utility has been controversial. The difference in the results reported is probably due to the relatively small number of patients in each study, and the lack of appropriate control groups. Failure to ensure that patients have employed an adequate training stimulus when using resistive breathing also contributes to inconsistencies in outcomes. Belman and associates[22] studied the effect of the breathing pattern used during resistive training, on the actual magnitude of the training load. They demonstrated that the use of a breathing pattern characterized by long and deep breaths results in an improvement in endurance, since, with this pattern, inspiratory mouth pressure, and thus the magnitude of the load, is reduced. Several studies using resistive training devices, which are highly dependent on the magnitude of flow, have been done in COPD, without control of the breathing pattern.[23–31] It is likely that in some of these studies, patients might have spontaneously adopted breathing strategies which minimize the effort sensation but also reduce the stimulus, to induce muscle remodelling. This certainly could be one cause for the variability in VMT effects that has been reported.

The following analysis of the effect of VMT in COPD patients will consider only those studies that have controlled both the load and the breathing pattern when using resistive training, or those that have employed a threshold device in which the magnitude of the load is practically flow independent.[6,7,32–45] Isocapnic hyperpnea will also be considered although it has been utilized much less frequently as a training stimulus in patients.[46,47]

TARGET RESISTIVE TRAINING

Table 42-1 summarizes the characteristics and outcomes of the studies that have controlled the load during resistive training.

Belman and Shadmehr[7] trained patients with a PFLEX device (Healthscan, Cedar Grove, NJ) and used a targeted feedback device to control pressure and pattern of breathing. Patients in the study group trained with a high intensity stimulus (target pressure as high as tolerated) whereas controls used a low intensity stimulus (7.5 to 10 cmH$_2$O). VMT for 6 weeks led to an increase in strength (PImax) and in

TABLE 42-1 Resistive Target Training in COPD

Reference	Sample Size	Training Characteristics	Duration	Outcome[a]
Belman and Shadmehr[7]	8 subjects 9 controls	High intensity Low intensity	6 weeks	↑ Pımax ↑ MSVC ↑ PIFR ↑ sustainable work
Harver et al[32]	10 subjects 8 controls	High intensity Low intensity	8 weeks	↑ Pımax ↓ Dyspnea
Heijdra et al[33]	10 subjects 10 controls	60% Pımax 10% Pımax	10 weeks	↑ Pdimax ↑ Pımax ↑ SIPmax ↑ Endurance time ↑ Nocturnal saturation

[a] Outcome: compared to control group
NOTE: Pımax, maximal inspiratory pressure; MSVC, maximal sustainable ventilatory capacity; PıFR, peak inspiratory flow rate; Pdimax, maximal transdiaphragmatic pressure; SIPmax, maximal sustainable inspiratory pressure.

endurance (MSVC) in both groups, but with a significantly larger effect in the high intensity load group, which also showed a significant increase in maximal sustainable mouth pressure (SIPmax), peak inspiratory flow, and maximal sustained work during loaded breathing. Harver and associates[32] also trained their patients using feedback. Eight weeks of training resulted in an increase in Pımax measured from FRC in their study group, although differences from the control group were not significant. These investigators also evaluated, the effect of VMT on dyspnea and found a significant improvement in the study group as compared to the control group. They found a significant correlation between the improvement in Pımax measured from residual volume and the improvement in dyspnea for both groups. As far as we know, this was the first study showing a clear evidence of improvement in dyspnea with VMT.

Another interesting effect of VMT has been recently reported by Heijdra and coworkers.[33] Using target-flow inspiratory training, they demonstrated that VMT improves Sa_{O_2} during sleep, probably related to the improvement in Pdimax, maximal sustainable inspiratory pressure (SIP), and endurance time.

In summary, studies that control the training load, report a significant increase in IM strength or endurance. Beneficial effect on dyspnea and on nocturnal desaturation are other reported positive outcomes.

THRESHOLD INSPIRATORY TRAINING

The studies that have used threshold inspiratory loads for training are summarized in Table 42-2.

Threshold inspiratory load training has the advantage over other methods since the applied load is flow-independent within a wide range of flow rates.[6] Therefore, the breathing strategy used by the patients while on the load is not critical to the success of the training.

Larson and associates[6] trained patients with 30 percent Pımax and controls with loads that were 15 percent Pımax. Eight weeks later, patients with the highest load had increased Pımax, endurance time, and the distance walked in 12 min (12 MWD) with no changes in respiratory symptoms or quality of life. The improvement in inspiratory muscle function with threshold training was confirmed by Flynn and

associates.[34] They also reported that their patients changed respiratory pattern during breathing on the threshold load to one that had a shorter inspiratory time as a fraction of total breath time (TI/Ttot) and a higher tidal volume to inspiratory time ratio after training. This permits a longer expiratory time (TE), possibly affording a larger resting period for the muscles and more time to return to a lower FRC. No effect on exercise tolerance was observed. Similar results have been reported by Lisboa and associates[35] employing two different training loads. They demonstrated that VMT with a load of 30 percent of Pımax produces a significant increase in Pımax, inspiratory muscle power output, endurance and dyspnea as compared to a load of 10 percent Pımax. After training, patients in the study group had changed their breathing pattern during loaded breathing in the same way as described by Flynn and coworkers.[34]

Preusser and colleagues[36] used even higher training loads in a supervised setting. The high intensity group trained with a load of approximately 52 percent of Pımax, while the low intensity group developed 22 percent of Pımax. They evaluated changes in strength, endurance, external work and symptoms during an endurance test and also the 12 MWD. Pımax increased only in the high load group whereas all the other indices showed a similar level of improvement in both groups. These results suggest that it is possible to obtain similar effects on respiratory muscle function and exercise capacity using different training loads. It is necessary to point out that the training load considered by Preusser and coworkers[36] to be low, ranged from 18 to 27 percent Pımax. This load is equivalent to the loads used by some other investigators who found positive training effects with them. Furthermore, several authors have reported some improvement in respiratory muscle function with even lower loads.[7,35]

The clinical effects of VMT for 10 weeks using a load of 30 percent of Pımax, were assessed by Lisboa and associates[37] in a group of COPD patients (FEV₁: 37 ± 3 percent of predicted). They observed a significant reduction in dyspnea transition index[38] and in the sensation of respiratory effort (Borg score) after walking for 6 min, as compared to a group trained with a load of 10 percent of Pımax. Both groups increased Pımax and the number of daily living activities they were able to perform. In a second phase the training loads were crossed over and patients trained for another 10

TABLE 42-2 Threshold Training in COPD

Reference	Sample Size	Training Characteristics	Duration	Outcome[a]
Larson et al[6]	10 subjects 12 controls	30% Pımax 15% Pımax	8 weeks	↑ Endurance ↑ Pımax ↑ 12 MD No changes in Q of L or symptoms
Flynn et al[34]	8 subjects 7 controls	High intensity None	6 weeks	↑ Pımax No changes in exercise performance
Lisboa et al[35]	10 subjects 10 controls	30% Pımax 10% Pımax	5 weeks	↑ Pımax ↑ Inspiratory muscle power ↑ Vımax ↓ Dyspnea
Preusser et al[36]	12 subjects 8 controls	52% Pımax 22% Pımax	12 weeks	↑ Pımax No significant differences in endurance and 12 MD between groups
Lisboa et al[37]	10 subjects 10 controls	30% Pımax 10% Pımax	10 weeks and cross over	↑ Pımax ↑ 6 MD ↓ Dyspnea

[a] Outcome: compared to control group

NOTE: 12 MD, 12-min walking distance; Q of L, quality of life; Vımax, maximal inspiratory flow; 6MD, 6-min walking distance.

weeks. The group that initially trained with a load of 30 percent of Pımax and then changed to a load of 10 percent of Pımax, showed no significant deterioration in either dyspnea, distance covered by walking for 6 min (6MWD), although a significant fall in Pımax was observed. There was no change reported in the quality of life. The group changing from the low to the high load showed a significant reduction in dyspnea and an increase in Pımax and 6MWD, which reached similar values to the group initially trained with the highest load. Figures 42-1, 42-2, and 42-3 show the changes in Pımax, transition dyspnea index, and in 6MWD in the two groups.

Two different hypothesis may explain the lack of clinical deterioration during the period in which a lower load was used: (1) the duration of the study might have been too short to show a loss in clinical effects, and (2) the use of a low load (10 percent Pımax) might be high enough to maintain the improvements gained with the higher training load.

That VMT is able to improve the power output of inspiratory muscles in COPD patients can be inferred from the data of Belman and Shadmehr[7] who measured endurance during loaded resistive breathing on resistive loads. They found a significantly greater rise in mean pressure, peak inspiratory flow rate, and work rate in the high intensity trained group as compared to the low intensity group. These changes are consistent with an improvement in power output and in the

FIGURE 42-1 Mean Pımax values + 1 SE in COPD patients before and after 10 weeks of VMT, followed by crossing the loads over for another 10 weeks. Patients initially trained with 30 percent Pımax (group 1) are represented by squares and those with 10 percent Pımax (group 2) by closed circles. After the first 10 weeks of VMT a significant increase in Pımax was observed in both groups. After crossing the loads over, Pımax fell in group 1 and continued to improve in group 2. (Anova for repeated measures). (From Lisboa et al.,[39] with permission.)

FIGURE 42-2 Effect of VMT on 6 MD using the same protocol as in Fig. 42-1. After VMT, 6 MD increased significantly in group 1. No deterioration when this load was lowered was observed. A significant improvement after increasing the load was observed in group 2. (Modified from Lisboa et al.,[39] with permission.)

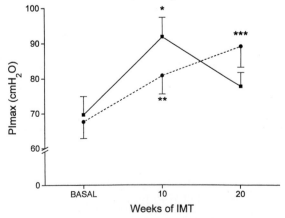

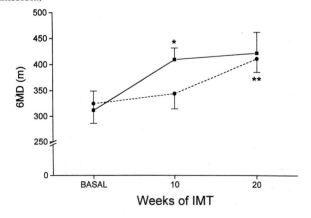

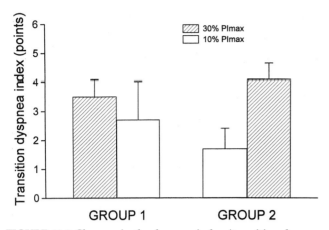

FIGURE 42-3 Changes in the dyspnea index (transition dyspnea index) in both groups after crossing the loads over. This index grades changes in dyspnea based on effort task, and effort on daily activities.[38] Patients in group 1 exhibited a nonsignificant deterioration, whereas in patients of group 2 a significant improvement in dyspnea was observed. (From Lisboa et al.,[39] with permission.)

velocity of shortening of inspiratory muscles, which may be beneficial when coping with the ventilatory demands of exercise. Lisboa and coworkers[35,39] have also reported improvement in inspiratory muscle power output with training with low and high threshold loads, mainly due to an increase of inspiratory flow. The patients who trained with the lower load, also increased power output, but chiefly by increasing the maximal sustainable pressure.[39]

We have evaluated the effects of VMT on exercise performance and found a reduction in both ventilation and V_{O_2} for the same level of exercise. A significant correlation between the fall in V_E and the reduction of V_{O_2} was also found, suggesting that the reduction in the metabolic cost of exercise might be related to the lower ventilation during exercise.[40] We speculated that dyspnea improved because of VMT. These patients could have increased their daily physical activity, achieving some degree of general training which, in turn, could have decreased lactic acid production for the same level of exercise, inducing a lower stimulus for ventilation.

All these studies demonstrate that threshold inspiratory training, with loads of different magnitude, improves inspiratory muscle strength, with variable effects on endurance or on exercise capacity. Two studies[34,35] have shown that after VMT, patients change their breathing pattern during loaded breathing to one with a shorter inspiratory time. This is associated with an increase in mean inspiratory flow. These results suggest that the velocity of shortening of inspiratory muscles becomes greater with VMT. The improvement in inspiratory flow and in V_T/T_I might be a convenient strategy to overcome the increased loads that arise during exacerbations.

ISOCAPNIC HYPERVENTILATION

Isocapnic hyperventilation has been infrequently used as a training stimulus for respiratory muscles in COPD.

Levine and coworkers[46] compared the effects of this type of VMT with those of intermittent positive pressure breathing (IPPB). Training was performed in the laboratory for 6 weeks and its effects were assessed through changes in pulmonary function tests, activities of daily living in endurance, psychological status, and exercise tests. Patients in the VMT group exhibited a significant increase in endurance (23 percent) as compared to the IPPB group, with no difference in the improvement of other parameters.

Ries and Moser[47] compared the effect of isocapnic hyperventilation training with that of walking exercise training. The VMT group showed a significant increase in both V_E and V_{O_2}max, associated to a nonsignificant improvement in inspiratory muscle endurance. No changes were observed in the control group. These few available studies do not allow us to draw definitive conclusions regarding this method of training.

VMT AS PART OF A MORE GLOBAL EXERCISE REHABILITATION PROGRAM

Table 42-3 summarizes the reported results of protocols combining the two interventions.

Goldstein and associates[41] studied the effect of combining threshold inspiratory training and physical rehabilitation in a small group of six patients using the highest load they could endure for 10 min. The control group trained with a very low load. Although an increase in endurance was observed in the study group, no additional effect on exercise tolerance was obtained. In contrast, Dekhuijzen and associates[42] demonstrated favorable effects using target flow inspiratory training as an additional procedure in a rehabilitation program consisting of 2 h of exercise training 5 days a week. Both groups increased P_{Imax} and the 12MWD, with a significantly larger improvement in the study group. Maximal work during exercise, V_{O_2}max and activities of daily living improved in both groups with no significant differences between them. In the study of Weiner and colleagues,[43] the effect of combining general exercise reconditioning (GER) with VMT was compared to GER alone and with a control group which received no training at all. Patients who received VMT added to GER, significantly improved inspiratory muscle performance and exercise tolerance as compared to those patients who received GER alone. A similar study was conducted by Wanke and coworkers.[44] Patients in the combined training group showed a significant improvement in diaphragm strength and endurance. Both groups increased maximal power output and oxygen uptake during exercise, but the improvement was significantly greater in the group with VMT. These results show that VMT, added to an exercise program using cycle ergometer for example, may enhance the beneficial effects of exercise training. According to the authors, the improvement in pressure generating capacity of the inspiratory muscles may enable patients to tolerate high levels of ventilation during exercise.

Different results and conclusions were reported by Berry and associates[45] when comparing the effect of combining VMT with general exercise reconditioning. They failed to find significant differences between groups. The authors' conclusion was that VMT does not provide additional clinically significant improvement in exercise performance. However, it is likely that the lack of difference between groups might be due to the use of a sham load of 15 percent P_{Imax} which could be high enough to produce some improvement in inspiratory muscles.

TABLE 42-3 Ventilatory Muscle Training Added to Exercise Reconditioning in COPD

Reference	Sample Size	Protocol	Type of VMT	Duration	Outcome[a]
Goldstein et al[41]	6 subjects 5 controls	RP + VMT RP + Sham VMT	Threshold	4 weeks	↑ IM endurance No difference in exercise tolerance
Dekhuijzen et al[42]	20 subjects 20 controls	RP + VMT 70% Pimax RP	Target flow	10 weeks	↑ Pimax ↑ 12 MD as compared to RP
Weiner et al[43]	12 subjects 12 controls 12 controls	GER + VMT 60% Pimax GER + Sham VMT No GER + No VMT	Threshold	6 months	↑ Pimax ↑ Endurance ↑ 12 MD as compared to GER
Wanke et al[44]	21 subjects 21 controls	Exercise + VMT Exercise	Threshold maximal in- spiratory maneuver	8 weeks	↑ Pimax ↑ Pdimax ↑ Exercise performance as compared to exercise alone
Berry et al[45]	8 subjects 9 controls 9 controls	GER + VMT 80% Pimax GER + VMT 15% Pimax VMT 15% Pimax	Threshold	12 weeks	No differences between groups in Pimax ↑ 12 MD similar to exercise group

[a] Outcome: compared to exercise

NOTE: RP, rehabilitation program; VMT, ventilatory muscle training; GER, general exercise reconditioning; IM, inspiratory muscles.

In summary, these studies seem to demonstrate that VMT added to an exercise training protocol in a general rehabilitation program improves exercise capacity in patients with COPD.

Neuromuscular Diseases

RATIONALE FOR TRAINING RESPIRATORY MUSCLES

Neuromuscular diseases can affect the ventilatory system at several levels resulting in weakness of the respiratory muscles and impairment of force generation. It has been shown that the inability of the inspiratory muscle to adequately expand the thorax results in stiffening of the costovertebral joints with a reduction in chest wall compliance.[48] In addition, the absence of deep breathing leads to microatelectasis and decreased pulmonary compliance. The reduction in both chest wall and lung compliance elevates the load on the inspiratory muscles and the work of breathing. Thus, on the one hand the capacity to generate force is diminished and on the other hand, higher pressures are necessary to overcome the increased loads. Therefore, inspiratory muscle reserve is reduced leading to fatigue and respiratory failure, which are the most important causes of death in these patients. Impaired cough, due to weakness of expiratory muscles together with the microatelectasis, contribute to frequent respiratory infections.[13] Training the respiratory muscles with the aim of improving their strength and endurance may prevent the development of these complications.

VMT IN NEUROMUSCULAR DISORDERS

The effects of VMT on strength and endurance of inspiratory muscles in these patients have been studied mainly in patients with Duchenne's muscular dystrophy (DMD). Most of the studies, however, do not have a control group and results are not definitive. No effect on IM strength after 8 weeks of VMT using resistive training was reported by Martinez and coworkers,[49] although an increase in endurance was found. Smith and colleagues[50] employed isocapnic hyperpnea as a

training stimulus, and found no changes in strength or in maximal voluntary ventilation after 5 weeks of training. A lack of improvement of VMT in this disease has also been reported by Rodillo and associates[51] in a double-blind cross-over trial using a resistive device with no control of the load. Different results were obtained by Wanke and associates[52] in a recent ramdomized controlled study. In 15 patients they used a special inspiratory resistive training device that provided visual control of the patients' performance. After 1 month of VMT, they found an improvement in inspiratory muscle strength and endurance (assessed by changes in Pdi and Tlim) with a subsequent increment at 3 and 6 months. Five of these patients discontinued VMT after 1 month because inspiratory muscle function was not better. These five patients had vital capacities less than 25 percent predicted and/or a Pa_{CO_2} over 45 mmHg. No significant improvements in respiratory muscle function were found in the control group. The authors conclude that in patients with Duchennes's muscular dystrophy, respiratory muscles, and the diaphragm in particular, are trainable for strength and endurance, provided that their ventilatory function is not already extremely limited. These findings are in agreement with those reported by Vilozni and associates[53] in a recent study with no control group. They employed hyperventilation as a stimulus and found a significant improvement in endurance only in patients with a moderate impairment of lung function, or in those who were recently immobilized or still ambulatory. Wanke and coworkers[52] studied whether training very weak inspiratory muscles caused them to fatigue. Their results show that the most severely affected patients do not show evidence of inspiratory muscle exhaustion with VMT, at least for 1 month.

In summary, the studies that have controlled the training load in patients with moderately severe DMD have found improved respiratory muscle function.

Quadriplegia is another condition in which the function of respiratory muscle, and the expiratory muscles in particular, can be severely impaired. It has been shown that patients with traumatic tetraplegia use the clavicular portion of the pectoralis major to expire actively. Estenne and associates[54] demonstrated that training with intermittent submaximal isometric contractions increased pectoralis muscle strength and expiratory reserve volume, as compared to patients in the control group undergoing conventional rehabilitation. From a clinical point of view the improvement of expiratory muscle function is very important in improving the effectiveness of cough. In 1980, Gross and coworkers[55] showed that the diaphragm in patients with quadriplegia is predisposed to fatigue due to reduced strength and endurance. They also demonstrated that VMT using resistive supervised inspiratory training increases both strength and endurance and protects against fatigue.

VMT in Patients with Chronic Heart Disease and Failure

Respiratory muscle function is impaired in some cardiac diseases, such as mitral valve disease[56] and chronic heart failure (CHF).[57] It has also been shown that inspiratory muscle weakness correlates with dyspnea in these patients.[58] McParland and associates demonstrated a reduction in inspiratory muscle strength in CHF, despite normal expiratory and limb muscle strength.[59]

Recently Mancini and associates[60] used VMT in patients with chronic congestive heart disease. They showed that training improved exercise capacity in these patients. Their VMT protocol was performed in the laboratory 3 days per week, using three different stimuli: isocapnic hyperventilation, resistive training, and strength training. Three months of VMT produced a significant increase in endurance, respiratory muscle strength, and exercise capacity measured by the 6MWD and peak V_{O_2}. Improvement in dyspnea and in the activities of daily living were also found. As compared to VMT studies in other diseases, this program was more intense and the authors evaluated its effects not only on respiratory muscle in function, but also on symptoms and exercise capacity. The improvement in dyspnea was attributed either to an increase in inspiratory muscle strength with a consequent improvement in respiratory muscle reserve or to dyspnea desensitization. The increase in V_{O_2} was believed to be caused by an increment in consumption of the inspiratory muscles as a result of training. As no changes in resting and exercise heart rate, as well as in V_{O_2} at the anaerobic threshold, were found, a systemic training effect was discarded. No cardiac complications related to VMT were observed. From this study it appears that VMT is safe in these patients, with no deleterious effects.

Conclusions

In spite of some controversial results, VMT seems to be a useful tool for rehabilitation of respiratory patients.

In our experience and in the literature reviewed, when a proper load is used respiratory muscle function improves with VMT, both in normal subjects and in patients with COPD. Moreover, there are encouraging data showing positive effects in other conditions such as neuromuscular diseases and chronic cardiac failure. The inconsistent results, which have discouraged clinical use, arise mainly from studies using resistive devices without an adequate control of the target load. Another confounding factor is that the loads used for control groups in many studies, are sufficient to induce a mild degree of training, thus reducing the differences between compared groups.

There is a correlation between the improvement in P_{Imax} and the reduction in dyspnea that has been demonstrated in some studies. VMT added to general physical training also appears to be beneficial in COPD patients. Larger studies, however, are necessary prior to widespread clinical application.

Regarding the training regime, there is not enough information to recommend one in particular, but we think that programs using intermediate loads (30 to 50 percent P_{Imax}) appear to be the most convenient. They not only increase strength and endurance of inspiratory muscles, but also inspiratory flow and power output, which are important factors in coping with the increased ventilatory demands of exercise. This can be achieved using threshold devices which are commercially available and can be effectively used for home training. A scheme of 15 min twice a day, 5 days a week, for at least 5 weeks, seems reasonable. It has not been established which is the minimum stimulus required to maintain the effects obtained with VMT.

The criteria for selecting patients for training are not defined. From a theoretical point of view, if a patient with COPD has few symptoms, and his or her respiratory muscle function is preserved, VMT may not be useful. On the other side, if there is severe muscle dysfunction, VMT could be detrimental. Therefore, we consider that the patients most likely to show positive effects are those presenting with dyspnea during daily living activities and moderately severe inspiratory muscle dysfunction. In neuromuscular disease, other criteria have to be developed, since the symptoms and goals of treatment are different.

References

1. Leith DE, Bradley M: Ventilatory muscle strength and endurance training. *J Appl Physiol* 41(4):508–516, 1976.
2. Goldstein RS: Ventilatory muscle training. Pulmonary rehabilitation in chronic respiratory insufficiency 3. *Thorax* 48:1025–1033, 1993.
3. Smith K, Cook D, Guyatt G, et al: Respiratory muscle training in chronic airflow limitation: A meta-analysis. *Am Rev Respir Dis* 145:533–539, 1992.
4. Gosselink R, Decramer M: Inspiratory muscle training: Where are we? *Eur Respir J* 7:2103–2105, 1994.
5. Faulkner JA: New perspectives in training for maximum performance. *JAMA* 205:741–746, 1968.
6. Larson JL, Kim MJ, Sharp JT, Larson DA: Inspiratory muscle training with a pressure threshold breathing device in patients with chronic obstructive pulmonary disease. *Am Rev Respir Dis* 138:689–696, 1988.
7. Belman MJ, Shadmehr R: Targeted resistive ventilatory muscle training in chronic obstructive pulmonary disease. *J Appl Physiol* 65(6):2726–2735, 1988.
8. Belman MJ, Botnick WC, Nathan SDF, Chon KIH: Ventilatory load characteristics during ventilatory muscle training. *Am J Respir Crit Care Med* 149:925–929, 1994.
9. Clanton TL, Dixon G, Drake J, Gadek JE: Inspiratory muscle conditioning using a threshold loading device. *Chest* 87(1):62–66, 1985.
10. Belman MJ, Gaesser GA: Ventilatory muscle training in the elderly. *J Appl Physiol* 64:899–905, 1988.

11. Tzelepis GF, Vega DL, Cohen D, et al: Pressure-flow specificity of inspiratory muscle training. *J Appl Physiol* 77(2):795–801, 1994.

12. Reid WD, Samrai B: Respiratory muscle training for patients with chronic obstructive pulmonary disease. *Phys Ther* 75:996–1005, 1995.

13. McCool FD, Tzelepis GE: Inspiratory muscle training in the patient with neuromuscular disease. *Phys Ther* 75:1006–1014, 1995.

14. Rochester DF, Arora NS, Braun NMT, Goldberg SK: The respiratory muscles in chronic obstructive pulmonary disease (COPD). *Bull Euro Physiopath Respir* 15:951–975, 1979.

15. Rochester DF: Effects of COPD on the respiratory muscles, in Cherniack NS (ed): *Chronic Obstructive Pulmonary Disease.* Philadelphia, Saunders, 1991:134–155.

16. Rochester DS, Braun NMT, Arora NS: Respiratory muscle strength in chronic obstructive pulmonary disease. *Am Rev Respir Dis* 119:151–154, 1979.

17. Gallagher CG: Exercise limitation and clinical exercise testing in chronic obstructive pulmonary disease. *Clin Chest Med* 15:305–326, 1994.

18. Dodd DS, Brancatisano T, Engel LA: Chest wall mechanics during exercise in patients with severe airflow obstruction. *Am Rev Respir Dis* 129:33–38, 1984.

19. O'Connell JM, Campbell AH: Respiratory mechanics in airways obstruction associated with inspiratory dyspnea. *Thorax* 31:669–676, 1976.

20. Killian KJ, Jones NL: Mechanisms of external dyspnea. *Clin Chest Med* 15:247–257, 1994.

21. Bégin P, Grassino A: Inspiratory muscle dysfunction and chronic hypercarbia in chronic obstructive pulmonary disease. *Am Rev Respir Dis* 143:905–912, 1991.

22. Belman MJ, Thomas SG, Lewis MI: Resistive breathing training in patients with chronic obstructive pulmonary disease. *Chest* 90:662–669, 1986.

23. Belman MJ, Mittman C: Ventilatory muscle training improves exercise capacity in chronic obstructive pulmonary disease patients. *Am Rev Respir Dis* 121:273–280, 1980.

24. Pardy R, Rivington RN, Despas P, Macklem PT: The effects of inspiratory muscle training on exercise performance in chronic airflow limitation. *Am Rev Respir Dis* 123:426–433, 1981.

25. Moreno R, Moreno R, Giugliano C, Lisboa C: Entrenamiento muscular inspiratorio en pacientes con limitación crónica del flujo aéreo. *Rev Méd Chile* 111:647–653, 1983.

26. Sonne LJ, Davis JA: Increased exercise performance in patients with severe COPD following inspiratory resistive training. *Chest* 81:436–439, 1982.

27. Jederlinic P, Muspratt JA, Miller MJ: Inspiratory muscle training in clinical practice. Physiologic conditioning or habituation to suffocation. *Chest* 86(6):870–873, 1984.

28. Ambrosino N, Paggiaro PL, Roselli MG, Contini V: Failure of resistive breathing training to improve pulmonary function tests in patients with chronic obstructive pulmonary disease. *Respiration* 84:455–459, 1984.

29. Patessio A, Rampulla C, Fracchia C, et al: Relationship between the perception of breathlessness and inspiratory resistive loading: Report on a clinical trial. *Eur Respir J* 2(suppl 7):587s–591s, 1989.

30. Guyatt G, Keller J, Singer J, et al: Controlled trial of respiratory muscle training in chronic airflow limitation. *Thorax* 47:598–602, 1992.

31. Chen H-I, Dukes R, Martin B: Inspiratory muscle training in patients with chronic obstructive pulmonary disease. *Am Rev Respir Dis* 131:251–255, 1985.

32. Harver A, Mahler DA, Daubenspeck JA: Targeted inspiratory muscle training improves respiratory muscle function and reduces dyspnea in patients with chronic obstructive pulmonary disease. *Ann Intern Med* 111:117–124, 1989.

33. Heijdra YF, Dekhuijzen PNR, Van Herwaarden CLA, Folgering HThM: Nocturnal saturation improves by target-flow inspiratory muscle training in patients with COPD. *Am J Respir Crit Care Med* 153:260–265, 1996.

34. Flynn MG, Barter CE, Nosworthy JC, et al: Threshold pressure training, breathing pattern, and exercise performance in chronic airflow obstruction. *Chest* 95:535–540, 1989.

35. Lisboa C, Muñoz V, Beroiza T, et al: Inspiratory muscle training in chronic airflow limitation: Comparison of two different training loads with a threshold device. *Eur Respir J* 7:1266–1274, 1994.

36. Preusser BA, Winningham ML, Clanton TL: High- vs low-intensity inspiratory muscle interval training in patients with COPD. *Chest* 106:110–117, 1994.

37. Lisboa C, Villafranca C, Pertuzé J, et al: Efectos clínicos del entrenamiento muscular inspiratorio en pacientes con limitación crónica del flujo aéreo. *Rev Méd Chile* 123:1108–1115, 1995.

38. Mahler DA, Weinberg DH, Wells CK, Feinstein AR: The measurement of dyspnea. Contents, interobserver agreement and physiologic correlates of two new clinical indexes. *Chest* 85:751–758, 1984.

39. Lisboa C, Villafranca C, Leiva A, et al: Inspiratory muscle training improves inspiratory muscle power output during loaded breathing in patients with COPD. *Am J Respir Crit Care Med* 151(4): A807, 1995.

40. Lisboa C, Villafranca C, Leiva A, et al: Inspiratory muscle training in chronic airflow limitation: Effect on exercise performance. *Eur Respir J* 10:537–542, 1997.

41. Goldstein R, De Rosie J, Long S, et al: Applicability of a threshold loading device for inspiratory muscle testing and training in patients with COPD. *Chest* 96:564–571, 1989.

42. Dekhuijzen PNR, Folgering HThM, Van Herwaarden CLA: Target-flow inspiratory muscle training during pulmonary rehabilitation in patients with COPD. *Chest* 99:128–133, 1991.

43. Weiner P, Azgad Y, Ganam R: Inspiratory muscle training combined with general exercise reconditioning in patients with COPD. *Chest* 102:1351–1356, 1992.

44. Wanke Th, Formanek D, Lahrmann H, et al: Effects of combined inspiratory muscle and cycle ergometer training on exercise performance in patients with COPD. *Eur Respir J* 7:2205–2211, 1994.

45. Berry MJ, Adair NE, Sevensky KS, et al: Inspiratory muscle training and whole-body reconditioning in chronic obstructive pulmonary disease. A controlled ramdomized trial. *Am J Respir Crit Care Med* 153:1812–1816, 1996.

46. Levine S, Weiser P, Gillen J: Evaluation of a ventilatory muscle endurance training program in the rehabilitation of patients with chronic obstructive pulmonary disease. *Am Rev Respir Dis* 133: 400–406, 1986.

47. Ries AL, Moser KM: Comparison of isocapnic hyperventilation and walking exercise training at home in pulmonary rehabilitation. *Chest* 90:285–289, 1986.

48. De Troyer A, Pride NB: The respiratory system in neuromuscular disorders, in Roussos C, Macklem PT: *The Thorax.* New York, Marcel Dekker, 1985; pp 1089–1121.

49. Martínez AJ, Stern L, Yeates J, et al: Respiratory muscle training in Duchenne muscular dystrophy. *Dev Med Child Neurol* 28:314–318, 1986.

50. Smith PM, Coahly JM, Edwards RHT: Respiratory muscle training in Duchenne muscular dystrophy. *Muscle Nerve* 11:784–785, 1988.

51. Rodillo E, Noble-Jamieson CM, Aber V, et al: Respiratory muscle training in Duchenne muscular dystrophy. *Arch Dis Child* 64:736–738, 1989.

52. Wanke T, Toifl K, Merkle M, et al: Inspiratory muscle training in patients with duchenne muscular dystrophy. *Chest* 105:475–482, 1994.

53. Vilozni D, Bar-Yishay E, Gur I, et al: Computerized respiratory muscle training in children with duchenne muscular dystrophy. *Neuromusc Disord* 4:249–255, 1994.

54. Estenne M, Knoop C, Vanvaerenberg J, et al: The effect of pecto-

ralis muscle training in tetraplegic subjects. *Am Rev Respir Dis* 139:1218–1222, 1989.

55. Gross D, Ladd HW, Riley EJ, et al: The effect of training on strength and endurance of the diaphragm in quadriplegia. *Am J Med* 68:27–35, 1980.

56. De Troyer A, Estenne M, Yernault JC: Disturbance of respiratory muscle function in patients with mitral valve disease. *Am J Med* 69:867–873, 1980.

57. Hammond MD, Bauer KA, Sharp JT, Rocha RD: Respiratory muscle strength in congestive heart failure. *Chest* 98:1091–1094, 1990.

58. McParland C, Krishnan B, Wang Y, Gallagher CG: Respiratory muscle weakness and dyspnea in chronic congestive heart failure. *Am Rev Respir Dis* 148:467–472, 1992.

59. McParland C, Resch EF, Krishnan B, et al: Inspiratory muscle weakness in chronic heart failure: Role of nutrition and electrolyte status and systemic myopathy. *Am J Respir Crit Care Med* 151:1101–1107, 1995.

60. Mancini DM, Henson D, La Manca J, et al: Benefit of selective respiratory muscle training on exercise capacity in patients with chronic congestive heart failure. *Circulation* 91:320–329, 1995.

Chapter 43

EXPERIENCES WITH SURGERY FOR CHRONIC LUNG DISEASE IN JAPAN

TAKAYUKI SHIRAKUSA

AKINORI IWASAKI

MINORU YOSHIDA

HIDEO TOYOSHIMA

Pulmonary emphysema, one kind of chronic lung disease, has been considered to be a completely irreversible disease. Until now, the most common treatment regimen for this disease has been a variety of medications, oxygen therapy, and pulmonary rehabilitation. Surgical treatment was initially reported in the 1950s by Dr. Brantigan,[1,2] however, his results were heavily criticized. Recently, Wakabayashi and coworkers[3,4] and Keenan and colleagues[5] have described performing laser ablation under a thoracoscope for chronic emphysema which has resulted in the improvement of subjective and objective symptoms. Moreover, Cooper and associates[6,7] have performed a direct resection of the damaged surface of an emphysematous lung, which was introduced as a pneumectomy in 1995[6] and has been referred to as a so-called "volume reduction surgery." Mckenna and coworkers[8] have utilized the technique of the thoracoscope for lung volume reduction, with results similar to that of a pneumectomy. Currently, the thoracoscopic volume reduction surgery is being used worldwide.[8–10] In addition, however, lung plication, a method to reduce emphysematous lesions of the lung surface with thoracoscopic resection, has recently been introduced as another surgical approach. Each of these procedures has its own merits and demerits. We have used all of these therapeutic approaches and have compared the results.

Indications for Surgical Treatment

In our unit, volume reduction surgery (VRS) is indicated for those who match the following criteria: (1) those in whom, despite strong medical treatment and management, dyspnea has not improved, (2) those who have been correctly diagnosed with pulmonary emphysema by a respiratory physician, (3) who have not experienced severe cardiac dysfunction, (4) who have no past history of thoracotomy, (5) who are under 80, (6) who have not experienced any other lung disease, (7) whose dyspnea is above grade III in the Hugh-Jones classification, and (8) for whom, on chest computerized tomogram and a pulmonary blood flow scintigram, the destructive lesion is heterogeneous. In addition, the patients with respiratory infection, that is, chronic bronchitis or bronchiectasis are avoided. Surgery in patients who smoke is also contraindicated. Figure 43-

1 shows the flow chart for the treatment of pulmonary emphysema, and Table 43-1 shows the summarized selection criteria for absolute and relative indications of surgical treatment for pulmonary emphysema.

Preoperative Patient Management

Preoperatively, chest radiograph, chest computed tomography, pulmonary blood flow scintigraphy, spirogram, precise lung function with emphysema, blood gas analyses, and cardiac function including cardiac catheterization data are necessary.

To determine whether surgical treatment is indicated or not, close cooperation between the respiratory physicians and the chest surgeons is indispensable. Smoking must be strictly prohibited for at least 3 months preoperatively. After thoracoscopic volume reduction surgery, various kinds of physiotherapy are necessary because of the effects of the surgical treatment. The most annoying complication of VRS is prolonged air leakage after the operation. Intractable air leaks may become a trigger of life threatening pneumonia or pyothorax. In fact, we lost one patient due to delayed air leakage following severe pyothorax after VRS. Great care must be taken to avoid injury of the lung surface or laceration during operation because the emphysematous lung has structural alterations which make it prone to the development of air leaks.

Surgical Procedures

VRS UNDER MEDIAN STERNOTOMY[6,7,12]

Generally, the operation for emphysema is performed under general anesthesia, making necessary one-lung ventilation using a double-lumen tube. A standard median sternotomy is made in the supine position, and the mediastinal pleura on the left or right side is opened longitudinally. The lung on the operative side is deflated, and one-lung ventilation is directed to the contralateral side. Excision is directed to parts which are detected as bullous or as severely damaged by lesion through preoperative CT and a blood flow scintigram. Cooper and coworkers[6] have indicated that their goal in VRS has been to reduce the overall volume of each lung by 20 to 30 percent. Usually, stapling devices are used successively for the resection of the lung. At this time, the use of some kind of buttress is necessary to prevent prolonged air leakage. Cooper[12] has obtained good results using bovine pericardial strips to buttress the staple line.

THORACOSCOPIC VRS[9,10]

In thoracoscopic VRS, under general anesthesia one-lung ventilation during the operation is also necessary. Initially, the first trocar is located at the fifth intercostal space on the midaxillary line. The trocar should not be inserted roughly, because violent handling of the trocar can sometimes lacerate the lung, causing prolonged air leakage. The second trocar should be inserted under thoracoscopic observation through the first trocar port. In addition, one or two ports should be made for the camera and the clamp in the anterior or posterior chest wall. The camera port should usually be placed at the seventh or eighth intercostal space on the midaxillary

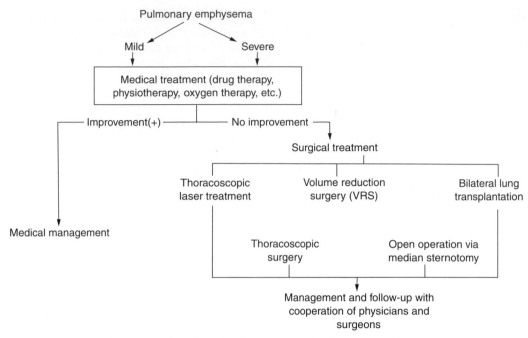

FIGURE 43-1 Flow chart for the treatment of pulmonary emphysema.

line. Using this procedure, the upper lobe and the basilar segment can be totally visualized. VRS usually begins from the apical area. A ring forceps or endoscopic clamp is inserted into the thoracic cavity, and the lung parenchyma is grasped at the apex of the lung.

The appropriate area of lung for resection is selected by inspecting the video monitor. An endoscopic stapler is introduced into the thoracic cavity, and a total of 20 to 30 percent of the lung may be resected by serial use of the stapler. Two drainage tubes, one for air leakage and the other for drainage of exudated fluid, are placed through the anterior and posterior incisions made for the ports. VRS on the contralateral side should be continued after changing the position of the patients in whom bilateral thoracoscopic VRS has been planned preoperatively.

TABLE 43-1 Selection Criteria of Fukuoka University for Indication of Surgical Treatment of Pulmonary Emphysema

Absolute criteria for operation
1. Established diagnosis of pulmonary emphysema based on clinical evaluation of respiratory function
2. Persistent dyspnea despite adequate medical therapy
3. Grade III or more advanced dyspnea according to Hugh-Jones classification
4. Heterogenous distribution of affected lung tissue demonstrated by CT scans and pulmonary blood flow scintigraphy

Relative criteria for operation
5. Absence of complications such as infection (bronchiectasia, pneumonia, etc.)
6. Strict abstinence from smoking
7. Under age 80 years
8. Absence of advanced cardiac dysfunction
9. Absence of extensive adhesions due to previous thoracotomy
10. Overinflation of the lung and flat diaphragm on chest x-ray films

SOURCE: The Second Department of Surgery, Fukuoka University.

LASER ABLATION[3–5,13]

Laser ablation is usually performed using a contact-type Nd-YAG laser at 5 to 10 W until the ablated lung surface becomes whitish. Although the entire pleural surface of the lung can be treated with laser ablation, this can also be combined with resection using an endoscopic stapler for apparent bullous lesions. After these procedures, the maximal shrinkage may be obtained; however, precautions should be taken to avoid excessive ablation which can often lead to perforation of the lung. The ablation of the contralateral side can also be performed thoracoscopically.

LUNG PLICATION[11]

The techniques for a thoracoscopic lung plication have recently been developed. This surgical procedure is performed using some specific endoscopic devices. Under the same anesthesia as used for thoracoscopic VRS, three or four ports are placed at the anterior, lateral, and posterior chest walls for camera and forceps. The thoracoscope is introduced through the camera port, and the assessment for plication is performed over the whole lung on video. After the lung plicating clamp is inserted into the thoracic cavity, the lung surface is grasped with the ring forceps. The appropriate amount of lung is rotated 180 degrees to allow compression of the lung parenchyma against the underlying lung tissue. The compressed lung tissue is stapled at its base by the endoscopic stapler.

Effect of Surgical Treatment on Lung Function

At present the 6-min walking distance is often used to assess the effects of surgical treatment. Cooper and coworkers[6] have reported that, at the time patients were first referred to them

TABLE 43-2 Results of FEV$_{1.0}$ (mL) before and after the Surgical Treatment of Pulmonary Emphysema

Author	No. of Patients	FEV$_{1.0}$ (mL)		Statistical Significance (p)
		Preoperative	Postoperative	
Cooper[6]	20	770 (25%)	1400 (44%)	<.001
Keenan[16]	67	820 ± 50 (30%)	1040 ± 60 (39%)	<.001
Keller[10]	25	800 ± 330	1050 ± 410	<.001
Little[19]	28	740 ± 70	850 ± 60	<.01
Miller[14]	40	560	1100	<.05
Nauheim[18]	25	710 ± 310	860 ± 530	<.001
Roue[20]	13	592 ± 143 (18 ± 5%)	896 ± 265 (27 ± 8%)	<.05
Teschler[15]	17	800 ± 70 (31 ± 2%)	1100 ± 80 (41 ± 2%)	<.001
Wakabayashi[4]	202	23.6 ± 10.8%	31.0 ± 9.6%	<.01
Shirakusa	35	859 ± 385 (39 ± 17%)	1203 ± 531 (54 ± 22%)	<.001

for treatment, the mean distance covered in 6 min was only 958 ft. This distance increased to approximately 1500 ft 6 months after the operation. Keller and colleagues[10] have described that in 25 patients with VRS, the 6-min walk distance increased from 934 ft preoperatively to 1071 ft postoperatively. Miller and coworkers[14] and Teschler and associates[15] have also reported that the postoperative distance for the 6-min walk increased significantly compared to the preoperative distance. In our unit, we have performed VRS in 35 patients by thoracoscope or under median sternotomy. The average volume of the FEV$_{1.0}$ was 860 mL preoperatively. Three months after the operation, this increased to 1200 mL (average), which is a significant improvement ($p < .001$) (Table 43-2) (Fig. 43-2). The forced vital capacity also increased significantly from 2500 mL (average) to 2950 mL (average). We evaluated the percent improvement of FEV$_{1.0}$, {[postoperative FEV$_{1.0}$ (mL)] − [preoperative FEV$_{1.0}$ (mL)]} / [preoperative FEV$_{1.0}$ (mL) × 100%] 3 months postoperatively in patients who had different surgical procedures. The improvement averaged 27 percent after unilateral thoracoscopic

VRS, 54 percent by VRS performed by median sternotomy, and 63 percent with bilateral thoracoscopic VRS. Based on these results, we concluded that results after thoracoscopic VRS are similar to those of VRS under median sternotomy.

Pulmonary function was also assessed by an exercise tolerance test with a bicycle ergometer, and by measurement of lung volume including the residual volume (Table 43-3) (Fig. 43-3), elastic recoil, dynamic compliance, and by the respiratory muscle function. The postoperative data in all those tests were better than those before VRS. As for DLCO (pulmonary diffusing capacity), two different results have been reported. Keenan and coworkers[16] and Wakabayashi and colleagues[4] have reported postoperative elevation of DLCO; however, Martinez and associates[17] have found that of no significant use after VRS. The evaluation of blood gas analysis is also somewhat controversial. Although in some reports[15,18–20] postoperative improvement of Pa$_{O_2}$ has been shown; other authors[4,14] have not observed these positive changes. Our results showed no significant change in Pa$_{O_2}$, postoperatively.

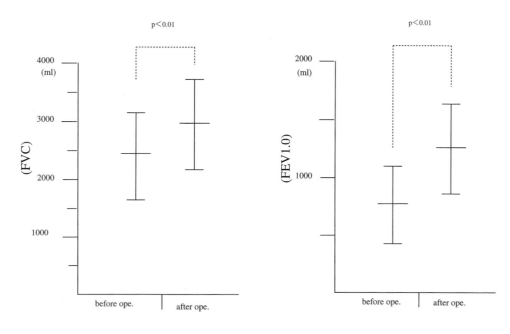

FIGURE 43-2 FVC (mL) and FEV$_{1.0}$ (mL) before and after surgical treatment of pulmonary emphysema ($n = 35$).

TABLE 43-3 Results of Residual Volume (RV) before and after the Surgical Treatment of Pulmonary Emphysema

Author	No. of Patients	RV (mL)		Statistical Significance (p)
		Preoperative	Postoperative	
Cooper[6]	20	5900 ± (288%)	3600 (177%)	<.001
Keenan[16]	28	5070 ± 350	4440 ± 350	<.01
Keller[10]	25	4840 ± 1610	4170 ± 1060	<.05
Little[19]	20	4500 ± 510	4070 ± 490	<.05
Nauheim[18]	15	6210 ± 1960	4160 ± 1270	n.s.
Teschler[15]	17	337 ± 31%	250 ± 21%	<.001
Wakabayashi[4]	125	201.0 ± 59.0%	174.9 ± 62.1	<.001
Shirakusa	20	5450 ± 1030 (324 ± 63%)	4620 ± 910 (276 ± 58%)	<.001

Current Problems of VRS and a View of the Future

Currently, the morbidity and mortality caused by COPD are increasing in European countries, as well as in the United States and Japan. In the past lung transplantation had been the sole surgical treatment for patients with a severe type of chronic emphysema. However, it has been difficult to perform large numbers of lung transplantations, and especially double lung transplantations because of a scarcity of donations of lungs from brain dead patients. Although in Japan organ transplantation is still legally permitted as of October

1997, the chances of performing a double lung transplantation are relatively small because of problems with using donations from brain dead patients. Under the current circumstances, surgical treatment is expected to become a much more common solution for patients with chronic emphysema in Japan, in particular for the over 10,000 patients who receive home oxygen therapy.

Until now, four types of surgical treatments have been introduced to us from America. Laser ablation has the benefit of its being less invasive for patients, however, the functional improvements are smaller than for other types of VRS. The frequency of applying laser ablation as a treatment for emphysema is declining in Japan, including in our unit. Lung

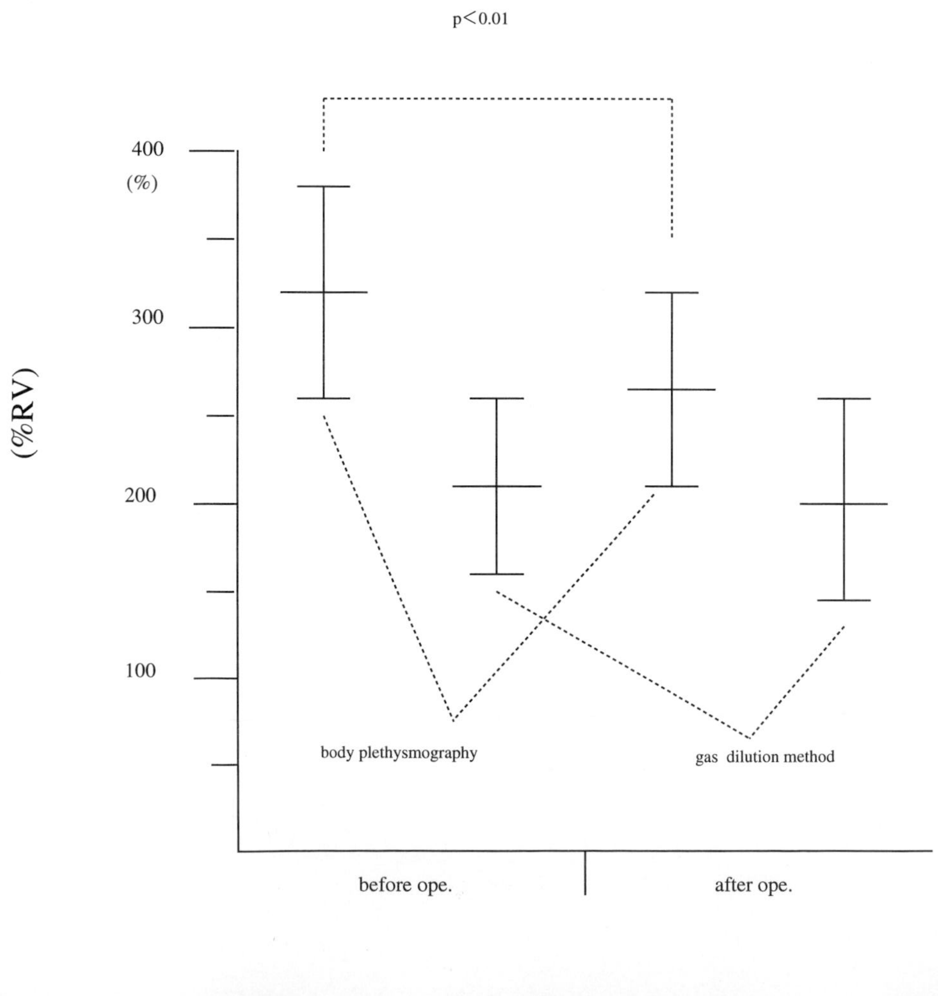

FIGURE 43-3 Percent residual volume before and after surgical treatment of pulmonary emphysema ($n = 20$).

plication also has the advantages of reducing the frequency of prolonged air leakage, however, the procedure is occasionally difficult because plicating devices are not appropriate for handling the slender physique of Japanese patients. There are two kinds of VRS accepted worldwide nowadays. VRS under median sternotomy has the following advantages: (1) it is an easy and accurate procedure for resecting destroyed lung, and (2) VRS under median sternotomy is a safe surgical treatment because air leakage during the operation can be confirmed by direct visualization and repaired correctly. We consider that the main disadvantages of this procedure are its invasiveness from the perspective of blood loss during the operation and postoperative pain. The dehiscence of the sternal attachment has been observed occasionally, and if it does occur, can be a serious complication in aged patients. Thoracoscopic VRS is less invasive than VRS under midsternotomy. The total doses of analgesic drugs administered postoperatively is less than that after VRS under median sternotomy. The blood loss during the operation is usually under 50 mL in a bilateral operation. VRS under median sternotomy is also more useful in resecting the lesions from the apex to the anterior part of the lung. On the other hand, by thoracoscopic VRS, the whole lung is resectable. For these reasons, we consider that thoracoscopic VRS is more favorable for aged patients with a poor performance status, and we like to use VRS under median sternotomy for patients who are younger and whose target areas for resection are in the apex to the anterolateral field of lung. As to the extent of volume reduction, Cooper and coworkers[6] have described their goal is to reduce the overall volume of each lung by 20 to 30 percent. McKenna and coworkers[8] have reported that their reduction volume was 46 ± 16 g in unilateral thoracoscopic VRS and 98 ± 28 g in bilateral thoracoscopic VRS. In our unit, the mean lung volume resected was 121.6 ± 43.2 g (average) under bilateral thoracoscopy and 122.2 ± 61.7 g (average) under median sternotomy.

Summary

Although the physiologic mechanism responsible for the clinical and functional improvements is still not well understood, it is an undisputed fact that volume reduction of overinflated lung tissue in emphysema patients significantly improves the overall quality of life. Further studies are necessary to evaluate the long-term effectiveness in prognosis after surgical treatment, compared with former methods of management.

References

1. Brantingan OC, Mueller E, Kress MB: A surgical approach to pulmonary emphysema. *Am Rev Respir Dis* 80:194, 1959.
2. Brantigan OC, Kress MB, Mueller EA: The surgical approach to pulmonary emphysema. *Dis Chest* 39:485, 1961.
3. Wakabayashi A, Brenner M, Wilson BF, et al: Thoracoscopic laser ablation of diffuse bullous emphysema. *Lancet* 337:881, 1991.
4. Wakabayashi A: Thoracoscopic laser pneumoplasty in the treatment of diffuse bullous emphysema. *Ann Thorac Surg* 60:936, 1995.
5. Keenan RJ, Landreneau RJ, Hazelrigg SR: Video-assisted thoracic surgical resection with the Nd:YAG laser. *J Thorac Cardivasc Surg* 110:363, 1995.
6. Cooper JD, Trulock EP, Triantefillow AN, et al: Bilateral pneumectomy (volume reduction) for chronic obstructive pulmonary disease. *J Thorac Cardiovasc Surg* 109:106, 1995.
7. Cooper JD, Patterson GA, Sumdaresan RS, et al: Results of 150 consecutive bilateral lung volume reduction procedures in patients with severe emphysema. *J Thorac Cardiovasc Surg* 112:1319, 1996.
8. Mckenna RJ, Brenner M, Gelb AF, et al: A randomized prospective trial of stapled lung reduction versus laser bullectomy for diffuse emphysema. *J Thorac Cardiovasc Surg* 111:317, 1996.
9. Shirakusa T: Video-assisted thoracoscopic surgery for pulmonary emphysema and bullous lung disease. *Asian Med J* 40:513, 1997.
10. Keller CA, Ruppel G, Hibbett A, et al: Thoracoscopic lung volume reduction surgery reduces dyspnea and improves exercise capacity in patients with pulmonary emphysema. *Am J Respir Crit Care Med* 156:60, 1997.
11. Crosa-Dorado VL, Pomi J, Perez-Penco EJ, et al: Treatment of dyspnea in emphysema: Pulmonary remodeling. Hemo- and pneumostatic suturing of the emphysematous lung. *Res Surg* 4:No3, 1992.
12. Cooper JD: Technique to reduce air leaks after resection of emphysematous lung. *Ann Thorac Surg* 57:1038, 1994.
13. Brenner M, Kayaleh RA, Milne EN, et al: Thoracoscopic laser ablation of pulmonary bullae. *J Thorac Cardiovasc Surg* 107:883, 1994.
14. Miller JI, Lee RB, Mansour KA, et al: Lung volume reduction surgery: Lessons learned. *Ann Thorac Surg* 61:1464, 1996.
15. Teschler H, Stamtis G, El-Raouf Farhat AA, et al: Effect of surgical lung volume reduction on respiratory muscle function in pulmonary emphysema. *Eur Respir J* 9:1779, 1996.
16. Keenan RJ, Landreau RJ, Sciurba FC: Unilateral thoracoscopic surgical approach for diffuse emphysema. *J Thorac Cardiovasc Surg* 111:308, 1996.
17. Martinez FJ, Whyte RI: Lung-volume reduction improves dynamic hyperinflation and respiratory muscle function. *Am J Respir Crit Care Med* 155:1984, 1997.
18. Nauheim KS, Keller CA, Krucylak PE, et al: Unilateral video-assisted thoracic surgical lung reduction. *Ann Thorac Surg* 61:1092, 1996.
19. Little AG, Swain JA, Nino JJ, et al: Reduction pneumoplasty for emphysema, early results. *Ann Surg* 222:365, 1995.
20. Roue C, Mal H, Sleiman C, et al: Lung volume reduction in patients with severe diffuse emphysema. *Chest* 110:28, 1996.

Chapter 44

ELECTRICAL STIMULATION OF RESPIRATORY MUSCLES

ARIE OLIVEN

The concept of artificial respiration by electrical stimulation of the phrenic nerve was first suggested over 200 years ago by Caldani, who demonstrated movement of the diaphragm upon phrenic nerve stimulation (PNS).[1] In 1818 Ure, using a battery, stimulated the phrenic nerve of a criminal immediately after execution. He reported strong contractions of the diaphragm and suggested that PNS could be used for resuscitation.[2] Successful resuscitation using PNS was recorded in the second half of the 19th century,[3-5] when moistened sponges were placed over the sternocleidomastoid muscles, serving as electrodes. In 1872, Duchenne asserted that PNS was the best way of limiting natural respiration.[6]

The clinical application of PNS was abandoned, however, when methods for negative- and positive-pressure ventilatory support became available. Only in 1948 to 1949 did Sarnoff and coworkers demonstrate that percutaneous PNS could sustain ventilation in animals and in patients with bulbar poliomyelitis and coined the term "electrophrenic respiration."[7,8] It was through the work of Glenn and coworkers, however, that diaphragm pacing achieved clinical importance. They introduced radiofrequency in the early 1960s to stimulate the phrenic nerve[9] and used the new device successfully on an intermittent, long-term basis to assist ventilation in a patient with primary, chronic hypoventilation.[10] During the next 25 years, this group of physicians, basic scientists, and engineers designed a system that optimized implant equipment and electrode characteristics, improved patient selection and surgical procedures, and evaluated the most effective and least damaging mode of PNS. As a result of their work and the expertise gained in other centers, today PNS offers a viable alternative to those patients for whom conventional modes of therapy have been deemed inadequate. Throughout the world, more then 1200 patients, ranging in age from 1 month to 80 years, have now had diaphragm pacemakers implanted, some of which have been pacing for more than 20 years. Despite many limitations that have so far restricted its wider application, patients and their families often welcome this more physiologic modality of respiratory support because it enables independence from the ventilator, is less intimidating and easier to handle, and may facilitate speech.

Triggered by the successful application of PNS, electrical stimulation was also attempted on other respiratory muscles. Stimulation of intercostal and expiratory muscles has not yet gained clinical application, although it is effective in canine experiments. Recently, stimulation of upper airway dilator muscles has been proposed for the treatment of obstructive sleep apnea. These treatment modalities are currently under investigation and will be discussed at the end of this chapter.

Phrenic Nerve Stimulation

METHODS OF PNS

PNS was originally applied transcutaneously, at the base of the neck, during resuscitations. This method is no longer used as a means of artificial respiration but is reserved for testing the viability of the phrenic nerve. Goldenthal described transcutaneous PNS using a glass electrode filled with argon gas, to which surges of high voltage were delivered at low amperage,[11] but this method has been abandoned. Similarly, the transvenous route has been explored for unilateral and bilateral PNS by several investigators.[12-15] This technique has been used to test phrenic nerve function and pace the diaphragm for short periods postoperatively and was proposed for long-term respiratory assistance. The difficulty of maintaining close contact with the phrenic nerve and the use of external stimulators precluded clinical use of this technique.

Although a totally implantable nuclear battery-powered unit has been described,[14] reports of chronic transvenous PNS have not been published. A different approach has been tested by Nochomovitz and coworkers, who inserted multi-stranded helical wire electrodes directly into the diaphragm of dogs. They achieved efficient diaphragm contractions when the electrodes were placed in the vicinity of the main phrenic trunk.[16] Clinical reports have not been published, however, on this method, which uses laparoscopic techniques and could be helpful in cases with damage to the phrenic nerve.

For many years, the standard clinical technique for PNS has been direct stimulation of the phrenic nerve, with electrodes placed in the thorax. The electrode most used today is a ribbon electrode of platinum, which is implanted against the mediastinal surface of the phrenic nerve, below the heart, and embedded in silicon for isolation.[17] Monopolar electrodes are preferred, but bipolar electrodes are available for patients with cardiac pacemakers, the signal of which may interfere with that of the phrenic stimulator. The electrode should not encircle the nerve, as this may confine developing scar tissue and may constrict the nerve. The electrode area is 0.2 cm², and the generally applied current of 1.5 mA is well below the charge that may damage neural tissue.[18] Light and electron microscopy of phrenic nerves taken from dogs subjected to long-term PNS of varying frequencies, as well as pathologic examination of human phrenic nerves taken from patients after chronic PNS for respiratory assistance, did not reveal damage to the nerve attributable to electrical stimulation.[19,20] Therefore, more sophisticated electrodes, designed to change the stimulation fields periodically, have not achieved popularity.

EQUIPMENT

Due to the high energy required for stimulation, implanted batteries have not yet been applied for clinical use. Therefore, all PNS systems use radiofrequency with an external power source, the transmitter, that transfers energy to an implanted radio receiver. Three PNS systems are currently available. Each costs approximately $20,000, but, unlike mechanical ventilators, they do not require expensive maintenance or disposable supplies. Detailed instructions for the operation, maintenance, and trouble shooting of the apparatus are provided by the commercial suppliers. The most widely used system is that of Avery Laboratories, Commack, NY, which was developed by Glenn and coworkers, with work beginning in 1960. It is simple to implant, reimbursed by the major insurance plans in the United States, and includes transtelephonic monitoring.[21] The PNS system of Atrotech Oy, Finland, has been in use in many countries since 1980.[22] It employs a quadripolar electrode which stimulates portions of the phrenic nerve sequentially to lessen the risk of diaphragm fatigue. Med-Implant Biotechnisches Labor, Austria, provides a system that requires a complex microsurgical technique for electrode implantation, providing as many as 16 combinations of stimulation.[23] The system was introduced in 1984 and has been used mainly in Austria and Germany.

INDICATIONS AND PATIENT SELECTION

Candidates for PNS are chronic respiratory insufficient patients requiring long-term ventilatory assistance, who have no significant impairment of phrenic nerves or the diaphragm and have near-normal lung function. The main group suitable for PNS are quadriplegic patients with high cervical cord lesions, usually due to traumatic injury.[17,24] Subjects with central hypoventilation syndrome, either primary (Ondine's curse) or secondary to organic brain lesions, constitute a second large group of patients treated with PNS.[25] PNS was also proposed for patients with COPD who hypoventilate during oxygen administration,[26] but simpler alternative techniques are usually more effective. PNS was attempted on a few patients with chronic refractory singultus,[27,28] without much benefit.

Considering the surgical procedure and the high costs involved, accurate diagnosis and the exclusion of the causes of hypoventilation not manageable by PNS are crucial. In particular, significant lung disease and lower motoneuron and primary muscular diseases need to be ruled out. Once chronic respiratory insufficiency has become stable, with no further improvement expected, several months after an injury or disease, the candidate should undergo meticulous screening to evaluate lung, upper airway, respiratory center, phrenic nerves, and diaphragm function. Complete pulmonary evaluation, as feasible and/or indicated by the patient's condition, should include imaging, blood gas evaluation at rest and during exercise, lung function tests including volumes and diffusion, and/or ventilation-perfusion scan. A sleep study is essential in patients who are only ventilated part-time. Respiratory responses to hypercapnia and hypoxia should also be evaluated whenever indicated. In addition, diaphragm function can be evaluated by fluoroscopy, inspiratory pressure measurement, or most accurately by measuring transdiaphragmatic pressure.

Obviously, successful PNS requires good phrenic nerve and diaphragm function. Therefore, accurate tests to assess phrenic nerve viability are required before electrode implantation. The best technique for the evaluation of the phrenic nerves is to document the contractile response of the diaphragm to transcutaneous PNS by surface electrodes in the neck.[29] The phrenic nerve can be stimulated transcutaneously, at the posterior border of the sternocleidomastoid muscle at the level of the cricoid cartilage. One-Hertz pulses should produce vigorous hiccup-like contractions of the hemidiaphragm, visible as outward movements of the anterior abdominal wall and rib cage. The movement of the diaphragm can also be visualized by radiography or ultrasound. Forceful contraction or descent of the diaphragm of 5 cm or more usually indicates that pacing will be successful. No response of the diaphragm usually indicates nonviability of the lower motoneurons and precludes the use of pacing.[29] With partial responses, additional tests can be performed. Nerve conduction time can be assessed by measuring the time span between the electrical spike and the corresponding muscle action potential recorded from surface electrodes placed over the eighth intercostal space. Normal conduction time in healthy adults is 8.4 ± 0.8 ms (it is shorter in children), but moderate prolongation (up to 14 ms) does not preclude successful PNS.[30] The same intercostal electrodes can be used to record diaphragm EMG, whose presence indicates adequate nerve and muscle function. Also, transdiaphragmatic pressure (Pdi) recording can be used to assess neuromuscular function by measuring the pressure difference between the esophagus and the stomach during PNS.[31] Whenever false-negative results due to inadequacy of electrical PNS is suspected, magnetic stimulation of the phrenic nerve roots may be useful.[32,33] However, interpretation of partial or equivocal responses remain a concern despite all tests: Technical failure in locating the nerve (for example, in obese patients) is difficult to distinguish from phrenic lower neuron damage, which is quite common in paraplegic patients. Also, certain forms of partial, even serious nerve damage, can be dealt with by adequate adjustment of stimulation parameters[34] or intercostal to phrenic anastomoses.[35,36] Finally, contraction response may be markedly reduced solely due to disuse atrophy, which is reversible by diaphragm conditioning with PNS.[37]

CHOICE OF UNILATERAL AND BILATERAL PNS

For adults with central hypoventilation, particularly those who need nocturnal ventilatory support alone, unilateral PNS is often satisfactory. For adequate ventilation, the hemidiaphragm needs to be paced forcefully, at a relatively high frequency (usually about 20 Hz) at a rate of 12 to 14 per minute. Relief of chronic hypoxemia and hypercapnia can usually be achieved by unilateral pacing for 10 to 12 h nightly. Tracheostomy was often required for upper airway obstruction, but nasal CPAP may solve this problem. Usually, the patient with PNS for central hypoventilation may be discharged from the hospital 1 month after implantation.[38]

Bilateral PNS is required for all children with central hypoventilation and most quadriplegics, as paradoxical movement of the rib cage and the contralateral diaphragm reduces the effectiveness of unilateral PNS. Also, the high stimulation intensity and frequency needed with unilateral PNS increase the risk of neuromuscular fatigue. Bilateral PNS is also required when 24-h ventilatory support is indicated, in the presence of partial nerve damage, and whenever pulmonary and/or chest wall compliance is reduced. Usually, simultaneous bilateral PNS is used, although alternate side stimulation is also possible. Alternate breath stimulation of each hemidiaphragm has been tried in the past, but this method was not found to be advantageous. Alternate PNS of each side for periods up to 12 h was used in patients with central hypoventilation who started with only unilateral PNS and some time later needed contralateral PNS.[38]

SURGICAL PROCEDURE

Surgical techniques have been developed and used extensively for both the cervical and the thoracic implantation approaches.[17,38–40] Electrode implantation in the neck is simpler to perform, but accessory branches which join the main trunk in the thorax are not stimulated. Also, the vicinity to the brachial plexus may cause contractions due to current spread to the latter. There is also the possibility of electrode displacement by neck movements. Therefore, this approach is usually reserved only for patients with contraindications to thoracotomy. The usual thoracic approach is through the second interspace anteriorly,[38,40] but other approaches are used as well. Meticulous caution must be taken to avoid infection, the occurrence of which may damage the nerve and usually requires removal of the entire implanted system. For this reason, Glenn recommends avoiding the commonly undertaken simultaneous implantation of bilateral electrodes and prefers two operations separated by at least 2 weeks, to avoid the greater danger of infection from the longer operation.[39] For most cases, a monopolar electrode is placed behind the nerve, as this technique is less traumatic than that of a bipolar electrode. Traumatic damage to the nerve is the most common cause for PNS failure in patients with intact nerves. A detailed description of the surgical procedure is given elsewhere.[39,40]

PNS SCHEDULE

Diaphragm pacemaker function is tested before closure of the chest, by holding the transmitter antenna over the implanted receiver. A stimulation threshold above 2 mA indicates inadequate contact of electrode and nerve that should be improved. Short stimulations should also be performed during the first postoperative days in order to reveal malfunctions which may require immediate correction.

Diaphragm excursions should be measured under fluoroscopy about 2 weeks after the operation, by which time postoperative inflammation around the nerve will have settled. Descent of the paced diaphragm ought to be greater than that produced by healthy volunteers during maximal voluntary efforts (about 10 cm). If the dome of a hemidiaphragm moves less than 5 cm during maximal PNS, either some damage to the phrenic nerve or the diaphragm can be assumed, or not all nerve fibers have been stimulated. Stimulation threshold (the minimal current intensity eliciting visible diaphragm contraction) should be monitored. This threshold tends to rise slightly over the first 6 months but may decline later on. With bilateral PNS, stimulation intensity and threshold of each hemidiaphragm are different, and each side needs to be tested separately.[39] Pacing schedule must be tailored for each patient individually, depending on diagnosis, severity of hypoventilation, the presence of unilateral or bilateral electrodes, the need for either continuous or nighttime only stimulation, and individual response and complications. In patients with central hypoventilation, diaphragm atrophy is not present, PNS is usually unilateral, and diaphragm fatigue is less common, and 8- to 10-h pacing can begin in the third week postoperatively. For patients with bilateral PNS, most of whom are quadriplegics who were ventilated many weeks prior to PNS, the diaphragm needs first to be conditioned. PNS is initiated with 10- to 15-min stimulation per hour during wakefulness, and the

stimulation periods are gradually lengthened. A stimulation frequency of 10 to 12 Hz is used, which is gradually decreased as conditioning of the diaphragm adjusts to the lower stimulation frequency. Due to muscle plasticity, chronic low-frequency stimulation results in conversion of the high glycolytic, fast but fatigue-sensitive type II fibers to the oxidative, slow-twitch fatigue-resistant type I fibers.[41] The normal diaphragm contains about an equal percentage of type I and type II fibers, and conversion of a fast-twitch to a slow-twitch muscle during chronic stimulation is known to require a few weeks. Therefore, the initial vibrating diaphragm contraction during PNS changes to a smooth movement once slowing of twitch-responses results in fusion of contractions.[39] This conditioning makes it possible to further lower stimulation frequency to 7 to 8 Hz and eventually enables continuous PNS without fatigue.[42] Current intensity and respiratory frequency are set to the lowest level which enables adequate ventilation. All parameters are changed gradually, over many weeks, while respiratory parameters are continuously monitored. Mechanical ventilation is substituted whenever signs of fatigue are noted. A snug abdominal binding and change in respiratory rate are always required for sitting. Obviously, even without complications, achievement of full-time, fatigue-free pacing is a complicated process that requires a specialized center with a professional and experienced team to optimize the results. It usually takes 14 to 18 weeks to achieve optimal results, but considerably longer periods are required in children or whenever PNS-associated or unrelated complications slow the process. The upfront sum requested by centers which offer PNS is about $200,000, but the total expenses for equipment and training may exceed this. In addition, full patient cooperation and a highly motivated and dedicated family are indispensable.

COMPLICATIONS

A long list of complications has been reported since the introduction of PNS 30 years ago. Technical improvements and experience have enabled the reduction or have even eliminated many of these complications. However, most statistics include early patients and their complications.

SURGICAL COMPLICATIONS

Iatrogenic injury to the phrenic nerve is the most common cause of failure to pace a normal nerve. The nerve is easily damaged, and the injury may not be recognized initially, requiring a later surgical reexploration. In a multicenter report, phrenic nerve injury appeared to occur in 18 of 115 (16 percent) of bipolar cuff-electrodes implantations.[43] Introduction of the monopolar electrodes reduced this risk to 7 percent, and if patients in whom the thoracic approach was used are analyzed separately, nerve compromise was considered to be probable in only 2/54 (3.7 percent).[43] Infection at the site of any of the implanted components is a serious complication, as it usually requires removal of the whole system.[39] Antiseptic bath, careful antiseptic preparation of the skin, double gloves and double masks for all surgeons, systemic and local antibiotics, careful sterilization of implanted components and their separation from the skin incision and chest tubes, and separation of left and right side electrode implantation are all recommended to reduce the risk of infection[39] and may have reduced the 4.5 percent early infections reported for 265 implantations before 1986.[43]

STIMULATION-INDUCED DAMAGE

Whenever cuff electrodes are used (usually bipolar electrodes), late entrapment of the phrenic nerve by the surrounding scar tissue may occur. This complication, as well as stimulation-induced nerve injury, is probably rare, particularly after the introduction of the monopolar electrodes. On light- and electron-microscopic examination, chronically stimulated phrenic nerves of dogs appear to be well preserved.[19,20] Histologic examination of the chronically stimulated canine diaphragm, however, may show degenerative changes if relatively high stimulation frequencies are used for prolonged periods.[44,45] Autopsy data on 13 phrenic nerves and 7 diaphragms from patients who died during or following pacing have shown abnormalities in 7 and 5 patients, respectively, but the pathologic studies were considered to be insufficient to provide accurate assessment of possible pacing-related damage.[43]

LATE INFECTIONS

As implanted devices have an increased likelihood of infection with the passing of time, late infection of the PNS device may occur and was reported to develop as late as 4 years after implantation.[46]

EQUIPMENT FAILURE

Pacemaker failure in a quadriplegic patient can be disastrous. Malfunction (other than battery exhaustion) results most commonly from breakage of the wire from the battery to the transmitter or from a broken antenna cable, but any part of the device may fail, including component failure in the receiver, circuit failure in the radio-transmitter, or, occasionally, electrode lead wire breakage.[43] Failure of the radio-receiver, usually due to ingress of body fluid into the electrical components, was reported by Glenn to be an almost routine occurrence about 5 years after implantation.[47] This problem has been dealt with by improving the epoxy cover. Failure of an internal component necessitates surgical reexploration. Fodstad reported that 11 operations were required in seven patients for receiver failure, electrode breakage, fibrosis around the nerve, and skin necrosis over the receiver.[28] Twenty-six internal component malfunctions, 15 of which were receiver failure, were reported in 33 children, on average about 6 years after implantation.[46,48] Vanderlinden and coworkers reported 10 receiver failures in 14 patients with bilateral implants, 5 of which occurred in the same subject, with failures occurring after 2 to 9 years.[49]

Equipment failure is often gradual, enabling early recognition and repair, but may occur suddenly. The true occurrence of the latter complication in PNS-dependent quadriplegics is difficult to assess, because some of the reported sudden deaths of such patients at home could be due to sudden equipment failure. Therefore, continuous patient supervision and monitoring is mandatory. An individualized patient-activated alarm system needs to be an intrinsic part of the equipment, and a mechanical ventilator should always be at hand.

COMPLICATIONS RELATED TO TRACHEOSTOMY

Almost all patients treated by PNS require tracheostomy. During normal breathing, activation of upper airway dilator muscles precedes inspiratory muscle activity to maintain pharyngeal patency. The lack of this synchrony in PNS-treated patients results in obstructive apneas, unless tracheostomy is present. The tracheostomy is also useful whenever mechanical ventilation should be resumed. Complications due to tracheostomy are not unique for patients with PNS, and the same precautions as with any tracheostomy should be undertaken. However, if a PNS candidate can be ventilated by an external device without tracheostomy, this modality should be preferred to PNS.[50]

ANALYSIS OF PATIENTS AND OUTCOME

It is difficult to assess the true success rate of PNS, as many patients were implanted in centers that did not report their results. In the larger published reports,[28,43,46,48,49,51–54] important information often cannot be ascertained. This includes data on accurate assessment of unassisted breathing capacity over the first years after spinal cord injury, because sufficient recovery of the phrenic nerve to enable weaning from mechanical ventilation may require 2 years or longer.[55] Glenn and coworkers collected and reported cumulative data on 477 patients who had pacemakers implanted up to 1985.[43] He noted that because of the complexity of the data accumulated, no meaningful statistical analysis was feasible. Most information was available on 165 patients only, who were implanted in six centers (about half by Glenn's group in Yale): The mean age of the patients was 34 years but ranged from a few months to 83 years. Almost half of the patients had cervical cord injury, more than a quarter had brain stem lesions, and most of the others had idiopathic or congenital central hypoventilation. The mean time from diagnosis to PNS was about 3.5 years. Four patients were paced for more than 15 years, including one with full-time, bilateral PNS. There was one operative death, and two patients had spontaneous recovery of respiration. Pacing was applied for overnight support in half of the patients and all the time in a quarter of them.

In half of the patients, PNS was considered as successful, providing sufficient respiratory support, albeit the ventilatory deficit was not always completely corrected. In another third, PNS provided "significant support," defined as substantial respiratory improvement, but additional mechanical support was also required.

Success rate was not affected by the patient's diagnosis or the use of unilateral or bilateral electrodes. In the elderly, however, reduced lung and chest wall compliance and possibly reduced adaptability of the diaphragm may reduce PNS effectiveness.[30] By the time of the study, 40 percent of the patients were dead. PNS was considered to have been successful or provided significant support in 80 percent of those who have died, a rate similar to that calculated for the survivors. The main causes of death were respiratory or cardiac failure, as well as infections which were not considered to be related to pacing. Two thirds of the patients were living at home. About 40 percent of them were working or learning.

In a retrospective analysis, about half of the patients assessed as PNS failures should not have been chosen for pacing. At least half of the early complications could now be prevented.[43]

PNS IN CHILDREN

Results on diaphragm pacing in infants and children have been reported mainly by one group,[46,56–59] and Hunt and coworkers summarized and reported their experience in 1988.[48] Thirty-four infants and children had a diaphragm pacer implanted throughout a 10-year period. Of these patients 26 had central hypoventilation syndrome (mostly congenital), and only 5 were quadriplegics. In children with congenital hypoventilation, PNS was started, in the mean, at the age of 5 months.

Although PNS equipment has to be modified for children's size, the system is the same as for adults. Similar complications were reported, with the exception that electrode wires need to sustain substantially greater stress. However, PNS in children differs from that in adults in several aspects. High compliance of the lung and the chest wall and the free mobility of the mediastinum in young age enable paradoxical movement of the contralateral hemidiaphragm and the chest wall whenever unilateral PNS is attempted. Hence, bilateral stimulation is always necessary in the first years of life. In addition, the endurance of the infant's diaphragm is relatively low. Conditioning requires much longer periods, the results are inferior to those achieved in adults, and only seldom can the diaphragm be stimulated for more than 12 h/day. Therefore, only children who need ventilatory support during sleep alone can become fully independent of mechanical ventilation. Those who require continuous ventilatory support need mechanical assistance during sleep for many years. Tracheostomy is practically always required in all children. Despite all these limitations, the increased mobility and ambulation of paced children may substantially improve quality of life and can be taken into consideration also in children who require awake ventilatory support.

PNS COMPARED TO MECHANICAL VENTILATION

Primary central hypoventilation syndrome can be treated by PNS,[60] but the new IPPV, CPAP, and BiPAP systems may provide an adequate solution for most patients with sleep hypopnea.[61] PNS is no longer indicated for COPD and hiccups. The incidence of spinal injuries that require ventilatory support is increasing, however, due to vehicle accidents. About 4 percent of surviving spinal cord injury patients are admitted with a neurologic level of C3 or above and are essentially apneic on admission.[51] As a result of improvements in equipment and training of emergency teams and trauma centers, more apneic patients are surviving. In about a third of these patients respiratory function never recovers enough, and they need full-time ventilatory support on discharge from the rehabilitation center.

Carter and coworkers compared the outcome of 37 patients requiring full-time ventilatory support on discharge from the spinal cord injury center.[51] Eighteen were on PNS, and the groups, although not randomized, were similar in most parameters. Mortality was similar in both groups (32 and 39 percent for the ventilator and PNS groups, respectively), as were the causes of death. Differences in survival were probably due to selection bias. Comparison of quality of life and expenses was not given, and the authors concluded that a multicenter collaborative work is needed to answer the relevant questions. Other publications tended to favor PNS for subjective or practical considerations: nursing care is simplified, mobility is enhanced, and normal speech may be possible.[54] The PNS system is much smaller and lighter than a ventilator and has simpler maintenance.[52] The patients wel-

come pacing as a means to free them from a ventilator, whereas the families may find the PNS less intimidating and easier to handle.[49] On the other hand, Glenn estimated that 10 to 15 of his patients discontinued PNS either because they did not believe it was a help, or because they found the maintenance of the equipment too complicated.[43] Bach and O'Connor reviewed the most complete reports on PNS and argue that the absence of important documentation makes the relative success of PNS difficult to assess.[50] Being supporters of noninvasive methods of ventilation,[55] they concluded that PNS should be reserved for those for whom noninvasive methods have not been well tolerated.

FUTURE GOALS

The present experience has defined patient selection, surgical technique, and optimal pattern and schedule of PNS that have proved effective in the management of paralytic respiratory failure. For further improvement, several steps have been suggested:

1. Designation of centers for patient selection, surgery, and long-term rehabilitation, follow-up, and monitoring by teams of physicians, engineers, and paramedical personnel knowledgeable in pacing.[43]
2. Synchronization of PNS with upper airway dilator muscle activity would enable diaphragm pacing without tracheostomy. This handicap of PNS has been recognized for many years, but no solution has proved to be effective.
3. Development of a totally implantable, battery-powered pacemaker would further improve patient's mobility and independence. An experimental device was produced over 20 years ago,[62] but is not yet available for clinical use.

CONCLUSIONS

PNS is an effective method of providing ventilatory support. Its use, however, is confined primarily to the small group of quadriplegics with high cervical cord injury and selected patients with central hypoventilation, who have normal phrenic nerves, diaphragm contractility, and lung function. In addition, the assistance available for the patient must be carefully evaluated. Institutionalized patients usually deteriorate, and support of a highly motivated family, capable and ready to undertake the difficult burden of all aspects of daily care of the ventilated and paced quadriplegic patient at home,[52] is invaluable. Even under ideal conditions, commitment of great amount of time, effort, and financial resources are essential for PNS to be successful.[30,31,39,50]

Electrical Stimulation of Other Respiratory Muscles

INTERCOSTAL MUSCLES

In animal experiments performed over 30 years ago, electrical stimulation of the spinal cord has been shown to contract the muscles of respiration and cause sufficient air exchange to sustain ventilation for many hours.[63] DiMarco and coworkers performed several studies to assess the utility of inspiratory intercostal muscles stimulation to provide ventilatory support.[64-67] This mode of pacing was intended for quadriplegic patients with phrenic nerves inadequate for PNS and applied with epidural electrodes to the thoracic spinal cord. Adequate ventilation could be maintained by this mode of stimulation in anesthetized dogs,[65] but in quadriplegics sufficient tidal volume generation was maintained for a few hours only.[64] Combined alternate stimulation of inspiratory intercostal muscles and expiratory abdominal muscles has recently been shown to maintain eucapnia in anesthetized dogs.[64] Because the anervation of the expiratory muscles is usually intact in quadriplegia and the fact that these muscles can be activated by spinal stimulation,[68] it is possible that this technique may be useful in some patients with ventilator-dependent quadriplegia.

UPPER AIRWAY DILATOR MUSCLES

Attempts to use upper airway dilating muscles electrical stimulation (UAMS) as a treatment modality for patients with obstructive sleep apnea have been undertaken ever since the respiratory importance of these muscles' action began to be appreciated. Obstructive sleep apnea is a common disorder, affecting about 2 to 4 percent of the adult population. It is characterized by recurrent episodes of upper airway obstruction during sleep, resulting in sleep fragmentation, daytime fatigue, and substantial morbidity associated with hypoxemia and hypertension. Despite considerable research effort over the last two decades, the pathophysiologic mechanisms leading to pharyngeal obstruction during sleep are not well understood, and treatment modalities are only partially effective and/or poorly tolerated.

Although many anatomic abnormalities have been implicated in the pathogenesis of obstructive sleep apnea, the role of functional mechanisms is obvious, since apneas occur only during sleep. Upper airway patency during inspiration depends largely on the balance between the negative intraluminal pharyngeal pressure and the forces exerted by the dilating muscles that support its walls. Contraction of upper airway muscles maintain pharyngeal patency by both dilating the upper airway and by stiffening its walls. It is believed that diminution in the level of dilator muscle tone and inspiratory activity during the transition from wakefulness to sleep is manifested by increased pharyngeal resistance and collapsibility. Accordingly, restoring awake dilator muscle tone by UAMS should improve upper airway conductance and stability during sleep. Indeed, many animal studies,[69–75] as well as studies in healthy humans during wakefulness[76] and sleep,[77] have shown that UAMS effectively improves pharyngeal patency.

Reports on unpublished trials who used intramuscular electrodes for UAMS in patients with obstructive sleep apnea date back 20 years, with a variety of results having been described.[78,79] More recently, researchers from Sendai, Japan, reported a significant reduction in apnea index with the use of submental UAMS.[80,81] Submental stimulation was applied when an apnea lasted for 5 s, and stopped with the resumption of breathing. Although EEG was not recorded during UAMS and, hence, arousals could not be excluded, they found improvement in multiple sleep latency tests following stimulation nights. These findings were supported by other studies of small numbers of subjects.[82,83] However, subsequent larger studies, using improved techniques to record EEG during UAMS, failed to induce significant changes in

upper airway patency or apnea index without prior induction of EEG arousals.[84,85] Moreover, even high-intensity submental stimulation during wakefulness does not appear to affect the tongue muscles.[86] In other studies in patients with sleep apnea, the genioglossus muscle was stimulated directly with either intramuscular electrodes[87] or sublingual surface electrodes,[88] and pharyngeal resistance and collapsibility were measured. Although improved pharyngeal conductance and stability, and occasional interruption of apneas, could be documented during UAMS without any sign of arousal, it is obvious that the level of locally applicable UAMS, and, hence, its clinical applicability, is limited by pain-induced arousals.

Several animal experiments documented substantial improvements in pharyngeal patency during hypoglossus nerve stimulation.[89,90] In patients with sleep apnea, hypoglossus nerve stimulation has been shown to dilate the pharynx[85] and increase inspiratory airflow during sleep.[91] Since 1995, a few patients have been implanted with a hypoglossus nerve stimulator similar to the one used for PNS, in a clinical feasibility study.[92]

References

1. Caldani LMA: Institutiones physiologicae, Venezia, 1786. Cited by Schechter DC: Application of electrotherapy to noncardiac thoracic disorders. *Bull NY Acad Med* 46:932, 1970.
2. Ure A: Experiments made on the body of a criminal immediately after execution, with physiological and philosophical observations. *J Sci Arts* 12:1, 1818. Cited by Schechter DC: Application of electrotherapy to noncardiac thoracic disorders. *Bull NY Acad Med* 46:932, 1970.
3. Beard GM, Rockwell AD: A practical treatise on the medical & surgical uses of electricity, including localized and general faradization; localized and central galvanization: electrolysis and galvano-cautery. New York, William Wood & Co, 1875, p 663.
4. Ferguson. Cited by Schechter DC: Application of electrotherapy to noncardiac thoracic disorders. *Bull NY Acad Med* 46:932, 1970.
5. Hufeland CW: *De usu vis electricae in asphyxia experimentis illustrato. Inauguraldissert, Gottingae,* 1873. Cited by Schechter DC: Application of electrotherapy to noncardiac thoracic disorders. *Bull NY Acad Med* 46:932, 1970.
6. Duchenne G: *De l'électrisation localisée et de son application a la pathologie et a la therapeutique par courants induits et par courants galvaniques interompus et continus.* Paris, Librairie J.B. Bailliere, 1872, p 914.
7. Sarnoff SJ, Hardenberg E, Whittenberger JL: Electrophrenic respiration: *Am J Physiol* 155:1, 1948.
8. Whittenberger JL, Sarnoff SJ, Hardenberg E: Electrophrenic respiration: II. Its use in man. *J Clin Invest* 28:124, 1949.
9. Glenn WWL, Hageman JH, Mauro A, et al: Electrical stimulation of excitable tissue by radio-frequency transmission. *Ann Surg* 160:338, 1964.
10. Judson JP, Glenn WWL: Radiofrequency electrophrenic respiration: Long-term application to a patient with primary hypoventilation. *JAMA* 203:1033, 1968.
11. Goldenthal S: Bilateral and unilateral activation of the diaphragm in the intact human: External electrical stimulation by capacitive coupling as recorded by cineradiography. *Conn Med* 25:236, 1961.
12. Daggett WM, Piccinini JC, Austen WG: A percutaneous wire electrode for chronic research use. *IEEE Trans Biomed Eng* 22:429, 1975.
13. Daggett WM, Shanahan EA, Kazemi H, et al: Intracaval electrophrenic stimulation: II. Studies on pulmonary mechanics, sur-

face tension, urine flow, and bilateral phrenic nerve stimulation. *J Thorac Cardiovasc Surg* 60:98, 1970.

14. Furman S, Koerner SK, Escher DJW, et al: Transvenous stimulation of the phrenic nerves. *J Thorac Cardiovasc Surg* 62:743, 1971.

15. Wanner A, Sackner MA: Transvenous phrenic nerve stimulation in anesthetized dogs. *J Appl Physiol* 34:489, 1973.

16. Nochomovitz ML, DiMarco AF, Mortimer JT, Cherniack NS: Diaphragm activation with intramuscular stimulation in dogs. *Am Rev Respir Dis* 127:325, 1983.

17. Glenn WWL, Hogan JF, Phelps ML: Ventilatory support of the quadriplegic patient with respiratory paralysis by diaphragm pacing. *Surg Clin North Am* 60:1055, 1980.

18. Pudenz RH: Adverse effects of electrical energy applied to the nervous system. *Neurosurgery* 1:190, 1977.

19. Kim JH, Manuelidis EE, Glenn WWL, Kaaneyuki T: Diaphragm pacing: Histopathological changes in the phrenic nerve following long-term electrical stimulation. *J Thorac Cardiovasc Surg* 72:602, 1976.

20. Kim JH, Manuelidis EE, Glenn WWL, et al: Light and electron microscopic studies of phrenic nerves after long-term electrical stimulation. *J Neurosurg* 58:84, 1983.

21. Auerbach A, Albert A, Dobelle WH: Transtelephonic monitoring of patients with implanted neurostimulators. *Lancet* 1:224–225, 1987.

22. Baer GA, Talonen PP, Shneerson JM, et al: Phrenic nerve stimulation for central ventilatory failure with bipolar and four-pole electrode systems. *PACE* 19:1061, 1990.

23. Thoma H, Gerner H, Holle J, et al: The phrenic pacemaker: Substitution of paralyzed functions in tetraplegia. *Trans Am Soc Artif Intern Organs* 33:472, 1987.

24. Glenn WWL, Hogan JF, Loke JSO, et al: Ventilatory support by pacing of the conditioned diaphragm in quadriplegia. *N Engl J Med* 310:1150, 1984.

25. Glenn WWL, Gee JBL, Cole DR, et al: Combined central alveolar hypoventilation and upper airway obstruction: Treatment by tracheostomy and diaphragm pacing. *Am J Med* 64:50, 1978.

26. Glenn WW, Gee JBL, Schacter EN: Diaphragm pacing: Application to a patient with chronic obstructive lung disease. *J Thorac Cardiovasc Surg* 75:273, 1978.

27. Fodstad H, Blom F: Phrenic nerve stimulation (diaphragm pacing) in chronic singultus. *Neurochirurgia* 27:115, 1984.

28. Fodstad H: The Swedish experience in phrenic nerve stimulation. *PACE* 10:246, 1987.

29. Shaw RK, Glenn WWL, Hogan JF, Phelps ML: Electrophysiological evaluation of phrenic nerve function in candidates for diaphragm pacing. *J Neurosurg* 53:345, 1980.

30. Glenn WWL, Sairenji H: Diaphragm pacing in the treatment of chronic ventilatory insufficiency, in Roussos C, Macklem PT (eds): *The Thorax: Lung Biology in Health and Disease,* vol 29. New York: Marcel Dekker, 1985, p 1407.

31. Moxham J, Shneerson JM: Diaphragmatic pacing. *Am Rev Respir Dis* 148:533, 1993.

32. Simolowski T, Fleury B, Launois S, et al: Cervical magnetic stimulation: A painless method for bilateral phrenic nerve stimulation in conscious humans. *J Appl Physiol* 67:1311, 1989.

33. Aquilina R, Wragg S, Moran J, et al: Magnetic stimulation as a simple and reliable method for stimulating the phrenic nerves in the neck. *Thorax* 46:754, 1991.

34. Dobelle WH: 200 cases with a new breathing pacemaker dispel myths about diaphragm pacing. *Trans Am Soc Artif Intern Organs* 40:244, 1994.

35. Krieger AJ, Danetz I, Wu SZ, et al: Electrophrenic respiration following anastomosis of the phrenic with the brachial nerve in the cat. *J Neurosurg* 59:262, 1983.

36. Krieger AJ, Gropper MR, Adler RJ: Electrophrenic respiration after intercostal to phrenic nerve anastomosis in a patient with anterior spinal artery syndrome: Technical case report. *Neurosurgery* 35:760, 1994.

37. Nochomovitz M, Hopkins M, Brodkey J, et al: Conditioning of the diaphragm with phrenic nerve stimulation after prolonged disuse. *Am Rev Respir Dis* 129:685, 1984.

38. Glenn WWL, Phelps ML: Diaphragmatic pacing by electrical stimulation of the phrenic nerve. *Neurosurgery* 17:974, 1985.

39. Glenn WWL, Holcomb WG, Hogan J, et al: Diaphragm pacing by radiofrequency transmission in the treatment of chronic ventilatory insufficiency: Present status. *J Thorac Cardiovasc Surg* 66:505, 1973.

40. Glenn WWL, Hogan JF: Technique of transthoracic placement of phrenic nerve electrodes for diaphragm pacing. Chicago, Film Library, American College of Surgeons, 1982.

41. Salmons S, Henriksson J: The adaptive response of skeletal muscle to increased use. *Muscle Nerve* 4:94, 1981.

42. Oda T, Glenn WWL, Fukuda Y, et al: Evaluation of electrical parameters for diaphragm pacing: An experimental study. *J Surg Res* 30:142, 1981.

43. Glenn WWL, Brouillette RT, Dents B: Fundamental considerations in pacing of the diaphragm for chronic ventilatory insufficiency: A multi-center study. *PACE* 11:2121, 1988.

44. Clerlolak TB, Fukuda Y, Glenn WWL, et al: Response of the diaphragm muscle to electrical stimulation of the phrenic nerve. A histochemical and ultrastructural study. *J Neurosurg* 58:92, 1983.

45. Sairenf H, Hogan H, Glenn WWL: Influence of phrenic nerve stimulation on diaphragm blood flow. *Prog Artif Org* 46:952, 1983.

46. Weese-Mayer DE, Morrow AS, Brouillette RT, et al: Diaphragm pacing in infants and children: A life-table analysis of implanted components. *Am Rev Respir Dis* 139:974, 1989.

47. Glenn WWL, Phelps ML, Electerades JA, et al: Twenty years experience in phrenic nerve stimulation to pace the diaphragm. *PACE* 9:781, 1986.

48. Hunt CE, Brouillette RT, Weese-Mayer DE, et al: Diaphragm pacing in infants and children. *PACE* 11:2135, 1988.

49. Vanderlinden RG, Epstein SW, Hyland RM, et al: Management of chronic ventilatory insufficiency with electrical diaphragm pacing. *Can J Neuro Sci* 15:63, 1988.

50. Bach R, O'Connor K: Electrophrenic ventilation: A different perspective. *J Am Parapl Soc* 14:9, 1991.

51. Carter RE, Dono WH, Halstead L, Wilkerson MA: Comparative study of electrophrenic nerve stimulation and mechanical ventilatory support in traumatic spinal cord injury. *Paraplegia* 25:86, 1987.

52. Lee MY, Kirk PM, Yarkony GM: Rehabilitation of quadriplegic patients with phrenic nerve pacers. *Arch Med Rehabil* 70:549, 1989

53. McMichan JC, Megran DG, Gracey DR, et al: Electrophrenic respiration. *Mayo Clin Prog* 54:662, 1979.

54. Oaker DD, Wilmot CB, Halverson D, Hamilton RD: Neurogenic respiratory failure: A 5-year experience using implantable phrenic nerve stimulators. *Ann Thor Surg* 30:118, 1980.

55. Bach JR, Alba AS: Noninvasive options for ventilatory support of the traumatic high level qudriplegic. *Chest* 98:13, 1990.

56. Ilbawi MN, Idriss S, Hunt E, et al: Diaphragmatic pacing in infants: Techniques and results. *Ann Thorac Surg* 40:323, 1985.

57. Hunt CE, Matalon SV, Thompson TR: Central hypoventilation syndrome. Experience with bilateral phrenic nerve pacing in 3 neonates. *Am Rev Respir Dis* 118:23, 1978.

58. Brouillette RT, Ilbawi MN, Hunt CE: Phrenic nerve pacing in infants and children: A review of experience and report on the usefulness of phrenic nerve stimulation studies. *J Pediatr* 102:32, 1983.

59. Brouillette RT, Ilbawi MN, Klemka-Walden L: Stimulus parameters for phrenic nerve pacing in infants and children. *Pediatr Pulmonol* 4:33, 1988.

60. Glenn WWL, Phelps ML, Gersten LM: Diaphragm pacing in the management of central alveolar hypoventilation, in Guilleminault C, Dement W, (eds): *Sleep Apnea Syndromes.* Krock Found Series, vol 2. New York, Alan R. Liss, 1978, p 333.

61. Bach JR, Alba AS: Management of chronic alveolar hypoventilation by nasal ventilation. *Chest* 97:52, 1990.

62. Oda T, Hogan JF, Glenn WWL, et al: A totally implantable diaphragm pacemaker for experimental studies: Effect of stimulating current level on diaphragm fatigue. *Trans Int Soc Artif Organs Suppl* 3:484, 1979.

63. Osterholm JL, Lemmon WM, Hooker TB, Pyneson J: Electrorespiration by stimulation of thoracic spinal cord. *Surg Forum* 17:421, 1966.

64. DiMarco AF, Supinski GS, Petro JA, Takaoca Y: Evaluation of intercostal pacing to provide artificial ventilation in quadriplegics. *Am J Respir Crit Care Med* 150:934, 1994.

65. DiMarco AF, Budzinsda K, Supinski GS: Artificial ventilation by means of electrical activation of the intercostal/accessory muscles alone in anesthetized dogs. *Am Rev Respir Dis* 139:961, 1989.

66. DiMarco AF, Altose M, Cropp A: Activation of the inspiratory intercostal muscles by electrical stimulation of the spinal cord. *Am Rev Respir Dis* 136:1385, 1987.

67. DiMarco AF, Romaniuk R, Kowalski E, Supinski GS: Efficacy of combined inspiratory intercostal and expiratory muscle pacing to maintain artificial ventilation. *Am J Respir Crit Care Med* 156:122, 1997.

68. DiMarco AF, Romaniuk JR, Supinski GS: Electrical activation of the expiratory muscles to restore cough. *Am J Respir Crit Care Med* 151:1466, 1995.

69. Strohl K, Wolin AD, Van Lunteren E, Fouke JM: Assessment of muscle action on upper airway stability in anesthetized dogs. *J Lab Clin Med* 110:221, 1987.

70. Miki H, Hida W, Shindoh C, et al: Effects of electrical stimulation of the genioglossus on upper airway resistance in anesthetized dogs. *Am Rev Respir Dis* 140:1279, 1989.

71. Van de Graaff WB, Gottfried SB, Mitra J, et al: Respiratory function of hyoid muscles and hyoid arch. *J Appl Physiol* 57:197, 1984.

72. Roberts JL, Read WR, Thach BT: Pharyngeal airway stabilizing function of sternohyoid and sternothyroid muscles in the rabbit. *J Appl Physiol* 57:1790, 1984.

73. Odeh M, Schnall R, Gavriely N, Oliven A: Effects of upper airway muscle contraction on supraglottic stability and pressure-flow relationship. *Respir Physiol* 92:139, 1993.

74. Odeh M, Schnall R, Gavriely N, Oliven A: Dependency of upper airway patency on head position: The effect of muscle contraction. *Respir Physiol* 100:239, 1995.

75. Bishara S, Odeh M, Schnall R, et al: Electrically activated dilator muscles reduce pharyngeal resistance in anesthetized dogs with upper airway obstruction. *Eur Respir J* 8:1537, 1995.

76. Schnall R, Pillar G, Kelsen SG, Oliven A: Dilatory effects of upper airway muscle contraction induced by electrical stimulation in awake humans. *J Appl Physiol* 78:1950, 1995.

77. Oliven A, Schnall R, Odeh M, Pillar G: Reduction of transpharyngeal resistance in sleeping humans by electrically induced genioglossus contraction. *Am Rev Respir Dis* 145:A170, 1992.

78. Harper RM, Saurland EK: The role of the tongue in sleep apnea, in Guilleminault C, Dement WC (eds): *Sleep Apnea Syndromes*, Kroc Foundation Series, vol 11. New York, Alan R. Liss, 1975.

79. Guilleminault CN, Powell N, Bowman B, Stoohs R: The effect of electrical stimulation on obstructive sleep apnea syndrome. *Chest* 107:67, 1995.

80. Miki H, Hida W, Chonan T, et al: Effects of submental electrical stimulation during sleep on upper airway patency in patients with obstructive sleep apnea. *Am Rev Respir Dis* 140:1285, 1989.

81. Hida W, Okabe S, Miki H, et al: Effects of submental stimulation for several consecutive nights in patients with obstructive sleep apnea. *Thorax* 49:446, 1994.

82. Hillarp B, Rosen I, Wickstrom O: Videoradiography at submental electrical stimulation during apnea in obstructive sleep apnea syndrome. *Acta Radiologica* 32:256, 1991.

83. Fairbanks DW, Fairbanks DNF: Neurostimulation for obstructive sleep apnea investigation. *ENT J* 93:52, 1993.

84. Edmonds LC, Daniels BK, Stanson AW, et al: The effects of transcutaneous electrical stimulation during wakefulness and sleep in patients with obstructive sleep apnea. *Am Rev Respir Dis* 146:1030, 1992.

85. Decker M, Haaga J, Arnold L, et al: Functional electrical stimulation and respiration during sleep. *J Appl Physiol* 75:1053, 1993.

86. Oliven A, Schnall R, Kelsen SG: Tongue muscle contraction and fatigability in obstructive sleep apnea. *Am J Respir Crit Care Med* 153:A532, 1996.

87. Schwartz AR, Eisele DW, Hari A, et al: Electrical stimulation of the lingual musculature in obstructive sleep apnea. *J Appl Physiol* 81:643, 1986.

88. Oliven A, Schnall R, Tov N, Kelsen SG: Sublingual electrical stimulation for obstructive sleep apnea. *Am J Respir Crit Care Med* 155:A676, 1997.

89. Schwartz AR, Thut D, Russ DB: Effect of electrical stimulation of the hypoglossal nerve on airflow dynamics in the isolated upper airway. *Am Rev Respir Dis* 147:1144, 1993.

90. Oliven A, Schnall R, Odeh M: Improved upper airway patency elicited by electrical stimulation of the hypoglossus nerves. *Respiration* 63:213, 1996.

91. Eisele DW, Smith PL, Alam DS, Schwartz AR: Direct hypoglossal nerve stimulation in obstructive sleep apnea. *Arch Otolaryngol Head Neck Surg* 123:57, 1997.

92. Podszus T, Schwartz AR: Electrical hypoglossal nerve stimulation in obstructive sleep apnea. *Am J Respir Crit Care Med* 151:A538, 1995.

Chapter 45
RESPIRATORY CARE IN SPINAL CORD INJURY

STEVEN L. LIEBERMAN
ROBERT BROWN

In the United States, there are approximately 200,000 people living with spinal cord injuries.[1,2] Of cases reported since 1990, the male-to-female ratio was slightly greater than 4:1, and the mean age at injury was 34 years, with 9 percent over the age of 60 years. Most injuries result from vehicular accidents, acts of violence, falls, and sports-related mishaps.

During the first half of the twentieth century, the spinal cord injury (SCI) victim usually died within a few years of injury.[3] Since then, the mortality rate has declined continually. This has been attributed to progress in trauma care, the advent of SCI treatment centers, newer antibiotics, and advances in neuroradiology. As a result of such gains, the mean life expectancy for those who survive the first 24 h is 85 to 90 percent that of the general population.[4–6] The risk of death is greatest during the first year after SCI and is especially high during the first 3 months after injury. The poorest prognosis is observed in those over the age of 50 years with complete tetraplegia. Leading causes of death in SCI are pneumonia, pulmonary embolism (PE), sepsis, and coronary artery disease.[1,7] Because of improved survival, the prevalence of persons with SCI is expected to increase about 20 percent by the year 2004.[7]

Pulmonary dysfunction accounts for the largest portion of morbidity in the SCI population.[8] In one multicenter study of acute SCI patients, the most prevalent chest complications in decreasing order were atelectasis, pneumonia, ventilatory failure, pleural effusions, and pneumothoraces/hemothoraces.[5] In addition, in many individuals with chronic SCI, in particular in individuals with tetraplegia, symptomatic breathlessness occurs both at rest and during activities of daily living.[9,10]

Pathophysiology

Injuries to the spinal cord are defined clinically as either complete or incomplete. For complete injuries, functional motor output and sensory feedback are absent below the SCI level, whereas for incomplete injuries, some neurologic activity persists below the injury site. Since 1991, the breakdown of reported SCI cases by neurologic category has been 29 percent complete paraplegia, 28 percent incomplete tetraplegia, 23 percent incomplete paraplegia, and 19 percent complete tetraplegia.[1] The extent of ventilatory muscle impairment depends on the location and completeness of the SCI. For complete injuries, ventilatory muscle function innervated below the level of injury is lost. In those with incomplete injuries, the degree of ventilatory muscle compromise is variable.

CERVICAL SCI

C1–C3

Since the phrenic nerve is derived from the third to fifth cervical segments, complete injuries above C3 produce nearly total ventilatory muscle paralysis. Those with such an injury cannot ventilate adequately and do not survive unless manual ventilation is instituted immediately. Not surprisingly, such patients have the largest incidence of respiratory complications, take the longest time to recover from such complications, and have the highest mortality when compared with all other SCI levels.[4,5,8] In acute SCI patients with injuries to levels C1–C4, the most common respiratory complications during the initial hospitalization are pneumonia, ventilatory failure, and atelectasis. If little respiratory muscle function recovers, patients with such injuries need chronic ventilatory support.

C3–C5

Injuries at levels C3 to C5 cause variable diaphragm impairment. Spontaneous ventilation is often inadequate following injury, and ventilatory support is frequently necessary. In most persons with injuries at this level, subsequent ventilatory muscle recovery usually results in permanent ventilatory support not being necessary.[11–13] The risk of remaining dependent on mechanical ventilation is greatest for those with injuries at level C3, underlying lung disease, and age over 50 years.[13] Temporal improvements in pulmonary function following SCI are attributed to descent of neurologic injury level as spinal cord inflammation resolves, enhanced recruitment of accessory muscles of ventilation, retraining of deconditioned muscles, and the change from flaccid to spastic paralysis.[11–16] As in other systemic neuromuscular disorders, some patients with injuries at this level may, with aging, insidiously develop chronic hypoventilation that may first become apparent decades after SCI and can necessitate chronic ventilatory support.[17]

In able-bodied individuals, the abdominal contents descend toward the pelvis when a seated or standing posture is assumed. In most persons with SCI, this descent is exaggerated because abdominal muscle paralysis increases abdominal compliance.[18,19] Although diaphragm operational length and the zone of apposition of the diaphragm to the rib cage are reduced in these positions when compared with supine,[20] in those with intact diaphragm function, ventilation is maintained by compensatory increases in neural output to the diaphragm (operational length compensation).[21,22] With marked diaphragm weakness, operational length compensation is inadequate to overcome the sequelae of the upright position, and ventilation can decline adversely.[23]

Exhalation from functional residual capacity (FRC) to residual volume (RV) requires contraction of the muscles of exhalation. To the extent that these muscles are paralyzed in SCI, the expiratory reserve volume (ERV = FRC − RV) is diminished, and this is particularly so in tetraplegia (paralyzed internal intercostal and abdominal muscles). Due to the effect of the abdominal contents pushing on the diaphragm, a change from the seated to the supine posture results in a substantial decrease in FRC (typically 0.5 to 1.0 L depending on subject size). However, the different postures do not affect total lung capacity (TLC) appreciably. Thus, in SCI, both the inspiratory capacity (IC = TLC − FRC) and the vital capacity

543

(VC = TLC − RV) are greatest in the supine posture. This improvement in VC has important implications in individuals being weaned from assisted ventilation. The advantage of a greater VC must be weighed against the possibility of gas-exchange problems arising from tidal breathing at low respiratory system volumes at which airways resistance is increased and airway closure may occur.

C5–C8

In complete injuries to levels C5 through C8, inhalation is supported by the diaphragm and accessory muscles in the neck, whereas exhalation depends primarily on the passive recoil of the chest wall and lungs, although some active exhalation may result from activity in the clavicular portions of the pectoralis major muscles.[24,25] In the C5 to C8 injury group, the most common respiratory complications during initial hospitalization are atelectasis, pneumonia, and ventilatory failure.[5]

During inhalation in the able-bodied, the rib cage moves outward due to the action of the external intercostal and other rib cage muscles and due to the effect on the lower rib cage of the diaphragm acting via its muscular insertions and the zone of apposition. These actions depend critically on increases in abdominal pressure during inhalation. In tetraplegia, the upper rib cage often moves paradoxically inward during inhalation.[20,26] This is due partly to paralysis of the external intercostals. Also, in tetraplegia the diaphragm is an ineffective elevator of the rib cage because high abdominal compliance leads to a small zone of apposition and to small abdominal pressure changes during inhalation.[20,27]

THORACIC SCI

Although more ventilatory muscle function is preserved in those with thoracic (T) level injuries, respiratory complications are still a problem during the acute hospitalization, probably because of the increased incidence of chest trauma in this group.[5,8] The most frequent chest complications are pleural effusions, atelectasis, and pneumothoraces/hemothoraces. Other morbid conditions in which chest trauma may result include rib fractures with flail chest, tracheobronchial or esophageal rupture, lung or myocardial contusion, and aortic transection. Additionally, fat emboli syndrome may occur in those with long bone fractures. The lower incidence of pneumonia in this group is probably attributable to better expiratory muscle function leading to a more effective cough.

VENTILATORY CONTROL

Individuals with tetraplegia have a blunted ventilatory and "air hunger" response to hypercapnia.[26,28,29] The causes are uncertain, but the reduction in the ventilatory response to hypercapnia is dramatic and unexplained solely by ventilatory muscle weakness or changes in respiratory system mechanics. The clinical consequences of such alterations in ventilatory control are unknown.

Clinical Aspects of SCI

LUNG DISEASE

Several sequelae of SCI lead to the high prevalence of retained secretions, atelectasis, pulmonary infections, and respiratory failure.[8,11] Expiratory muscle weakness causes ineffective coughing. Additional factors that may interfere with coughing are rib fractures, thoracoabdominal surgery, and an altered level of consciousness from head trauma or use of sedating medications. In addition, gastric distention and ileus following SCI can progress to aspiration of gastric contents.[30,31] About 20 percent of acute cervical level SCI patients also experience a syndrome of bronchial mucus hypersecretion, which is characterized by production of excessive amounts of a tenacious mucus and possibly results from an impaired peripheral sympathetic nervous system.[32] Furthermore, some complete tetraplegics have been found not to sigh spontaneously.[33] Such persons may have an increased incidence of atelectasis and respiratory infections when compared with individuals who do sigh, although this has not been studied prospectively.

THROMBOEMBOLI

Without preventive measures, the incidence of deep venous thrombosis (DVT) is 50 to 100 percent during the first 3 months after SCI, with the greatest risk occurring during the first 2 weeks.[34,35] The risk of DVT appears to be small during the first 72 h following SCI. Not only does the stasis from lower extremity paralysis and immobility increase the risk of DVT, but also platelet and coagulation abnormalities favoring clot formation occur during the acute SCI.[36–38] Some investigators also suggest that vascular intimal injury contributes to DVT formation in acute SCI.[35] Even with prophylaxis, pulmonary embolism remains a common cause of death, especially during the first year after injury.[7] The risk of a fatal pulmonary embolism is greatest for those with cervical injury levels, obesity, and an absence of spasticity.[39]

Current preventive measures are based upon only a small number of controlled studies. When used alone, standard low-dose heparin is inadequate for DVT prophylaxis in acute SCI.[40,41] Although both adjusted-dose heparin, in which the activated partial thromboplastin time is maintained at about 40 s, and low-dose warfarin reduce the risk of DVT, both have an associated bleeding risk thought to be particularly great in SCI.[40] Preliminary evidence suggests that low-molecular-weight heparin has similar or better efficacy than standard heparin while having the additional benefits of once-a-day dosing and a lower risk of bleeding.[42] Intermittent pneumatic compression boots work not only by decreasing venous stasis but also by altering coagulation and fibrinolysis.[43] When used alone for prevention of DVT, they are unreliable, but when combined with low-dose anticoagulant therapy, such devices are potentially more beneficial and are now the standard of care.[34,44] Whenever compression modalities are delayed for longer than 24 h after SCI or when there is clinical evidence of a DVT, then we recommend that testing should be performed to exclude the presence of a DVT prior to employment of such devices because leg compression can dislodge clots and cause pulmonary embolism. Based upon prevailing data, it is recommended that preventive therapy be continued for at least 2 to 3 months following SCI in those with persistent lower extremity paralysis.[34,35] The merits of preventive therapy beyond 3 months have not been studied adequately.

If leg trauma precludes use of compression boots, then a

vena cava filter should be inserted.[34,44] Even following filter insertion, heparin prophylaxis should be provided. In several medical centers, vena cava filters are inserted routinely in acute SCI patients in an attempt to minimize the risk of pulmonary embolism.[45] Data to support this approach are lacking.

The SCI clinician must maintain a low threshold for evaluation of thromboembolic disease, since associated clinical findings are often absent.[38,46] Diagnostic testing and treatment of thromboemboli in the SCI patient are otherwise similar to other patient groups, in whom therapy should last for at least 3 months following DVT or pulmonary embolism.[47] Once the patient is anticoagulated with either intravenous or adjusted-dose subcutaneous heparin, warfarin can be started (to a target INR of 2 to 3). Adjusted-dose heparin is an option particularly well suited for the patient undergoing rehabilitation, in whom the intravenous catheter and infusion pump can be quite cumbersome. A vena cava filter should be inserted when anticoagulation is contraindicated, for recurrent pulmonary embolism during appropriate anticoagulation, or when the sequelae of a pulmonary embolism would be particularly morbid. There appears to an increased risk of migration of a Greenfield filter in SCI patients.[48] It has been proposed that the migration is secondary to pressure transmitted to the vena cava during activities such as abdominal thrusting for cough assistance and frequent patient turning for pressure sore prevention. Due to the bleeding potential, thrombolytic therapy probably should only be considered in acute SCI patients for life-threatening pulmonary embolism.[47]

The incidence of DVT decreases in association with the transition from acute to chronic SCI.[34,46] Proposed mechanisms to explain this include increased mobility with rehabilitation, atrophy of lower extremity veins, and resolution of the hypercoagulable state. Although the risk of fatal pulmonary embolism is greater in those without spasticity, as mentioned previously, lower extremity spasticity does not prevent the development of DVT. Although the risk of DVT is lower in chronic SCI, it is not zero. Such patients should be considered for DVT prophylaxis, particularly when treatment results in bed rest.

CARDIOVASCULAR CONTROL

Disruption of autonomic pathways by injuries at or above level T6 can lead to bradyarrhythmias and hypotension, especially during the acute SCI phase.[49] Patients undergoing tracheal suctioning are at particular risk for such derangements in cardiovascular function.[50,51] For example, during suctioning, tracheal vagal afferents are stimulated, causing increased vagal efferent output to the heart, which in upper-level SCI patients is unopposed by sympathetic nerve activity. Hypoxia augments such vagal activity. Correction of hypoxia with supplementary oxygen usually prevents such arrhythmias. When this is unsuccessful, atropine may be given prior to suctioning. Rarely, cardiac pacemakers have been required because affected individuals have developed syncope during suctioning.[13] A similar reflex, which also is usually preventable with atropine, may occur during endotracheal intubation. In the chronic SCI population, there does not appear to be an increased incidence of cardiac dysrhythmias.[52]

NONCARDIOGENIC PULMONARY EDEMA

As a consequence of chest trauma or aspiration, acute SCI patients may develop adult respiratory distress syndrome.[5,30] Also, neurogenic pulmonary edema may occur during both the acute and chronic phases of SCI.[53-55] This protein-rich alveolar edema is believed to result from increased centrally mediated sympathetic activity, possibly leading to a combination of pulmonary venoconstriction, reduced pulmonary vascular compliance, enhanced pulmonary capillary permeability, lymphatic constriction, and elevated systemic vascular resistance.[56,57] This may occur in autonomic dysreflexia, a syndrome characterized by profound systemic hypertension, headaches, diaphoresis above the SCI level, and ocular changes.[58,59] This syndrome is triggered by sympathetic reflexes initiated by noxious stimulation in the distribution of spinal segments below the SCI level (usually only in those with injuries at or above T6). Such stimuli include bladder or bowel distention, anal fissures, urinary tract infections, decubitus ulcers, and even DVT or pulmonary embolism. When untreated, autonomic dysreflexia can lead to considerable morbidity and death. Primary management is to treat any precipitating factors. Antihypertensive medications should be used only in those with persistently severe hypertension in order to avoid the subsequent development of hypotension as the autonomic dysreflexia subsides.

AIR TRAVEL

Following SCI, some patients need air transport to a spinal cord center. When transported by flight, mucus plugging can be especially problematic if the patient breathes dry air cycled from outside the airplane.[60] The risk of this is probably decreased by humidification of inspired air. In addition, supplemental oxygen should be considered to avoid the hypoxemia that may develop at higher altitudes. Suctioning equipment and atropine also should be readily accessible during transport of such patients.

SLEEP

Some reports suggest an increased incidence of sleep apnea in SCI patients, predominantly of the obstructive or mixed obstructive and central types.[61,62] Possible mechanisms for this include neck muscle hypertrophy, ventilatory muscle spasticity, antispasm medications, obesity, or an effect of injury to some undefined spinal cord pathway involved with control of sleep. Snoring is a sign associated with sleep apnea in the able-bodied population. Using a health questionnaire, we found that 84 of 197 (43 percent) SCI subjects reported loud snoring during 1 or more nights per week, similar to that reported in studies of the able-bodied.[63] While there was no association between snoring and level or completeness of injury, there was an association with an elevated mean body mass index and the use of antispasticity medications (e.g., diazepam and/or baclofen).

As in other neuromuscular disorders, those with severe ventilatory muscle weakness that includes the diaphragm are prone to develop hypoxemia during the rapid eye movement (REM) stage of sleep.[64,65] This may relate to a combination of worsened ventilation-perfusion mismatch, upper airway narrowing, and REM-related inhibition of inspiratory muscles other than the diaphragm.

SYRINGOMYELIA

One long-term complication of SCI, which when undiagnosed can lead to ventilatory failure and death, is syringomyelia, a cystic degeneration of the spinal cord.[66,67] Although not understood well, many believe that a syrinx cavity forms in the spinal cord either by liquefaction necrosis of cord tissue or hematoma formation at the site of injury. While small cyst formation may be found in about 50 percent of patients soon after SCI, progressive cavitary enlargement occurs in the range of 0.3 to 8.0 percent of SCI patients.[66,68] The cavity is usually less than 1 cm wide but can be up to 10 vertebral segments long.

Syringomyelia must be suspected in any patient who after a period of stability begins to develop new neurologic findings. Although symptoms begin most commonly years after SCI, they may occur as early as 2 months postinjury. The most common first symptom is pain at or above the SCI level that may radiate to the neck and upper extremities. The pain is often potentiated by coughing, sneezing, straining, and assuming an upright position. Unless diagnosed early, sensory and motor deficits ensue, usually in ascending fashion. Ventilatory failure results from the consequences of progressive cervical spine or brain stem involvement.

The preferred diagnostic test is magnetic resonance imaging (MRI). Patients with asymptomatic cysts or minor symptoms should be followed by serial physical examinations and MRI studies. For those with progressive symptoms, MRI-guided needle aspiration of the syrinx provides only temporary relief, whereas longer-lasting therapy entails surgical decompression with possible insertion of a drainage shunt.[67,69]

THERMOREGULATION

Temperature control is altered by SCI, especially in those with injuries at or above T6, where damage to the autonomic nervous system impairs sweating, shivering, and the ability to constrict or dilate the peripheral vasculature in response to changes in environmental temperature.[70,71] Such persons have difficulty maintaining basal temperature, and body temperature may change in the direction of variations in the environmental temperature. Although SCI patients do mount febrile responses during infections, they have lost the ability to compensate for fever. Maneuvers such as removing blankets and clothing and lowering the environmental temperature often are necessary to diminish a fever. In SCI, body temperature may rise substantially during exercise.[72] Reduction of room temperature and light exercise clothing may be helpful in this situation.

Diagnostic Tests

PULMONARY FUNCTION TESTING

Height is used to calculate predicted pulmonary function, but in SCI patients, such a measurement is often not feasible.[73] In order to assess stature accurately in SCI patients, it is best to measure supine length, perhaps during a prior physical examination. Although convenient, use of arm span or recalled height for stature has an associated risk of considerable error in predicted values in some subjects and should not be used in research.[73]

It appears to be difficult for many complete SCI patients, especially those with injury at the cervical level, to meet the acceptability and reproducibility spirometry standards set by the American Thoracic Society (ATS).[74] The most common reason for unacceptable blows is high back extrapolation volumes,[75] which presumably result from ventilatory muscle weakness. Ashba and coworkers[74] recommended that less stringent acceptability standards be used for SCI patients. When such criteria were instituted, the FVC and the forced expiratory volume in the first second (FEV_1) were no more than 4 percent greater than values obtained using the ATS criteria. These small differences are not clinically significant. Furthermore, data using the modified criteria were reproducible. Thus the modified criteria can be used for assessing changes in individuals over time.

Pulmonary function testing of SCI patients has demonstrated that most of those with complete cervical level injuries and some persons with complete upper thoracic level injuries have a restrictive ventilatory defect.[11,15,25,33,76,77] Typically, this is characterized by reductions in TLC, VC, IC, and ERV and an increase in RV, the latter due to expiratory muscle weakness. Measures of airflow, such as the FEV_1, are reduced in proportion to the reduction in VC. In those with injuries to lower thoracic and lumbosacral areas, pulmonary function measurements usually have been within normal limits.[77] Limitations in these studies included small study groups; use of mostly hospitalized patients, which may have biased the results due to inclusion of sicker patients; a lack of measurement of stature; an absence of consideration of tobacco use; and a failure to adhere to accepted criteria for pulmonary function testing. These limitations may have led to overestimation of pulmonary function abnormalities in SCI patients.

In uncontrolled studies of airway responsiveness in tetraplegics, FEV_1 increased by 12 percent or more in 40 to 50 percent of those tested following inhalation of a beta agonist or an anticholinergic agent.[78,79] Furthermore, during bronchoprovocation testing, the dose of methacholine required to cause a decrease in FEV_1 by 20 percent in tetraplegics was much less than for individuals without hyperreactive airways.[80] Neither abnormalities of the sympathetic or parasympathetic nervous systems have been found to be responsible for the observed airway hyperresponsiveness, and the mechanism remains unclear.

As in other generalized neuromuscular disorders, reductions in maximal inspiratory and expiratory static pressures (PImax and PEmax) exist in SCI patients.[11,28] Prior studies have used flange-style mouthpieces, which led to an underestimation of PEmax.[81] For accuracy, measurements should be made with a tube-style mouthpiece. Data obtained in this fashion demonstrate PEmax values that are much greater than previously reported in SCI patients.

RADIOGRAPHY

Due to spinal instability, erect chest radiographs are often contraindicated in acute SCI patients. Instead, supine films are used for evaluation of the lung parenchyma and pleura. The clinician must be aware that the supine chest radiograph is neither sensitive nor specific for diagnosing lung consolidation, atelectasis, or pleural effusions in this population.[82] Plain supine films may have some utility for screening, but in general, computed tomography (CT) or MRI scanning should be performed whenever a clinical situation suggests that chest radiography results are erroneous, for example, during evaluation of fever of unknown etiology.

Therapy

CHEST PHYSIOTHERAPY

Chest physiotherapy appears to decrease the risk of mucus retention, atelectasis, and pneumonia; decreases the frequency with which ventilatory support is needed; and improves survival in the acutely injured SCI patient.[11] Since atelectasis is nearly as common in those with thoracic injuries, both cervical and thoracic SCI patients should undergo such therapy.[5] This may include deep breathing efforts, frequent position changes, postural drainage of secretions, nasotracheal suctioning, and manually assisted coughing using forceful upper abdominal thrusts in a posterior and cephalad direction.[83] Although there are no data demonstrating clinical efficacy, many clinicians also use beta-agonist bronchodilator therapy to enhance mucociliary clearance. Hypoxemia may develop during postural drainage when persons in the acute phase of intercostal muscle paralysis are tilted in a head-down position.[84] It has been demonstrated that expiratory muscles innervated by segments C5 to C7 can be trained in SCI patients,[24,25] but it is not yet known if such training improves cough sufficiently to reduce mucus retention and its numerous consequences. Insufflation-exsufflation devices also may be of help with the management of secretions,[17,85] but controlled trials have not been done to assess this rigorously. Of note, intermittent positive-pressure breathing has not been shown to be of clinical benefit in SCI patients.[86,87] When other forms of pulmonary hygiene fail, a therapeutic bronchoscopy should be performed. To assist with mobilization of pulmonary secretions during bronchoscopy, we find it particularly helpful to perform intermittent abdominal thrusts on the patient.

Functional electrical stimulation devices are being used in the research laboratory to develop ways to improve the cough of SCI patients. One technique used in dogs is to stimulate electrically the lower thoracic spinal cord to activate expiratory muscles, including the abdominal muscles and the lower internal intercostals.[88] Another approach to enhancing cough has been surface electrical stimulation of abdominal muscles.[89] In 14 tetraplegics, the cough generated by surface electrical stimulation was similar to the cough produced by manually assisted abdominal thrusting, as assessed by peak expiratory flow rates.[89] The safety and clinical utility of these electrical stimulation techniques need further investigation, but the potential for benefit appears great.

VENTILATORY SUPPORT

A number of techniques may augment ventilation in those with respiratory muscle weakness. Intermittent glossopharyngeal breathing in high cervical level SCI patients uses oral, pharyngeal, and laryngeal muscles to enhance ventilation.[90,91] This may be especially helpful during disconnection from mechanical ventilation. With marked diaphragm weakness or paralysis, a rocking bed may be useful to augment ventilation. In addition, external abdominal compression with an elastic binder[27,92] or pneumobelt[93,94] may improve ventilation

when individuals with abdominal muscle paralysis and diaphragm weakness assume an upright position. Inspiratory muscle training has been shown to improve the strength and endurance of the ventilatory muscles in SCI patients.[95–97] The clinical benefits of such training are unknown.

When inadequate gas exchange persists, a variety of mechanical ventilatory devices can be used.[85] Acute respiratory decompensation requires intubation and positive-pressure ventilation. Once intubated, such patients should be tilted with the head upright at a 45-degree angle to diminish the risk of aspiration of gastric contents.[98] Unless extubation appears imminent, tracheostomies usually are performed within 7 to 10 days of intubation to improve patient comfort and to obviate the risk of laryngeal damage.

With chronic ventilatory failure, support is often provided with a positive-pressure mechanical ventilator applied via a tracheostomy tube. In those requiring chronic ventilatory assistance, survival data vary markedly from study to study. In one study of individuals who survived the first 24 h of SCI and remained ventilator-dependent by hospital discharge, the survival rate was 25 percent after 1 year.[99] Of the survivors at 1 year, the survival rate over the next 14 years was 60 percent. In another study, this time of acute SCI patients who were ventilator-dependent at hospital discharge, the survival rates were 90 percent at 1 year, 56 percent at 3 years, and 33 percent at 5 years postinjury.[13] Pneumonia remains the leading cause of death in mechanically ventilated SCI patients.[99]

One consideration for ventilatory support in those with chronic complete injuries rostral to C3 (above the takeoff level of the phrenic nerve) is surgical implantation of an electrophrenic pacemaker.[100–102] Patients appear to prefer phrenic pacemaker systems to positive-pressure ventilation. The reasons include that the systems are small and can be kept out of view, that ventilation through the mouth feels more natural, and that taste and smell are enhanced by ventilation through the mouth and nose.[103] Furthermore, speech via a phrenic pacemaker system may be more continuous and contain fewer and shorter pauses when compared with that achieved during positive-pressure mechanical ventilation.[104] Prior to surgical implantation of such a system, intact phrenic nerves should be confirmed by electrophrenic or magnetic stimulation of the nerve in the neck with verification of hemidiaphragm contraction by electromyography and fluoroscopy or ultrasonography. Although not instituted at all centers, we recommend maintenance of a tracheostomy in case of pacemaker failure, to avoid upper airway obstruction during sleep,[105] and for suctioning. Although it is suboptimal for prolonged periods when used alone, intercostal nerve pacing may have clinical utility in the future to enhance inspiratory capacity in tetraplegics with insufficient ventilation due to unilateral phrenic nerve paralysis or inadequate phrenic nerve pacing.[106]

Other devices can be used for ventilatory support in patients with high cervical injuries.[85,90] Negative-pressure body ventilators (including the tank, cuirass, and poncho) are options. Such devices are cumbersome and may result in upper airway obstruction during sleep.[105] Another form of support that obviates upper airway obstruction is positive-pressure ventilation via an oral or nasal mask. Contraindications to such devices include altered mental status, facial trauma, and copious airway secretions.

IMMUNIZATIONS

Published guidelines for pneumococcal pneumonia and influenza prophylaxis do not include specific reference to individuals with SCI.[107,108] Nevertheless, the risk of prolonged morbidity or death from pneumonia is so great in SCI patients that we recommend that they be vaccinated. It appears, however, that vaccination is not always common practice.[109]

SPEECH THERAPY

Expiratory muscle weakness in spontaneously breathing tetraplegics may cause speech abnormalities such as reduced vocal amplitude and a lower number of syllables per breath when compared with able-bodied individuals.[110] During speech, many tetraplegics appear to compensate for expiratory muscle weakness first by inhaling maximally and then by terminating speech at higher than usual lung volumes. This pattern of ventilation is probably chosen to optimize the recoil pressure of the respiratory system driving flow across the vocal cords.

Whenever possible, a fenestrated, cuffed tracheostomy tube should be used in mechanically ventilated patients to provide the psychological benefit of communication by voice. The presence of the fenestration and deflation of the cuff can lead to substantial loss of tidal volume through the mouth. If necessary, the tidal volume can be increased accordingly. During the daytime, patients can minimize the "leak" by controlling glottal patency and by use of accessory muscles of ventilation and have the advantage of being able to speak. These compensatory mechanisms are lost during sleep. Therefore, during the night, the inner cannula should be inserted (thereby occluding the fenestration), and the cuff should be inflated.

In mechanically ventilated individuals, phonation occurs during most of ventilator-driven inhalation and during the early part of exhalation.[111] The time for speech per breath is often short and accompanied by a long intervening period of silence, making it difficult to partake in activities such as group conversation or using a telephone. By decreasing inspiratory flow and adding positive end-expiratory pressure, the time that tracheal pressure exceeds what is necessary for phonation is augmented, and a smoother tracheal pressure waveform is promoted.[112] Such easy ventilator manipulations improve speech timing, stabilize loudness, and result in a more pleasant voice quality.

EXERCISE

Now that survival has improved, increasing interest has focused on the role of exercise for persons with SCI.[113–115] Although nearly all individuals undergo rehabilitation following the acute SCI, most do not undergo further formal rehabilitation following hospital discharge. In many individuals with chronic SCI, in particular, in individuals with tetraplegia, symptomatic breathlessness occurs both at rest and during activities of daily living.[9,10] In many of them, exercise intolerance may limit the ability to perform basic activities such as transfers in and out of bed and motor vehicles and the ability to negotiate physical barriers such as ramps.[116] In such individuals, this may have an impact on functional independence and quality of life.

Currently, important research is being carried out on the association between physical fitness in SCI patients and psychological abnormalities, insulin resistance, reduced high-density lipoprotein levels, and other complications of SCI such as urinary tract infections, decubitus ulcers, and bone demineralization.[115,117,118] It still needs to be determined whether physical fitness reduces the risk of these complications or if, instead, those with SCI who are able to become physically fit are from the healthiest of the SCI population. It is reasonable to expect that as in the able-bodied population, participation in regular exercise will reduce the risk for cardiovascular disease in the SCI population.

An obvious cause of exercise intolerance in SCI patients is paresis/paralysis of muscles below the level of injury. However, factors other than injury level may contribute to exercise intolerance in SCI patients, even when the exercise is being performed by trained muscles above the injury level.[114–116,119] During exercise in SCI, abnormalities of the peripheral sympathetic nervous system impair arteriolar constriction and venoconstriction in nonexercising muscles and in the abdominal viscera.[120] This leads to reduced venous return, which ultimately reduces blood flow to exercising muscles. This is also a likely cause for the blood pressure decrease that often occurs in SCI patients exercising at higher workloads. In addition, in some tetraplegics, loss of sympathetic control of the heart leads to chronotropic insufficiency, whereby the heart rate peaks at 110 to 130 beats per minute during exercise.[121–123] Furthermore, ventilatory muscle paralysis also may limit exercise performance, especially in tetraplegics.[123,124] Other potential problems may arise from impairments in thermoregulation and the adrenal catecholamine response to exercise.[72]

Even with all the aforementioned limitations during exercise, regular upper extremity aerobic exercise improves exercise capacity in acute and chronic SCI patients.[114,123,125] Although exercise programs with the best training effects need to be designed, the most aerobically challenging forms of exercise for persons with lower extremity paralysis appear to be arm-crank ergometry, swimming, and wheelchair sports such as basketball and wheelchair propulsion on a track. One newer option for voluntary arm exercise is the Wheelchair Aerobic Fitness Trainer (WAFT; Packer Engineering, Inc., Naperville, IL).[126] This is a computer-controlled treadmill that easily connects to most wheelchairs. Changes in wheelchair propulsion workload are determined by variations in speed and resistance. Effective, yet safe, upper extremity exercise regimens still need to be defined. Cardiac performance may be enhanced and hypotension avoided during exercise by application of positive-pressure pneumatic devices to the lower extremities and abdomen, thereby redistributing blood away from these locations to the central circulation.[127]

Other newer modes of exercise have been used primarily at regional/SCI centers. Electrical stimulation across muscle motor points leads to muscle contraction, which, when resulting in coordinated limb movements, is known as *functional electrical stimulation* (FES).[113,115,128–130] Activities using FES include walking, lower extremity ergometry, and weight lifting. Walking is most successful in those with injuries at T3 to T12. Lower extremity FES ergometry training, especially when combined with voluntary upper extremity exercise, offers the ability to exercise a larger muscle mass, potentially leading to a greater physiologic challenge to the cardiopulmonary system and thereby a greater training effect. Whether

FES actually provides a sufficient stimulus to accomplish this has not been established yet. Although it appears to have benefits for rehabilitation, FES may be impractical because of cost, the time and technical support needed for setup, discomfort in incomplete injuries, and the possibility of provoking unwanted reflexes. Ideal exercise regimens and the long-term effects of FES on the body still need to be determined.

The Future

Current active areas of scientific investigation in SCI medicine include strategies to minimize spinal cord damage,[131] mechanisms to promote restoration of spinal cord function via nerve cell regeneration or spinal cord grafting,[132] and ways in which to improve quality of life.[115] It is the hope that someday there may be a cure for SCI. In the meantime, although the life span of SCI patients has increased, the mortality rate is still unacceptably high.[7] In order to improve life expectancy further, additional research is needed in the prevention and management of pneumonia, pulmonary embolism, and sepsis.

References

1. National Spinal Cord Injury Statistical Center: *Spinal Cord Injury: Facts and Figures at a Glance.* Birmingham: The University of Alabama at Birmingham, 1996.
2. Lasfargues JE, Custis D, Murrone F, et al: A model for estimating spinal cord injury prevalence in the United States. *Paraplegia* 33:62–68, 1995.
3. Whiteneck GG, Charlifue SW, Frankel HL, et al: Mortality, morbidity, and psychosocial outcomes of persons spinal cord injured more than 20 years ago. *Paraplegia* 30:617–630, 1992.
4. DeVivo MJ, Stover SL, Black KJ: Prognostic factors for 12-year survival after spinal cord injury. *Arch Phys Med Rehabil* 73:156–162, 1992.
5. Jackson AB, Groomes TE: Incidence of respiratory complications following spinal cord injury. *Arch Phys Med Rehabil* 75:270–275, 1994.
6. Samsa GP, Patrick CH, Feussner JR: Long-term survival of veterans with traumatic spinal cord injury. *Arch Neurol* 50:909–914, 1993.
7. DeVivo MJ, Black KJ, Stover SL: Causes of death during the first 12 years after spinal cord injury. *Arch Phys Med Rehabil* 71:197–200, 1990.
8. Fishburn MJ, Marino RJ, Ditunno JF: Atelectasis and pneumonia in acute spinal cord injury. *Arch Phys Med Rehabil* 71:197–200, 1990.
9. Ayas N, Garshick E, Lieberman SL, Brown R: Breathlessness in spinal cord injury depends on injury level. *Am J Respir Crit Care Med* 155:A173, 1997.
10. Spungen AM, Grimm DR, Lesser M, et al: Self-reported prevalence of pulmonary symptoms in subjects with spinal cord injury. *Spinal Cord* 35:652–657, 1997.
11. McMichan JC, Michel L, Westbrook PR: Pulmonary dysfunction following traumatic quadriplegia. *JAMA* 243:528–531, 1980.
12. Ledsome JR, Sharp JM: Pulmonary function in acute cervical cord injury. *Am Rev Respir Dis* 124.41–44, 1981.
13. Wicks AB, Menter RR: Long-term outlook in quadriplegic patients with initial ventilator dependency. *Chest* 90:406–410, 1986.
14. Axen K, Pineda H, Shunfenthal I, Haas F: Diaphragmatic function following cervical cord injury: Neurally mediated improvement. *Arch Phys Med Rehabil* 66:219–222, 1985.
15. Haas F, Axen K, Pineda H, et al: Temporal pulmonary function changes in cervical cord injury. *Arch Phys Med Rehabil* 66:139–144, 1985.
16. Pichurko B, McCool FD, Scanlon P, et al: Factors related to respiratory function recovery following acute quadriplegia. *Am Rev Respir Dis* 131:A337, 1985.
17. Bach J: Inappropriate weaning and late onset ventilatory failure of individual with traumatic spinal cord injury. *Paraplegia* 31:430–438, 1993.
18. Estenne M, de Troyer A: The effects of tetraplegia on chest wall statics. *Am Rev Respir Dis* 134:121–124, 1986.
19. Goldman J, Morgan MDL, Denison DM: The measurement of abdominal wall compliance in normal subjects and tetraplegic patients. *Thorax* 41:513–518, 1986.
20. Urmey W, Loring S, Mead J, et al: Upper and lower rib cage deformation during breathing in quadriplegics. *J Appl Physiol* 60:618–622, 1986.
21. Banzett RB, Ingbar GF, Brown R, et al: Diaphragm electrical activity during negative lower torso pressure in quadriplegic men. *J Appl Physiol* 51:654–659, 1981.
22. McCool FD, Brown R, Mayewski RJ, Hyde RW: Effects of posture on stimulated ventilation in quadriplegia. *Am Rev Respir Dis* 138:101–105, 1988.
23. Danon J, Druz WS, Goldberg NB, Sharp JT: Function of the isolated paced diaphragm and the cervical accessory muscles in C1 quadriplegics. *Am Rev Respir Dis* 119:909–919, 1979.
24. De Troyer A, Estenne M, Heilporn A: Mechanism of active expiration in tetraplegic subjects. *N Engl J Med* 314:740–744, 1986.
25. Estenne M, Knoop C, Vanvaerenbergh J, et al: The effect of pectoralis muscle training in tetraplegic subjects. *Am Rev Respir Dis* 139:1218–1222, 1989.
26. Bergofsky EH: Mechanism for respiratory insufficiency after cervical cord injury. *Ann Intern Med* 61:435–447, 1964.
27. McCool FD, Pichurko M, Slutsky AS, et al: Changes in lung volume and rib cage configuration with abdominal binding in quadriplegia. *J Appl Physiol* 60:1198–1202, 1986.
28. Manning HL, Brown R, Scharf SM, et al: Ventilatory and $P_{0.1}$ response to hypercapnia in quadriplegia. *Respir Physiol* 89:97–112, 1992.
29. Lieberman SL, Schwartzstein RM, Harrington RM, et al: Role of spinal cord in ventilatory and sensory response to hypercapnia. *Am J Respir Crit Care Med* 153:A119, 1996.
30. Reines HD, Harris RC: Pulmonary complications of acute spinal cord injuries. *Neurosurgery* 21:193–196, 1987.
31. Sutton RA, Macphail I, Bentley R, Nandy MK: Acute gastric dilatation as a relatively late complication of tetraplegia due to very high cervical cord injury. *Paraplegia* 19:17–19, 1981.
32. Bhaskar KR, Brown R, O'Sullivan DD, et al: Bronchial mucus hypersecretion in acute quadriplegia. *Am Rev Respir Dis* 143:640–648, 1991.
33. McKinley AC, Auchincloss JH, Gilbert R, Nicholas JJ: Pulmonary function, ventilatory control, and respiratory complications in quadriplegic subjects. *Am Rev Respir Dis* 100:526–532, 1969.
34. Consortium for Spinal Cord Medicine: Prevention of thromboembolism in spinal cord injury. *Spinal Cord Med* 1:20, 1997.
35. Merli GJ, Crabbe S, Paluzzi RG, Fritz D: Etiology, incidence, and prevention of deep vein thrombosis in acute spinal cord injury. *Arch Phys Med Rehabil* 74:1199–1205, 1993.
36. Myllynen P, Kammonen M, Rokkanen P, et al: The blood F VIII:Ag/F VIII:C ratio as an early indicator of deep venous thrombosis during post-traumatic immobilization. *J Trauma* 27:287–290, 1987.
37. Petaja J, Myllynen P, Rokkanen P, Nokelainen M: Fibrinolysis and spinal injury. *Acta Chir Scand* 155:241–246, 1989.
38. Rossi EC, Green D, Rosen JS, et al: Sequential changes in factor VIII and platelets preceding deep vein thrombosis in patients with spinal cord injury. *Br J Haematol* 45:143–151, 1980.

39. Green D, Twardowski P, Wei R, Rademaker AW: Fatal pulmonary embolism in spinal cord injury. *Chest* 105:853–855, 1994.

40. Green D, Lee MY, Ito VY, et al: Fixed- vs adjusted-dose heparin in the prophylaxis of thromboembolism in spinal cord injury. *JAMA* 260:1255–1258, 1988.

41. Merli GJ, Herbison GJ, Ditunno JF, et al: Deep vein thrombosis: Prophylaxis in acute spinal cord injured patients. *Arch Phys Med Rehabil* 69:661–664, 1988.

42. Green D, Chen D, Chmiel JS, et al: Prevention of thromboembolism in spinal cord injury: Role of low-molecular-weight heparin. *Arch Phys Med Rehabil* 75:290–292, 1994.

43. Weitz J, Michelsen J, Gold K, et al: Effects of intermittent pneumatic calf compression on postoperative thrombin and plasmin activity. *Thromb Haemost* 56:198–201, 1986.

44. Merli GJ, Crabbe S, Doyle L, et al: Mechanical plus pharmacological prophylaxis for deep vein thrombosis in acute spinal cord injury. *Paraplegia* 30:558–562, 1992.

45. Wilson JT, Rogers FB, Wald SL, et al: Prophylactic vena cava filter insertion in patients with traumatic spinal cord injury: Preliminary results. *Neurosurgery* 35:234–239, 1994.

46. Kim SW, Charallel JT, Park KW, et al: Prevalence of deep venous thrombosis in patients with chronic spinal cord injury. *Arch Phys Med Rehabil* 75:965–968, 1994.

47. Merli GJ: Management of deep vein thrombosis in spinal cord injury. *Chest* 102:652S–657S, 1992.

48. Balshi JD, Cantelmo NL, Menzoian JO: Complications of caval interruption by Greenfield filter in quadriplegics. *J Vasc Surg* 9:558–562, 1989.

49. Mathias CJ, Frankel HL: Cardiovascular control in spinal man. *Am Rev Physiol* 50:577–592, 1988.

50. Berk JL, Levy MN: Profound reflex bradycardia produced by transient hypoxia or hypercapnia in man. *Eur Surg Res* 9:75–84, 1977.

51. Mathias CJ: Bradycardia and cardiac arrest during tracheal suction mechanisms in tetraplegic patients. *Eur J Intensive Care Med* 2:147–156, 1976.

52. Leaf DA, Bahl RA, Adkins RH: Risk of cardiac dysrhythmias in chronic spinal cord injury patients. *Paraplegia* 31:571–575, 1993.

53. Brown BT, Carrion HM, Politano VA: Guanethidine sulfate in the prevention of autonomic hyperreflexia. *J Urol* 122:55–57, 1979.

54. Kiker JD, Woodside JR, Jelinek GE: Neurogenic pulmonary edema associated with autonomic dysreflexia. *J Urol* 128:1038–1039, 1982.

55. Poe RH, Reisman JL, Rodenhouse TG: Pulmonary edema in cervical spinal cord injury. *J Trauma* 18:71–73, 1978.

56. Malik AB: Mechanisms of neurogenic pulmonary edema. *Circ Res* 57:1–18, 1985.

57. Samuels MA: Neurally induced cardiac damage. *Neurol Clin* 11:273–292, 1993.

58. Colachis SC III: Autonomic hyperreflexia with spinal cord injury. *J Am Paraplegia Soc* 15:171–186, 1992.

59. Lee BY, Karmakar MG, Herz BL, Sturgill RA: Autonomic dysreflexia revisited. *J Spinal Cord Med* 18:75–87, 1995.

60. Armitage JM, Pyne A, Wiliams SJ, Frankel H: Respiratory problems of air travel in patients with spinal cord injuries. *Br Med J* 300:1498–1499, 1990.

61. McEvoy RD, Mykyryn I, Sajkov D, et al: Sleep apnoea in patients with quadriplegia. *Thorax* 50:613–619, 1995.

62. Short DJ, Stradling JR, Williams SJ: Prevalence of sleep apnea in patients over 40 years of age with spinal cord lesions. *J Neurol Neurosurg Psychiatry* 55:1032–1036, 1992.

63. Ayas N, Garshick E, Epstein L, et al: Predictors of snoring in spinal cord injury. *J Spinal Cord Med* 20:461, 1997.

64. Braun SR, Giovannoni R, Levin AB, Harvey RF: Oxygen saturation during sleep in patients with spinal cord injury. *J Phys Med* 61:302–309, 1982.

65. Bye PTP, Ellis ER, Issa FG, et al: Respiratory failure and sleep in neuromuscular disease. *Thorax* 45:241–247, 1990.

66. Biyani A, Masry WSE: Post-traumatic syringomyelia: A review of the literature. *Paraplegia* 32:723–731, 1995.

67. Sgouros S, Williams B: Management and outcome of posttraumatic syringomyelia. *J Neurosurg* 85:197–205, 1996.

68. Backe HA, Betz RR, Mesgarzadeh M, et al: Post-traumatic spinal cord cysts evaluated by magnetic resonance imaging. *Paraplegia* 29:607–612, 1991.

69. Wiart L, Dautheribes M, Pointillart V, et al: Mean-term follow-up of a series of post-traumatic syringomyelia patients after syringo-peritoneal shunting. *Paraplegia* 33:241–245, 1995.

70. Attia M, Engel P: Thermoregulatory set point in patients with spinal cord injuries (spinal man). *Paraplegia* 21:233–248, 1983.

71. Schmidt KD, Chan CW: Thermoregulation and fever in normal persons and in those with spinal cord injuries. *Mayo Clin Proc* 67:469–475, 1992.

72. Petrofsky JS: Thermoregulatory stress during rest and exercise in heat in patients with a spinal cord injury. *Eur J Appl Physiol* 64:503–507, 1992.

73. Garshick E, Ashba J, Tun CG, et al: Assessment of stature in spinal cord injury. *J Spinal Cord Med* 20:36–42, 1997.

74. Ashba J, Garshick E, Tun CG, et al: Spirometry: Acceptability and reproducibility in spinal cord injured subjects. *J Am Paraplegia Soc* 16:197–203, 1993.

75. American Thoracic Society: ATS statement: Snowbird workshop on standardization of spirometry. *Am Rev Respir Dis* 119:831–838, 1979.

76. Almenoff PL, Spungen AM, Lesser M, Bauman WA: Pulmonary function survey in spinal cord injury: Influences of smoking and level and completeness of injury. *Lung* 173:297–306, 1995.

77. Hemingway A, Bors E, Hobby RP: An investigation of the pulmonary function of paraplegics. *J Clin Invest* 37:773–782, 1958.

78. Almenoff PL, Alexander LR, Spungen AM, et al: Bronchodilatory effects of ipratropium bromide in patients with tetraplegia. *Paraplegia* 33:274–277, 1995.

79. Spungen AM, Dicpinigaitis PV, Almenoff PL, Bauman WA: Pulmonary obstruction in individuals with cervical spinal cord lesions unmasked by bronchodilator administration. *Paraplegia* 31:404–407, 1993.

80. Dicpinigaitis PV, Spungen AM, Bauman WA, et al: Bronchial hyperresponsiveness after cervical spinal cord injury. *Chest* 105:1073–1076, 1994.

81. Tully K, Koke K, Garshick E, et al: Maximal expiratory pressures in spinal cord injury using two mouthpieces. *Chest* 112:113–116, 1997.

82. Bain G, Rodley R, Jamous A, et al: A comparison of the chest radiograph and computerized tomography in assessing lung changes in acute spinal injuries: An assessment of their prevalence and the accuracy of the chest x-ray compared with CT in their assessment. *Paraplegia* 33:121–125, 1995.

83. Kirby NA, Barnerias MJ, Siebens AA: An evaluation of assisted cough in quadriparetic patients. *Arch Phys Med Rehabil* 47:705–710, 1966.

84. Goldman AL, George J: Postural hypoxemia in quadriplegic patients. *Neurology* 26:815–817, 1976.

85. Bach JR: Alternative methods of ventilatory support for the patient with ventilatory failure due to spinal cord injury. *J Am Paraplegia Soc* 14:158–174, 1991.

86. McCool FD, Mayewski RF, Shayne DS, et al: Intermittent positive pressure breathing in patients with respiratory muscle weakness. *Chest* 90:546–551, 1986.

87. Stiller K, Simionato R, Rice K, Hall B: The effect of intermittent positive pressure breathing on lung volumes in acute quadriparesis. *Paraplegia* 30:121–126, 1992.

88. DiMarco AF, Romaniuk JR, Supinski GS: Electrical activation of the expiratory muscles to restore cough. *Am J Respir Crit Care Med* 151:1466–1471, 1995.

89. Jaeger RJ, Turba RM, Yarkony GM, Roth EJ: Cough in spinal cord injured patients: Comparison of three methods to produce cough. *Arch Phys Med Rehabil* 74:1358–1361, 1993.

90. Bach JR, Alba AS: Noninvasive options for ventilatory support of the traumatic high level quadriplegic patient. *Chest* 98:613–619, 1990.

91. Montero JC, Feldman DJ, Montero D: Effects of glossopharyngeal breathing on respiratory function after cervical cord transection. *Arch Phys Med Rehabil* 48:650–653, 1967.

92. Maloney FP: Pulmonary function in quadriplegia: Effect of a corset. *Arch Phys Med Rehabil* 60:261–265, 1979.

93. Miller HJ, Thomas E, Wilmot CB: Pneumobelt use among high quadriplegic population. *Arch Phys Med Rehabil* 69:369–372, 1988.

94. Weingarden SI, Belen JG: Alternative approach to the respiratory management of the high cervical spinal cord injury patient. *Int Disabil Stud* 9:132–133, 1987.

95. Gross D, Ladd HW, Riley EJ, et al: The effect of training on strength and endurance of the diaphragm in quadriplegia. *Am J Med* 68:27–35, 1980.

96. Kogan I, McCool FD, Lieberman SL, et al: The diaphragm hypertrophies during inspiratory muscle training in quadriplegia. *Am J Respir Crit Care Med* 153:A25, 1996.

97. Weissman AR, Rutchik A, Grimm DR, et al: Inspiratory muscle training improves lung function, inspiratory pressure and dyspnea in persons with chronic quadriplegia. *J Spinal Cord Med* 19:41, 1996.

98. Torres A, Serra-Batlles JS, Ros E, et al: Pulmonary aspiration of gastric contents in patients receiving mechanical ventilation: The effect of body position. *Ann Intern Med* 116:540–543, 1992.

99. DeVivo MJ, Ivie CS: Life expectancy of ventilator-dependent persons with spinal cord injuries. *Chest* 108:226–232, 1995.

100. Creasey G, Elefteriades J, DiMarco A, et al: Electrical stimulation to restore respiration. *J Rehabil Res Dev* 33:123–132, 1996.

101. Dobelle WH, D'Angelo MS, Goetz BF, et al: 200 cases with a new breathing pacemaker dispel myths about diaphragm pacing. *ASAIO J* 40:M244–M252, 1994.

102. Nochomovitz ML, Peterson DK, Stellato TA: Electrical activation of the diaphragm. *Clin Chest Med* 9:349–358, 1988.

103. Esclarin A, Bravo P, Arroyo O, et al: Tracheostomy ventilation versus diaphragmatic pacemaker ventilation in high spinal cord injury. *Paraplegia* 32:687–693, 1994.

104. Hoit JD, Shea SA: Speech production and speech with a phrenic nerve pacer. *Am J Speech Pathol* 5:53–60, 1996.

105. Bach JR, Penek J: Obstructive sleep apnea complicating negative-pressure ventilatory support in patients with chronic paralytic/restrictive ventilatory dysfunction. *Chest* 99:1386–1393, 1991.

106. DiMarco AF, Supinski GS, Petro JA, Takaoka Y: Evaluation of intercostal pacing to provide artificial ventilation in quadriplegics. *Am J Respir Crit Care* 150:934–940, 1994.

107. Centers for Disease Control and Prevention: Prevention of pneumococcal disease: Recommendations of the advisory committee on immunization practices. *MMWR* 46(RR-8):1–24, 1997.

108. Centers for Disease Control and Prevention: Prevention and control of influenza: Recommendations of the advisory committee on immunization practices. *MMWR* 46(RR-9):1–25, 1997.

109. Darouiche RO, Groover J, Rowland J, Musher DM: Pneumococcal vaccination for patients with spinal cord injury. *Arch Phys Med Rehabil* 74:1354–1357, 1993.

110. Hoit JD, Banzett RB, Brown R, Loring SH: Speech breathing in individuals with cervical spinal cord injury. *J Speech Hear Res* 33:798–807, 1990.

111. Hoit JD, Shea SA, Banzett RB: Speech production during mechanical ventilation in tracheotomized individuals. *J Speech Hear Res* 37:53–63, 1994.

112. Hoit JD, Banzett RB: Simple adjustments can improve ventilator-supported speech. *Am J Speech Pathol* 6:87–96, 1997.

113. Figoni SF: Exercise responses and quadriplegia. *Med Sci Sports Exerc* 25:433–441, 1993.

114. Hoffman MD: Cardiorespiratory fitness and training in quadriplegics and paraplegics. *Sports Med* 3:312–330, 1986.

115. Noreau L, Shepard RJ: Spinal cord injury, exercise and quality of life. *Sports Med* 20:226–250, 1995.

116. Janssen TWJ, Van Oers AJM, Van der Woude LHV, Hollander AP: Physical strain in daily life of wheelchair users with spinal cord injuries. *Med Sci Sports Exerc* 6:661–670, 1994.

117. Bauman WA, Spungen AM: Disorders of carbohydrate and lipid metabolism in veterans with paraplegia or quadriplegia: A model of premature aging. *Metabolism* 43:749–756, 1994.

118. Young JS, Burns PE, Bower AM, McCutcheon R: Spinal cord injury statistics: Experience of regional spinal cord injury systems. Pheonix, AZ, Good Samaritan Medical Center, 1982.

119. Wicks JR, Oldridge NB, Cameron BJ, Jones NL: Arm cranking and wheelchair ergometry in elite spinal cord-injured athletes. *Med Sci Sports Exerc* 15:224–231, 1983.

120. King ML, Lichtman SW, Pelicone JT, et al: Exertional hypotension in spinal cord injury. *Chest* 106:1166–1171, 1994.

121. Coutts KE, Rhodes EC, McKenzie DC: Maximal exercise response of tetraplegics and paraplegics. *J Appl Physiol* 55:479–482, 1983.

122. Eriksson P, Lofstrom L, Ekblom B: Aerobic power during maximal exercise in untrained and well-trained persons with quadriplegia and paraplegia. *Scand J Rehabil Med* 20:141–147, 1988.

123. Hjeltnes N: Control of medical rehabilitation of para- and tetraplegics by repeated evaluation of endurance capacity. *Int J Sports Med* 5(suppl):171–174, 1984.

124. Silver JR: The oxygen cost of breathing in tetraplegic patients. *Paraplegia* 1:204–214, 1963.

125. Davis G, Plyley MJ, Shepard RJ: Gains of cardiorespiratory fitness with arm-crank training in spinally disabled men. *Can J Sports Sci* 16:64–72, 1991.

126. Langbein WE, Fehr LS, Edwards LC: A new wheelchair exercise test to assess anaerobic power and anaerobic work capacity of persons 55 years of age and older, in Langbein WE, Wyman DJ (eds): *Health Related Physical Activity.* National Veterans Golden Age Games Research Monograph. Chicago, Hines VA Hospital, 1994; pp 56–63.

127. Pitetti KH, Barrett PJ, Campbell KD, Malzahn ED: The effect of lower body positive pressure on the exercise capacity of individuals with spinal cord injury. *Med Sci Sports Exerc* 26:463–468, 1994.

128. Cybulski GR, Penn RD, Jaeger RJ: Lower extremity functional neuromuscular stimulation in cases of spinal cord injury. *Neurosurgery* 15:132–146, 1984.

129. Hooker SP, Figoni SF, Glaser RM, et al: Physiologic responses to prolonged electrically stimulated leg-cycle exercise in the spinal cord injured. *Arch Phys Med Rehabil* 71:863–869, 1990.

130. Pollack SF, Axen K, Spielolz N, et al: Aerobic training effects of electrically induced lower extremity exercise in spinal cord injured people. *Arch Phys Med Rehabil* 70:214–219, 1989.

131. Tator CH: Experimental and clinical studies of the pathophysiology and management of acute spinal cord injury. *J Spinal Cord Med* 19:206–214, 1996.

132. Bernstein JJ, Goldberg WJ: Experimental spinal cord transplantation as a mechanism of spinal cord regeneration. *Paraplegia* 33:250–253, 1995.

Chapter 46

MANAGEMENT OF SLEEP-DISORDERED BREATHING

AHMED BAHAMMAM

MEIR KRYGER

Most patients with disorders of the respiratory system have worsening of physiologic abnormalities during sleep that needs to be considered when planning a rehabilitation program. Patients with sleep disorders can be incapacitated by sleepiness and can be unable to work, adversely affecting their quality of life. With readily available treatment, patients without other cardiopulmonary diseases may regain their usual lifestyle completely. This chapter will review the management of obstructive sleep apnea (OSA), central sleep apnea (CSA), and sleep problems in patients with heart failure, chronic obstructive pulmonary disease (COPD), and asthma.

Evaluation

The most common symptoms of sleep disorders are excessive daytime sleepiness, snoring, insomnia (i.e., difficulty in sleep onset and sleep maintenance), and disrupted sleep. Other symptoms (e.g., morning headaches, impotence in males) and comorbidities (e.g., arterial hypertension and accelerated cardiovascular disease) can affect normal function as seriously. Laboratory testing is used to confirm the diagnosis of sleep disorders. The most widely used test (and currently the "gold standard") is comprehensive polysomnography. This involves an overnight laboratory study that monitors sleep (stages, continuity, movements), respiratory variables (Sa_{O_2}, chest wall movement, abdominal movement, and airflow), and the electrocardiogram. The polysomnogram is analyzed to obtain indexes of sleep structure and disruption and indexes of respiratory abnormalities. The most important of the latter is the *apnea index* (AI), the number of apneic events that occur during each hour of sleep.

Obstructive Sleep Apnea (OSA)

Obstructive sleep apnea (OSA) is a relatively common medical problem affecting 2 to 4 percent of middle-aged adults.[1] Only a minority of this group have sought medical attention, because the public is unaware of the problem, and many of these remain undiagnosed because most physicians do not include an assessment of sleep in the medical history.[2] This disorder is characterized by repetitive obstruction of the upper airway during sleep that results in daytime hypersomnolence, snoring, sleep disruption, hypoxemia, and cardiac arrhythmias. Treatment decisions are guided by clinical features and laboratory findings.[3]

INDICATIONS FOR TREATMENT

It has been shown that an apnea index (AI) > 20 results in a much higher mortality than an AI < 20 in untreated patients.[4] Thus many clinicians believe that patients with an AI > 20 should be treated. The decision to treat patients with fewer apneic episodes depends on the overall assessment of the patient. It has been reported that an AI > 5 is associated with an increased risk for myocardial infarction.[5] Our practice is to treat patients with an AI of 5 to 20 if they have an additional cardiovascular risk factor (high blood pressure, high cholesterol, and cigarette smoking). In addition, we treat those patients with an AI < 20 if daytime sleepiness can be confirmed.

REDUCING FACTORS PROMOTING APNEA

Obesity is the main risk factor in patients with obstructive sleep apnea. Recent work has demonstrated that body fat tends to be distributed in the upper body (neck and pharynx) in OSA patients. This narrows the upper airway and predisposes to obstruction when the pharyngeal muscles relax during sleep.[6,7] In obese patients, weight loss can significantly decrease the severity of apnea.[8] However, weight reduction by diet is often difficult to achieve and even more difficult to sustain. Despite this, weight loss should be considered a major goal for overweight patients with OSA, since even slight weight loss may lead to significant improvement in some patients.

In all patients (especially those who are not obese), other causes of apnea should be considered, including hypothyroidism, acromegaly, and skeletal abnormalities of the jaw (e.g., retrognathia).

Factors that are known to increase the severity of upper airway obstruction should be avoided, such as alcohol and sedatives that produce pharyngeal muscle relaxation.[9,10] Ethanol ingestion prior to sleep may precipitate obstructive events in nonapneic snorers and aggravate apnea in patients with OSA. In addition, ethanol may raise the arousal threshold and prolong apnea. Benzodiazepines and other sedatives may have similar effects. Therefore, patients with OSA ideally should abstain from alcohol. However, not all patients will be compliant with this recommendation. Patients also should be made aware that alcohol may make them even more sleepy during the daytime.

In some patients, upper airway dysfunction and the frequency of apnea are greater in the supine position than in the lateral recumbent position. Although training patients to sleep in the lateral recumbent position may be useful,[11] long-term effects are not clear.

POSITIVE AIRWAY PRESSURE

Since the introduction of nasal continuous positive airway pressure (CPAP) by Sullivan and colleagues[12] in 1981, it has become the treatment of choice for OSA. CPAP works by introducing positive pressure into the upper airway, counteracting the negative inspiratory pressure that causes the pharynx to collapse during an obstructive apnea event. This prevents apneas and hypopneas, oxygen desaturation, and apnea-related sleep fragmentation in most patients.

There are many manufacturers of CPAP systems. The units are small, portable, and reliable. The most commonly used units maintain a fixed pressure. Some automated systems make measurements that reflect airway resistance and deliver just enough pressure to keep the airway open. Some units deliver high pressures during inspiration (BiPAP bilevel positive airway pressure) and lower pressure during expiration. Some units ramp up the pressure slowly. These modifications have been introduced to improve patient comfort and therefore compliance. It is unclear whether compliance is actually improved by these modifications.[13] Machines for generating positive airway pressure run on household electrical current, weigh approximately 2 kg (5 lb), and fit on a bedside table.[14] CPAP pressure is usually delivered by nasal mask. For certain patients, a nasal mask may not work well because an adequate seal cannot be achieved or the mouth opens and pressure cannot be maintained. For some of these patients, nasal pillows or a mask that covers both the nose and the mouth may be appropriate. Patients should be studied in the sleep laboratory to determine the optimal positive pressure required to maintain patency of the upper airway during sleep. This can be accomplished in one or two nights of testing. CPAP pressures in the range of 8 to 12 cmH$_2$O are usually required.

Patients usually experience a rebound increase in both rapid eye movement (REM) sleep and stages III and IV sleep and are harder to awaken immediately after the initiation of CPAP therapy.[15] Gradually, the sleep pattern returns to normal over the first few weeks of therapy. This is usually associated with dramatic improvement in alertness and daytime somnolence.[16] During the REM rebound period, life-threatening hypoxemia can occur, particularly in patients with severe sleep apnea and hypercapnia.[17] For this reason, initiation of CPAP therapy in the hospital should be considered in patients with congestive heart failure, severe nocturnal hypoxemia, carbon dioxide retention, and other medical problems such as unstable coronary artery disease.[18]

CPAP COMPLIANCE

On discontinuation of CPAP therapy without weight loss, the OSA returns to its previous degree of severity within days.[19] Accordingly, it is very important that the patient uses CPAP all night every night, since poor compliance is likely to influence outcome significantly. Long-term compliance remains the major problem with nasal CPAP therapy. Earlier studies of compliance, based on patient reports, demonstrated a good compliance rate.[20,21] However, recent studies using objective methods (e.g., built-in timers on the nasal CPAP compressors or pressure sensors within the mask that determine the number of hours of nasal CPAP use) have not confirmed such good compliance levels.[22-26] The minimum number of hours per night of CPAP use required to ameliorate OSA symptoms is not known and probably varies from patient to patient. Patients thus should be advised to use the machines for the maximum amount of time that they can tolerate.

Patient education and regular follow-up, especially in the first few weeks of therapy, may improve patient compliance. It has been reported that the frequency of nasal CPAP use may be predicted by its use in the first few weeks of prescription.[26] Nasal CPAP units now have systems built in to monitor compliance.[27]

EFFECTS OF CPAP

Apart from its effect on snoring, apnea, and somnolence, nasal CPAP has other significant effects with regular long-term use.[18] Nasal CPAP has been shown to improve survival in patients with obstructive sleep apnea when compared with the conservative management of weight loss.[4,28] Mood changes and cognitive psychological functioning improve with the treatment of OSA by nasal CPAP.[29] Long-term use of nasal CPAP has some hormonal effects as well. Low serum testosterone has been demonstrated in male patients with OSA, which may explain the loss of libido often seen in these patients. Use of nasal CPAP for 3 months led to normalization of testosterone levels.[30] Somatomedin C (insulin-like growth factor, which reflects 24-h growth hormone secretion), which can be depressed in OSA, also was found to normalize after treatment of OSA with nasal CPAP.[30] This may explain the impaired growth reported in the pediatric population with sleep apnea and the subsequent increase in growth rate after treatment. Right-sided heart function improves after CPAP with diuresis and resolution of peripheral edema.[18] CPAP treatment also may reduce elevated systemic blood pressure in OSA.[31]

UNWANTED EFFECTS

Nasal CPAP is a relatively safe mode of therapy. Most side effects are minor and localized to the nose. These include (in the order of frequency) dryness of the upper airway (65 percent), sneezing and nasal drip (35 percent), local skin irritation (30 percent), nasal congestion (25 percent), eye irritation (20 percent), aerophagia (16 percent), sinusitis (8 percent), and epistaxis (4 percent).[32] Serious complications are rare and include corneal abrasion, pneumocephalus, massive epistaxis, and bacterial meningitis.[27]

Side effects should be recognized and treated promptly. Dryness of the oral and nasopharyngeal mucosa may respond to the addition of humidification to the nasal CPAP system. Eye irritation is usually secondary to air leak around the mask and may be prevented by using a well-fitting mask. Patients with nasal congestion and irritation may benefit from nasal anticholinergic agents, decongestants, or steroid nasal sprays.[18] In some patients, chin straps prevent drying of the upper airway by correcting a major source of leak through the open mouth.

Patients who still cannot tolerate nasal CPAP because of nasal irritation and congestion despite medical treatment or those with persistent mouth leak may benefit from using oronasal CPAP with the mask covering both nose and mouth.[27]

INTRAORAL APPLIANCES

Oral appliances offer an alternative that may be attractive for some OSA patients dissatisfied with nasal CPAP.[33] An *intraoral appliance* is a device that is used during sleep in the mouth to modify the position of the mandible, the tongue, and other structures in the upper airway in order to relieve snoring or sleep apnea.

Types of Appliances

Currently there are approximately 40 different intraoral devices,[27] which can be grouped into two main types: dental appliances and tongue retainers.[34]

DENTAL APPLIANCES Most of the currently available intraoral appliances are of this group. They move the lower mandible upward and forward. Cephalometric radiographic studies have demonstrated an increase in various upper airway dimensions when the patients are awake.[35-37] The American Sleep Disorders Association recently has published practice guidelines for the use of dental appliances.[38]

TONGUE-RETAINING DEVICES   These devices have been designed to keep the tongue in an anterior position during sleep. They secure the tongue by means of negative pressure in a soft plastic bulb, which fits between the lips and the teeth and holds the device and tongue anteriorly in the oral cavity.[39]

Efficacy

Analysis of several studies showed that OSA improves in the majority of patients. Approximately half the patients who improved achieved an AI < 20, but as many as 40 percent were left with notably elevated AIs. At present, the data are too limited to formulate any general recommendation about which patients are likely to benefit and what is the optimal device. A recent review of literature from the American Sleep Disorders Association[38] concluded that snoring is improved in most cases and is often eliminated.

Side Effects

Side effects are considered minor in most patients. Excessive salivation and transient discomfort for a brief time after awakening are the most common initial complaints. With regular use and adjustment of fit, these symptoms usually subside. Temporomandibular joint (TMJ) discomfort and tenderness and changes in occlusive alignment may present as late complications and may necessitate cessation of treatment.[39]

SURGICAL TREATMENT

INDICATIONS

It is unusual to find an anatomic lesion as the cause of OSA; in one series of 200 patients with OSA, a specific space-occupying lesion was found in 3 patients only.[40] In such rare cases, specific surgery is corrective. In the remainder, no such lesion is identifiable, and apnea results from a disproportionate anatomy of the upper airway structures.[41] Attempts to identify the specific site of obstruction in OSA using different techniques from radiographic to direct visualization suggest that patients with OSA have different patterns of narrowing of the pharynx.[42] This has led to the conclusion that the pharynx can be functionally divided into two portions: the retropalatal pharynx and the retrolingual pharynx.[43] Several procedures have been developed for the treatment of OSA. The goal of these procedures is to augment the upper airway, and each procedure is designed to alter specific portions of that compromised region.

TYPES OF PROCEDURES

A detailed discussion of different surgical procedures is beyond the scope of this chapter, but we will briefly review some techniques (for details, the reader is referred to a recently published review from the American Sleep Disorders Association[30]).

Uvulopalatopharyngoplasty (UPPP) is the most widely used technique. It aims at enlarging the retropalatal airway through excision of tonsils, trimming and reorientation of the posterior and anterior tonsillar pillars, and excision of the uvula and posterior portion of the palate.[34] In general,

this procedure is effective in half of patients.[3] However, there is no evidence that UPPP improves survival.[4] It is presently not possible to accurately predict which patients will benefit from the procedure.

Laser-assisted uvulopharyngoplasty and radiofrequency volume reduction have been developed as outpatient treatments.[44,44a] However, little evidence is available to assess the efficacy of these procedures, and there are no long-term published follow-up studies. Further published studies are needed before these approaches can be recommended for treating patients with OSA.

Midline glossectomy, an operation that reduces the bulk of the tongue, has been used in patients who do not respond to UPPP, as well in those who demonstrate narrowing of the airway at the base of the tongue.[45] The long-term effect of this procedure is not known, and so it is not widely done.

Another procedure that increases the size of the retrolingual pharynx is mandibular advancement, performed with or without maxillary advancement. Success with this procedure, which is done in only a few centers for OSA, has been variable.[3]

Rarely, tracheostomy may be required in the patient with severe sleep apnea not responding to the treatment just outlined.

Central Sleep Apnea (CSA)

Central sleep apnea is not a disease but represents the final pathway in a large group of heterogeneous disorders.[46] Control of normal breathing during sleep relies on a finely coordinated metabolic control system that consists of the chemoreceptors, vagal intrapulmonary receptors, and numerous brain stem mechanisms. An episode of central apnea in adults is defined as cessation of breathing for 10 s or more due to loss of respiratory effort. In less than 10 percent of apneic patients, central apnea is the predominant component. A useful clinical approach to CSA is one based on the presence or absence of hypercapnia during wakefulness. Hypercapnic CSA is usually secondary to central hypoventilation, chest wall disease, or neuromuscular disease. Nonhypercapnic CSA, on the other hand, occurs in patients with Cheyne-Stokes respiration secondary to medical disorders (discussed below) or idiopathic central sleep apnea. The first group is characterized by an elevated awake Pa_{CO_2} and reduced hypercapnic respiratory ventilatory response. The predominant clinical findings are those of respiratory failure, cor pulmonale, and daytime hypersomnolence. The nonhypercapnic group, on the other hand, is characterized by an awake Pa_{CO_2} that is low or normal and an elevated hypercapnic ventilatory response. The complaint of this group tends to be insomnia or sleep disruption and frequent awakening during the night.

TREATMENT

Because the pathophysiology causing the central apneas is different, the specific treatment is different for the hypercapnic and nonhypercapnic groups.

HYPERCAPNIC CSA

The priority in this group is to support ventilation. Patients must be cautioned against the use of sedatives that can readily induce acute respiratory failure.

Oxygen Therapy

Low-flow nocturnal oxygen may improve hypoxemia and in some cases may decrease the periods of apnea.[47] However, hypercapnia and the frequency of obstructive apnea may increase.[48]

Respiratory Stimulants

Acetazolamide is a carbonic anhydrase inhibitor known to induce metabolic acidosis that probably lowers Pa_{CO_2} apnea threshold. Although this drug may work acutely, there is no evidence that it is effective in the long-term management of patients with hypercapnic CSA. There is an increased risk of the development of obstructive apneas after acetazolamide administration in some patients previously demonstrated to have central events.[49] Hence, follow-up sleep studies are necessary in patients being treated with acetazolamide. Isolated reports of the use of other medications, such as theophylline, naloxone, and medroxyprogesterone acetate, imply that these drugs have little efficacy in the treatment of central apnea.[50]

Assisted Ventilation

If the preceding fail, consideration should be given to some form of assisted ventilation. Nasal CPAP has been shown to improve both ventilation and hypoxemia in some patients with CSA.[51,52] The mechanism of this improvement is not clear. It is possible that during sleep, these patients have pharyngeal airway collapse or closure that may initiate a reflex inhibition of ventilation that may cause central apnea.[50] With nasal CPAP, airway closure is prevented, and such "reflex" apnea is abolished. If nasal CPAP fails, other forms of assisted nocturnal ventilation via the nasal airway may be used, including nasal BiPAP with timed backup or a conventional home ventilator. Diaphragmatic pacing, negative-pressure ventilation using a cuirass, or positive-pressure ventilation through tracheostomy are used less commonly.

NONHYPERCAPNIC CSA

We will review treatment of CSA patients with heart failure in the following section. In nonhypercapnic CSA patients without heart failure, the priority is to reduce arousals and improve sleep quality and consequently daytime function. Since idiopathic central sleep apnea (ICSA) is rarely associated with hypoxemia, oxygen therapy is not usually helpful.

Because arousal from sleep may be an important factor in propagating ICSA, sedative agents that reduce arousals also may reduce the tendency for central sleep apnea. Benzodiazepines have been used in such patients and have resulted in a significant reduction in the number of central apneas and arousals.[53] However, since sedatives can inhibit ventilation and worsen the problem in some patients, this therapeutic intervention must be approached cautiously, and the possibility of hypoventilation must be completely ruled out.

Acetazolamide has been reported to improve sleep and decrease central sleep apnea index in patients with nonhypercapnic CSA after prolonged treatment.[54]

HEART FAILURE AND CHEYNE-STOKES RESPIRATION (CSR)

Cheyne-Stokes respiration (CSR) is a variant of CSA that consists of repetitive cycles of apnea or hypopnea followed by periods of hyperpnea. The ventilatory phase is characterized by a crescendo-decrescendo pattern of tidal volume. The association with congestive heart failure (CHF) has been known for many years; however, only in the past few years has it become apparent that CSR may indeed constitute a clinical problem in patients. Significant degrees of hypoxemia can develop in patients with CSR as a result of apnea even when oxygenation is relatively normal during wakefulness.[55] Due to hypoxemia and disruption of sleep, patients with CHF who have CSR experience daytime sleepiness much more than patients with CHF but without CSR.[56] Patients with CHF with CSR may have higher mortality rates than patients without CSR,[57,58] which stresses the importance of investigating and treating sleep-related respiratory disturbances in patients with CHF.

THERAPY

Treatment of CSR should be considered in symptomatic patients (i.e., insomnia, sleep disruption, daytime sleepiness) and patients with nocturnal hypoxemia. The first goal is to maximize treatment of the heart failure. This by itself may reverse the CSR.

Nocturnal hypoxemia can be improved and the number of CSR events reduced in patients with CHF and CSR with supplementation of oxygen at low flow (2 to 3 L/min by nasal prongs).[59]

The effects of nasal CPAP on CSR, sleep quality, and daytime sleepiness in patients with heart failure are inconclusive. The results of the few studies that addressed this subject are contradictory.[60-63] Furthermore, in one study it was demonstrated that nasal CPAP may even be detrimental in some patients with heart failure.[63] Until definitive trials are done, we believe that nasal CPAP is indicated in patients with congestive heart failure only if they have confirmed obstructive sleep apnea. If a trial of nasal CPAP is contemplated, the patient should be assessed carefully for the adequacy of left ventricular filling pressure, because the positive intrathoracic pressure induced by CPAP reduces the preload (venous return) and may result in a significant reduction in stroke volume (Starling's law).

Since frequent arousals and insomnia are seen commonly in patients with heart failure and CSR, the idea of using hypnotics to eliminate arousal or induce sleep appears intriguing. However, the available data in the literature that addresses the use of hypnotics in this group of patients are very limited. Two studies with a small number of patients have found that the administration of benzodiazepines at night reduced arousals and improved daytime somnolence but did not reduce CSR or central sleep apneas.[64,65] In the preceding studies, the use of benzodiazepines was safe, with no worsening of nighttime oxygen saturation.

From the preceding data, we believe that a short-acting benzodiazepine may be prescribed for patients with sleep-onset insomnia and an intermediate-acting agent for sleep maintenance insomnia. Obstructive sleep apnea and hypoventilation should be ruled out before prescribing any hypnotic.

COPD and Sleep

Patients with COPD are prone to develop hypoxemia during sleep, especially during REM sleep. This phenomenon is more pronounced in patients who have hypoxemia when awake.[66] This is particularly true in patients with an elevated Pa_{CO_2}. However, patients with COPD may develop nocturnal desaturation even if their awake arterial oxygen tension is above 60 mmHg.[67] Hypoventilation is the major cause of hypoxemia during sleep in COPD patients. Hypoxemia is most severe during the phasic manifestation of REM sleep. This finding may be related to the loss of tone of accessory respiratory muscles during REM. Reduction in functional residual capacity (FRC) and ventilation-perfusion mismatch may contribute as well. Although patients with COPD sleep poorly when compared with healthy subjects, there is no objective evidence of daytime somnolence in patients with COPD on multiple sleep latency testing.[68]

INDICATIONS

Treatment should be considered in all patients with an awake Pa_{O_2} of less than 55 mmHg or in those who have cor pulmonale or polycythemia or who develop nocturnal hypoxemia.[69,70] Optimizing treatment of the lung disease is the first step. Long-term domiciliary oxygen therapy remains the only treatment shown by controlled clinical trials to significantly prolong survival in COPD.[69,70] The oxygen dose used for the treatment of hypoxemia in COPD patients is that which maintains Sa_{O_2} (awake) or during exercise above 90 percent. At the present, there are no data available to indicate the minimum level of nocturnal oxygenation required to improve survival. Two reports in patients with daytime Pa_{O_2} values greater than 60 mmHg, but with nocturnal desaturation, have found that nocturnal oxygen therapy did not improve survival.[71,72] Some but not all reports found that correction of nocturnal hypoxemia improves sleep quality in patients with COPD.[68]

RESPIRATORY STIMULANTS

There is currently no convincing scientific evidence that long-term use of any respiratory stimulant improves survival in patients with hypoxic COPD. Thus their use must remain experimental.

INTERMITTENT POSITIVE-PRESSURE VENTILATION (IPPV) BY NASAL MASK

This technique has a theoretical advantage over long-term oxygen therapy of reducing rather than increasing arterial carbon dioxide tension, but there are relatively few data on the use of IPPV in COPD. Early reports on this technique are encouraging.[73,74] However, long-term results and data on survival are not available.

INSPIRATORY MUSCLE TRAINING

A significant correlation between respiratory muscle strength (maximum inspiratory mouth and transdiaphragmatic pressures) and nocturnal desaturation has been described.[75] On the other hand, it is known that respiratory muscle training can improve respiratory muscle strength.[76] Recently, Heijdra and coworkers[77] have shown that target-flow inspiratory muscle training improves nocturnal saturation in patients with severe COPD by increasing respiratory muscle strength and endurance. Further studies are needed before this approach can be recommended.

Asthma

Nocturnal asthma is a manifestation of bronchial hyperreactivity. Normally, the airways narrow slightly at night. Whereas normal people have an overnight fall in peak flow of 8 percent, peak flow rate changes are far greater especially in poorly controlled asthmatics (50 percent).[78] Well-controlled asthmatics may have normal diurnal variation. A difference between early morning peak flow and bedtime peak flow of greater than 15 percent suggests poor control. Thus nocturnal asthma can be looked at as representing an exaggeration of normal circadian patterns. The causes of these circadian changes are incompletely understood. Circadian changes in epinephrine, adenosine monophosphate (AMP), histamine and other inflammatory mediators, cortisol, vagal tone, body temperature, and airway secretions are potential mechanisms that favor nocturnal bronchoconstriction.[79,80] Other factors that have been suggested include interruption of bronchodilator therapy and other treatment, allergens in the bedding, sinusitis and rhinitis, and gastroesophageal reflux.

Patients with nocturnal asthma tend to have interrupted sleep, decreased daytime mental function, and increased daytime somnolence compared with healthy control persons.[81]

THERAPY

The treatment of nocturnal asthma is based on an understanding of the circadian rhythms and the chronotherapeutic aspects of each medication, that is, directing more intense therapy to when the disease is the worst.

PHARMACOLOGIC TREATMENT

The majority of patients with nocturnal asthma will need pharmacologic intervention to control their symptoms. The first step in this part of the management is to optimize the dosage of the patient's current daytime asthma medication for better overall asthma management. In general, good control of symptoms during the day will improve control during the night.

Corticosteroids

The mainstay of therapy of asthma is the regular use of inhaled steroids. Through their anti-inflammatory action, inhaled corticosteroids are very effective in controlling nocturnal symptoms and reducing the circadian variations in airway hyperresponsiveness.[82] The response should be assessed, and if needed, the dose can be built up gradually until optimal response is achieved. In asthmatics who are on oral corticosteroids, the time of administration of the steroid has been shown to affect the severity of nocturnal asthma. It has been demonstrated that administering prednisone at 3 P.M. is superior to 8 A.M. or 8 P.M. dosing in improving asthma.[83] The same concept may hold true as well for inhaled corticosteroids.[84] Nocturnal asthma generally will be controlled in most asthmatics with the use of 400 to 1000 μg of inhaled beclomethasone, budesonide, flunisolide, fluticasone, or triamcinolone.

β_2-Adrenergic Agonists

Longer-acting inhaled β_2-agonists may be beneficial. Salmeterol xinfoate (Serevent) can be tried in a dose of 50 μg twice daily.[85] It has a 12-h duration and holds promise in the treatment of nocturnal asthma.

Theophylline

Sustained-release theophylline preparations have been shown to produce improvement in nocturnal asthma.[86] A chronopharmacologic approach to achieve higher serum concentration during the night (at the time of greatest airflow limitation) has been shown to be helpful. Martin and colleagues[87] demonstrated that achieving a higher serum theophylline concentration, through the use of a long-acting theophylline preparation in a single daily dose given at 7 P.M., produced significant improvement in the awakening FEV_1 compared with lower therapeutic levels observed with twice-daily dosing. This approach did not adversely affect sleep quality. Time of administration should be individualized on the basis of the absorption profile of the chosen agent and the rate of elimination. Preparations administered once daily are usually most efficacious if used at about 6 or 7 P.M. rather than at bedtime.

POTENTIALLY REVERSIBLE FACTORS

One should always rule out any possible reversible causes of nocturnal asthma. Possible reversible causes include the following:

ENVIRONMENTAL

The possibility of an extrinsic allergen should be considered. Treatment is thus preventative, and the first approach is to ensure that the patient's sleeping environment is allergen-free. Occupational asthma may present initially with nocturnal symptoms, so inquiry about the work environment may be helpful.

SINUSITIS

Good control of sinusitis may help in the prevention of nocturnal asthma.[88] Nasal saline washes, oral decongestants, and nasal steroid preparations may improve nocturnal asthma in this group of patients.[89] Exacerbations of sinusitis should be treated with appropriate antibiotics.

GASTROESOPHAGEAL REFLUX (GER)

The possibility of GER should be considered in all patients with nocturnal asthma, and patients should be asked carefully about the presence of any of the symptoms of GER, especially water brash or "heartburn" during the day or night. Occasionally, a patient is not symptomatic but still has the problem. If this possibility is considered, 24-h esophageal pH monitoring may be considered.

If the patient is considered to have GER, general measures should be considered first, which include weight loss, decreasing the size of meals, avoidance of foods that may reduce the tone of the lower esophageal sphincter (e.g., chocolate, fat), elevation of the head of the bed, avoidance of alcohol and smoking, especially at night, avoidance of recumbency for 3 h after eating, and avoidance of tight-fitting garments. Usually these measures are not enough on their own, and patients require pharmacotherapy. Proton pump inhibitors (e.g., omeprazole) are the most effective treatment for GER.[90] However, the clinical experience with such agents in the treatment of nocturnal asthma is limited. Standard doses of H_2 blockers are usually inadequate for the management of

GER, and higher doses (two- to fourfold) may be required.[91] The main problem of H_2 blockers is the high relapse rate after stopping treatment. Prokinetic agents (e.g., cisapride) are comparable to H_2 blockers for treating GER but have not been studied well in asthmatic patients.

SLEEP APNEA IN THE PATIENT WITH ASTHMA

A number of patients with OSA have coexisting bronchial asthma. Treatment of the sleep apnea with nasal CPAP can produce marked improvement in both nocturnal and daytime asthma control.[92]

References

1. Young T, Palta M, Dempsey J, et al: The occurrence of sleep-disordered breathing among middle aged adults. *N Engl J Med* 328:1230, 1993.
2. Rosen RC, Rosekind M, Rosevear C, et al: Physician education in sleep and sleep disorders: A national survey of U.S. medical schools. *Sleep* 16:249, 1993.
3. Hudgel DW: Treatment of obstructive sleep apnea: A review. *Chest* 109:1346, 1996.
4. He J, Kryger MH, Zorick FJ, et al: Mortality and apnea index in obstructive sleep apnea: Experience in 385 male patients. *Chest* 94:9, 1988.
5. Hung J, Whiteford EG, Parsons RW, et al: Association of sleep apnea with myocardial infarction in men. *Lancet* 336:261, 1990.
6. Horner RL, Mohaiddin RH, Lowell DG, et al: Sites and sizes of fat deposits around the pharynx in obese patients with obstructive sleep apnea and weight matched controls. *Eur Respir J* 2:613, 1989.
7. Shelton KE, Woodson H, Gay S, et al: Pharyngeal fat in obstructive sleep apnea. *Am Rev Respir Dis* 148:462, 1993.
8. Smith PL, Gold AR, Meyers DA, et al: Weight loss in mildly to moderately obese patients with obstructive sleep apnea. *Ann Intern Med* 103:850, 1985.
9. Bonora M, Shields GI, Knuth SL, et al: Selective depression by ethanol of upper airway respiratory motor activity in cats. *Am Rev Respir Dis* 130:156, 1984.
10. Bonora M, St John WM, Bledsoe TA: Differential elevation by protriptyline and depression by diazepam of upper airway respiratory motor activity. *Am Rev Respir Dis* 131:41, 1985.
11. Cartwright R, Ristanovic R, Diaz F, et al: A comparative study of treatments for positional sleep apnea. *Sleep* 14:546, 1991.
12. Sullivan CE, Berthon-Jones M, Issa FG, et al: Reversal of obstructive sleep apnea by continuous positive airway pressure applied through the nares. *Lancet* 1:862, 1981.
13. Reeves-Hoche MK, Hudgel DW, Meck R, et al: Continuous versus bi-level positive airway pressure for obstructive sleep apnea. *Am J Respir Crit Care Med* 151:443, 1995.
14. Strollo PJ, Rogers RM: Obstructive sleep apnea. *N Engl J Med* 334:99, 1996.
15. Issa FG, Sullivan CE: The immediate effects of nasal continuous positive airway pressure treatment on sleep pattern in patients with OSA syndrome. *Electroencephalogr Clin Neurophysiol* 63:10, 1986.
16. Hoffstein V, Viner S, Mateika S, et al: Treatment of obstructive sleep apnea with nasal continuous positive airway pressure. *Am Rev Respir Dis* 145:841, 1992.
17. Krieger J, Weitzenblum E, Monassier JP: Dangerous hypoxemia during continuous positive airway pressure treatment of obstructive apnea. *Lancet* 2:1429, 1983.
18. Sullivan CE, Grunstein RR: Continuous positive airway pressure in sleep-disordered breathing, in Kryger M, Roth T, Dement W (eds): *Principles and Practice of Sleep Medicine*, 2d ed. Philadelphia, Saunders, Co 1994; pp 694–705.

19. Lamphere J, Roehrs T, Witting R, et al: Recovery of alertness after CPAP in apnea. *Chest* 96:1364, 1989.

20. Waldhorn RE, Herrick TW, Nguyen MC, et al: Long-term compliance with nasal continuous positive airway pressure therapy of obstructive sleep apnea. *Chest* 97:33, 1990.

21. Rolfe I, Olson LG, Saunder NA: Long-term acceptance of continuous positive airway pressure in obstructive sleep apnea. *Am Rev Respir Dis* 144:1130, 1991.

22. Krieger J: Long-term compliance with nasal continuous positive airway pressure in obstructive sleep apnea patients and nonapneic snorers. *Sleep* 15:S42, 1992.

23. Kribbs NB, Pack AI, Kline LR, et al: Objective measurement of patterns of nasal CPAP use by patients with obstructive sleep apnea. *Am Rev Respir Dis* 147:887, 1993.

24. Meurice JC, Dore P, Paquereau J, et al: Predictive values of long-term compliance with nasal continuous positive airway pressure treatment in sleep apnea syndrome. *Chest* 105:429, 1994.

25. Reeves-Hoche MK, Meck R, Zwillich CW: Nasal CPAP: An objective evaluation of patient compliance. *Am J Respir Crit Care Med* 149:149, 1994.

26. Engleman HM, Martin SE, Douglas NJ: Compliance with CPAP therapy in patients with the sleep apnea/hypopnea syndrome. *Thorax* 49:263, 1994.

27. Wali SO, Kryger MH: Medical treatment of sleep apnea. *Curr Opinion Pulmonary Med* 1:498, 1995.

28. Keenan SP, Burt H, Ryan CF, et al: Long-term survival of patients with obstructive sleep apnea treated by uvulopalatopharyngoplasty or nasal CPAP. *Chest* 105:155, 1994.

29. Engleman HM, Martin SE, Deary IJ, et al: Effect of continuous positive airway pressure treatment on daytime function in sleep apnea/hypopnea syndrome. *Lancet* 343:572, 1994.

30. Grunstein RR, Handelsman DJ, Lawrence S, et al: Neuroendocrine dysfunction in sleep apnea: Reversal by continuous positive airway pressure. *J Clin Endocrinol Metab* 68:352, 1989.

31. Wilcox I, Grunstein RR, Hender JA, et al: Effect of nasal continuous positive airway pressure during sleep on 24-hour blood pressure in obstructive sleep apnea. *Sleep* 16:539, 1993.

32. Pepin JL, Leger P, Veale D, et al: Side effects of nasal CPAP therapy in sleep apnea syndrome. *Chest* 107:375, 1995.

33. Ferguson K, Takashi O, Lowe AA, et al: A randomized crossover study of an oral appliance vs nasal-continuous positive airway pressure in the treatment of mild–moderate obstructive sleep apnea. *Chest* 109:1269, 1996.

34. Lowe AA: Dental appliances for the treatment of snoring and obstructive sleep apnea, in Kryger M, Roth T, Dement W (eds): *Principles and Practice of Sleep Medicine*, 2d ed. Philadelphia, Saunders, 1994; pp 722–735.

35. Bonham PE, Currier GF, Orr WC, et al: The effect of modified functional appliances on obstructive sleep apnea. *Am J Orthod Dentofacial Orthop* 94:384, 1988.

36. Schmidt-Nowara WW, Mead TE, Hays MB: Treatment of snoring and obstructive sleep apnea with a dental orthosis. *Chest* 99:1378, 1991.

37. Johnson LM, Arnett GW, Tamborello JA, et al: Airway changes in relationship to mandibular posturing. *Otolaryngol Head Neck Surg* 106:143, 1992.

38. Practice parameters for the treatment of snoring and obstructive sleep apnea with oral appliances (American Sleep Disorders Association Report). *Sleep* 18:511, 1995.

39. Schmidt-Nowara W, Lowe A, Wiegand L, et al: Oral appliances for the treatment of snoring and obstructive sleep apnea: A review. *Sleep* 18:501, 1995.

40. Sher AE: Obstructive sleep apnea syndrome: A complex disorder of upper airway. *Otolaryngol Clin North Am* 23:593, 1990.

41. Rojewski TE, Schuller DE, Clark RW, et al: Videoscopic determination of the mechanism of obstruction in obstructive sleep apnea. *Otolaryngol Head Neck Surg* 92:127, 1984.

42. Launois SH, Feroah TR, Campell WN, et al: Site of pharyngeal narrowing predicts outcome of surgery for obstructive sleep apnea. *Am Rev Respir Dis* 147:182, 1993.

43. Sher AE, Schechtman KB, Piccirillo JF: The efficacy of surgical modifications of the upper airway in adults with obstructive sleep apnea syndrome. *Sleep* 19:156, 1996.

44. Walker RP, Grigg-Damberger MM, Gopalsami C, et al: Laser-assisted uvulopalatoplasty for snoring and obstructive sleep apnea: Results in 170 patients. *Laryngoscope* 105:938, 1995.

44a. Powell NB, Riley RW, Troell RJ, et al: Radiofrequency volumetric tissue reduction of the palate in subjects with sleep-disordered breathing. *Chest* 113:1163–1174, 1998.

45. Woodson BT, Fujita S: Clinical experience of lingual plasty as part of the treatment of severe obstructive sleep apnea. *Otolaryngol Head Neck Surg* 107:40, 1992.

46. Bradley TD, McNicholas WT, Rutherford R, et al: Clinical and physiological heterogeneity of the central sleep apnea syndrome. *Am Rev Respir Dis* 134:217, 1986.

47. McNicholas W, Carter JL, Rutherford R, et al: Beneficial effect of oxygen in primary alveolar hypoventilation and central sleep apnea. *Am Rev Respir Dis* 125:773, 1982.

48. Gold AR, Bleecker ER, Smith PL: A shift from central and mixed sleep apnea to obstructive sleep apnea resulting from low-flow oxygen. *Am Rev Respir Dis* 132:220, 1985.

49. Sharp J, Druz W, D'Souza V, et al: Effect of metabolic acidosis upon sleep apnea. *Chest* 87:619, 1985.

50. White DP: Central sleep apnea, in Kryger M, Roth T, Dement W (eds): *Principles and Practice of Sleep Medicine*, 2d ed. Philadelphia, Saunders, 1994; pp 630–641.

51. Sullivan C, Berthon-Jones M, Issa FG: Remission of severe obesity-hypoventilation syndrome after short-term treatment during sleep with nasal CPAP. *Am Rev Respir Dis* 128:177, 1983.

52. Issa F, Sullivan C: Reversal of central apnea using nasal CPAP. *Chest* 90:165, 1986.

53. Bonnet MH, Dexter JR, Arand DL: The effect of triazolam on arousal and respiration in central sleep apnea patients. *Sleep* 13:31, 1990.

54. De Backer WA, Verbraecken J, Willemen M, et al: Central apnea index decreases after prolonged treatment with acetazolamide. *Am J Respir Crit Care Med* 151:87, 1995.

55. Bradley TD: Right and left ventricular functional impairment and sleep apnea. *Clin Chest Med* 13:459, 1992.

56. Hanly P, Zuberi-Khokhar N: Daytime sleepiness in patients with congestive heart failure and central sleep apnea. *Chest* 107:952, 1995.

57. Findley LJ, Zwillich CW, Ancoli-Israel S, et al: Cheyne-Stokes breathing during sleep in patients with left ventricular heart failure. *South Med J* 178:11, 1985.

58. Hanly PJ, Zuberi-Khokhar N: Increased mortality associated with Cheyne-Stokes respiration in patients with congestive heart failure. *Am J Respir Crit Care Med* 153:272, 1996.

59. Hanly PJ, Miller TW, Steljes DG, et al: The effect of oxygen on respiration and sleep in patients with congestive heart failure. *Ann Intern Med* 111:777, 1989.

60. Takasaki Y, Orr D, Popkin J, et al: Effects of nasal CPAP on sleep apnea in congestive heart failure. *Am Rev Respir Dis* 140:1578, 1989.

61. Naughton MT, Lin PP, Benard DC, et al: Treatment of congestive heart failure and Cheyne-Stokes respiration during sleep by continuous positive airway pressure. *Am J Respir Crit Care Med* 151:92, 1995.

62. Buckle P, Millar T, Kryger M: The effect of short-term nasal CPAP on Cheyne-Stokes respiration in congestive heart failure. *Chest* 102:31, 1992.

63. Davies RJO, Harrington KJ, Ormerod OJM, et al: Nasal continuous positive airway pressure in chronic heart failure with sleep-disordered breathing. *Am Rev Respir Dis* 147:630, 1993.

64. Biberdorf DJ, Steens R, Millar TW, Kryger MH: Benzodiazepines

in congestive heart failure: Effects of temazepam on arousability and Cheyne-Stokes respiration. *Sleep* 16:529, 1993.

65. Guilleminault C, Clerk A, Labanowski M, et al: Cardiac failure and benzodiazepines. *Sleep* 16:524, 1993.

66. Fleetham JA, Mezon B, West P, et al: Chemical control of ventilation and sleep arterial oxygen desaturation in patients with COPD. *Am Rev Respir Dis* 122:583, 1980.

67. Fletcher EC, Miller J, Devine GW, et al: Nocturnal oxyhemoglobin desaturation in COPD patients with arterial oxygen tension above 60 mmHg. *Chest* 92:604, 1987.

68. Douglas NJ: Nocturnal hypoxemia in patients with chronic obstructive lung disease. *Clin Chest Med* 13:523, 1992.

69. Medical Research Council Working Party Report: Long-term domiciliary oxygen therapy in chronic hypoxic cor pulmonale complicating chronic bronchitis and emphysema. *Lancet* 1:681, 1981.

70. Nocturnal Oxygen Therapy Trial Group: Continuous nocturnal oxygen therapy in hypoxemic chronic obstructive pulmonary disease: A clinical trial. *Ann Intern Med* 93:391, 1980.

71. Fletcher EC, Donner CF, Midgren B, et al: Survival in COPD patients with the daytime $Pa_{O_2} > 60$ mmHg, with or without nocturnal desaturation. *Chest* 101:649, 1992.

72. Fletcher EC, Luckett RA, Goodnight-White S, et al: A double blind trial of nocturnal supplemental oxygen for sleep desaturation in patients with COPD and daytime Pa_{O_2} above 60 mmHg. *Am Rev Respir Dis* 145:1070, 1992.

73. Carroll N, Branthwaite MA: Control of nocturnal hypoventilation by nasal intermittent positive pressure ventilation. *Thorax* 43:349, 1988.

74. Elliot MW, Simmonds AK, Carrol MP, et al: Domiciliary nocturnal nasal intermittent positive pressure ventilation in hypercapnic respiratory failure due to chronic obstructive lung disease: Effects on sleep and quality of life. *Thorax* 47:342, 1992.

75. Heijdra YF, Dekhuijzen PNR, Van Herwaarden CLA, et al: Nocturnal saturation and respiratory muscle function in patients with COPD. *Thorax* 50:610, 1995.

76. Haver A, Mahler DA, Daubenspeck A: Targeted inspiratory muscle training improves respiratory muscle function in patients with COPD. *Ann Intern Med* 111:117, 1989.

77. Heijdra YF, Dekhuijzen PNR, Van Herwaarden CLA, et al: Nocturnal saturation improves by target-flow inspiratory muscle training in patients with COPD. *Am J Respir Crit Care Med* 153:260, 1996.

78. Hetzel MR, Clark TJH: Comparison of normal and asthmatic

circadian rhythms in peak expiratory flow rate. *Thorax* 35:732, 1980.

79. Martin RJ: Nocturnal asthma: Circadian rhythm and therapeutic interventions. *Am Rev Respir Dis* 147:S25, 1993.

80. Postma DS, Oosterhoff Y, Van Aalderen MC, et al: Inflammation in nocturnal asthma? *Am J Respir Crit Care Med* 150:S83, 1994.

81. van-Keimpema AR, Ariaan SZM, Nauta JJ, et al: Subjective sleep quality and mental fitness in asthmatic patients. *J Asthma* 32:69, 1995.

82. Wempe JB, Tammeling EP, Postma DS, et al: Effects of budesonide and bambuterol on circadian variation of airway responsiveness and nocturnal symptoms of asthma. *J Allergy Clin Immunol* 90:349, 1992.

83. Beam WR, Weiner DE, Martin RJ: Timing of prednisone and alternation of airway inflammation in nocturnal asthma. *Am Rev Respir Dis* 146:1524, 1992.

84. Pincus D, Szefler S, Ackerson L, et al: Chronotherapy of asthma with inhaled steroids: The effect of dosage timing on drug efficacy. *J Allergy Clin Immunol* 95:1172, 1995.

85. Fitzpatrick MF, Mackay T, Driver H, et al: Salmeterol in nocturnal asthma: A double-blind, placebo-controlled trial of a long-acting inhaled beta-2 agonist. *Br Med J* 301:1365, 1990.

86. Zwillich CW, Neagley SR, Cicutto LC, et al: Nocturnal asthma therapy: Inhaled Bitolterol versus sustained-release theophylline. *Am Rev Respir Dis* 139:470, 1989.

87. Martin RJ, Cicutto LC, Ballard RD, et al: Circadian variations in theophylline concentration and the treatment of nocturnal asthma. *Am Rev Respir Dis* 139:475, 1989.

88. Hamilos DL: Gastroesophageal reflux and sinusitis in asthma. *Clin Chest Med* 16:683, 1995.

89. Corren J, Adinoff AD, Buchmeier AD, et al: Nasal beclomethasone prevents the seasonal increase in bronchial responsiveness in patients with allergic rhinitis and asthma. *J Allergy Clin Immunol* 90:250, 1992.

90. Vigneri S, Termini R, Leandro G, et al: A comparison of five maintenance therapies for reflux esophagitis. *N Engl J Med* 333:1106, 1995.

91. Hixon LJ, Kelley CL, Jones WN, et al: Current trends in the pharmacotherapy of gastroesophageal reflux disease. *Arch Intern Med* 152:717, 1992.

92. Chan CS, Woolcock AJ, Sullivan CE: Nocturnal asthma: Role of snoring and obstructive sleep apnea. *Am Rev Respir Dis* 137:1502, 1988.

Chapter 47

PERIOPERATIVE PULMONARY CARE

LOUTFI S. ABOUSSOUAN

JAMES K. STOLLER

The prevalence of pulmonary complications after surgery ranges from 6 to 76 percent and depends on the preoperative condition of the surgical candidate, the surgical procedure, and the type of postoperative complications considered. The purposes of a preoperative evaluation and therapy include

1. To minimize the surgical risk by implementing interventions before, during, and after surgery.
2. To identify patients at prohibitive risk and to avert surgery in such individuals.
3. To suggest alternative approaches such as local anesthesia or analgesia, limited lung resection, or laparoscopic surgery.
4. To reduce costs associated with management of complications and prolonged hospital stay.

In addressing these considerations, this chapter will first explore the effects of anesthesia and surgery on lung function. Next, pre-, intra-, and postoperative interventions that can lessen the rate of severity of postoperative pulmonary complications will be reviewed. Finally, the risk factors and predictors for postoperative pulmonary complications will be reviewed for both resectional and nonresectional surgery.

Effects of Surgery on Lung Function

EFFECTS OF ANESTHETIC AGENTS

Anesthetic agents may have several deleterious effects on pulmonary function. These may include a decrease in functional residual capacity, cephalad excursion of the dependent portions of the diaphragm, worsening ventilation-perfusion mismatch due to inhibition of hypoxic pulmonary vasoconstriction, and impairment of mucociliary clearance.

The effects of anesthesia on lung volumes may be mediated by alterations in the tonic and phasic activity of the respiratory muscles when spontaneous breathing is maintained or total elimination of this activity when paralysis with mechanical ventilation is initiated. In anesthetized patients, there is a cephalad shift of the most dorsal part of the diaphragm in both supine and prone positions.[1] This may promote the rapid (i.e., within 5 min of induction) formation of atelectasis in dependent portions of the lung, as documented by computed tomographic (CT) scanning.[2] Similarly, the functional

residual capacity (FRC) may decrease by 20 percent (approximately 500 mL).[3] This effect is now thought to be secondary to chest wall relaxation and resulting decrease in the rib cage transverse diameter and possibly to shift of central blood to the abdomen[4] rather than motion of the diaphragm.[5] As a consequence of decreased FRC, patients with an increased closing capacity (i.e., due to obesity, smoking, or increased age) may have increased airway closure.[1] However, the effect on gas exchange may be minimal.[1]

Anesthetic agents and vasodilators also may prevent hypoxic pulmonary vasoconstriction and therefore increase venous admixture from atelectatic or hypoxic areas of the lung. Intravenous anesthetic agents appear to preserve the normal hypoxia-induced pulmonary vasoconstriction, but controversy surrounds the effects of inhalational anesthetic agents.[1]

Also, mucociliary flow may be impaired for 2 to 6 days after anesthesia, potentially contributing to postoperative pulmonary complications. Both impairment in ciliary flow and impairments in ion and water transport have been implicated.[6,7]

EFFECTS OF SURGERY

The supine posture is the one most likely to be adopted in surgery and, in the awake patient, may result in a decrease in forced vital capacity (FVC) approaching 20 percent.[8] This drop can be higher in obese patients and those with neuromuscular disease, diaphragmatic dysfunction, or chronic obstructive pulmonary disease (COPD).

Most surgery will cause a decline in lung function. The vital capacity (VC) is the most reduced lung compartment, and the magnitude of its decline varies with the type of surgery[9] (Fig. 47-1). Typically, upper abdominal surgery causes the greatest decline in VC, to between 37 and 53 percent of preoperative values,[9–14] followed by lower abdominal surgery (58 to 75 percent of preoperative value) and nonresectional thoracotomy (58 percent of preoperative value).[9,13] Among upper abdominal procedures, subcostal incisions exert less impact on postoperative lung function than midline incisions.[9]

The low point in postoperative VC occurs on the first postoperative day for most procedures and on the second postoperative day for nonresectional thoracotomy.[9] The return to preoperative baseline VC may be delayed 7 to 10 days for upper abdominal surgery.[9] A more severe pulmonary restrictive defect of longer duration (6 to 17 weeks) has been reported after coronary revascularization surgery.[15–18] For instance, Braun and coworkers[16] have shown that mean VC remained 34 percent below baseline at 2 weeks and 17 percent below baseline at 17 weeks after coronary bypass grafting. Similarly, Wahl and associates[18] found that a severe restrictive pulmonary impairment occurs in subjects undergoing coronary artery bypass grafting, from a VC reduced to 61 percent of its preoperative value on day 3 to 76.4 percent of the preoperative value on day 7. Lung function returned to its preoperative baseline 3 months after bypass surgery.[18] Respiratory muscle weakness, as determined by measurements of inspiratory and expiratory mouth pressures, has been shown to contribute to the immediate post-bypass grafting pulmonary restrictive defect, whereas structural alterations in chest wall mechanics may account for the persistence of a late restrictive impairment.[15]

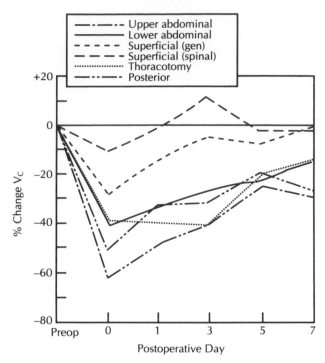

FIGURE 47-1 Changes in VC relative to preoperative values in different surgical groups. The VC was depressed from day 0 through day 7 after upper abdominal surgery. The depression was less marked and less prolonged after lower abdominal procedures. The least marked but still significant change in VC was noted in patients with superficial incisions receiving general anesthesia from day 0 through day 3. The thoracotomy and posterior incision groups are included for comparison. The posterior group contained only three patients (two undergoing bilateral adrenalectomy and one bilateral nephrectomy), which were too few for statistical evaluation. The thoracotomy group differed from the other groups with regard to operative time, use of pump oxygenator, and postoperative ventilatory assistance. The skew of the populations in all groups does not allow use of conventional statistical parameters such as standard deviation or standard error. (From Ali J, Weisel RD, Layug AB, et al: Consequences of postoperative alterations in respiratory mechanics. *Am J Surg* 128:376–382, 1974; used by permission.)

Preoperative Preparation of the Patient

RATIONALE

The rationale for preoperative intervention is to lessen the risk of surgery and to identify patients with specific remediable risk factors for postoperative complications.

PREOPERATIVE TREATMENT OF AIRFLOW OBSTRUCTION

Chronic obstructive pulmonary disease (COPD) may predispose to postoperative pulmonary complications such as atelectasis, pneumonia,[19] ventilatory failure,[19,20] and prolonged stay in the intensive care unit.[21] Several studies have indicated that aggressive preoperative treatment of airflow obstruction decreases the rate of postoperative complications. For instance, in a retrospective study of COPD patients undergoing general anesthesia, preoperative treatment with bronchodilators, systemic corticosteroids, and/or antibiotics signifi-

cantly reduced the rate of postoperative pulmonary complications from 43 percent in untreated patients to 24 percent in treated patients.[22] Similar findings were seen in another study, where preoperative treatment with bronchodilator therapy, smoking cessation, antibiotics, and/or chest physiotherapy reduced the prevalence of postoperative pulmonary complications from 60 percent in controls to 22 percent in the treatment group.[23]

The individual impact of each intervention is unknown. Corticosteroids may result in a greater than 15 percent improvement in forced expiratory volume in 1 s (FEV_1) in about 15 to 56 percent of patients with COPD.[24] Further, preoperative hydrocortisone in patients with severe asthma may reduce the rate of postoperative pulmonary complications to that of nonasthmatic patients.[25] Also, preoperative wheezing is associated with a higher rate of postoperative complications, suggesting that adequate treatment with corticosteroids may reduce this risk.[25] Overall, it appears reasonable to pretreat patients with COPD or asthma with corticosteroids. Although concerns may be raised about the risk of wound dehiscence in patients on steroids, a study of factors influencing wound dehiscence after abdominal surgery did not find steroids to be a significant risk factor.[26] As a guideline, it has been our practice to treat patients with COPD or asthma who have active wheezing at their preoperative evaluation with prednisone or an equivalent corticosteroid drug at a dose of 1 mg/kg for 1 to 2 weeks before elective surgery. This regimen also may be appropriate in patients who have required systemic or inhaled corticosteroids within 6 months prior to surgery.[27] Stable patients without wheezing may be treated with steroids starting the night preceding the surgery (i.e., hydrocortisone 100 mg parenterally every 8 h). Caution is recommended in using corticosteroids in other patients. For instance, in one study, pretreatment of patients undergoing cardiac surgery with a single massive dose of methylprednisolone (30 mg/kg) was associated with increased intraoperative blood loss, higher incidence of low cardiac output, and increased requirement for postoperative mechanical ventilation.[28]

Similarly, the magnitude of reduction of postoperative risk attributed to bronchodilators is unknown. Indeed, some authors have associated the perioperative use of bronchodilators with an increased risk of cardiac and serious pulmonary complications,[29] although bronchodilator use in these studies simply may have been a marker of more serious pulmonary disease.[29] Furthermore, the preoperative use of salbutamol was not found to decrease the rates of postoperative chest infection in patients undergoing elective upper abdominal surgery.[30] Notwithstanding these concerns, the preoperative use of bronchodilators such as ipratropium bromide and/or beta agonists seems appropriate to optimize the pulmonary function of patients with evidence of airflow obstruction. In one study of patients with reactive airway disease, prophylactic preoperative inhalation of bronchodilators effectively reduced intraoperative bronchospasm.[31]

PREOPERATIVE ANTIBIOTICS FOR COPD AND BRONCHIECTASIS

Preoperative antibiotics in patients with COPD are best reserved for those with evidence of active bacterial infection. A sputum examination may be necessary to determine whether bacterial infection is present and antibiotic therapy is warranted.[32] A simple Gram's stain of expectorated sputum will allow an estimation of neutrophil and bacteria numbers, both expected to increase over baseline in bacterial exacerbations.[32] Alternatively, exacerbations characterized by an increase in dyspnea, sputum volume, and sputum purulence or any two of these three clinical indices probably should be treated with antibiotics.[33,34]

PREOPERATIVE SMOKING CESSATION

The potential adverse effects of smoking on the respiratory system are numerous and include impairment of mucociliary clearance, mucus hypersecretion, airflow obstruction, and elevation of carboxyhemoglobin and a consequent decrease in oxygen-carrying capacity. Smoking is associated with an increase in the rate of decline of FEV_1 in susceptible smokers,[35,36] and smoking cessation can be expected to cause an actual increase in FEV_1 in subjects younger than 35 years of age and to return the rate of decline in lung function to normal.[36] Other beneficial effects of smoking cessation on lung function include improvement in measures of small airways function such as the ratio of closing volume to VC or total lung capacity (TLC) and the slope of phase 3 on a nitrogen washout curve.[37]

Cigarette smoking has been identified as a risk factor for the development of postoperative pulmonary complications.[20,38–41] For instance, in a prospective study of 111 patients undergoing elective surgery, the risk of postoperative pulmonary complications increased steadily with increased smoking from 8 percent in nonsmokers to 43 percent in very heavy smokers.[38] As a corollary, smoking cessation before surgery has been credited with decreasing the risk of postoperative pulmonary complications from 57 percent for those who quit smoking for 2 months or less to 15 percent for those who stopped smoking more than 2 months prior to surgery.[42]

The reduction in postoperative complications in relation to smoking cessation parallels the time frame in improvement of physiologic parameters. For instance, smoking cessation for only 1 week does not improve small airways function,[43] whereas smoking cessation for 1 month causes an improvement in the phase 3 slope on a nitrogen washout curve.[44] Similarly, the risk of developing postoperative complications decreases only after 4 weeks of smoking cessation[42] and becomes statistically significant after 8 weeks.[42] Moreover, a plateau in the improvement of pulmonary function is seen after 6 to 8 months of smoking cessation and corresponds to the time frame at which the rate of postoperative pulmonary complications reaches that of never smokers (11 percent).[42]

With these observations in mind, it is reasonable to recommend smoking cessation for as long as possible before surgery and at least 2 months before an elective procedure.

PREOPERATIVE DEEP VENOUS THROMBOSIS PROPHYLAXIS

Different preoperative modalities for the prevention of deep venous thrombosis have been recommended in moderate-to high-risk surgery. These include elastic stockings, intermittent pneumatic compression, low-dose unfractionated heparin, or warfarin[45–47] (Table 47-1). The recommendations from the American College of Chest Physicians consensus conference on antithrombotic therapy are summarized in Table 47-1[45] and will be discussed further below.

Intraoperative Factors

IMPACT OF ANESTHESIA TYPE

General anesthesia impairs diaphragmatic function and respiratory drive in response to hypercarbia and hypoxemia, reduces FRC, worsens ventilation-perfusion mismatch, and promotes atelectasis and dead space. Epidural anesthesia may impair expiratory efforts (e.g., cough) due to denervation of the anterior abdominal muscles and may impair FRC. Although conventional wisdom asserts that postoperative mortality and morbidity are lower in patients receiving epidural anesthesia compared with general anesthesia, adequate documentation has been lacking, and several studies have had conflicting results.[1] Overall, there appears to be no advantage of epidural anesthesia over general anesthetic techniques for the prevention of pulmonary complications. However, it is noteworthy that epidural or spinal anesthesia has been credited with a significant decrease in the risk of deep venous thrombosis compared with general anesthesia for hip surgery.[48,49] However, these two studies used prophylactic measures against deep venous thrombosis that would be considered inadequate by current standards (see Table 47-1). The advantage of regional anesthesia for preventing deep venous thrombosis when current prophylactic measures are used therefore remains to be determined.

In patients with reactive airways disease, general anesthesia with endotracheal intubation can be associated with a higher frequency of perioperative bronchospasm (8.9 percent) compared with both general anesthesia using mask (0 percent) and regional anesthesia (2.2 percent).[31,50] Such bronchospasm may be effectively avoided by the preoperative use of bronchodilators[31] or avoiding general anesthesia with tracheal intubation.[50]

SURGICAL CONSIDERATIONS

Surgical procedures with shorter durations may be associated with a lower risk of complications and shorter intensive care unit stays.[50–52] In a study of operations performed in patients with severe chronic obstructive pulmonary impairment, the rates of postoperative pulmonary complications were 4, 23, 38, and 73 percent as surgical time increased from less than 1 h, 1 to 2 h, 2 to 4 h, and more than 4 h, respectively.[51] However, this may be a reflection of more severe surgical disease rather than of the duration of the procedure.[50]

More recently, advances in surgical techniques have allowed the performance of less invasive surgery. These techniques include thoracoscopy for chest procedures and laparoscopy for abdominal procedures. For instance, laparoscopic cholecystectomy causes less profound and less prolonged lung dysfunction than open cholecystectomy.[14,53,54] In one study, laparoscopic cholecystectomy was found to reduce postoperative atelectasis, analgesic requirements, and length of stay.[14] Alternatively, other investigators found an increase in surgical time for laparoscopic compared with small incision cholecystectomy and no significant reduction in hospital stay or postoperative recovery.[55] Laparoscopic techniques have been extended to other types of surgery such as hernio-

TABLE 47-1 Prevention of Venous Thromboembolism in Surgical Patients

Type of Surgery[a]	Prophylactic Measure[b]	Grade of Recommendation[c]
Low-risk general surgery: uncomplicated, minor, <40 years, no risk factors	Early ambulation	C
Moderate-risk general surgery: major, >40 years, no other risk factors	ES, LDUH (2 h before and q12h after surgery), or IPC; IPC and ES pre- and postop if possible	A
High-risk general surgery: major, >40 years, other risk factors or MI	LDUH (q8h) or LMWH; IPC as alternative if prone to hematoma or infection	A
Very high-risk general surgery: major, >40 years, previous thromboembolism or malignant disease or stroke or spinal cord injury	LDUH or LMWH started preop, or dextran started intraop; all combined with IPC started intraop; Periop warfarin in some patients[d]	B (A for warfarin)
Total hip replacement	Postop SC LMWH twice-daily fixed dose, or oral anticoagulation started pre- or postop,[d] or adjusted-dose unfractionated heparin preop; ±adjuvant ES or IPC	A
Total knee replacement	Postoperative SC, twice daily, unmonitored, fixed dose LMWH, or IPC	A
Hip fracture surgery	Preoperative, SC fixed dose, unmonitored LMWH, or oral anticoagulation,[d] ±adjuvant IPC	A
Intracranial neurosurgery	IPC (±ES) or LDUH (±IPC if high risk)	A

[a] Classification of level of risk based on Salzman et al.[46]
[b] Source: Clagett et al.[45]
[c] Grades A and B: Recommendations based on randomized trials or meta-analyses in which the lower limit of the confidence interval exceeds (grade A) or overlaps (grade B) the minimal clinically important benefit. Grade C: Recommendations based on nonrandomized cohort or case series. SOURCE: Cook et al.[47]
[d] Goal of warfarin or anticoagulation is INR 2.0 to 3.0 (low intensity).
NOTE: ES, elastic stockings; IPC, intermittent pneumatic compression; LDUH, low-dose unfractionated heparin; LMWH, low-molecular-weight heparin; SC, subcutaneous.

laparotomy,[56] appendectomy,[57] and radical nephrectomy[58] with variable results. The advantages of a laparoscopic approach for these other procedures remain to be defined.

Thoracoscopy also was found to be a safe and effective procedure with a low rate of postoperative complications[59] and a significant shortening of hospital stay.[60] The use of thoracoscopy for resecting primary lung cancer carries the risk of a compromised operation, and its role in this setting remains to be defined.[61] In some patients with lung carcinoma or with large benign lesions, the procedure may need to be converted to a thoracotomy.[59] Esophagectomy also has been performed through a thoracoscopic approach, thus far without reducing postoperative or anastomotic complications.[62]

Postoperative Care

CHEST PHYSICAL THERAPY AND MECHANICAL AIDS

Chest physiotherapy (e.g., deep breathing exercises, coughing, postural drainage, percussion, and vibration) and lung expansion techniques (e.g., incentive spirometry, intermittent positive-pressure breathing, mask CPAP) are used frequently for the prevention and treatment of postoperative pulmonary complications. These complications include sputum retention, radiographic changes, atelectasis, or signs or symptoms of bronchopulmonary infections. Overall, studies have shown that incentive spirometry, intermittent positive-pressure breathing (IPPB), and deep breathing exercises are equally effective in preventing pulmonary complications after abdominal surgery.[63–65] Similarly, in a recent randomized clinical trial in patients undergoing abdominal surgery, equal rates of respiratory complications (12 to 15 percent) were found in patients receiving incentive spirometry alone versus those receiving a mixed regimen consisting of deep breathing exercises for low-risk patients and incentive spirometry and physiotherapy in high-risk patients.[66] On the other hand, whether these modalities improve ventilation and clearance of secretions[64] or prevent radiographic changes postoperatively remains unclear.[63,67] Some studies cast doubt on the utility of breathing and coughing exercises alone in preventing fever, hypoxemia, radiographic abnormalities, or clinically significant postoperative pulmonary complications.[67] Several reports have attributed adverse effects to IPPB, including decreased VC after administration,[68] decreased Pa_{O_2},[69] and an 18 percent rate of complications due to abdominal distention.[63] Incentive spirometry has been favored over other techniques of lung expansion in the United States because of its putative beneficial effects (e.g., prevention of pulmonary complications, lack of complications associated with therapy, decreased length of hospitalization) and ease of administration.[63]

Nasal continuous airway pressure (CPAP), and possibly bilevel positive airway pressure, may have several beneficial effects, including reversal or prevention of postoperative atelectasis, reversal of hypoxemia, and averting the need for intubation. Administered postoperatively, nasal CPAP can normalize pulmonary function,[70] including FRC.[70–72] Nasal CPAP for up to 12 h after surgery has been observed to improve hypoxemia in the immediate postoperative period[73,74] but did not prevent the late development of hypoxemia or atelectasis.[73–75] Further, comparison of CPAP with bottle blowing,[71] positive expiratory pressure (PEP) mask,[76,77] or simple coughing or deep breathing exercises[72] suggests no advantage of nasal CPAP over these other modalities in preventing postoperative pulmonary complications.

In conclusion, notwithstanding some discrepant conclusions from available studies, incentive spirometry is the preferred therapy for preventing pulmonary complications after upper abdominal or thoracic surgery. Intermittent positive-pressure breathing may be used as salvage therapy for patients who have failed chest physiotherapy or incentive spirometry. Moreover, IPPB may be the first-line therapy for patients with chest wall deformities or neuromuscular weakness. Other modalities such as CPAP or bilevel positive airway pressure may be useful for treating atelectasis and hypoxemia and averting intubation if the cause for respiratory failure is readily reversible.[78] Preoperative instructions are necessary to familiarize the patient with the proper use of incentive devices.

IMPACT OF POSTOPERATIVE PAIN MANAGEMENT

EPIDURAL VERSUS PARENTERAL ANALGESIA

Several studies document better postoperative pain control with epidural opioid analgesics compared with parenteral analgesia,[79] although most studies indicate no significant difference between those two options regarding the effects on pulmonary function, rate of complications, or ventilation and oxygenation.[79] For example, a recent prospective, randomized study showed that epidural analgesia provides adequate pain relief but did not reduce pulmonary complications, radiographic chest abnormalities, or hospital stay.[80] In contrast, Kilbride and coworkers[81] have reported a significantly lower rate of pneumonia and atelectasis after major abdominal procedures in patients receiving epidural anesthesia compared with intramuscular or patient-controlled analgesia. Similarly, Liu and associates[82] reported a lower rate of postoperative pulmonary complications after high-risk surgeries when postoperative pain control was achieved with epidural analgesia compared with systemic opioids. In a study of patients undergoing elective cholecystectomy or total hip replacement surgery, intravenous morphine analgesia was associated with greater oxygen desaturation, more central and obstructive apneas, and paradoxic breathing compared with regional (epidural or intercostal) analgesia.[83] Overall, recommendations for postoperative epidural analgesia for low- to moderate-risk surgery should be individualized and tempered by the finding of more episodes of systolic hypotension compared with parenteral opioids in one study.[80] However, in high-risk surgery, the advantages of postoperative epidural analgesia are clearer.[81–83]

PATIENT-CONTROLLED ANALGESIA

Patient-controlled analgesia (PCA) allows the patient to self-administer a set dose of drug intravenously. In one study, Bennett and colleagues[84] reported smaller declines in peak expiratory flow rates after upper abdominal surgery in patients receiving PCA compared with those receiving intramuscular injections on an as-needed basis. Alternatively, Welchew[85] found no differences in FVC, FEV_1, or peak expiratory flow rates between patients treated with these two modalities. Lung function after coronary artery bypass graft surgery also was found to be equally reduced in patients receiving PCA versus as-needed intramuscular analgesia.[86] Postthoracotomy lung function was found to be less impaired in patients receiving epidural analgesia compared with those receiving PCA.[87] In a study of patients undergoing major abdominal procedures, PCA was associated with significantly lower rates of postoperative pneumonia than intra-

muscular analgesia (4.5 versus 21 percent, respectively).[81] However, epidural analgesia was associated with a significantly lower rate of atelectasis (13 percent) compared with either PCA (45 percent) or intramuscular analgesia (47 percent).[81]

PREVENTION OF VENOUS THROMBOEMBOLISM

Deep venous thrombosis and its associated risk of pulmonary embolism are a preventable cause of postoperative mortality and morbidity. Prophylaxis is justified by its low risk, the clinically silent nature of these disorders, the difficulty of clinical detection, and the high risk of pulmonary embolism. Clinical risk factors include advanced age (over 40 years), prolonged immobility or paralysis, prior venous thromboembolism, malignancy, major surgery (particularly involving abdomen, pelvis, lower extremities), obesity, varicose veins, congestive heart failure, myocardial infarction, stroke, fracture of the pelvis, hip, or leg, or possibly high estrogen use.[45]

Despite the identification of risk factors for venous thromboembolism, the recognition of its silent nature, and the availability of prevention methods, appropriate prophylactic measures remain underutilized. Recognizing this shortcoming, the American College of Chest Physicians issued a clinical consensus statement with a goal to encourage use and to tailor the available prophylactic measures to the specific clinical risk factors of the patient[45–47] (see Table 47-1). Of note, aspirin is not recommended as a prophylactic measure in general surgical patients.[45]

Somewhat unappreciated is the fact that the risk of deep venous thrombosis may persist for at least 2 months after elective total hip replacement surgery.[88,89] Recent studies have confirmed that prolonged (i.e., 4 to 6 weeks) prophylaxis with either low-molecular-weight heparin[88] or oral anticoagulation[89] reduces the risk of deep venous thrombosis and pulmonary embolism by more than half compared with prophylaxis given during hospitalization only. For instance, enoxaparin (a low-molecular-weight heparin) reduced the rate of thromboembolism from 39 percent in patients who received prophylaxis during their hospitalization only to 18 percent in those who received a 1-month course.[88] Further, a cost-analysis model suggested that a strategy of 6 weeks of oral anticoagulation after total hip replacement was cost-effective.[89] However, extending this period to 12 weeks would increase the risk of bleeding beyond the benefit of reducing thromboembolic events and is costly.[89]

Predictors and Risk Factors for Postoperative Pulmonary Complications

In evaluating patients for surgery, an important distinction is whether the surgery involves lung resection or is nonresectional surgery. For example, although the value of pulmonary function testing is argued in evaluating the nonresectional surgery candidate,[41,50,51,90–92] there is consensus that pulmonary function testing is an important aspect of the preoperative evaluation of the lung resection candidate.

NONRESECTIONAL SURGERY

As reviewed in Table 47-2, many studies have evaluated the risk factors for pulmonary complications of nonresectional

TABLE 47-2 Postoperative Pulmonary Complications in Selected Large Series: Prevalence and Risk Factors

Author	Surgery	PPC Prevalence and Type	Risk Factors
Stein[93]	Varied	35% all respiratory	A, T; lung function: MEFR, N_2 slope, FEV_1/FVC, Pa_{CO_2}, RV/TLC.
Wightman[39]	Varied	6.2% C, fever, new physical findings	UA; chronic respiratory disease; smoking; male. Not obesity
Latimer[40]	EUA	76% all respiratory	>110% IBW, smoking, airflow obstruction, anesthesia >3.5 h
Cain[21]	ET, EUAV	29% ICU stay >5 days	Airflow obstruction
Gracey[19]	Varied	19% all respiratory, 2% pneumonia, 2% ventilated >48 h, 2% atelectasis, 4% retained secretions	FVC <75%, $FEF_{25-75\%}$ < 50%, MVV < 50%; UA
Garibaldi[52]	ET, EA	17.5% pneumonia	>250 lb; duration of preoperative stay and surgery; ASA class; T, UA; albumin. Not male gender
Poe[94]	EC	14.8% atelectasis, pneumonia, or purulent bronchitis	FVC, $FEF_{25-75\%}$, closing volume, N_2 slope. Not age, weight, FEV_1, or smoking
Warner[42]	ECABG	18.7% all respiratory, 5.7% segmental lobe collapse, 2.6% purulent sputum and temperature >38.5°C, 8.3% bronchospasm, 4.2% chest tube	FEV_1, days since quitting smoking, enflurane
Svensson[20]	AA repair	60% all respiratory, 43% ventilated >48 h, 15% tracheostomy	COPD, smoking history, FEV_1, Pa_{CO_2}
Hall[95]	Laparotomy	23.2% atelectasis or pneumonia	ASA > 2; UA incision; residual intraperitoneal infection; >59 years; >25 kg/m^2; preoperative stay >4 days, gastroduodenal, colonic surgery.
Kispert[98]	Vascular	12.9% pneumonia, ventilated >48 h, ARDS; 30.7% for AA, 8% for PV, and 4.7% for carotid surgery	Abdominal procedure, $FEV_1 \leq 2$ L/s, $FEV_1/FVC \leq 0.65$
Pedersen[96]	Varied	4% all respiratory	>70 years, major abdominal or emergent surgery, COPD, anesthesia >180 min with pancuronium
Calligaro[97]	AAo	16% pneumonia, reintubation, or ventilator >24 h, 38% atelectasis, 1.7% mortality	ASA class, FVC < 80%, $FEF_{25-75\%}$ < 60%, >150% ideal body weight, >70 years, >5 L crystalloids during surgery
Kroenke[29]	T, A	10% pneumonia, reintubation, or ventilatory failure; 6.1% mortality	Abnormal chest radiograph, perioperative bronchodilator use, ASA class, age > 70 years. Not spirometry
Lawrence[91]	E,A	3% cardiopulmonary complications	Abnormal lung exam, abnormal preoperative CXR, Goldman cardiac risk index, Charlson comorbidity index. Not spirometry.
Spivack[41]	CABG	8.3% ventilated >48 h	Abnormal LVEF, comorbidity (CHF, angina, smoking, diabetes)

NOTE: AA, aortic aneurysm surgery; A, abdominal surgery; AAo, abdominal aortic surgery; C, cholecystectomy; CABG, coronary artery bypass graft surgery; COPD, chronic obstructive pulmonary disease; E, elective surgery; IBW, ideal body weight; PV, peripheral vascular; T, thoracic surgery; UA, upper abdominal surgery; UAV, upper abdominal vascular surgery.

SOURCE: Adapted from Stoller JK, Holden DH, Matthay MA: Preoperative evaluation, in Bone RC (ed): *Pulmonary and Critical Care Medicine*. Chicago, Mosby–Year Book, 1993; used by permission.

surgery.[19–21,29,39–42,52,91,93–98] Although the types of pulmonary complications evaluated in these studies vary widely, most recent studies have focused on serious complications, such as prolonged postoperative mechanical ventilation and mortality.[92]

Among available studies, the weight of evidence suggests several definite risk factors for pulmonary complications, such as abdominal and thoracic sites of surgery and COPD. Although not universally accepted,[99] other widely cited risk factors include composite scores, such as the ASA (American Society of Anesthesiology) score.[29,50,95,97] Also, the presence of cardiac morbidity appears to be a significant determinant of postoperative pulmonary complications[41,91,100] (Table 47-3).

Probable risk factors are those suggested by partial agreement between studies and include obesity, advanced age, history of cigarette smoking, and the presence of hypercapnia (see Table 47-3).

Finally, possible risk factors include those which are occa-

sionally mentioned, including male gender, duration of surgery, extended hospital stay before surgery, and hypoalbuminemia (see Table 47-3).

INDICATIONS FOR PREOPERATIVE PULMONARY FUNCTION TESTING

Current recommendations from the American College of Physicians position paper concerning nonresectional surgery emphasize the need for a thorough preoperative evaluation based on a general history and physical examination.[101,102] According to these recommendations, factors that should prompt pulmonary function testing to assess the degree and nature of pulmonary impairment before surgery include

1. History of cigarette smoking
2. Presence of dyspnea
3. Evidence of uncharacterized lung disease, that is, pulmo-

TABLE 47-3 Risk Factors for Postoperative Pulmonary Complications

Definitive risk factors (general agreement among studies)
   Site of operation (especially upper abdominal and thoracic)
   General illness of the patient (e.g., ASA classification)
   Chronic obstructive pulmonary disease
   Cardiac morbidity (e.g., Goldman index)
Probable risk factors (partial agreement among studies)
   Obesity (e.g., >250 lb, body mass index > 25)
   Advanced age (e.g., >59 years)
   Ever smoked cigarettes
   Hypercapnia
Possible risk factors (occasionally cited)
   Male gender
   Duration of surgery
   Extended hospital stay before surgery
   Hypoalbuminemia

SOURCE: Adapted from Stoller JK, Holden DH, Matthay MA: Preoperative evaluation, in Bone RC (ed): *Pulmonary and Critical Care Medicine.* Chicago, Mosby–Year Book, 1993; used by permission.

nary symptoms or history of pulmonary disease but no pulmonary function testing within 60 days
4. Expectedly long or extensive surgical procedure
5. Expected need for postoperative rehabilitation

Specific recommendations for different types of surgery are outlined below.

Cardiac Surgery
Because recent series suggest that smoking history does not predict prolonged intensive care unit stay and only an elevated Pa_{CO_2} (but not spirometric measurements) predicts mortality, the current recommendation is to perform preoperative arterial blood gas determinations and spirometry in candidates for coronary artery bypass surgery with a history of tobacco use and dyspnea.[101,102]

Upper Abdominal Surgery
Routine preoperative spirometry adds little to a thorough clinical evaluation in identifying postoperative pulmonary complications after upper abdominal surgery. Again, spirometry and arterial blood gas determinations are best reserved for patients with a history of tobacco use and dyspnea.[102]

Lower Abdominal Surgery
The risk of postoperative complications following lower abdominal surgical incisions diminishes with distance from the diaphragm. Preoperative spirometry may be indicated in patients with uncharacterized pulmonary disease and expectedly prolonged or extensive surgery.[102]

Other Surgeries
Recommendations for preoperative pulmonary spirometry are again dictated by clinical suspicion of uncharacterized pulmonary disease and by possible strenuous postoperative rehabilitation, as might be expected after orthopedic surgery.[102]

Although these recommendations are widely employed, limitations must be considered and may explain the incomplete compliance with these guidelines (i.e., up to 39 percent of preoperative pulmonary spirometry requests do not satisfy ACP guidelines).[103] For example, critical reviews have emphasized that the predictive value of spirometry before abdominal operations is unproved[90] and perhaps not helpful.[91] Even patients with severe chronic obstructive pulmonary impairment, defined as an FEV_1 of less than 50 percent of predicted, may undergo surgery successfully.[51] Other challenges to the guidelines are that clinical variables other than spirometry measurements [i.e., age over 70, American Society of Anesthesiology (ASA) class above 3, abnormal chest radiograph, and perioperative bronchodilator administration] have been observed to be better predictors of cardiopulmonary complications than spirometry.[29] In a prospective analysis of factors associated with pulmonary complications after noncardiothoracic surgery in patients with severe COPD ($FEV_1 \leq 1.2$ L and $FEV_1/FVC < 0.75$), composite classification systems such as the ASA physical status and the Shapiro score were better predictors than pulmonary risk factors (e.g., smoking history, FEV_1, or FEV_1/FVC).[50] The same study also identified nonpulmonary factors such as anesthesia duration, emergency surgery, abdominal incision, and general anesthesia as single risk factors associated with postoperative pulmonary complications.[50] Similarly, other studies have found no value to preoperative spirometry in predicting postoperative complications after elective abdominal surgery[91,92] or cardiac surgery.[41] Again, more important predictive variables included abnormal findings on lung examination or chest radiograph, cardiac morbidity (as evaluated by the Goldman cardiac risk index), and overall comorbidity (as evaluated by the Charlson comorbidity index).[91] In one prospective evaluation of patients undergoing coronary artery bypass graft surgery, pulmonary diagnosis, spirometry measurements, and blood gas determinations did not predict postoperative respiratory outcome,[41] whereas reduced left ventricular ejection fraction and the presence of a preexisting comorbid condition (e.g., congestive heart failure, angina, active smoking, diabetes) did.[41]

In summary, pulmonary function studies need not be performed routinely before nonresectional surgery because they are unlikely to alter the decision as to whether to proceed with the planned procedure or to affect postoperative care. The clinical decisions should still be based on a careful clinical assessment including physical examination, review of the chest radiograph, and assessment of comorbid conditions. As discussed earlier, composite scores such as the ASA score,[29,50,95,97] Shapiro score,[50] and Charlson's index[91] are more important predictors than spirometric variables. Particular attention should be paid to evaluating cardiac morbidity, because cardiac risk factors relate closely to postoperative pulmonary complications.[41,51,91,100] Spirometry measurements may be reserved to assist in decision making in case of upper abdominal surgery, particularly where a full clinical evaluation is incomplete (i.e., impaired functional ability due to lower extremity disability or uncertainty about physical or radiographic findings).[104]

RESECTIONAL SURGERY
Resectional surgery poses a greater risk for postoperative complications because thoracotomy impairs lung function more than other procedures (see Fig. 47-1) and because lung function is expected to be lost after resection. The American

College of Physicians recommendations for lung resection surgery candidates suggest performing (in sequence) spirometry and arterial blood gas determinations, split lung function studies, and exercise testing.[102]

CONVENTIONAL TESTS OF LUNG FUNCTION

Maximum Voluntary Ventilation (MVV)

The MVV represents the maximal volume of repetitively inhaled and then exhaled air over a period of 12 to 15 s, with the result expressed in liters per minute. Alternatively, the MVV can be estimated by multiplying FEV_1 times 35. Early reports have studied low MVV in combination with other parameters (i.e., FVC or RV/TLC) as a predictor of poor outcome (either mortality or postoperative complications).[105,106] In a more recent study that used a combination of pulmonary artery pressure and perfusion scan–predicted FEV_1 as a standard for determining resectability, an MVV of less than 50 percent was found in 5 of 6 patients deemed nonresectable but in only 2 of 23 patients deemed resectable.[107]

1-Second Forced Expiratory Volume

The FEV_1 is a commonly used criterion for operability. Overall, multiple studies have assessed the value of measuring FEV_1 in determining resectability. Preoperative values below 2 L typically have been associated with an increased risk,[108–110] but the positive predictive value of a low FEV_1 is poor. For instance, in one study, a preoperative FEV_1 less than 1 L was not found to predict postoperative complications.[111] In attempting to identify a specific threshold value above which the surgical risk of complications or death is low, an FEV_1 > 2 L for a male adult (or >60 percent of predicted) is proposed for lobectomy[110] and >80 percent for pneumonectomy.

Predicted postoperative FEV_1 appears to be a better predictor of postoperative complications.[111–113] Because hypercapnia has been described in COPD patients whose FEV_1 was under 800 mL,[114] Olsen and associates[107] and Kristerssen and colleagues[115] proposed a predicted postpneumonectomy FEV_1 <800 mL as precluding surgery. This arbitrary estimate appears to have been based on personal experience[116] and may be too conservative in older patients and women, whose smaller size dictates that an FEV_1 of 800 mL is a larger percentage of predicted.[110] To account for these gender and age effects on the threshold value for FEV_1, a predicted postoperative threshold value of FEV_1 that is 35 to 40 percent of predicted has been proposed and found to be a better criterion than the absolute value of FEV_1.[112,116–118]

Forced Vital Capacity

Although an FVC below 1.7 to 2 L also has been proposed, there is no cutoff value for FVC. In one study, FVC was not a significant predictor of morbidity or mortality.[119]

Diffusion Capacity (DLCO)

The DLCO may provide a more accurate representation of the physiologic impairment in patients undergoing lung resection because it reflects the gas-exchange function of the lung. Advantages of measuring DLCO include detecting emphysema even when spirometric variables are normal[120] and representing the gas-exchange response under stress or exercise, like a formal exercise test.[110] Although not all studies have found the DLCO to be a useful discriminator of those at risk for postoperative complications,[118,121,122] several studies have identified the diffusion capacity as an important predictor of postoperative morbidity and mortality.[112,113,120] For instance, using a cutoff value of 60 percent of predicted, Ferguson and coworkers[120] observed positive and negative predictive values of the diffusion capacity for the development of pulmonary complications of 45 and 81 percent, respectively.[120] At the same cutoff level, the positive and negative predictive values for death were 25 and 95 percent, respectively.[120]

As with the FEV_1, the predicted postoperative diffusion capacity (DLCO-PPO) may be a more significant independent predictor of pulmonary complications, morbidity, and death after lung resection.[112,113,118,119] For instance, a DLCO-PPO <40 percent was associated with a mortality rate of 33 percent.[112] Similarly, the DLCO-PPO was found to be significantly lower in patients who subsequently developed complications.[112,118] The predicted postoperative DLCO and the predicted postoperative FEV_1 appear to be independent predictors of risk.[112,120] Although not confirmed in all series,[119] the product of predicted postoperative FEV_1% and predicted postoperative DLCO% (PPP) was found to be the best predictor of postoperative mortality in one report where a PPP of less than 1650 identified six of eight deaths.[113]

Arterial Blood Gases

An elevated preoperative Pa_{CO_2} (i.e., >45 mmHg) is often considered a predictor of pulmonary complications.[101] For instance, in one series, two of four patients with preoperative hypercapnia required prolonged postoperative mechanical ventilation.[123] On the other hand, Morice and associates[124] have observed that high-risk patients with maximal oxygen consumption values greater than 15 mL/kg per minute tolerated resectional surgery despite preoperative hypercapnia. Also, in one prospective analysis, hypercapnia was not found to predict postoperative complications.[111] Therefore, hypercapnia itself does not pose an absolute contraindication to resection.

SPLIT LUNG FUNCTION STUDIES

Split lung function studies allow estimation of postoperative lung function based on preoperative measurements. These determinations have been applied to a variety of lung function measurements such as FEV_1,[111–113] FVC,[112,125] TLC,[112] MVV,[125] diffusion capacity,[112,113,119] and even oxygen consumption on exercise testing.[126] Available split lung function studies are considered below.

Split Spirometry

This technique requires intubation with a double-lumen endotracheal tube, with each lumen connected to a separate spirometer delivering 100% oxygen. In this way, independent lung ventilation (by measurement of individual minute ventilation or VC) and perfusion (by measurement of individual slope of oxygen uptake) can be assessed. Using this method, the correlation between actual postpneumonectomy and predicted VC has been found to be high ($r = 0.86$).[125,127] Although the technique of split spirometry is rarely used now, it did allow the validation of noninvasive radionuclide studies that are currently used in evaluating high-risk lung resection candidates.[128]

Lateral Position Test

This test measures the increase in the FRC during tidal breathing between supine and each lateral decubitus position. The increase is due to expansion of the uppermost lung, and the combined increase (the sum of each individual change in FRC) is proportional to total lung function. The individual contribution of each lung can then be expressed in relative terms as the ratio of each individual FRC change to the sum of the FRC changes. Although less invasive than split spirometry, the test may not be well tolerated in patients with COPD in need of study and is associated with significant variability in the same patient.[129] Thus the lateral position test is rarely used.

Pulmonary Artery Occlusion

Occlusion of the pulmonary artery on the side to be resected can be induced by inflating a balloon catheter and allows an assessment of pulmonary artery pressure proximal to the occlusion as well as the resulting systemic arterial oxygenation. The development of significant pulmonary hypertension or hypoxemia, either at rest or with exercise, has been considered a contraindication to surgery. Formal evaluation of this technique was performed by Uggla[130] and by Olsen and colleagues,[107] who identified threshold values during exercise of 35 mmHg for mean pulmonary pressure and 45 mmHg for systemic oxygenation. Values below these thresholds were felt to be associated with prohibitive surgical risk. The lack of consensus in the medical literature as to the usefulness of pulmonary artery catheter measurements for this specific purpose and its invasive nature has prevented widespread acceptance of this test in clinical practice.

Calculated Postoperative FEV$_1$

A simple assessment of residual lung function can be obtained by assuming that all 19 pulmonary segments contribute equally to lung function. With this assumption, the predicted postoperative lung function (FEV$_1$ or FVC) would be equal to preoperative lung function times $(1 - S/19)$, where S is the number of segments expected to be removed at surgery.[131] Regression equations indicate a good correlation between predicted and actual postoperative values of FVC and FEV$_1$.[132] However, there is an overall tendency of predicted postoperative FEV$_1$ to underestimate actual values (by 265 mL in lobectomies and by 475 mL in pneumonectomies).[132] A more elaborate prediction equation assumes the presence of 42 subsegments and factors in an estimation of subsegments occluded by tumor.[133] As with the other estimate, a good correlation between expected and predicted postoperative values was observed, but this method also underestimated the correct postoperative values by 286 mL.

Radionuclide Studies

Estimates of the individual contribution of each lung to total function can be obtained by radionuclide studies. Both ventilation[115,134] and perfusion[135] lung scanning methods have been found to achieve good correlation between predicted and actual postoperative values for FVC or FEV$_1$. As with the calculated method, these predicted values also have been found to underestimate actual postoperative values, adding a margin of safety to the assessments.[135] This technique is now one of the most commonly used for determining expected postoperative lung function.

EXERCISE TESTING

The rationale for using these methods lies in the assumption that exercise testing better evaluates the physiologic status and reserve of the cardiopulmonary system than static measurements.[110] As will be reviewed, this assumption enjoys considerable, though not unanimous, support.[110]

Stair Climbing

Stair climbing is a simple preoperative test that may be of value in evaluating the lung resection candidate preoperatively. For example, Holden and coworkers[117] used 44 steps as a cutoff and observed positive and negative predictive values for 90-day postoperative mortality of 91 and 80 percent, respectively. Another retrospective review found that two of four patients unable to climb one flight of stairs without dyspnea died after lung resection.[136] In another retrospective study, postoperative intubation hours, hospital stay, and cardiopulmonary complications after lung resection were all greater in patients unable to climb 75 steps compared with those who could.[137]

Walk Distance

A similar and frequently used test is the 6- or 12-min walking distance. In the same study cited earlier by Holden and coworkers,[117] a cutoff 6-min walk distance of 1000 ft (305 m) had positive and negative predictive values for 90-day postoperative mortality of 85 and 100 percent, respectively. Similarly, in a study by Pierce and colleagues,[113] the 6-min walk distance was significantly lower in patients who subsequently developed respiratory failure. Alternatively, in another study, the 12-min walk distance tended to be lower in patients who subsequently had postoperative complications compared with those who did not, but the difference failed to achieve statistical significance (1018 versus 905 m; $p = .2$).[112] Therefore, further validation of this test is required before it can be endorsed as a predictive variable.

Cardiopulmonary Exercise Testing

A reduced oxygen uptake at maximal exercise (V$_{O_2}$ max) also has been identified as a risk factor for postoperative complications[112,117,118,121,122,124,126,138–145] (Table 47-4), although this risk may be conferred by general cardiopulmonary functional impairment. Specifically, a cardiopulmonary index (CPRI) derived from clinical cardiac and pulmonary parameters has been observed to be more sensitive and specific than oxygen uptake in predicting cardiopulmonary complications[143] (Table 47-5). The CPRI adopts a modification of the Goldman risk index[146] and appends a pulmonary risk index.[143] At a threshold score of 4 or greater, the positive and negative predictive values of the CPRI for cardiopulmonary complications were 79 and 86 percent, respectively.[143] Further, a multiple logistic regression model incorporating V$_{O_2}$ and CPRI indicated that V$_{O_2}$ was not a significant independent predictor and does not add to an assessment of risk based on clinical parameters.[143] Simple historic information based on age, smoking, dyspnea, and cancer status overlaps some characteristics of the CPRI and also was found to predict postoperative morbidity.[144] Overall, most recent studies evaluating the role of maximal oxygen uptake support its use in predicting postoperative mortality and morbidity (see Table 47-4) and justify its incorporation in a decision analysis for surgical risk. Nevertheless, marked variation among available studies

TABLE 47-4 Results from Exercise Studies in Predicting Postoperative Complications

Author	V_{O_2}[a]	Does V_{O_2} Below Threshold Predict?		Predictive Values for Complications		Predictive Values for Death	
		Complications	Death	PPV	NPV	PPV	NPV
Eugene[138]	1.0 L/mn	NA	Yes	NA	NA	75	100
Colman[139]	NA	No[b]	No[b]	NA	NA	NA	NA
Smith[121]	15 mL/kg/min	Yes	No	100	69	17	94
Bechard[140]	10 mL/kg/min	Yes	Yes	71	93	29	100
Miyoshi[141]	NA[c]	No	Yes	NA	NA	NA	NA
Markos[112]	15 mL/kg/min	No	No	38	70	6	96
Olsen[142]	9 mL/kg/min[d]	No	Yes[f]	NA	NA	63	94
Holden[117]	10 mL/kg/min	Yes	Yes	100	63	50	100
Morice[124]	15 mL/kg/min	NA	NA	NA	75	NA	NA
Nakagawa[122]	401 mL/min/m²[c]	Yes	Yes	67	75	27	100
Epstein[143]	500 mL/min/m²	Yes	NA	64	77	NA	NA
Dales[144]	1.25 L	Yes	NA	50	81	NA	NA
Walsh[145]	15 mL/kg/min	No	No	60	60	20	100
Bolliger[118]	60%	Yes	Yes	89	89	50	100
Bolliger[126]	10 mL/kg/min[e]	Yes	Yes	100	86	100	100

[a] At maximal exercise unless otherwise specified.
[b] Includes surgical complications.
[c] At arterial lactate level of 20 mg/dL.
[d] Calculated V_{O_2} at 40 W.
[e] Expected postoperative value.
[f] Includes ventilatory support for more than 30 days from preoperative intubation.
NOTE: NA, not available from data provided.
SOURCE: Adapted from Stoller JK, Holden DH, Matthay MA: Preoperative evaluation, in Bone RC (ed): *Pulmonary and Critical Care Medicine*. Chicago, Mosby–Year Book, 1993; Used by permission.

exists regarding patient selection, definitions of complications (as with possible inclusion of nonpulmonary or surgical complications), or threshold values of V_{O_2} (e.g. <10 to >15 mL/kg/min). Also, most studies lack proof that a maximal V_{O_2} value was actually reached. Attempts to circumvent this difficulty have included measurements of V_{O_2} at a specific effort (i.e., 40 W)[142] or standardized by interpolation to a specific lactate level (typically around 20 mg/dL).[122,141] More recently, Bolliger and associates[118] have suggested that values for V_{O_2} expressed as a percentage of expected predicted values have greater sensitivity than absolute values. It is noteworthy that refinements in surgical technique, such as less invasive approaches (e.g., video-assisted thoracoscopy) and limited resections, may allow these threshold values to be lowered further.[118]

Oxygen Delivery

Oxygen delivery measurements during exercise also have, been used to predict postresectional morbidity and mortality. The oxygen delivery at 40 W of exercise was found to be significantly lower in patients who experienced complications of surgery (i.e., death or prolonged intubation) compared with those who did not.[142] Similarly, Nakagawa and colleagues[122] found that a threshold oxygen delivery of 500 mL/m² per minute during exercise (standardized at a body lactate level of 20 mg/dL) was 100 percent sensitive and specific in predicting mortality. These authors further incorporated this parameter in an algorithm for surgical resectability.[147]

Pulmonary Vascular Resistance

This technique consists of measurements of pulmonary vascular resistance (PVR) during treadmill exercise using a flow-directed catheter. It assumes that the loss of pulmonary vas-

cular compliance with lung resection is a greater determinant of postoperative complications than the loss of diffusion surface. At a threshold value for PVR with exercise of 190 dyn/s/cm^{-5}, Fee and associates[148] found positive and negative predictive values for death after lung resection of 42 and 100 percent, respectively. Of interest, all five patients who died in this study had PVR values above the threshold, but only one would have been expected based on conventional preoperative spirometry and blood-gas criteria.[148] Alternatively, Olsen and associates[142] found no evidence that pulmonary vascular pressures or resistance with exercise predicts intolerance to lung resection.

CONCLUSIONS REGARDING PREDICTING CANDIDACY FOR LUNG RESECTION SURGERY

Overall, available studies support several conclusions regarding the risk of pulmonary complications after lung resection. First, it appears that low preoperative values are not as helpful as estimates of postoperative values.[111,119,126] Also, values expressed as a percentage of predicted have been more helpful than values using absolute thresholds.[118,142] Finally, three parameters emerge as significant high-risk indicators, including low estimated postoperative FEV$_1$,[111] low estimated postoperative DLCO,[119] and low oxygen uptake at peak exercise.[143] An algorithm incorporating preoperative and postoperative (determined by quantitative perfusion scans) FEV$_1$% and DLCO% with exercise oxygen uptake is proposed (Fig. 47-2).

Summary

Pulmonary complications after surgery occur commonly, especially after upper abdominal surgery and thoracic proce-

TABLE 47-5 Cardiopulmonary Risk Index (CPRI) in Pulmonary Resection

Cardiac Risk Index		Pulmonary Risk Index	
Variable	Points	Variable	Points
1. Congestive heart failure (S_3, jugular venous distention, LVEF ≤40%)[a]	11	1. Obesity (body mass index ≥ 27 kg/m²)	1
2. Myocardial infarction during previous 6 months	10	2. Cigarette smoking within 8 weeks of surgery	1
3. Greater than 5 PVCs/min (noted at anytime preoperatively)	7	3. Productive cough within 5 days of surgery	1
4. Rhythm other than NSR or PACs (on preoperative ECG)	7	4. Diffuse wheezing or rhonchi noted within 5 days of surgery	1
5. Age > 70 years	5	5. $FEV_1/FVC < 70\%$	1
6. Important valvular aortic stenosis[a]	3	6. $Pa_{CO_2} > 45$ mmHg	1
7. Poor general medical condition[a]	3		

Cardiac risk index points = 3–47[b]
CRI score: 1 (0–5 points), 2 (6–12 points),
  3 (12–25 points), 4 (> 25 points)

Cardiac risk index score (CRI) = 1–4	Pulmonary risk index score (PRI) = 0–6

Cardiopulmonary risk index score (CPRI) = CRI + PRI = 1–10

[a] As defined by Goldman et al.[146]
[b] CRI points start at 3 because 3 points are assigned for the thoracic procedure.
NOTE: S_3, third heart sound; LVEF, left ventricular ejection fraction; PVC, premature ventricular contractions; NSR, normal sinus rhythm; PAC, premature atrial contractions.
SOURCE: Adapted from Epstein et al.,[143] with permission.

dures. Extremity surgery is also associated with an increased risk of postoperative deep venous thrombosis and its attendant risk of pulmonary embolism. Beneficial steps in lessening the risk of postoperative complications are summarized in Table 47-6. Preoperative interventions that may lessen the rate of postoperative pulmonary complications include treatment of airflow obstruction (with smoking cessation, bronchodilators, steroids, and possibly antibiotics), deep venous thrombosis prophylaxis in selected patients, and instructions on the use of incentive spirometry. Intraoperative factors to lessen the risk of pulmonary complications include laparoscopic surgery where possible, particularly for cholecystectomy, shorter surgical procedures if attainable, and possibly epidural or local anesthesia. Beneficial postoperative steps include the conscientious use of incentive spirometry, initiation or continuation of deep venous thrombosis prophylaxis for up to 4 to 6 weeks in selected patients, and possibly epidural analgesia, particularly in high-risk pa-

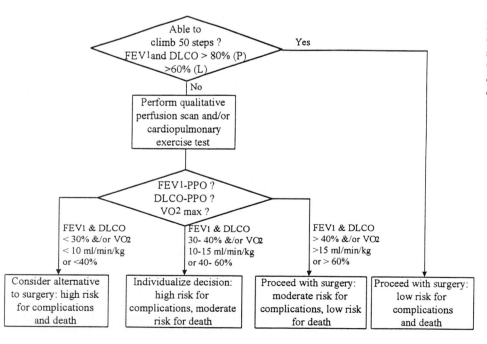

FIGURE 47-2 Algorithm for the preoperative evaluation of the lung resection candidates. P, pneumonectomy; L, lobectomy; V_{O_2}, oxygen consumption; PPO, predicted postoperative.

TABLE 47-6 Beneficial Steps in Lessening the Pulmonary Risks of Surgery

Preoperative
  Smoking cessation for at least 2 months preoperatively if possible
  Treatment of airflow obstruction: bronchodilators, steroids, antibiotics
  Deep venous thrombosis prophylaxis in selected patients
  Instruction on the use of incentive devices
Intraoperative
  Laparoscopic procedure (particularly cholecystectomy)
  Shorter surgical procedure
  Epidural or local anesthesia (to reduce the thrombosis risk or bronchospasm)
Postoperative
  Deep venous thrombosis prophylaxis (for up to 6 weeks in selected patients)
  Incentive spirometry
  Epidural analgesia (particularly for high-risk surgery)

tients. The preoperative evaluation of the surgical candidate must include a careful general clinical assessment including ASA class and particularly cardiac morbidity that contributes significantly to postoperative pulmonary complications for both resectional and nonresectional surgery. Pulmonary function studies are not indicated routinely in the preoperative evaluation, except for lung resectional surgery. In resectional surgery, the FEV_1, DLCO, oxygen consumption at maximal exercise, and their corresponding predicted postoperative values appear to be significant indicators of postoperative pulmonary complications.

References

1. Sykes LA, Bowe EA: Cardiorespiratory effects of anesthesia. *Clin Chest Med* 14:211–226, 1993.
2. Brismar B, Hedenstierna G, Lundquist H, et al: Pulmonary densities during anesthesia with muscular relaxation: A proposal of atelectasis. *Anesthesiology* 62:422–428, 1985.
3. Wiener-Kronish JP, Matthay MA: Preoperative evaluation, in Murray JF, Nadel JA (eds): *Textbook of Respiratory Medicine.* Philadelphia, WB Saunders, Co. 1988; pp 683–698.
4. Hedenstierna G, Strandberg A, Brismar B, et al: Functional residual capacity, thoracoabdominal dimensions, and central blood volume during general anesthesia with muscle paralysis and mechanical ventilation. *Anesthesiology* 62:247–254, 1985.
5. Krayer S, Rehder K, Vetterman J, et al: Position and motion of the human diaphragm during anesthesia-paralysis. *Anesthesiology* 56:298–303, 1982.
6. Rubin BK, Finegan B, Ramirez O, King M: General anesthesia does not alter the viscoelastic or transport properties of human respiratory mucus. *Chest* 98:101–104, 1990.
7. Pizov R, Takahashi M, Hirshman CA, Croxton T: Halothane inhibition of ion transport of the tracheal epithelium: A possible mechanism for anesthetic-induced impairment of mucociliary clearance. *Anesthesiology* 76:985–989, 1992.
8. Allen SM, Hunt B, Green M: Fall in vital capacity with posture. *Br J Dis Chest* 79:267–271, 1985.
9. Ali J, Weisel RD, Layug AB, et al: Consequences of postoperative alterations in respiratory mechanics. *Am J Surg* 128:376–382, 1974.
10. Meyers JR, Lombeck L, O'Kane H, et al: Changes in functional residual capacity of the lung after operation. *Arch Surg* 110:576–583, 1975.
11. Hansen G, Drablos PA, Steinert R: Pulmonary complications, ventilation, and blood gases after upper abdominal surgery. *Acta Anaesthesiol Scand* 21:211–215, 1977.
12. Dohi S, Gold MI: Comparison of two methods of postoperative care. *Chest* 73:592–595, 1978.
13. Dureuil B, Cantineau JP, Desmonts JM: Effects of upper or lower abdominal surgery on diaphragmatic function. *Br J Anaesth* 59:1230–1235, 1987.
14. Schauer PR, Luna J, Ghiattas AA, et al: Pulmonary function after laparoscopic cholecystectomy. *Surgery* 114:389–399, 1993.
15. van Belle AF, Wesseling GJ, Penn OC, Wouters EF: Postoperative pulmonary function abnormalities after coronary artery bypass surgery. *Respir Med* 86:195–199, 1992.
16. Braun SR, Birnbaum ML, Chopra PS: Pre- and postoperative pulmonary function abnormalities in coronary artery revascularization surgery. *Chest* 73:316–320, 1978.
17. Taggart DP, El-Fiky M, Carter R, et al: Respiratory dysfunction after uncomplicated cardiopulmonary bypass. *Ann Thorac Surg* 56:1123–1128, 1993.
18. Wahl GW, Swinburne AJ, Fedullo AJ, et al: Effect of age and preoperative airway obstruction on lung function after coronary artery bypass grafting. *Ann Thorac Surg* 56:104–107, 1993.
19. Gracey DR, Divertie MB, Didier EP: Preoperative pulmonary preparation of patients with chronic obstructive pulmonary disease: A prospective study. *Chest* 76:123–129, 1979.
20. Svensson LG, Hess KR, Coselli JS, et al: A prospective study of respiratory failure after high-risk surgery on the thoracoabdominal aorta. *J Vasc Surg* 14:271–282, 1991.
21. Cain HD, Stevens DM, Adaniya R: Preoperative pulmonary function and complications after cardiovascular surgery. *Chest* 76:130–135, 1979.
22. Tarhan S, Moffitt EA, Sessler AD, et al: Risk of anesthesia and surgery in patients with chronic bronchitis and chronic obstructive pulmonary disease. *Surgery* 74:720–726, 1973.
23. Stein M, Cassara EL: Preoperative pulmonary and evaluation for surgery patients. *JAMA* 211:787–780, 1970.
24. Stoller JK, Gerbarg ZB, Feinstein AR: Corticosteroids in stable chronic obstructive pulmonary disease: Reappraisal of efficacy. *J Gen Intern Med* 2:29–35, 1987.
25. Pien LC, Grammer LC, Patterson R: Minimal complications in a surgical population with severe asthma receiving prophylactic corticosteroids. *J Allergy Clin Immunol* 82:696–700, 1988.
26. Makela JT, Kiviniemi H, Juvinen T, Laitinen S: Factors influencing wound dehiscence after midline laparotomy. *Am J Surg* 170:387–390, 1995.
27. Dunlap NE, Fulmer JD: Corticosteroid therapy in asthma. *Clin Chest Med* 5:669–683, 1984.
28. Coffin LH, Shinozaki T, DeMeules JE, et al: Ineffectiveness of methylprednisolone in the treatment of pulmonary dysfunction after cardiopulmonary bypass. *Am J Surg* 130:555–550, 1975.
29. Kroenke K, Lawrence VA, Theroux JF, et al: Postoperative complications after thoracic and major abdominal surgery in patients with and without obstructive lung disease. *Chest* 104:1445–1451, 1993.
30. Dilworth JP, Warley AR, Dawe C, White RJ: The effect of nebulized salbutamol therapy on the incidence of postoperative chest infection in high risk patients. *Respir Med* 88:665–668, 1994.
31. Kumeta Y, Hattori A, Mimura M, et al: A survey of perioperative bronchospasm in 105 patients with reactive airway disease. *Masui* 44:396–401, 1995.
32. Chodosh S: Treatment of acute exacerbations of chronic bronchitis: State of the art. *Am J Med* 91(suppl 6A):87S–92S, 1991.
33. Murphy TF, Sethi S: Bacterial infection in chronic obstructive pulmonary disease. *Am Rev Respir Dis* 146:1067–1083, 1992.
34. Anthonisen NR, Manfreda J, Warren CPW, et al: Antibiotic therapy in exacerbations of chronic obstructive pulmonary disease. *Ann Intern Med* 106:196–204, 1987.

35. Fletcher C, Peto R: The natural history of chronic airflow limitation. *Br Med J* 1:1645–1648, 1977.

36. Camilli AE, Burrows B, Knudson RJ, Lebowitz MD: Longitudinal changes in forced expiratory volume in one second in adults: Effects of smoking and smoking cessation. *Am Rev Respir Dis* 135:794–799, 1987.

37. Buist AS, Nagy JM, Sexton GJ: The effect of smoking cessation on pulmonary function: A 30-month follow-up of two smoking cessation clinics. *Am Rev Respir Dis* 120:953–957, 1979.

38. Chalon J, Tayyab MA, Ramanathan S: Cytology of respiratory epithelium as a predictor of respiratory complications after operation. *Chest* 67:32–35, 1975.

39. Wightman JAK: A prospective study of the incidence of postoperative pulmonary complications. *Br J Surg* 55:85–91, 1968.

40. Latimer RG, Dickman M, Day WC, et al: Ventilatory patterns and pulmonary complications after upper abdominal surgery determined by preoperative and postoperative computerized spirometry and blood gas analysis. *Am J Surg* 122:622–632, 1971.

41. Spivack SD, Shinozaki T, Albertini JJ, Deane R: Preoperative prediction of postoperative respiratory outcome: Coronary artery bypass grafting. *Chest* 109:1222–1230, 1996.

42. Warner MA, Offord KP, Warner ME, et al: Role of preoperative cessation of smoking and other factors in postoperative pulmonary complications: A blinded prospective study of coronary artery bypass. *Mayo Clin Proc* 64:609–616, 1989.

43. Chodoff P, Margand PM, Knowles CL: Short term abstinence from smoking: Its place in preoperative preparation. *Crit Care Med* 3:131–133, 1975.

44. Buist AS, Sexton GJ, Nagy JM, Ross BB: The effect of smoking cessation and modification of lung function. *Am Rev Respir Dis* 114:115–122, 1976.

45. Clagett GP, Anderson FA, Heit J, et al: Prevention of venous thromboembolism. *Chest* 108(suppl 4):312S–334S, 1995.

46. Salzman EW, Hirsh J: Prevention of venous thromboembolism, in Colman RW, Hirsh J, Marder VJ, et al (eds): *Hemostasis and Thrombosis: Basic Principles and Clinical Practice,* 3d ed. Philadelphia, Lippincott, 1994; p 1332.

47. Cook DJ, Guyatt GH, Laupacis A, et al: Clinical recommendations using levels of evidence for antithrombotic agents. *Chest* 108(suppl 4):227S–230S, 1995.

48. Wille-Jørgensen P, Christensen SW, Bjerg-Nielsen A, et al: Prevention of thromboembolism following elective hip surgery: The value of regional anesthesia and graded compression stockings. *Clin Orthop* 247:163–167, 1989.

49. Sorenson RM, Pace NL: Anesthetic techniques during surgical repair of femoral neck fractures. *Anesthesiology* 77:1085–1104, 1992.

50. Wong DH, Weber EC, Schell MJ, et al: Factors associated with postoperative pulmonary complications in patients with severe chronic obstructive pulmonary disease. *Anesth Analg* 80:276–284, 1995.

51. Kroenke K, Lawrence VA, Theroux JF, Tuley MR: Operative risk in patients with severe obstructive pulmonary disease. *Arch Intern Med* 152:967–971, 1992.

52. Garibaldi RA, Britt MR, Coleman ML, et al: Risk factors for postoperative pneumonia. *Am J Med* 70:677–680, 1981.

53. Frazee RC, Roberts JW, Okeson GC, et al: Open versus laparoscopic cholecystectomy: A comparison of postoperative pulmonary function. *Ann Surg* 213:651–654, 1991.

54. Putensen-Himmer G, Putensen C, Lammer H, et al: Comparison of postoperative respiratory function after laparoscopy or open laparotomy for cholecystectomy. *Anesthesiology* 77:675–680, 1992.

55. Majeed AW, Troy G, Nicholl JP, et al: Randomised, prospective, single-blind comparison of laparoscopic versus small-incision cholecystectomy. *Lancet* 347:989–994, 1996.

56. Lawrence K, McWhinnie D, Goodwin A, et al: Randomised

57. Lejus C, Delile L, Plattner V, et al: Randomized, single-blinded trial of laparoscopic versus open appendectomy in children: Effects on postoperative analgesia. *Anesthesiology* 84:801–806, 1996.

58. McDougall E, Clayman RV, Elashry OM: Laparoscopic radical nephrectomy for renal tumor: The Washington University experience. *J Urol* 155:1180–1185, 1996.

59. Krasna MJ, Deshmukh S, McLaughlin JS: Complications of thoracoscopy. *Ann Thorac Surg* 61:1066–1069, 1996.

60. Ferson PF, Landreneau RJ, Dowling RD, et al: Comparison of open versus thoracoscopic lung biopsy for diffuse infiltrative pulmonary disease. *J Thorac Cardiovasc Surg* 106:194–199, 1993.

61. Miller JI Jr: Limited resection of bronchogenic carcinoma in the patients with impaired pulmonary function. *Ann Thorac Surg* 56:769–771, 1993.

62. Robertson GS, Lloyd DM, Wicks AC, Veitch PS: No obvious advantages for thoracoscopic two-stage oesophagectomy. *Br J Surg* 83:675–678, 1996.

63. Celli BR, Rodriguez KS, Snider GL: A controlled trial of intermittent positive pressure breathing, incentive spirometry, and deep breathing exercises in preventing pulmonary complications after abdominal surgery. *Ann Rev Respir Dis* 130:12–15, 1984.

64. Stiller KR, Munday RM: Chest physiotherapy for the surgical patient. *Br J Surg* 79:745–749, 1992.

65. Thomas JA, McIntosh JM: Are incentive spirometry, intermittent positive pressure breathing, and deep breathing exercises effective in the prevention of postoperative pulmonary complications after upper abdominal surgery? A systematic overview and meta-analysis. *Phys Ther* 74:3–16, 1994.

66. Hall JC, Tarala RA, Tapper J, Hall JL: Prevention of respiratory complications after abdominal surgery: A randomized clinical trial. *Br Med J* 312:148–153, 1996.

67. Stiller K, Montarello J, Wallace M, et al: Efficacy of breathing and coughing exercises in the prevention of pulmonary complications after coronary artery surgery. *Chest* 105:741–747, 1994.

68. Ali J, Serrette C, Wood LDH, et al: Effect of postoperative intermittent positive pressure breathing on lung function. *Chest* 85:192–196, 1984.

69. Gale GD, Sanders DE: Incentive spirometry: Its value after cardiac surgery. *Can Anaesth Soc J* 27:475–480, 1980.

70. Lindner KH, Lotz P, Ahnefeld FW: Continuous positive airway pressure effect on functional residual capacity, vital capacity and its subdivisions. *Chest* 92:66–70, 1987.

71. Heitz M, Holzach P, Dittmann M: Comparison of the effect of continuous positive airway pressure and blowing bottles on functional residual capacity after abdominal surgery. *Respiration* 48:277–284, 1985.

72. Stock MC, Downs JB, Gauer PK, et al: Prevention of postoperative pulmonary complications with CPAP, incentive spirometry, and conservative therapy. *Chest* 87:151–157, 1985.

73. Jousela I, Rasanen J, Verkkala K, et al: Continuous positive airway pressure by mask in patients after coronary surgery. *Acta Anaesthesiol Scand* 38:311–316, 1994.

74. Pinilla JC, Oleniuk FH, Tan L, et al: Use of nasal continuous positive airway pressure mask in the treatment of postoperative atelectasis in aortocoronary bypass surgery. *Crit Care Med* 18:836–840, 1990.

75. Carlsson C, Sonden B, Thylen U: Can postoperative continuous positive airway pressure (CPAP) prevent pulmonary complications after abdominal surgery? *Intensive Care Med* 7:225–229, 1981.

76. Ricksten SE, Bengtsson A, Sodeberg C, et al: Effects of periodic positive airway pressure by mask on postoperative pulmonary function. *Chest* 89:774–781, 1986.

77. Ingerwersen UM, Larsen KR, Bertelsen MT, et al: Three different mask physiotherapy regimens for prevention of post-operative

pulmonary complications after heart and pulmonary surgery. *Intensive Care Med* 19:294–298, 1993.

78. Stoller JK: Respiratory effects of positive and expiratory pressure. *Respir Care* 36:454–463, 1988.

79. Simpson T, Wahl G, DeTraglia M, et al: The effects of epidural versus parenteral opioid analgesia on postoperative pain and pulmonary function in adults who have undergone thoracic and abdominal surgery: A critique of research. *Heart Lung* 21:125–140, 1992.

80. Jayr C, Thomas H, Rey A, et al: Postoperative pulmonary complications: Epidural analgesia using bupivacaine and opioids versus parenteral opioids. *Anesthesiology* 78:666–676, 1993.

81. Kilbride MJ, Senagore AJ, Mazier WP, et al: Epidural analgesia. *Surg Gynecol Obstet* 174:137–140, 1992.

82. Liu S, Carpenter RL, Neal JM: Epidural anesthesia and analgesia: Their role in postoperative outcome. *Anesthesiology* 82:1474–1506, 1995.

83. Catley DM, Thornton C, Jordan C, et al: Pronounced, episodic oxygen desaturation in the postoperative period: Its association with ventilatory pattern and analgesic regimen. *Anesthesiology* 63:20–28, 1985.

84. Bennett R, Batenhorst RL, Foster TS, et al: Postoperative pulmonary function with patient-controlled analgesia. *Anesth Analg* 61:171, 1982.

85. Welchew EA: On-demand analgesia: A double-blind comparison of on-demand intravenous fentanyl with regular intramuscular morphine. *Anaesthesia* 38:19–25, 1983.

86. Searle NR, Bergeron G, Perrault J, et al: Hydromorphone patient-controlled analgesia (PCA) after coronary artery bypass surgery. *Can J Anaesth* 41:198–205, 1994.

87. Slinger P, Shennib H, Wilson S: Postthoracotomy pulmonary function: A comparison of epidural versus intravenous meperidine infusions. *J Cardiothorac Vasc Anesth* 9:128–134, 1995.

88. Bergqvist D, Benoni G, Björgell O, et al: Low-molecular-weight heparin (enoxaparin) as prophylaxis against venous thromboembolism after total hip replacement. *N Engl J Med* 335:696–700, 1996.

89. Sarasin FP, Bounameaux H: Antithrombotic strategy after total hip replacement. *Arch Intern Med* 156:1661–1668, 1996.

90. Lawrence VA, Page CP, Harris GD: Preoperative spirometry before abdominal operations: A critical appraisal of its predictive value. *Arch Intern Med* 149:280–285, 1989.

91. Lawrence VA, Dhanda R, Hilsenbeck SG, Page CP: Risk of pulmonary complications after elective abdominal surgery. *Chest* 110:744–750, 1996.

92. Jayr C, Matthay MA, Goldstone J, et al: Preoperative and intraoperative factors associated with prolonged mechanical ventilation: A study in patients following major abdominal vascular surgery. *Chest* 103:1231–1236, 1993.

93. Stein M, Kotta GM, Simon M, et al: Pulmonary evaluation of surgical patients. *JAMA* 181:765–770, 1962.

94. Poe RH, Kelley MC, Dass T, et al: Can postoperative pulmonary complications after elective cholecystectomy be predicted? *Am J Med Sci* 295:29–34, 1988.

95. Hall JC, Tarala RA, Hall JL, et al: A multivariate analysis of the risk of pulmonary complications after laparotomy. *Chest* 99:923–927, 1991.

96. Pedersen T, Viby-Mogensen J, Ringsted C: Anesthetic practice and post-operative pulmonary complications. *Acta Anaesthesiol Scand* 36:812–818, 1992.

97. Calligaro KD, Azurin DJ, Dougherty MJ, et al: Pulmonary risk factors of elective abdominal aortic surgery. *J Vasc Surg* 18:914–921, 1993.

98. Kispert JF, Kazmers A, Roitman L: Preoperative spirometry predicts perioperative pulmonary complications after major vascular surgery. *Am Surg* 58:491–495, 1992.

99. Vodinh J, Bonnet F, Touboul C, et al: Risk factors of postoperative pulmonary complications after vascular surgery. *Surgery* 105:360–365, 1989.

100. Williams-Russo P, Charlson ME, MacKenzie R, et al: Predicting postoperative pulmonary complications: Is it a real problem? *Arch Intern Med* 152:1209–1213, 1992.

101. Zibrak JD, O'Donnell CR, Marton K: Indications for pulmonary functions testing. *Ann Intern Med* 112:763–771, 1990.

102. American College of Physicians: Position paper: Preoperative pulmonary function testing. *Ann Intern Med* 112:793–794, 1990.

103. Hnatiuk OW, Dillard TA, Torrington KG: Adherence to established guidelines for preoperative pulmonary function testing. *Chest* 107:1294–1297, 1995.

104. Macpherson DS: Pulmonary function tests before surgery. *Chest* 110:587–589, 1996.

105. Gaensler EA, Cugell DW, Lindgren I, et al: The role of pulmonary insufficiency in mortality and invalidism following surgery for pulmonary tuberculosis. *J Thorac Cardiovasc Surg* 29:163–187, 1955.

106. Mittman C: Assessment of operative risk in thoracic surgery. *Am Rev Respir Dis* 84:197–207, 1961.

107. Olsen GN, Block AJ, Swenson EW, et al: Pulmonary function evaluation of the lung resection candidate: A prospective study. *Am Rev Respir Dis* 111:379–387, 1975.

108. Boushy SF, Billig DM, North LB, Helgason AH: Clinical course related to preoperative and postoperative pulmonary function in patients with bronchogenic carcinoma. *Chest* 59:383–391, 1971.

109. Boysen PG, Block AJ, Moulder PV: Relationship between preoperative pulmonary function tests and complications after thoracotomy. *Surg Gynecol Obstetr* 152:813–815, 1981.

110. Marshall MC, Olsen GN: The physiologic evaluation of the lung resection candidate. *Clin Chest Med* 14:305–320, 1993.

111. Kearney, DJ, Lee TH, Reilly JJ, et al: Assessment of operative risk in patients undergoing lung resection: Importance of predicted pulmonary function. *Chest* 105:753–759, 1994.

112. Markos J, Mullan BP, Hillman DR, et al: Preoperative assessment as a predictor of mortality and morbidity after lung resection. *Am Rev Respir Dis* 139:902–910, 1989.

113. Pierce RJ, Copland JM, Sharpe K, Barter CE: Preoperative risk evaluation for lung cancer resection: Predicted postoperative product as a predictor of surgical mortality. *Am J Respir Crit Care Med* 150:947–955, 1994.

114. Segall JJ, Butterworth BA: Ventilatory capacity in chronic bronchitis in relation to carbon dioxide retention. *Scand J Respir Dis* 47:215–224, 1966.

115. Kristersson S, Lindell S, Sranberg L: Prediction of pulmonary function loss due to pneumonectomy using ^{133}Xe-radiospirometry. *Chest* 62:694–698, 1972.

116. Gass GD, Olsen GN: Preoperative pulmonary function testing to predict postoperative morbidity and mortality. *Chest* 89:127–135, 1986.

117. Holden DA, Rice TW, Stelmach K, Meeker DP: Exercise climbing, 6-min walk, and stair climb in the evaluation of patients at high risk for pulmonary resection. *Chest* 102:1774–1779, 1992.

118. Bolliger CT, Jordan P, Solèr M, et al: Exercise capacity as a predictor of postoperative complications in lung resection candidates. *Am J Respir Crit Care Med* 151:1472–1480, 1995.

119. Ferguson MK, Reeder LB, Mick R: Optimizing selection of patients for major lung resection. *J Thorac Cardiovasc Surg* 109:275–283, 1995.

120. Ferguson MK, Little L, Rizzo L, et al: Diffusion capacity predicts morbidity and mortality after pulmonary resection. *J Thorac Cardiovasc Surg* 96:894–900, 1988.

121. Smith TP, Kinasewitz GT, Tucker WY, et al: Exercise capacity as a predictor of post-thoracotomy morbidity. *Am Rev Respir Dis* 129:730–734, 1984.

122. Nakagawa K, Nakahara K, Miyoshi S, Kawashima Y: Oxygen

transport during incremental exercise load as a predictor of operative risk of lung cancer patients. *Chest* 101:1369–1375, 1992.

123. Milledge JS, Nunn JF: Criteria of fitness for anesthesia in patients with chronic obstructive lung disease. *Br Med J* 3:670–673, 1975.

124. Morice RC, Peters EJ, Ryan MB, et al: Exercise testing in the evaluation of patients at high risk for complications from lung resection. *Chest* 101:356–361, 1992.

125. Neuhaus H, Cherniack NS: A bronchospirometric method of estimating the effect of pneumonectomy on the maximum breathing capacity. *J Thorac Cardiovasc Surg* 55:144–148, 1968.

126. Bolliger CT, Wyser C, Roser H, et al: Lung scanning and exercise testing for the prediction of postoperative performance in lung resection candidates at increased risk for complications. *Chest* 108:341–348, 1995.

127. Snider GL, Shaw AR: A critical evaluation of bronchospirometric measurement in predictive loss of ventilatory function due to thoracic surgery. *J Lab Clin Med* 64:321–328, 1964.

128. Isawa T, Shiraishi K, Oka S: Postoperative effects on ventilation-perfusion relationships in operated lungs. *Am Rev Respir Dis* 96:411–419, 1967.

129. Jay SJ, Stonehill RB, Kiblani SO, et al: Variability of the lateral position test in normal subjects. *Am Rev Respir Dis* 121:165–167, 1980.

130. Uggla LG: Indications for and results of thoracic surgery with regard to respiratory and circulatory function tests. *Acta Chir Scand* 111:197–213, 1956.

131. Juhl B, Frost N: A comparison between measured and calculated changes in the lung function after operation for pulmonary cancer. *Acta Anaesthesiol Scand* 57(suppl):39–45, 1975.

132. Zeiher BG, Gross TJ, Kern JA, et al: Predicting postoperative pulmonary function in patients undergoing lung resection. *Chest* 108:68–72, 1995.

133. Nakahara K, Monden Y, Ohno K, et al: A method of predicting postoperative lung function and its relation to postoperative complications in patients with lung cancer. *Ann Thorac Surg* 39:260–265, 1985.

134. Ali MK, Mountain CF, Ewer MS, et al: Predicting loss of pulmonary function after pulmonary resection for bronchogenic carcinoma. *Chest* 77:337–342, 1980.

135. Olsen GN, Block AJ, Tobias JA: Prediction of postpneumonectomy pulmonary function using quantitative macroaggregate lung scanning. *Chest* 66:13–16, 1974.

136. Van Nostrand D, Kjelsberg MO, Mumphrey EW: Preresectional evaluation of risk from pneumonectomy. *Surg Gynecol Obstet* 127:306–312, 1968.

137. Olsen GN, Bolton JWR, Weiman DS, Hornung CA: Stair climbing as an exercise test to predict the postoperative complications of lung resection. *Chest* 99:587–590, 1991.

138. Eugene J, Brown SE, Light RW, et al: Maximum oxygen consumption: A physiologic guide to pulmonary resection. *Surg Forum* 33:260–262, 1982.

139. Colman NC, Schraufnagel DE, Rivington RN, Pardy RL: Exercise testing in evaluation of patients for lung resection. *Am Rev Respir Dis* 125:604–606, 1982.

140. Bechard D, Wetstein L: Assessment of exercise oxygen consumption as a preoperative criterion for lung resection. *Ann Thorac Surg* 44:344–349, 1987.

141. Miyoshi S, Nakahara K, Ohno K, et al: Exercise tolerance test in lung cancer patients: The relationship between exercise capacity and postthoracotomy hospital death. *Ann Thorac Surg* 44:487–490, 1987.

142. Olsen GN, Weiman DS, Bolton JWR, et al: Submaximal invasive exercise testing and quantitative lung scanning in the evaluation for tolerance of lung resection. *Chest* 95:267–273, 1989.

143. Epstein SK, Faling J, Daly BDT, Celli BR: Predicting complications after pulmonary resection: Preoperative exercise testing vs a multifactorial cardiopulmonary risk index. *Chest* 104:694–700, 1993.

144. Dales RE, Dionne G, Leech JA, et al: Preoperative prediction of pulmonary complications following thoracic surgery. *Chest* 104:155–159, 1993.

145. Walsh GL, Morice RC, Putnam JB, et al: Resection of lung cancer is justified in high-risk patients selected by exercise oxygen consumption. *Ann Thorac Surg* 58:704–711, 1994.

146. Goldman L, Caldera D, Nussbaum SR, et al: Multifactorial index of cardiac risk in noncardiac surgical procedures. *N Engl J Med* 297:845–850, 1977.

147. Nakahara K, Miyoshi S, Nakagawa K: A method for predicting postoperative lung function and its relation to postoperative complications in patients with lung cancer, 1992 update. *Ann Thorac Surg* 54:1016–1017, 1992.

148. Fee HJ, Holmes EC, Gewirtz HS, et al: Role of pulmonary resistance measurements in preoperative evaluation of candidates for lung resection. *J Thorac Cardiovasc Surg* 75:519–524, 1978.

Chapter 48

MANAGEMENT OF CYSTIC FIBROSIS

STANLEY B. FIEL

Cystic fibrosis (CF) is the most common inherited disease among Caucasians, with an incidence of approximately 1 in 2500 births.[1] The disease is seen much less frequently in blacks and Asians.[2] When the constellation of symptoms was first described in 1938, it presaged death at an early age—the average life expectancy was only 1 year.[3] In contrast, the advent of progressively more effective therapies and diagnostic methods over the past decades has increased the average life expectancy to roughly 30 years.[4] As a consequence of the survival of CF patients into adulthood, the optimization of disease management strategies has assumed considerably more importance in an attempt to preserve an acceptable level of social functioning and quality of life for the patient.

The primary causes of morbidity and mortality with CF are cardiorespiratory in nature, despite additional manifestations of the disease in other body systems, including the gastrointestinal tract.[1,5] The gastrointestinal complications of CF include several digestive abnormalities and nutritional deficiencies. In addition, there is an association between malnutrition and deteriorating lung function. Although the nutritional aspects of care are important, they are beyond the scope of this chapter. Maintenance of adequate pulmonary function determines the patient's prognosis, and precipitous deterioration of lung function is a harbinger of imminent death. Therefore, the discussion of therapeutics in this chapter will be confined to matters related to the respiratory system. A brief elaboration of the pathogenesis of CF is provided, followed by an outline of the current standards of treatment for maintenance of respiratory function and for acute exacerbations of disease. A section on the most recent therapeutic advances is provided, along with an examination of possible future trends in CF treatment.

Pathogenesis of Cystic Fibrosis

With the discovery of the particular genetic mutations underlying the symptoms of CF, research has at last provided a unified theory for the pathogenesis of the disease. Cystic fibrosis is an autosomal recessive disease. Heterozygous individuals are asymptomatic carriers; an individual must possess mutations on both alleles to express the basic physiologic defect leading to clinical symptoms. However, there are a multitude of different mutations within the gene itself that can cause CF.[5-7]

The primary defect in CF lies in the gene coding for the cystic fibrosis transmembrane (conductance) regulator (*CFTR*), a protein that acts as a transmembrane chloride channel in epithelial cells of lung, pancreas, liver, and sweat glands. This apical chloride conductance channel is sensitive to cyclic adenosine monophosphate (cAMP) and mediates the balance between secretion of chloride ions and absorption

of sodium ions, secondarily affecting water transport as well. Thus the abnormal functioning of the gene product CFTR directly affects the composition and viscosity of pulmonary secretions. Viscid, tenacious pulmonary secretions are the basis for the most serious of the clinical problems observed in CF; various methods for controlling these secretions form the core of standard CF therapy at the present time.[5-8]

The pulmonary expression of CF begins with secretion of mucus that is more viscous than normal as a result of the defect in chloride transport in pulmonary epithelium. Such thickened secretions, which can be seen quite soon after birth of an affected infant, are more difficult to expel from the lungs. Impairment of mucociliary clearance also may occur in CF patients. The end result is inspissated mucus in the airways, leading to airways obstruction and initiating a pathologic cascade of secondary events that further compromises respiratory function (Fig. 48–1).

Accumulation of thick, mucopurulent secretions in the airways provides a favorable environment for colonization by opportunistic pathogens.[9] Evidence of such colonization is present even in the neonate and becomes more extensive with increasing age.[7,10,11] The variety of organisms present varies as the infant matures, reflecting both environmental exposure and the overgrowth of increasingly more drug-resistant organisms as the individual undergoes successive courses of pharmacotherapy. Initially, *Hemophilus influenzae* and *Staphylococcus aureus* predominate; later, more virulent species such as *Pseudomonas aeruginosa, Xanthomonas maltophilia,* and *Burkholderia cepacia* become established. Other pathogens also may be present: *Klebsiella, Escherichia coli, Proteus, Enterobacter, Citrobacter, Candida, Aspergillus,* and nontuberculous mycobacteria such as *Mycobacterium avium-intracellulare.*[1,9-14]

In response to bacterial, fungal, and/or viral invasion, neutrophils are recruited into the lungs. The resulting cellular attack leads to release of inflammatory mediators and accumulation of cellular debris secondary to lysis of neutrophils and bacteria. The presence of large fragments of deoxyribonucleic acid (DNA) from the nuclei of lysed cells drastically increases the viscosity of pulmonary secretions. Chronic inflammation can cause permanent destruction or loss of elasticity of lung tissue—partly as a result of the action of neutrophil-derived enzymes such as elastase—reducing ventilatory efficiency. A vicious cycle is engendered by repeated cycles of infection and inflammation. Over time, the capacity of lung tissue to recover is decreased, and the damage becomes irreversible. Hypoxemia, increased vascular resistance, and pulmonary hypertension ensue, culminating in cor pulmonale, respiratory failure, and death.

Therapy of Cystic Fibrosis: Overview

Treatment strategies exist to target virtually every aspect of the pathophysiologic cascade of events in CF (Table 48–1). However, therapy for CF can be inconvenient and time-consuming for the patient; care must be taken to avoid drastically compromising the patient's level of psychosocial functioning insofar as the extent of disease permits.[7] The complex treatment regimens required are best managed by a multidisciplinary CF treatment facility that utilizes the services of pulmonary specialists, nurses, respiratory therapists, nutri-

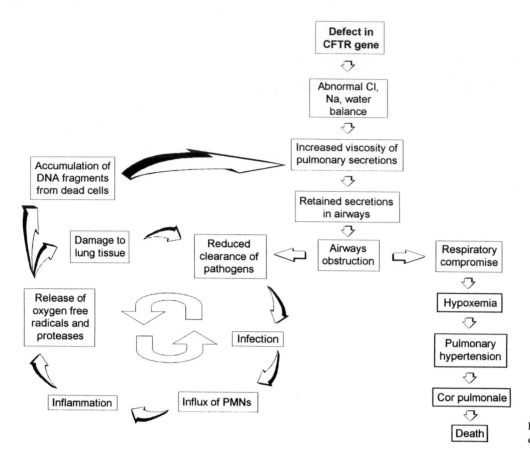

FIGURE 48-1 Pathogenesis of cystic fibrosis.

tional consultants, and social workers to continuously evaluate the patient's condition and adjust therapy accordingly.[7,10] The team approach also can provide valuable support for the patient and the caregiver as the disease progresses.

The primary aim of CF therapy is to facilitate the clearance of secretions from the tracheobronchial tree. Secondary objectives include reducing the rate of bacterial colonization of the respiratory system, decreasing the number and severity of acute exacerbations of the disease, and maintaining adequate oxygenation in the face of ever-decreasing pulmonary capacity. The strategies for accomplishing these ends are qualitatively similar during maintenance therapy and for acute episodes; the differences lie in the intensity of application of the various treatment modalities.

Colonization of the lungs with pathogenic organisms is inevitable in CF patients. Once this occurs, the organisms can never be completely eradicated, and this should not be seen as a goal of therapy. However, the establishment of chronic infection and subsequent inflammation should be delayed as long as possible by the prompt application of standard mechanical and pharmacologic measures. The patient's condition should be assessed frequently by means of clinical signs and symptoms, sputum cultures, and pulmonary function tests. Rapid intervention at the first sign of an

TABLE 48-1 Treatment Strategies for CF Airways Disease

	Abnormality	Solution	Approach
	• Abnormal CF gene	Provide normal gene	Gene therapy
	• Abnormal CFTR protein	Provide normal protein	Protein therapy:
		Activate mutant form	Phosphodiesterase inhibitors, phosphatase inhibitors, others?
			Butyrate, chaperonins, and CPX
	• Abnormal salt transport	Block Na^+ uptake	Amiloride
		Increase CL^- efflux	ATP/UTP
?	• Abnormal mucus	Decrease viscosity	DNase
?	• Impaired clearance	Augment ciliary action	Chest percussion
	• *Pseudomonas* infection	Reduce bacterial count	Antibiotics
	• Inflammatory response	Decrease host reaction	Antiproteases
			Anti-inflammatory drugs (steroids, ibuprofen)
	• Bronchiectasis	Replace irreversibly damaged areas	Lung transplantation

SOURCE: Adapted from Collins,[6] with permission.

TABLE 48-2 Chest Physiotherapy Techniques

Method	Apparent Advantages	Possible Disadvantages
Percussion and postural drainage (P&PD) is the "gold standard" of airway clearance techniques Forced expiratory technique (FET or "huffing") is sometimes used in addition to P&PD.	P&PD effectively clears the airways and may improve pulmonary function. Conventional P&PD appears superior to FET alone. P&PD is the only practical alternative for infants and very young children.	P&PD requires a partner for full treatment, takes time and energy to perform, and can be limited by chest deformities, pain, gastroesophageal reflux, or injuries.
Autogenic (i.e., self-generated) drainage (AD) utilizes expiratory airflow to mobilize secretions The active cycle of breathing (ACB) technique was developed in Britain, where it is used more than any other technique. It includes breathing control, thoracic exercises, and FET maneuvers. It is often used in conjunction with autogenic drainage. High-frequency chest compression (HFCC) is provided with an inflatable vest.	AD appeals to patients who cannot tolerate postural drainage because of gastroesophageal reflux or who have no one to assist them with percussion. Many patients find AD relaxing. AD seems an effective means of airway clearance for patients with sufficient airflow to propel mucus, provided that particular lobes do not need to be targeted. HFCC is less time-consuming than P&PD, and patients appreciate the autonomy provided by the inflatable vest. It may be useful in very ill patients.	AD is widely used in Europe, where it was first developed. It is time-consuming and requires intensive training and follow-up evaluation. In the United States it is not generally used for children <12 years of age. ACB is used more widely in Britain than any other technique.
Positive expiratory pressure (PEP) uses expiratory maneuvers to mobilize secretions without causing compression of unstable airways. The flutter is a hand-held device that combines the PEP technique with oscillations at the airway opening to facilitate clearance.	PEP is widely used in Europe. In the United States it is sometimes used as an adjunct to "huffing" maneuvers. Although its effectiveness is not clear, some patients and therapists like it. It can be used by patients who are very debilitated or very young (i.e., 3 years of age). Patients appreciate the benefits of the flutter and the ease of its use. In the short term, the device enhances sputum expectoration.	These newer techniques are promising, and they may be associated with higher patient satisfaction and compliance. However, there is limited evidence of their benefits relative to P&PD. Relative indications and contraindications have not yet been rigorously established.

exacerbation is essential to prevent precipitous deterioration of the patient's health status.[11,12,14] The following sections outline the currently accepted conventional treatments for CF, as well as newer therapies and possible future avenues for exploration.

Conventional Pulmonary Therapy of Cystic Fibrosis

CLEARANCE OF AIRWAY SECRETIONS

Defects in the clearance of sputum appear very early in the disease, and measures to enhance clearance should be instituted as soon as feasible for each patient. Various mechanical methods can be used for chest physiotherapy (CPT), although the long-term benefits of these procedures have yet to be proven in controlled clinical studies. However, it is intuitively obvious that any regimen that can reduce respiratory blockage by removing mucopurulent secretions should have a salutary effect on the overall health status of the CF patient.

Table 48–2 lists the most common forms of CPT, along with their advantages and disadvantages for certain patients. The older techniques, such as percussion and postural drainage, are time-consuming and often require assistance from another person. In contrast, newer methods such as autogenic drainage or the use of a positive expiratory pressure (PEP) mask or flutter device can be accomplished without assistance, thus increasing the patient's feelings of autonomy and

control over the disease.[1,5,12,14-16] For all these CPT methods, specific instruction is required for the patient and/or caregiver to perform the maneuvers correctly. Lastly, physical exercise in general can increase drainage and positively affect the patient's well-being.

Percussion/compression techniques are designed to loosen tenacious secretions and promote their subsequent clearance by coughing. Postural drainage, in association with percussion, uses gravity as an aid to move sputum from the small to the large airways for eventual expectoration. The flutter device produces rapid pressure oscillations in the airways, while the PEP mask can be used to force the airways open; both of these methods can facilitate clearance of secretions. Dynamic breathing techniques (forced expiratory technique, autogenic drainage) seek to open different areas of the lung to drainage by using periods of relaxed breathing combined with forcible "huffing" and alternating, controlled expansion of various areas of the lung. These techniques are thought to be useful in patients in whom the bronchi are prone to collapse when subjected to vigorous coughing.

The choice of CPT method depends on several factors, including the amount of sputum produced, the general physical fitness level of the patient (i.e., strength of respiratory muscles), the patient's age and likely degree of compliance with the regimen, the availability of assistance, the presence or absence of airway hyperreactivity, and the extent of respiratory compromise. Inhaled anticholinergic agents (i.e., ipratropium bromide) or β-adrenergic agonists (e.g., albuterol, terbutaline) can be useful adjuncts to CPT, since these agents will relax bronchial smooth muscle and open the airways for more effective mucus clearance.[14–17] However, the sensitivity of CF patients to the actions of β-adrenergic agonists may vary by individual and at different times in the same individual. Patients in whom wheezing and airway hyperreactivity are prominent features may benefit from standard types of asthma therapy (oral or inhaled corticosteroids and / or bronchodilators) in addition to CPT.

It is not only the volume of sputum produced by CF patients that is a problem but also the viscous nature of the secretions that makes them so difficult for the patient to expel. Therefore, decreasing sputum viscosity should facilitate the removal of mucus plugs by CPT and coughing. Sputum viscosity can be reduced by increasing the level of hydration of pulmonary secretions; several ways have been proposed to accomplish this, and many of them are currently undergoing clinical investigation. These approaches will be covered in a later section. Alternatively, viscosity can be reduced by altering one or more components of the purulent secretions—such as the long strands of DNA that accumulate as a result of cell death following the influx of neutrophils into infected or inflamed lung tissue.

Recombinant gene techniques have been employed to synthesize human deoxyribonuclease (rhDNase, dornase alfa), an enzyme that hydrolyzes and depolymerizes DNA.[17,18] Long strands of DNA are cleaved to form shorter strands, a process that has been shown to drastically decrease the elasticity, adhesiveness, and viscosity of infected sputum.[7,14,17,18] In vitro studies demonstrated the conversion of the purulent sputum of CF patients from a nonflowing gel to a fluid when dornase alfa was added. These promising initial investigations were followed by clinical trials that reported improvements in pulmonary function tests and the number of acute exacerbations of disease in patients given aerosolized dornase alfa on a daily basis. The drug is given at a dosage of 2.5 mg, once or twice daily, depending on the clinical response.

Another important but indirect way to reduce sputum viscosity is to prevent or limit colonization of the lungs by pathogenic organisms, thereby limiting the resulting inflammation and its adverse sequelae. The next subsection will examine the basic tenets of judicious antibiotic use in CF patients.

ANTIBIOTIC THERAPY

Antibiotic therapy is the pharmacologic mainstay of CF treatment.[19] Because of the hospitable environment provided to pathogens by retained mucoid secretions, lung infections are a constant and inescapable fact of life for CF patients. Antibiotic regimens of varying composition and intensity must be used intermittently, either on an outpatient or inpatient basis, to slow the rate of deterioration in pulmonary function that occurs secondary to chronic infection and inflammation of the lungs.

Penetration of antibiotics into lung tissue is low in the presence of copious sputum and conditions of chronic inflammation.[4,12] Cystic fibrosis patients often exhibit altered pharmacokinetics as well, including reduced absorption, higher clearance rates, and larger-than-normal volumes of distribution. Therefore, drug doses must be increased to achieve the required therapeutic concentrations. An unfortunate consequence of the frequent, albeit necessary, use of large doses of antibiotics in CF patients is the development of multi-drug-resistant strains of bacteria. To add to the difficulty of choosing an appropriate antibiotic, the standard methods of sensitivity testing may not accurately reflect the in vivo susceptibilities of the infecting organisms.[14]

Pseudomonas infections, which are common in CF patients, are notoriously difficult to treat. Effective treatment may require high doses of antibiotics with low therapeutic indices and great potential for toxic reactions such as nephrotoxicity or ototoxicity (e.g., aminoglycosides). In addition, *Pseudomonas* colonies can assume mucoid forms that grow in biofilms and secrete a polysaccharide that greatly reduces the penetration of antibiotics and thus reduces their efficacy.[4,9,10,13] Some species, such as *B. cepacia* and *X. maltophilia*, are resistant to virtually all currently available antibiotics. Resistant organisms can be spread from patient to patient by close interpersonal contact or by patient contact with contaminated surfaces.

Despite the growing problem of bacterial resistance, the therapeutic advantages of antibiotic use are incontrovertible. The steady increase in projected life span for CF patients over the last half-century is owed primarily to the availability of antibiotics. These drugs may be given orally, intravenously, or by aerosol depending on the pharmacokinetic properties of the individual drugs and the severity of the infection.

The therapeutic armamentarium of antibiotics used in CF remains relatively constant (see Table 48–3),[19] but the doses, combinations, methods of administration, and dosing schedules will vary depending on the goals of treatment. Cystic fibrosis patients alternate between periods of stable disease, where maintenance therapy is sufficient to maintain ade-

TABLE 48-3 Major Pathogens Identified in CF Patients

Organism	Antibiotics
Pseudomonas aeruginosa	β-Lactams (ticarcillin,[a] piperacillin,[a] carbenicillin,[a] ceftazidime, cefsulodin, aztreonam, imipenem) Aminoglycosides (tobramycin, amikacin, gentamicin) Fluoroquinolones (ciprofloxacin, norfloxacin, ofloxacin)
Burkholderia cepacia	Fluoroquinolones (ciprofloxacin, norfloxacin, ofloxacin)
Haemophilus influenzae	β-Lactams (ampicillin, amoxicillin,[a] cephalosporins) Chloramphenicol TMP-SMX[b] Fluoroquinolones (ciprofloxacin, norfloxacin, ofloxacin)
Staphylococcus aureus	β-Lactams (oxacillin, nafcillin, dicloxacillin) Fluoroquinolones (ciprofloxacin, norfloxacin, ofloxacin) Macrolides (azithromycin, clarithromycin, erythromycin)

[a] With or without a β-lactamase inhibitor such as clavulanic acid, sulbactam, or taxobactam.
[b] TMP-SMX, trimethoprim-sulfamethoxazole.
SOURCE: Adapted from Rosenstein,[19] with permission.

quate pulmonary function, and acute exacerbations, in which the patient's clinical status will deteriorate rapidly and aggressive, intravenous antibiotic treatment is mandatory.[4]

ACUTE EXACERBATIONS OF PULMONARY INFECTION

Sudden worsening of respiratory symptoms may occur in response to environmental irritants or allergens or as a result of a bacterial or viral infection (Table 48–4). Because of the precarious health status of most CF patients, treatment of an acute episode usually requires hospitalization to provide continuous monitoring of the results of therapeutic interventions, including rapid changes in strategy if sufficient improvement is not achieved within the desired time frame. Treatment is usually for a minimum of 10 days; longer intervals may be required, however, and treatment should be continued until clinical improvement is observed.[8,4,10,12,14] High-dose intravenous combination antibiotic therapy is the norm under these circumstances. While monotherapy was used in the past, it has a greater tendency to foster development of antibiotic resistance and has lost favor in recent years as a result. Table 48–5 lists the most common causative organisms and their recommended treatments.

Because acute exacerbations of disease requiring parenteral therapy occur so frequently in CF patients, many physicians advocate the placement of a permanent indwelling catheter to provide ready intravenous access. Use of such catheters implies, of course, a commitment by the patient and/or primary caregiver to proper hygiene to avoid complications (e.g., thrombosis, sepsis). A well-maintained permanent catheter, combined with adequate social support, may enable the patient to be treated at home rather than in the hospital. This has the advantage of avoiding patient exposure to hospital-acquired nosocomial infections, as well as reducing the disruption of the patient's life that is inevitably caused by frequent hospitalizations. Cost considerations also favor home treatment over inpatient care.

MAINTENANCE ANTIBIOTIC THERAPY

Once the acute episode has been brought under control and pulmonary function tests show a return to acceptable levels, maintenance therapy can be resumed. Although the lungs of CF patients are in a state of chronic inflammation and bacterial colonization, attempts nonetheless should be made to reduce the bacterial burden and, by inference, the likelihood of repeated acute exacerbations.[8,10,12,20] Table 48–6 lists some recommended regimens for maintenance treatment. Some physicians have advocated prophylactic use of antibiotics for this purpose, either on a daily basis (orally or by inhalation) or by means of recurrent cycles (e.g., every 3 months) of intensive intravenous treatment.

Although this type of regimen again raises concerns about the development of resistant strains of pathogens, it makes eminent clinical sense to try to attenuate the multiple adverse effects of chronic infection in CF. At present, well-controlled clinical trial data are lacking for this approach. However, as more CF patients survive to adulthood, the need for antibiotic maintenance/prophylaxis will only increase, and the safest and most efficacious means for providing it should be carefully explored.

INHALED ANTIBIOTIC THERAPY

Inhalation therapy with antibiotics may offer advantages over systemic administration. The drugs are delivered directly to the pulmonary epithelium via aerosolization, bypassing the liver and first-pass metabolism. Direct delivery also somewhat obviates the problem of poor drug penetration into lung tissue after oral or parenteral dosing; therefore, smaller total amounts of drug can be used to achieve the same effect. Systemic absorption is greatly reduced when drugs are inhaled, lessening the possibility of adverse effects or drug interactions with concomitant medications given by other routes.[4,5,8,14,21] Table 48–7 lists some of the antibiotics currently used for inhalation therapy.

However, not all antibiotics can be given via inhalation techniques. Some antibiotics or antibiotic solutions are unstable when exposed to nebulizers that generate heat or that use ultrasonic vibration to aerosolize particles. Combinations of antibiotics may not be physically or chemically compatible for use together in an aerosol form. Drugs that are highly irritating to epithelial surfaces are likewise not good candidates for this mode of administration, and some may precipitate bronchoconstriction. The type of nebulizer employed is also critically important; the particles produced must be of a size (1 to 8 μm) that will reach the smaller airways before being deposited. The possibility of spreading resistant microorganisms by the use of inadequately sterilized nebulizers also must be considered with this type of treatment. On the other hand, the development of antibiotic resistance should be no more likely with aerosol therapy than with other routes of administration.

A number of clinical trials of aerosol antibiotics for maintenance therapy have demonstrated clinical improvement, reduced hospital admissions, and reductions in sputum colony counts. In a recent study,[22] tobramycin was delivered as a 300 mg bid dose (Tobi Tobramycin solution for inhalation, Pathogenesis Corporation, Seattle, WA) by Pari LC plus nebulizer for 4 weeks alternating with 4 weeks off treatment for a total of three treatment cycles (24 weeks total). Patients in the Tobramycin group had an average increase in FEV of 10 percent at week 20 compared with a 2 percent decline in the placebo group. Additionally, patients in the Tobramycin group were 26 percent less likely to be hospitalized and 36 percent less likely to be treated with IV antibiotics than patients in the placebo group. Inhaled antibiotic therapy used in conjunction with a CPT session always must be administered after CPT, or the inhaled drug will merely be expectorated with the sputum.

A summary of general considerations for antibiotic treatment in CF patients is provided in Table 48–8.

TABLE 48-4 Clinical Signs of an Acute Exacerbation of Pulmonary Infection in CF

- A change in the volume, color, and/or appearance of sputum
- Increased cough, dyspnea, or respiratory rate
- Deterioration in pulmonary function tests
- Hypoxemia
- New findings on chest physical examination and/or x-ray
- Onset of fever, fatigue, anorexia, weight loss, and decreased exercise tolerance

SOURCE: Adapted from Bye,[1] with permission.

TABLE 48-5 Recommended Antibiotics and Dosages for Treatment of Acute Exacerbations of Disease in CF Patients

Prevalent Bacteria	FIRST CHOICE			ALTERNATIVE		
	Antibiotic	DOSE Child	DOSE Adult	Antibiotic	DOSE Child	DOSE Adult
S. aureus	Cephalothin Nafcillin[b]	25–50 mg/kg q6h 25–50 mg/kg q6h	1 g q6h 1 g q6h	Vancomycin[a]	15 mg/kg q6h	500 mg q6h
H. influenzae and S. aureus	Ticarcillin[c]-clavulanate plus gentamicin[d]	100 mg/kg ticarcillin and 3.3 mg/kg clavulanate q6h; 3 mg gentamicin q8h	3 g ticarcillin and 0.1 g clavulanate q6h; 3 mg/kg gentamicin q8h	Nafcillin[b] plus gentamicin[d]	25–50 mg/kg q6h 3 mg/kg q8h	1 g q6h 3 mg/kg q8h
S. aureus and P. aeruginosa	Ticarcillin[c]-clavulanate plus tobramycin[d]	100 mg/kg ticarcillin and 3.3 mg/kg cla-vulanate q6h; 3 mg/kg tobramycin q8h	3 g ticarcillin and 0.1 g clavulanate q6h; 3 mg/kg tobramycin q8h			
P. aeruginosa only	Ticarcillin[c] plus tobra-mycin[d]	100 mg/kg q6h 3 mg/kg q8h	3 g q6h 3 mg/kg q8h	Tobramycin[d] plus ceftazidime, piperacillin, or imipenem[e] Aztreonam[f] plus amikacin[g]	3 mg/kg q8h 50 mg/kg q8h 100 mg/kg q6h 15–25 mg/kg q6h 50 mg/kg q6h 5–7.5 mg/kg q8h	3 mg/kg q8h 2 g q8h 3 g q6h 0.5–1 g q6h 2 g q8h 5–7.5 mg/kg q8h
P. aeruginosa and Burkhold-eria cepacia	Ceftazidime plus ciprofloxacin	50–75 mg q8h 15 mg/kg q12h	2 g q8h 400 mg q12h IV	Ceftazidime plus chlor-amphenicol or TMP-SMX[i]	50–75 mg/kg q8h 15–20 mg/kg q6h 5 mg/kg TMP IV and 25 mg/kg SMX q6h	2 g q8h 5 mg/kg TMP IV and 25 mg/kg SMX q6h 15–20 mg/kg q6h
B. cepacia only	Chloramphenicol[h] or TMP-SMX[i] or both	15–20 mg/kg q6h 5 mg/kg TMP and 25 mg/kg SMX q6h	15–20 mg/kg q6h 5 mg/kg TMP and 25 mg/kg SMX q6h			

[a] Vancomycin should be infused slowly to avoid histamine release. Serum concentrations should be monitored; the peak concentration ranges from 20–30 μg/mL and the trough concentration from 5–10 μg/mL.
[b] Nafcillin should be diluted to a concentration <20 mg/mL to minimize phlebitis.
[c] Ticarcillin may be associated with occasional platelet dysfunction. Its use is limited by concern about the possibility of selection for resistant organisms such as Stenotrophomonas maltophilia and B. cepacia.
[d] Serum concentrations should be monitored. Peak concentrations range from 8–12 μg/mL; trough concentration is <2 μg/mL.
[e] This drug is for patients with a sensitivity to cephalosporin or multidrug-resistant organisms.
[f] Frequent antibiotic susceptibility testing is recommended to ensure treatment with the optimal combination of antibiotics.
[g] Serum concentrations should be monitored. Peak concentrations range from 15–25 μg/mL; trough concentration is <5 μg/mL.
[h] Serum concentrations should be monitored. Peak concentrations range from 10–25 μg/mL; trough concentrations range from 5–10 μg/mL.
[i] TMP-SMX, trimethoprim-sulfamethoxazole.
SOURCE: Adapted from Ramsey,[8] with permission.

Newer Therapies for Cystic Fibrosis

As our knowledge of the pathogenesis of CF has increased, so has the number and variety of hypothetical points of intervention (see Table 48–1). Current research is targeting some of these processes by exploring the use of biologic response modifiers to alter the disease process at the level of the respiratory epithelium. Another approach would be to supplement the natural defenses of lung tissue against destruction by neutrophil-derived enzymes by exogenous administration of inhibitors of enzyme synthesis or activity. The most drastic interventional strategy consists of insertion of a fully functional native CFTR gene to compensate for the dysfunctionality of the mutated form in CF patients. More traditional approaches include development of vaccines against common pathogens or the use of anti-inflammatory agents.

CORRECT ABNORMAL CFTR

One approach is to facilitate the correct intracellular processing of the abnormal CFTR protein, assisting it in reaching the membrane in individuals with the delta F508 and other similar trafficking mutations (e.g., butyrate and chaperonins). Another approach is to induce a high level of chloride channel activity in the small number of CFTR molecules that are correctly localized (e.g., CPX, milrinone, and phosphodiesterase inhibitors). A final strategy aims to compensate for the CFTR channel defect by altering chloride and sodium flux through other membrane channels (e.g., UTP).

ANTI-INFLAMMATORY THERAPY

The state of chronic inflammation and progressive destruction of tissue that exists in the lungs of CF patients might be susceptible to inhibition by a number of agents having

TABLE 48-6 Recommended Oral Antibiotics and Dosages for Maintenance Treatment of CF Patients

| Pathogen | Antibiotic | DOSE | |
		Child	Adult
S. aureus	Dicloxacillin	6.25 mg/kg q6h	250–500 mg q6h
	Cephalexin	12.5 mg/kg q6h	500 mg q6h
	Amoxicillin-clavulanate[a]	10–15 mg/kg amoxicillin and 2.5–3.75 mg/kg clavulanate q8h	250–500 mg amoxicillin and 125 mg clavulanate q8h
	Erythromycin	15 mg/kg q8h	250 mg q8h
	Clarithromycin	7.5 mg/kg q12h	500 mg q12h
H. influenzae	Cefaclor	10–15 mg/kg q8h	250–500 mg q8h
	Amoxicillin	20–40 mg/kg q8h	500 mg q8h
S. aureus and H. influenzae	Cefixime	8 mg/kg/d	400 mg/d
	Amoxicillin-clavulanate[a]	10–15 mg/kg amoxicillin and 2.5–3.75 mg/kg clavulanate q8h	250–500 mg amoxicillin and 125 mg clavulanate q8h
	TMP-SMX[b]	4 mg/kg TMP and 20 mg/kg SMX q12h	160 mg TMP and 800 mg SMX q12h
	Cefpodoxime	5 mg/kg q12h	200 mg q12h
	Cefuroxime	20 mg/kg q12h	250–500 mg q12h
P. aeruginosa	Ciprofloxacin[c]	Not indicated	500–750 mg q12h
	Ofloxacin[c]	Not indicated	400 mg q12h
B. cepacia	TMP-SMX	4 mg/kg TMP and 20 mg/kg SMX q12h	160 mg TMP and 800 mg SMX q12h

[a] Higher doses of clavulanate are frequently associated with diarrhea.
[b] TMP-SMX, trimethoprim-sulfamethexazole.
[c] Ciprofloxacin and ofloxacin are not indicated for use in patients <18 years of age.
NOTE: List is not intended to be exhaustive.
SOURCE: Adapted from Ramsey,[8] with permission.

a variety of mechanisms of action. The nonsteroidal anti-inflammatory agent ibuprofen is currently under investigation for this purpose. Ibuprofen has been shown to inhibit neutrophil migration and release of proteolytic enzymes.[4,7,8,12,14,23] Efficacy has been demonstrated in pediatric patients with mild disease in one study. One advantage of ibuprofen is its long history of safe use and its relative lack of serious adverse effects. Pentoxifylline, a xanthine derivative, has been shown to reduce adhesiveness of activated neutrophils and decrease the release of lysosomal enzymes and toxic oxygen free radicals, as well as having other anti-inflammatory effects. Corticosteroids have potent anti-inflammatory effects, but these drugs have serious side effects when given in oral doses that will control inflammatory processes in CF patients.[17,24] Inhaled corticosteroids might offer a suitable, and safer, alternative, however.

FUTURE DIRECTIONS IN THERAPY OF CYSTIC FIBROSIS

Newer methods aimed at decreasing sputum viscosity include the use of amiloride, adenosine triphosphate (ATP),

TABLE 48-7 Antibiotics Used for Inhalation Therapy

Antibiotic	Dose
Amikacin	200 mg/d
Ceftazidime	2 g/d
Colistin	150–300 mg/d
Gentamicin	160 mg/d
Tobramycin	160–1800 mg/d

SOURCE: Adapted from Wallace et al.,[4] with permission.

uridine triphosphate (UTP), gelsolin, neutrophil protease inhibitors, secretory leukocyte protease inhibitors, or immunotherapy against *Pseudomonas* species.

Amiloride is a diuretic that works by blocking sodium transport in epithelial cells. The drug must reach the apical surface of the pulmonary epithelium and is therefore effective only when used as an aerosol.[2,16,17,25] Large amounts of sputum will block access of the drug to the epithelial cells; thus amiloride may only be useful in patients with relatively mild disease who produce nonpurulent sputum. When sodium transport into the epithelial cell is inhibited, the obligatory water molecules surrounding the sodium ion increase the hydration level of bronchial secretions, reducing sputum viscosity and facilitating mucociliary clearance. Some studies have demonstrated that amiloride can slow deterioration of pulmonary function, but documentation of long-term overall health benefits is generally lacking to date for this drug treatment.

Chloride secretion can be augmented by aerosol administration of nucleotide triphosphates (ATP, UTP) to stimulate an alternate, calcium-dependent chloride channel in the epithelial membrane. This effectively bypasses the defective CFTR chloride channel. However, ATP is rapidly metabolized to adenosine, which is an irritant and may cause bronchospasm. Use of UTP eliminates this problem.[16,17] Clinical trials are in progress to evaluate this type of treatment.

Gelsolin is a plasma protein that cleaves actin filaments that are a component of purulent sputum and contribute to its increased viscosity. Thus this compound might be useful as a mucolytic in CF patients. In addition, gelsolin acts synergistically with DNase to reduce sputum viscosity.[17] The potential therapeutic merit of gelsolin is under investigation.

TABLE 48-8 Special Considerations in Antibiotic Treatment for CF Patients

Goal	Return the patient to baseline in terms of symptoms, sputum reduction, and lung function (FEV₁); eradication of *P. aeruginosa* is not possible.
Targets	Multiple organisms and multiple strains of *P. aeruginosa, S. aureus, H. influenzae,* and *B. cepacia.*
Dose	Dose must be significantly higher than for non-CF patients due to (1) altered pharmacokinetics, (2) inactivation of some drugs (i.e., tobramycin) which bind to free DNA, (3) coexistent strains of *P. aeruginosa* with varying susceptibilities, and (4) presence of alginate strains of *P. aeruginosa.* Optimal dosing is based on monitoring of peak and trough serum concentrations.
Duration	2–3 weeks.
Choice of drugs	Synergistic drug combinations can prevent, or override, development of resistance. Antipseudomonal combinations are generally comprised of aminoglycosides (e.g., tobramycin, gentamicin) and β-lactams. Among the latter, cephalosporins (i.e., ceftazidime) are preferred over the semisynthetic penicillins for their dosing convenience. Imipenem is not recommended for routine treatment, as it readily induces resistance. Drug choice is based on sputum bacteriology and, when necessary, in vitro synergy testing.
Intravenous drugs	IV drug delivery is used for (1) moderate to severe exacerbations and (2) subacute clinical or pulmonary deterioration. Home therapy, which is less disruptive to patients and is also less costly, may be considered if other traditional benefits of hospital care are not required. Midline catheters and long-term indwelling venous catheters provide useful alternatives to patients requiring frequent venous access. Otherwise, arrangements must be made for placing an IV line at home or in the hospital.
Oral drugs	Oral drugs (primarily ciprofloxacin or other quinolones) are used for (1) mild to moderate exacerbations and (2) maintenance therapy. Quinolones are not indicated for use in children <18 years of age, but ciprofloxacin has been administered to >1000 children on a compassionate basis with no clear increase in arthropathy. Broad-spectrum antibiotics may be useful against nonpseudomonal bacteria, and they may reduce the release of bacterial toxins, limiting inflammation.
Inhaled drugs	Aerosolized drugs (tobramycin, colistin) are commonly used for maintenance therapy following CPT. They are thought to provide high concentrations of drug in the airways with limited toxicity. High-dose tobramycin (300 mg 2× daily) delivered by ultrasonic nebulizer improved lung function and decreased *P. aeruginosa* density in a multicenter double-blind crossover study. Decisions to use aerosolized drugs are made on a case-by-case basis.
Indications	Signs and symptoms that may indicate the necessity for IV treatment are discussed above.
Monitoring	Careful monitoring is necessary to avoid renal or ototoxicity. Aminoglycosides have a narrow therapeutic/toxic window. Ciprofloxacin is generally well tolerated, although arthropathy is sporadically reported. Intermittent use is desirable, and long-term use is discouraged because drug resistance can occur after 3–4 weeks of therapy.
Allergy	Desensitization may be necessary in cases of allergy to aminoglycosides or semi-synthetic penicillins.
Multidrug resistance	Strategies for minimizing or overcoming multidrug resistance include (1) avoiding overuse, (2) avoiding monotherapy, (3) using in vitro synergy test results to guide drug choice, and (4) using high doses of drugs.
Maintenance therapy	Maintenance antibiotic therapy with oral or aerosolized agents to prevent a decline in lung function is common, but the effectiveness of this practice is now being questioned and is being increasingly scrutinized for its possible role in the development of multidrug-resistant organisms.

Another novel method of reducing sputum viscosity employs liposomes of distearoyl phosphatidylglyerol (DSPG) to correct lipid imbalances in secretions of CF patients. These surface-active liposomes can improve mucociliary transport and clearance and also may reduce the adherence of *Pseudomonas* to respiratory epithelium.

Part of the inflammatory process in CF involves the accumulation of by-products of cellular damage caused by endogenous proteases. This cellular debris also contributes to the thickening of pulmonary secretions. If the action of proteases could be inhibited, damage to lung tissue might be alleviated, and part of the increase in sputum viscosity could be prevented as well. Aerosol administration of α_1-antitrypsin or secretory leukocyte protease inhibitor has been shown to restore the balance between naturally occurring proteases and antiproteases in the lung, reducing the activity of chemotactic cytokines and decreasing the influx of neutrophils into lung tissue.[2,5,11,16,26] Both of these substances are found in normal lung tissue but are probably overwhelmed by the disease process in CF. Synthetic inhibitors of elastase are also being developed; these drugs could prevent the loss of lung elasticity due to damage by naturally occurring proteases.

Gene therapy is perhaps the most ambitious method postulated to date for treatment of CF. The methodology for achieving transfer of normal *CFTR* genes into a host organism has only recently become available and is still being perfected. The theory behind this approach is to insert a fully functional, wild-type *CFTR* gene into the pulmonary epithelial cell as a means of compensating for the defective gene already present. It is hoped that this would normalize chloride transport sufficiently to ameliorate the symptoms of CF at the level of the epithelium, thereby preventing the initiation of the pathologic cascade of events culminating in airways obstruction, chronic infection and inflammation, tissue destruction, and ultimate respiratory failure.[6,17,27–29] Many problems remain to be solved before this approach is feasible from a therapeutic perspective. One of these is the method of introduction of the gene into the human host cell. Early attempts used viral vectors, such as adenoviruses, that normally infect the host cell. Both the safety and ultimate efficacy of this system remain to be fully explored. Other methods for introduction of the gene exist, including the use of cationic lipid preparations and molecular conjugate forms that can facilitate DNA entry into the cell by receptor-mediated endocytosis. All these methods are still highly experimental.

Because *Pseudomonas* species are frequently found in CF patients and are often resistant to multiple drugs, these bacteria are prime targets for vaccines or immunotherapy directed toward preventing or inhibiting their colonization of the respiratory tract.[11] Difficulties arise because these bacteria are confined to the epithelial surface of the lungs and do not often produce systemic infection. Therefore, a vaccine would have to confer local protection for the pulmonary epithelium over a long period of time. In addition, colonization with *Pseudomonas* occurs fairly early in the patient's life; any vaccine aimed at preventing such an occurrence therefore would have to be safe enough to administer to young patients. At the present time, no vaccine has been developed that fulfills these requirements. Passive immunotherapy with hyperimmune globulin is another avenue of investigation currently under study. Administration of this product may facilitate the host's defenses against *Pseudomonas*, particularly when infection is due to drug-resistant strains.[5,14] Early results have been promising, but extensive clinical testing will still be required to establish the efficacy of this approach.

Summary

Recent advance in the treatment of CF are cause for hope to physicians and patients who must deal with the effects of the disease on a daily basis. However, the disease is still ultimately fatal for those afflicted, although life expectancy has increased tremendously over the last half century. It is important for the physician to treat the manifestations of CF aggressively, since failure to do so may result in rapid and irreversible deterioration in the patient's clinical status. Cystic fibrosis involves many body systems other than the respiratory system, and treatment objectives must focus not only on reducing the pathophysiologic effects but also on maintaining the patient's quality of life and psychosocial functioning. Respiratory complications are the primary determinant of morbidity and mortality in CF; as such, their treatment assumes primacy in the overall clinical scheme. Chest physiotherapy to clear the copious secretions and antibiotic treatment of chronic pulmonary infections are the twin pillars of clinical management in CF. Future therapies may be able to target processes earlier in the course of disease and thus prevent the complications commonly observed at present.

References

1. Bye MR, Ewig JM, Quittell LM: Cystic fibrosis. *Lung* 172:251, 1994.
2. Wilmott RW, Fiedler MA: Recent advances in the treatment of cystic fibrosis. *Pediatr Clin North Am* 41:431, 1994.
3. Anderson DH: Cystic fibrosis of the pancreas and its relation to celiac disease: A clinical and pathologic study. *Am J Dis Child* 56:344, 1938.
4. Wallace CS, Hall M, Kuhn RJ: Pharmacologic management of cystic fibrosis. *Clin Pharm* 12:657, 1993.
5. Fiel SB: *Cystic Fibrosis.* St Louis, Year Book Medical Publishers, 1995; p 1.
6. Collins FS: Cystic fibrosis: Molecular biology and therapeutic implications. *Science* 256:774, 1992.
7. Davis PB, Drumm M, Konstan MW: Cystic fibrosis. *Am J Respir Crit Care Med* 154:1229, 1996.
8. Ramsey B: Management of pulmonary disease in patients with cystic fibrosis. *Drug Ther* 335:179, 1996.
9. Hoiby N: Cystic fibrosis and endobronchial *Pseudomonas* infection. *Curr Opin Pediatr* 5:247, 1993.
10. Webb AK: The treatment of pulmonary infection in cystic fibrosis. *Scand J Infect Dis* (suppl 96):24, 1995.
11. Zach MS: Lung disease in cystic fibrosis: An updated concept. *Pediatr Pulmonol* 8:188, 1990.
12. Burns JL, Ramsey BW, Smith AL: Clinical manifestations and treatment of pulmonary infections in cystic fibrosis. *Adv Pediatr Infect Dis* 8:53, 1993.
13. Buret A: *Pseudomonas aeruginosa* infections in patient with cystic fibrosis: New immunomodulatory strategies. *Clin Immunol* 2:261, 1994.
14. Fiel SB: Clinical management of pulmonary disease in cystic fibrosis. *Lancet* 341:1070, 1993.
15. Sanchez I, Guiraldes E: Drug management of noninfective complications of cystic fibrosis. *Drugs* 50:626, 1995.
16. Konstan MW, Stern RC, Doershuk CF: Efficacy of the flutter device for airway mucus clearance in patients with cystic fibrosis. *J Pediatr* 124:689, 1994.
17. Sexauer WP, Fiel SB: New treatment modalities for cystic fibrosis. *Curr Opin Pulmonary Med* 1:457, 1995.
18. Wagner JA, Chao AC, Gardner P: Molecular strategies for therapy of cystic fibrosis. *Ann Rev Pharmacol Toxicol* 35:257, 1995.
19. Rosenstein BJ: Molecular basis, diagnosis, and treatment of cystic fibrosis. *Pediatr Rounds* 4:5, 1995.
20. Hodson ME: Maintenance treatment with antibiotics in cystic fibrosis patients: Sense or nonsense? *Neth J Med* 46:288, 1995.
21. Touw DJ, Brimicombe RW, Hodson ME, et al: Inhalation of antibiotics in cystic fibrosis. *Eur Respir J* 8:1594, 1995.
22. Ramsey BW, Pepe MS, Oth KL, et al: Efficacy and safety of chronic intermittent inhaled Tobramycin in patients with CF. To be published, 1998.
23. Konstan MW, Vargo KM, Davis PB: Ibuprofen attenuates the inflammatory response to *Pseudomonas aeruginosa* in a rat model of chronic pulmonary infection: Implications for anti-inflammatory therapy in cystic fibrosis. *Am Rev Respir Dis* 141:186, 1990.
24. Eigen H, Rosenstein BJ, FitzSimmons S, Schidow DV: A multicenter study of alternate-day prednisone therapy in patients with cystic fibrosis. *J Pediatr* 126:515, 1995.
25. Suter S: New perspectives in understanding and management of the respiratory disease in cystic fibrosis. *Eur J Paediatr* 153:144, 1994.
26. Stromatt SC: Secretory leukocyte protease inhibitor in cystic fibrosis, in *Proteases, Protease Inhibitors and Protease-Derived Peptides.* Basel, Birkhäuser Verlag, 1991; p 103.
27. Rosenfeld MA, Ronald G, Crystal RG: Gene therapy for pulmonary diseases. *Pathol Biolerol* 41:677, 1993.
28. Crystal RG: In vivo gene therapy: A strategy to use human genes as therapeutics, in *Transactions of the American Clinical Climatological Association*, Gordon Wilson Lecture, 1994; pp 87–90.
29. Smith AE: Treatment of cystic fibrosis based on understanding CFTR. *J Inher Metab Dis* 18.508, 1995.

Chapter 49

NONINVASIVE VENTILATION IN NEUROMUSCULAR DISEASE

NICHOLAS S. HILL
SIDNEY S. BRAMAN

The second half of the twentieth century has seen an explosive rise in the use of invasive devices to prolong life in the critically ill respiratory patient. This is best exemplified by the rapid increase in the use of translaryngeal intubation and tracheostomy to assist in the mechanical ventilatory support of patients with respiratory failure. Although these methods have unquestionably improved survival, they have done so at a cost, both in terms of morbidity and financially. Invasive mechanical ventilation is accompanied by a myriad of problems, not only those related directly to the intubation or placement of the tracheostomy such as laryngeal trauma or hemorrhage but also those secondary to prolonged intubation such as recurrent pneumonias related to macro- and microaspiration, atelectasis, and the need for repeated suctioning.[1] Invasive mechanical ventilation also increases patient discomfort and anxiety, interfering with normal speech and swallowing functions, necessitating sedation, and contributing to the prolongation of ventilatory support.[2] In addition, invasive ventilation is usually administered at great expense in acute care hospitals and highly skilled nursing facilities. Even when delivered in the home, invasive mechanical ventilation is costly, and favorable cost-benefit analyses have not been performed to justify these expenditures.

These problems associated with the use of invasive ventilatory techniques have stimulated increasing interest among practitioners in noninvasive ventilatory techniques that offer less morbid and lower-cost alternatives to invasive ventilation in appropriate patients. For long-term ventilatory support of neuromuscular disease patients, these techniques that obviate the need for an invasive artificial airway have largely supplanted invasive techniques as the ventilatory modes of first choice. Initially, negative-pressure devices that were developed during the poliomyelitis epidemics of the 1920s through 1950s were the most frequently used noninvasive ventilators. More recently, noninvasive positive-pressure techniques have shown great promise in patients with respiratory failure due to a variety of neuromuscular diseases. This chapter presents a historical perspective on the development of noninvasive ventilators and a brief overview of the types of ventilators now available, focusing on their advantages and limitations. The chapter then discusses mechanisms of chronic respiratory failure and considers how intermittent ventilatory assistance might work in patients with neuromuscular disease. The chapter also considers issues relating to the initiation and selection of an appropriate regimen of mechanical ventilation and specific applications of mechanical ventilatory assistance in the more common neuromuscular disorders that benefit from noninvasive ventilation.

Historical Perspective

The first description of noninvasive ventilatory support was in 1832 by a Scottish physician, John Dalziel.[3] He described a prototype of the negative-pressure ventilator or "iron lung" as an airtight box in which the subject sat with his or her head protruding outside the box. A negative inspiratory pressure was generated inside the box with the use of a pair of hand-operated bellows that were synchronized with the subject's respirations. In 1918, the first electrically driven negative-pressure ventilator was developed by Dr. Steuart of South Africa and applied to patients suffering from polio-induced respiratory paralysis.[3] The iron lung ventilator used widely for neuromuscular respiratory failure during the poliomyelitis epidemics was developed during the late 1920s by Drinker,[4] an engineer at the Harvard School of Public Health, and later modified by J. H. Emerson. These devices immediately gained widespread use as polio mortality from respiratory paralysis was reduced from 100 to 50 percent.

A modified fiberglass version of the iron lung was introduced in the late 1970s by an individual with respiratory paralysis from poliomyelitis who had used the larger version of the iron lung for many years. This device, called the *Portalung*, is smaller and lighter than the iron lung (weighing only 45 kg as opposed to 325 kg), although it still requires two persons for portage.[5] Other more portable negative-pressure devices had been developed during the polio epidemic of the 1950s such as the Tunnicliffe jacket,[6] now referred to as a "wrap" or "poncho" ventilator, and the chest cuirass or "tortoise shell."[7]

Other ingenius approaches to ventilatory support appeared during the first half of this century in response to the polio epidemics and later were adapted to treat a wide variety of neuromuscular disorders. These included the rocking bed, first introduced as a resuscitative device by Eve in 1932,[8] who used a rocking chair to resuscitate a child who was dying of diptheritic diaphragmatic paralysis, and the intermittent abdominal pressure respirator, or "pneumobelt," developed during the 1950s.[9] Both devices function by exerting an intermittent force on the abdomen that displaces a weakened diaphragm upward and downward, thereby assisting ventilation. Another approach to combating neuromuscular respiratory failure is exemplified by phrenic nerve stimulation in patients with high cervical cord lesions that was developed by Glenn and coworkers during the 1960s.[10] Also during the 1960s, certain centers used noninvasive positive-pressure devices for long-term support of neuromuscular patients with respiratory failure, applying intermittent positive pressure to the upper airway via mouthpieces and face masks.[11] However, after control of the poliomyelitis epidemics and despite the wide availability of noninvasive techniques, end-stage neuromuscular patients who developed respiratory failure during the 1970s and early 1980s most often received either invasive ventilatory assistance or no assistance at all.[12]

With the development of the nasal mask for administration

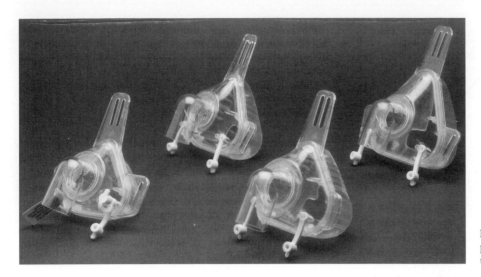

FIGURE 49-1 Standard nasal continuous positive airway pressure (CPAP) masks used for delivery of nasal ventilation.

of continuous positive airway pressure (CPAP) to patients with obstructive sleep apnea during the early 1980s, a wide variety of comfortable and more tolerable interfaces became available commercially. Investigators rapidly learned that application of positive-pressure ventilation nocturnally via these nasal masks would ameliorate symptoms and gas-exchange disturbances in neuromuscular disease patients with chronic respiratory failure.[13,14] Since then, use of noninvasive positive-pressure ventilation in patients with respiratory failure due to neuromuscular disease has burgeoned, greatly reducing the need for tracheostomy placement or for alternative modes of noninvasive ventilation.

The current interest in noninvasive ventilation for neuromuscular disease also has been fueled by the worldwide movement to keep chronic respiratory failure patients at home whenever possible. Invasive ventilation has been used to treat respiratory failure in numerous neuromuscular disease patients for many years, unquestionably prolonging survival. However, use of invasive ventilation greatly complicates delivery of mechanical ventilation in the home, necessitating a higher skill level among caregivers and adding to costs. Because of its relative ease of administration and lower cost, noninvasive ventilation offers a very attractive alternative to invasive ventilation for home use. However, noninvasive ventilation is not entirely equivalent to invasive ventilation, permitting no direct access to the airway in patients with severe swallowing or cough impairment. Thus patients with neuromuscular disease who are being considered for noninvasive ventilation must be evaluated carefully to make certain that they are appropriate candidates, taking into consideration their specific neuromuscular impairments as well as their desires relating to aggressiveness of care.

Options for Noninvasive Ventilation

NONINVASIVE POSITIVE-PRESSURE VENTILATION

Noninvasive positive-pressure ventilation (NPPV), the most commonly used noninvasive method presently, consists of a positive-pressure ventilator that delivers intermittent positive pressure to the lungs through a mask (or interface) that is affixed to the nose, mouth, or both. During the past decade, NPPV has replaced invasive positive-pressure ventilation as

the ventilatory mode of first choice for neuromuscular patients with chronic respiratory failure by virtue of its greater convenience, portability, and lower cost. For these reasons, it is desirable to switch patients to noninvasive ventilation and remove the artificial airway if possible.

INTERFACES

At the present time, many different nasal masks are available, including standard plastic masks that fit over the nose (Respironics, Inc., Murrysville, PA; Healthdyne, Inc., Marietta, GA; and Nellcor-Puritan-Bennett, Lenexa, KS) (Fig. 49-1), masks that have soft silicone "bubbles" or "comfort flaps" that reduce the strap tension necessary to maintain a tight airseal (Sullivan Bubble Mask, Resmed, Inc., San Diego, CA; Respironics), nasal "pillows" or "seals" that consist of small cones inserted into the nostrils (Adams Circuit, Puritan-Bennett, Healthdyne) (Fig. 49-2), custom molding kits (Respiro-

FIGURE 49-2 Nasal "pillows" (Nellcor-Puritan-Bennett, Inc., Lenexa, KS) used for nasal ventilation.

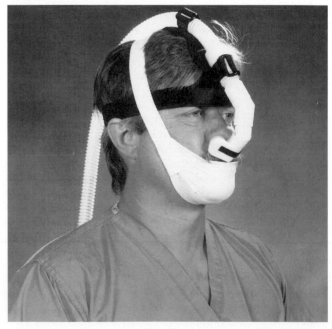

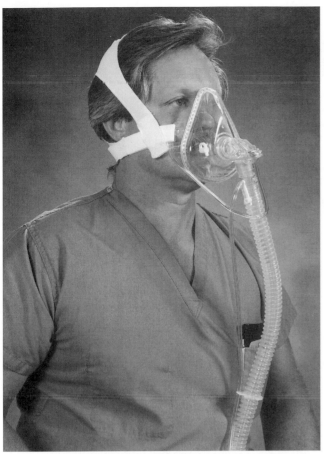

FIGURE 49-3 Oronasal mask (Spectrum, Respironics, Inc., Pittsburgh, PA) designed for use with noninvasive ventilation. It includes an "antiasphyxia" valve and quick-release strap.

nics), and newer more compact masks that appeal to patients with claustrophobia (Monarch mask, Respironics).

Oronasal masks are also available to serve as interfaces for the delivery of NPPV. The availability of these masks actually antedated that of nasal masks, but until recently, these were designed mainly for use in the anesthesia suite (Vital Signs, Inc., Totowa, NJ) and were not often well tolerated for chronic use. However, newer oronasal masks designed specifically for the administration of NPPV have become available and are quite suitable for chronic use (Spectrum, Respironics) (Fig. 49-3). These may be preferred in patients who have excessive air leaking through the mouth. They are equipped with anti-rebreathing valves and rapid removal straps to minimize the risks of asphyxiation in the event of ventilator failure or aspiration due to vomiting.

Mouthpiece interfaces are also suitable for chronic administration of NPPV. These consist of commercially available mouthpieces held in place by plastic lipseals (Nellcor-Puritan-Bennett) or devices that are custom fitted by an orthodontist.[15] These have been used to administer round-the-clock ventilatory assistance to patients with little or no vital capacity by using a strapped-on or orthodontic device during sleep and a mouthpiece connected to a gooseneck clamp on a wheelchair for daytime use.[15] Mouthpieces may be useful in patients who have excessive air leaking through the mouth

while using nasal masks, but air leaking through the nose may still pose problems. Patients using mouthpieces also may have difficulty with oral accumulation of saliva or orthodontic problems after prolonged use.[15]

A wide variety of positive-pressure ventilators may be used to deliver NPPV. The earlier reports on the use of NPPV in neuromuscular disease employed standard portable volume ventilators in the assist/control mode and relatively large tidal volumes (>15 mL/kg) to compensate for air leaks.[13,14] More recently, portable pressure-limited ventilators, referred to as *bilevel positive airway pressure (BPAP) devices* (BiPAP, Respironics, Quantum, Healthdyne, 335, Nellcor-Puritan-Bennett, VPAP, Resmed, Inc.), have been used to deliver NPPV[16] (Fig. 49-4). These devices cycle between two levels of positive airway pressure using either flow or time triggering. Originally developed to lower mean airway pressure and improve tolerance in patients requiring high levels of nasal CPAP for obstructive sleep apnea, these devices function effectively as ventilators.[17] They are particularly advantageous for home delivery of nocturnal nasal ventilation because of simplicity of operation, portability (weights range from 5 to 12 kg), quietness, ability to compensate for air leaks, and relatively low cost.[17] They lack alarms, which are unnecessary and may disturb sleep in patients requiring only nocturnal assistance, and usually have no internal battery. However, for these reasons, they are unsuitable for patients requiring continuous ventilation unless appropriate alarms and backup systems are added.

Because few studies have compared ventilator modes and

FIGURE 49-4 Example of "bilevel" positive-pressure ventilator used for noninvasive ventilation (BiPAP S/T, Respironics, Inc.).

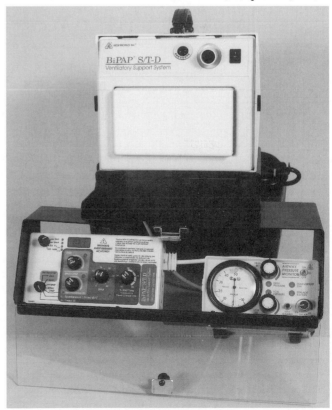

interfaces directly, selection of the interface-ventilator combination depends largely on patient needs and practitioner and patient preferences. Available evidence on the use of NPPV in acute respiratory failure demonstrates that although volume- and pressure-limited ventilator modes have similar efficacy, patient tolerance is better with the pressure-limited modes.[18] However, as will be discussed in more detail later, success can be achieved with many combinations of interfaces and ventilators.

NEGATIVE-PRESSURE VENTILATION

Negative-pressure ventilators create an intermittent subatmospheric pressure outside the thorax and abdomen, facilitating chest wall and abdominal expansion and thereby assisting inhalation. Exhalation occurs as the elastic recoil of the lung and chest wall passively reduces lung volume when pressure within the device rises to atmospheric levels. The efficiency of the negative-pressure ventilator, that is, the tidal volume generated for a given negative pressure, is determined by the compliance of the chest wall and abdomen and the surface area over which the negative pressure is applied. For this reason, the tank ventilator is more effective because it applies negative pressure to the entire chest wall and abdomen, and the chest shell ventilator is less effective because it applies negative pressure only to the smaller area beneath the shell. As would be expected, studies also have shown that shells applying negative pressure to both the chest wall and abdomen are much more efficient than those applying negative pressure to the chest wall alone.[7] Although the wrap ventilator is usually more efficient than the shell ventilator, collapse of the jacket onto the upper chest wall and lower abdomen during use may compromise efficiency. Problems with air leaking also may reduce efficiency of the wrap and chest shell ventilators and, to a lesser extent, the iron lung.

Despite its effectiveness and reliability, the tank ventilator has a number of drawbacks, including bulk (3 m long) and weight (300 kg). It also may induce claustrophobic reactions and interferes with nursing care, although it does have portholes on the sides to facilitate access. The Portalung, chest shell, and wrap are far more portable than iron lungs, but the negative-pressure generators used with them still weigh 15 to 30 kg. The tank and wrap ventilators also often induce musculoskeletal back and shoulder pain because they require that the patient remain supine. The chest shell may be used in the sitting position, but it often causes discomfort and pressure sores at points of skin contact, particularly if fit is not optimal.

Of even greater concern, obstructive apneas associated with severe oxygen desaturations are common in patients with neuromuscular disease using negative-pressure ventilators and may necessitate a switch to alternative forms of ventilation.[19,20] This problem is likely related to the lack of preinspiratory contraction of pharyngeal muscles that prevents collapse of upper airway structures during normal patient-initiated breathing.[21] Traditional negative-pressure ventilators lack patient-triggered modes, making the upper airway susceptible to collapse prior to ventilator-triggered breaths. It remains to be seen whether newer negative-pressure ventilators with a patient-triggered mode, such as the NEV-100 (Respironics, Inc., Westminster, CO), will alleviate this problem. Because of these limitations, negative-pressure ventilators have become second-line choices for delivery of noninvasive ventilation.

ABDOMINAL DISPLACEMENT VENTILATORS

The rocking bed[22] and intermittent abdominal pressure respirator (pneumobelt)[9] both rely on displacement of the abdominal viscera to assist diaphragm motion and hence ventilation. The rocking bed consists of a mattress on a motorized platform that oscillates in an arc of approximately 40 degrees on a fulcrum at hip level. The patient lies supine with the head and knees raised slightly to prevent sliding. When the head moves down, the abdominal contents and diaphragm slide cephalad, assisting exhalation. When the head rises, the abdominal contents and diaphragm slide caudad, assisting inhalation. The rocking rate is between 12 and 24 times per minute, adjusted to optimize patient comfort and minute volume, as measured with a hand-held spirometer or magnetometer. The chief advantages of the rocking bed are ease of operation, lack of encumbrances, and patient comfort. Limitations include bulkiness and lack of portability.

The pneumobelt consists of a corset-like device that wraps around the patient's midsection and holds an inflatable rubber bladder firmly against the anterior abdomen.[9] A positive-pressure ventilator intermittently inflates the bladder, compressing the abdominal contents, forcing the diaphragm cephalad, and actively assisting exhalation. During bladder deflation with the patient seated or standing, gravity pulls the abdominal contents and diaphragm back to the original position, assisting inhalation. Bladder inflation pressures are usually between 35 and 50 cmH$_2$O, higher pressures yielding larger tidal volumes. Desired minute volume is then achieved by adjusting ventilator rate, usually between 12 and 22 inflations per minute. The pneumobelt can be mounted easily on a wheelchair and leaves the hands and face unencumbered, facilitating desk work. Cosmetically pleasing to patients, it is easily hidden under clothing. Because it requires gravity to pull the diaphragm down during bladder deflation, the patient must sit at an angle of at least 30 degrees. Hence nocturnal use is limited to patients who can sleep sitting up.[23] The most useful application of the pneumobelt is to serve as a daytime adjunct to other forms of noninvasive ventilation nocturnally.

Both the rocking bed and pneumobelt are especially well suited for use in patients with bilateral diaphragmatic paralysis because their main action is to assist diaphragm motion.[5] However, they are both relatively ineffective ventilators and are of limited use in patients suffering from acute worsening of their respiratory failure, particularly if complicated by secretion retention. Furthermore, efficacy depends on abdominal compliance, so patients with severe kyphoscoliosis or excessive obesity may not be ventilated adequately.

OTHER METHODS OF VENTILATORY ASSISTANCE FOR NEUROMUSCULAR DISEASES

Diaphragm pacing and glossopharyngeal breathing are used in selected patients to enhance independence from mechanical ventilation. Diaphragm pacing consists of a radiofrequency transmitter and antenna that send stimulatory signals to an internal receiver and electrode placed surgically near the phrenic nerve, usually in the supraclavicular region.[10] Use of diaphragm pacing is limited to patients who have an intact diaphragm and phrenic nerve such as those with quadriplegia due to high spinal cord lesions or with central hypoventilation. Recent advances in NPPV have virtually eliminated the need for diaphragm pacing in patients with central hypoventilation.[24]

Diaphragm pacing has a number of limitations, including high cost, a lack of alarms despite the potential to fail abruptly, and the tendency to produce upper airway obstruction by the same mechanism as negative-pressure ventilators, preventing closure of the tracheostomy in 90 percent of users.[25] In addition, there are no controlled studies that demonstrate long-term efficacy. Nonetheless, diaphragm pacers are very easy to use, highly portable, and free patients from the need to be connected to positive-pressure ventilators. Thus occasional patients with high cord lesions may still prefer diaphragm pacing to other types of ventilatory assistance. Its chief application at the present time appears to be in children who have difficulty adapting to other forms of ventilation.[24]

Glossopharyngeal or "frog" breathing uses intermittent gulping motions of the tongue and pharyngeal muscles to force air into the trachea.[26] When initiating a "gulp," the patient lowers and then raises the tongue against the palate in a piston-like fashion, injecting air into the trachea. With practice, each gulp injects approximately 50 to 150 mL of air in approximately 0.5 s. The patient closes the glottis after each gulp to prevent escape of air and rapidly repeats the gulping until a "tidal volume" of approximately 500 or 600 mL is achieved. The air is then exhaled and the series of gulps repeated 8 to 10 times per minute so that a normal minute volume can be achieved. The technique can be used instead of mechanical ventilatory assistance for periods of up to several hours, even in patients with severely weakened lower respiratory muscles. It also can be used to augment individual breaths in patients with low tidal volumes or to achieve inhaled volumes of 2 to 2 1/2 L to assist in coughing. The obvious advantage of the technique is that it requires no mechanical appliances, but its use is limited to patients who have relatively intact upper airway musculature and more or less normal lungs. Some patients have difficulty learning the technique, and aerophagia may be a problem. Good candidates include those with high spinal cord injuries or postpolio syndrome and selected patients with other neuromuscular diseases.[27]

ASSISTING COUGH IN NEUROMUSCULAR DISEASES

Most neuromuscular diseases cause weakness of both inspiratory and expiratory muscles. The approaches to ventilatory assistance described earlier serve mainly as aids to inspiration. However, weakened expiratory muscles in combination with a markedly reduced vital capacity lead to severe cough impairment. The inability to cough effectively is tolerable for patients who have minimal airway secretions, but the onset of acute bronchitis may precipitate a life-threatening crisis. In this situation, or in others where secretions must be mobilized, strategies to assist expiratory function should be employed.

Cough effectiveness depends on the ability to generate adequate cough airflows. In addition to sufficient inspiratory (to achieve a vital capacity > 1.5 L) and expiratory muscle

function, this necessitates adequate airway conductance and intact glottic function so that explosive release of intrathoracic pressure can generate high peak expiratory cough flows.[28] Bach and coworkers[29] have demonstrated that tracheostomies can be removed succesfully when peak cough flows of more than 3 L/s can be achieved. Considering that many patients with severe neuromuscular disease are too weakened to achieve cough flows in this range spontaneously, cough-assistive techniques should be applied to augment cough flows.

The simplest maneuver to augment cough flow is manually assisted or "quad" coughing. This consists of firm, quick thrusts applied to the subcostal area using the palms of the hands, timed to coincide with the patient's cough effort. This technique should be taught to caregivers of patients with severe neuromuscular disease to be used in the event of acute bronchitis or any time the patient is afflicted by secretion retention. With practice, this technique can be applied effectively and with minimal discomfort to the patient. The patient should be semiupright when manually assisted coughing is applied, but regurgitation of gastric contents may still be a concern, and caution should be exercised after meals.

Although manually assisted coughing may enhance expiratory force, it does not augment inspired volume. Patients with severely restricted volumes, therefore, may still achieve insufficient cough flows, even when assisted by skilled caregivers. To overcome this problem, mechanically assisted breaths may be necessary.[30] One approach is to "stack" breaths using glossopharyngeal breathing or volume-limited ventilation and then to cough using manual assistance. Another is to use a cough inexsufflator (J.H. Emerson, Inc., Cambridge, MA) that delivers positive pressure of 30 to 40 cmH₂O via a face mask and then rapidly switches to an equal negative pressure.[30] The positive pressure assists delivery of an adequate tidal volume, and the negative pressure has the effect of simulating the rapid expiratory flows generated by a cough. The increase in expiratory flows may be potentiated by combination with manually assisted coughing.

Other devices, such as the percussive ventilator and Hayek oscillator, have theoretical advantages over some of the other techniques for assisting secretion removal[29] and may be tried, but evidence to support their use in neuromuscular disease is virtually nonexistent. Whatever approach is adopted, it is extremely important for practitioners caring for patients with chronic respiratory failure due to neuromuscular disease to be cognizant of the various approaches for enhancing secretion removal. Particularly when noninvasive ventilation is being employed and there is no direct access to the airway, these cough-assistive techniques are critical in maintaining airway patency and permitting long-term support in nonhospital settings.

Pathophysiology of Respiratory Failure in Neuromuscular Disease

The mechanisms responsible for respiratory failure in neuromuscular diseases are summarized in Fig. 49-5. Ultimately, the root cause of respiratory failure in neuromuscular diseases is muscle weakness, but the rate of progression, severity, and distribution of involvement lead to a variety of pre-

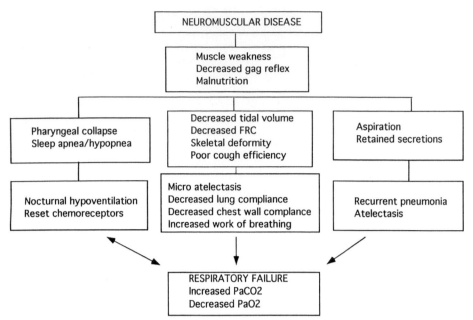

FIGURE 49-5 Schema depicting pathogenesis of respiratory failure in neuromuscular disease. See text for details.

sentations. Also, respiratory center involvement may occur primarily as a component of the disease process (myotonic dystrophy or some cases of poliomyelitis) or secondarily as a consequence of resetting of the respiratory center sensitivity for CO_2 because of progressive hypercapnia.

Conceptually, three groups of muscles can be considered as critically important for breathing. First are the inspiratory muscles, including the diaphragm, external intercostals, and accessories, that are essential for sustaining ventilation. Indexes of inspiratory muscle function in common use include the maximal inspiratory pressure (PImax) and inspiratory capacity. These are only rough indicators, but severe reductions are predictive of ventilatory failure. For instance, when the PImax falls below 30 percent of predicted or the ratio of tidal volume to vital capacity rises above 60 percent, respiratory muscle fatigue and incipient hypercapnia are likely.[31,32] This failure to adequately ventilate is potentiated by other consequences of prolonged neuromuscular weakness, including kyphoscoliosis and atelectasis that reduce chest wall and lung compliance, further exacerbating the restriction.

The expiratory muscles, including the abdominals and internal intercostals, are also commonly involved in neuromuscular diseases. Impairment of these muscles reduces the vital capacity and, most important, compromises cough efficiency. Indexes of expiratory muscle performance include the maximal expiratory pressure (PEmax) and expiratory reserve volume. Significant reductions in these measures correspond with the inability to generate an adequate cough airflow, placing the patient at risk for secretion retention.[29] This, in combination with impairment of the bulbar muscles, the third major group, leads to a potentially lethal scenario, where the patient aspirates because of swallowing impairment and then develops respiratory failure due to mucus plugging because of an ineffective cough.

Respiratory failure in this setting may occur acutely, often as a consequence of a respiratory infection that increases the volume of secretions, or it may be insidious, with the gradual retention of CO_2. The pathogenesis of this slow process is not fully understood, but it is thought to be related to a resetting of the respiratory center sensitivity for CO_2. Partly as a result of upper respiratory tract weakness that predisposes to sleep-disordered breathing and partly related to "central fatigue," the patient hypoventilates nocturnally, with retention of bicarbonate and a progressive blunting of respiratory drive.[32] *Central fatigue* is a hypothetical downregulation of the respiratory center in response to severe respiratory muscle weakness that is thought to avert the development of frank peripheral muscle fatigue. Symptoms associated with hypercapnia and poor sleep quality subsequently occur, including restless sleep, fatigue, morning headache, and daytime hypersomnolence, often in the absence of dyspnea or symptoms directly attributable to the respiratory system.

These mechanisms that contribute to the development of respiratory failure also highlight the therapeutic avenues taken to support such patients. First, ventilation is provided to assist the inspiratory muscles and alleviate hypoventilation. This ventilation is usually intermittent, often just nocturnal, unless the patient is incapable of breathing spontaneously during the daytime. Second, expiratory muscles are assisted, using physical maneuvers or mechanical devices, as described previously. Third, severe bulbar involvement is treated with positioning to avoid aspiration, anticholinergics to minimize saliva, and gastric tube placement to maintain adequate nutrition. Fortunately, many neuromuscular diseases involve only one or two of the major muscle groups and may progress very slowly, so prognosis can be favorable. Specific attributes of particular neuromuscular diseases will be discussed later. The next section examines the evidence for the utility of some of the therapeutic approaches.

Evidence for the Efficacy of Noninvasive Ventilation in Neuromuscular Diseases

Numerous uncontrolled trials have reported efficacy of noninvasive ventilation for many types of neuromuscular dis-

TABLE 49-1 Studies on the Use of Noninvasive Positive-Pressure Ventilation[a] in Chronic Respiratory Failure

References, First Author, Year	Types of Mask/Ventilator	DIAGNOSIS		Symptom Relief	ARTERIAL BLOOD GASES				Duration
		COPD[b]	RTD[b]		BASELINE		AFTER TRIAL		
					P_{CO_2}	P_{O_2}	P_{CO_2}	P_{O_2}	
Kerby, 1987[14]	Nasal/VOL		5	Yes	58.8	63.0	44.3	77.8	>3 mos
Bach, 1987[13]	Nasal/VOL		5	Yes					
Ellis, 1987[37]	Nasal/VOL		5	Yes	70.0	61.0	46.0	83	3–12 mos
Carroll, 1988[87]	Nasal/VOL	4	6	Yes	61.5	45.8	51.0	60.8	3–18 mos
Leger, 1989[40]	Nasal/VOL		29 (5)	Yes	52.3	58.0	41.0	71.0	12 mos
Bach, 1990[36]	Nasal/VOL		52	Yes	68.0[c]	46.0[c]			19.8 mos
Heckmatt, 1990[39]	Nasal/VOL		14 (4)	Yes	61.5	50.3			18 mos
Gay, 1991[38]	Nasal/VOL	4 (1)	22 (4)	Yes	64.0	52.0	51.0	68	5.8 mos
Goldstein, 1991[45]	Nasal/VOL		6	Yes	60.3	43.5	51.6	64.2	14 mos
Mean					61.7	53.5	47.7	69.8	
Total		8 (1)	144 (13)						
Percentage success		88	92						

[a] BiPAP, bilevel positive airway pressure; COPD, chronic obstructive pulmonary disease; RTD, restrictive thoracic disease; VOL, volume ventilator.
[b] Number of patients (number of failures).
[c] End-tidal P_{CO_2} data from 10 patients studied overnight.
SOURCE: From Meyer TJ, Hill NS: Noninvasive positive pressure ventilation to treat respiratory failure. *Ann Intern Med* 120:760–770, 1994, with permission.

ease. Experience from the polio epidemics demonstrated that noninvasive ventilatory techniques could be used for decades to support patients with chronic respiratory failure.[33] During the early 1980s, studies reported that nocturnal ventilatory assistance using mainly negative-pressure ventilation improved gas exchange and symptoms of hypoventilation for extended periods of time.[34,35] Beginning in 1987, studies appeared showing similar results using NPPV[13,16,36–40] (Table 49-1). Several of these studies also demonstrated that when patients were switched from negative-pressure ventilation to NPPV, rapid eye movement (REM) sleep–related oxygen desaturations were ameliorated, and patients generally preferred NPPV.[37,39] Although no prospective, randomized, controlled trials were reported, all the uncontrolled trials were favorable.

In view of the uniformly favorable results of the uncontrolled trials, investigators were reluctant to perform randomized, prospective trials that would include unventilated controls. Instead, two groups of investigators[16,41] observed the effect of temporary withdrawal of NPPV from patients with chronic respiratory failure due to neuromuscular disease (or chest wall deformities) who had been previously stabilized by it. They reasoned that if NPPV in fact improved daytime and nocturnal gas exchange and symptoms, deterioration in these variables should occur during temporary withdrawal. Both studies demonstrated a substantial worsening of nocturnal hypoventilation accompanied by deterioration of sleep quality or symptoms of sleepiness after an average of 1 week of withdrawal. There was no deterioration in daytime pulmonary function, but trends toward worsening of daytime gas exchange were detected. Using patients as their own controls, these studies provide the strongest evidence available that nocturnal noninvasive ventilation ameliorates nocturnal hypoventilation and improves sleep quality, symptoms, and daytime gas exchange in patients with chronic respiratory failure due to neuromuscular disease. Despite the lack of randomized, controlled trials, the uniformly favorable evidence from uncontrolled and tempo-

rary withdrawal trials is considered by most authorities in the field to be sufficient.

Mechanisms of Action

The mechanism of action for noninvasive ventilatory support in conscious, cooperative patients with neuromuscular disease seems straightforward. The patient positions upper airway structures and suppresses breathing efforts to allow the ventilator to intermittently increase the transpulmonary gradient, inflate the lungs, and assume part or even all of the breathing work. How adaptation of noninvasive ventilation during sleep occurs is not so clear, however. In sleeping patients using NPPV, the respiratory neurons must maintain upper airway patency to permit air entry into the lungs while suppressing inspiratory muscle activity so that the ventilator is able to assist ventilation. Although this process is poorly understood, recent studies on normal sleeping subjects demonstrate that the size of the glottic aperture is important during use of NPPV.[42] With controlled ventilation, the glottis narrows when the patient falls asleep and then narrows further when minute volume is increased, perhaps as a protective mechanism against hyperventilation.[42] During spontaneous breathing modes such as pressure-support ventilation, glottic aperture is not as important in determining airway patency.[42] These findings suggest that upper airway control mechanisms are important in determining the efficacy of NPPV and that merely increasing tidal volume to compensate for air leaking may be counterproductive. Much remains unknown about the role of physiologic responses of the upper airway and respiratory control center in determining the success of NPPV. Changes in nasal resistance and the ability to minimize escape of air through the mouth while suppressing inspiratory muscle activity may be important, but further studies evaluating these and other possible factors are needed.

It is also unclear how reversal of chronic hypoventilation

occurs, sometimes after as little as 4 to 6 h of ventilatory assistance nightly. Two main theories have been proposed to explain this improvement. The first, often referred to as the *rest hypothesis,* posits that inspiratory muscles in patients with respiratory insufficiency are chronically fatigued.[32,43] Intermittent ventilatory assistance rests the fatigued muscles, improving daytime respiratory muscle function and allowing improved rates of ventilation during ventilator-free periods. Studies supporting this theory have demonstrated that inspiratory muscles do indeed rest during use of negative- or positive-pressure ventilation[31,44] and that, at least in some studies, inspiratory muscle strength or endurance improves after periods of mechanical ventilatory assistance.[43,45,46] However, chronic respiratory muscle fatigue has never been defined adequately, nor has it been demonstrated consistently in patients with neuromuscular disease and chronic respiratory failure.[32] Also, many studies have found no improvement in inspiratory muscle strength after successful application of noninvasive ventilation.[38,39,47]

The second theory proposes that patients with respiratory insufficiency undergo a gradual resetting of the respiratory *setpoint* for CO_2. Particularly during sleep, hypoventilation worsens, leading to a progressively higher CO_2 setpoint and increasing daytime CO_2 retention.[32] Nighttime assisted ventilation reduces nocturnal hypoventilation, lowering the CO_2 setpoint and thereby daytime Pa_{CO_2}. One study supporting this theory demonstrated that after daytime CO_2 had been lowered by several weeks of nocturnal assisted ventilation, hypoventilation was less severe during a night without assisted ventilation than it had been before nocturnal ventilation was started, suggesting a lowering of the CO_2 setpoint.[48] Another study demonstrated that after temporary discontinuation of nocturnal nasal ventilation in patients with chronic respiratory failure previously stabilized by it, nocturnal hypoventilation and daytime symptoms recurred without evidence of respiratory muscle dysfunction.[16]

Although these latter studies favor the second theory, neither theory has been proven beyond doubt. Further, the theories are not mutually exclusive, and both may apply to a greater or lesser degree depending on the patient. Of course, exceptions to both theories undoubtedly exist, such as occasional patients with central hypoventilation who continue to hypoventilate if ventilator assistance is applied only intermittently.

Evaluation of the Neuromuscular Patient with Suspected Respiratory Failure

Table 49-2 depicts the evaluation of respiratory impairment in patients with neuromuscular disease. With the exception of neuromuscular syndromes known to cause primary impairment of central respiratory drive, neuromuscular diseases rarely cause respiratory failure until pulmonary function has become severely impaired. Thus serial measurement of pulmonary functions including spirography, lung volume measurements, and maximal inspiratory and expiratory pressures is sufficient, initially, to monitor patients.[49] The frequency of monitoring is determined by the rapidity of progression of the neuromuscular syndrome and may range from every 1 to 2 months to yearly. In addition, symptoms and signs that suggest daytime hypoventilation or a sleep

TABLE 49-2 Commonly Used Tests for Evaluation of Respiratory Impairment in Neuromuscular Diseases

History and physical examination
  Laboratory evaluation
  Spirometry, supine and upright
  Peak expiratory flow
  Lung volumes
  Maximal inspiratory and expiratory pressures
  Arterial blood gases
Sleep evaluation
  Nocturnal oximetry
  Multichannel recording
  Full polysomnography
Other
  Transdiaphragmatic pressures (in selected patients)
  Thyroid function tests
  Chemistries, including potassium, phosphate, magnesium

disturbance should be sought, including morning headache, daytime hypersomnolence, nightmares, inability to concentrate, enuresis, and increased daytime fatigue (Table 49-3).

Once vital capacity drops below 1.2 to 1.5 L (or <40 to 50 percent of predicted) or maximal inspiratory pressure is less than 30 percent of predicted, daytime blood gases should be monitored periodically as well. We do not believe that noninvasive determinations of oxygen saturation or P_{CO_2} are sufficiently accurate to replace blood gas determinations, although they may be used as part of a serial monitoring program to assess responses to therapy. Close attention also should be paid to the pattern of respiratory muscle involvement. Pulmonary function tests may reveal greater involvement of inspiratory than expiratory muscles, or vice versa, dictating different therapeutic approaches. Diaphragm weakness or paralysis, which may be the sole presenting manifestation of some neuromuscular syndromes, also should be sought. Orthopnea and abdominal paradox during breathing in the supine position and reduction in supine vital capacity strongly suggest this diagnosis, but esophageal and gastric pressure monitoring may be indicated for confirmation. Practitioners also should consider possible aggra-

TABLE 49-3 Symptoms of Respiratory Impairment in Neuromuscular Diseases

Constitutional
  Generalized fatigue
  Weakness
Cardiopulmonary
  Dyspnea
  Lower-extremity edema
  Orthopnea
  Secretion retention
CNS
  Early morning headaches
  Daytime hypersomnolence
  Mood disturbances
  Psychiatric problems
Sleep
  Restless sleep
  Nightmares
  Enuresis
  Frequent arousals

vating conditions that may contribute to hypercapnia, such as obstructive sleep apnea, hypothyroidism, congestive heart failure, or electrolyte disturbances.[49]

Sleep monitoring is indicated in the presence of symptoms that suggest a sleep disturbance, particularly when pulmonary functions are diminished. Other comorbid conditions that justify performance of a sleep study include obesity and a history of snoring. Sleep-disordered breathing almost always precedes the onset of daytime hypoventilation in these patients, and sleep monitoring of oximetry or P_{CO_2} may detect evidence of nocturnal hypoventilation, even in the absence of daytime hypercapnia. The need for routine full polysomnography has not been established in the evaluation of patients with neuromuscular disease; overnight oximetry or multichannel recording (oximetry, oronasal airflow, chest wall impedance) in the home may be adequate to detect nocturnal breathing disorders in many patients.

All practitioners should be aware that patients with neuromuscular disease, particularly those with severe limb weakness, may have no dyspnea or other symptoms directly attributable to the respiratory system, even after they have developed severe hypercapnia. As shown in Table 49-3, the symptoms associated with severe pulmonary dysfunction in these patients may be quite subtle and are often related to sleep disturbance. Such symptoms in patients with neuromuscular weakness should prompt measurement of blood gases and consideration of a sleep evaluation. Hypnotics and tranquilizers should never be given as initial therapies for these patients because these drugs may aggravate the respiratory failure or even precipitate respiratory arrest.

Indications for Noninvasive Ventilatory Assistance in Neuromuscular Disease

Based on the available evidence, the best established indication for noninvasive ventilation in patients with neuromuscular diseases is gradually worsening symptomatic hypercapnia (Table 49-4). Other contributing reversible conditions should be optimally treated, secretions should be controllable, and the patient should be able to adequately protect the upper airway. Bulbar involvement is not an absolute contraindication to noninvasive ventilation, as long as cough is not too severely impaired, although outcomes are poorer

TABLE 49-4 Indications and Contraindications for Noninvasive Ventilation in Neuromuscular Diseases

Indications
  Gas exchange
    Daytime hypercapnia ($Pa_{CO_2} > 45$)
               or
    Nocturnal hypoventilation (sustained O_2 saturation <88%)
               and
    Symptom or signs (see Table 49-3)
    Cor pulmonale
Relative contraindications
  Swallowing or cough impairment
  Need for continuous ventilation
Absolute contraindications
  Uncontrollable secretion retention
  Inability to cooperate

than in patients with intact upper airway function.[50] Other acceptable indications for noninvasive ventilation in patients with neuromuscular disease include exacerbations caused by acute respiratory infections. During these episodes, noninvasive ventilation may be tried initially, or if secretion retention is problematic, temporary translaryngeal intubation may be necessary. However, once secretions have diminished, noninvasive ventilation may be useful in expediting extubation. Depending on subsequent recovery of pulmonary function, some of these patients will continue to use noninvasive ventilation on a long-term basis, whereas others may no longer need ventilatory assistance, at least temporarily. Should such patients develop a pattern of repeated hospitalizations for respiratory failure, noninvasive ventilation may be useful in reducing the need for rehospitalization and permitting management of some acute exacerbations in the home. No controlled studies have established the efficacy of noninvasive ventilation for these latter indications, but recent studies, mainly in patients with chronic obstructive pulmonary disease (COPD), suggest that noninvasive positive-pressure ventilation for acute respiratory failure improves gas exchange and reduces the need for intubation.[51,52] Patients receiving noninvasive ventilation for acute respiratory failure must be monitored closely, and invasive ventilation should be readily available in the event of further decompensation.

More controversial issues with regard to indications for noninvasive ventilation in patients with neuromuscular disease include its role in patients who have only nocturnal hypoventilation without frank daytime hypercapnia and the question of whether noninvasive ventilation should be started "prophylactically" before the onset of hypercapnia or symptoms in the hope that the progression of respiratory impairment can be slowed. As discussed earlier, sleep-disordered breathing and nocturnal hypoventilation probably precede daytime CO_2 retention in many neuromuscular disease patients. Thus symptoms to suggest sleep-disordered breathing should prompt a sleep evaluation, and if significant obstructive sleep apnea or nocturnal hypoventilation (sustained O_2 saturation < 88 percent) is found, therapy with CPAP or noninvasive ventilation is indicated.

The issue of whether to treat neuromuscular disease patients before the onset of daytime hypercapnia or symptoms has not been resolved. Partly based on the results of the randomized, controlled study[53] on the "prophylactic" use of NPPV in Duchenne muscular dystrophy patients that was stopped early because of excess mortality in the NPPV group, most practitioners now await the onset of symptoms before recommending initiation of noninvasive ventilation. This is also a pragmatic issue, because compliance is usually poor unless the patient is motivated by the desire for symptom relief.

Noninvasive ventilation is relatively contraindicated for some neuromuscular disease patients (see Table 49-4). Invasive ventilation is preferred when the patient has severe impairment of swallowing and is unable to adequately clear secretions or protect the airway. Inability to cooperate with noninvasive ventilation is another reason to consider invasive ventilation, such as in very small children or patients with severe intellectual impairment. The need for continuous ventilatory assistance is another potential indication for invasive ventilation. Some investigators report success with noninvasive ventilatory techniques, even when patients have little or no measurable vital capacity,[54] but this should be considered only in patients with intact upper airway function, such as those with high spinal cord lesions, and only when a staff highly skilled in noninvasive ventilatory and cough-assistive techniques is available. Ethical issues also may preclude the use of mechanical ventilation. Some patients may decline the use of any form of assisted ventilation but more often are willing to try noninvasive ventilation rather than invasive ventilation. Practitioners must discuss such issues before the onset of severe respiratory failure, making certain that patients are fully informed about the potential consequences of their decisions and that they and their loved ones are prepared and supported as much as possible for the anticipated outcomes.

Initiation of Noninvasive Ventilation in Patients with Neuromuscular Disease

Before initiating assisted ventilation, the practitioner should review the goals, as exemplified in Table 49-5, which may vary among patients and which may influence the choice of ventilator system. For instance, a patient who feels that portability and convenience are priorities may prefer a compact system with few monitoring features, whereas someone who wishes to maximize safety and reliability may desire greater monitoring capabilities or even consider switching to an invasive system if airway protection becomes compromised.

Although many ventilator options are available to patients with neuromuscular disease, NPPV has become the modality of first choice for most patients because of comfort, convenience, and portability advantages. NPPV is initiated by selecting a properly fitting, comfortable interface. Most often this consists of a standard nasal mask connected to a positive-pressure ventilator. For acutely hospitalized patients, a standard "critical care" ventilator in the assist/control or pressure-support mode may be used, but for long-term use, a portable positive-pressure ventilator is preferred. The best method for optimizing ventilator settings has not been established, but we prefer the assist/control setting for either pressure- or volume-limited modes because many neuromuscular patients breathe at the controlled backup rate while asleep. The backup rate is therefore set at slightly below the awake spontaneous breathing rate to let the patient "trigger" during wakefulness and permit controlled breathing when the spontaneous rate slows during sleep.

The tidal volume (or inspiratory pressure) is then gradu-

ally increased until the patient's limit of tolerance is reached or a physiologic target is met. The latter could be an increase in assisted tidal volume to 30 to 50 percent over baseline or a 5 to 10 cmH$_2$O drop in Pa$_{CO_2}$, as determined by arterial blood gases or end-tidal CO$_2$ monitoring after the first 30 to 60 min of ventilation. These targets may not be attainable in many patients who sense mask or air-pressure discomfort before meeting them. It is important to prioritize patient comfort over arbitrary physiologic targets, particularly in the chronic setting, in order to encourage patient compliance. For patients needing O$_2$ supplementation, many ventilators have oxygen blenders. However, bilevel-type ventilators lack these, so oxygen tubing is connected directly to the mask or to a T-connector in the ventilator tubing, with liter flow titrated to oximetry readings or arterial blood gas results.

Initially, coaching is necessary to encourage patients to breathe in synchrony with the ventilator and to allow it to assist their breathing. Fortunately, most patients learn to synchronize with the ventilator fairly rapidly. The initial duration of ventilatory assistance depends on patient tolerance and the severity of the respiratory impairment. In patients with acute respiratory failure, ventilatory assistance may be required initially for more than 20 h per day,[52] with mask removal only for communication or ingestion of meals. Duration of use is then tapered as the patient is stabilized. For patients with stable chronic respiratory failure, initial use may amount to only a few hours a night. After the initial trial, the patient is encouraged to begin nocturnal use for as long as tolerated. The amount of time needed before patients are able to sleep through the night using the device is highly variable, ranging from a few days to a few months.[16] A minority of patients may be unable to adapt at all, and these patients should be given trials of alternative noninvasive ventilators, or if indicated and desired, tracheostomy placement should be contemplated.

Noninvasive ventilators besides NPPV are now considered second-line choices, indicated when patients fail to tolerate or respond favorably to NPPV or express a strong initial preference for them. They function less well than NPPV in patients with severe chest wall deformities and should not be used for patients with significant obstructive sleep apnea unless combined with CPAP.[20] Initiation follows guidelines similar to those used for NPPV, but of course, specific approaches depend on the device being applied and patient need for and tolerance of ventilatory assistance. In general, these devices, when selected, are used on patients with chronic respiratory failure, and the initial trial should be performed in a relaxed, daytime setting. Although our current practice with NPPV is to use outpatient initiation in most patients with chronic respiratory failure who are otherwise stable and satisfy requirements for home mechanical ventilation (Table 49-6), we still prefer a brief hospitalization for other noninvasive ventilators to encourage thorough familiarization with the function and application of the device. As with NPPV, respiratory rate is usually set at approximately slightly below spontaneous breathing rate, although exceptions include the rocking bed, in which rates exceeding 16 may reduce tidal volume,[55] and diaphragm pacing, where the lowest tolerated rate minimizes the potential for the development of diaphragm fatigue.[10] With negative-pressure ventilators and the pneumobelt, inspiratory pressures are begun at minimal levels to facilitate patient adaptation and

TABLE 49-5 Goals of Noninvasive Ventilation in Neuromuscular Diseases

1. Stabilize and reverse hypoventilation
2. Improve nocturnal ventilation and sleep quality
3. Enhance quality of life
4. Improve physical/psychological function
5. Reduce complications of respiratory failure (polycythemia, cor pulmonale)
6. Avoid invasive ventilation/tracheostomy
7. Provide cost benefit to long-term care
8. Prolong survival

TABLE 49-6 Requirements for Home Mechanical Ventilation

1. Motivated patient who is clinically stable
2. Adequate financial resources
3. Adequate home care team
   a. Trained family members and/or caregivers
   b. Home respiratory therapy company
   c. Visiting nurses
   d. Home health aides
   e. Physician
4. Physical therapy program
5. Psychological counseling and support for patient and family
6. Vocational rehabilitation as needed

are increased gradually to the limit of patient tolerance or to a preestablished end point, as discussed earlier. After the initial trial, nocturnal ventilation is begun as with NPPV. If the patient fails to adapt to one device, trials with others may still be successful. Whatever ventilator or combination of ventilators is selected, the aim should be to optimize patient comfort, independence, and safety, taking patient preferences into account. Typical initial settings for the various ventilators are shown in Table 49-7.

Monitoring and Follow-Up

Patients should be seen frequently during the early adaptation period to assisted ventilation. A respiratory therapist should visit the patient at home to reinforce proper use of the equipment and to make further adjustments to optimize fit and comfort. The patient also should have physician follow-up to check on symptoms and gas exchange, using arterial blood gases or end-tidal CO_2 monitoring with oximetry. The Pa_{CO_2} usually falls gradually over a period of weeks as duration of nocturnal use increases. Symptoms of hypoventilation usually resolve over a similar period of time. There is no consensus on optimal daytime blood gas values in patients with neuromuscular disease receiving nocturnal ventilatory assistance, but complete normalization of Pa_{CO_2} is not necessary in our experience. Daytime Pa_{CO_2} values in the high 40s or even middle 50s mmHg are acceptable as long as signs of cor pulmonale and symptoms are absent. However, should symptoms persist, further adjustments should be made. In addition, nocturnal monitoring of oximetry, airflow, and chest wall motion should be performed after the patient has begun using the ventilator for at least a few hours nightly.

This is particularly important in patients using negative-pressure ventilators because of the frequent occurrence of obstructive sleep apneas and severe desaturations. However, it is also important in patients using other devices including NPPV who may be ventilated inadequately because of insufficient inflation pressures or excessive air leaking. Inspiratory pressures or tidal volumes may be adjusted gradually upward as tolerated by the patient, and air leaking may be controlled by refitting the mask and use of chin straps or nose pledgets, depending on the type of interface and the source of the leak. Oxygen supplementation is usually unnecessary once hypoventilation has been reversed.

Once gas exchange has been brought into the desired range and symptoms have been controlled adequately, patients with very slowly progressive neuromuscular syndromes may be seen as infrequently as two or three times yearly. At these follow-up visits, gas exchange should be reassessed using arterial blood gas determinations or noninvasive monitoring devices. Patients should be taught to recognize symptoms of hypoventilation and to contact the physician should these recur. In the event of recurrence, a daytime arterial blood gas should be checked, and if the Pa_{CO_2} has climbed, stabilization often can be restored by increasing inspiratory pressure, backup rate, or the duration of ventilatory assistance, including daytime naps. If these maneuvers are unsuccessful, nocturnal monitoring should be repeated seeking oxygen desaturations or evidence of excessive air leaking. Rebreathing of exhaled air has been proposed as one mechanism for failure to improve Pa_{CO_2} in patients using bilevel-type ventilators that have single ventilator tubes.[56] This problem can be minimized by using expiratory pressures of at least 4 cmH_2O that maintain adequate ventilator airflow during exhalation and by using exhalation valves that minimize rebreathing.

Complications

Complications of noninvasive ventilation depend on the type of ventilator and/or interface selected, and although a complete discussion is beyond the scope of this chapter, practitioners should familiarize themselves with the potential pitfalls associated with whichever device is chosen. With regard to NPPV, the most common complications are usually minor in nature and are related to the interface, airflow or pressure, or the ventilator itself.[57] These include nasal or oral congestion or dryness, skin ulcers over the bridge of the

TABLE 49-7 Usual Settings for Noninvasive Ventilation

	Pressure or Volume	Rate
Portable positive-pressure ventilator		
Bilevel	10–18 cmH_2O (inspiratory)	12–20
	2–5 cmH_2O (expiratory)	
Volume	10–15 mL/kg	12–22
Negative-pressure ventilators		
Tank	−12 to −18 cmH_2O	12–16
Wrap	−25 to −35 cmH_2O	14–20
Cuirass	−30 to −40 cmH_2O	14–20
Rocking bed	—	12–20
Pneumobelt	30–50 cmH_2O	12–22

TABLE 49-8 Complications of Noninvasive Ventilation

Common
  Air leaking
  Nasal/oral congestion/dryness
  Eye irritation
  Gastric insufflation
  Nasal bridge redness/ulceration
Less common
  Failure to tolerate or ventilate
Unusual
  Aspiration
  Pneumothorax

nose, ear or sinus pain, eye irritation due to air leakage underneath the mask, and gastric insufflation (Table 49-8). These problems are treated with local measures, including refitting of masks or headgear, using alternative interfaces, or adjusting delivered pressures or volumes. To minimize the risk of skin ulceration, proper mask fitting is essential, and use of the manufacturer's fitting gauges is encouraged. The problem is treated by reducing strap tension, placing protective materials on the ulcerated area, or switching to alternative interfaces such as nasal pillows or mouthpieces. Excessive air leaking around the mask or through the mouth can interfere with efficacy. This problem may be ameliorated by refitting of the mask, use of chin straps, or switching to an alternative interface.

Applications of Noninvasive Ventilation in Specific Neuromuscular Diseases

Most studies on the use of noninvasive ventilation in neuromuscular diseases have included patients with a variety of neuromuscular syndromes (Table 49-9). If only one or two patients have been described within a larger series, it is difficult to dissect out the unique responses of a specific neuromuscular disease to noninvasive ventilation. On the other hand, a few series have focused on single neuromuscular diseases, or larger series have had sufficient numbers of patients with the more common neuromuscular diseases to warrant specific commentary. The following will focus on the more commonly encountered neuromuscular diseases

TABLE 49-9 Neuromuscular Disorders Commonly Treated with Noninvasive Ventilation

Stable or slowly progressive
  Postpolio syndrome
  High spinal cord lesion
  Muscular dystrophies
    Duchenne
    Beckers
    Limb girdle
    Myotonic dystrophy
  Multiple sclerosis
Rapidly progressive
  Motoneuron disease (amyotrophic lateral sclerosis)
  Bilateral diaphragm paralysis
  Guillain-Barré ⎫ Noninvasive ventilation
  Myasthenia gravis ⎰ rarely used

that are managed with noninvasive ventilation and will draw on the literature as well as our personal experience in discussing relevant management issues.

STABLE OR SLOWLY PROGRESSIVE NEUROMUSCULAR DISEASES

POLIOMYELITIS AND POSTPOLIO SYNDROME
A great deal of experience was gained in the management of neuromuscular respiratory failure during the worldwide polio epidemics that occurred during the 1920s through the 1950s. Thousands of patients were managed with tank ventilators during their acute crises, sometimes including tracheostomies if bulbar function became significantly impaired. Most patients either recovered sufficiently to become independent from mechanical ventilation or died. However, some continued to use noninvasive ventilatory devices, including tank ventilators, the more portable cuirass or wrap ventilators, rocking beds, or pneumobelts, sometimes in combination.[5] Some patients went home and continued successful use of these devices for decades, even when vital capacity was severely reduced.[33]

More recently, additional patients who had recovered from their acute respiratory paralysis have developed chronic respiratory failure due to the occurrence of postpolio syndrome. In this syndrome, previously affected muscles develop progressive weakness, presumably due to gradual neuronal loss, often two or three decades after the initial illness.[15] The development of respiratory failure as a consequence of postpolio syndrome is unusual in patients who had no respiratory involvement during their acute episode of poliomyelitis, but some patients were very young at the time and may not recall the extent of respiratory involvement. The onset of respiratory failure in these patients can be precipitated by acute respiratory infections, or it can be subtle, with the insidious development of symptoms of chronic hypoventilation, such as easy fatigability, daytime hypersomnolence, and morning headaches. Physicians must have a heightened awareness of this possibility in patients who previously have suffered respiratory complications of acute poliomyelitis.

The use of nocturnal negative-pressure ventilation to stabilize respiratory failure in these patients was first reported during the late 1970s.[7] Subsequently, Curran and Colbert[58] described the nocturnal use of cuirass ventilators or mouthpiece NPPV to reverse hypoventilation in 6 patients with postpolio syndrome, none of whom died during follow-up periods ranging up to 56 months. The largest group of patients with respiratory failure due to polio was reported by Bach and colleagues.[54] Among 257 patients with various causes of respiratory failure, 101 had polio and were managed successfully using mouthpiece ventilation for at least part of the day. Sixty-one of these patients used the mouthpiece for more than 20 h daily. Forty-six of these had minimal vital capacities and were capable of less than 10 min of spontaneous unassisted breathing. Despite this severe impairment, survival rates were excellent, with two-thirds using the ventilators for more than 10 years. Long-term outcomes are also excellent for polio patients managed with invasive ventilation, with 10-year survival rates approaching 90 percent.[59] The favorable outcomes regardless of the mode of ventilation used are most likely related to the stable nature of the neurologic defects that often progress minimally over a 10-year period. Based on these results, postpolio patients are often ideal candidates for the application of a variety of forms of noninvasive ventilation, as long as bulbar involvement has not severely impaired the ability to protect the airway. However, considering that the last large polio epidemic in the United States occurred more than 40 years ago, respiratory failure due to the complications of poliomyelitis will become a less common indication for the application of noninvasive ventilation in the future.

SPINAL CORD INJURY

The need for assisted ventilation in patients with spinal cord injury is determined largely by the level and acuity of the lesion. Patients with high cervical lesions (C1–C3) almost invariably require continuous ventilatory support because they lose all but accessory and bulbar muscle function. The diaphragm is innervated from C3 to C5, so patients with lesions between C3 and C5 have variable requirements for ventilatory support, some retaining partial diaphragm function after initial injury.[60] Patients with C5–C6 or lower lesions have intact diaphragm function and rarely need long-term ventilatory support. During the period immediately following the injury and for several weeks or months thereafter, patients with high spinal cord injuries commonly require invasive ventilatory support. Subsequently, a number of adaptations occur that can promote weaning. These include improved conditioning of the diaphragm so that it can sustain a greater workload, increased rigidity of paralyzed chest wall and abdominal muscles that reduces paradoxical movements and improves ventilatory efficiency, recovery of neurologic function that may occur in some patients, and introduction of techniques to enhance removal of secretions.[61] Because of these adaptations, 50 to 80 percent of patients with lesions at C3–C5 who initially require mechanical ventilation eventually will wean entirely.[62] As would be expected, the higher the level of the lesion, the older the patient, and the more numerous the associated injuries, the lower is the likelihood of weaning.

Because patients with high spinal cord lesions are usually left with intact bulbar function and have near-normal lung, chest wall, and abdominal compliances, the options for ventilatory support are numerous.[63,64] Following the acute injury, endotracheal intubation, via tracheostomy if the neck is too unstable, is the treatment method of first choice. Respiratory complications are common during this period, including atelectasis, pneumonia, and pulmonary embolism, and direct airway access is advantageous. However, once stabilization has occurred, attempts to wean the patient from mechanical ventilation or to switch to noninvasive modes of ventilation are indicated. If the patient has an inadequate vital capacity or fatigues easily during weaning trials, aggressive further weaning attempts may be counterproductive. Positive-pressure ventilation via a tracheostomy is usually continued in this setting,[62] but trials of noninvasive ventilation also should be considered.[63]

Positive-pressure ventilation, via either the nose or mouth, is the noninvasive method of first choice for nocturnal ventilatory assistance in qudriplegics.[54,64] For daytime ventilatory assistance, pneumobelts may be preferred by patients with very low vital capacities because they provide continuous assistance without limiting use of the face or hands.[65] Mouth-piece positive-pressure ventilation for daytime use seems to be preferred by patients with slightly more ventilatory reserve if they can turn their heads enough to use a mouthpiece attached to a gooseneck apparatus on a wheelchair.[63,64] Patients who are unable to tolerate NPPV also may be managed successfully with negative-pressure ventilation both nocturnally and during the daytime,[66] when a chest shell ventilator can be used in the sitting position. However, nocturnal monitoring should be done in these patients to assess the frequency and severity of obstructive apneas.

In patients who wish to be free of any mechanical encumbrances but have severe reductions in vital capacities, glossopharyngeal breathing can be taught, even in patients with C1–C3 lesions, and this can provide up to several hours of free time from the ventilator.[27] Some patients may be interested in having diaphragm pacers implanted as a means of freeing themselves from other mechanical ventilators, but this usually precludes removal of the tracheostomy and is quite expensive, at least initially. Very few comparative data are available to help in weighing the various options, so patient and physician preferences usually determine the specific modes of ventilatory support used. Regardless of the ventilatory mode chosen, a severely weakened cough mechanism is universal in patients with high spinal cord lesions, so secretion removal must be a top priority. Close attention to assisting cough has decreased the incidence of pulmonary complications and the need for ventilatory support after acute quadriplegia.[67]

MUSCULAR DYSTROPHIES AND OTHER PROGRESSIVE MYOPATHIES

The muscular dystrophies are among the most common progressive neuromuscular disorders that affect the respiratory muscles (see Table 49-9). The age at onset of respiratory failure varies widely between the various entities, with the onset for Duchenne muscular dystrophy averaging 20 years, that for Becker's roughly 43 years, and others such as limb-girdle or scapulohumeral dystrophies rarely causing respiratory failure before 40 or 50 years.[68] Patients with advanced muscular dystrophies commonly have sleep-disordered breathing, leading to nocturnal hypoxemia and hypoventilation prior to the onset of respiratory failure.[69] Therefore, overnight polysomnography or, at least, oximetry may be indicated when significant respiratory muscle weakness has occurred. If desaturations are found, oxygen supplementation alone may prolong the sleep-disordered breathing events or exacerbate hypoventilation,[70,71] so institution of nasal CPAP or BiPAP is recommended.

Kyphoscoliosis is also common in the muscular dystrophies, affecting 50 to 80 percent of patients with Duchenne muscular dystrophy and virtually all patients with spinal muscular atrophies.[72] Spinal stabilization surgery may be effective in halting the progression of scoliosis, but this must be used selectively and timed appropriately. Significant kyphoscoliosis decreases chest wall compliance, contributing to the restrictive ventilatory defect. In patients without neuromuscular disease, angles of curvature exceeding 90 and 130 degrees are associated with dyspnea on exertion and respiratory failure, respectively, and in combination with weakness, smaller angles may predispose to ventilatory failure. If ventilatory assistance is deemed warranted, the presence of kyphoscoliosis places special constraints on the choice of ventilator modes. Without customizing, most negative-pressure ventilators fail to fit adequately, and the reduced chest wall compliance interferes with their efficiency. Accordingly, devices such as the cuirass and rocking bed are rarely acceptable in patients with severe kyphoscoliosis.

Despite the preceding problems, negative-pressure ventilation has been used extensively in patients with muscular dystrophies, mainly those without significant kyphoscoliosis. Daytime hypercapnia and symptoms are reversed in patients with Duchenne muscular dystrophy treated with iron lungs or wrap ventilators overnight.[34,35] Alexander and coworkers[73] reported 10 patients with Duchenne muscular dystrophy who survived an average of 3.4 years beyond the onset of respiratory failure by using a variety of noninvasive ventilators. Bach and associates[54] reported a similar experience with 31 patients with Duchenne muscular dystrophy, 23 of whom were still alive 7 years after initiating mouth intermittent positive-pressure breathing. This approach was successful in allowing patients to lead active lives at home despite the need for continuous ventilatory support.

Long-term follow-up studies of Duchenne muscular dystrophy patients using noninvasive ventilators have revealed that noninvasive ventilation is temporizing and that the underlying illness progresses despite ventilatory assistance. Of eight patients using mainly negative-pressure ventilation in one series,[47] three died within 48 months, and three needed to have tracheostomies and positive-pressure ventilation because of progressive respiratory deterioration. In another series,[58] 23 patients with Duchenne muscular dystrophy used negative-pressure ventilation, initially only at night, but as vital capacity continued to drop, patients had to increase duration of ventilation by an average of 0.95 h/day per year. Survival was extended an average of 6.3 years beyond the onset of respiratory failure, but six of the patients died, four suddenly while using their ventilators. This suggests that cardiovascular events related to the associated cardiomyopathy may become an important cause of mortality, even after respiratory failure has been stabilized.

Among Duchenne muscular dystrophy patients using negative-pressure ventilators, sleep-disordered breathing with severe oxygen desaturations occurs commonly.[20] This may reflect the underlying sleep-disordered breathing defects found in these patients,[69] but it also may be potentiated by negative-pressure ventilation. Ellis and coworkers[37] demonstrated that oxygen desaturations occurring with negative-pressure ventilation could be ameliorated by switching to nasal positive-pressure ventilation. Thus NPPV is now preferred over other noninvasive modalities in patients with muscular dystrophy requiring ventilatory assistance, even when weakness is severe. However, tracheostomy for delivery of positive-pressure ventilation may be preferred by some patients requiring round-the-clock ventilation or in patients who develop recurrent aspiration or difficulty coping with airway secretions.

Although most series have focused on patients with Duchenne muscular dystrophy, applications of mechanical ventilators have been described for most other progressive myopathies and neuropathies as well, usually as single or multiple case reports.[38–40,54,58] These uncontrolled series have reported improved gas exchange and symptoms after use of negative- and positive-pressure ventilators in limb girdle muscular dystrophy, polyneuropathies, myotonic dystro-phy, the spinal muscular atrophies, and acid maltase deficiency.

Survival of patients with muscular dystrophies who have developed symptomatic hypercapnia is almost certainly prolonged substantially with NPPV, but no prospective, controlled studies have examined this question, largely for ethical reasons. Vianello and coworkers[74] observed that of five patients with Duchenne muscular dystrophy who received nasal NPPV, all were alive 2 years later, whereas four of five similar patients who declined any ventilatory assistance had died. The study on prophylactic use of NPPV by Raphael and colleagues[53] showing increased mortality among NPPV users has raised some concerns, but most practitioners believe that although prophylactic use of NPPV may not be beneficial, therapeutic use in hypercapnic patients prolongs survival. A similar effect on survival is seen with iron lungs, with case reports describing Duchenne muscular dystrophy patients who have used them for up to 12 years after the onset of ventilatory failure.[34] Despite this evidence that various forms of ventilatory assistance, particularly NPPV, prolong survival in patients with muscular dystrophies, as many as 24 percent of muscular dystrophy clinics in the United States were not offering mechanical ventilatory assistance to their patients with respiratory failure according to a survey conducted during the mid-1980s.[12] It is possible that tracheostomy extends survival in Duchenne muscular dystrophy even longer than NPPV, once severe quadriparesis and cough impairment have occurred. Robert and associates[59] have reported survivals averaging 7 years after the onset of ventilatory failure in tracheostomized patients with muscular dystrophy. However, controlled comparisons have never been done, and the decision to use tracheostomy PPV is one that should be made with very careful consideration of patient desires and caregiver capabilities.

MULTIPLE SCLEROSIS

Respiratory failure in multiple sclerosis is usually a late manifestation of a disease that progresses in fits and starts, sometimes rapidly, sometimes slowly, with variable respiratory involvement. Although cases of acute respiratory failure have been reported,[75] patients with multiple sclerosis who develop chronic respiratory failure usually experience an insidious onset. The choice of ventilator for patients with multiple sclerosis is determined mainly by the severity of bulbar involvement. When bulbar function is intact, nasal or mouth noninvasive ventilation may be successful, even in patients with profound respiratory insufficiency.[54] Negative-pressure ventilation also has been used successfully.[66] However, patients with significant bulbar involvement usually require tracheostomy PPV.

The decision to initiate mechanical ventilation raises ethical issues in patients with multiple sclerosis because the course of the disease is difficult to predict,[76] and tracheostomy eventually may be needed if significant bulbar involvement develops. On the other hand, many patients with multiple sclerosis are still ambulatory when they develop respiratory failure, and the initiation of noninvasive ventilation is well accepted by patients and their families. As the disease progresses and patients become more dependent, some may decline the step to invasive PPV. These issues should be discussed with patients and their families well in advance so that emotional turmoil can be minimized. If invasive PPV is declined, referral to a home-based hospice program is advisable as patients approach the end-stages of their disease.

RAPIDLY PROGRESSIVE NEUROMUSCULAR DISEASES

AMYOTROPHIC LATERAL SCLEROSIS

Respiratory failure is usually a manifestation of advanced amyotrophic lateral sclerosis (ALS), occurring infrequently in patients who are still ambulatory. However, occasional patients present with bilateral diaphragmatic paralysis and require ventilatory assistance early on. Once respiratory failure occurs, further deterioration in global functioning may progress rapidly,[77] so ethical aspects of ventilatory support in patients with amyotrophic lateral sclerosis must be addressed promptly. In a survey of 38 patients presenting with ALS, the vast majority preferred to hear as much information as possible about ventilator options.[78] Initially, slightly over half the patients wished cardiopulmonary resuscitation in the event of an acute deterioration. However, 6 months later, fewer than 10 percent expressed this desire. The authors concluded that ethical issues should be addressed early before a crisis occurs and that discussions should be repeated periodically to detect changes in patient wishes. In another survey of 99 ALS patients with respiratory failure, only 10 percent opted for mechanical ventilation, mainly invasive.[79] However, among those patients who chose to be ventilated, 90 percent were happy with the decision.

Noninvasive ventilation has been used increasingly in patients with ALS, so the proportion of patients trying mechanical ventilation will likely increase. Gay and colleagues[38] reported success in seven of nine patients with ALS as part of a larger series of patients using nasal ventilation. These seven patients had improvements in gas exchange and symptoms, and one patient remained stable after 26 months. However, three of the seven died within 6 months, and most of the survivors had been ventilated for a year or less. More recently, Aboussouan and coworkers[50] found that nasal NPPV was tolerated in 18 of 39 (46 percent) patients with respiratory insufficiency due to ALS. Risk of death was reduced by a factor of 3.1 if patients tolerated NPPV, and even though swallowing dysfunction is ordinarily considered a relative contraindication to the use of noninvasive ventilation, patients with bulbar involvement who tolerated NPPV also had improved survival. Bulbar involvement halved the likelihood of tolerating the device, however.

The preceding studies support using NPPV in patients with ALS who meet initiation criteria (see Table 49-4), even when bulbar structures are involved. Survival is likely to be prolonged, although the modality is, admittedly, temporizing. Patients will have to decide whether or not to proceed to invasive PPV when bulbar and cough function further deteriorate. In our experience, most decide to use NPPV for as long as possible but refrain from tracheostomy placement. If patients opt for a tracheostomy, the aim should still be to return them to their home and maximize independence. Placing a portable ventilator on an electric wheelchair allows them to remain mobile. However, home ventilation of such patients can be successful only if the patient and family/caregivers are highly motivated and capable and if they receive adequate support from personal attendants, visiting nurses, physicians, home respiratory therapy vendors, and

insurers. Before embarking on such a course, all concerned must be aware of how stressful and demanding invasive home mechanical ventilation can be.

MYASTHENIA GRAVIS AND GUILLAIN-BARRÉ SYNDROME

Myasthenia gravis and Guillain-Barré syndrome both usually present acutely, with the need for temporary respiratory support in approximately 10 to 20 percent of patients until the process reverses. For this reason, and because the pharyngeal muscles are usually involved, standard endotracheal intubation with positive-pressure ventilation is usually the ventilatory mode of choice. Among 22 patients with respiratory failure due to myasthenia gravis, Gracey and coworkers[80] reported that the average duration of mechanical ventilation after intubation was 8 days, and the longest was 32 days. Only one patient required tracheostomy. In Guillain-Barré syndrome, the average duration of ventilatory assistance is a bit longer (37 days in one study[81]), and most patients receive a tracheostomy. In both conditions, intubation should be performed for airway protection before the onset of frank respiratory failure, and patients must be monitored closely for swallowing difficulty, cough impairment, and aspiration. Vital capacity and maximal inspiratory and expiratory pressures also must be monitored closely, since a vital capacity of less than 10 to 20 mL/kg (or twice the predicted tidal volume) or a maximal inspiratory pressure of less than 20 to 25 cmH$_2$O is the usual indication for intubation.[80–83]

Only exceptional cases of patients with respiratory insufficiency due to these syndromes would be appropriately managed using noninvasive ventilation. A patient with relative sparing of upper airway musculature and with borderline reduction in vital capacity could conceivably be managed noninvasively, in the hope that the condition would stabilize. Endotracheal intubation and the accompanying morbidity that includes pneumonia in up to 30 percent of patients with Guillain-Barré syndrome[83] could thereby be potentially avoided. On the other hand, it should be borne in mind that no controlled trials support such an approach, and patients given a trial of noninvasive ventilation should be observed closely. Practitioners should be prepared to intubate if further deterioration occurs, preferably before the development of frank respiratory failure.

BILATERAL DIAPHRAGMATIC PARALYSIS

Bilateral diaphragmatic paralysis causes chronic respiratory failure that is characterized by sleep-disordered breathing, nocturnal hypoventilation, and orthopnea. It may occur in association with other neuromuscular conditions such as ALS or multiple sclerosis, as a consequence of surgery or trauma, or as an idiopathic process. A number of different noninvasive ventilator modes may be used to treat bilateral diaphragmatic paralysis. Negative-pressure ventilation has been used successfully, and rocking beds have particular appeal because they maintain diaphragm motion during sleep. In one series of patients with bilateral diaphragmatic paralysis occurring after cardiac surgery, the rocking bed was used to assist nocturnal ventilation until diaphragm function returned after 4 to 27 months.[84] Among noninvasive positive-pressure modes, CPAP may be useful by shifting the active phase of the respiratory cycle to the expiratory muscles. However, more recently, nasal NPPV has been the main modality used.[85]

OTHER NEUROMUSCULAR CONDITIONS OCCASIONALLY TREATED WITH NPPV

Many other common neuromuscular conditions affect upper or lower respiratory muscle function, including cerebrovascular disease and Parkinson's disease. However, these are usually not treated with noninvasive ventilation. Strokes commonly predispose to chronic aspiration but rarely involve lower respiratory muscles enough to cause hypoventilation. Nocturnal hypoxemia from obstructive sleep apnea is a common problem in patients with Parkinson's disease. Irregular contractions of the glottic and supraglottic muscles leading to upper airway obstruction have been reported in a third of patients. Alveolar hypoventilation has been described in the familial form of Parkinson's disease and has been postulated to be a factor in the cognitive deficits seen.[86] However, trials using CPAP, BiPAP, or other types of noninvasive ventilation have not been reported in Parkinson's patients. Nevertheless, if respiratory insufficiency is present, nasal or oral NPPV would be preferable to negative-pressure ventilation in view of the high incidence of nocturnal upper airway obstruction.[87]

PEDIATRIC APPLICATIONS

Although a complete discussion of the pediatric applications of noninvasive ventilation is beyond the scope of this chapter, it must be recognized that many neuromuscular syndromes become evident during the childhood years, particularly the muscular dystrophies and atrophies. Few studies have focused on pediatric issues per se, but most of the observations made earlier with regard to the congenital neuromuscular syndromes apply to children as well, particularly those old enough to cooperate and comprehend the purpose of the therapy. If ventilatory support is indicated in younger children, the efficacy of noninvasive ventilation may be limited by the inability to cooperate and the higher nasal resistance of small children compared with older children and adults who may require relatively high mask pressures.

Summary and Conclusions

Most neuromuscular diseases affect the respiratory muscles, impairing pulmonary function and leading to respiratory insufficiency that may present abruptly or insidiously. Because of the variety of neuromuscular conditions, both congenital and acquired, it is difficult to generalize about the onset of respiratory compromise. Depending on the specific entity, presentation may occur at any age and with a variety of manifestations. If the inspiratory muscles are involved primarily, hypoventilation is commonly the first manifestation. However, some patients present with more involvement of the expiratory muscles, in which case cough is impaired, and a crisis may occur when an acute respiratory infection leads to secretion retention. With some neuromuscular conditions, bulbar involvement leads to chronic aspiration and increased risk for pneumonia. Significant involvement of all three is usually lethal without invasive ventilatory support.

Noninvasive ventilation has been used for many decades for patients with neuromuscular diseases, starting with negative-pressure ventilation during the polio epidemics. More recently, noninvasive positive-pressure (NPPV) has become the modality of first choice for most of these patients because of comfort, convenience, portability, and cost advantages.

Consisting of a portable positive-pressure ventilator connected by either a nasal, oronasal, or mouthpiece interface, this mode directs intermittent positive pressure to the upper airway and actively assists inspiration. Although it usually requires time (several weeks) and effort on the part of the patient for successful adaptation, nocturnal NPPV can sustain adequate alveolar ventilation for many years in patients with stable or slowly progressive neuromuscular diseases and is very conducive to use in the home. Controlled trials documenting its efficacy and ability to prolong survival are lacking, but for ethical reasons, these are unlikely to be done. The optimal time for initiation has not been established. Also, the mechanism by which intermittent ventilatory assistance (for as few as 4 h/day) stabilizes gas exchange is not fully understood, but the reversal of severe hypoventilation particularly during sleep and "resetting" of the respiratory center sensitivity to CO_2 probably play a role.

Despite these gaps in the scientific basis for application, NPPV has been widely accepted as the therapy of choice for most patients with stable or slowly progressive neuromuscular disorders. Appropriate patients must be selected using accepted guidelines, and methods for initiation should be optimized to enhance the chances for success. Attention should be paid to individual characteristics such as cough impairment that would necessitate the use of cough-assistive devices. Practitioners also should monitor pulmonary functions, daytime blood gases, and nocturnal oxygenation periodically so that progression of the underlying disease or worsening of daytime gas exchange can be detected and stability maintained, often by adding to the hours of daily ventilation. Successful management of home NPPV is an ongoing process that requires communication and close cooperation of the patient, physician, home respiratory therapy vendor, and caregivers. When administered with a conscientious but optimistic and supportive approach, noninvasive ventilation can enhance the quality and quantity of life for individuals severely afflicted with neuromuscular disease and greatly broaden their options for ventilatory assistance.

References

1. Stauffer JL, Olsen DE, Petty TL: Complications and consequences of endotracheal intubation and tracheostomy: A prospective study of 150 critically ill patients. *Am J Med* 70:65–76, 1981.
2. Bonnaro P: Swallowing dysfunction after tracheostomy. *Ann Surg* 174:29–33, 1971.
3. Woollam CHM: The development of apparatus for intermittent negative respiration, 1832–1918. *Anaesthesia* 31:666–685, 1976.
4. Drinker P, Shaw LA: An apparatus for the prolonged administration of artificial respiration: I. Design for adults and children. *J Clin Invest* 7:229–247, 1929.
5. Hill NS: Clinical applications of body ventilators. *Chest* 90:897–905, 1986.
6. Spalding JMK, Opie L: Artificial respiration with the Tunnicliffe breathing-jacket. *Lancet* 1:613–615, 1958.
7. Collier CR, Offeldt JE: Ventilatory efficiency of the cuirass respirator in totally paralyzed chronic poliomyelitis patients. *J Appl Physiol* 6:532–538, 1954.
8. Eve FC: Actuation of the inert diaphragm. *Lancet* 2:995, 1932.
9. Adamson JP, Lewis L, Stein JD: Application of abdominal pressure for artificial respiration. *JAMA* 169:1613–1617, 1959.
10. Glenn WWL, Holcomb WG, Hogan J, et al: Diaphragm pacing by radiofrequency transmission in the treatment of chronic ventilatory insufficiency. *J Thorac Cardiovasc Surg* 66:505–520, 1973.

11. Alba A, Khan A, Lee M: Mouth IPPV for sleep. *Rehabil Gaz* 24:47–49, 1981.
12. Colbert AP, Schock NC: Respirator use in progressive neuromuscular disease. *Arch Phys Med Rehabil* 66:760–762, 1985.
13. Bach JR, Alba A, Mosher R, Delaubier A: Intermittent positive pressure ventilation via nasal access in the management of respiratory insufficiency. *Chest* 94.168–170, 1987.
14. Kerby GR, Mayer LS, Pingleton SK: Nocturnal positive pressure ventilation via nasal mask. *Am Rev Respir Dis* 135:738–740, 1987.
15. Bach JR, Alba AS, Bahatiuk G, et al: Mouth intermittent positive pressure ventilation in the management of post-polio respiratory insufficiency. *Chest* 1:859–864, 1987.
16. Hill NS, Eveloff SE, Carlisle CC, Goff SG: Efficacy of nocturnal nasal ventilation in patients with restrictive thoracic disease. *Am Rev Respir Dis* 145:365–371, 1992.
17. Strumpf DA, Carlisle CC, Millman RP, et al: An evaluation of the Respironics BiPAP bilevel CPAP device for delivery of assisted ventilation. *Respir Care* 35:415–422, 1990.
18. Vitacca M, Rubini F, Foglio K, et al: Noninvasive modalities of positive pressure ventilation improved the outcome of acute exacerbations in COLD patients. *Intensive Care Med* 19:450–455, 1993.
19. Bach JR, Penek J: Obstructive sleep apnea complicating negative pressure ventilatory support in patients with chronic paralytic restrictive ventilatory dysfunction. *Chest* 99:1386, 1991.
20. Hill NS, Redline S, Carskadon MA, et al: Sleep-disordered breathing in patients with Duchenne muscular dystrophy using negative pressure ventilators. *Chest* 102:1656–1662, 1992.
21. Peltier LF: Obstructive apnea in artificially hyperventilated subjects during sleep. *J Appl Physiol* 5:614–618, 1953.
22. Plum F, Whendon DG: The rapid-rocking bed: Its effect on the ventilation of poliomyelitis patients with respiratory paralysis. *JAMA* 245:235–241, 1951.
23. Yang GFW, Alba A, Lee M, Khan A: Pneumobelt for sleep in the ventilator user: Clinical experience. *Arch Phys Med Rehabil* 70:707–711, 1989.
24. Moxham J, Shneerson JM: Diaphragmatic pacing. *Am Rev Respir Dis* 148:533–536, 1993.
25. Bach JR, O'Connor K: Electrophrenic ventilation: A different perspective. *J Am Paraplegia Soc* 14:9–17, 1991.
26. Dail CW, Affeldt JE, Collier CR: Clinical aspects of glossopharangeal breathing. *JAMA* 158:445–449, 1953.
27. Bach JR, Alba AS, Bodofsky E, et al: Glossophrayngeal breathing and noninvasive aids in the management of post-polio respiratory insufficiency. *Birth Defects* 23:99–113, 1987.
28. Barach AL, Beck GJ, Smith RH: Mechanical production of expiratory flow rates surpassing the capacity of human coughing. *Am J Med Sci* 226:241–248, 1994.
29. Bach JR: Update and perspectives on noninvasive respiratory muscle aids: 2. The expiratory muscle aids. *Chest* 105:1538–1544, 1994.
30. Bach JR: Mechanical insufflation-exsufflation: Comparison of peak expiratory flows with manually assisted and unassisted coughing techniques. *Chest* 104:1553–1564, 1993.
31. Rochester DF, Braun NMT, Lane S: Diaphragmatic energy expenditure in chronic respiratory failure. *Am J Med* 63:223–232, 1977.
32. Roussos C: Function and fatigue of respiratory muscles. *Chest* 88:1245–1315, 1985.
33. Sternburg L, Sternburg D: *View from the Seesaw.* New York, Dodd, Mead, 1986.
34. Curran FJ: Night ventilation by body respirators for patients in chronic respiratory failure due to late stage Duchenne muscular dystrophy. *Arch Phys Med Rehabil* 62:270–274, 1981.
35. Garay SM, Turino GM, Goldring RM: Sustained reversal of chronic hypercapnia in patients with alveolar hypoventilation syndromes: Long-term maintenance with noninvasive mechanical ventilation. *Am J Med* 70:268–274, 1981.
36. Bach JR, Alba AS: Management of chronic alveolar hypoventilation by nasal ventilation. *Chest* 97:52–57, 1990.
37. Ellis ER, Bye PTP, Bruderer JW, Sullivan CE: Treatment of respiratory failure during sleep in patients with neuromuscular disease. *Am Rev Respir Dis* 1135:148–152, 1987.
38. Gay PC, Patel AM, Viggiano RW, Hubmayr RD: Nocturnal nasal ventilation for treatment of patients with hypercapneic respiratory failure. *Mayo Clin Proc* 144:1234–1239, 1991.
39. Heckmatt JZ, Loh L, Dubowitz V: Nighttime nasal ventilation in neuromuscular disease. *Lancet* 335:579–581, 1990.
40. Leger P, Jennequin J, Gerard M, Robert D: Home positive pressure ventilation via nasal masks in patients with neuromuscular weakness and restrictive lung or chest wall disease. *Respir Care* 34:73–79, 1989.
41. Jimenez JFM, de Cos Escuin JS, Vicente CD, et al: Nasal intermittent positive pressure ventilation: Analysis of its withdrawal. *Chest* 107:382–388, 1995.
42. Jounieaux V, Aubert G, Dury M, et al: Effects of nasal positive-pressure hyperventilation on the glottis in normal sleeping subjects. *J Appl Physiol* 79:186–193, 1995.
43. Braun NMT, Faulkner J, Hughes RL, et al: When should respiratory muscles be exercised? *Chest* 84:76–84, 1983.
44. Carrey Z, Gottfried SB, Levy RD: Ventilatory muscle support in respiratory failure with nasal positive pressure ventilation. *Chest* 97:150–158, 1990.
45. Goldstein RS, De Rosie JA, Avendano MA, Dolmage TE: Influence of noninvasive positive pressure ventilation on inspiratory muscles. *Chest* 99:408–415, 1991.
46. Cropp A, Dimarco AF: Effects of intermittent negative pressure ventilation on respiratory muscle function in patients with severe chronic obstructive pulmonary disease. *Am Rev Respir Dis* 135:1056–1061, 1987.
47. Mohr CH, Hill NS: Long-term follow-up of nocturnal ventilatory assistance in patients with respiratory failure due to Duchenne-type muscular dystrophy. *Chest* 97:91–96, 1990.
48. Goldstein RS, Molotiu N, Skrastins R, et al: Reversal of sleep-induced hypoventilation by nocturnal negative pressure ventilation in patients with restrictive ventilatory impairment. *Am Rev Respir Dis* 135:1049–1055, 1987.
49. Strumpf DA, Millman RP, Hill NS: The management of chronic hypoventilation. *Chest* 98:474–480, 1990.
50. Aboussouan LS, Khan SU, Meeker DP, et al: Effect of noninvasive positive pressure ventilation on survival in amyotrophic lateral sclerosis. *Ann Intern Med* 6:450–453, 1997.
51. Brochard L, Mancebo J, Wysocki M, et al: Noninvasive ventilation for acute exacerbations of chronic obstructive pulmonary disease. *N Engl J Med* 333:817–822, 1995.
52. Kramer N, Meyer TJ, Meharg J, et al: Randomized, prospective trial of noninvasive positive pressure ventilation in acute respiratory failure. *Am J Respir Crit Care Med* 151:1799–1806, 1995.
53. Raphael JC, Chevret S, Chastang C, et al: French multicenter trial of prophylactic nasal ventilation in Duchenne muscular dystrophy. *Lancet* 343:1600–1604, 1994.
54. Bach JR, Alba AS, Saporito LR: Intermittent positive pressure ventilation via the mouth as an alternative to tracheostomy for 257 ventilator users. *Chest* 103:174–182, 1993.
55. Gordon AS, Fainer DC, Ivy AC: Artificial respiration. *JAMA* 144:1455–1464, 1950.
56. Ferguson GT, Gilmartin M: CO_2 rebreathing during BiPAP ventilatory assistance. *Am J Respir Crit Care Med* 151:1126–1135, 1995.
57. Hill NS: Complications of noninvasive positive pressure ventilation. *Respir Care* 42:432–442, 1997.
58. Curran FJ, Colbert AP: Ventilator management in Duchenne muscular dystrophy and post poliomyelitis syndrome: Twelve years' experience. *Arch Phys Med Rehabil* 70:180–185, 1989.
59. Robert D, Gerard M, Leger P, et al: La ventilation mechanique a domicile definitive par tracheotomie de l'insufficient respiratoire chronique. *Rev Fr Mal Respir* 11:923–926, 1983.

60. Detroyer A, Deboyd DZ, Thirion J: Function of the respiratory muscles in acute hemiplegia. *Am Rev Respir Dis* 123:631–632, 1981.

61. Mansel JK, Norman JR: Respiratory complications and management of spinal cord injuries. *Chest* 97:1446–1452, 1990.

62. Wicks AB, Menter RR: Long-term outlook in quadriplegic patients with initial ventilator dependency. *Chest* 90:406–410, 1986.

63. Bach JR, Alba AS: Noninvasive options for ventilatory support of the traumatic high level quadraplegic. *Chest* 98:613–619, 1990.

64. Bach JR: Alternative methods of ventilatory support for the patient with ventilatory failure due to spinal cord injury. *J Am Paraplegia Soc* 14:158–174, 1991.

65. Bach JR, Alba AS: Total ventilatory support by the intermittent abdominal pressure ventilator. *Chest* 99:630–636, 1991.

66. Splaingard ML, Frates RC, Jefferson LS, et al: Home negative pressure ventilation: Report of 20 years of experience in patients with neuromuscular disease. *Arch Phys Med Rehabil* 66:239–243, 1985.

67. McMichan JC, Mitchell W, Westbrook PR: Pulmonary dysfunction following traumatic quadriplegia. *JAMA* 243:528–531, 1980.

68. Rideau Y, Jankowski LW, Grellet IJ: Respiratory function in the muscular dystrophies. *Muscle Nerve* 4:155–164, 1981.

69. Smith PEM, Calverley PMA, Edwards RHT: Hypoxemia during sleep in Duchenne muscular dystrophy. *Am Rev Respir Dis* 137:884–888, 1988.

70. Gay PC, Edmonds LC: Severe hypercapnia after low-flow oxygen therapy in patients with neuromuscular disease and diaphragmatic dysfunction. *Mayo Clin Proc* 50:327–330, 1995.

71. Smith PEM, Edwards THT, Calverley PMA: Oxygen treatment of sleep hypoxemia in Duchenne muscular dystrophy. *Thorax* 44:997–1001, 1989.

72. Smith PEM, Calverley PMA, Edwards PHT, et al: Practical problems in the respiratory care of patients with muscular dystrophy. *N Engl J Med* 316:1197–1205, 1987.

73. Alexander MA, Johnson EW, Petty J, Stauch D: Mechanical ventilation of patients with late stage Duchenne muscular dystrophy: Management in the home. *Arch Phys Med Rehabil* 60:289–292, 1978.

74. Vianello A, Bevilacqua M, Vittorino S, et al: Long-term nasal intermittent positive pressure ventilation in advanced Duchenne's muscular dystrophy. *Chest* 105:445–448, 1994.

75. Yamamoto T, Imai T, Yamasaki M: Acute ventilatory failure in multiple sclerosis. *J Neurol Sci* 89:313–324, 1989.

76. Kelly B, Luce JM: The diagnosis and management of neuromuscular disease causing respiratory failure. *Chest* 99:1485–1494, 1991.

77. Sivak ED, Gipson WT, Hanson MR: Long-term management of respiratory failure in amyotrophic lateral sclerosis. *Ann Neurol* 12:18–23, 1982.

78. Silverstein MD, Stocking CB, Antel JP: Amyotrophic lateral sclerosis and life-sustaining therapy: Patients' desires for information, participation in decision making, and life-sustaining therapy. *Mayo Clin Proc* 66:906–913, 1991.

79. Moss AH, Casey P: Home ventilation for amyotrophic lateral sclerosis patients: Outcomes, costs and patient, family and physician attitudes. *Neurology* 43:438–443, 1993.

80. Gracey DR, Divertie MB, Howard FM: Mechanical ventilation for respiratory failure in myasthenia gravis. *Mayo Clin Proc* 58:597–602, 1983.

81. Gracey DR, McMichan JC, Divertie MB, Howard FM: Respiratory failure in Guillain-Barré syndrome. *Mayo Clin Proc* 57:742–746, 1982.

82. Newton J: Prevention of pulmonary complications in severe Guillain-Barré syndrome by early assisted ventilation. *Br Med J* 142:444–445, 1985.

83. Ropper AH: Guillain-Barré syndrome. *N Engl J Med* 326:1130–1136, 1992.

84. Abd AG, Braun NMT, Baskin MI, et al: Diaphragmatic dysfunction after open heart surgery: Treatment with a rocking bed. *Ann Intern Med* 111:881–886, 1991.

85. Lin MC, Liaw MY, Huang CC, et al: Bilateral diaphragmatic paralysis: A rare cause of acute respiratory failure managed with nasal mask bilevel positive airway pressure (BiPAP) ventilation. *Eur Respir J* 10:1922–1924, 1997.

86. Kimura D, Hahn A, Burnett HJM: Attentional and perseverative impairment in two cases of familial fatal Parkinsonism with cortical sparing. *Can J Neurosci* 14:597–599, 1987.

87. Carroll N, Branthwaite MA: Control of nocturnal hypoventilation by nasal intermittent positive pressure ventilation. *Thorax* 43:349–353, 1988.

Chapter 50
REHABILITATION OF LUNG CANCER PATIENTS

NATHAN LEVITAN

There are thousands of publications related to the screening, prevention, or treatment of patients with lung cancer. An abundance of literature also exists related to the symptomatic management of terminally ill patients whose disease has recurred despite treatment efforts. In recent years, there has been a renewed focus on the importance of patient comfort during the course of cancer treatment, and a variety of techniques have been developed to measure and to maintain quality of life.[1,2] However, little has been written pertaining specifically to the rehabilitation of lung cancer patients. This chapter will focus on opportunities for the lung cancer patient to regain lost functionality during each phase of disease management.

In order to provide a broad clinical overview of lung cancer, this chapter will begin with a review of the epidemiology and state-of-the-art management of this disease. The focus will then shift to the rehabilitation of patients who have undergone these treatments. Disabilities caused by activities that may have predisposed to the development of cancer, those related to the lung tumor itself, and the adverse effects of surgical, radiation, and chemotherapy treatments will be considered. The effectiveness of selected rehabilitation efforts in the care of terminally ill cancer patients will be addressed as well.

Overview of Lung Cancer Management

LUNG CANCER EPIDEMIOLOGY

Cancer is second only to cardiovascular disease as a cause of death among adults in the United States.[3] Annually in the United States, approximately 1.4 million people are diagnosed with cancer (excluding nonmelanoma skin cancer and in-situ carcinoma of the cervix), and approximately 560,000 deaths occur. Although prostate cancer occurs more commonly in men than lung cancer, and breast cancer occurs more commonly in women, lung cancer is the most common cause of cancer deaths among men and women (Table 50-1). Lung cancer causes 28 percent of cancer deaths each year in the United States. In 1990, the age-adjusted mortality rates per 100,000 population were 75.6 for men and 31.7 for women. Among individuals 55 to 74, the mortality rates were >500 per 100,000 and >200 per 100,000 population among men and women, respectively.

Tobacco exposure is by far the most important risk factor for lung cancer.[4,5] Accordingly, trends in lung cancer incidence follow trends in smoking with a 20 to 30 year lag time. Per capita cigarette consumption peaked in 1963 and has been gradually declining since that time. Between 1973 and 1990, the incidence of lung cancer has increased by 9 percent in men and by 110 percent in women. Lung cancer rates among men peaked in the mid-1980s and have begun to decline. Lung cancer rates among women are expected to peak in the year 2001. In Asia and Africa, rates of cigarette consumption and lung cancer continue to rise. Several investigators have recently demonstrated the importance of second hand smoke exposure as a cause of lung cancer.[6] It is estimated that 5 percent of lung cancer among nonsmokers is related to environmental tobacco smoke.[7]

LUNG CANCER PATHOLOGY AND STAGING

The vast majority (>95 percent) of malignancies arising in the lung are epithelial in origin; they are designated as carcinomas. Lung carcinomas are grouped into non-small cell or small cell tumors. The former are subclassified as squamous cell, adenocarcinoma, large cell, undifferentiated, or bronchoalveolar. Approximately 80 percent of lung cancers are non-small cell type, and approximately 20 percent are small cell.[8] When assigning a tumor stage and selecting a management approach, the important distinction is between non-small cell and small cell histology. Patients with different subtypes of non-small cell lung cancer are generally managed in a similar fashion.

Newly diagnosed non-small cell lung cancers are classified in accordance with the International TNM Tumor Staging System.[9] The details of lung cancer staging are beyond the scope of this chapter. However, in order to facilitate a discussion of tumor management, a brief overview of this system will be presented. The primary tumor is described as T1–4, depending on size and extent of local invasion. The nodal status is described as N1 (hilar), N2 (ipsilateral mediastinal), or N3 (contralateral mediastinal or supraclavicular). The presence or absence of distant metastatic disease is described as M0 (no distant metastatic disease) or M1 (distant metastatic disease present). A distinction is often made between staging that is based on *clinical* information (such as physical examination and radiograph results) versus *pathologic* information obtained at the time of biopsy or surgical exploration.

Depending on the details of the TNM categories, the tumor is then assigned a global tumor stage I, IIA, IIB, IIIA, IIIB, or IV.[10] These categories are utilized to guide the clinician in selecting a treatment approach. An overview of the staging categories is shown in Table 50-2. Stage I tumors are of small size and have no detectable tumor within resected lymph nodes. Stage II tumors are somewhat larger and may involve ipsilateral hilar nodes. Stage IIIA tumors are locally advanced but are generally technically resectable. Stage IIIB tumors are locally advanced and are unresectable. Stage IV tumors have demonstrable distant metastases separate from the primary tumor and regional nodes; they are uniformly unresectable.

Small cell lung cancers are staged as limited or extensive. Limited stage small cell lung cancers are confined to one hemithorax (generally excluding those with malignant pleural effusion). All other small cell lung cancers are classified as extensive stage. Approximately 20 percent of small cell lung cancers are limited stage at the time of diagnosis. The frequency of each tumor stage and the associated prognosis for both non-small cell and small cell lung cancer are shown in Table 50-3.

TABLE 50-1 Incidence and Mortality of Cancer among Men and Women

PREDICTED NEW CASES OF CANCER AMONG ADULTS IN THE UNITED STATES 1997				PREDICTED DEATHS FROM CANCER AMONG ADULTS IN THE UNITED STATES 1997			
Men		Women		Men		Women	
Prostate	334,500	Breast	180,000	Lung	98,000	Lung	67,000
Lung	111,000	Lung	83,000	Prostate	42,000	Breast	44,000
Colorectal	66,400	Colorectal	64,800	Colorectal	27,000	Colorectal	28,000

CONVENTIONAL TREATMENT OF LUNG CANCER

State-of-the-art treatment of non-small cell lung cancer has changed considerably during the middle and late 1990s, due largely to the discovery of effective ways to combine chemotherapy, radiation therapy, and surgery. These innovations, many of which should now be considered standard practice in the management of lung cancer patients, are discussed below in the section entitled, "New Developments in Lung Cancer." In contrast to the complex arena of multimodality therapy, the conventional treatment of non-small cell lung cancer has been relatively simple. Surgical resection alone has been utilized whenever this procedure is technically feasible (i.e., for most stage I, II, or IIIA tumors).

A tumor that has spread to liver, bone, brain, supraclavicular nodes, or contralateral lung is clearly unresectable. The presence of a malignant pleural effusion renders a tumor unresectable. If chest radiograph or chest CT scan show evidence of mediastinal adenopathy, then CT-guided needle biopsy and/or mediastinoscopy are utilized to clarify the extent of mediastinal involvement with tumor. A tumor involving contralateral mediastinal nodes or bulky ipsilateral mediastinal nodes is considered unresectable.[11,12]

If the tumor appears to be resectable based on these criteria, then the general medical condition of the patient is considered. Pulmonary function tests and split function ventilation/perfusion studies are utilized to predict the patient's postresection pulmonary reserve. Noting that the extent of obstructive disease is predictive of the likelihood of postoperative complications, the FEV_1 is a particularly important parameter.[13] Patients must have a predicted postoperative FEV_1 of 750 to 800 cc in order to be considered eligible for surgical resection.[14]

At the time of surgery, the extent of local invasion of a tumor is determined. An attempt is made to remove the tumor along with regional intrapulmonary and/or hilar nodes en bloc. Mediastinal lymph node dissection is carried out as well. If a tumor is found at the time of thoracotomy to involve mediastinum, heart, great vessels, trachea, esophagus, carina, vertebral body, or contralateral mediastinal nodes, then resection is often not carried out. Although a discussion of the management of superior sulcus cancers is beyond the scope of this chapter, such tumors may be considered resectable despite considerable local extrapulmonary invasion.[15]

The surgeon determines the extent of resection that is necessary to obtain negative surgical margins and to optimize long-term outcome. Tumors less than 1 cm in diameter may be removed by wedge resection or segmental resection. Investiga-

tors have shown that occult tumor spread to regional lymphatics occurs in 17 percent of tumors measuring 1.1 to 2 cm and 38 percent of tumors larger than 2 cm. As a result, resection of most tumors with curative intent necessitates the removal of at least an entire lobe.[16,17] Resection of larger tumors requires the removal of one or more lobes or an entire lung.

Preoperative staging studies are utilized in an effort to identify patients whose tumors are unresectable prior to thoracotomy, thus sparing them the morbidity of unnecessary surgery. However, some patients are determined to have advanced disease only on the basis of direct tumor visualization at the time of surgery. When surgical resection cannot be utilized due to the presence of a locally advanced tumor without a malignant pleural effusion, conventional treatment in the past has consisted of radiation therapy. Such treatment has little impact on long-term survival, but it can have some impact on local tumor control.[18,19] Patients with a large malignant pleural effusion benefit symptomatically from chest tube drainage followed by sclerosis. When residual tumor remains following attempted resection, radiation therapy has been used to reduce the likelihood of local recurrence and the associated morbidity.

In the past, patients with non-small cell lung cancer have received chemotherapy only for palliation of symptoms in the presence of locally advanced or distant metastatic disease. Several prospective randomized trials have compared chemotherapy with supportive care in this population. Chemotherapy can achieve tumor shrinkage and palliation of symptoms in 20 to 25 percent of patients. Among those studies that demonstrated a survival advantage in association with chemotherapy, the median prolongation of survival was approximately 4 months.[20-22] For patients with stage IV non-small cell lung cancer, the use of chemotherapy remains highly individualized. Treatment is generally reserved for palliation symptoms among patients with advanced disease. Each patient must decide whether chemotherapy-related toxicity is justified by the potential for symptom control and a modest prolongation of survival.

The conventional treatment of small cell lung cancer consists of chemotherapy administered either prior to or concurrently with radiation for patients with limited stage disease and chemotherapy alone for patients with extensive stage disease. It is assumed that hematogenous dissemination of cancer has occurred in nearly all patients with small cell lung cancer prior to diagnosis, regardless of tumor stage. Accordingly, surgical resection of small cell lung cancer is seldom performed. When a solitary pulmonary nodule is resected and is found to contain small cell lung cancer, such patients receive chemotherapy following surgery.[23]

TABLE 50-2 Overview of Lung Cancer Staging

Non-Small Cell Lung Cancer

Stage I
  Tumor ≤3 cm
  Negative hilar and mediastinal nodes
  No malignant pleural effusion
  No distant metastatic disease
Stage II
  Tumor may be >3 cm
  Ipsilateral hilar nodes may be involved
  No mediastinal node involvement, malignant pleural effusion,
    or distant metastatic disease
Stage IIIA
  Locally advanced and resectable
  Ipsilateral mediastinal nodes may be involved
  No direct invasion of mediastinal structures
  No malignant pleural effusion or distant metastatic disease
Stage IIIB
  Locally advanced and unresectable
  Contralateral mediastinal nodes may be involved
  Malignant pleural effusion may be present
Stage IV
  Distant metastatic disease

Small Cell Lung Cancer

Limited
  Tumor limited to one hemithorax (excluding malignant pleural
    effusion)
Extensive
  Tumor beyond one hemithorax (including malignant pleural ef-
    fusion)

PROGNOSIS FOLLOWING CONVENTIONAL TREATMENT

The prognosis associated with each stage of non-small cell lung cancer is shown in Table 50-3. Note that 60 percent of patients with non-small cell lung cancer have stage IIIB or IV disease at the time of diagnosis. Such patients are unlikely to survive for 5 years following diagnosis.[24] However, even patients with stages I and II non-small cell lung cancer, whose tumors appear to be small in size and easily resectable, have a 20 to 60 percent likelihood of dying from lung cancer within 5 years. Why is it that patients who appear to have early stage disease and undergo "curative" resection still face such a high risk of dying from disseminated disease? This occurs because non-small cell lung cancers are several years old by the time they become large enough to detect on a chest film or CT scan. During this lengthy period of occult tumor growth prior to diagnosis, there has been an opportunity for the release of cancer cells through the blood stream to other parts of the body.[25] Even for many patients with early stage tumors, non-small cell lung cancer may be a systemic disease.

Patients with small cell lung cancer have a generally poor prognosis as well. Despite a greater than 60 percent likelihood of tumor shrinkage with chemotherapy, most tumors eventually become resistant to chemotherapy. Between 10 and 20 percent of patients with limited small cell lung cancer are cured of their disease. Most other patients succumb to their disease within 2 years of diagnosis. The survival statistics for patients with small cell lung cancer are shown in Table 50-3.[26]

NEW DEVELOPMENTS IN LUNG CANCER TREATMENT

Newer techniques allow the surgeon to carry out both more limited and more extensive resections than in the past. Precision tumor dissection can be accomplished in a patient with limited pulmonary reserve. Other procedures (including intrapericardial pneumonectomy, sleeve pneumonectomy, sleeve lobectomy, and extended anterior/posterior resections) permit the judicious resection of locally advanced tumors.[27] Video-assisted thoracoscopy is now available for tumor diagnosis, lysis of adhesions within the pleural space, and for biopsy or resection of peripheral nodules.[28,29]

Radiotherapy innovations include the use of twice-daily radiotherapy, conformal radiotherapy, and brachytherapy.[30,31] Although the benefits relative to conventional radiotherapy remain to be proven, twice-daily radiation permits the delivery of higher radiation doses over a shorter period of time, with less opportunity for tumor cell repair between treatments. Conformal radiation refers to the use of sophisticated treatment planning techniques in order to deliver radiation in a precise fashion to match the 3-dimensional shape of the tumor. This technique maximizes dose delivery to the tumor, while sparing surrounding healthy lung. Brachytherapy refers to radiation that is applied directly to the tumor either intraoperatively or through a catheter. High doses can be delivered locally, while sparing surrounding tissue.

In recent years, the use of chemotherapy has been broadened in the management of non-small cell lung cancer. Studies have evaluated the efficacy of chemotherapy alone, prior to surgery, following surgery, or concurrently with radiotherapy.[32,33] As discussed below, the efficacy of chemotherapy in locally advanced and metastatic disease has been demonstrated. Many new chemotherapeutic agents and combinations have been developed. Hematopoietic growth factors and agents that specifically protect the patient from several of the toxic effects of chemotherapy are available as well.[34,35]

Surgical resection continues to be the treatment of choice for patients with stages I and II non-small cell lung cancer. A recent study has investigated the role of therapy with vitamin A derivatives in an effort to prevent the development of second primary lung cancers; the results of this trial are not yet available. Studies are also under way to evaluate the role of postoperative (adjuvant) chemotherapy in such patients. It is now recognized that the survival of patients with stage III non-small cell lung cancer can be prolonged with initial chemotherapy and/or radiotherapy.[36-38] Such treatment appears to be superior to surgery alone for stage

TABLE 50-3 Frequency of Each Tumor Stage at Diagnosis

Tumor Type and Stage	Frequency at Diagnosis (%)	Five Year Survival (%)
Non-Small Cell Lung Cancer		
Stage I	20	70–80
Stage II	20	40–60
Stage III	25	20
Stage IV	35	<5
Small Cell Lung Cancer		
Limited Stage	20	15
Extensive Stage	80	<5

IIIA disease or to radiotherapy alone for IIIB disease. It remains unclear whether surgical resection following chemoradiotherapy further improves survival among patients with IIIA disease. Patients with IIIB disease are generally treated with chemoradiotherapy alone.[39,40]

The treatment of patients with stage IV non-small cell lung cancer has changed in recent years as a result of the availability of new types of chemotherapy. Agents including carboplatin, paclitaxel, docetaxel, vinorelbine, and gemcitabine can achieve tumor response rates of 20 to 25 percent.[41-44] There is some evidence that treatment with the combination carboplatin and paclitaxel can result in prolonged survival for a subset of patients.[45] Vinorelbine and gemcitabine are active as single agents; their efficacy in combination with other agents is under active investigation.[46]

Due to the paucity of objective data concerning the efficacy of these new agents in comparison to older drugs and the absence of truly effective treatment for stage IV non-small cell lung cancer, such patients should be encouraged to participate in clinical research trials. Such trials provide patients with access to innovative agents and drug combinations. The results of treatment contribute to the development of new therapeutic approaches to this disease.

Patients with limited stage small cell lung cancer are now treated with concurrent chemotherapy and radiotherapy. This type of treatment has resulted in higher rates of local control and disease-free survival as compared to the same treatments delivered in a sequential fashion.[47,48] The impact of innovative radiotherapy techniques and the value of new drugs and drug combinations continue to be investigated.

ADVERSE EFFECTS OF TREATMENT

As noted above, the three primary modalities of treatment that are utilized alone or in combination for lung cancer treatment include surgery, radiation, and chemotherapy. The side effects of each type of therapy will be briefly considered in this section.

The primary adverse effect of surgical resection of a lung tumor pertains to the loss of healthy lung parenchyma. Resection of larger tumors often necessitates removal of more than one lobe or even an entire lung. The burden of providing adequate oxygen exchange during periods of peak demand is, therefore, shifted to a smaller volume of lung. For many lung cancer patients with a long history of cigarette smoking, the remaining lung may be severely impaired. The patient with adequate healthy remaining lung parenchyma may experience dyspnea only with moderate to extreme exertion. The more severely affected patient may become hypoxic with minimal activity such as having a bowel movement or brushing his/her teeth.

Blood loss during surgery may render the patient anemic. A young patient without heart disease will generally experience reduced exercise tolerance with a hematocrit below 25 percent. A patient in his/her late 60s or 70s, or a patient with heart disease, may become symptomatic if the hematocrit drops below 30 percent.

Another side effect of lung surgery pertains to the deconditioning that occurs during the sedentary postoperative period and during convalescence. Patients who have undergone resection of a portion of one lung (i.e., in whom pneumonectomy was not performed) generally require a chest tube for 1 to 3 days following surgery to expand the remaining lung. This tube can cause pain with movement and often restricts the patient's activity level. The sedentary patient may have partial collapse (atelectasis) of healthy lung tissue, which reduces the efficiency of oxygen exchange. Accessory muscles of respiration (such as the intercostal muscles) may become weakened through inactivity, thus further limiting the patient's exercise tolerance.

Thoracic radiation therapy is generally delivered over a period of 5 to 6 weeks in cumulative doses of 4500 to 6000 cGy. Treatment may be directed to the "tumor bed" and surrounding nodes if resection has already taken place. If radiotherapy is used as the primary modality of treatment, the tumor and a margin of healthy surrounding lung tissue are included in the field. During conventional radiotherapy, some healthy lung tissue is unavoidably included in the treatment field. As noted above, new techniques such as conformal radiotherapy and/or brachytherapy permit the delivery of radiation to a more limited pulmonary field, thereby reducing the likelihood of complications.[49]

The most important and irreversible adverse effect of thoracic radiotherapy is impaired respiratory function secondary to pulmonary fibrosis.[50] This process begins 4 to 8 weeks following the completion of radiotherapy and continues for up to 2 years. Pulmonary alveoli located within the radiation field are rendered incapable of oxygen exchange. In addition, the scarring process can restrict large portions of the remaining healthy lung from full expansion, thereby impairing efficient oxygen exchange.[51]

There are several reversible forms of toxicity associated with radiation therapy to the lung. When a large volume of lung is treated, generalized fatigue can occur. This symptom begins after several treatments have been administered and may persist for days to weeks following the completion of treatment. An acute inflammatory process (radiation pneumonitis) can occur 2 to 4 months following the completion of radiotherapy. Fever, dyspnea, and hypoxia may occur, along with a pulmonary infiltrate within the radiation field. This condition responds well to treatment with high doses of glucocorticoid medications.[52]

Patients who develop metastatic disease may receive palliative radiation to other parts of the body. Adverse effects of such treatment depend upon the anatomic location of the treatment field. If radiation therapy is delivered to the spinal cord in a dose exceeding 4000 cGy, 2 percent of patients will develop deterioration of the cord 9 to 12 months following treatment.[53] Conventional doses of radiation can cause generalized pain and stiffness in the pelvis and hips. If the radiation field includes multiple vertebral bodies or large bones such as the pelvis and femurs, myelosuppression (particularly anemia and/or thrombocytopenia) may result. These effects usually resolve within a few weeks of the completion of treatment.

Chemotherapy can produce a wide variety of toxic effects, depending on the specific agents used. It is beyond the scope of this chapter to review the specific side-effect profile of every agent used in the treatment of patients with lung cancer. A brief summary of some of the toxic effects associated with several of the more commonly utilized chemotherapeutic agents is provided in Table 50-4. In general, side effects such as nausea, diarrhea, or allergic reactions occur within hours of chemotherapy administration and are transient.

TABLE 50-4 Common Side Effects of Selected Chemotherapeutic Agents Used in the Treatment of Lung Cancer

Drug	Side Effects Likely to Resolve within 4 Weeks of Discontinuing Chemotherapy	Side Effects That May Be Long Lasting or Irreversible
Cisplatin	Nausea Fatigue	Nephrotoxicity Ototoxicity Peripheral neuropathy
Etoposide	Constipation Fatigue Myelosuppression Alopecia	Peripheral neuropathy
Paclitaxel	Allergic reaction Myalgias Myelosuppression Alopecia	Peripheral neuropathy
Carboplatin	Nausea Fatigue Myelosuppression Alopecia	
Vinorelbine	Nausea Fatigue Myelosuppression Alopecia	Peripheral neuropathy
Gemcitabine	Diarrhea Myelosuppression Skin rash Flu-like symptoms Alopecia Edema	

Mouth soreness, fatigue, anorexia, hair loss, anemia, or neutropenia may be delayed by several weeks and are also temporary. Certain agents cause neurotoxicity, cardiotoxicity, nephrotoxicity, or pulmonary fibrosis; these effects tend to be long lasting and are often irreversible.[54]

DISABILITY RELATED TO PROGRESSIVE TUMOR GROWTH

The risks and benefits of specific types of treatment have been discussed above. Those patients who are fortunate enough to be cured of their disease may be entirely healthy, or they may have some residual symptoms related to prior treatment. Those patients who are not cured with initial treatment will eventually develop progressive disease and die. The tumor itself can cause disability related to a variety of local and distant effects.

The presence of the tumor in the lung may cause respiratory dysfunction. Metastatic tumor in other organs may cause pain, bone fractures, hepatic failure, or neurologic dysfunction. Generalized effects attributable to the underlying tumor include fatigue, anorexia, weight loss, and disuse-related muscular atrophy. Non-small cell lung tumors (particularly squamous cancers) can produce a PTH-like protein that causes hypercalcemia and related complications. Small cell lung tumors can cause a paraneoplastic muscle weakness similar to myasthenia gravis (Eaton-Lambert syndrome).[55] Patients who become terminally ill are most likely to be troubled with pain, dyspnea, fatigue, and malnutrition. At any point, lung cancer patients may have difficulty with anxiety and/or depression.

MULTIDISCIPLINARY APPROACH TO THE REHABILITATION OF THE PATIENT WITH LUNG CANCER

Lung cancer patients are a heterogeneous group, including "healthy" individuals who have undergone a curative thoracotomy, patients undergoing intensive chemotherapy and/or radiotherapy, and those who are receiving comfort care near the end of life. As discussed above, symptoms experienced by the lung cancer patient can be related to the tumor or to treatment; they can be generalized or organ specific. Disorders include but are not limited to those that are respiratory, neurologic, musculoskeletal, metabolic, constitutional, and/or psychiatric.

Accordingly, opportunities for rehabilitation of the lung cancer patient are broad ranging. The development of a rehabilitation program requires a multidisciplinary team with expertise in the underlying disorder as well as a variety of therapeutic interventions. The disciplines of physical medicine and rehabilitation provide diagnostic and therapeutic services directed at specific types of neurologic and musculoskeletal dysfunction. Physical, occupational, and recreational therapy can be directed at restoring the function of specific muscle groups as well as global conditioning and adaptation to activities of daily living.

Pulmonary rehabilitation can focus on disabilities related to the underlying lung tumor or pulmonary complications of treatment or tumor growth. Attention to the patient's nutritional state, emotional/psychiatric symptoms, and an understanding of pain control technology are also important components of a multidisciplinary approach. These interventions will be discussed in greater detail in the sections that follow.

THE IMMEDIATE POSTOPERATIVE PERIOD

Following surgery, the patient should be encouraged to ambulate as soon as possible. Even if a chest tube remains in place, the patient need not be bed-bound. If the patient experiences pain with movement, the judicious use of analgesics may be helpful. Incentive spirometry may help to expand atelectatic lung tissue and has been shown to be superior to purely expiratory exercises.[56] Pulse oximetry should be used to follow oxygen saturation at rest and with exertion. Oxygen saturation should be maintained at a level of 90% or above. A postoperative hematocrit should be checked. An elderly patient or a patient with heart disease may require transfusion of packed red cells if the hematocrit remains below 30 percent. Younger patients and those without heart disease generally do not receive blood transfusions unless the hematocrit falls below 25 percent. Interventions include postoperative positional drainage, chest percussion, and chest percussion, as well as more vigorous programs to strengthen muscles of respiration and improve endurance.[57]

LOSS OF PULMONARY FUNCTION

When a lung tumor cannot be eradicated and remains within the thorax, its presence may cause compressive atelectasis of surrounding lung and may obstruct adjacent airways. Tumor resection results in loss of that portion of lung occupied by the tumor itself and a variable portion of surrounding healthy lung. As discussed above, radiation therapy damages some portion of normal lung and can cause a restrictive pattern of lung disease. The loss of pulmonary function associated with each of these events is generally irreversible. Pulmonary parenchyma cannot regenerate, and these damaged tissues do not regain function following exercise therapy. However, the function of the remaining healthy lung can be optimized. Rehabilitation activities that eliminate atelectasis in healthy lung and strengthen accessory muscles of respiration can significantly improve a patient's functional status.

GENERALIZED AND/OR FOCAL MUSCLE WEAKNESS

Patients who undergo surgical resection of a lung tumor experience a period of enforced bed rest during the postoperative period. As discussed above, unless a pneumonectomy is performed, a chest tube is left in place for 2 to 3 days following surgery. The presence of a chest tube can restrict mobility. Patients who do not have a chest tube are still limited by the presence of a large and painful thoracotomy incision. To a lesser extent, patients may adopt a sedentary lifestyle during chemotherapy or radiotherapy treatments. These events can result in generalized loss of muscle conditioning and strength.

Patients who receive treatment with glucocorticoids during irradiation for brain metastases or as an appetite stimulant may develop weakness of muscles within the hips and shoulders (proximal myopathy). Depending on the location of brain metastases, focal muscle weakness of an upper and/or lower extremity may occur. Chemotherapeutic agents such as the vinca alkaloids, cisplatin, and paclitaxel can produce neuropathy. These effects occur most often in distal lower and upper extremities in a symmetrical fashion. Sensory neuropathy is most common, although loss of motor function may occur as well.

Patients with either generalized or specific muscle weakness can benefit from rehabilitation services. Depending on the extent of disability, the specific loss of function, and the patient's ability to participate in rehabilitation efforts, an appropriate program of physical, occupational, and/or recreational therapy can be designed.

DISABILITY FOLLOWING TREATMENT OF BONE METASTASES AND FRACTURES

Among patients with metastatic lung cancer, symptomatic bone involvement occurs commonly at some point in their illness. Bone metastases from lung cancer may be blastic or lytic. The presence of bone metastases can result in disability as a result of pain alone or as a result of fractures in compromised bone. External beam radiotherapy is used to treat focal painful bone metastases. If surgical fixation is needed following pathologic fracture of a weight-bearing bone, radiotherapy is generally used postoperatively. When bone involvement is widespread, either systemic chemotherapy or systemic radiotherapy (with Strontium-89, for example) are used for palliation. If the patient is strong enough to participate in physical, occupational, or recreational therapy, such intervention can help him/her to regain lost function following treatment of bone metastases.

ANOREXIA AND MALNUTRITION

At every point in the management of patients with lung cancer, attention to appetite, body weight, and nutrition are of great importance. During the period following lung resection and during chemotherapy or radiotherapy, patients often experience diminished appetite. The tumor itself can profoundly suppress appetite regardless of the patient's nutritional state.[58,59] A persistent state of malnutrition further complicates the management of a patient with cancer, in that malnutrition can cause fatigue, susceptibility to infection, and it can increase the likelihood of toxicity in association with chemotherapy or radiotherapy.

The management of anorexia can be challenging, as the patient may experience a powerful aversion to food. Noting that this aversion often takes the form of early satiety, patients can be instructed to ingest six to eight small meals daily. High-calorie supplements and liquid forms of nutrition can be used. Patients are instructed to avoid high volume, low-calorie foods such as vegetables and fruits, and they are advised to disregard concerns about intake of sodium, cholesterol, or saturated fats. The patient can often benefit from an individualized nutritional plan developed together with a dietician.

Several pharmacologic agents have been used in an effort to reverse tumor-related anorexia.[60,61] Megestrol acetate is among the most effective appetite stimulants, although this medication is also associated with lower-extremity edema and a risk of thromboembolic disease.[62,63] Patients who appear to be depressed in association with their anorexia may experience an improvement in appetite following treatment with antidepressant medications. Glucocorticoids may also increase appetite, but significant complications may occur with long-term use (see below).

FATIGUE

This general symptom may occur at any point in the management of patients with lung cancer. Fatigue is a common constitutional symptom related to the underlying malignancy, the pathophysiology of which is poorly understood. However, it can also result from anemia or from disorders such as hypercalcemia, hypothyroidism, or adrenal insufficiency. Treatments including surgery, radiotherapy, and chemotherapy can result in fatigue; it can also occur as a manifestation of malnutrition or depression.

Postoperative fatigue and that associated with chemotherapy and/or radiotherapy is generally self-limited and does not require specific intervention. If properly identified, fatigue that is secondary to disorders such as anemia, hypercalcemia, hypothyroidism, or adrenal insufficiency can usually be managed with appropriate pharmacologic intervention. The treatment of malnutrition is discussed above. The management of depression is discussed below.

Fatigue that is related to an untreatable underlying malignancy is difficult to manage. Treatment with amphetamine medications may be extremely effective. Common side effects include agitation, insomnia, and diminished appetite. Glucocorticoid therapy can also provide a sense of increased energy. Immediate side effects may include agitation, insomnia, hyperglycemia, and an increase in appetite. With long-term use, proximal myopathy and osteopenia can occur.

PAIN

Patients with lung cancer may experience chest pain as an initial sign of lung cancer. They may undergo surgical resection of the tumor and experience postoperative pain. Chemotherapy-induced neuropathy can occur in the form of painful paresthesias. Metastatic disease in liver, bone, or brain can produce abdominal discomfort, bone pain, or headaches.

The optimal approach to pain management in a cancer patient is one in which multiple disciplines are involved in the assessment of the etiology of pain and in the development of a comprehensive management strategy.[64,65] The specific treatment of pain varies according to its etiology. Musculoskeletal pain may respond to thermal or cryotherapy, electrical stimulation, massage therapy, or traction devices. Neurogenic pain may be treated with electrical stimulation; localized injection of nerves, roots, or plexi; and occasionally with surgical ablation procedures.

A medication regimen can be carefully selected for pain of different types.[66] For example, bone pain will often respond to nonsteroidal anti-inflammatory agents (such as ibuprofen). Neurogenic pain will often respond to certain antiseizure medications (such as gabapentin or carbamazepine), antidepressants (such as amitriptyline), and benzodiazepines (such as lorazepam or diazepam). Long-acting narcotics (such as sustained-release oral morphine, sustained-release oral oxycodone, or transdermal fentanyl) and short-acting narcotics (such as morphine, oxycodone, hydromorphone, hydrocodone, or codeine) have broad utility, although they have the potential to cause sedation, constipation, dry mouth, and nausea. Glucocorticoids are also useful for pain management, although osteopenia, hyperglycemia, and mental status changes can occur. Considerable expertise is needed in the development of an analgesic medication regimen that will achieve maximal efficacy while minimizing side effects.

The presence of pain can result in loss of the ability to ambulate and carry out activities of daily living. Specific types of physical therapy intervention are often needed in order to teach the patient to accomplish these activities in an alternative fashion. In addition, muscles that lose strength as a result of pain-related disuse may benefit from specific strengthening programs.

Psychological assessment of the patient with pain is of great importance. Underlying anxiety or depression can profoundly alter the patient's experience of pain. In addition, the presence of pain can result in both anxiety and depression. An understanding of the impact of the patient's pain and disability on his/her social situation can lead to alterations in the management plan.

There is no doubt that physical and occupational therapy can be of benefit to many patients with pain. This approach can be used to develop new ways to accomplish activities of daily living without precipitating a pain crisis. In addition, it is often possible to regain musculoskeletal and neurologic functions that have been lost as a result of pain and/or its underlying etiology. However, the use of physical therapy to provide a direct analgesic effect is more controversial. Despite the belief of many authors that exercise therapy is effective in this regard, there are few clinical trials that support this conclusion. Koltyn and coworkers studied pain perception following aerobic exercise and found that this activity resulted in a statistically significant elevation of pain threshold and a reduction of pain ratings.[67] Nichols and Glenn evaluated the effect of aerobic walking on the pain and disability of patients with fibromyalgia. There was a trend (without statistical significance) suggesting an improvement in pain as a result of physical activity.[68] Barkin and associates suggest that the reason for the paucity of supporting clinical trial data pertain to inherent difficulties in the conduct of research of this type.[69,70]

DEPRESSION AND ANXIETY DISORDERS

Studies of psychological symptoms in patients with cancer indicate that over 40 percent of patients develop clinical depression and/or an anxiety disorder.[71,72] Factors that contribute to such symptoms might include a hereditary predisposition to affective disorders, medication side effects, and/or the patient's situational reaction to potential mortality, loss of autonomy, and sudden alteration in lifestyle. The debilitating effects of surgery, radiation therapy, and chemotherapy can have a significant psychological impact.

Specific pharmacologic agents used in the course of cancer treatment (including general anesthetics, glucocorticoids, narcotics, and benzodiazepines) can complicate the evaluation of a patient who exhibits signs of depression and/or anxiety. General anesthetics can result in lingering sedation and confusion. Glucocorticoid therapy can result in a sense of well-being and increased energy; it can also cause insomnia, agitation, confusion, and anxiety. The process of glucocorticoid withdrawal causes fatigue and depression. Narcotics can cause sedation, confusion, and visual hallucinations. Benzodiazepines frequently cause sedation; however, some individuals experience disinhibition and an increase in symptoms of agitation and anxiety.

Multiple approaches can be utilized in the management of psychological symptoms that are troubling to the cancer patient. An initial attempt should be made to clarify the cause of these symptoms. Elimination of environmental precipitants and/or offending medications can be useful. Individual psychotherapy, family therapy, group therapy, and/or behavioral modification techniques may be appropriate for patients who are receptive to such interventions.

Pharmacologic therapy for depression and anxiety can be highly effective. Results are often achieved far more quickly than with psychotherapeutic or behavior modification techniques. Benzodiazepines (such as lorazepam and diazepam), tricyclic antidepressants (such as amitriptyline and desipramine), and newer serotonin reuptake inhibitors (such as fluoxetine and paroxetine) can be used individually or in combination to treat anxiety disorders. The latter two categories of medications are used to treat depression. Trazodone hydrochloride, a newer antidepressant medication that is chemically unrelated to both the tricyclic antidepressants and the serotonin reuptake inhibitors can be effective in treating patients with both depression and anxiety.

It is important to note that these medications have side effects of their own. Many patients require the use of multiple psychoactive drugs in combination, thereby compounding the risk of treatment-related adverse reactions. Such medications should be prescribed with the assistance of an experienced psychopharmacologist.

Occupational therapy, physical therapy, and other types of rehabilitation medicine can indirectly help to treat anxiety and depression as a result of their impact on patient autonomy and normalization of lifestyle. A more challenging and controversial question is whether physical exercise can be used to specifically treat anxiety and depression in cancer patients.

Many studies have been conducted to investigate the efficacy of exercise in the treatment of depression.[73,74] A meta-analysis of 15 such studies of depression in patients with heart disease revealed that exercise exerts a statistically significant beneficial effect.[75] Martinsen reviewed 12 studies of exercise intervention to treat depression and again showed a beneficial effect.[76] Ruuskanen and Ruoppila showed that exercise can promote perceptions of psychological well-being among the elderly.[77] Palmer and colleagues reviewed the effects of exercise in the treatment of depression in recovering substance abusers.[78] The specific type (aerobic versus anaerobic) and duration of exercise varied widely among these studies.[79,80] A 2-year longitudinal study of patients with one or more chronic illnesses (including diabetes mellitus, hypertension, and heart disease) demonstrated a correlation between higher levels of physical activity and a sense of well-being.[81]

Fewer studies have investigated the effectiveness of physical activity as a treatment for anxiety disorders. In their study of patients with heart disease, Kugler and coworkers found that physical activity was a beneficial intervention in the treatment of anxiety disorders as well as depression.[75] Petruzello and associates found that physical activity can improve anxiety disorders. They concluded that the exercise must be aerobic; it must last for more than 20 min and must continue for more than 10 weeks.[82]

These data provide evidence that physical activity may be an effective component of treatment for affective disorders, including some patients with underlying medical illness. One can infer from these data that rehabilitation medicine may be useful in treating anxiety and depression in some cancer patients. However, the specific type of rehabilitation therapy, the duration, and frequency are not well defined.

Conclusion

An overview of the staging and prognosis associated with small cell and non-small cell lung cancer has been presented above. Conventional treatments as well as newer multimodality approaches to the management of this disease have been described. Despite many recent innovations in the treatment of patients with lung cancer, the long-term prognosis of such patients remains disappointing. In the absence of curative treatments for the majority of patients with lung cancer, the management of symptoms is of paramount importance.

For patients with all stages of lung cancer, opportunities exist to reverse or ameliorate disability related to the underlying tumor or to the effects of treatment. A comprehensive, multidisciplinary approach to the rehabilitation of lung cancer patients should include appropriate utilization of postoperative pulmonary rehabilitation, physical, occupational, and recreational therapy techniques, as well as treatment of anxiety and depression, fatigue, malnutrition, and pain. These interventions can have a major impact on quality of life experienced by patients with lung cancer, regardless of the outcome of specific anticancer therapy.

References

1. Hopwood P, Thatcher N: Current status of quality of life measurement in lung cancer patients. *Oncology* 5:159, 1991.
2. Tchekmedyian NS, Cells DF (eds): Quality of life in current oncology practice and research. *Oncology* 4:1, 1990.
3. Parker SL, Tong T, Bolden S, et al: Cancer statistics, 1997. *CA Cancer J Clin* 47:5, 1997.
4. Doll RE, Hill AB: A study of the etiology of carcinoma of the lung. *Br Med J* 2:1271, 1952.
5. Hammond EC: Smoking in relation to the death rates of one million men and women. *Natl Can Institut Monogr* 19:127, 1966.
6. Trichopoulos D: Risk of lung cancer and passive smoking, in DeVita VD, Hellman S, Rosenberg SA (eds): *Important Advances in Oncology 1995.* Philadelphia, J.B. Lippincott, 1995; p 77.
7. Schottenfeld D: Epidemiology of lung cancer, in Pass HI, Mitchell JB, Johnson DH et al (eds): *Lung Cancer: Principles and Practice.* Philadelphia, Lippincott-Raven, 1996; pp 305–321.
8. Colby TV, Koss MN, Travis WD: *Tumors of the Lower Respiratory Tract, Armed Forces Institute of Pathology Fascicle,* 3d series. Washington, DC. Armed Forces Institute of Pathology, 1995.
9. *Manual for Staging of Cancer, American Joint Committee on Cancer,* 4th ed. J.B. Lippincott, 1993.
10. Mountain CF: Revisions in the international system for staging lung cancer. *Chest* 111:1710, 1997.
11. Patteson GA, Ginsberg Rj, Poon PY, et al: A prospective evaluation of MRI, CT, and mediastinoscopy in preoperative assessment of mediastinal node status in bronchogenic carcinoma. *J Thorac Cardiovasc Surg* 94:679, 1987.
12. Bollen ECM, Van Duin CJ, Theunessen PHMH, et al: Mediastinal lymph node dissection in resected lung cancer: Morbidity and accuracy of staging. *Ann Thorac Surg* 55:961, 1993.
13. Stein M, Koota GM, Simon M, et al: Pulmonary evaluation of surgical patients. *JAMA* 181:765, 1962.
14. Smith PK, Wolfe WG: Preoperative assessment of pulmonary function: Quantitative evaluation of ventilation and blood gas exchange, in: *Surgery of the Chest,* 6th ed. Philadelphia, WB Saunders, 1995; pp 1–21.
15. Temeck B, Okunieff PG, Pass HI: Chest wall disease including superior sulcus tumors, in Pass HI, Mitchell JB, Johnson DH, et al (eds): *Lung Cancer: Principles and Practice.* Philadelphia, Lippincott-Raven, 1996; pp 585–601.
16. Ginsberg RJ, Rubinstein LV: Randomized trial of lobectomy versus limited resection for T1N0 non-small cell lung cancer. *Ann Thorac Surg* 60:615, 1995.
17. Ishida T, Yano T, Maeda K: Strategy for lymphadenopathy in lung cancer 3 cm or less in diameter. *Ann Thorac Surg* 50:708, 1991.
18. Johnson DH, Einhorn LH, Bartolucci A, et al: Thoracic radiotherapy does not prolong survival in patients with locally advanced unresectable non-small cell lung cancer: *Ann Intern Med* 113:33, 1990.
19. Perez CA, Pajak TF, Rubin P, et al: Long-term observations of the patterns of failure in patients with unresectable non-oat cell carcinoma of the lung treated with definitive radiotherapy. Report by the Radiation Therapy Oncology Group. *Cancer* 59:1874, 1987.
20. Non-Small Cell Lung Cancer Collaborative Group: Chemotherapy in non-small cell lung cancer: A meta-analysis using updated data on individual patients from 52 randomized clinical trials. *Br Med J* 311:899, 1995.
21. Johnson DH: Chemotherapy for metastatic non-small-cell lung cancer—can that dog hunt? *J Nat Can Instit* 85:766, 1993.
22. Cartei G, Caragei F, Cantone A, et al: Cisplatin-cyclophosphamide-mitomycin combination chemotherapy with supportive care versus supportive care alone for treatment of metastatic non-small-cell lung cancer. *J Natl Can Instit* 85:794, 1993.

23. Sandler AB: Current management of small cell lung cancer. *Semin Oncol* 24:463, 1997.

24. Naruke T, Goya T, Tsuchiya R, et al: Prognosis and survival in resected lung carcinoma based on the new international staging system. *J Thorac Cardiovasc Surg* 96:440, 1988.

25. Steel GG: *Growth Kinetics of Tumors.* Oxford, Clarendon Press, 1977.

26. Sagman U, Maki E, Evans WK, et al: Small-cell carcinoma of the lung: Derivation of a prognostic staging system. *J Clin Oncol* 9:1639, 1991.

27. Warren WH, Faber LP: Extended resections for locally advanced pulmonary carcinomas, in Pass HI, Mitchell JB, Johnson DH, et al (eds): *Lung Cancer: Principles and Practice.* Philadelphia, Lippincott-Raven, 1996; pp 567–584.

28. McKneally MR: Video-assisted thoracic surgery: Standards and guidelines. *Chest Surg Clin North Am* 3:345, 1993.

29. McKenna RJ: Lobectomy by video-assisted thoracic surgery with mediastinal node sampling for lung cancer. *J Thorac Cardiovasc Surg* 107:879, 1994.

30. Fowler JF: Carcinoma of the lung: Hyperfractionation or resection and chemotherapy? *Int J Radiat Oncol Biol Phys* 20:169, 1991.

31. Mendiondo OH, Dillon M, Beach LJ: Endobronchial brachytherapy in the treatment of recurrent bronchogenic carcioma. *Int J Radiat Oncol Biol Phys* 9:579, 1983.

32. Ihde DC: Chemotherapy of lung cancer. *N Engl J Med* 327:1434, 1992.

33. Ruckdeschel JC: Combined modality therapy of non-small cell lung cancer. *Semin Oncol* 24:429, 1997.

34. Vose JM, Armitage JO: Clinical applications of hematopoietic growth factors. *J Clin Oncol* 13:1023, 1995.

35. Alberts DS: Introduction: Applications of amifostine in cancer treatment. *Semin Oncol* 23:1, 1996.

36. Albain KS, Rusch VW, Crowley JJ, et al: Concurrent cisplatin/etoposide plus chest radiotherapy followed by surgery for stages IIA (N2) and IIIB non-small-cell lung cancer: Mature results of Southwest Oncology Group phase II study 8805. *J Clin Oncol* 13:1880, 1995.

37. Rosell T, Gomez-Codina J, Camps C, et al: A randomized trial comparing preoperative chemotherapy plus surgery with surgery alone in patients with non-small-cell lung cancer. *N Engl J Med* 330:153, 1994.

38. Roth JA, Fosella F, Komaki R, et al: A randomized trial comparing preoperative chemotherapy and surgery with surgery alone in resectable stage IIIA non-small-cell lung cancer. *J Natl Can Inst* 86:673, 1994.

39. Schaake-Koning C, van den Bogaert W, Dalesio O, et al: Effects of concomitant cisplatin and radiotherapy on inoperable non-small-cell lung cancer. *N Engl J Med* 326:524, 1992.

40. Dillman RO, Seagren SL, Propert KJ, et al: A randomized trial of induction chemotherapy plus high-dose radiation versus radiation alone in Stage III non-small-cell lung cancer. *N Engl J Med* 323:940, 1990.

41. Langer CJ, Leighton JC, Comis RL, et al: Paclitaxel and carboplatin in combination in the treatment of advanced non-small-cell lung cancer: A phase II toxicity, response, and survival analysis. *J Clin Oncol* 13:1860, 1995.

42. Ramanathan RK, Belani CP: Chemotherapy for advanced non-small cell lung cancer: Past, present, and future. *Semin Oncol* 24:440, 1997.

43. Le Chevalier T, Pujol JL, Douillard JY, et al: A three-arm trial of vinorelbine plus cisplatin, vindesine plus cisplatin, and single-agent vinorelbine in the treatment of non-small cell lung cancer: An expanded analysis. *Semin Oncol* 21(Suppl 10):28, 1994.

44. Takimoto CH: Clinical status and optimal use of topotecan. *Oncology* 11:1635, 1997.

45. Langer C, Rosvold E, Millenson M, et al: Paclitaxel by 1 to 24 hour infusion combined with carboplatin in advanced non-small

46. cell lung carcinoma: A comparative analysis. *Proc Am Soc Clin Oncol* 16:452a, 1997.

46. Eastern Cooperative Oncology Group protocol #E1594.

47. Johnson DH, Kim K, Turrisi AT, et al: Cisplatin and etoposide and concurrent thoracic radiotherapy administered once versus twice daily for limited-stage small cell lung cancer: Preliminary results of an intergroup trial. *ASCO Abstracts* 1994 #1105.

48. Sandler AB: Current management of small cell lung cancer. *Semin Oncol* 24:463, 1977.

49. Sause WT, Turrisi AT: Principles and application of preoperative and standard radiotherapy for regionally advanced non-small cell lung cancer, in Pass HI, Mitchell JB, Johnson DH, et al (eds): *Lung Cancer: Principles and Practice.* Philadelphia, Lippincott-Raven, 1996; pp 697–710.

50. Maasilta P: Radiation-induced lung injury from the chest physician's point of view. *Lung Canc* 7:367, 1991.

51. Marks L: The pulmonary effects of thoracic irradiation. *Oncology* 8:89, 1994.

52. Roberts CM, Foulcher E, Zaunders JJ, et al: Radiation pneumonitis: A possible lymphocyte-mediated hypersensitivity reaction. *Ann Intern Med* 118:696, 1993.

53. Coy P, Baker S, Dolman CL: Progressive myelopathy due to radiation. *Can Med Assoc* 100:1129, 1969.

54. Perry MC: *The Chemotherapy Source Book.* Baltimore, Williams and Wilkins, 1992.

55. Stephansson K, Arnason GW: Paraneoplastic syndromes of the brain, spinal cord, nerves, and the striated muscle, in Moosa AR, Robson D, Schimpft (ed): *Comprehensive Textbook of Oncology.* Baltimore, Williams and Wilkins, 1986; pp 410–416.

56. Bartlett RH, Brennon ML, Gazzaniga AB, et al: Studies on the pathogenesis and prevention of postoperative pulmonary complications. *Surg Gynecol Obstet* 137:925, 1975.

57. Helmholz HF, Stonnington HH: Rehabilitation of respiratory function, in Kotke FJ, Lehmann JF (eds): *Krusen's Handbook of Physical Medicine and Rehab,* 4th ed. Philadelphia, WB Saunders, 1990; pp 858–873.

58. Tracey K, Vlassara H, Cerami A: Cachetin/tumour necrosis factor. *Lancet* May 20:1122, 1989.

59. Tisdale MJ: Biology of cachexia. *J Natl Cancer Inst* 89:1763, 1997.

60. Bruera E: Current pharmacological management of anorexia in cancer patients. *Oncology* 6:125, 1992.

61. Chlebowski RT, Bulcavage L, Grosvenor M, et al: Hydrazine sulfate influence on nutritional status and survival in non-small cell lung cancer. *J Clin Oncol* 8:9, 1990.

62. Von Roenn JH: Randomized trial of megestrol acetate for AIDS-associated anorexia and cachexia. *Oncology* 51 (Suppl 1):19, 1994.

63. Loprinzi CL, Ellison NM, Schaid DJ, et al: Controlled trial of megestrol acetate for the treatment of cancer anorexia and cachexia. *J Natl Cancer Inst* 82:1127, 1990.

64. Rosen NB: Physical medicine and rehabilitation approaches to the management of myofacial pain and fibromyalgia syndromes. *Balliere's Clinical Rheumatology* 8:881–916, 1994.

65. Flor H, Fydrick T, Backman E, et al: Efficacy of multidisciplinary pain treatment centers: A meta-analytic view. *Pain* 49:221, 1992.

66. Levy MH: Pharmacologic treatment of cancer pain. *N Engl J Med* 335:1124, 1996.

67. Koltyn K, Garvin W, Gardiner RL, et al: Perception of pain following aerobic exercise. *J Am Coll Sports Med* 28:1418, 1996.

68. Nichols DS, Glenn TM: Effects of aerobic exercise on pain perception, affect, and level of disability in individuals with fibromyalgia. *Phys Ther* 74:327, 1994.

69. Barkin RL, Lubenow TR, Bruehl S et al: Management of chronic pain. Part II. *Disease-A-Month.* Volume 42, Number 8, 1996.

70. Deyo RA: Conservative therapy of low back pain. *JAMA* 250:1057, 1983.

71. Derogatis LB, Morrow GR, Fetting J, et al: The prevalence of psychiatric disorders among cancer patients. *JAMA* 249:751, 1983.

72. Stoudemire A, McDaniel JS: Psychiatric factors affecting medical conditions (psychosomatic disorders), in Kaplan HI, Sadock BJ (eds): *Comprehensive Textbook of Psychiatry VI.* Baltimore, Williams and Wilkins, 1995; pp 1463–1604.

73. Gauvin L, Spence JC: Physical activity and psychological well-being: Knowledge base, current issues, and caveats. *Nutrit Rev* 54:S53, 1996.

74. Plante TG: Getting physical—does exercise help in the treatment of psychiatric disorders? *J Psychoasoc Nurse* 34:38, 1996.

75. Kugler J, Seelback H, Kruskemper GM: Effects of rehabilitation exercise programs on anxiety and depression in coronary patients. A meta-analysis. *Br J Clin Psychol* 33:401, 1994.

76. Martinsen EW: Physical activity and depression: Clinical experience. *Acta Psychiatr Scand Suppl* 377:23, 1994.

77. Ruuskanen JM, Ruoppila I: Physical activity and psychological well-being among people aged 65–84 years. *Age and Aging* 24:292, 1995.

78. Palmer JA, Palmer LK, Michaels K, et al: Effects of type of exercise on depression in recovering substance abusers. *Percept Motor Skills* 80:523, 1995.

79. Doyne J, Ossip-Klein DJ, Bowman ED, et al: Running versus weight lifting in the treatment of depression. *J Counsel Clin Psychol* 55:748, 1987.

80. Martinsen EW, Hoffart A, Solbert O: Comparing aerobic and nonaerobic forms of exercise in the treatment of clinical depression: A randomized trial. *Comprehen Psych* 30:324, 1989.

81. Stewart AL, Hays RD, Wells KB et al: Long-term functioning and well-being outcomes associated with physical activity and exercise in patients with chronic conditions in the medical outcomes study. *J Clin Epidemiol* 47:719, 1994.

82. Petruzzello SJ, Landers DM, Hatfield BD, et al: A meta-analysis on the anxiety-reducing effects of acute and chronic exercise. Outcomes and mechanisms. *Sports Med* 11:143, 1991.

Chapter 51

LUNG VOLUME REDUCTION SURGERY IN THE UNITED STATES

ARTHUR F. GELB

MATTHEW BRENNER*

ROBERT J. MCKENNA, JR.

RICHARD FISCHEL

NOE ZAMEL

MARK J. SCHEIN

Symptomatic patients with severe airflow limitation due to chronic obstructive pulmonary disease (COPD) including emphysema have a poor prognosis. Despite optimal medical therapy including oxygen, antibiotics, corticosteroids, oral and inhaled bronchodilators, and physical rehabilitation, relief from dyspnea and a markedly impaired lifestyle is often elusive. When the forced expiratory volume in 1 s (FEV_1) is $\leq .075$ liter or ≤ 30 percent predicted, 2-year mortality of 30 to 55 percent and 3-year mortality of 40 to 60 percent has been reported.[1-5] A recent study[6] of patients admitted to the intensive care unit for exacerbation of underlying COPD reported 1 year mortality of 30 percent, whereas it doubled in patients aged > 65 years, irrespective of the need for assisted ventilation. Patients with severe COPD with FEV_1 ≤ 0.51 or ≤ 20 percent predicted who have the rare opportunity to undergo unilateral lung transplantation still face a 2-year mortality of 30 percent in addition to the multiple problems related to chronic immunosuppression.[7]

Rehabilitation

The pertinent issues and role of pulmonary rehabilitation have been addressed previously.[8-10] In a statement by the American Thoracic Society[8] it is "(1) to lessen airflow limitation, (2) to prevent and treat secondary medical complications such as hypoxemia and infections, and (3) to decrease respiratory symptoms and improve quality of life." In patients with severe end stage COPD in whom polypharmacy has been optimized, the role of pulmonary rehabilitation as redefined by an NIH workshop[11] is to provide "a multidimensional continuum of services directed to persons with pulmonary disease and their families, usually by an interdisciplinary team of specialists, with the goal of exceeding and maintaining the individual's maximum level of independence and functioning in the community." It is important that adequate emphasis be placed on patient education, oxygen usage, nutritional support, large muscle group aerobic exercise training, and breathing retraining including purse lip, diaphragmatic, and relaxation.[8-11] Just as important is to address the social and psychological problems of anxiety and depression and feelings of dependency and helplessness in dyspneic patients with marked physical impairment and greatly altered lifestyles.

Casaburi[12] reviewed the outcome of 900 patients with symptomatic COPD who underwent physical rehabilitation. Measurements of quality of life, relief of dyspnea, and physical and walking endurance were reported to be improved in selected patients, despite no improvement in either lung function studies and/or oxygen dependency. Similar observations were also reported by Ries and coworkers,[3] Goldstein and colleagues,[14] Celli,[13] and others.[8-11] Moreover, following pulmonary rehabilitation, decreased hospital usage was noted by some but not all observers.[13]

The role of pulmonary rehabilitation prior to lung volume reduction surgery (LVRS) is to maximize all potential benefits. In a small subset of patients with severe airflow limitation, successful pulmonary rehabilitation may temporarily preclude or obviate the need for LVRS. However, in the vast majority of patients with severe airflow limitation, successful pulmonary rehabilitation and increased physical endurance should provide potential LVRS candidates a better outcome with reduced surgical morbidity and mortality. Alternatively, patients with an unsuccessful pulmonary rehabilitation experience may not be good candidates for LVRS.

Pathophysiology of COPD

Emphysema is destruction of lung parenchyma distal to the terminal airways.[15,16] There is physiologic loss of lung elastic recoil forces that normally provide both radial traction support of peripheral airways as well as the driving pressure during forced expiration. Peripheral airways collapse more easily and expiratory airflow limitation occurs prematurely resulting in lung dynamic hyperinflation and intrinsic PEEP.[17] Marked hyperinflation causes shortening and downward displacement of the diaphragm, resulting in impaired inspiratory muscle function.[18-21] The compliant chest wall accommodates the hyperinflated lung, but at the expense of its normal inspiratory expansive properties. In severe airflow limitation, the rib cage inspiratory muscles may contribute more to the tidal volume than the diaphragm. Tidal breathing at rest shifts to higher lung volume and this together with respiratory muscle dysfunction contributes to the sensation of dyspnea in symptomatic patients.[22] Progressive severe hyperinflation may also lead to impaired cardiac function.[23]

Emphysema in association with chronic cigarette smoking is also accompanied by intrinsic small airways abnormalities. The classic work by Hogg and coworkers[24] and more recent studies[25-27] confirm that the major cause of airflow limitation in cigarette-related severe COPD and emphysema is increased airway resistance from intrinsic small airways obstruction rather than loss of lung elastic recoil due to parenchymal destruction. However, the contributory role of loss of lung elastic recoil to causing expiratory airflow limitation should not be underestimated.

Detection of Emphysema

A reduced diffusing capacity is anticipated in any disease that disrupts the alveolar capillary surface area. However, it should be emphasized that a spuriously low diffusing

* Supported in part by Department of Energy (DOE) grant DE-f603-91ER61227 and NIH grant RO 1192 (MB).

capacity may occur in patients with severe airflow limitation with $FEV_1 < 1$ liter who have predominantly intrinsic small airways disease and no or trivial morphologic emphysema.[26,27] Similarly, we[27a] and others[28] have also noted a marked reduction in static lung elastic recoil pressure at total lung capacity < 12 cmH_2O in the presence of severe airflow limitation and no or trivial morphologic emphysema. Furthermore, there is no correlation between airflow limitation and anatomic extent and distribution of emphysema.[25-27] Previous radiologic and morphologic correlative studies[16,27] noted that high resolution, 2-mm thin-section computed tomography (CT) lung scans closely corroborate the extent, distribution, and severity of whole lung morphologic emphysema. As previously described,[16,27] we use a modification of the picture-grading system[16,29,30] adapted for lung CT[16,28,31-33] to score areas of low attenuation and vascular obliteration for emphysema. When we evaluated 81 consecutively seen patients with severe airflow limitation, that is, $FEV_1 < 50$ percent predicted, only 24 (30 percent) had CT scored severe grade of emphysema ≥ 60.[27] Thus, emphysema is not the major cause of airflow limitation in severe COPD. Paradoxically, similar to the observations of Hogg and coworkers,[25] we also noted generalized emphysema scores ≥ 60 in 2 of 11 patients (18 percent) with $FEV_1 \geq 70$ percent predicted.[27]

History of Lung Volume Reduction Surgery

Previous surgical interventions in severe emphysema were based on the presumption that the lungs were too large for the chest cavity. Attempts were made to compress the hyperinflated lung or to increase the chest cavity, but no long-standing, significant benefits were documented.[34] In 1957, Brantigan and Mueller[35] reported the near equivalent of LVRS to decrease the volume of the hyperinflated lung. They hypothesized an increase in the circumferential pull on the bronchioles would result in greater airway stability. Unfortunately, no supporting objective data was documented and an 18 percent mortality led to abandonment of the procedure.[35]

In 1991, Wakabayashi and coworkers[36] used contact and free beam laser techniques to shrink the lung volume in emphysema. Despite overall poor follow-up, they demonstrated dramatic clinical and functional improvement in selected patients with bullous lung disease and generalized emphysema. Cooper and colleagues,[37] in a classic paper, reevaluated LVRS by resecting targeted areas of emphysematous lung destruction bilaterally that had no or little perfusion using a median sternotomy incision. Air leaks were reduced with bovine pericardium.[37,38] Follow-up at > 24 months reported very significant mean improvement in clinical and lung function parameters.[38] Subsequently, McKenna and associates,[39] using video-assisted thoracoscopic techniques in a randomized prospective study, concluded that unilateral lung stapled resection was better than unilateral lung laser shrinkage and that bilateral lung stapling offered superior results to unilateral stapling.[40] Furthermore, results and safety of bilateral video-assisted thoracoscopic techniques[40] were similar to median sternotomy (< 5 percent 90-day mortality).[38] McKenna and coworkers[41] and Cooper and

colleagues[37,38] also noted that upper or lower targeted lung resection was better than resecting diffuse emphysema. Both[37-41] emphasized optimal results following resection of targeted emphysematous destruction in the upper lung fields compared to the lower lung fields. Published reports[38-48] of bilateral LVRS in over 700 patients, all of whom had had medical treatment and pre-LVRS physical rehabilitation, noted a 37 to 83 percent mean increase in FEV_1 (liter), 26 to 62 percent increase in 6-min walk test and up to 60 percent reduction in partial or complete oxygen dependence at 6 months postprocedure. Ninety-day mortality was 2.5 to 10 percent with mean length of hospital stay 10 to 17 days. Dramatic improvements in quality of life were reported, yet some patients had only a modest increase in workload post-LVRS despite significant increase in FEV_1.[38] Of interest, it was reported that although there was significantly greater improvement in FEV_1 following bilateral lung transplantation compared to unilateral, both patients achieved a similar maximal oxygen consumption,[49] and 6-min walk test.[50] This paradox suggests a limit to work performance despite improved lung mechanics that may be related to chronic muscle deconditioning and decreased peripheral oxygen extraction.[51]

Following LVRS with a decrease in hyperinflation and increased lung elastic recoil,[52-55a] there is significantly greater inspiratory muscle strength and transdiaphragmatic pressure.[22,56-58] Relief from dyspnea is associated with breathing slower at lower lung volumes with increased inspiratory time,[22,57,57a,58] but with variable effects on arterial blood gases[58a] and exercise.[58b]

Improvements in lifestyle and lung function ≥ 2 years post-LVRS are now documented.[38,55a,59]

Patient Selection

CLINICAL

Based on our previous studies,[39-41,53-55a,60-61b] potential patient candidates for LVRS should be symptomatic with at least grade 3 dyspnea,[62] that is, shortness of breath on walking less than 100 yards despite maximal medical therapy. The patients should not be acutely ill or have any comorbid illness that would preclude at least 3 years survival. There should be no recent tobacco usage for at least 3 months and no evidence for substance abuse. Corticosteroid dosage usually is < 20 mg prednisone equivalent daily. Presence of chronic bronchitis and bronchiectasis are relative contraindications. There should be evidence for fixed, severe airflow limitation, that is, $FEV_1 < 1$ liter and/or < 35 percent predicted. Also, there is marked hyperinflation using correct plethysmographic techniques[63] for measurements of functional residual capacity. Our preoperative FEV_1 has been 0.7 liters ± 0.06 (mean $\pm$ SEM) (24 $\pm$ 2 percent predicted); FVC, 2.3 liters $\pm$ 0.2 (55 $\pm$ 5 percent predicted); FRC, 7.5 liters $\pm$ 0.3 (195 $\pm$ 9 percent predicted); RV, 6.8 liters $\pm$ 0.3 (275 $\pm$ 11 percent predicted); TLC, 9.5 liters $\pm$ 0.3 (148 $\pm$ 5 percent predicted); single breath diffusing capacity, 5.0 mL/min/mmHg $\pm$ 1.0 (18 $\pm$ 4 percent predicted).[53,54] Chest roentgenogram and high-resolution thin-section lung CT should demonstrate severe, bilateral, nongiant bullous, generalized emphysema with a visual score ≥ 60.[26,27] There should be a heterogeneous emphysematous distribution with predominance in either

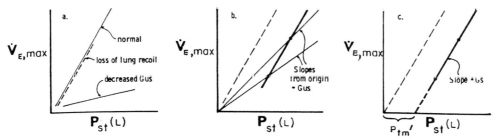

FIGURE 51-1 Schematic maximum flow-static recoil plots. *A.* Loss of lung recoil does not affect the maximum flow-static recoil slope. A decrease in the maximum flow-static recoil slope indicates a decrease in upstream conductance. *B.* Parallel displacement of maximum flow points (heavy continuous line) to higher values of static recoil pressure. In the analysis of Mead and coworkers[66] this change is also interreted as a decrease in upstream conductance. Interrupted line indicates a normal maximum flow-static recoil curve. *C.* Graphical interpretation of the maximum flow-static recoil curve (heavy continuous line) shown in *B* using the analysis of Pride and associates.[67]

upper or, less optimally, lower lung fields. Perfusion lung scans should demonstrate an absence or paucity of perfusion corresponding to the worst targeted emphysematous areas, with relatively good perfusion to the lung fields with relatively less emphysema. The matching defects on lung CT and perfusion scans are crucial for best LVRS selection.

Arterial blood gases will always demonstrate an increased $(A\text{-}a)O_2$ gradient and part- or full-time oxygen dependency is not unusual. Arterial Pa_{CO_2} should be ≤ 50 mmHg, although selected patients with $Pa_{CO_2} > 50$ mmHg have been reported to have done well post- LVRS.[42] Cycle ergometry performed to symptom limited maximum demonstrates maximal oxygen consumption invariably < 10 mL/kg/min. Measurements of static lung elastic recoil at TLC are < 12 cmH$_2$O.

The presence of an undiagnosed concomitant localized coin lesion < 2 cm diameter in the anticipated surgical resection area is not a contraindication to surgery. McKenna and coworkers[64] have reported successful concomitant LVRS and resection of malignant nodules.

Prior to surgical intervention, echocardiography should demonstrate adequate left ventricular function. The presence of significant pulmonary hypertension (mean pulmonary artery pressures > 35 mm) is unusual and Keller and Naunheim[65] have shown that routine preoperative right-sided cardiac catheterization is unnecessary.

PHYSIOLOGIC

In order to determine the mechanism(s) of expiratory airflow limitation in COPD, it is important to construct maximum expiratory flow–static lung elastic recoil pressure curves (MFSR).[66,67] Maximum expiratory flow volume loops obtained only from a pressure compensated flow or volume plethysmograph are used to plot airflow against static lung elastic recoil pressure at isovolume points. The slope of the line over the effort-independent relatively linear 50 to 30 percent expired part of the forced vital capacity is the conductance (G_s) of the small airways (s) segment according to the model proposed by Pride and colleagues.[67] The s segment extends from the alveoli to and includes the collapsible flow limiting segment.[67] The critical transmural pressure (Ptm') in the collapsible flow limiting segment is determined by extrapolating the slope of the MFSR to zero $\dot{V}$max.[67] This intercept at $\dot{V}$max = 0 is the difference between lateral intraluminal pressure of the collapsible flow limiting segment and the extraluminal (pleural) pressure. Thus $\dot{V}$max = [Pst (liters) − Ptm'] G_s.[67] The s airway segment is equal to the length of the upstream airway segment of Mead and coworkers[66] if the Ptm' = 0. However, in emphysema with both loss of lung elastic recoil and concomitant intrinsic small airways abnormalities[24-27] as the flow limiting small airways segment migrate peripherally upstream, Ptm' invariably is positive because of increased airway collapse and/or intrinsic luminal narrowing.[53,54,68] Hence, the s-airway segment of Pride and colleagues[67] is shorter than the upstream segment of Mead and associates[66] (Fig. 51-1).

Maximum expiratory flow volume loops obtained at the mouth are grossly distorted in severe airflow obstruction due to intrathoracic gas compression.[69] Therefore, they do not provide reliable data to construct MFSR curves to study the mechanism(s) of airflow limitation.

We have previously noted using the MFSR model of Pride and coworkers[67] that in asymptomatic patients who have clinically unsuspected but proven anatomic emphysema (mean grade 50 visual score) with normal or borderline forced expiratory volume in 1 s (FEV$_1$), that airflow limitation can be completely accounted for by loss of lung elastic recoil despite morphologic evidence of small airways abnormalities.[68,70] However, in symptomatic patients who have alpha$_1$-antitrypsin deficiency with overt airway obstruction and mild to moderate cigarette usage Black and colleagues[71] reported that only half the patients had airflow limitation that could be accounted for by loss of lung elastic recoil. The remaining half had airflow limitation due to both loss of lung elastic recoil as well as decreased small airways conductance. Presumably this was due to intrinsic small airway abnormalities and/or collapse since no morphologic studies were available. Black and colleagues[71] noted that this last pattern was also characteristic of chronic cigarette smokers with overt airway obstruction without alpha$_1$-antitrypsin deficiency. This pattern is also typical of the patients who undergo lung volume reduction surgery, despite chest roentgenogram, CT, and morphologic evidence of severe generalized emphysema.[53,54] We have repeatedly demonstrated that airflow limitation is due to both loss of lung elastic recoil as well as markedly reduced conductance of the s airway segment and increased airway collapsibility.[53,54,55a] These findings should not be unexpected since almost all patients are chronic cigarette smokers and morphologic studies have documented extensive intrinsic small airways abnormalities in COPD, despite severe emphysema.[24,25,27]

Following bullectomy in bullous lung disease with or without accompanying generalized emphysema, we[72,73] and others[74–77] have been able to demonstrate that the improvement in both expiratory airflow limitation and airway conductance could be accounted for by the measured increase in lung elastic recoil.[72–75,77] This results in both greater driving pressure during forced exhalation as well as increased circumferential tethering of small airways, thereby helping to maintain airway caliber. We believe that this same mechanism is operant following lung volume reduction surgery for generalized emphysema. The surgical removal of nonfunctioning destroyed emphysematous lung causes an absolute increase in lung elastic recoil 6 months following unilateral LVRS,[52] and at 6 to 24 months,[55a] extending to 24 months (unpublished) following bilateral LVRS. We believe that the reduction in lung volume together with increase in lung elastic recoil is responsible for the increased expiratory airflow and airway conductance[53,54,55a] and the increased inspiratory muscle and diaphragm function.[22,56–58]

Furthermore, those patients who had the greatest increase in FEV_1 post-LVRS not only increased their lung elastic recoil, but also their conductance of the s airway segment as evidenced by a steeper slope in their MFSR curve.[53,54] They also had the greatest increase in the coefficient of retraction, that is, lung elastic recoil at TLC divided by TLC.[78] However, the increase in FEV_1 and airway conductance post-LVRS could not be correlated with any preoperative lung function study or with extent of heterogenous distribution of emphysema on chest roentgenogram or lung CT.[53,54] We also noted discrepancies between post-LVRS end points, with varying improvement in clinical status, oxygen dependence, exercise tolerance, and improvement in lung function.[53,54,55a]

Operative Technique and Postoperative Care

As previously described,[39–41,53–55,63] after obtaining informed consent and approval of the Institutional Human Investigation Committee at Chapman Medical Center, Orange or Cedars-Sinai Medical Center, Los Angeles, patients undergo sequential bilateral video-assisted thoracoscopic surgery at the same operative sitting under vecuronium paralysis and isoflurane general anesthesia with fraction of inspired oxygen of 1.0 using a left-sided 39 F double-lumen endotracheal tube (Mallincrodt Anesthesia, St. Louis, MO). After single-dependent lung ventilation has been achieved, the contralateral upside deflated lung is examined. Visually, the most distended, destroyed, emphysematous areas previously targeted by the preoperative lung CT and lung perfusion scan, usually in the upper and middle lung fields, is excised and linear staple lines are reinforced with bovine pericardium (Peri-Strips, Bio-Vascular Inc., St. Paul, MN) or bovine collagen (Instat, Johnson and Johnson, New Brunswick, NJ) to minimize air leaks. It is estimated that the excised lung volume is approximately 15 to 20 percent of each lung. Actual weight of each resected lung is 30 to 120 g with a mean of 60 g. Following lung excision, apical pleural tents and/or talc pleurodesis is not required. Operative time is from 1 to 2 h. In selected patients, alternative median sternotomy incisions are used.[37,38]

Following reversal of neuromuscular blockade, patients are extubated as rapidly as possible despite permissive hypercapnia in selected patients. Aggressive pulmonary toilet, intravenous aminophylline, corticosteroids in selected patients, aerosolized beta$_2$-agonists, and ipratropium bromide are used to achieve maximal bronchodilation. Lethargic patients with increasing respiratory acidosis (pH < 7.20) may require noninvasive ventilatory support using a face mask and pressure support ventilation to avoid reintubation.

Keller and coworkers[65] have detailed the postoperative management of LVRS patients and the reader is encouraged to review their experiences. Despite bilateral chest tubes, close attention must be given to look for air leaks, subcutaneous emphysema and pneumothoraces. Chest tube water seal drainage without negative suction often suffices. McKenna and colleagues[79] have shown that patients who are clinically stable but have persistent air leaks (25 of 109 patients) can be safely discharged with a small chest tube and a Heimlich valve, thereby, markedly reducing the need and costs of hospitalization. However, beginning postoperatively as soon as possible, aggressive pulmonary rehabilitation and physical conditioning is initiated and is similar but to lesser physical intensity to that which the patient underwent preoperatively. Aggressive ambulation and cycle ergometry together with respiratory physiotherapy are cardinal tenets of postoperative care and complement medical treatment. With aggressive but excellent postoperative care, most patients can be discharged safely with < 5 percent 90-day mortality.[39–41,53–55,63] Our 1-year mean survival for bilateral stapled LVRS averaged 85 ± 2.3 percent (±SEM), mean 2-year survival averaged 81 ± 2.7 percent, and mean 3-year survival averaged 72 ± 4.4 percent.[79a]

Future

Despite results of numerous publications[37–48,50,52–61,63,64,78] evidence supporting the clinical and physiologic efficacy of LVRS, using the patient as their own control, the Health Care Financing Administration (HCFA) has had a nonreimbursement policy for LVRS for generalized emphysema in Medicare beneficiaries since December 1995. They[80] stated "it cannot reasonably be concluded at this time that the objective data permit a logical and a scientifically defensible conclusion regarding the risks and benefits of LVRS as currently provided." Subsequently, the NHLBI and HCFA have developed a clinical trial to begin in late 1997 to establish the risks and benefits of LVRS in Medicare patients with lung CT scores of moderate to severe generalized emphysema who have physiologic evidence of severe hyperinflation and airflow limitation (FEV_1 < 1 liter). This joint clinical research effort will be known as the National Emphysema Treatment Trial (NETT). It will be conducted in 18 clinical centers to prospectively randomize approximately 5000 patients over 5 years between best medical therapy and best medical therapy plus LVRS. End points will include survival, lung function, cost, quality of life, oxygen dependence, and exercise capacity. The relative role(s) of median sternotomy versus video-assisted thoracoscopic surgery for bilateral LVRS will be evaluated. It is hoped, this and other ongoing or soon to be initiated trials will resolve the future treatment role of LVRS in patients with generalized emphysema who have received maximum therapy and the issues of Medicare reimbursement.

References

1. Anthonisen NR: Prognosis in chronic obstructive pulmonary disease: Results from multicenter clinical trials. *Am Rev Respir Dis* 140:595–599, 1989.

2. Burrows B, Earle RH: Course and prognosis of chronic obstructive lung disease. A prospective study of 200 patients. *N Engl J Med* 280:397–404, 1969.

3. Ries AI, Kaplan RM, Limbery TM, Prewitt L: Effects of pulmonary rehabilitation on physiologic and psychosocial outcome in patients with chronic obstructive pulmonary disease. *Ann Intern Med* 12:823–832, 1995.

4. Boushy SF, Thompson HK Jr, North LB, et al: Prognosis in chronic obstructive pulmonary disease. *Am Rev Respir Dis* 108:1373–1383, 1973.

5. Traver GA, Cline MG, Burrows B: Predictors of mortality in chronic obstructive pulmonary disease. *Am Rev Respir Dis* 119:895–902, 1979.

6. Seneff MG, Wagner DP, Wagner RP, et al: Hospital and 1-year survival of patients admitted to intensive care units with exacerbation of chronic obstructive pulmonary disease. *JAMA* 274:1852–1857, 1995.

7. 1995 Annual report of the US scientific registry of transplant recipients and the organ procurement and transplantation network: Transplant data: 1988–1994, Richmond, VA, United network for organ sharing. Rockville MD, U.S. Department of the Health and Human Services, 1995.

8. American Thoracic Society: Comprehensive outpatient management of COPD. *Am J Respir Crit Care Med* 152:592–597, 1995.

9. Canadian Thoracic Society Workshop Group: Guidelines for the assessment and management of COPD. *Can Med Assoc J* 147:420–428, 1992.

10. Donner CF, Muir JF. Rehabilitation and chronic care scientific group of the European Respiratory Society: Selection criteria and programs for pulmonary rehabilitation in COPD patients. *Eur Respir J* 10:744–757, 1997.

11. Pulmonary rehabilitation research NIH workshop summary. *Am Rev Respir Dis* 49:825–893, 1994.

12. Casaburi R: Exercise training in chronic obstructive lung disease, in Casaburi R, Petty TL (eds): *Principles and Practice of Pulmonary Rehabilitation*. Philadelphia, WB Saunders, 1993:204–224.

13. Celli BR: Pulmonary rehabilitation in patients with COPD. *Am J Respir Crit Care Med* 152:861–864, 1995.

14. Goldstein RS, Gort EH, Stubbing, et al: Randomized controlled trial of respiratory rehabilitation. *Lancet* 334:1394–1397, 1994.

15. Snider GL: Emphysema: The first two centuries and beyond. *Am Rev Respir Dis* 146:1334–1344,1615–1622, 1992.

16. Thurlbeck WM, Muller NL: Emphysema: Definition, imaging and of quantification. *Am J Roentgenol* 163:1017–1025, 1994.

17. Smith TC, Marini JJ: Impact of PEEP on lung mechanics and work of breathing in severe airflow obstruction. *J Appl Physiol* 65:1488–1499, 1988.

18. Similowski T, Yan S, Gautheir AP, et al: Contractile properties of the human diaphragm during chronic hyperinflation. *N Engl J Med* 325:917–923, 1991.

19. Decramer M: Hyperinflation and respiratory muscle interaction. *Eur Respir J* 10:934–941, 1997.

20. Martinez FJ, Cooper JI, Celli BR: Factors influencing ventilatory muscle recruitment in patients with chronic airflow obstruction. *Am Rev Respir Dis* 142:276–282, 1990.

21. DeTroyer A. Effect of hyperinflation on the diaphragm. *Eur Respir J* 10:708–713, 1997.

22. Martinez FJ, Montes de Oca M, Whyte RI, et al: Lung volume reduction improves dyspnea, dynamic hyperinflation, and respiratory muscle function. *Am J Respir Crit Care Med* 155:1984–1990, 1997.

23. Scharf SM, Cassidy SS (eds): *Heart–Lung Interactions in Health and Disease*. New York, Marcel Dekker, 1989.

24. Hogg JC, Macklem PT, Thurlbeck WM: Site and nature of airway obstruction in chronic obstructive lung disease. *N Engl J Med* 278:1355–1360, 1968.

25. Hogg JC, Wright JL, Wiggs BL, et al: Lung structure and function in cigarette smokers. *Thorax* 49:473–478, 1994.

26. Gelb AF, Schein M, Kuei J, et al: Limited contribution of emphysema in advanced chronic obstructive pulmonary disease. *Am Rev Respir Dis* 147:1157–1161, 1993.

27. Gelb AF, Hogg JC, Muller NL, et al: Contribution of emphysema and small airways in COPD. *Chest* 109:353–359, 1996.

27a. Gelb AF, Zamel N, Hogg JC, et al: Pseudo physiologic emphysema due to severe small airways disease. *Am J Respir Crit Care Med* 158:in press, 1998.

28. Morrison NJ, Abboud RT, Ramadan F, et al: Comparison of single-breath carbon monoxide diffusing capacity and pressure-volume curves in detecting emphysema. *Am Rev Respir Dis* 139:1179–1187, 1989.

29. Wright JL, Wiggs B, Pare PD, et al: Ranking the severity of emphysema on whole lung slices: Concordance of upper lobe, lower lobe and entire lung ranks. *Am Rev Respir Dis* 133:136–145, 1986.

30. Thurlbeck WM, Dunnel MS, Hartung W, et al: A comparison of three methods of measuring emphysema. *Hum Pathol* 1:215–226, 1970.

31. Jamal K, Cooney TP, Fleetham JA, et al: Chronic bronchitis: Correlation of morphologic findings to sputum production and flow rates. *Am Rev Respir Dis* 129:719–722, 1984.

32. Kuwano K, Matsuba K, Ikeda T, et al: The diagnosis of mild emphysema: Correlation of computed tomography and pathology scores. *Am Rev Respir Dis* 141:169–178, 1990.

33. Hruban RH, Meziane MA, Zerhouni EA, et al: High resolution computed tomography of inflation-fixed lungs: Pathologic-radiologic correlation of centrilobular emphysema. *Am Rev Respir Dis* 136:935–940, 1987.

34. Deslauriers J: History of surgery for emphysema. *Semin Thorac Cardiovasc Surg* 8:43–51, 1996.

35. Brantigan OC, Mueller E: Surgical treatment of pulmonary emphysema. *Am Surg* 23:789–804, 1957.

36. Wakabayashi A, Brenner M, Kayaleh RA, et al: Thoracoscopic carbon dioxide laser treatment of bullous emphysema. *Lancet* 337:881–883, 1991.

37. Cooper JD, Trulock EP, Triantafillou AN, et al: Bilateral pneumectomy (volume reduction) for chronic obstructive pulmonary disease. *J Thorac Cardiovasc Surg* 109:106–116, 1995.

38. Cooper JD, Patterson GA, Sundaresan RS, et al: Results of 150 consecutive bilateral lung volume reduction procedures in patients with severe emphysema. *J Thorac Cardiovasc Surg* 112:1319–1330, 1996.

39. McKenna RJ Jr, Brenner M, Gelb AF, et al: A randomized prospective trial of stapled lung reduction versus laser bullectomy for diffuse emphysema. *J Thorac Cardiovasc Surg* 111:317–321, 1996.

40. McKenna RJ Jr, Brenner M, Fischel RJ, Gelb AF: Should lung

volume reduction surgery be unilateral or bilateral? *J Thorac Cardiovasc Surg* 112:1331–1339, 1996.

41. McKenna RJ Jr, Brenner M, Fischel RJ, et al: Patient selection for lung volume reduction surgery. *J Thorac Cardiovasc Surg* 114:957–967, 1997.

42. Argenziano M, Moazami N, Thomashaw B, et al: Extended indications for volume reduction pneumoplasty in advanced emphysema. *Ann Thorac Surg* 62:1588–1597, 1996.

43. Bingisser R, Zollinger A, Hauser M, et al: Bilateral volume reduction for diffuse pulmonary emphysema by video-assisted thoracoscopy. *J Thorac Cardiovasc Surg* 112:875–882, 1996.

44. Daniel M, Chan BK, Bhaskar V, et al: Lung volume reduction surgery: Case selection, operative technique, and clinical results. *Ann Thorac Surg* 61:526–532, 1996.

45. Kotloff RM, Tino G, Bavaria JE, et al: Bilateral lung volume reduction surgery for advanced emphysema. *Chest* 110:1399–1406, 1996.

46. Miller JL, Lee RB, Mansour KA: Lung volume reduction surgery: Lessons learned. *Ann Thorac Surg* 61:1464–1469, 1996.

47. Wisser W, Tschernko E, Senbaklavaci O, et al: Functional improvement after volume reduction: Sternotomy versus videoendoscopic approach. *Ann Thorac Surg* 63:822–828, 1997.

48. Szekely LA, Oelberg DA, Wright C, et al: Preoperative predictors of operative morbidity and mortality in COPD patients undergoing bilateral lung volume reduction surgery. *Chest* 111:550–558, 1997.

49. Orens JB, Becker FS, Lynch JP III, et al: Cardiopulmonary exercise testing following allogenic lung transplantation for different underlying disease states. *Chest* 107:144–149, 1995.

50. Gaissert HA, Trulock EP, Cooper JD, et al: Comparison of early functional results after volume reduction or lung transplantation for chronic obstructive pulmonary disease. *J Thorac Cardiovasc Surg* 111:296–305, 1996.

51. Ross DJ, Waters PF, Mohsenifar Z, et al: Hemodynamic responses to exercise after lung transplantation. *Chest* 103:46–53, 1993.

52. Sciurba FC, Rogers RM, Keenan RJ, et al: Improvement in pulmonary function and elastic recoil after lung reduction surgery for diffuse emphysema. *N Engl J Med* 334:1095–1099, 1996.

53. Gelb AF, Zamel N, McKenna RJ Jr, et al: Mechanism of short-term improvement in lung function following emphysema resection. *Am J Respir Crit Care Med* 154:945–951, 1996.

54. Gelb AF, Brenner M, McKenna RJ Jr, et al: Lung function 12 months following emphysema resection. *Chest* 110:1407–1415, 1996.

55. Gelb AF, Zamel N, McKenna RJ, et al: Contribution of lung and chest wall mechanics following emphysema resection. *Chest* 110:1711–1714, 1996.

55a. Gelb AF, Brenner M, McKenna RJ Jr, et al: Serial lung function and elastic recoil 2 years after lung volume reduction surgery for emphysema. *Chest* 113:1497–1506, 1998.

56. Teschler H, Stamatis G, El-Raouf Farhat AA, et al: Effect of surgical lung volume and respiratory muscle function in pulmonary emphysema. *Eur Respir J* 9:1779–1784, 1996.

57. O'Donnell DE, Webb KA, Bertley JC, et al: Mechanism of relief of exertional breathlessness following unilateral bullectomy and lung volume reduction surgery in emphysema. *Chest* 110:18–27, 1996.

57a. Laghi F, Jubran A, Topeli Arzu, et al: Effect of lung volume reduction surgery on neuromechanical coupling of the diaphragm. *Am J Respir Crit Care Med* 157:475–483, 1998.

58. Benditt JO, Wood DE, McCool FD, et al: Changes in breathing and ventilatory muscle recruitment patterns induced by lung volume reduction surgery. *Am J Respir Crit Care Med* 155:279–284, 1997.

58a. Albert RK, Benditt JO, Hildebrandt J, et al: Lung volume reduction surgery has variable effects on blood gases in patients with emphysema. *Am J Respir Crit Care Med* 158:71–76, 1998.

58b. Ferguson GT, Fernandez E, Zamora MR: Improved exercise performance following lung volume reduction surgery for emphysema. *Am J Respir Crit Care Med* 157:1195–1203, 1998.

59. Roué C, Mal H, Sleiman C, et al: Lung volume reduction in patients with severe diffuse emphysema. *Chest* 110:28–34, 1996.

60. Brenner M, McKenna RJ Jr, Gelb AF, et al: Objective predictors of response for staple versus laser emphysematous lung reduction. *Am J Respir Crit Care Med* 155:1295–1301, 1997.

61. Brenner M, Yusen R, McKenna RJ Jr, et al: Lung volume reduction surgery for emphysema. *Chest* 110:205–218, 1996.

61a. Brenner M, McKenna RJ Jr, Gelb AF, et al: Dyspnea response following bilateral thoracoscopic staple lung volume reduction surgery. *Chest* 112:916–923, 1997.

61b. Brenner M, McKenna RJ Jr, Gelb AF, et al: Rate of FEV, change following lung volume reduction surgery. *Chest* 113:652–659, 1998.

62. Task Group on Screening for Respiratory Disease in Occupational Settings: Official statement of the American Thoracic Society. *Am Rev Respir Dis* 126:952–956, 1982.

63. Coates AL, Peslin AL, Rodenstein D, Stocks J: Measurement of lung volumes by plethysmography. *Eur Respir J* 10:1415–1427, 1997.

64. McKenna RJ Jr, Fischel R, Brenner M, Gelb AF: Combined operation for lung volume reduction surgery and lung cancer. *Chest* 110:885–888, 1996.

65. Keller CA, Naunheim KS: Perioperative management of lung volume reduction patients in surgical approaches to end-stage disease: Lung transplantation and volume reduction, in Maurer J (ed): *Clinics in Chest Medicine*. Philadelphia, W.B. Saunders, 1997:285–300.

66. Mead J, Turner JM, Macklem PT, et al: Significance of the relationship between lung recoil and maximum expiratory flow. *J Appl Physiol* 22:95–108, 1967.

67. Pride NB, Permutt S, Riley RL, et al: Determinants of maximum expiratory flow from the lungs. *J Appl Physiol* 23:646–662, 1967.

68. Zamel N, Hogg J, Gelb AF: Mechanisms of maximal expiratory flow limitation in clinically unsuspected emphysema and obstruction of the peripheral airways. *Am Rev Respir Dis* 113:337–345, 1976.

69. Ingram RH Jr, Schilder DP: Effects of thoracic gas compression on the flow volume curve of the forced vital capacity. *Am Rev Respir Dis* 94:56–62, 1966.

70. Gelb AF, Gold WM, Wright RR, et al: Physiologic diagnosis of subclinical emphysema. *Am Rev Respir Dis* 107:50–63, 1973.

71. Black LF, Hyatt RE, Stubbs SE: Mechanism of expiratory airflow limitation in chronic obstructive pulmonary disease associated with alpha₁-antitrypsin deficiency. *Am Rev Respir Dis* 105:891–899, 1972.

72. Gelb AF, Gold WM, Nadel JA: Mechanism limiting airflow in bullous lung disease. *Am Rev Respir Dis* 107:571–578, 1973.

73. Gelb AF, Gold WM, Nadel JA: Mechanism of expiratory airflow limitation in bullous lung disease. *Am Rev Respir Dis* 105:1005, 1972.

74. Boushy SF, Billig DM, Kohen R: Changes in pulmonary function after bullectomy. *Am J Med* 47:916–923, 1969.

75. Pride NB, Barter CE, Hugh-Jones P: The ventilation of bulla and the effect of their removal on thoracic gas volumes and tests of overall pulmonary function. *Am Rev Respir Dis* 107:83–98, 1973.

76. Rogers RM, DuBois AB, Blakemore WS: Effects of removal of bullae on airway conductance and conductance volume ratios. *J Clin Invest* 47:2569–2579, 1968.

77. Fitzgerald MX, Keelan PJ, Cugell DW, et al: Long-term results of surgery for bullous emphysema. *J Thorac Cardiovasc Surg* 68:566–587, 1974.

78. Schlueter DP, Immekus J, Stead WW: Relationship between maximal inspiratory pressure and total lung capacity (correlation of retraction) in normal subjects and in patients with emphy-

sema, asthma, and diffuse pulmonary infiltration. *Am Rev Respir Dis* 96:656–665, 1967.

79. McKenna RJ Jr, Fischel RJ, Brenner M, Gelb AF: Use of Heimlich valve to shorten hospital stay after lung reduction surgery for emphysema. *Ann Thorac Surg* 61:1115–1117, 1996.

79a. Brenner M, McKenna RJ Jr, Chen JC, et al: Survival following bilateral staple lung volume reduction surgery for emphysema. *Chest*: accepted 1998.

80. AHCPR: *Lung volume reduction surgery for end-stage chronic obstructive pulmonary disease.* Publication No. 96-0062.

Chapter 52

THE PULMONARY CONSEQUENCES OF ABDOMINAL SURGERY

GARY W. RAFF

BERNARD GARDNER

The patients undergoing pulmonary rehabilitation are not immune from abdominal diseases such as appendicitis, or colon cancer. This chapter will review the changes in pulmonary performance which occur as a result of surgical procedures within the abdominal cavity. Much literature has been generated on this topic since 1908, when Pasteur first described paradoxical breathing movements in a patient after abdominal surgery.[1-2] A brief discussion of some historic contributions will be followed by review of the physiologic changes which occur after abdominal surgery. Explanations for the derangements in lung function will be presented and risk factors for complications, as well as strategies used to combat these, will be discussed. This will be followed by considerations of anesthetic and surgical techniques and their impact on lung function. Postoperative considerations will also be reviewed.

History

One of the most insightful contributors to the understanding of perioperative pulmonary physiology was Pasteur. He was the first to recognize paradoxic abdominal wall movement during breathing after abdominal surgery. He surmised correctly that reflex inhibition of the "direct extenders of the lung" (diaphragm and intercostals) was likely responsible for this condition. In addition, he was the first to show data confirming a differential incidence of complications depending on the location of the surgery.[1] He showed that operations above the umbilicus were almost three times more likely to result in complications than those performed below the umbilicus.

The next major contribution in this area of investigation occurred with the ability to measure changes in total lung volumes and its segments after surgical procedures. In the mid-1800s Hutchinson discussed using the spirometer to measure lung capacity and attempted to correlate disease processes with alterations in spirometry.[3] Later, Beecher measured lung volumes after laparotomy. In this landmark paper he identified the fundamental changes in residual volume, functional residual capacity, total lung capacity, and vital capacity that occur after abdominal surgery. He demonstrated that although there is minimal change in minute ventilation, breathing becomes more shallow, and there is a compensatory increase in respiratory rate. In addition, he showed that the changes in lung volumes are worse after upper abdominal surgical procedures as compared to those done in the lower abdomen.[3]

During the poliomyelitis epidemics of the late 1940s and early 1950s, more work on pulmonary dynamics was completed. Great advances in modes of ventilation were made, including recognition of improved survival with the use of negative-pressure devices (iron lung), followed by the acceptance and use of positive pressure ventilation. Many investigations in the late 1950s to 1970s looked at the interrelationship of the cardiac and pulmonary systems. Pioneers such as West and others described the effect of changes in blood flow on gas exchange and the fundamental physiology governing normal cardiopulmonary function.[4]

More recent research had examined factors which predispose patients to decompensation after surgery and techniques to prevent or diminish pulmonary dysfunction postoperatively.[5,6]

Physiologic Changes in the Perioperative Period

Unless specific therapy for respiratory or cardiac disorders is given prior to surgery, the first major changes occur when the patient is put under general anesthesia. Later changes occur during surgery and the postoperative period. The postoperative changes which occur are likely to continue for at least 7 to 14 days from the time of surgery. This section will deal specifically with changes which occur during and immediately after surgery while a later section will address specific preoperative and postoperative considerations.

There are multiple adverse affects which occur as a result of general anesthetics, as well as other agents used during general anesthesia. Endotracheal intubation, pooling of secretions, interruption of mucocillary function, V/Q mismatch, atelectasis, reduced compliance and lung volumes, and length of time under anesthesia affect pulmonary function adversely. Respiratory muscle dysfunction after upper abdominal surgery also contributes to the derangements seen.

Intubation of the trachea initiates multiple detrimental events which worsen lung function beginning with increasing physiologic and anatomic dead space. In all patients there is reduced tracheobronchial clearance and atelectasis, as well as the other changes described above. In patients with reactive airway disease, there is the potential to cause or worsen bronchospasm leading to intrapulmonary shunting and V/Q mismatch.

Normally, the mucociliary elevator is able to keep the airways clear of secretions. There is evidence that not only is mucociliary function impaired by intubation, but also alveolar macrophage dysfunction after general anesthesia.[7] Although the individual contributions of decreased alveolar macrophage function and diminished mucociliary transport to postoperative and intraoperative dysfunction are not clear, there is an increase in postoperative pulmonary complications with increasing anesthesia and operative times.[8-10] The anatomic location of the operation may also affect tracheobronchial clearance. A study in humans by Gamsu and coworkers compared clearance of radiopaque particles from the lungs of patients undergoing abdominal procedures versus lower extremity procedures.[11] In this study tracheobronchial clearance took more than twice as long (>100 h) in the group undergoing abdominal surgery. Of note, the abdominal procedures tended to be much longer in duration because of a multitude of factors; the primary reason for this was not clear.[11] Another study looking at the relationship between lower respiratory tract contamination at operation found an increased incidence of postoperative chest infection after general anesthesia, presumably as a result of inadequate ability to clear tracheal secretions.[12] Other factors such as humidification and temperature of the inspired gas during general anesthesia also can affect mucosal function. In a model of the effects of different levels of humidity and temperature on mucosal function, there appears to be an optimal temperature and level of humidity above or below which mucosal function is impaired.[13] Ideal temperature, as one might surmise, seems to be core temperature, while the ideal level of humidity is 100 percent relative humidity. However, there is no prospective randomized trial available which has tested this. Most volitile anesthetics have been shown to affect alveolar macrophage function and/or tracheobronchial clearance. Halothane, isoflurane, and enflurane are known to reduce alveolar macrophage antimicrobial activity at clinically relevant concentrations.[14,15] Whether the effect is primarily one of reduction in cytotoxic, or phagocytic ability, or viability of alveolar macrophages is not clear. In addition, release of inflammatory mediators and endotoxin during surgery can result in activation of alveolar macrophages and alteration of their activity, as well as causing decrements in pulmonary function.

Inability to clear secretions, displacement of nitrogen by volitile anesthetics, and high concentrations of oxygen during general anesthesia contribute to the development of resorption atelectasis during and after general anesthesia.[16,17] Nitrogen helps to prevent alveolar collapse when oxygen diffuses down its concentration gradient into the alveolar capillaries. When nitrogen is washed out, and the partial pressure of oxygen is decreased, the resultant pressure in the alveolus is reduced, leading to atelectasis. This propensity to develop atelectasis is worsened since most patients breath closer to their closing volume during anesthesia and also postoperatively.[6] Any time spent below closing volume increases the likelihood of atelectasis developing. Discussion concerning atelectasis during anesthesia would not be complete without considering the effects of changes in lung volumes under general anesthesia. The most important of these to consider in this context is decreases in expiratory reserve volume.[3,18] Reductions in expiratory reserve volume promote small airway closure and subsequent atelectasis. In normal subjects closing volume is below end-expiratory volume resting breathing (expiratory reserve volume). When expiratory reserve volume decreases, it gets closer to closing volume. In the elderly and in smokers, it falls to levels below closing volume. Most atelectasis occurs in dependent areas where gravitational and anatomic forces cause secretions to pool, and pulmonary blood flow tends to be greater.[19] This was first observed in dogs in the 1940s.[20] Investigators found that after hours under anesthesia without compensatory sighs, ventilation to the dependent lung zones was greatly diminished.[20] This in turn heightened shunt fraction and contributed to hypoxemia. Hypoxemia also contributes to decreased clearance of microbial agents and altered alveolar macrophage cytotoxity and phagocytosis.[6,7]

As mentioned above, there are decreases in lung volumes following abdominal procedures. Besides the formation of atelectasis, there is also decreased lung compliance. The mechanism is as follows: During normal ventilation, at end expiration, recoil in the lung and expansile force in the chest wall are balanced. This balance point is usually at the point of optimal compliance for each individual. When lung volume decreases, this relationship is altered. The balance point shifts away from the expansile recoil of the chest wall, making it more difficult to expand the lungs since end expiratory recoil no longer matches the expansile forces in the chest wall. This is further aggravated by postoperative pain and abdominal splinting.[21] In studies looking at the effects of local anesthetics, smaller derangements in lung function seem to occur when postoperative pain control is optimized and it has been recognized that many abnormalities in postoperative ventilatory function can be decreased by using adequate local anesthesia.[22–25] Good control of pain seems to reduce or prevent reflex inhibition of muscles involved in ventilation. Diaphragmatic EMG amplitude increases by 50 percent or greater,[26] and vital capacity increases as well.[27] However, there is still no convincing evidence available to show prevention or reversal of these changes to baseline through the use of local anesthesia alone.

Anesthetic Considerations

There are many derangements in respiratory muscle function as a result of both anesthesia and the surgical procedure. General anesthesia results in decreased ventilatory drive and muscle function.[28] This is a direct result of the anesthetic agent and muscle relaxant used during general anesthesia. Using special techniques to evaluate diaphragmatic function in humans, it has been shown that handling of the upper abdominal viscera can result in reflex inhibition of respiratory drive.[29–31] These changes slowly return to baseline during the early postoperative period (during the first week or so). In nonabdominal/nonthoracic procedures these changes rapidly return to baseline.[6] Interestingly, if you control postoperative pain after surgery with epidural analgesia there is still measurable diaphragmatic dysfunction. Therefore, postoperative pain alone is not responsible for diaphragmatic dysfunction after upper abdominal surgery.[5] Using changes in gastric pressure as compared with changes in transdiaphragmatic pressure, Dureuil was able to show in 1986 that after upper abdominal surgery, the major mechanism responsible for diaphragmatic dysfunction are likely reflex in nature, originating from the abdominal or chest wall.[30] As mentioned above, these changes are most severe and longest lasting in operations close to the diaphragm. In operations distant from the diaphragm the changes return toward normal within days while in upper abdominal surgery, it may take up to 2 weeks before diaphragmatic function returns to baseline. This process contributes to diminished cough, postoperative pulmonary restriction, and possibly to postoperative pulmonary complications.

Prevention of Pulmonary Complications after Surgery

The incidence of pulmonary complications in patients with upper abdominal surgery has been reported to be as high as 70 percent.[20] However, there is wide variation,[32] in part

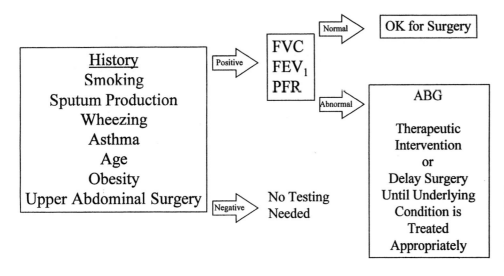

FIGURE 52-1 Preoperative pulmonary evaluation. FVC, functional vital capacity; FEV_1, forced expiratory volume in 1 s; PFR, peak flow rate. (Modified from Celli,[5] with permission.)

because of the lack of a uniform definition of what constitutes a complication. In any case, there is no doubt that pulmonary complications are a leading cause of morbidity and mortality in the postoperative patient.

Preoperative Evaluation

Identification of patients at risk begins with a thorough history and physical examination. Important points in the history include a history of smoking, prior lung resection or abnormal lung function, history of tuberculosis or other pulmonary pathogens, history of asthma or chronic obstructive pulmonary disease, chronic bronchitis, productive cough, or history of cardiac dysfunction. In addition, the patient should be questioned about previous radiologic and physiologic tests of cardiopulmonary function, such as x-rays, CT scans, and exercise tests. On physical examination special attention should be paid to weight (obesity is a risk factor), evidence of abnormal breathing pattern or respiratory rate, and chest wall, lung, and cardiac examinations. Other factors such as generalized wasting or ascites should be noted since they can cause abnormalities in lung or abdominal/thoracic wall muscle function postoperatively. The type of operation and approach selected should also be considered. For example, there is evidence that pulmonary dysfunction is more common after minilaparotomy versus laparoscopic cholecystectomy[33] and that complications are more prevalent in upper abdominal and thoracic procedures.[34] Whenever possible the procedure should be tailored to the individual patient to minimize physiologic derangements as a result of surgery.

Once a thorough history and physical examination are completed, a reasonable discussion can be made about further evaluation as shown in Fig. 52-1.

There is much evidence that the degree of abnormality on spirometry correlates with the incidence of postoperative pulmonary complications.[6,35–38] Because of the relatively low cost, simplicity and availability, and noninvasive nature, spirometry is used to help stratify patients with risk factors identified on history and physical examination. If a patient has risk factors but normal spirometry, then their risk for postoperative pulmonary complications should be quite low.[32,39] A past history of smoking and orthopnea are impor-

tant correlates of postoperative pulmonary complications. However, if pulmonary function testing is abnormal, then the patient is at significant risk for pulmonary complication postoperatively and will benefit from preoperative preparation.[20]

Preoperative Preparation

Smokers should be encouraged strongly to stop since smoking clearly increases the incidence of postoperative pulmonary complications.[40] Smoking results in an increase in postoperative complications, including reduction of tracheobronchial clearance, increased secretions from chronic bronchitis, and increased carboxyhemoglobin concentration. Postoperative hypoxemia is poorer in smokers compared to nonsmokers. In addition, the risk of pneumonia is twice that seen in nonsmokers.[41–43] Preoperative optimization to help minimize the effect of smoking must include cessation of smoking. Although there is no prospective study of the duration necessary to maximize this effect, as much as 4 to 8 weeks may be necessary to see the full benefit from this.[41] It is interesting to note that this time period corresponds with that required for tracheobronchial clearance to improve, implying that impairment of tracheobronchial clearance is a major contributor to smoking's effect on postoperative complications.[44] This may be one of the principle mechanisms by which the cessation of smoking helps to minimize pulmonary complications postoperatively.

Patients with active wheezing or poorly controlled asthmatics are at increased risk for pulmonary complications after surgery such as bronchospasm, atelectasis, and pneumonia.[44] Severe bronchospasm must be anticipated and the patient should be optimized with pharmacologic therapy and spirometry prior to surgery. Markers of optimal preoperative preparation include minimizing of symptoms, decreasing or elimination of wheezing, and improved pulmonary functions. The first-line medications are the β-agonists.[45] Theophylline is useful more as a respiratory muscle stimulant than a bronchodilator when considering how good the β-agonists are. In this role they may be especially useful in COPD patients.[46,47] Corticosteroids may also be helpful in the symptomatic asthmatic or recalcitrant COPD patient.[48] Usually these are begun 12 to 24 h prior to surgery since they achieve their maximal benefits hours after administration.

Cardiac function may need to be improved, and obesity and respiratory infections treated. There are a wide range of physiologic derangements which occur as a result of morbid obesity including decreased diaphragmatic function, decreased chest wall compliance from increased body mass, and sleep apnea syndrome.[32,49] Because of this, elective surgery should be postponed if possible while a regimented weight loss program is begun. In addition, pulmonary "training" based on lung expansion maneuvers should be started as soon as practical.

Cardiac function, especially if there are symptoms of early heart failure, should be optimized prior to any operative intervention as it can adversely impact on pulmonary function and on other multiple organ systems. Respiratory infection should be treated prior to elective surgical procedures. In COPD patients, productive cough with purulent sputum appears to be a significant risk factor for pneumonia. In patients with positive tracheal aspirates after tracheal intubation there is an almost 30-fold increase in the incidence of postoperative lower respiratory tract infection.[50,51] These patients should be treated with appropriate antibiotics until the productive cough has resolved and sputum is clear.

Intraoperative Considerations

Other modifiable factors include choices of anesthetic agents, duration of operation, and type of incision. Epidural anesthesia with postoperative epidural analgesia has been associated with a significantly decreased incidence of postoperative respiratory failure in high-risk patients.[25] Some studies have been reported showing no difference in complication rate after epidural anesthesia but most do not specifically address high-risk pulmonary patients. Other confounding variables, such as choice of anesthetic agent, type of postoperative analgesic regimen, hemoglobin concentration, and presence of aspiration, are also rarely considered.[24,52–56] Duration of operation is directly correlated with postoperative pulmonary complication.[57] Although intuitive, it is worth stating that an expedient, well performed operation should be the goal to help decrease pulmonary derangements postoperatively. Other operative factors include the approach chosen and incision used to gain access to body cavities.

Upper abdominal procedures have a much higher incidence of pulmonary complications in the postoperative period than lower abdominal operations or operations on the extremities.[34] There has also been some literature looking at the type of incision and its effect on postoperative morbidity. Vertical laparotomies are thought to have a higher incidence of postoperative pulmonary complications than horizontal incisions.[58,59] It is hypothesized that since horizontal laparotomies involve fewer dermatomes, they may result in less pain and less reflex inhibition of the diaphragm, although hard data to support this theory is lacking in our review of the topic. Operative approaches which are thought to result in fewer postoperative complications include retroperitoneal approaches and laparoscopic procedures.

The retroperitoneal approach has been best studied for operations on the aorta and its branches. In a randomized prospective study of transabdominal versus retroperitoneal incisions for abdominal aortic surgery in 145 patients, there was no difference in pulmonary complications although overall there were fewer complications in the retroperitoneal group.[60] The literature is however not clear on this matter. The definition for what constitutes a pulmonary complication in each study and variable use of continuous epidural analgesia postoperatively, as well as intensive respiratory therapy, play a role in determining the incidence of postoperative pulmonary complications in these studies. In the majority of studies, the general feeling is that there is some improvement in postoperative recovery, including pulmonary function.[56,61–65]

Laparoscopic surgery has been shown to decrease the incidence of postoperative pulmonary complications after cholecystectomy in nonrandomized trials.[66–68] In a randomized study of 133 patients FVC, FEV_1, and peak expiratory flow rates were all significantly better at 24 and 48 h postoperatively compared to mini-laparotomy.[33] This study also showed a significant difference in oxygen saturation between the two groups, even when taking smoking into account. The number of pulmonary complications however was too small to make any firm conclusions as to whether or not this will translate into decreased incidence of respiratory complications.

Postoperative Considerations

Upper abdominal surgery and thoracic surgery result in a restrictive pattern of pulmonary function that persists for a period of more than 2 weeks.[69] This is one of the primary mechanisms of pulmonary dysfunction in the postoperative period and is thought to impact negatively in the incidence of sputum retention, atelectasis, and pulmonary infection. There are many factors which can worsen this pattern including pain, narcotic use, alveolar hypoventilation, V/Q mismatch, electrolyte abnormalities, muscle weakness and other preoperative abnormalities in pulmonary function.

General anesthesia reduces FRC and pulmonary function by the mechanisms already discussed such as reduced tracheobronchial clearance, increased secretions, and increased alveolar dead space and altered cardiac output. In addition, during the initial postextubation phase there is arterial hypoxemia not related to the mechanical factors of ventilation.[70,71] Alveolar hypoventilation in patients who are not completely recovered from the effects of general anesthetics results in worsening of V/Q mismatch since compensatory hypoxic pulmonary vasoconstriction is impaired by many general anesthetics.[72] Most general anesthetics are cardiac depressants and there is potential for decrement of cardiopulmonary function as well. Shivering in hypothermic patients worsens oxygenation as a result of increases in the work of breathing and oxygen consumption.

Postoperative pain has been shown to contribute to a number of abnormalities in pulmonary function including reducing or eliminating deep sighs, decreasing tidal volume, reducing the effectiveness of the cough to clear the airways of secretions, and increasing nonpulmonary morbidity.[73] There has been a large body of literature which addresses the multiple and sometimes complex delivery systems for medications available to help reduce postoperative pain in order to reduce pulmonary complications postoperatively. This includes patient controlled analgesia (PCA), epidural analgesia, intermittant IV or IM analgesia, narcotic and nonnarcotic analgesia, and different types of narcotics and other analgesics, making it difficult to compare these studies. The following statements are probably reasonable in this regard. One might suspect that continuous levels of analgesic are better than intermittent bolus injections but this may not be the case.[74] This is likely a result of multiple factors which do not relate to the inability of intermittent bolus medication to alleviate pain. For example, some patients will not seek pain relief, even when faced with severe pain.[75] In addition, staff have been shown to be more apt to administer narcotics on the basis of their own perception of a patient's pain than the patient's own perception.[76] Although most studies show improvement in pain control and many show improved pulmonary function with epidural analgesia, fewer show less pulmonary complications. No major study shows increased pulmonary complications with epidural use. It is probably beneficial in reducing pulmonary complications, although there is no large prospective randomized study which adequately addresses this issue. Other modalities such as continuous wound perfusion and transcutaneous electrical stimulation require further study before any meaningful appraisal of their worth can be made.

Postoperative Strategies to Prevent Pulmonary Complications

The foundation of postoperative pulmonary care is continued treatment of preoperative derangements in pulmonary function, including asthma, COPD, and infection. In addition, the alterations brought about by general anesthesia, the surgical procedure, and postoperative pain must be considered. In order to assess the adequacy of intervention it is necessary to properly monitor the patients postoperatively.

Assessment of pulmonary function in the postoperative patient can include modalities as continuous pulse-oximetry, pulmonary function testing, arterial blood gas analysis, chest x-rays, pulmonary artery catheters and even continuous oximetric pulmonary artery catheters.

The value of postoperative chest x-rays and pulse-oximetry is intuitive. Identification of atelectasis or lobar collapse, pneumothorax, pulmonary infiltrates, congestive heart failure are all useful in making therapeutic decisions in the postoperative patient. In addition, in all patients after general anesthesia, the use of transcutaneous pulse-oximetry is mandatory until fully recovered from anesthesia. In patients with preexisting pulmonary dysfunction pulse-oximetry should be utilized to monitor the continued effectiveness of treatment. Arterial blood gas analysis can be a useful adjunct in the management of these patients as well. They are more sensitive to changes in oxygenation than saturation alone and can also offer information about acid-base balance and in some hospitals can offer electrolyte and lactate measurements, all of which can greatly impact pulmonary function. In addition, there are a subset of patients who will probably benefit from use of specialized monitoring. Septic patients or patients with cardiopulmonary compromise often can benefit from cardiac optimization to help to improve oxygen delivery to the tissues and treat right heart failure and cardiogenic shock.

COPD

It is a formidable challenge to minimize complications in patients with obstructive pulmonary disease who undergo abdominal surgery because of the extensive and severe changes in the function of lung, circulation, and respiratory muscle that can occur. Work of breathing is increased and oxygenation is impaired and the ability to compensate for the additional problems caused by the surgery may be extremely limited.

Postoperatively they may exhibit respiratory failure for a variety of reasons such as failure to oxygenate. Pulmonary edema, pneumonia or pneumonitis, atelectasis or pulmonary embolism, respiratory insufficiency, and carbon dioxide retention may occur as a result of poor ventilatory drive or weakened respiratory musculature. Injudicious use of narcotics or sedative hypnotics in these patients can contribute to inadequate ventilatory drive. Avoidance of high oxygen concentrations and use of minimal narcotics necessary to control pain will help to reduce complications in these patients after abdominal surgery.

Bronchodilators, incentive spirometry, and maneuvers to increase inspiratory capacity and functional residual capacity, treating atelectasis, pleural effusion, congestive heart failure, and retained secretions is the mainstay of treatment postoperatively.

Summary

Pulmonary complications after abdominal surgery are common particularly after upper abdominal procedures. The physiologic alterations that affect lung function perioperatively include the formation of atelectasis hypoxia and diaphragmatic dysfunction. Atelectasis occurs mainly from reduction of functional expiratory capacity and diminished tracheobronchial clearance. Diaphragm dysfunction is mainly due to reflex inhibition which is incompletely blocked with epidural analgesia.

Patients should be carefully stratified as to their risk prior to surgery with careful history and physical, followed by specialized pulmonary function tests if indicated. Preoperative efforts should focus on patient education, improving tracheobronchial clearance, and treating infection, asthma, and COPD. In addition, lung expansion pulmonary therapy and pulmonary function tests should be done prior to elective procedures. The procedure itself should be tailored to the patient's surgical disorder.

References

1. Pasteur W: Massive collapse of the lung. *Br J Surg* 1:587–601, 1914.
2. Pasteur W: Active lobar collapse of the lung after abdominal operations. *Lancet* 2:1080–1083, 1910.
3. Beecher HK: The measured effect of laparotomy on the respiration. *J Clin Invest* 12:639–650, 1933.
4. West JB, Jones NL: Effect of changes in topographical distribution of lung blood flow on gas exchange. *J Appl Physiol* 20:825, 1965.
5. Celli BE: What is the value of preoperative pulmonary function testing? *Med Clin North Am* 77:309–325, 1993.
6. Tisi GM: Preoperative evaluation of pulmonary function. Validity, indications, and benefits. *Am Rev Resp Dis* 119:293–310, 1979.

7. Kotani N, Lin CY, Wang JS, et al: Loss of alveolar macrophages during anesthesia and operations in humans. *Anesth Analg* 81:1255–1262, 1995.

8. Modell JH, Moya F: Postoperative pulmonary complications. Incidence and management. *Anesth Analg* 45:432–439, 1966.

9. Wightman JAK: A prospective survey of the incidence of postoperative pulmonary complications. *Br J Surg* 55:85–91, 1968.

10. Otto CW: Respiratory morbidity and mortality. *Int Anesthiol Clin* 18:85–106, 1980.

11. Gamsu G, Singer MM, Vincent HH, et al: Postoperative impairment of mucous transport in the lung. *Am Rev Respir Dis* 114:673–679, 1976.

12. Morran GG, McNaught W, Mcardle CS: The relationship between intraoperative contamination of the lower respiratory tract and postoperative chest infection. *J Hosp Infect* 30:31–37, 1995.

13. Williams R, Rankin N, Smith R, et al: Relationship between the humidity and temperature of inspired gas and the function of the airway mucosa. *Crit Care Med* 24:1920–1929, 1996.

14. Welch WD: Halothane inhibits the microbicidal oxidative activity of pulmonary alveolar macrophages. *Anesth* 58:456–459, 1983.

15. Welch WD: Enflurane and isoflurane inhibit the oxidative activity of pulmonary alveolar macrophages. *Respiration* 47:24–29, 1985.

16. Coryllos PN, Birnbaum GI: Studies in pulmonary gas absorption in bronchial obstruction: Behavior and absorption times of oxygen, carbon dioxide, nitrogen, hydrogen, helium, ethylene, nitrous oxide, ethyl chloride and ether in the lung. *Am J Med Sci* 183:347–357, 1932.

17. Dale WA, Rahn H: Rate of gas absorption during atelectasis. *Am J Physiol* 170:606–610, 1953.

18. Anascombe AR, Buxton R: Effect of abdominal operations on total lung capacity and its subdivisions. *Br Med J* 2:84–89, 1958.

19. West JB, Dollery CT, Naimark A: Distribution of blood flow in the isolated lung; relation to vascular and alveolar pressures. *J Appl Physiol* 19:713–717, 1964.

20. Drinker CK, Hardenberg E: Effects of the supine position upon the ventilation of the lungs of dogs. *Surgery* 24:113–120, 1948.

21. Ali J, Weisel RD, Layug AB, et al: Consequences of postoperative alterations in respiratory mechanics. *Am J Surg* 128:376–382, 1974.

22. Wahba RWM: Perioperative functional residual capacity. *Can J Anaesth* 38:384–400, 1991.

23. Weissman C: Perioperative respiratory physiology. *J Crit Care* 6:160–171, 1991.

24. Baron JP, Bertrand M, Barre E, et al: Combined epidural and general anesthesia versus general anesthesia for abdominal aortic surgery. *Anesthesiology* 75:611–618, 1991.

25. Yeager MP, Glass DD, Neff RK, et al: Epidural anesthesia and analgesia in high risk surgical patients. *Anesthesiology* 66:729–736, 1987.

26. Pansard JL, Philip Y, Bahnini A, et al: Effects of thoracic extradural block on diaphragmatic activity after upper abdominal surgery. *Anesthesiology* 67:A537–544, 1987.

27. Mankikian B, Cantineau JP, Bertrand M, et al: Improvement of diaphragmatic function by a thoracic extradural block after upper abdominal surgery. *Anesthesiology* 68:379–383, 1988.

28. Laws AK: Effects of induction of anesthesia and muscle paralysis on functional residual capacity of the lungs. *Can Anaesth Soc J* 15:325–331, 1968.

29. Simonneau G, Vivien A, Sartene R, et al: Diaphragm dysfunction induced by upper abdominal surgery. *Am Rev Respir Dis* 128:899–903, 1983.

30. Dureuil B, Viires N, Cantineau JP, et al: Diaphragmatic contractility after upper abdominal surgery. *J Appl Physiol* 61:1775–1780, 1986.

31. Ford GT, Whitelaw W, Rosenal TW, et al: Diaphragmatic function after upper abdominal surgery in humans. *Am Rev Respir Dis* 127:431–436, 1983.

32. Latimer RG, Dickman M, Day WC, et al: Ventilatory patterns and pulmonary complications after upper abdominal surgery determined by preoperative and postoperative computerized spirometry and blood gas analysis. *Am J Surg* 122:622–632, 1971.

33. McMahon AJ, Russell IT, Ramsay G, et al: Laparoscopic and minilaparotomy cholecystectomy: A randomized trial comparing postoperative pain and pulmonary function. *Surgery* 115:533–539, 1994.

34. Pedersen T, Eliasen K, Henriksen E: A prospective study of risk factors and cardiopulmonary complications associated with anaesthesia and surgery: Risk indicators of cardiopulmonary morbidity. *Acta Anaesthesiol Scand* 34:144–155, 1990.

35. Miller WR, Wu N, Johnson RL Jr: Convenient method of evaluating pulmonary ventilatory function with a single breath test. *Anesthesiology* 17:480–486, 1956.

36. Williams CD, Brenowitz JB: "Prohibitive" lung function and major surgical procedures. *Am J Surg* 132:763–766, 1976.

37. Stein M, Koota GM, Simon M, Frank HA: Pulmonary evaluation of surgical patients. *JAMA* 181:765–770, 1962.

38. Stein M, Cassara E: Preoperative pulmonary evaluation and therapy for surgery patients. *JAMA* 211:787–790, 1970.

39. Collins C, Darke C, Knowelden J: Chest complications after upper abdominal surgery: Their anticipation and prevention. *BMJ* 1:401–406, 1968.

40. Morton HJV, Camb DA: Tobacco smoking and pulmonary complications after operation. *Lancet* 1:368–370, 1944.

41. Warner MA, Offord KP, Warner ME, et al: Role of preoperative cessation of smoking and other factors in postoperative complications. A blinded prospective study of coronary bypass patients. *Mayo Clin Proc* 64:609–616, 1989.

42. Tait AR, Kyff JV, Crider B, et al: Changes in arterial oxygen saturation in cigarette smokers following general anesthesia. *Can HJ Anesth* 37:423–428, 1991.

43. Davies JM: Preoperative respiratory evaluation and management of patients for upper abdominal surgery. *Yale J Biol Med* 64:329–349, 1991.

44. Gold ML, Helrich A: A study of the complications related to anesthesia in asthmatic patients. *Anesth Analg* 42:283–293, 1963.

45. Celli BE: Perioperative respiratory care of the patient undergoing upper abdominal surgery. *Clin Chest Med* 14:253–261, 1993.

46. Murciano D, Auclair MH, Pariente R, et al: A randomized trial of theophylline in patients with severe chronic obstructive pulmonary disease. *N Engl J Med* 320:1521–1525, 1989.

47. Dureuil B, Desmonts JM, Mankikian B, et al: Effects of aminophylline on diaphragmatic dysfunction after upper abdominal surgery. *Anesthesiol* 62:242–246, 1985.

48. Oh SH, Patterson R: Surgery in corticosteroid-dependent asthmatics. *J Allergy Clinical Immunol* 53:345–351, 1974.

49. Vaughan RW, Engelhart RC, Wise L: Postoperative hypoxemia in obese patients. *Ann Surg* 180:877–882, 1974.

50. Carrel T, Schmid ER, von Segesser L, et al: Preoperative assessment of the likelihood of infection of the lower respiratory tract after cardiac surgery. *Thorac Cardiovas Surg* 39:85–88, 1991.

51. Chalon J, Tayyab MA, Ramanathan S: Cytology of respiratory epithelium as a predictor of respiratory complications after operation. *Chest* 67:32–35, 1975.

52. Jayr C, Thomas H, Rey A, et al: Postoperative pulmonary complications. Epidural analgesia using bupivacaine and opioids versus parenteral opioids. *Anesthesiology* 78(4):666–676, 1993.

53. Pecoraro JP, Dardik H, Mauro A, et al: Epidural anesthesia as an adjunct to retroperitoneal aortic surgery. *Am J Surg* 160:187–191, 1990.

54. Raggi R, Dardik H, Mauro AL: Continuous epidural anesthesia and postoperative epidural narcotics in vascular surgery. *Am J Surg* 154:192–197, 1987.

55. Cunningham FO, Egan JM, Inahara R: Continuous epidural anesthesia in abdominal vascular surgery. A review of 100 consecutive cases. *Am J Surg* 139:624–627, 1980.

56. Rosenbaum, GJ, Arroyo PJ, Sivina M: Retroperitoneal approach

used exclusively with epidural anesthesia for infrarenal aortic disease. *Am J Surg* 168:136–139, 1994.

57. Kroenke K, Lawrence VA, Theroux JF, et al: Operative risk in patients with severe obstructive pulmonary disease. *Arch Intern Med* 152:967–971, 1992.

58. Mohr DN, Lavender RC: Preoperative pulmonary evaluation. Identifying patients at increased risk for complications. *Postgrad Med* 100:241–256, 1996.

59. Halasz NA: Vertical vs. horizontal laparotomies. *Arch Surg* 88:911–914, 1964.

60. Sicard GA, Reilly JM, Rubin BG, et al: Transabdominal versus retroperitoneal incision for abdominal aortic surgery: Report of a prospective randomized trial. *J Vasc Surg* 21:174–183, 1995.

61. Cambria RP, Brewster DC, Abbott WM, et al: Transperitoneal versus retroperitoneal approach for aortic reconstruction: A randomized prospective study. *J Vasc Surg* 11:314–325, 1990.

62. Rob C: Extraperitoneal approach to the abdominal aorta. *Surgery* 53:87–89, 1963.

63. Taheri SA, Nowakowski PA, Stoesser FG: Retroperitoneal approach for aortic surgery: Experience with 75 consecutive cases. *Vasc Surg* 3:144–148, 1969.

64. Helsby R, Moossa AR: Aortoiliac reconstruction with special reference to the extraperitoneal approach. *Br J Surg* 62:596–600, 1975.

65. Shepherd AD, Scott GR, Mackey WE, et al: Retroperitoneal approach to high-risk abdominal aortic aneurysms. *Arch Surg* 121:444–449, 1986.

66. Frazee RC, Roberts JW, Okeson GC, et al: Open versus laparoscopic cholecystectomy: A comparison of postoperative pulmonary function. *Ann Surg* 213:651–653, 1991.

67. Joris J, Cigarini I, Legrand M, et al: Metabolic and respiratory changes after cholecystectomy performed via laparotomy or laparoscopy. *Br J Anaesth* 69:341–345, 1992.

68. Mealy K, Gallagher H, Barry M, et al: Physiological and metabolic responses to open and laparoscopic cholecystectomy. *Br J Surg* 79:1061–1064, 1992.

69. Joris JL, Sottiaux TM, Chiche JD, et al: Effect of bi-level positive airway pressure (BIPAP) nasal ventilation on the postoperative pulmonary restrictive syndrome in obese patients undergoing gastroplasty. *Chest* 111:665–670, 1997.

70. Craig DB: Postoperative recovery of pulmonary function. *Anesth Analg* 60:46–52, 1981.

71. Klineberg PL, Bagshaw RJ: Hypoxemia and general anesthesia: An analysis of distribution of ventilation and perfusion. *Intern Anesth Clin* 19:123–167, 1981.

72. Mathers JM, Benumof JL, Wahrenbrock EA: General anesthetics and regional hypoxic pulmonary vasoconstriction. *Anesthesiology* 46:111–114, 1977.

73. Lewis KS, Whipple JK, Michael KA, Quebbeman EJ: Effect of analgesic treatment on the physiological consequences of acute pain. *Am J Hosp Pharm* 51:1539–1554, 1994.

74. Egbert AM, Parks LH, Short LM, et al: Randomized trial of postoperative patient controlled analgesia vs intramuscular narcotics in frail elderly men. *Arch Intern Med* 150:1897–1903, 1990.

75. Sriwatanakul K, Weis OF, Allonza JL, et al: Analysis of narcotic analgesic usage in the treatment of postoperative pain. *JAMA* 250:926–929, 1983.

76. Cohen FL: Postsurgical pain relief: Patient's status and nurses' medication choices. *Pain* 9:265–274, 1980.

Chapter 53

PULMONARY REHABILITATION IN PEDIATRIC PATIENTS

SUSHMITA MIKKILINENI

Pediatric pulmonary rehabilitation is still in its infancy and although a well-established practice in adult medicine, little information is available on the field of pediatric pulmonary rehabilitation. A few inpatient rehabilitation facilities do exist, but there are almost no organized outpatient programs. Modern technology and treatments have improved survival and increased the life span of many infants and children who would have otherwise succumbed to their disease much earlier. As a result of this, there is an emerging group of patients whose needs are not yet well established and there is no consensus on the management of these patients. While it is well accepted that individualized treatment plans and close follow-up improves outcome there is a paucity of literature on the diagnoses, complications, treatment, and outcomes in this group of patients.

As described by the American Thoracic Society, pulmonary rehabilitation means providing comprehensive respiratory care for patients with pulmonary disease and includes optimization of physical and mental capabilities such that the individual is capable of the highest possible functional capacity at the societal level.[1] For the pediatric patient, this can be a daunting task, for, not only does the program have to be individualized for the particular disease and its complications but also to the individual's developmental stage, potential for lung growth, and family dynamics which is even more important in the pediatric setting, because a child cannot be rehabilitated into society unless the family is willing to take on the responsibility of the child. Incorporating the child into the family with the least possible disruption in its lifestyle should be the primary goal of a pediatric rehabilitation program. Rehabilitation of the child with pulmonary problems encompasses a wide age range, from the neonatal patients with bronchopulmonary dysplasia (BPD) to the young adults with cystic fibrosis (CF), and diseases with variable prognosis. In diseases such as muscular dystrophy (MD) and CF there is a progressive deterioration of lung function in spite of good care and the goal here would be to delay the deterioration and improve quality of life; in other diseases such as in BPD the prognosis is excellent and the child can be expected to have a normal and relatively healthy life span and the ultimate goal in this case would be aggressive weaning of support while minimizing developmental delay, and short-term invasive measures such as tracheostomies and gastrostomies may be undertaken at the cost of increasing the burden to the child and caregiver in order to achieve long-term goals. Pediatric pulmonary rehabilitation, therefore, deals with a diverse population with vastly different outcomes and, therefore, different goals and these issues need to be considered when planning such a program.

The basic principles of any rehabilitative program include patient selection, medical and psychosocial evaluation, determining goals, instituting a program to include any or all of the following—physical therapy, exercise conditioning, respiratory therapy, education, and finally assessment of patient progress and long-term follow-up.[1] Pediatric specific issues regarding some common pediatric pulmonary diseases will be discussed in this chapter.

Pediatric Asthma

Asthma is the most common pediatric pulmonary disorder. Approximately 11 to 15 percent of children less than 18 years of age suffer from repeated wheezing episodes. Although the majority of the patients suffer from what can be clinically classified as mild asthma, pediatric asthma poses a significant burden to the society. While mild asthmatics may be considered under adequate control by conventional clinical measures, these patients may have significant functional impairment. Furthermore, the burden of pediatric asthma is difficult to quantify because the concept of adequate control may have different meanings to the physician, the patient, and the family.[2] Thus, patient evaluation should include not only history, physical exam, and pulmonary function testing, but also assessment of health-related quality of life,[3] as clinical indices only weakly correlate with the child's feeling and functional capabilities in everyday situations. The pediatric asthma quality of life questionnaire (PAQLQ)[4] and the pediatric asthma caregiver's quality of life questionnaire[5] were recently developed and should be used more frequently in pediatric asthma centers. An individualized care plan should be developed depending on the medical, social, and psychological needs of the patients.

Goals of a pediatric asthma rehabilitation program should be to ensure that every asthmatic child leads as normal a lifestyle as possible, has minimal symptoms and infrequent exacerbations with the least possible side effects from medications. Minimal restriction of physical activity and preservation of lung growth and function is an important aspect of the management of pediatric patients.

Although the above goals seem simple and achievable, studies have shown that they are not reached in the majority of children.[6,7] One of the major problem is the fact that infants and toddlers are not able to verbalize their discomfort and older children are often used to their symptoms and have changed their lifestyle to a more sedentary one and do not perceive their state as "abnormal." Parents also do not want their children to be on chronic medications and will restrict their activities so the child can be "symptom free." These factors lead to undertreatment and may actually increase airway hyperresponsiveness over time.

LUNG GROWTH AND ASTHMA

Several studies on the long-term effects of persistent asthma in childhood are available. Retrospective studies have shown that lung function is reduced in symptom-free adults with a past history of asthma in childhood.[8] Significantly reduced lung growth has been reported in asthmatic children,[9] and spirometric measurements were found to worsen over time among children with persistent wheezing,[10] bronchial hyper-responsiveness,[11] or asthma.[12] Gold and coworkers prospectively studied a cohort of approximately eleven thousand white American children of ages 6 to 18 years with annual spirometries between 1974 and 1989. FEV_1 values were 6 percent and FEF_{25-75} values were 17 percent lower in these children as compared to the normal population.[13] Martinez and coworkers studied children in the first 6 years of their life and reported that children with persistent wheezing had significantly reduced increase in lung function.[14]

In a recent long-term study, Agertoft and Pedersen[15] reported that significantly greater improvement in lung function occurred in children who started inhaled steroid treatment within 2 years after the onset of their asthma symptoms. In addition, better lung function was achieved at a lower total dose of inhaled steroid in children who started these medications within the first 4.5 years of the onset of their symptoms than in those that started them after 5 years of symptoms. Also, in the group of children that did not receive inhaled steroids, lung function did not increase as well as in those that received inhaled steroids. Konig and Shaffer[16] conducted a retrospective study to evaluate the effect of stepwise therapy on the long-term outcome of childhood asthma. Significant improvement in symptoms and hospitalizations were observed in the group treated with an inhaled anti-inflammatory medication (sodium cromoglycate or steroids). Analysis of the pulmonary function tests revealed that children treated with only bronchodilators had significant decreases in FVC and FEV_1, while a trend toward improvement was seen in both groups treated with the inhaled anti-inflammatory drugs. In this study, however, delay in starting sodium cromoglycate and not inhaled corticosteroid had a negative outcome on both clinical symptoms and pulmonary function.

TREATMENT

From the above observations, it is clear that anti-inflammatory drugs are disease modifiers and need to be introduced early in the course of the disease. Based on the observation that mild asthmatics treated with only bronchodilators tend to have worse pulmonary function than those with more severe disease but treated with inhaled anti-inflammatory drugs, and given the fact that children and their families tend to underestimate symptoms, children should be given maximal therapy early on in the disease. The latest guidelines of the Global Initiative for Asthma[17] have recommended earlier use of inhaled nonsteroidal anti-inflammatory drugs in mild asthmatics. The present recommendations are to start inhaled sodium cromoglycate in children with symptoms >1 day per week as compared to the previous recommendations of starting these drugs in children with symptoms >3 days per week. There is also a trend toward earlier use of oral and inhaled steroids but the benefits and side effects need to be carefully weighed prior to including them into a chronic treatment regime. Recent prospective studies on the use of long-term use of inhaled steroids have shown evidence for growth suppression, more evident in the prepubertal age.[18] In all cases a step-wise management should be instituted and medications added and discontinued according to symptoms and lung function measurements.

ASSESSMENT OF LUNG FUNCTION

Periodic measurement of lung function provides an objective assessment of the control of the child's asthma and may sometimes justify a step-up of treatment even in the absence of reported symptoms. Exercise testing is useful not only to diagnose exercise-induced asthma but also for exercise prescription and reassurance to the parent and child that pretreatment with medications can provide effective control of symptoms. Peak expiratory flow rate (PEFR) measurements can be carried out in children as young as 3 years old although it is more reliable in the older child. Although commonly prescribed, the use of peak-flow meters at home may not be a reliable indicator of the child's lung function. Normal PEFR values may be obtained even in the presence of severe small airways obstruction.[19,20] Furthermore, PEFR is an effort-dependent measure and can therefore be variable depending on the technique. Careful attention to technique should be given to avoid unnecessary increase of treatment or to prevent school absenteeism particularly in adolescents who may alter their measurements to stay home from school.

DELIVERY SYSTEMS

A metered-dose inhaler (MDI) and a spacer combination is the most effective way of delivering treatment to infants, children, and adolescents.[21] Different kinds of spacers are available and the choice depends on the comfort and familiarity of the physician, child, and caregiver with a particular device. In general, in children less than 6 years of age, a spacer with a face mask is preferred. The number of breaths per puff depends on the tidal volume of the child, thus, the younger the child, the more breaths, as well as more puffs, are needed for better lung deposition. In the older child, an MDI with spacer combination is still the recommended choice but a spacer with mouth piece should be used. Adolescents will choose their own device and are most likely to be compliant with only an MDI, therefore they should receive instruction on its proper use and their technique should be supervised. Nebulizers are cumbersome to use and not any more effective than the MDI-spacer combination.[22] However, it still remains a useful delivery system in acute asthma exacerbations in children when there are severe reductions in vital capacity, and the nebulizers can deliver oxygen and drug without the need for patient cooperation.

ASTHMA EDUCATION

Asthma education is the single most important factor in improving compliance for better control of asthma. Education should involve the patient and/or caregiver. Children as young as 2 or 3 years old can be involved in the education process. The education materials should be geared to the different age groups. In most cases noncompliance is due to poor understanding of the pathophysiology of the disease process and the need for ongoing medications even when symptoms are absent. Education should be aimed at improving the understanding of the pathophysiology of the disease, different triggers and means to avoid them, the appropriate use of medications and their actions, and use and cleaning of their respiratory equipment. One of the most important aspects of education is early recognition of signs and symptoms of worsening disease. Parents of infants should be taught to appreciate tachypnea, nasal flaring, and retractions. Cough is often the only symptom of pediatric asthma and caregivers should be sensitized to the fact that a lingering cough is not just a "cold" and nocturnal cough in a patient with asthma signifies worsening of disease state. An individualized protocol of treatment should be made out, and written instructions regarding acute exacerbations and emergency management should be given to caregivers as well as older children. Above all, asthma management should be approached as a team effort with the patient and the family playing a central role. Psychosocial needs should be addressed and school nurses and teachers should be informed of the child's condition so that he/she is accommodated in school, particularly in regards to serious allergies to food and animals. The patient should be allowed to spend as much time in school as is safely possible and should not be sent home at the first sign of a cough. Asthma support groups, asthma education classes and updates for school nurses and teachers can be provided at the asthma center and will be helpful in better management of the patient.

ASTHMA AND EXERCISE

Exercise is often overlooked as an important component in the diagnosis and management of asthma. It is estimated that between 40 to 95 percent of asthmatics will show evidence of exercise-induced bronchospasm given sufficient exercise stimulus.[23] Therefore, it is not uncommon that many children with asthma are reluctant to participate in sports and other strenuous activities. This leads to a vicious cycle of decreased physical fitness, deconditioning, and worsened exercise-induced dyspnea which is not necessarily related to bronchospasm. Exercise training is beneficial for all asthmatics, but particularly so for the moderate to severe asthmatics who tend to be more sedentary. In addition to psychological benefits, enhancement of self-esteem, and weight control, exercise training has been shown to improve aerobic fitness in asthmatic children. This allows the patient to perform a given work load with less ventilation and thereby less exercise-induced bronchospasm.[24] Given an adequate treatment regime and exercise training most children with asthma should be able to participate in any sports or activity of their choice.

Exercises such as dancing, karate, and swimming that improve thoracic cage mobility, strengthen trunk extensor and shoulder girdle muscles are useful in improving posture and preventing the rounded shoulders and kyphotic appearance of patients with severe asthma. In addition ventilatory muscle training such as abdominal breathing may be useful. Relaxation therapy may be useful in patients who tend to panic during acute exacerbations.

Cystic Fibrosis

Cystic fibrosis (CF) is the most common genetic disease in the Caucasian population, occurring in 1 in 2500 live births.[25] The genetic defect leads to the absence of a protein, cystic fibrosis transmembrane conductance regulator (CFTR), which is responsible for transport of chloride ions across epithelial cell membranes. The CFTR gene defect leads to a reduced chloride conductance at the apical surface of epithelia; in the sweat ducts, this causes a failure of chloride *reabsorption* which leads to excessive chloride losses in sweat,

which is characteristic of this disease. In the airways there is abnormal chloride *secretion* which leads to excessive sodium and water reabsorption leading to extracellular dehydration and thick, inspissated mucus. Mucous plugging occurs and airway clearance is significantly reduced. A vicious cycle of bacterial trapping, infection, inflammation, and tissue destruction ensues, leading to bronchiectasis, fibrosis, and progressive deterioration of lung function. Pancreas is the other organ most commonly involved in CF. Blockage of pancreatic ducts, prevents pancreatic enzymes from reaching the intestines and malabsorption and poor nutritional status are common in the absence of adequate pancreatic enzyme supplementation.

Although CF is a multisystem disease, pulmonary and nutritional status determine the overall prognosis for a patient. In recent years comprehensive and aggressive treatment and newer therapeutic modalities aimed at improving airway clearance, controlling airway infection, and improving nutritional status have raised the median survival age from about 18 years in 1976 to about 29 years in 1994.[26]

QUALITY OF LIFE IN CF

With improved survival, the number of patients with moderate to severe disease is increasing and quality of life issues in these patients are becoming increasingly important. Progressive worsening of pulmonary function leads to impaired exercise capacity and this may have a significant impact on quality of life (QOL). QOL is affected by physical as well as psychosocial functioning. Studies evaluating psychosocial functioning in CF children suggested that children with relatively severe CF have very little psychosocial impairment compared to their healthy peers and are able to cope quite well with life's tasks.[27] Similarly, when psychosocial functioning of adult CF patients was compared to healthy adults, although a higher degree of impairment was seen in CF patients, no statistical difference was found as compared to their healthy peers.[28,29] QOL measures such as the Quality of Well-Being Scale[30,31] and Sickness Impact Profile[32] have been used in various studies and it has been suggested that these scales should be used to assess outcome of various treatments in the CF patients.[33] When the Sickness Impact Profile was used to assess QOL issues, the overall QOL of CF patients was found to be diminished when compared to normal population but was mainly due to limitation of physical functioning and in categories of sleep and rest, eating, home management, recreational activities, and employment.[32] Dyspnea, measured by the Dyspnea Scale played a significant role in impaired physical, psychosocial, and overall functioning. While in some studies, FEV_1 correlated significantly with QOL,[30] in the study of De Jong and coworkers,[32] exercise capacity as measured by the maximal workload (Wmax) rather than pulmonary function correlated with QOL, suggests that CF patients cope well with severe impairments in pulmonary function but diminished exercise performance is more closely related to diminished QOL. However, whatever may be the perceived problem, diminished pulmonary function ultimately leads to decreased exercise capacity and these are all interrelated causes leading to diminished QOL.

Most studies on QOL have included mainly adult patients with moderate to severe impairment of pulmonary function. With modern treatment and early diagnosis, children usually have good pulmonary function and their physical performance may be no different from their healthy peers. However, developmental and behavioral issues play a pivotal role in the care of the preschool child and routine therapy with nebulized bronchodilator treatments, chest physiotherapy, pancreatic enzyme supplementation, and maintaining adequate nutritional status may prove to be an enormous psychosocial burden to the family, significantly affecting the QOL of the family. Behavioral issues need to be addressed and strategies advised so that these routine treatments are the least disruptive to the daily routine of family life.

CF AND EXERCISE

Exercise limitation in CF patients is related to diminished pulmonary function, particularly airflow obstruction.[34,35] Cardiovascular adaptations to exercise are normal in patients with mild disease and although peak heart rate may be low in those with more severe disease, it is not due to cardiovascular limitations but rather ventilatory limitations and dyspnea.[35] Patients with severe disease may have arterial desaturation during exercise[35,36] and careful exercise testing should be carried out prior to recommending any form of an exercise regimen. Conventional exercise testing on cycle ergometer and treadmill using standard protocols is generally used but more recently the 6-min walking test has been used to test younger patients with CF.[37] Gulmans and colleagues showed that the maximal walking distance correlated well with the maximal work capacity and concluded that the 6-min walking test can reliably assess exercise capacity and arterial desaturation in children with mild to moderate disease.[37] This test simulates normal childhood activities, does not require specialized equipment, and, when *properly* administered, can be a useful tool for testing children.

Exercise should be an integral part of daily life of the CF patient. In addition to having a positive impact on QOL, Nixon and associates have shown that the probability of 8-year survival in patients with higher aerobic fitness was 83 percent as compared to 28 percent in CF patients with lower aerobic fitness even when controlled for pulmonary function and nutritional status[38] (Fig. 53-1). Exercise training programs incorporating jogging,[34] swimming,[39] and upper body strengthening,[40] have in general failed to show a consistent improvement in pulmonary function, although there is a significant improvement in aerobic fitness, which in turn is associated with better quality of well-being.[30] Similar benefits are seen with a home exercise training program with bicycle training.[41] Specific ventilatory muscle training including biofeedback-assisted breathing retraining[42] and inspiratory muscle conditioning[43] may be useful as well. Training programs that can be easily integrated into daily living, are likely to be more successful in producing lasting benefits, as patients may continue with the exercise regime even after the end of the training session. In addition to physical and psychosocial benefits, exercise may improve sputum clearance.[44,45]

Children with CF need special consideration in regard to exercise-induced bronchospasm and excessive salt and fluid losses and dehydration during exercise. Many patients may need preexercise bronchodilators; exercising in the heat should be avoided; and children should take plenty of fluids and salt supplements when exercising. Supplemental oxygen

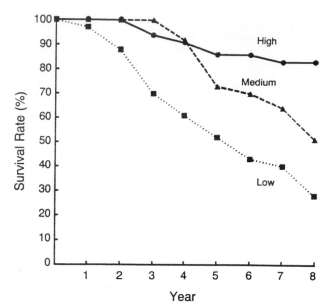

FIGURE 53-1 Survival among 109 patients with cystic fibrosis, according to fitness level. (Reprinted with permission, from Nixon et al., N Engl J Med 327:1785–1788, 1992.)

should be prescribed for patients who have arterial desaturation with exercise as this may enable the patient to carry on submaximal exercise and thus improve cardiopulmonary efficiency.[46]

CF AND CHEST PHYSIOTHERAPY

In CF most of the morbidity and mortality are associated with pulmonary complications caused by reduced airway clearance. Clearing the airways of thick, sticky, and potentially infected secretions has been the mainstay of CF therapy for many years. Chest physiotherapy (CPT) techniques are aimed at improving bronchial drainage from the various bronchopulmonary segments and generally consist of postural drainage with manual or mechanical percussion and vibration followed by deep breathing and coughing. While conventional CPT is the most commonly used technique, it requires the presence and commitment of parents or caregivers and can be time consuming, as well as tiring. More recently, newer modalities of CPT have been tried with the idea of providing independence while maintaining effective bronchial clearance and thereby improving compliance. Table 53-1 lists the various bronchial drainage techniques available.

The newer techniques of active cycle breathing (forced expiratory technique), autogenic drainage, and positive ex-

TABLE 53-1 Bronchial Drainage Techniques

Postural drainage with percussion (conventional chest PT)
  Manual vs. mechanical
Active cycle breathing (Forced expiration technique)
Autogenic drainage
Positive expiratory pressure (PEP)
Oscillating PEP-flutter devices
High-frequency chest-wall oscillation
High-frequency mouth oscillation

piratory pressure breathing are more useful for older patients as they require active breathing techniques which are more difficult to learn and require concentration to perform. In addition, there is confusion about the exact techniques even among physiotherapists and may not be properly taught or properly performed by the patients, leading to ineffective sputum production.[47] The high-frequency chest wall oscillation or "vest" therapy is another technique designed for self-administration of airway clearance therapy and it allows the patient to receive therapy to all areas of the lung simultaneously. This form of therapy has gained popularity among CF patients. It is simple to use and has been found to be at least as useful as standard CPT.[48,49] High-frequency mouth oscillation devices function on similar principles and have recently become available.[50] Another small and portable device is the "Flutter," which generates controlled oscillating positive pressure and interrupts expiratory flow when one breathes through it and has been shown to be effective in increasing sputum production.[51]

Conflicting reports are available in literature on the efficacy of the different CPT modalities in clearing bronchial secretions. While most studies have shown an increase in sputum production with different CPT modalities, long-term benefits, including improvement in pulmonary function, improved QOL, and decreased morbidity are not known. A recent metaanalysis of CPT in the management of patients with CF showed that standard CPT (STD) results in significantly greater sputum expectoration than no treatment at all and that the addition of exercise to STD resulted in statistically increased FEV_1 over STD alone, but no significant difference between sputum production or FEV_1 was noted between STD and other CPT modalities.[52]

Whatever the mode of CPT used, it should be well suited to the lifestyle of the patient. When CPT is introduced in early infancy, it is more easily incorporated into the daily routine of the patient and family, thus leading to the least disruption and improved compliance in the toddler and early childhood years. The older CF patient should be allowed to choose a modality that he/she feels most comfortable with and would be most likely to use. Aerobic exercises, such as swimming, karate, and dancing should be encouraged in addition to CPT.

CF AND NUTRITION

Management of nutritional status is an important aspect of ongoing CF care. There is a strong relationship between nutritional status and lung disease in the CF patient. There is evidence to show that as the lung disease deteriorates, nutritional status worsens.[53] On the other hand, improved nutritional status positively impacts pulmonary function and survival. Zemel and coworkers obtained data on 1405 children between the ages of 6 to 8 years from the Cystic Fibrosis Patient Registry, and prospectively studied the relationship between growth, nutritional status, and pulmonary function for 2 years. They found that children who gain more in weight and body mass index experience milder declines in FEV_1.[54] The impact of nutrition on survival was described by Corey and associates in a comparative study of two clinic populations in Boston and Toronto.[55] They found that the Toronto group had improved survival, which was related to their better nutritional status. In addition improved nutri-

tional status has a positive impact on respiratory, diaphragmatic, and skeletal muscle strength and, therefore, on the exercise capacity and ultimately the quality of life in CF patients.

Nutritional assessment should be an important part of regular health maintenance of the CF patient. Pancreatic insufficiency is present in about 85 percent of patients with CF and regular weight checks and history pertaining to ongoing insufficiency and malabsorption should be obtained. The presence of any of the following: frequent, bulky, loose and malodorous stools; abdominal pain or distention; or flatulence may indicate the need for adjustment of pancreatic enzymes. Often, failure to gain weight is the result of pulmonary exacerbation and the need for aggressive antibiotic therapy and CPT, rather than malabsorption.

Dietary assessment should be periodically carried out and the enzyme dosages checked. Routine biochemical evaluation including serum protein, albumin, hemoglobin, and, when indicated, vitamin A and E levels and fecal fat evaluation should be done. Pancreatic enzyme replacement should be determined and adjusted on an individual basis. Some patients may need H_2-blockers in addition to pancreatic supplements. Very high doses of pancreatic enzymes should be avoided as they have been associated with fibrosing colonopathy.[56] As the disease progresses, the endocrine function of the pancreas may be affected and diabetes may develop. In addition, CF patients are at risk for developing gastroesophageal reflux and patients, especially those with advanced disease, should be evaluated for the need for insulin and H_2-blockers.

Despite treatment advances in CF, suboptimal nutritional status continues to be problematic for most patients. Although pancreatic insufficiency is an important cause of this malnutrition, negative energy balance is an important component. CF patients have an increased resting energy expenditure due to abnormal pulmonary mechanics, increased oxygen costs of breathing, and chronic infection and inflammation.[57] It is recommended, that CF patients consume a diet with normal to high fat, and one that provides them with calories at 120 to 150 percent of the recommended daily allowance (RDA), and sufficient salt replacement. They need double the RDA of fat-soluble vitamins, A, D, E, K,[58] and this is usually provided with vitamin supplements. Critical stages for nutritional impairment occur during infancy, adolescence, and pregnancy; in addition patients are at particular risk for malnutrition when lung disease is advanced and when diabetes develops. Increased caloric supplements during these periods are usually necessary. If patients cannot keep up with oral intake because of anorexia, nasogastric or gastrostomy-tube feedings may be needed, but parental nutritional is rarely necessary.

PSYCHOSOCIAL ISSUES IN CF

CF is a chronic, progressive, and life-shortening disease, and patients and families experience several stresses throughout their life. During early years of infancy, the family usually bears the major brunt of psychosocial and financial stresses, but, as the child gets older and becomes more independent, a variety of additional emotional and psychological factors impact upon the physical well-being of the patient.

The diagnosis of CF in a child is invariably stressful for

the family. Initial feelings of denial and shock are soon replaced by grief and then acceptance. Parents tend to become emotionally closer to the CF child, being overprotective and focused on physical symptoms.[59] Almost as soon as the diagnosis is made, families are expected to handle a whole careplan which can be stressful. Siblings often feel neglected and become jealous of the attention given to their brother or sister. In hopes of maintaining a normal life, parents tend to overcompensate, which magnifies the usual stresses of daily living. Children are particularly prone to infections in the first few years of their life and a great deal of anxiety exists about avoiding infections and parents who have to send their children to day-care often feel guilty, or give up their jobs to stay home, adding to their emotional and financial burdens. Behavioral issues compound the difficulty parents have in keeping up with the daily regimen of respiratory treatments, CPT, and enzyme supplementation.

Parental care-giving can produce marital strain. This may cause marriages to breakup in some whereas, in many, the relationship strengthens. Quittner and associates found that in couples who have children with CF, wives reported significantly higher conflict over child-rearing and greater depression, and husbands reported significantly lower social and sexual intimacy. Mothers were usually dissatisfied with the amount of help received from their spouses.[60] Parents usually benefit from psychosocial support provided by the CF center and interventions focusing on above conflicts should be developed for them.

As the child gets older, personal stresses in the child's life increase. Adolescence is a particularly stressful period. Self-image issues become important and patients begin to have adjustment difficulties. Adolescents typically become less compliant, often deny reality, and are prone to wishful thinking as a coping method. Thompson and coworkers reported that over 50 percent of adolescents with CF meet criteria for a DSM-III diagnosis.[61] This includes oppositional disorder and phobic and anxiety disorders. They suggested that interventional strategies should promote better coping and adaptive methods. They should be counseled on better problem-solving methods and encouraged to seek out social support.

The psychosocial stresses of the adult CF patient are similar to those of other patients with chronic debilitating pulmonary diseases and are discussed in detail in Chap. 48.

Neuromuscular Diseases

Neuromuscular problems in children can be hereditary, such as in spinal muscular atrophy and Duchenne muscular dystrophy, or acquired, as in spinal cord injuries. Respiratory complications from decreased ventilatory reserves are the main cause of mortality in these children. Since the advent of home mechanical ventilation, the survival of children with these diseases has significantly improved. Early intervention directed toward prevention of thoracic and spinal deformities and improved ventilation, enhances lung growth and reduces the frequency of pneumonia and atelectasis. Orthopedic braces help prevent severe scoliosis, and when present early correction by spinal fusion should be undertaken. Physical therapy and breathing exercises help maintain the mobility of the sternocostal joints, in addition to preventing orthopedic deformities. Routine chest physical therapy is usually

not indicated, as these patients do not have increased secretions, but therapy becomes necessary during episodes of respiratory infections. Breathing techniques such as glossopharyngeal breathing and neck breathing should be instituted, if and when the child is able. Glossopharyngeal breathing is usually a difficult technique for younger children but neck breathing can be learned by children as young as 3 years old.[62] The latter is a useful technique in patients with high spinal cord injuries who have strong neck muscles but have diaphragmatic paralysis. Bulbar involvement occurs in many patients with progression of disease and gastrostomy tubes for feeding are necessary in patients with swallowing difficulties.

When respiratory insufficiency sets in, support can be provided by the use of various noninvasive methods of ventilation. Nasal mask positive pressure support or ventilation, or negative pressure ventilation via cuirasse can be used. Tracheostomy with mechanical ventilation will be necessary in some patients. Although advocated by some, the early use of mechanical ventilation to prevent chest wall deformities has not been found to be beneficial.[63] The use of long-term ventilation in patients with neuromuscular disease is controversial because of ethical issues and that decision has to be made together with the family and the patient if possible.

The goal of pulmonary rehabilitation in children with neuromuscular diseases is to extend life expectancy while maintaining quality of life and providing comfort with respiratory support.

Rehabilitation of the Low-Birth-Weight Infant

Recent advances in technology has reduced morbidity and mortality, and consequently resulted in improved survival of the low-birth-weight (750 to 1500 g) and very-low-birth-weight infant (<750 g).[64,65] Various studies have shown that severe disability occurs in 26 percent of infants weighing <750 g, in 17 percent of infants weighing 750 to 1000 g, and in 11 percent of infants weighing 1000 to 1500 g at birth.[66,67] Although the rates are relatively low, this represents a large number of children who will require various levels of lifelong technologic support. In addition, there is another group of infants who do not have long-term disability, but are still relatively smaller and sicker at discharge and continue to be dependant on some form of technology. The financial burden of caring for these children is enormous and because of the recent trend toward managed care, there is a thrust toward earlier discharge and parents are called upon to assume increasing responsibilities for the child in their home. While it is developmentally and psychosocially good for the child to be home, not all parents are ready for it and a lot of planning and education have to take place before a child can be sent home.

BRONCHOPULMONARY DYSPLASIA (BPD)

BPD is described as chronic lung disease secondary to neonatal respiratory disease and is based on radiologic, clinical, and pathologic criteria.[68] Premature infants who require mechanical ventilation and have the prolonged need for oxygen may develop BPD. The incidence varies depending on the centers reporting it, but usually, the smaller and more premature the infant, the higher the incidence. In a multicenter study published by Avery and coworkers, the incidence was reported to be 76.9 percent for infants with a birth weight of 700 to 800 g and 12.9 percent in infants with birth weight of 1250 to 1500 g.[69] With newer modes of mechanical ventilation and the use of surfactant at birth, the severity of BPD has reduced but it continues to be a significant cause of morbidity and mortality in premature infants.

BPD is usually not an isolated problem in the premature neonates. A higher incidence of cardiopulmonary and central nervous system complications are seen in these children.[70] Frequent respiratory infections and reactive airways disease are common and pulmonary hypertension with or without cor pulmonale commonly occur in the more severe patients. Neurodevelopmental delay occurs from prolonged ventilatory support, poor nutritional status, lack of sensory stimulation, and neurologic insults secondary to intraventricular hemorrhage. These infants have decreased energy and respiratory reserves and tend to decompensate with the least provocation leading to arterial desaturation during what is often termed a BPD "spell." Frequent hypoxic spells can further aggravate neurologic and cardiac problems making the care of these infants extremely difficult in the first few months of life. Hypoxia, increased work of breathing, poor intake because of discoordinated suck and swallow leads to poor nutritional status, which adds to the increased morbidity.

A comprehensive, multidisciplinary follow-up program is essential for the successful rehabilitation of premature infants into the family unit. Assessment of the child, family, and home is necessary prior to discharge, and establishing realistic goals and expectations is important. The complexity of the care required at home will depend on individual clinical situations. This may range from simply careful monitoring to the need for ventilatory support and gastrostomy feedings. The out-patient follow-up program for the child should ideally begin prior to discharge from the nursery. The pediatrician, neonatologists, and a team of nurses and involved specialists should plan the follow-up program, such that continuity of care is available. The need for home nursing should be assessed at the time of discharge. If skilled nursing is not necessary, home visiting nurses for a few hours per day can provide the support necessary during the initial transition phase. Several interventions, such as occupational, speech, and physical therapy, can be provided at home. This can reduce the number of trips to the hospital, in addition to providing care in a more comfortable and familiar environment.

The out-patient program should consist of routine well-baby care including immunizations, as well as frequent assessment of respiratory, nutritional, and neurodevelopmental status. The parents should be made aware of their child's potential disabilities and limitations, and should learn to recognize signs of their child's respiratory distress and response to stress, and interventions needed to deal with the particular situation. Many patients with BPD are discharged home on diuretics and oxygen which are weaned on an out-patient basis. Most infants requiring oxygen at discharge are also discharged with an apnea monitor. Bronchodilators, antireflux medications, and anticonvulsants may also be required. Parents need to become familiar with all medications

and their doses and side-effects. The importance of avoiding respiratory infections should be stressed and influenza vaccine should be recommended to children older than a corrected age of 6 months. Nutritional status is often compromised in children with BPD, as they have a high caloric requirement, and depending on their cardiovascular status, will often need fluid restriction. High-calorie formula and fortification of available formulas to provide even higher calorie per ounce of fluid, is often necessary to provide the adequate calories without increasing the volume consumed.

HOME O$_2$ THERAPY

Infants and children require oxygen for a variety of reasons. The need for oxygen can be short- or long-term, ranging from months to years. Premature infants with BPD may require oxygen for many months. Children with chronic lung diseases from other causes, such as interstitial lung disease and advanced cystic fibrosis may have a chronic oxygen requirement. In the past these children would have to remain hospitalized in an acute or rehabilitation facility. With the availability of newer catheters and oxygen delivery devices these children can be safely managed at home.

In BPD infants, Donn and coworkers reported an estimated savings of $60,000 per patient by providing home care instead of hospital care.[71] Rosen and colleagues reported a reduction of 25 patient months of hospitalization in 1 year.[72] Home oxygen therapy is thus cost-effective and reduces hospital stay. Hospitalization is disruptive to the family and can be psychologically stressful to the infant and child. Home care enhances the psychosocial and physical growth and development of the child.

The primary requisite for discharge of a patient on oxygen is that their lung disease is stable and that the parents are willing to manage the oxygen therapy at home. A stable and reliable home environment with good support systems should be available. Prior to discharge the home has to be prepared and parents and other caregivers should be instructed on the care of the child and the use of the equipment. The child's room should be well ventilated, smoke-free, and no smoking should be allowed in the house. These infants and children are prone to respiratory decompensations, and caregivers should be taught to anticipate changes in the needs of the child. A home-care agency that is reliable and can provide supplies promptly when needed should be available, and the family should have access to a physician and emergency services at all times.

The most common method of delivering oxygen to infants and children is via a nasal cannula. Small catheters that fit infant nares are now available but they can be easily plugged with mucus and care should be taken to keep them clean. In older children, adult cannulas with the prongs cut off, can be used. As children will usually grab at their tubing and pull it off, it is often necessary to secure the cannulas by taping it to the cheeks. Infants are rarely sent home on more than 2 liters/min of oxygen via nasal cannula, and a portable liquid oxygen container is usually all that is necessary. In the older child requiring higher flows of oxygen, an oxygen concentrator should be prescribed for home, while portable liquid oxygen is reserved for travel. Oxygen is provided via a tracheostomy mask for those children who have a tracheostomy. While humidification is not necessary when oxygen

TABLE 53-2 Common Causes of Chronic Respiratory Failure/ Ventilator-Dependency in Children

A. Severe restrictive chest wall diseases
    Severe scoliosis
    Kyphoscoliosis
B. Neurologic
  1. Central
    a. Congenital hypoventilation syndrome
    b. Central nervous system injury/asphyxia
    c. Arnold-Chiari malformation
    d. Obesity-hypoventilation syndrome
  2. Peripheral
    a. High spinal cord injury
    b. Phrenic nerve lesions/diaphragmatic paralysis
C. Muscular
    Congenital or acquired myopathy
    Werdnig-Hoffman disease
    Duchenne muscular dystrophy
    Infant botulinism
    Myasthenia gravis
D. Respiratory
    Chronic lung disease
    Bronchopulmonary dysplasia
    Tracheobronchial abnormalities
    Sleep-apnea syndromes
E. Cardiovascular
    Complex congenital heart disease with pulmonary artery hypertension

is provided via the nasal cannula, a heated humidifier should always be used for oxygen therapy via the tracheostomy.

Weaning from oxygen occurs as the lung disease improves. It is usually a gradual process based on clinical symptoms, but home pulse oximetry can also guide the weaning process. Weaning is usually started after the infant has been stable for a while, is gaining weight, and there has been no need for an increase in their respiratory medications, or diuretics as in the case of BPD. There is no fixed protocol for weaning, but it is always started during the day while the child is awake. Oxygen is continued at previous levels during feeding and sleep till the child is completely weaned to room air during the day. Once this is accomplished, weaning during feeds and at nights is attempted, while monitoring the child's color, respiratory rate and effort, and pulse oximetry. Weaning is continued until the child is on minimal oxygen at night. Prior to completely weaning the child off oxygen, the child should have a normal overnight pulse oximetry study. Often an infant will require only as little as 0.125 liter of oxygen, but will desaturate without it. Even low flows of oxygen, when mixed in the infant's small tidal volume, can provide a significantly high fraction of inspired oxygen.

APNEA MONITORS

Cardiorespiratory monitoring at home, although controversial, is most commonly used in the low-birth-weight infants, in whom there is a high incidence of apnea of prematurity. Due to the immaturity of the central nervous system, apnea and bradycardia may continue even after the stabilization of the cardiorespiratory status, and is often exacerbated during periods of illness. An apnea monitor is a relatively simple piece of equipment, and does not require any special skills for its use. However, it is a source of tremendous anxiety for the parents and caregivers because the consequences of a true alarm can be life-threatening. Studies of infants with home apnea monitors[73,74] have demonstrated that family life can be impacted with home monitoring. Parents report feeling isolated and unable to get adequate baby-sitting services. Their biggest concern is their response to an alarm and their ability to perform cardiopulmonary resuscitation (CPR). Ongoing teaching and close contact with an apnea program may help alleviate some of these fears.

Parents need to learn the use of the apnea monitor, including proper placement of the leads. Parents must learn CPR prior to discharge. Most importantly they must learn to assess the infant's pulse and respirations. It should be emphasized that when an alarm sounds, assessment of the infant is the first step, as most alarms sound because of loose leads caused by the movement of the child. The wires should be placed under clothing, away from the child's reach, to prevent the child from dislodging leads by pulling at them and also to avoid inadvertent strangulation. The parents should be within hearing distance of the monitor and should be able to reach the baby within 10 to 15 s if the monitor alarms. Emergency telephone numbers and names of contact persons should be clearly posted near telephones at home.

The infant is assessed clinically during routine physician visits. In addition, the monitor is downloaded at periodic intervals or when the recording capacity is full. The tracings are evaluated for the presence of apnea and bradycardia and oxygen desaturation. The frequency and duration of each

FIGURE 53-2 A 3-year-old child with spinal muscular atrophy receiving physical therapy at home.

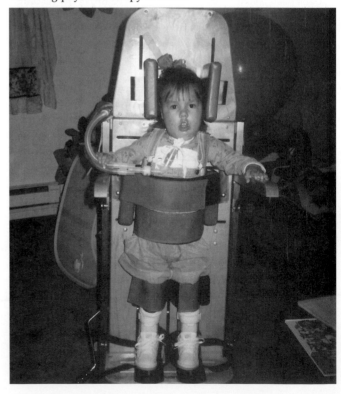

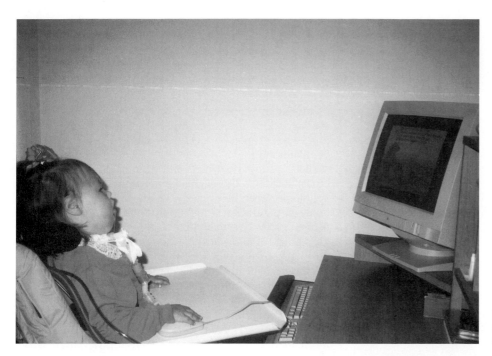

FIGURE 53-3 A child with spinal muscular atrophy using a computer with specially equipped "mouse."

event is noted. Depending on the abnormality noted, further workup for gastroesophageal reflux or increased medications such as caffeine may be needed. Monitors are usually discontinued after the infants have had no real events for a period of 2 to 3 months and are off oxygen.

Children with Tracheostomy

Tracheostomy is being performed on a more frequent basis in the pediatric age group. This increase seems to be related to the improved survival of preterm infants, and children with craniofacial anomalies and pulmonary and neurologic disorders. In the pre-term infants, the usual indications for performing a tracheostomy are to bypass upper airway obstruction, and for pulmonary toilet. Upper airway obstruction in infants can result from subglottic stenosis due to prolonged intubation, congenital tracheal anomalies, or pharyngeal hypotonia, which results from poor muscle tone in neurologically devastated children. In addition to pharyngeal hypotonia, infants with severe neuromotor retardation often chronically aspirate, and tracheostomy aids in tracheal suctioning and decreasing the frequency of aspiration pneumonias. In the older child, tracheostomy is usually needed to provide prolonged mechanical ventilation in patients with chronic lung disease and neuromuscular disease.

Bringing a child home with a tracheostomy raises several anxiety provoking concerns for the caregiver.[75–77] The infant and child's speech is often the biggest concern. Parents worry that they would be unable to hear their infant's cry or that their child would be unable to summon help. As a result parents reorganize their homes and have significantly altered lifestyles so that they are close to the child at all times. In the older child, speech development and their ability to return to school and communicate with peers is a big concern. Communication in these children can be improved with the use of the Passy-Muir speaking valves.[78] In infants, bells tied to

the ankles, can be used to serve as a means of communication, and children soon learn that making noise gets the attention of their parents.[79] It is recommended that parents and children learn to use sign language to enhance communication and social development.[80] Caring for a tracheotomized child requires specialized skills, and friends and families are often reluctant to care for the child. Lack of medically trained babysitting services adds to the psychosocial burden and feeling of social isolation. In regard to the child, parents are concerned about being able to maintain a patent airway and the probability of increased infections. In the Wills study, mothers felt that they needed more support in areas of (1) homemaker services, (2) communication with professionals, and (3) the opportunities to interact with other parents of infants/children with tracheostomies.[77]

A lot of literature exists about home care of the tracheotomized child and the reader is referred to some of them.[79,81–83] Several family members should be involved in the discharge planning and predischarge training in tracheostomy care. They need to know about the equipment, its use, and how to clean it. Instructions regarding feeding and bathing of the child, skin care around the stoma, and guidance regarding avoiding fuzzy clothing and loose necklaces with tiny beads, are all important components of discharge training. Accidental decannulations and plugged tracheostomy tubes are the leading causes of mortality in these children[84] and competency regarding suctioning, tracheostomy changes, and cardiopulmonary resuscitation are essential prior to discharge.

While tracheostomy care is an integral part of the daily routine, most of these children have severe lung and/or neurologic disease, often with associated neurodevelopmental delays. Therefore, comprehensive care by a multidisciplinary team is essential. The child and the family form the central focus of the team and maintaining a stable family unit and integrating the child in that unit should be the

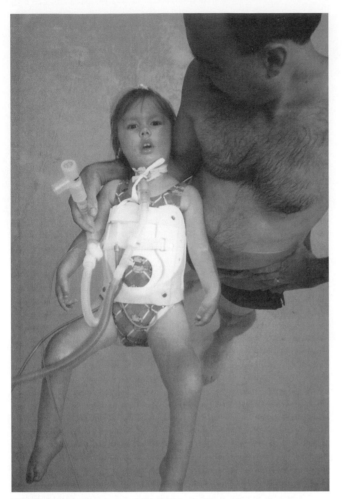

FIGURE 53-4 The same child taking a dip in the swimming pool. This has to be done very cautiously, so that water does not get into the tracheostomy and tubing, and the ventilator should be disconnected from the electric source and should be running on a battery.

primary goal. Global developmental issues including psychosocial development are an important part of the rehabilitation program.

Many of the above concerns and issues are common to ventilator-dependent children and their families.

Home Mechanical Ventilation

The Congressional Office of Technology Assessment (1988) suggested that there are as many as 2000 ventilator-dependent children and adolescents in the United States each year.[85] The etiology of pediatric ventilator dependence is variable and Table 53-2 lists some of the common causes. Some patients have rehabilitative disorders and the potential for weaning exists, but in many with chronic diseases, the need for ventilator support is lifelong. The need for ventilator assistance can be continuous or intermittent, with some patients requiring only night-time ventilation.

Ventilator-dependent children can be cared for in an acute care facility, extended care/rehabilitation facility, or at home. When the family is able, the best alternative is home care, but several obstacles may prevent a family from taking their

child home. It is well known that home care enhances psychosocial development and decreases respiratory infections and is cost-effective.[86] Improvements in technology have enabled these children to be discharged to their families while still requiring specialized care, but the availability and competence of home-care providers have not kept pace with the increasing need for skilled home care. As a result, home care is often suboptimal, costly, and not easily accessible, and this is a cause of major concern for families with children on ventilator support.

Lack of support systems and financial assistance are also crucial factors in deterring a family from home care for their ventilator-dependent child. Financial reimbursement of home care is dismal. Although it can be more cost effective, it often costs the *family* more to take a child home than to keep him/her in the hospital. Medicaid benefits may pay for hospital care, but will limit support if the child goes home.

The discharge planning team should help the family investigate alternate funding resources. Besides setting up nursing and respiratory services, help is often needed in rearranging the home environment to accommodate for equipment and supplies. Properly grounded electrical outlets and availability of manual ventilation and when appropriate a second ventilator unit allow for increased mobility of the child throughout the home. The local telephone and electric companies, as well as the fire and rescue services, should be notified of the child's dependence on life-support. Realistic goals should be defined for the child and the family and the team should work closely and professional services should be readily available to the family around the clock. After a period of time the family gains confidence in taking care of their child, requiring less support from the medical staff. This independence should be respected, as the family is already dealing with significant invasion of privacy and the enormous time commitment required in handling the care of their child. Once comfortable and stable at home, the family should be encouraged to embark on outings and trips with the backup support of the nursing and medical staff. Gilgoff and Helgren have shown that such outings can be safely carried out as long as they are well planned.[87] Figures 53-2 to 53-4 show a child with spinal muscular atrophy participating in routine activities at home, including working with a special computer and also taking a dip in the backyard swimming pool! Active participation in community and family activities is necessary for obtaining a high quality of life. It should be recognized that the family is undertaking a great responsibility, their only return being the joy of having their child in their midst. Every effort must be made in maintaining the family integrity and providing support when needed.

Discussions of ethical issues are equally important. These are difficult issues in pediatrics, as most often the child involved has little input into the decision. It is enormously difficult for a parent to opt for withdrawal or withholding of support. Feelings of guilt and failure to be realistic are usually the reasons for requesting ongoing support. It is often difficult to delineate quality of life of the child and that of the parents. While the parent may have great satisfaction and joy from having the child at home, it may only be prolonging life and suffering of the child. The medical team has an immense responsibility in helping the family make appropriate decisions. In controversial cases, ethics committees usually defer to the parents' wishes.

Conclusions

With improved outcome and survival, the socioeconomic burden of caring for children with chronic disabilities has increased. Great strides have been made in the field of pediatric rehabilitative medicine, but we have a long way to go. Organized programs and protocols need to be developed and financial and reimbursement issues need to be addressed. Specialized schools and day-care centers and skilled caregivers are urgently needed in optimizing the care for these medically fragile children. The society as a whole bears a tremendous responsibility for integrating these children into the community and improving their quality of life.

References

1. Hodgkin J, Farrell M, Gibson S, et al: Pulmonary rehabilitation, Official ATS statement. *Am Rev Respir Dis* 124:663–666, 1981.
2. Lenney W: The burden of pediatric asthma. *Pediatr Pulmonol* Suppl 15:13–16, 1997.
3. Juniper EF: How important is quality of life in asthma? *Pediatr Pulmonol* Suppl 15:17–21, 1997.
4. Juniper EF, Guyatt GH, Feeny DH, et al: Measuring quality of life in children with asthma. *Qual Life Res* 5:35–46, 1996.
5. Juniper EF, Guyatt GH, Feeny DH, et al: Measuring quality of life in the parents of children with asthma. *Qual Life Res* 5:27–34, 1996.
6. Speight AN, Lee DA, Hey EN: Underdiagnosis and undertreatment of asthma in childhood. *Br Med J* 286:1253–1256, 1983.
7. Anderson HR, Bailey PA, Cooper JS, et al: Morbidity and school absence caused by asthma and wheezing illness. *Arch Dis Child* 58:777–784, 1983.
8. Godden DJ, Ross S, Abdalla M, et al: Outcome of wheeze in childhood. *Am J Respir Crit Care Med* 149:106–112, 1994.
9. Kelly WJ, Hudson I, Raven J, et al: Childhood asthma and adult lung function. *Am Rev Respir Dis* 138:26–30, 1988.
10. Backer V, Urik CS: Development of lung function in relation to increased degree of bronchial responsiveness. *J Asthma* 29:331–341, 1992.
11. Sherill D, Sears MR, Lebowitz MD, et al: The effects of airway hyperresponsiveness wheezing and atopy on longitudinal pulmonary function in children: A 6-year follow-up study. *Pediatr Pulmonol* 13:78–85, 1992.
12. Weiss ST, Tosteson TD, Segal MR, et al: Effects of asthma on pulmonary function in children. *Am Rev Respir Dis* 145:58–64, 1992.
13. Gold DR, Wypij D, Wang X, et al: Gender and race-specific effects of asthma and wheeze on level and growth of lung function in children in six US cities. *Am J Respir Crit Care Med* 149:1198–1208, 1994.
14. Martinez FD, Wright AL, Taussig LM, et al: Asthma and wheezing in the first six years of life. *N Engl J Med* 332:133–138, 1995.
15. Agertoft L, Pedersen S: Effects of long-term treatment with an inhaled corticosteroid on growth and pulmonary function in asthmatic children. *Respir Med* 88:373–381, 1994.
16. König P, Shaffer J: The effect of drug therapy on long-term outcome of childhood asthma possible preview of the international guidelines. *J Allergy Clin Immunol* 85:190–194, 1996.
17. Global Initiative for Asthma: *Global strategy for Asthma Management and Prevention. NHLBI/WHO workshop report.* National Institutes of Health Publication No. 95-3659, National Institutes of Health, Bethesda, MD, January 1995.
18. Verberne AAPH, Frost C, Roorda RJ, et al: One year treatment with salmeterol compared with beclomethasone in children with asthma. *Am J Respir Crit Care Med* 156:688–695, 1997.
19. Akhter J, Gaspar MM, Newcomb RW: Persistent peripheral airway obstruction in children with severe asthma. *Ann Allergy* 63:53–58, 1989.
20. Gerritsen J, Koeter GH, Postma DS, et al: Prognosis of asthma from childhood to adulthood. *Am Rev Respir Dis* 140:1325–1330, 1989.
21. Agertoft L, Pederson S: Influence of spacer device on drug delivery to young children with asthma. *Arch Dis Child* 71:217–220, 1993.
22. Gillies J: Overview of delivery system issues in pediatric asthma. *Pediatr Pulmonol* Suppl 15:55–58, 1997.
23. Bar-Or O: *Pediatric Sports Medicine for the Practitioner.* New York, Springer-Verlag, 1983:89.
24. Nixon PA: Role of exercise in the evaluation and management of pulmonary disease in children and youth. *Med Sci Sports Exerc* 28(4):414–420, 1996.
25. Davis PB, Drumm M, Konstan MW: Cystic fibrosis. State of the art. *Am J Respir Crit Care Med* 154:1229–1256, 1996.
26. Cystic Fibrosis Foundation: *Patient Registry 1994 Annual Data Report.* Bethesda, MD, Cystic Fibrosis Foundation, 1995.
27. Drotar D, Doershuk CF, Stern RC, et al: Psychosocial functioning of children with cystic fibrosis. *Pediatrics* 67:338–343, 1981.
28. Blair C, Cull A, Freeman CP: Psychosocial functioning of young adults with cystic fibrosis and their families. *Thorax* 49:798–802, 1994.
29. Shepherd SL, Hovell MF, Harwood IR, et al: A comparative study of the psychosocial assets of adults with cystic fibrosis and their healthy peers. *Chest* 97:1310–1316, 1990.
30. Orenstein DM, Nixon PA, Ross EA, et al: The quality of well being in cystic fibrosis. *Chest* 95:344–347, 1989.
31. Dunlevy CL, Douce FH, Hill E, et al: Physiological and psychological effects of low-impact aerobic exercise on young adults with cystic fibrosis. *J Cardiopulmon Rehabil* 14:47–51, 1994.
32. De Jong W, Kaptein AA, Van der Schans CP, et al: Quality of life in patients with cystic fibrosis. *Pediatr Pulmonol* 23:95–100, 1997.
33. Orenstein DM, Pattishall EN, Nixon PA, et al: Quality of well-being before and after antibiotic treatment of pulmonary exacerbation in patients with cystic fibrosis. *Chest* 98:1081–1084, 1990.
34. Orenstein DM, Franklin BA, Doershuk CF, et al: Exercise conditioning and cardiopulmonary fitness in cystic fibrosis. The effects of a three month supervised running program. *Chest* 80:392–398, 1981.
35. Cropp GJ, Pullano TP, Cerny FJ, et al: Exercise tolerance and cardiorespiratory adjustment at peak work capacity in cystic fibrosis. *Am Rev Respir Dis* 126:211–216, 1982.
36. Henke K, Orenstein D: Oxygen saturation during exercise in cystic fibrosis. *Am Rev Respir Dis* 129:708–711, 1985.
37. Gulmans VAM, Van Veldhoven NHMJ, De Meer K, et al: The six-minute walking test in children with cystic fibrosis: Reliability and validity. *Pediatr Pulmonol* 22:85–89, 1996.
38. Nixon PA, Orenstein DM, Kelsey SF, et al: The prognostic value of exercise testing in patients with cystic fibrosis. *N Engl J Med* 327:1785–1788, 1992.
39. Edlund L, French R, Herbst J, et al: Effects of a swimming program on children with cystic fibrosis. *Am J Dis Child* 140:80–83, 1986.
40. Keens T, Kasten I, Wannmoler E, et al: Ventilatory muscle endurance training in normal subjects and patients with cystic fibrosis. *Am Rev Respir Dis* 116:853–866, 1977.
41. De Jong W, Grevink RG, Roorda RJ, et al: Effect of a home exercise training program in patients with cystic fibrosis. *Chest* 105:463–468, 1994.
42. Delk KK, Gevirtz R, Hicks DA: The effects of biofeedback assisted breathing retraining on lung functions in patients with cystic fibrosis. *Chest* 105:23–28, 1993.
43. Sawyer EH, Clanton TL: Improved pulmonary function and exercise tolerance with inspiratory muscle conditioning in children with cystic fibrosis. *Chest* 104:1490–1497, 1993.
44. Zach MS, Oberwaldner B, Hausler F: Cystic fibrosis: Physical

exercise versus chest physiotherapy. *Arch Dis Child* 57:587–589, 1982.

45. Zach MB, Purrer B, Oberwaldner B: Effect of swimming on forced expiration and sputum clearance in cystic fibrosis. *Lancet* 2:1201–1203, 1981.

46. Nixon PA, Orenstein DM, Curtis SE, et al: Oxygen supplementation during exercise in cystic fibrosis. *Am Rev Respir Dis* 142:807–811, 1990.

47. Partridge C, Pryor J, Webber B: Characteristics of the forced expiratory technique. *Physiotherapy* 75:193–194, 1989.

48. Kluft J, Beker L, Castagnino M, et al: A comparison of bronchial drainage treatments in cystic fibrosis. *Pediatr Pulmonol* 22:271–274, 1996.

49. Warwick WJ, Hansen LG: The long-term effect of high-frequency chest compression therapy on pulmonary complications of cystic fibrosis. *Pediatr Pulmonol* 11:265–271, 1991.

50. King M, Phillips DM, Zidulka A, et al: Tracheal mucus clearance in high-frequency oscillation II: Chest wall versus mouth oscillation. *Am Rev Respir Dis* 130:703–706, 1984.

51. Konstan MW, Stern RC, Doershuk CF: Efficacy of the Flutter device for airway mucus clearance in patients with cystic fibrosis. *J Pediatr* 124:689–693, 1994.

52. Thomas J, Cook DJ, Brooks D: Chest physical therapy management of patients with cystic fibrosis: A meta-analysis. *Am J Respir Crit Care Med* 151:846–850, 1995.

53. Pencharz P, Durie P: Nutritional management of cystic fibrosis. *Ann Rev Nutr* 13:131–136, 1993.

54. Zemel BS, Jawad A, Stallings VA: Longitudinal patterns of growth and pulmonary function in 6- to 8-year-old children with cystic fibrosis from the cystic fibrosis foundation patient registry. *Pediatr Pulmonol* Suppl 13:102–103, 1996.

55. Corey M, McLaughlin FJ, Williams M, et al: A comparison of survival, growth and pulmonary function in patients with cystic fibrosis in Boston and Toronto. *J Clin Epidemiol* 41:586–591, 1988.

56. Smyth RL, Van Velzen D, Smyth AR, et al: Strictures of ascending colon in cystic fibrosis and high-strength pancreatic enzymes. *Lancet* 343:85–86, 1994.

57. Bell SC, Saunders MC, Elborn JS, et al: Resting energy expenditure and oxygen cost of respiration in patients with cystic fibrosis. *Thorax* 51:126–130, 1995.

58. Ramsey B, Farrell P, Pencharz P, et al: Nutritional assessment and management in cystic fibrosis: A consensus report. *Am J Clin Nutr* 55:108–116, 1992.

59. Calvi AM, Anthony M, Helton J, et al: Psychosocial issues in families of infants with cystic fibrosis identified through newborn screening: The early years. *Pediatr Pulmonol* Suppl 13:148–149, 1996.

60. Quittner AL, Opipari LC, Regoli MJ, et al: The impact of caregiving and role strain on family life: Comparisons between mothers of children with cystic fibrosis and matched controls. *Rehabil Psych* 37:289–304, 1992.

61. Thompson RJ, Gustafson KE, Spock A: Adaptation to chronic illness: Adolescents and their parents. *Pediatr Pulmonol* Suppl 13:152–153, 1996.

62. Gilgoff IS, Barras DM, Jones MS, et al: Neck breathing: A form of voluntary respiration for the spine-injured ventilator-dependent quadriplegic child. *Pediatrics* 82:741–745, 1988.

63. Raphael JC, Chevret S, Chastang CI, et al: Randomized trial of preventive nasal ventilation in Duchenne muscular dystrophy. *Lancet* 343:1600–1604, 1994.

64. Kitchen W, Doyle L, Ford G, et al: Changing two-year outcome of infants weighing 500–999 grams at birth: A hospital study. *J Pediatr* 118:938–943, 1991.

65. McCormick M: Long-term follow-up of infants discharged from neonatal intensive care units. *JAMA* 261:1767–1772, 1989.

66. US Congress, Office of Technology Assessment: *Neonatal Intensive Care for Low Birth Weight Infants: Costs and Effectiveness.* Publication No. OTA-HCS.38. Washington, DC: Office of Technology Assessment, 1987.

67. Hack M, Horbar J, Malloy M, et al: Very low birth weight outcomes of the National Institutes of Child Health and Human Development Neonatal Network. *Pediatrics* 87:587–596, 1991.

68. Northway WH, Rosan RC, Porter DY: Pulmonary disease following respiratory therapy of hyaline membrane disease: Bronchopulmonary dysplasia. *N Engl J Med* 276:357–368, 1967.

69. Avery ME, Tooley WH, Keller JB, et al: Is chronic lung disease in low birth weight infants preventable? A survey of eight centers. *Pediatrics* 79:26–30, 1987.

70. Teberg AJ, Pena I, Finello K, et al: Prediction of neurodevelopmental outcome on infants with and without bronchopulmonary dysplasia. *Am J Med Sci* 301:369–374, 1991.

71. Donn S: Cost effectiveness of home management of bronchopulmonary dysplasia. *Pediatrics* 70:330–331, 1982.

72. Rosen C, Glaze D, Fost J: Home monitor follow-up of persistent apnea and bradycardia in preterm infants. *Am J Dis Child* 140:547–550, 1986.

73. Black L, Hersher L, Steinschneider A: Impact of the apnea monitor on family life. *Pediatrics* 62:681–685, 1978.

74. Cain L, Kelly D, Shannon D: Parents perceptions of the psychological and social impact of home monitoring. *Pediatrics* 66:37–41, 1980.

75. Newton L, Chambers H, Ruben R, et al: Home care of the pediatric patient with a tracheostomy. *Ann Otol Rhinol Laryngol* 91:633–640, 1982.

76. Aradine CR: Home care for young children with long-term tracheostomies. *Am J Matern Child Nurs* 5:121–125, 1980.

77. Wills J: Concerns and needs of mothers providing home care for children with tracheostomies. *Matern Child Nurs J* 12:89–108, 1983.

78. Passy V, Baydur A, Prentice W, et al: Passy-Muir® tracheostomy speaking valve on ventilator-dependent patients. *Laryngoscope* 103:653–658, 1993.

79. Dougherty JM, Parrish JM, Hock-Long L: Developing a competency-based curriculum for tracheostomy and ventilator care. *Pediatr Nurs* 21(6):581–584, 1995.

80. Hall SS, Weatherly KS: Using sign language with tracheotomized infants and children. *Pediatr Nurs* 15(4):362–367, 1989.

81. Hazinski MF: Pediatric home tracheostomy care: A parents guide. *Pediatr Nurs* 12:41–69, 1986.

82. Whitford KM: Health care needs of ventilator-dependent children. *Pediatr Nurs* 14:216–219, 1988.

83. Laraya-Cuasay L, Mikkilineni S: Respiratory conditions and care, in Rosenthal S, Sheppard JJ, Lotze M (eds): *Dysphagia and the Child with Developmental Disabilities,* San Diego, CA, Singular Publishing Group, 1995:227.

84. Schreiner MS, Donar ME, Kettrick RG: Pediatric home mechanical ventilation. *Pediatr Clin North Am* 34(1):47–60, 1987.

85. Office of Technology Assessment (1988): *Technology Dependent Children: Hospital versus Home Care* (OTA-M-H-38). Washington, DC: US Government Printing Office.

86. Stutts A: Selected outcomes of technology dependent children receiving home care and prescribed child care services. *Pediatr Nurs* 20(5):501–507, 1994.

87. Gilgoff IS, Helgren J: Planning an outing from hospital for ventilator-dependent children. *Development Med Child Neurol* 34:904–910, 1992.

Chapter 54

SMOKING CESSATION IN THE ELDERLY AND IN PATIENTS WITH RESPIRATORY DISEASE

E. PAUL CHERNIACK

The enormity of the morbidity and mortality from cigarette smoking as documented by a vast array of statistics, including 3 million deaths per year in the world, half of which occur in the elderly above 70,[1,2] and that deaths from smoking are the largest single category of preventable deaths in the United States impel the increasing interest in smoking cessation. While the mortality from smoking, although still substantial, has declined in the most developed countries among men, it continues rise in the developing countries and in women worldwide.[3] Many patients requiring pulmonary rehabilitation are elderly, particularly those with chronic respiratory diseases. To understand the desirability and feasibility of smoking cessation in the elderly and patients with respiratory disease, it is important to elucidate the characteristics of these populations of smokers.

The Aged Smoker

Smoking is less prevalent among the elderly than in younger individuals. According to one study 10 years ago, while 30.9 percent of those aged 45 to 64 are smokers, only 19 percent of those aged 65 to 74 smoked, and only 8.9 percent of people over 75 used tobacco products.[4–6] There are many possible explanations for this decline. Younger smokers may have increased mortality, leaving more nonsmokers alive at older ages.[7,8] Older smokers who survive may have more medical problems inducing them to stop. Half of all smokers are successful at spontaneously quitting over a lifetime, especially after multiple attempts,[8,9] and more of the elderly may have over their lifetimes been successfully able to quit.

For a number of reasons, getting the aged smoker to quit may be more difficult. The older nicotine-dependent person has a greater use and addiction to nicotine.[4,10–14] According to one survey, two-thirds smoke less than half an hour after waking and use more than 20 cigarettes a day, and a little more than one-third use cigarettes with a relatively high nicotine content.[4] The aged often are surrounded by others who smoke; 57 percent indicated that they had a smoking spouse, and 19.2 percent felt that most of those they socialize with also used tobacco.[4] Elderly smokers have beliefs about their health and smoking that impede their ability to quit. No more than one-third felt confident that they could quit, 47 percent did not accept that smoking would result in better health, and 45 percent stated that continuing to smoke would

In memory of Mr. Sam Aptman

not harm them.[4] Aged tobacco consumers are more socially isolated, precluding positive reinforcement that might aid in quitting, and are more "fatalistic," implying that they are more addicted, and more concerned with the development of potential withdrawal symptoms including craving, insomnia, anorexia, anxiety, anhedonia, weight gain, boredom, and inability to concentrate.[4,15] The sedentary lifestyles of many elderly may make certain withdrawal symptoms more likely, such as weight gain, anhedonia, and boredom.[10] They visit physicians less frequently and are less likely to participate in preventive health efforts, meaning they will be less likely to be offered assistance in quitting and be less likely to accept it.[10] A mere 39 percent had been offered physician assistance in cessation in one survey.[10] Sensory and cognitive dysfunction in the elderly may impair cessation efforts.[10]

Despite the barriers to cessation in the elderly, those who do quit still derive much benefit. There are clearly greater increased risks to continued smoking in the elderly. In an epidemiologic study of 35,000 physicians in England, the 70-year-old smoker who quit was twice as likely to live to age 85 as a smoker who did not (41 versus 21 percent).[16,17] A project in which 13,000 retired individuals were followed for almost 10 years revealed statistically significant greater mortality in current smokers for deaths from all causes, deaths from coronary heart disease, deaths from cerebrovascular disease, and smoking-induced cancers. These risks increased with the amount smoked, and decreased in former smokers with the time since quitting.[18]

While calculations of percent of population surviving at a given age do not show a much higher percentage survival among people quitting smoking at age 65 or above than that of smokers, there is evidence to suggest the reduction of the absolute number of deaths among quitters remains even into the eighth decade of life.[16,19]

Decreases in mortality and morbidity occur in the elderly for many disorders exacerbated by smoking. Those who quit after 65 can still expect a reduction in the increased risk of cardiovascular disease caused by smoking, probably related to less atherosclerosis in the former smoker.[16,20–23] Reduction in risk of stroke has been shown in quitters in studies not restricted to the elderly alone.[16,24,25] In research not limited to the elderly, mortality from peripheral vascular disease, amputations, decreased pain,[16,26–29] and increased graft survival,[16,29,30] improved ability to exercise,[16,31] and enhanced arterial pressures[16,31] were noted in the older individuals. The incidence of pulmonary neoplasms in the elderly can be cut through smoking cessation to a larger degree than in the young, as the elderly have more neoplasms.[16,32,33] A "younger" aged individual (60 to 64 years) was found in one study to cut in half the chance that he might develop lung cancer if he stayed abstinent for 10 to 15 years.[16,34] The individual over 60 who stops tobacco intake will still experience a loss in forced expiratory volume in 1 s (FEV_1) at a rate comparable to nonsmokers, but not as great a loss as that experienced by smokers.[16,35,36]

Smokers with Pulmonary Disease

While most workers in pulmonary rehabilitation list smoking cessation as an essential component of any program, the characteristics and motivations of the smoker with pulmonary disease have not been well defined. Individuals with heart and lung diseases are less likely to smoke than healthy individuals.[37–39] Dudley and coworkers found that a scale of psychosocial variables could significantly predict who would smoke among a chest clinic population, although there was not much difference between smokers and quitters.[37,39] Daughton and colleagues, in a group of 107 patients (mean age in the 50s) entering a pulmonary rehabilitation program, found that a scale of "psychosocial assets" predicted those who still smoked, but the accuracy of classification was only 63 percent.[37] Pederson and associates noted that 74 percent of the middle-aged smokers admitted to a pulmonary ward of a teaching hospital and entering a smoking cessation program had previously tried to quit.[40] The reasons patients gave for continued smoking were relaxation (35.2 percent), enjoyment (32.4 percent), habit (19.7 percent), and avoidance of withdrawal (12.7 percent).[40]

Smokers with COPD who quit experience less cough, sputum, and dyspnea, but do not decrease their forced expiratory volume in 1 s (FEV_1).[41–43] The Lung Health Study, which studied smokers with abnormalities in pulmonary function but who were not yet symptomatic (to be discussed in more detail later), showed improvement in FEV_1 after the first year for quitters, followed by a sightly smaller decrease in FEV_1 in exsmokers, than would be observed in nonsmokers.[44]

Nicotine Addiction

Addiction to nicotine is believed to be a manifestation of the binding of the drug to cholinergic receptors, most importantly the acetylcholine receptors of the brain, particularly in the thalamus, cortex, interpeduncular nucleus, amygdala, septum, and brain stem motor nuclei.[45,46] There may also be an effect on the afferent nerves of the carotid body chemoreceptors,[47–49] and there is stimulation of receptor sites on the spinal cord, adrenal medulla, and autonomic ganglion.[47]

Nicotine is extremely rapidly acting and accumulates in the blood rapidly, crossing into the brain from 7 to 19 s.[47,49] While blood levels quickly fall,[49] nicotine stores in the body can prolong the terminal half-life to at least 20 h.[47] Processing of the drug occurs in the liver, where 70 to 80 percent is converted to cotinine, the rate-limiting step in nicotine metabolism, and cotinine plasma levels are used as one method of assessing tobacco use.[48] Further metabolism results in urinary excretion.[48]

Smokers continue using nicotine for reasons of both positive and negative reinforcement.[45] Users obtain stress relief, relaxation, alertness, greater attention, increased reaction time, increased visual processing, and weight loss.[45,49–51] Performance on monotonous tasks is especially enhanced.[50,51] They also avoid manifestations of withdrawal which include hunger, loss of concentration, increase in weight, anxiety, and irritability.[45]

There is no data on aging effects on the distribution of nicotine after inhalation, or the manifestations of nicotine addiction or withdrawal. Theoretically, the volume of distribution could increase as the mass of the aged individual decreases, which might enhance the absorption of rapidly acting nicotine replacement products, for instance, nicotine spray and gum, but not alter nicotine absorption from slower acting replacement products, for instance, the nicotine patch.[16] Aged individuals have been shown to have the same blood levels of nicotine and cotinine during nicotine patch use.[16]

The Process of Smoking Cessation

The attitude smokers have toward quitting has been characterized into five stages by a model known as the Transtheoretical Model.[52–55] Individuals are considered to be in the precontemplation phase if they have no interest in quitting, the contemplation phase if they are considering stopping in the next 6 months, the preparation phase if they are preparing to quit in the next month, the action phase if they have quit for less than 6 months, and the maintenance phase if they have quit for more than 6 months. A recent survey polling smokers interviewed from different parts of the country showed approximately 40 percent of tobacco users in the precontemplation or contemplation stages, and 20 percent in the preparation stage, but there was a larger variation in stage in smokers who were older than 65 in different survey sites than there was in younger smokers.[52] The Transtheoretical model encompasses the continual changes in behavior a smoker undergoes, although it does not take into account the social and environmental influences on a smoker's behavior.[56]

Many smokers who quit on their own have relapses after 6 months of abstinence. In turn, they may make further attempts to quit. One survey of 630 smokers found a continuous abstinence rate of only 8 percent after 6 months of abstinence and 23 percent of those who did quit for a long time actually smoked a few cigarettes at some point during their "abstinence."[57] After multiple attempts 50 percent cease smoking.[58,59]

The Interpretation of Smoking Cessation Studies

Understanding of how efficacious are smoking cessation methods in an aged or respiratory-impaired smoker is complicated by the array of methods used to define whether or not a method is a success. Three commonly used methods include point prevalence, continuous (sustained), and prolonged abstinence.[60,61]

Point prevalence refers to percentage of smokers who have quit at some given point after the intervention. This period can vary among studies; the National Interagency Council on Smoking more than 20 years ago recommended at least 7 days.[60] If the period is 7 days or less, it can be verified biochemically, by methods which will be discussed later. If the period is months later, it can include smokers who relapsed after the intervention, but ultimately did quit.[60] However, since point prevalence only measures a small period of time during which a smoker stopped, there is always the possibility (which is greater for smaller intervals after the intervention at which the prevalence is measured) that a subject might resume smoking, and, in fact, be a treatment failure.[60,61] Since the point prevalence rate is very dependent on the length of time used between measurements, it is more variable over time and between studies.[60] Finally, it is less useful when measuring the potential health benefits of quitting if the period is relatively short.[60]

Continuous or sustained abstinence is the percentage of smokers who have completely stopped smoking for a given period of time. A number of studies have indicated that the longer exsmokers maintain abstinence, the more likely they are to never smoke again, and so a long period of sustained abstinence comes closer to indicating a definitive treatment for nicotine dependence.[60,62,63] This measure is more likely to be stable or comparable among studies, and it is easier to assess health benefits acquired by quitting through the use of sustained abstinence.[60] The disadvantages to the use of this measure is (1) that smokers often go through relapses until they ultimately quit; (2) since smokers will relapse, the percentage can only decrease over time as more relapses occur; and (3) it is more difficult to verify objectively, since the longest potential biochemical verification period is 1 week, and it is harder to follow a smoker continuously for longer time intervals.

Prolonged abstinence represents the sum of both continuous and point prevalence over longer periods of time, such as for months to years. It more stable and comparable between studies, accounts for relapses in quitters, can be used to study health effects, but is difficult to objectively verify.[61] Smokers have a high probability of relapse during the first 6 months.[60,64] Those who quit for a year have only a 5 percent relapse rate in the following year, but 37 percent will relapse at some later time.[60,65] After 5 years, the chance of relapse is minimal.[7,60]

There are a number of biochemical markers for verifying smoking cessation. Carbon monoxide, which has a half-life of 4 to 5 h, can be measured easily in expired gas, and has a specificity of 84 to 98 percent and has a sensitivity of 80 to 85 percent, which can be increased by the smoker's report of time since the last cigarette.[60,66–68] The time of day (late day measurements are more accurate), time since last cigarette, amount of environmental carbon monoxide present, and lactose intolerance affect specificity.[60,69,70] False negatives have been reported in 2 to 16 percent.[60,71–75]

The prime metabolite of nicotine by the liver, cotinine, has also been used for smoking verification. It can be assayed in the saliva, urine, or plasma, although the urine levels are not regarded as stable.[60,76,77] Test sensitivity is greater than 90 percent and specificity is 98 percent.[60] Cotinine has a half-life of between 15 to 40 h, and can detect light, occasional smoking, and smokeless tobacco.[60,78–81]

A less frequently used marker for tobacco is thiocyanate, a metabolite of hydrogen cyanide gas produced by cigarette smoke.[60] Although it has a half-life of 10 to 14 days, its low sensitivity and specificity are a major problem, since it is present in many vegetable products and beer.[60,82–84]

Smoking has also been assessed by subject or observer report. One of the most basic methods has been a count of cigarettes smoked. While it may be subject to inaccuracy because of differences within types of cigarettes, methods of smoking among subjects, and the way in which given cigarettes are inhaled, it is often the measure of choice.[60]

Questionnaires have been frequently used to determine the severity of nicotine addiction, motivations for smoking or cessation, and symptoms of withdrawal. These often vary between studies, and there has been little published analysis of the relative merits of different questionnaires used in smoking cessation studies. One of the most commonly used is the Fagerstrom Tolerance Questionnaire, an eight-question,

eleven-point survey (11, maximum nicotine dependence), which has been shown in some studies to correlate with carbon monoxide, nicotine, and cotinine levels, and more dependent subjects were shown to benefit from the use of nicotine gum, one of the methods of smoking cessation which will be discussed later.[83] Another questionnaire, the Horne-Russell scale, was used to ascertain which subjects benefited from a given dose of nicotine gum.[85,86] Smokers appear more likely to give reliable information to an investigator when there is a good relationship between investigator and subject. The accuracy of information retrieved through a face-to-face interview appears to be 98 to 99 percent.[61,87] The reliability of questionnaires administered by mail or phone can be as low as 26 percent.[61,88]

Another important consideration in the proper interpretation of smoking cessation is the use of appropriate placebo controls in studies of nicotine replacement devices. The ability of a subject to perceive differences between a treatment and a placebo creates expectations that interfere with the ability of a study to detect treatment effects.[89] If the placebo contains no nicotine, the subject using it may be able to guess this because he or she will miss the usual physiologic or psychological effects of the drug (such as tachycardia). Subjects who receive the usual positive reinforcing effects from nicotine substitution might correctly guess that they are receiving replacement and might deliberately smoke less and avoid a feared overdose.

Finally, many studies purporting to demonstrate the efficacy of primarily one intervention actually include several different methods of secondary intervention. In many studies of nicotine replacement, subjects may have been advised to quit by a health professional (which as we will also see later, will cause a small but significant number of smokers to quit) and have also been given self-help manuals and/or received counseling sessions. Descriptions of patient characteristics in the methods sections of most published reports do not indicate what other cessation methods subjects have been exposed to in the past, nor how recently they may have been exposed to other methods before starting a given trial, which theoretically might influence their propensity to quit in future. When a quit rate is given for an intervention, it is difficult, therefore, to know whether the primary or secondary components of the intervention were actually responsible for cessation. Interpreting the results of meta-analyses may be complicated by the variation in secondary interventions used in individual studies, and the way in which reviewers handled secondary interventions.

Methods of Smoking Cessation Which Are Potentially Useful in Respiratory Patients

The purpose of this section is to provide brief overview of potentially important methods of smoking cessation and their efficacies that have been investigated or might in future be investigated specifically either in the elderly or in respiratory patients. In fact, many of these methods, for example, nicotine patch/spray, have not been specifically studied in respiratory patients, although there is at least evidence that many of these methods do or might prove useful, when we are not yet really sure that they are.

ADVICE TO QUIT

One of the simplest methods of smoking cessation and one that has been shown to be effective, albeit in a small number of cases, is practitioner advice to quit. Two meta-analyses of studies have shown that this is an effective method, and the Agency for Health Care Policy and Research (AHCPR) of the U.S. Department of Health and Human Services and the National Cancer Institute advocate its implementation.[58,90,91] Advice alone has been shown to increase quit rates from 2 to 10 percent.[58,61,92–94] Advice to quit increases the odds ratio for quitting by 1.3 (1.1 to 1.6, 95 percent confidence intervals) and the advice is effective whether offered by a physician or another health professional.[91] The AHCPR recommends that all smokers be urged to quit in a "clear, strong, personalized" message.[91]

SELF-HELP MANUALS

The efficacy of self-help manuals is less clear. A meta-analysis by Law and Tang found an overall efficacy rate of 1.8 percent[93] and another by Viswesvaran assessed a rate of 15 percent.[94] The odds ratio for increased probability of cessation resulting from the use of such manuals is 1.2 (1.0 to 1.6, 95 percent confidence indexes).[91] Curry, in a review of self-help studies, noted an initial cessation rate of 4 to 44 percent and a long-term abstinence rate of from 2 to 38 percent.[95] There appears no great advantage to one type of manual over another.[95] The particular benefits of the self-help approach is that most smokers prefer them and at least one study found them cost-effective.[96]

BEHAVIORAL THERAPIES

Behavioral therapies are usually administered by mental health professionals and try to alter the learned behavior that contributes to the continuation of smoking.[58] Often interventions have offered trials of combinations of methods.[58] One such therapy is skills training or relapse prevention, which involves predicting situations in which one is likely to smoke.[58] The AHCPR meta-analysis gives a cessation rate for this therapy of 13.7 percent and a cessation odds ratio of 1.6 (95 percent confidence index of 1.2 to 2.2).[91] This method is also recommended in American Psychiatric Association practice guidelines.[58] Stimulus control involves the identification of stimuli which smokers believe induce them to smoke before a quit attempt and trying to avoid these stimuli.[58] Patients remove cigarettes and smoking paraphernalia, shun others who smoke, and distance themselves from situations they feel are likely to cause them to start.[58] Sachs, in his review of smoking cessation methods assigns a cessation rate for a combination of stimulus control and other behavioral techniques at 33 percent, although he admits that the studies do not include objective verification of quitting.[61]

Aversive therapies, such as rapid smoking, attempt to prevent smoking by guiding individuals to smoke in such quantities that they sense the undesirable side effects of nicotine.[58] Viswesvaran, in his meta-analysis, reports a cessation rate of 29 percent.[94] The AHCPR meta-analysis gives a quit rate of 17.5 percent, with an odds ratio for cessation over baseline of 2.1 (95 percent confidence interval, 1.04 to 4.2). The two main drawbacks to these methods are patient compliance and safety,[58] considerations which should be important in the elderly and patients with pulmonary disease. Other behavioral techniques deemed less effective include contingency management (rewarding or punishing smokers for their actions),[58,97–99] cue exposure (creating scenarios in which individuals develop strong desires to smoke and analyzing these),[58,100–103] nicotine fading (gradually decreasing the amount of nicotine used),[58,97,98,104,105] and physiologic feedback.[58,60,93]

NICOTINE REPLACEMENT THERAPIES

NICOTINE GUM

Although ingested nicotine is readily metabolized by the liver, nicotine gum allows buccal absorption with a peak after 30 min.[47,58] A number of meta-analyses, such as those of Lam and coworkers[106] did not find much efficacy in the gum, but others have found a small but statistically greater increase in quit rate of from 3 to 16 percent in smokers using nicotine gum over placebo gum, and an odds ratio of quitting using gum of 1.4 to 1.6.[58,91,93,94,107,108] However, reviews of studies in which the use of gum has been combined with other therapies, such as behavioral therapies, have shown an increase in cessation rates of 20 to 30 percent.[61,108–111] Nicotine supplied in a 4-mg nicotine polacrilex gum appears to be more efficacious than the 2-mg nicotine gum, especially in heavy smokers.[61,86] Nicotine gum may be a more problematic option in the elderly, as it can stick to dentures, require a great deal of chewing to reach optimal levels of nicotine, and require good cognition and motor skills to employ the proper chewing technique.[16]

NICOTINE PATCHES

Transdermal nicotine patches supply nicotine gradually, reaching a maximum dose after 6 to 10 h.[58] The starting dose depends on how many cigarettes smoked a day. Treatment continues over a month, and the dose is tapered over the next month.[91] Smokers who quit during the first 2 weeks in one study tended to remain abstinent during the entire 8 weeks.[112] The patch has been shown to be effective in numerous meta-analyses, with a 22 percent 6-month cessation rate (placebo, 9 percent and an odds ratio of 2.1 to 3.0.[91,112–114] Russell and coworkers, in heavy smokers (more than 31 cigarettes a day), found greater success with 44-mg patches (twice the normal initial starting dose).[115] Jorenby and associates observed a greater 1-month cessation quit rate, but also more frequent and severe side effects with the 44-mg patch.[116] Yudkin and colleagues found the patch to be more effective in young (ages 20 to 49) than in middle-aged to older patients (ages 50 to 69), but this was because the placebo group in the latter population was almost three times as likely to quit as in the former. All smokers were given a self-help manual.[117] The authors also noted that smokers who smoked between 20 to 29 cigarettes a day were more likely to be helped than those who smoked more or fewer cigarettes.[117] On the other hand, Paoletti and coworkers, who had a much smaller sample size (297 versus 1686 in the Yudkin study) and did not mention secondary interventions, found that subjects with lower baseline cotinine levels had a greater rate of cessation.[118]

OTHER THERAPIES

Fewer studies have been performed using other replacement methods, such as the nicotine spray, which was approved by the FDA in 1996, in which nicotine is absorbed from a nasal spray.[58,119] Several studies have reported benefit,[58,91,119–122] but the nasal spray is often irritating to the nose, and causes symptoms of rhinorrhea.[122] Nicotine inhalers (nicotine embedded in a plastic rod and inhaled as a vapor) produced a 28 percent cessation rate after 6 weeks (versus 12 percent placebo) and a 15 percent cessation rate (versus 5 percent placebo) after 1 year.[58,123] Other medications that have been reported to have some success in trials in recent years include clonidine (which has been shown in some studies to have greater effect in women),[58,124] citric acid inhalers,[125,126] capsaicin-enhanced cigarettes,[127] moclobemide,[128] and low-nicotine regenerated smoke aerosol.[129] Black pepper vapor[130] and smoking without nicotine[131] have been used to decrease withdrawal symptoms, and, in one study, exercise was used in women in a very small study to maintain abstinence.[132]

Studies in the Elderly

While many of the studies establishing the efficacy of smoking cessation programs included some "younger" elderly in their 60s, very few, and even fewer methodologically rigorous studies, have specifically examined methods to quit in the elderly or have explored the influence of age on a particular method or regimen. A number of large-scale trials that attempted to reduce the incidence of coronary artery disease by modifying risk factors, such as the Multiple Risk Factor Intervention Trial (MRFIT) and the Oslo Coronary Risk Reduction Trial, included a number of the smoking cessation interventions previously mentioned, but these trials were generally confined to middle-aged subjects.[61,133–136]

Several studies have used physician advice, telephone counseling, self-help guides, behavioral techniques, and nicotine replacement to help the elderly to quit. Vetter and Ford utilized practitioner advice to increase quit rates.[137] Approximately 400 elderly English smokers between 60 and 100 years old in a general practice who had been identified by a questionnaire mailed to them were divided into a control group and an intervention group. The latter group were urged by a physician in person to stop smoking and offered the services of a nurse who could be contacted to provide advice.[137] There is no mention of how the control group was treated. Six months later, a questionnaire was again sent to the individuals, and they were asked to undergo breath CO analysis.[137] There was no statistically significant difference in abstinence rates between the groups.[137]

The studies of Rimer and Orleans explored the use of self-help guides and telephone counseling. Rimer and coworkers divided approximately 1800 subjects into three groups: a group who received a standard self-help guide, a group who were given a guide specifically designed for the elderly called *Clear Horizons,* which also advised on the use of nicotine gum and some behavioral techniques, and a third group which received the *Clear Horizons* guide and two 10- to 15-min phone calls after 4 to 8 weeks, and again at 16 to 20 weeks after obtaining the guide.[138] Results, extracted from telephone interviews of the approximately 1500 subjects who the investigators were able to follow at 3 months indicated that 12 percent of those receiving the guide and counseling quit, while only 9 and 7 percent respectively of those receiving the *Clear Horizons* guide and the standard guide quit (p =

.006, if all nonrespondents were considered smokers, the numbers would be 10, 7, and 6 percent).[138] The authors state that "telephone counseling increased adherence to quitting plans and boosted quit rates by 50% among smokers in a large HMO"[138] but the article they cite as a reference includes no such data.[15]

Hill and associates attempted an intervention of behavioral therapy including information and education, setting a quit date and relapse prevention training.[139] Although the regimen was described as intended to show benefit for the "older" smoker, the average age of the participants was only 59.4 years. Eighty-two subjects were allocated to receive behavioral therapy for 12 90-min sessions over 3 months either alone, together with nicotine gum, or together with a physical exercise program.[139] Control subjects received only the exercise.[139] One year after the study was started, subjects in the behavioral therapy programs had cessation rates from 27.8 to 31.8 percent, whereas those who received exercise alone had an abstinence rate of 10 percent (p < .05 if the three different behavioral interventions are pooled versus exercise).[139]

Morgan and colleagues randomized 659 patients in primary care practices aged 50 to 75, mean age approximately 60, to "usual care" or one intervention group which received advice to stop smoking, the *Clear Horizons* guide, and possibly nicotine gum.[140] Approximately 60 percent of the interventional subjects received the gum, although it is not clearly stated what criteria were used to decide who obtained nicotine replacement.[140] Patient data was collected by telephone survey at 2 and 4 weeks and 6 months, and there was no objective verification of abstinence.[141] After 6 months, 15.41 percent of the intervention group and 8.16 percent of the group received usual care (p < .005).[140]

Orleans and coworkers did a telephone survey of the use of the nicotine patch by 1070 smokers aged 65 to 74, 6 months after they had filled prescriptions for nicotine patch.[141] In approximately 60 percent, it was the patient rather than the physician who suggested the use of the patch, and only 54 percent had received any advice on how to use them.[141] Forty-seven percent smoked at least once while using the patch (which patients should not do), but nevertheless, 29 percent still ultimately quit.[141]

Based on efficacy rates obtained from meta-analysis of studies using primarily but not exclusively smokers, the patch may be relatively cost-effective.[142] Costs for "younger" elderly, ages 60 to 69, were less than those predicted to be incurred from asymptomatic screening for hypertension at age 60.[142]

Transdermal nicotine has been found to be safe in patients with a history of cardiac disease, including some elderly patients.[143] In a survey of 584 outpatients mean age approximately 60 (range 45 to 82) who used the patch or a placebo for 10 weeks, there were no significant differences in cardiac deaths or admissions.[143]

However, while the 14-week cessation rate of those who wore the patch was significantly higher than for those who wore the placebo (21 versus 9 percent, p = .001), by 6 months the rates lost statistical significance (14 versus 11 percent).[143]

Among the elderly, age (the older the more likely to quit), number of cigarettes (the more cigarettes, the greater likelihood of relapse if the total was below 25 cigarettes a day), and age at quitting (with age over 65 then the greater probability of relapse) predict likelihood of quitting.[144] Depression may increase the probability that elderly women will quit.[145]

Smoking Cessation in Patients with Respiratory Disease

There is surprisingly little research attempting to determine the efficacy of smoking cessation methods in patients with chronic pulmonary disease.[146,147]

Physician advice as a cessation aid was considered in several studies. Raw noted that advice to stop smoking increased quit rates among patients with COPD, and, in interviewing patients who had just seen the pulmonary physician if a psychologist wore a white coat, smoking cessation increased further.[148,149] Williams obtained a 30 to 37 percent cessation rate after physician advice in an English pulmonary clinic.[148,150] When 160 of 372 patients with "respiratory disease" who were told to quit and were followed for 7 years returned a mailed questionnaire, slightly less than a third reported not smoking for the past year before being contacted, and another 5 percent had stopped smoking for less than 1 year.[151]

In an attempt to improve on the success rates afforded by providing physician advice alone, spirometry has been used as a device to motivate smokers to quit.[152–159] This should be especially relevant to individuals who already have pulmonary disease. In order to provide a more compelling incentive to give up nicotine, smokers were shown a comparison between their abnormal spirometry and what would be predicted for an individual of the same age. Several studies reported good success,[152–154,156,157,159] including one in which a questionnaire and report of spirometry results led to a 20 percent quit rate in an emphysema screening clinic,[152,155] and one in which better spirometry results after quitting were used to maintain abstinence.[153] However, some studies failed to find any improvement.[158–160]

Risser and Belcher studied the efficacy of a combination of advice, spirometry, and education.[159] They followed 238 outpatients who were invited and agreed to participate in a "health promotion clinic. They studied 90 smokers divided into a control group who received a brief lecture on the risks of smoking and methods of quitting, a self-help manual, and an invitation to attend nine individualized counseling sessions, and an intervention group who received all of the above plus spirometry with discussion of results.[159] After one year, 33 percent of the intervention group and 10 percent of the control group had stopped smoking as verified by CO breath analysis, $p = .015$ (if all subjects not contacted were counted as still smoking the quit rates were 20 versus 7 percent, $p = .06$).[159]

Pederson and coworkers examined the effect of advice, a self-help manual, and additional follow-up counseling on 74 patients admitted to a pulmonary ward.[161] All subjects were told to quit, and half (the intervention group) were randomly chosen to receive a self-help guide and alternate-day 15- to 20-min counseling sessions.[161] After 6 months, more of the intervention group quit smoking (33 versus 21 percent), but the difference was not statistically significant.[161]

Behavioral techniques have also been used specifically in patients with pulmonary illnesses. Sachs and associates, in a series of 16 patients with COPD or congestive heart failure used rapid smoking to achieve a smoking cessation rate of 50 percent at 6 months.[162] Hall and coworkers achieved a 50 percent 2-year abstinence rate using rapid smoking in 18 patients with cardiac and pulmonary disease, verified by self-report, CO, cotinine, and thiocyanate, while no one stopped smoking in a control group of other smokers who received no intervention.[87] No arrhythmias or ischemia occur as a consequence of rapid smoking.[87] Turner and coworkers used a combination of brand fading (changing to a lower-nicotine brand) on stimulus control on six patients with COPD, obtaining one quit after 6 months.[163]

Nicotine replacement therapy has also been examined in patients with pulmonary disease, in combination with other therapies. One of the earliest investigations was the British Thoracic Society trial, in which 1550 smokers with smoking-associated medical conditions including lung diseases, cardiovascular diseases, and peptic ulcer between 18 and 65 were randomized to receive advice to stop smoking, advice and a self-help booklet, or advice plus 2 mg nicotine gum or placebo gum.[164] Patients were followed for 1 year, and only received gum after 3 months if they requested it. Subjects were considered abstinent if they stated they were not smokers for 6 months and 1 year after the start of the study, and this assertion was verified by CO and thiocyanate monitoring.[164] A total of 9.7 percent of participants could be considered as successfully quitting smoking, but there was no significant difference between any of the groups.[164] The methodology of this trial has been criticized because the manner and average number of pieces of gum chewed by each patient is unknown and serum nicotine levels were not obtained. In addition, patients continued to smoke while taking the gum, which they should not have done, and the patients were recruited over a long period of time (13 months) raising the possibility of selection bias. Two-thirds of the patients were from the lowest socioeconomic groups, who are less likely to cease smoking on gum.[61]

Crowley and coworkers used a combination of gum and behavioral techniques in 49 outpatients with COPD for 3 months.[42] The participants were divided into two experimental groups and control groups who had home visits.[42] Each control patient was matched to a specific patient in one of the experimental groups.[42] The two experimental groups were given a CO breath analysis, a supply of nicotine gum, and a reinforcement of receiving lottery tickets for a self-report of not having smoked; one group was told the result of the CO analysis and reinforced if the CO analysis verified abstinence, the other group was not told the results of their CO analysis and reinforced only on the basis of their reported abstinence.[42] Sachs and coworkers treated 44 smokers with COPD by giving them advice to stop smoking and setting a quit date. This was reinforced by a personalized review of x-rays, spirometry, ECGs, and stress tests. In addition, patients were given nicotine gum and instructed in its use by a physician.[61,165] The physician continued to individually counsel the patients, who could use up to 30 pieces a day ad lib.[61,165] On average patients used the gum for 8.0 and 9.5 months. Twenty-seven other subjects, who had not been randomized, were put on a waiting list and were called every 6 months to verify smoking status.[61,165] Slightly more than 2 years later, 27 percent of the gum users were abstinent but none of the control smokers were.

In a large-scale study (the Lung Health Study) to prevent

the progression of COPD, with 1587 smokers aged 35 to 60, who had mild spirometric abnormalities suggestive of COPD (FEV_1 between 55 and 90 percent, FVC less than 0.7 liters), smoking cessation techniques were used.[44,166] The smokers receiving the intervention were also told to stop smoking by a physician, went to 12 group sessions over a 10-week period, and were taught behavioral techniques to quit smoking and the use of nicotine gum. About 40 percent of the participants had previously used nicotine gum before being enrolled in the study.[167] Patients were followed yearly for 5 years, with CO- and cotinine-validated cessation rates.[44,166] The combined sustained quit rate for the intervention groups after 5 years was 22 percent, while that for the control was 5 percent.[44,166]

Buproprion

In one recent trial, buproprion, has been used to achieve smoking cessation, albeit in middle-aged subjects.[168] Six hundred fifteen subjects were divided into groups receiving one of three different doses of buproprion or placebo. Depressed subjects were excluded from the study, but not those with just a history of depression.[168] Intention-to-treat analysis was performed and subjects were evaluated using both point prevalence and continuous abstinence.[168] Using the measurement of continuous abstinence, the cessation rate was significantly greater than placebo at the 300-mg dose 6 weeks after the quit date (24.4 versus 10.5 percent).[168] When point prevalence abstinence was measured, there was statistically significant abstinence in subjects treated with all of the three doses of buproprion used after one year.[168]

Conclusions

Pulmonary rehabilitation in the elderly patient and those with respiratory disease should include smoking cessation therapy. A number of techniques have been used successfully, but their relative efficacy has not been rigorously tested in well-designed studies. Reported results show that smoking cessation methods have at least as good a chance in these special patients as they do in the general population.

References

1. Wald NJ, Hackshaw AK: Cigarette smoking: An epidemiological overview. *Brit Med Bull* 52(1):3, 1996.
2. Peto R, Lopez AD, Boreham J, et al: Mortality from smoking in developed countries: 1950–2000. Oxford, Oxford University Press, 1993.
3. Peto R, Lopez AD, Boreham J, et al: Mortality from smoking worldwide. *Brit Med Bull* 52(1):12, 1996.
4. Cox JL: Smoking cessation in the elderly patient. *Clin Chest Med* 14(3):423, 1993.
5. Burns DM: Cigarettes and cigarette smoking. *Clin Chest Med* 12:631, 1991.
6. Giovino GA, Henningfield JE, Tomar SL, et al: Epidemiology of tobacco use and dependence. *Epidem Rev* 17(1):48, 1995.
7. U.S. Department Health and Human Services: The health consequences of smoking: A report of the Surgeon General, 1990. Rockville, MD: Centers for Disease Control, Center for Chronic Disease Prevention and Promotion, Office of Smoking and Health, 1989. DHHS publication no. 89-8411.
8. Fisher EB, Lichtenstein E, Haire-Joshu D, et al: Methods suc-
cesses and failures of smoking cessation programs. *Ann Rev Med* 44:481, 1993.
9. Curry SJ, McBride MM: Relapse prevention for smoking cessation: Review and evaluation of concepts and interventions. *Ann Rev Pub Health* 15:345, 1994.
10. Rimer BK, Orleans CT, Keintz MK, et al: The older smoker *Chest* 97(3):547, 1990.
11. Boyd NR: Smoking cessation: A four-step plan to help older patients quit. *Geriatrics* 51(11):52, 1996.
12. Rimer BK, Orleans CT: Older smokers, in Orleans CT, Slade J (eds): *Nicotine Addiction: Principles and Management.* New York, Oxford University Press, 1993; pp 385–395.
13. Centers for Disease Control. Cigarette smoking among adults. *MMWR* 43:925, 1994.
14. U.S. Department of Health and Human Services: Smoking and health: A national status report. Bethesda, MD: Public Health Service, Centers for Disease Control, Center for Health Promotion and Education. DHHS Publication (CDC) no.: 87-8396, 1990.
15. Orleans CT, Rimer BK, Cristinzio S, et al: A national survey of older smokers: Treatment needs of a growing population. *Health Psychol* 10(5):343, 1991.
16. Gourlay SG, Benowitz NL: The benefits of stopping smoking and the role of nicotine replacement therapy in older patients. *Drugs Aging* 9(1):8, 1996.
17. Doll R, Peto R, Wheatley K: Mortality in relation to smoking: 40 years' observations on male British doctors. *BMJ* 309:901, 1994.
18. Paganini-Hill A, Hsu G: Smoking and mortality among residents of a California retirement community. *Am J Pub Health* 84(6):992, 1994.
19. U.S. Department of Health and Human Services: The health benefits of smoking cessation: A report of the Surgeon General, 1990. U.S. Department of Health and Human Services, Public Health Service, Centers for Disease Control, Center for Chronic Disease Prevention and Health Promotion, Office on Smoking and Health, 1990. DHHS publication (CDC) no: 90-8416.
20. LaCroix AZ, Lang J, Scherr P, et al: Smoking and mortality among older men and women in three communities. *N Engl J Med* 324:1619, 1991.
21. Jajich CL, Ostfeld AM, Freeman DH, et al: Smoking and coronary heart disease mortality in the elderly. *JAMA* 252:2831, 1984.
22. Hermanson B, Omenn GS, Kronmal RA, et al: Beneficial six-year outcome of smoking cessation in older men and women with coronary artery disease. *N Engl J Med* 319:1365, 1988.
23. Tell GS, Howard G, McKinney WM, et al: Cigarette smoking cessation and extracranial carotid atherosclerosis. *JAMA* 261:1178, 1989.
24. Donnan GA, McNeill JJ, Adena MA, et al: Smoking as a risk factor for cerebral ischaemia. *Lancet* ii:643, 1989.
25. Rogot E, Murray JL: Smoking and causes of death among US veterans: 16 years of observation. *Pub Health Rep* 95:213, 1980.
26. Faulkner KW, House AK, Castleden WM: The effect of cessation of smoking on the accumulative survival rates of patients with symptomatic peripheral vascular disease. *Med J Austral* 1:217, 1993.
27. Jonason T, Bergstrom R: Cessation of smoking in patients with intermittent claudication. *Acta Med Scand* 221:253, 1987.
28. Lepantalo M, Lassila R: Smoking and occlusive peripheral artery disease. *Eur J Surg* 157:83, 1991.
29. Myers KA, King RB, Scott DF: The effect of smoking on the late patency of arterial reconstructions in the legs. *Br J Surg* 65:267, 1978.
30. Wetzig GA, Gough IR, Furnival CM: One hundred cases of arteriovenous fistula for haemodialysis access: The effect of cigarette smoking on patency. *Austral NZ J Surg* 55:551, 1985.
31. Quick CRG, Cotton LT: The measured effect of stopping smoking on intermittent claudication. *Br J Surg* 69:S24, 1982.
32. Lubin JH, Blot WJ: Lung cancer and smoking cessation: Patterns of risk. *J Natl Cancer Inst* 85:422, 1993.

33. Sobue T, Yamaguchi N, Suzuki T, et al: Lung cancer incidence rate for male ex-smokers according to age at cessation of smoking. *Jpn J Cancer Res* 84:601, 1993.

34. Halpern MT, Gillespie BW, Warner KE, et al: Patterns of absolute risk of lung cancer mortality in former smokers. *J Natl Cancer Inst* 85:457, 1993.

35. Higgins MW, Enright PL, Kronmal RA, et al: Smoking and lung function in elderly men and women. *JAMA* 269:2741, 1993.

36. Sherrill DL, Lebowitz MD, Knudson RJ: Longitudinal methods for describing the relationship between pulmonary function, respiratory symptoms, and smoking in the elderly subjects: The Tucson study. *Eur J Resp J* 6:342, 1993.

37. Daughton DM, Fix AJ, Kass I, Patil KD: Smoking cessation among patients with COPD. *Addict Behav* 5:125, 1980.

38. Ball KP, Kirby BV, Bogen C: First year's experience in an anti-smoking clinic. *BMJ* 5451:1651, 1965.

39. Dudley DL, Aickin M, Martin CV: Cigarette smoking in a chest clinic population-psychophysiologic variable. *J Psychosom Res* 21:367, 1977.

40. Pederson LL, Wanklin JM, Lefcoe NM: The effect of counseling on smoking cessation among patients hospitalized with chronic obstructive pulmonary disease: A randomized clinical trial. *Int J Addict* 26(1):107, 1991.

41. U.S. Department of Health and Human Services: The health consequences of smoking: Chronic obstructive lung disease. A report of the Surgeon General. US Public Health Service, DHHS (PHS) no: 84-50205, 1984.

42. Crowley TJ, Macdonald MJ, Walter MI: Behavioral anti-smoking trial in chronic obstructive pulmonary disease patients. *Psychopharmacology* 119:193, 1995.

43. Tashkin DP, Clark VA, Coulson AH, et al: The UCLA population studies of chronic obstructive respiratory disease. VIII. Effect of smoking cessation on lung function: A prospective study of a free-living population. *ARRD* 130:707, 1984.

44. Antonisen NR, Connett JE, Kiley JP, et al: Effects of smoking intervention and the use of an inhaled anticholinergic bronchodilator on the rate of decline of FEV_1. *JAMA* 272(19):1497, 1994.

45. Benowitz NL: Pharmacology of nicotine: Addiction and tolerance. *Ann Rev Pharm Toxicol* 36:597, 1996.

46. Clarke PBS, Schwartz RD, Paul SM, et al: Nicotinic binding in the rat brain: Autoradiographic comparison of [^{3}H] acetylcholine, [^{3}H] nicotine, and [^{125}I] α-bungarotoxin. *J Neurosci* 5:1307, 1985.

47. Benowitz NL: Pharmacologic aspects of cigarette smoking and nicotine addiction. *N Engl J Med* 319:1318, 1988.

48. Ginzel KH: The importance of sensory nerve endings as sites of dopamine action. *NaunynScmiedelbergs Arch Pharmacol* 288:29, 1975.

49. Comroe JH Jr: The pharmacological actions of nicotine. *Ann NY Acad* 90:48, 1960.

50. Pomerleau OF, Pomerleau CS: Neuroregulators and the reinforcement of smoking: Towards a biobehavioral explanation. *Neurosci Biobehav Rev* 8:503, 1984.

51. Wesnes K, Warburton DM: Smoking, nicotine, and human performance. *Pharmacol Ther* 21:189, 1983.

52. Velicer WF, Fava JL, Prochaska JO, et al: Distribution of smokers by stage in three representative samples. *Prev Med* 24:401, 1995.

53. DiClemente CC, Prochaska JO, Fairhurst SK, et al: The process of smoking cessation: An analysis of precontemplation, contemplation and preparation stages of change. *J Consult Clin Psychol* 59:295, 1991.

54. Prochaska JO, DiClemente CC: Stages and processes of self-change of smoking: Toward an integrative model of change. *J Consult Clin Psychol* 51:390, 1983.

55. Brown RA, Goldstein MG, Niaura R, et al: Nicotine assessment and management, in Stoudmeire A, Fogel BS (eds): *Psychiatric Care of the Medical Patient*. New York, Oxford University Press, 1993:877–901.

56. Fisher E, Haire-Joshu D, Morgan G, et al: State-of-the art review: Smoking and smoking cessation. *ARRD* 142:702, 1990.

57. Hughes JR, Gulliver SB, Fenwick JW, et al: Smoking cessation among self-quitters. *Health Psychol* 11(5):331, 1992.

58. American Psychiatric Association: Practice guidelines for the treatment of patients with nicotine dependence. *Am J Psychiat* 153(10)suppl:1, 1996.

59. U.S. Department of Health and Human Service: National trends in smoking cessation, in *The Health Benefits of Smoking Cessation: A Report of the Surgeon General*. U.S. Government Printing Office, 1990:580–616.

60. Velicer WF, Prochaska JO, Rossi JS, Snow MG: Assessing outcome in smoking cessation studies. *Psychol Bull* 111(1):23, 1992.

61. Sachs DPL: Advances in smoking cessation treatment. *Current Pulmonology* 12:139, 1991.

62. Hunt WA, Barnett LW, Branch LG: Relapse rates in addiction programs. *J Clin Psychol* 27:455, 1971.

63. Hunt WA, Bespalec DA: An evaluation of current methods of modifying smoking behavior. *J Clin Psychol* 30:431, 1974.

64. Cohen S, Lichtenstein E, Prochaska JO, et al: Debunking myths about self-quitting: Evidence from 10 prospective studies of persons quitting smoking by themselves. *Am Psychol* 44:1355, 1989.

65. Ockene JK, Hymowitz M, Sexton M, Broste SK: Comparison of patterns of smoking behavior change among smokers in the Multiple Risk Factor Intervention Trial (MRFIT). *Prev Med* 11:621, 1982.

66. Stewart RD: The effect of carbon monoxide on humans. *Ann Rev Pharm* 15:409, 1975.

67. Bauman KE, Koch GG, Bryan ES: Validity of self reports of adolescent cigarette smoking. *Int J Addict* 17:1131, 1982.

68. Benowitz NL: The use of biological fluid samples in assessing tobacco smoke consumption. *NIDA Res Monogr Ser* 48:6, 1983.

69. McNeil AS, Owen LA, Belcher M, et al: Abstinence from smoking and expired-air carbon monoxide levels: Lactose intolerance as a possible source of error. *Am J Pub Health* 80:1114, 1990.

70. Vogt TM, Selvin S, Widdowson G, Hulley SB: Expired air carbon monoxide and serum thiocyanate as object measures of cigarette exposure. *Am J Pub Health* 67:545, 1977.

71. Abrams DB, Folic MJ, Biener L, et al: Saliva cotinine as a measure of smoking status in field settings. *Am J Pub Health* 77:846, 1987.

72. Glynn SM, Gruder CL, Jegerski JA: Effects of biochemical validation of self-reported cigarette smoking on treatment success and on misreporting abstinence. *Health Psychol* 5:125, 1986.

73. Pojer R, Whitfield JB, Poulos V, et al: Carboxyhemoglobin, cotinine, and thiocyanate assay compared for distinguishing smokers from nonsmokers. *Clin Chem* 30:1377, 1984.

74. Pechacek TF, Murray DM, Luepker RV, et al: Measurement of adolescent smoking behavior. *J Behav Med* 7:123, 1984.

75. Jarvis M, Tunstall-Pedoe H, Feyerabend C, et al: Comparison of tests used to distinguish smokers from nonsmokers. *Am J Pub Health* 77:1435, 1987.

76. Etzel RA: A review of saliva cotinine as a marker of tobacco smoke exposure. *Prev Med* 19:190, 1990.

77. Carey KB, Abrams DB: Properties of saliva cotinine in young adult light smokers. *Am J Pub Health* 78:842, 1988.

78. Greenburg RA, Haley NJ, Etzel RA, Loda FA. Measuring the exposure of infants to tobacco smoke: Nicotine and cotinine in urine and saliva. *N Engl J Med* 310:1075, 1984.

79. Haley NJ, Sepkovic DW, Hoffman D: Elimination of cotinine from body fluids: Disposition in smokers and non-smokers. *Am J Pub Health* 79:1046, 1989.

80. Sepkovic DW, Haley NJ, Hoffman D: Elimination from the body of tobacco products by smokers and passive smokers. *JAMA* 256:863, 1986.

81. Langer P, Greer NH: *Antithyroid Substances and Naturally Occurring Goitrogens*. Basel, Karger, 1977.

82. U.S. Department of Health, Education, and Welfare. *Smoking*

and Health: A report of the Surgeon General. Washington DC: U.S. Department of Health, Education, and Welfare, Public Health Service. Publication no (PHS):79–50066.

83. Swan GE, Parker SD, Chesney MA, Rosenman RH: Reducing the confounding effects of environment and diet on saliva thiocyanate values in ex-smokers. *Addict Behav* 10:187, 1985.

84. Neaton J, Broate S, Cohen L, et al: The multiple risk factor intervention trial (MRFIT): VII: A comparison of risk factor changes between the two study groups. *Prev Med* 10:519, 1981.

85. Fagerstrom K, Schneider NG: Measuring nicotine dependence: A review of the Fagerstrom Tolerance Questionnaire. *J Behav Med* 12:159, 1989.

86. Tonnesen P, Fryd V, Hansen M, et al: Effect of nicotine chewing gum in combination with group counseling on the cessation of smoking. *N Engl J Med* 318:15, 1988.

87. Hall RG, Sachs DPL, Hall SM, et al: Two-year efficacy and safety of rapid smoking therapy in patients with cardiac and pulmonary disease. *J Consult Clin Psychol* 52:574, 1984.

88. Jamrozik K, Vessey M, Fowler G, et al: Controlled trial of three different anti-smoking interventions in general practice. *BMJ* 288:1499, 1984.

89. Sutton SR: Great expectations: Some suggestions for applying the balanced placebo design to nicotine and smoking. *Br J Addict* 86:659, 1991.

90. Glynn TJ, Manley MW: *How to help your patients stop smoking.* U.S. Government Printing Office, 1989.

91. U.S. Department of Health and Human Services: *Clinical Practice Guideline, No. 18: Smoking Cessation.* Rockville, MD: U.S. Department of Health and Human Services, Public Health Service, Agency for Health Care Policy and Research. Publication no (PHS): 96-0692.

92. Foulds J: Strategies for smoking cessation. *Br Med Bull* 52:157, 1996.

93. Law M, Tang JL: An analysis of the effectiveness of interventions intended to help people stop smoking. *Arch Intern Med* 155:1933, 1995.

94. Viswesvaran C, Schmidt FL: A meta-analytic comparison of the effectiveness of smoking cessation methods. *J Appl Psych* 77(4):554, 1992.

95. Curry SJ: Self-help interventions for smoking cessation. *J Consult Clin Psych* 61(5):790, 1993.

96. Altman DG, Flora JA, Fortmann SP, Farquhar JW: The cost-effectiveness of three smoking cessation programs. *Am J Pub Health* 77:162, 1987.

97. Schwartz JL: Methods of smoking cessation. *Med Clin North Am* 76:451, 1992.

98. Schwartz JL: *Review and Evaluation of Smoking Cessation Methods: The United States and Canada.* Washington, DC: U.S. Department of Health and Human Services, 1987.

99. U.S. Department of Health and Human Services: Treatment of tobacco dependence, in: *The Health Consequences of Smoking: Nicotine Addiction.* U.S. Government Printing Office, 1988:459–560.

100. Corty E, McFall R: Response prevention in the treatment of cigarette smoking. *Addict Behav* 9:405, 1984.

101. Lowe M, Green L, Kurtz S, et al: Self-initiated, cue extinction, and covert sensitization procedures in smoking cessation. *J Behav Med* 3:357, 1984.

102. Raw M, Jarvis M, Feyerabend C, Russell MAH: Comparison of nicotine chewing gum and psychological treatments for dependent smokers. *Br J Med* 281:481, 1980.

103. Raw M, Russell MAH: Rapid smoking, cue exposure, and support in the modification of smoking. *Behav Res Ther* 18:363, 1980.

104. Gould RA, Clum GA: A meta-analysis of self-help treatment approaches. *Clin Psychol Rev* 13:169, 1993.

105. Glascow RE, Lichtenstein E: Long-term effects of behavioral smoking cessation interventions. *Behav Ther* 18:297, 1987.

106. Lam WL, Sze PC, Sacks HS, Chalmer TC: Meta-analysis of randomized controlled trials of nicotine chewing gum. *Lancet* 2:27, 1987.

107. Baille A, Mattick RP, Hall W, Webster P: Meta-analytic review of the efficacy of smoking cessation interventions. *Drug Alcohol Rev* 13:157, 1994.

108. Hughes JR: Pharmacotherapy for smoking cessation: Unvalidated assumptions, anomalies, and suggestions for further research. *J Consult Clin Psych* 61:751, 1993.

109. Cepeda-Benito A: Meta-analytic review of the efficacy of nicotine chewing gum in smoking treatment programs. *J Consult Clin Psychol* 61:822, 1993.

110. Gourlay SG, McNeil JJ: Antismoking products. *Med J Austral* 153:699, 1990.

111. Tang JL, Law M, Wald N: How effective is nicotine replacement therapy in helping people to stop smoking? *Br J Med* 308:21, 1994.

112. Kenford SL, Fiore MC, Jorenby DE, et al: Predicting smoking cessation. *JAMA* 271(8):589, 1994.

113. Fiore MC, Smith SS, Jorenby DE, Baker TB: The effectiveness of the nicotine patch for smoking cessation. *JAMA* 271(24):1940, 1994.

114. Silagy C, Mant D, Fowler G, Lodge M: Meta-analysis on efficacy of nicotine replacement therapies in smoking cessation. *Lancet* 343:139, 1994.

115. Dale LC, Hurt RD, Offord KP, et al: High-dose nicotine patch therapy. *JAMA* 274(17):1353, 1995.

116. Fiore MC, Jorenby DE, Baker TB, Kenford SL: Tobacco dependence and the nicotine patch. *JAMA* 268(19):2687, 1992.

117. Yudkin PL, Jones L, Lancaster T, Fowler GH: Which smokers are helped to give up smoking using transdermal nicotine patches? Results from a randomized, double-blinded, placebo-controlled trial. *Br J Gen Prac* 46:145, 1996.

118. Paoletti P, Fornai E, Maggiorelli F, et al: Importance of baseline cotinine plasma values in smoking cessation: Results from a double-blind study with nicotine patch. *Eur Respir J* 9:643, 1996.

119. Sutherland G, Stapleton JA, Russell MAH, et al: Randomised controlled trial of nasal nicotine spray in smoking cessation. *Lancet* 340:324, 1992.

120. Hjalmarson A, Franzon M, Westin A, Wiklund O: Effect of nicotine nasal spray on smoking cessation. *Arch Intern Med* 154:2567, 1994.

121. Tonnesen P, Norregaard J, Sawe U, Simonsen K: Recycling with nicotine patches in smoking cessation. *Addiction* 88:533, 1993.

122. Perkins KA, Grobe JE, Stiller RL, et al: Nasal spray nicotine replacement suppresses cigarette smoking desire and behavior. *Clin Pharm Ther* 52:627, 1992.

123. Tonnesen P, Norregard J, Mikkelsen K, et al: A double-blind trial of a nicotine inhaler for smoking cessation. *JAMA* 269:1268, 1993.

124. Gourlay SG, Benowitz NL: Is clonidine an effective smoking cessation therapy? *Drugs* 50(2):197, 1995.

125. Westman EC, Behm FM, Rose JE: Airway sensory replacement combined with nicotine replacement for smoking cessation. *Chest* 107:1358, 1995.

126. Behm FM, Schur C, Levin ED, et al: Clinical evaluation of a citric acid inhaler for smoking cessation. *Drug Alcohol Depend* 31:131, 1993.

127. Behm FM, Rose JE: Reducing craving for cigarettes while decreasing smoke intake using capsaicin-enhanced low tar cigarettes. *Exper Clin Psychopharmacol* 2(2):143, 1994.

128. Berlin I, Said S, Spreux-Varoquaux O, et al: A reversible monoamine oxidase A inhibitor (moclobemide) facilitates smoking cessation and abstinence in heavy, dependent smokers. *Clin Pharm Ther* 58:444, 1995.

129. Behm FM: Low-nicotine regenerated smoke aerosol reduces desire for cigarettes. *J Substance Abuse* 2:237, 1990.

130. Rose JE, Behm FM: Inhalation of vapor from black pepper extract reduces smoking withdrawal symptoms. *Drug Alcohol Depend* 34:224, 1994.

131. Butschky MF, Bailey D, Henningfield JE, Pickworth WB: Smok-

ing without nicotine delivery decreased withdrawal in 12-hour abstinent smokers. *Pharm Biochem Behav* 50(1):91, 1995.

132. Marcus BH, Albrecht AE, Niaura RS, et al: Exercise enhances the maintenance of smoking cessation in women. *Addict Behav* 20(1):87, 1995.

133. Hughes GH, Hymowitz N, Ockene JK, et al: The Multiple Risk Factor Intervention Trial (MRFIT): V. Intervention on smoking. *Prev Med* 10:476, 1981.

134. Multiple Risk Factor Intervention Trial Research Group: Multiple Risk Factor Intervention Trial: Risk factor changes and mortality results. *JAMA* 248:1465, 1982.

135. Jarvis MJ, West R, Tunstall-Pedoe H, et al: An evaluation of the intervention against smoking in the Multiple Risk Factor Intervention Trial. *Prev Med* 13:501, 1984.

136. Hjermann I, Velve-Byre K, Holme I, et al: Effect of diet and smoking intervention on the incidence of coronary heart disease: Report from the Oslo Study Group of a randomised trial in healthy men. *Lancet* 2:1303, 1981.

137. Vetter NJ, Ford D: Smoking prevention among people aged 60 and over: A randomized controlled trial. *Age Aging* 19:164, 1990.

138. Rimer BK, Orleans CT, Fleisher L, et al: Does tailoring matter? The impact of a tailored guide on ratings and short-term smoking related outcomes for older smokers. *Health Educ Res* 9(1):69, 1994.

139. Hill RD, Rigdon M, Johnson S: Behavioral smoking cessation treatment for chronic older smokers. *Behav Ther* 24:321, 1993.

140. Morgan GD, Noll EL, Orleans CT, et al: Reaching midlife and older smokers: Tailored interventions for routine medical care. *Prev Med* 25:346, 1996.

141. Orleans CT, Resch N, Noll E, et al: Use of transdermal nicotine in a state-level prescription plan for the elderly. *JAMA* 271(8):601, 1994.

142. Fiscella K, Franks P: Cost-effectiveness of the transdermal nicotine patch as an adjunct to physicians' smoking cessation counseling. *JAMA* 275(16):1247, 1996.

143. Joseph AM, Norman SM, Ferry LH, et al: The safety of transdermal nicotine as an aid to smoking cessation in patients with cardiac disease. *N Engl J Med* 335:1792, 1996.

144. Salive ME, Coroni-Hutley J, LaCroix AZ: Predictors of smoking cessation and relapse in older adults. *Am J Pub Health* 82:1268, 1992.

145. Salive ME, Blazer DG: Depression and smoking cessation in older adults: A longitudinal study. *J Am Geriatr Soc* 41:1313, 1993.

146. Rodrigues JC, Illowite JS: Pulmonary rehabilitation in the elderly. *Clin Chest Med* 14(3):429, 1993.

147. Niederman MS, Clemente PH, Fein AM, et al: Benefits of a multidisciplinary rehabilitation program. *Chest* 99(4):798, 1991.

148. Campbell IA: Smoking cessation, in Hodgkin JE, Petty TL (eds): *Chronic Obstructive Pulmonary Disease: Current Concepts.* Philadelphia, WB Saunders, 1987:64–67.

149. Raw M: Persuading people to stop smoking. *Behav Res Therapy* 14:97, 1976.

150. Williams HO: Routine advice against smoking—A chest clinic pilot study. *Practitioner* 202:672, 1969.

151. Pederson LL, Wanklin JM, Lefcoe NM: Self-reported long term smoking cessation in patients with respiratory disease: Prediction of success and perception of health effects. *Int J Epidem* 17:804, 1988.

152. Morris JF, Sturman W: Spirometry and respiratory questionnaire: Value for screening and smoking cessation. *ARRD* 109:702, 1974.

153. Paxton R, Scott S: Nonsmoking reinforced by improvements in lung function. *Addict Behav* 6:313, 1981.

154. Petty TL, Cherniack RM: Let's identify COPD early! *Clin Notes Resp Dis* 21:8, 1982.

155. Morris JF, Temple W: Spirometric "lung age" estimation for motivating smoking cessation. *Prev Med* 14:660, 1985.

156. Petty TL, Pierson DJ, Dick NP, et al: Follow-up evaluation of a prevalence study for chronic bronchitis and chronic airway obstruction. *ARRD* 114:881, 1976.

157. Hepper NGG, Drage CW, Davies SF, et al: Chronic obstructive pulmonary disease: A community-oriented program including professional education and screening by a voluntary health agency. *ARRD* 121:97, 1980.

158. Loss RW, Hall WJ, Speers DM: Evaluation of early airway disease in smokers: Cost effectiveness of pulmonary function testing. *Am J Med Sci* 278:27, 1979.

159. Risser NL, Belcher DW: Adding spirometry, carbon monoxide, and pulmonary symptom results to smoking cessation counseling: A randomized trial. *J Gen Intern Med* 5:16, 1990.

160. Li VC, Kim YJ, Ewart CK, et al: Effects of physician counseling on the smoking behavior of asbestos-exposed workers. *Prev Med* 13:462, 1984.

161. Pederson LL, Wanklin JM, Lefcoe NM: The effects of counseling on smoking cessation among patients hospitalized with chronic obstructive pulmonary disease: A randomized clinical trial. *Int J Addict* 26(1):107, 1991.

162. Sachs PL, Hall RG, Sachs BL: Success of rapid smoking therapy in smokers with pulmonary and coronary heart disease. *Am Rev Respir Dis* 123:111, 1981.

163. Turner SA, Daniels JL, Hollandsworth JG: The effects of a multicomponent smoking cessation program with chronic obstructive pulmonary disease outpatients. *Addict Behav* 10:87, 1985.

164. British Thoracic Society: Comparison of four methods of smoking withdrawal in patients with smoking related diseases. *BMJ* 286:595, 1983.

165. Sachs DPL, Benowitz NL, Silver KJ: Effect of nicotine polacrilex (Nicorette) in patients with chronic obstructive pulmonary disease, in Aoki M, Hisamichi S, Tominaga S (eds): *Smoking and Health 1987: Proceedings of the 6th World Conference on Smoking and Health. Tokyo, 9–12 November 1987.* Amsterdam, Elsevier, 1988:793–796.

166. Kanner RE: Early intervention in chronic obstructive pulmonary disease. *Med Clin North Am* 80(3):523, 1996.

167. Murray RP, Bailey WC, Daniels V, et al: Safety of nicotine polacrilex gum used by 3094 participants in the Lung Health Study. *Chest* 109:438, 1996.

168. Hurt RD, Sachs DPL, Glover ED, et al: A comparison of sustained-release buproprion and placebo for smoking cessation. *N Engl J Med* 337(17):1195–1202, 1997.

PART VI
PSYCHOSOCIAL CONSIDERATIONS

Chapter 55

SOCIAL, PSYCHOLOGICAL, AND BEHAVIORAL FACTORS AND PATIENT MANAGEMENT OF LUNG DISEASE

NOREEN M. CLARK
FARYLE NOTHWEHR

While social and psychological factors are thought to be important in all lung diseases, for some conditions, for example, sarcoidosis, asbestoses, and white and black lung, virtually no studies have examined their influence on health behavior or health status. However, these factors have been studied to some extent in patients with asthma, COPD, and cystic fibrosis. This chapter perforce will first focus on these three conditions, and then move to issues in managing lung diseases in general. Available findings suggest that full control is dependent not only on the soundness of the therapeutic plan but on the ability of patients to manage disease supported by family members and others in the social environment. While similarities exist across the conditions to be considered, each has unique social, behavioral, and epidemiologic features and deserves individual attention.

Asthma

The first few years of life and early adulthood are the most likely times for symptoms of asthma to appear. Delayed diagnosis may occur because early symptoms were mild or atypical.[1] It has been documented that prevalence of asthma is higher in boys than in girls during childhood but that in adolescence and during adulthood the prevalence tends to be higher in women,[2] and health care utilization for asthma is also higher for them.[3,4] Numerous cohort studies have indicated that the onset of asthma is very often preceded by other allergic disease such as eczema, allergic rhinitis, positive skin test, or high blood IgE.[2] Family history of allergic disorders is considered a risk factor for asthma as atopy and bronchial reactivity seem to cluster in families.[1,5] Low birth weight which is often associated with maternal smoking and/or mechanical ventilation, and absence of breastfeeding

are also suspected to predispose one to asthma.[6] The highest risk populations for problems with asthma appear to be poor racial/ethnic minorities who reside in urban environments.[6] Socioeconomic status (SES) confounds the association between race/ethnicity and asthma prevalence. Conditions of poverty affect the development and management of asthma through many avenues such as access to high quality medical care, education, housing conditions, and the presence of stressful, competing demands.[6] Indoor allergens such as dust mites, cockroaches, animal dander, and molds are especially difficult to eradicate in inner city dwellings.[7,8] A small percentage of asthma is deemed related to occupational exposures. Agents suspected include metal salts, industrial chemicals, pharmaceutical agents, biological enzymes, animals, and vegetable dusts.[9]

GOALS OF THERAPY

Goals of asthma therapy include control of symptoms, full physical and psychosocial functioning, and no interference with social relationships and quality of life. In order to reach these goals, people with asthma (including children and/or their parents) must be able to identify and avoid the things that cause symptoms, use prescribed medications in the proper manner to prevent or control symptoms, maintain one's daily routine and participate in physical activity, develop or maintain family and other social support for these behaviors, and communicate effectively with health care providers. Complicating this process is the fact that, aside from some very basic or "core" management behaviors that are important for almost all people with asthma, the tasks of management are largely unique to each person based on the individual disease characteristics, personal attributes, and lifestyle considerations. There are differences among people with asthma regarding the factors that give rise to attacks, the medication regimens that are effective, and the social situations that affect one's ability to manage the condition. In addition, these factors may change over time for any individual. This means that people must develop their own repertoires of effective behavioral strategies and use a decision making process which allows them to change or refine these strategies as needed.[10] Further, as it is impossible for clinicians to provide direction for every contingency a patient may face, individuals must exercise a high degree of independent decision making about asthma, within the doctor's general guidelines.

INTERVENTIONS TO IMPROVE ASTHMA MANAGEMENT BY THE PATIENT

A first generation of patient disease management programs for school-aged children with asthma has shown that interventions based in clinical settings can result in outcomes including fewer episodes of symptoms, less emergency department (ED) use, fewer hospitalizations and/or improved adjustment and academic performance in school.[11-13] One study[11] provided data to suggest health care cost savings for children with a history of hospitalization offset program costs $14 to $1. A second generation of programs showed that education for parents of very young children (four and younger) could reduce a child's symptoms and increase parents' management efforts.[14,15] Studies have shown that a clinic-based disease management intervention can be successfully adapted to a school setting,[16] and for different populations of children.[17] At least one community-based program has also proven successful.[18]

A growing body of research has shown that adults with asthma can learn to improve their management techniques and realize greater control over the disruption asthma causes. Four teams of researchers[19–22] have demonstrated that disease management education for adults offered in the clinic setting can generate outcomes including control of symptoms, improved metered-dose inhaler (MDI) use, better environmental control, less ED use, fewer hospitalizations, and/or reduced health care costs. Two studies have focused education specifically on adults with a history of health care use. Bolton and coworkers[23] provided an intervention for emergency department users and Mayo and associates[24] for adults with a previous hospitalization for asthma. Both found education to be associated with reductions in subsequent use of health services. Even very brief educational programs have produced results. Yoon and colleagues[25] found reduced hospital readmissions and ED use from a three-hour intervention. Kelso and coworkers[26] provided emergency department patients with one hour of education on site and found subsequent reductions in ED visits.

Studies in asthma have shown that gains in asthma knowledge are not necessarily associated with behavior change. Heringa and associates[27] in their study found both intervention and control patients improved their asthma knowledge levels, yet only program participants increased their management skills. Rubin[28] showed that behavior change is associated only with moderate increases in asthma knowledge. Beyond moderate levels, knowledge ceases to be associated with adoption and use of disease management practices by the patient. Allen and coworkers,[29] as might be expected, noted that education without concurrent adequate clinical treatment did not improve patients' health status. Two teams have provided persuasive data to suggest education for adults based in the clinic or hospital is cost effective. Trautner and associates[30] showed education in the clinic generated a 1:2.28 cost benefit ratio. Two studies suggest that group formats are acceptable to many adult patients, save time, and generate the same behavioral benefit as individual counseling[19,31] and community-based education can be effective.[32]

Computer-assisted instruction has yielded positive results. Osman and colleagues[33] and Huss and coworkers[34] found adding interactive computer learning to patient disease management education resulted in reduced hospital admissions, less sleep disturbance, and better environmental control.

There is general agreement among clinicians that when recorded sequentially peak flow monitoring (PFM) can provide useful information for the physician in following the course of reversible airway obstructive lung disease, most notably asthma. Although data are limited, available studies suggest that flow rates decline with increasing symptoms.[35,36] Nevertheless, patients without symptoms can have reduced airflow,[37] and patients with normal peak flow readings may also have obstruction.[38] Such findings suggest that using only one indicator (for example, symptoms or PFM) as the cue to problems with asthma may increase the risk of underestimating the seriousness of the condition. At least one investigation has shown that patient ability to detect airflow subjectively is very limited.[39] On the other hand, other studies have suggested that some patients are very good at this[40] and better

than physicians.[41] Different peak flow meters have been shown to give different readings.[35]

Because PFM is dependent on the level of patient effort[42,43] and because it may be more sensitive to large airway than small airway resistance, its usefulness may be limited in some populations, for example, young children or individuals who are not highly motivated to give their best effort. If patients do not perceive clear-cut benefits to monitoring, adherence is likely to be poor. Some patients may find peak flow monitoring a simplification of their existing regimen, whereas others may find it too burdensome to be worth any benefits they derive. For example, the failure of patients with mild or intermittent disease to see changes in peak flow may serve as a disincentive for PFM. If patient adherence to PFM varies with severity or intermittency of asthma, then studies of PFM that do not control for these are likely to give ambiguous or conflicting results. Similarly, some physicians may not find patient peak flow monitoring worth the effort if clear-cut benefits for both patient and physician are not evident.

Four recent studies have examined patient education for peak flow monitoring (PFM) versus symptom monitoring in asthma. Malo and coworkers,[44] Charlton and colleagues,[45] the Grampian Study,[46] and Jones and associates[47] found no better outcomes (including MD visits, hospitalization, sleep disturbances, work interruptions) for groups using PFM than among patients using conventional symptom monitoring. Ignacio and Gonzalez,[48] however, reported that the PFM group patients in their study had better results related to days lost from work, symptoms, and ED visits than those who did not use PFM.

D-Souza and coworkers[49] found it was possible to combine management plans for both peak flow and symptom monitoring in a credit card sized format and found patients who used the card had improved PEFR, less interrupted sleep, and fewer days of limited activity.

THE SOCIAL ENVIRONMENT AND ASTHMA

As with other chronic conditions, factors in the social environment, including the workplace, are considered to be important to the successful management of asthma by patients, as well as to the emotional health of caregivers. Several studies explore influences on management by families of children with asthma. Mrazek and colleagues[50] suggest that problems in coping and parenting may contribute to the development of symptoms in children who are genetically at risk for asthma. In another study, some parents were found to have misconceptions about causes, triggers, symptoms, and treatment which could potentially diminish the effectiveness of management of their children's asthma.[51] Conversely, children with parents who are knowledgeable about asthma management have been found to feel more competent to handle the condition.[52] The extent and depth of family communication about asthma has been found to vary by culture and by the educational level of the mother.[53] Fathers may also play a significant role in asthma management in the family. One study concludes that when fathers share the tasks of caring for their child's asthma, whether or not they are living in the home, mothers experience less disruption in their daily lives.[54] Two studies[55,56] indicate that both mothers and fathers of children with asthma may be more overtly negative and critical of their children than parents of youngsters without the disease.

Although studied less, the social environment is also believed to play an important role in the management of asthma in adults. Using the critical incident technique, Wilson and colleagues compiled an extensive list of asthma patient management competencies necessary for adults.[57] This list includes taking actions to resolve significant personal problems or stressful life situations that may adversely affect asthma management. Data from focus groups of adults with asthma also suggest that family members or close friends can either help or hinder one's asthma management efforts.[58] A study[59] has shown that both the amount of perceived distress among adult patients and their appraisal of available social support predicted emergency department visits. Similarly, Strunk[60] and Sur and coworkers[61] suggest that slow onset fatal asthma can be predicted in part by the social psychological profile of the patient, for example, suffering psychological problems, being highly disorganized, or being unable to mobilize personal and family resources to care for the disease.

Chronic Obstructive Pulmonary Disease

Chronic obstructive pulmonary disease (COPD), here defined to include chronic bronchitis and emphysema, is found more frequently in men than women, and increases with age in both sexes.[62] It has been suggested that at least a portion of the gender difference is attributable to physician bias toward labeling male patients as having emphysema and female patients as asthmatic or bronchitic.[63] According to a 1984 Surgeon General's report, approximately 80 to 90 percent of deaths from COPD and allied conditions are attributable to smoking. This report also points to evidence that establishes alpha$_1$-antiprotease deficiency as an independent cause of COPD.[64] Rapid decline in lung function in smokers with COPD appears to terminate with smoking cessation, even in patients who already exhibit abnormal spirometry results,[65] making smoking cessation a high priority in treatment. Other suspected contributors to the disease include occupational exposures, outdoor and indoor pollution, climate, and acute respiratory infections.[62,66] A few dietary factors have been suggested as contributing to chronic lung disease including linoleic acid, alcohol, and fruit intake.[67] Racial differences in COPD prevalence and/or pulmonary function measures have been found with whites having higher rates of the disease than blacks and Native Americans. Confounding issues such as environmental exposures or differences in response to smoking must be considered in these comparisons.[68,69] Some social factors have been shown to be important in the epidemiology of COPD. For example, an inverse relationship between education and obstructive diseases has been found.[70–72]

GOALS OF THERAPY

People with COPD tend to have a continued, relatively rapid decline in lung function and a high mortality rate. Goals of treatment include control of symptoms, maximum exercise tolerance, and psychosocial well-being.[73] Smoking cessation is obviously important to reaching these goals as are pulmonary rehabilitation and medication for symptom management. COPD patients learn energy conservation techniques, and are encouraged to engage in an exercise regimen that will improve exercise tolerance and their ability to perform

daily activities.[74] Depression is fairly common among those with COPD and must be considered a factor in a comprehensive educational program. Effective management requires accounting for the social effects of the disease and its resultant disability and dependence.[74–76] It is important that people with this disease receive annual influenza vaccines, and augmentation therapy for severe alpha$_1$-antitrypsin deficiency is often recommended.[73]

INTERVENTIONS TO IMPROVE COPD DISEASE MANAGEMENT BY THE PATIENT

Several investigators have shown the effectiveness of pulmonary rehabilitation programs that combine disease management education and exercise training. Effects of these programs diminish after a few years indicating periodic subsequent education is needed. Mall,[77] for example, showed a program in an outpatient clinic of a community hospital produced improved treadmill performance and better understanding of disease, as well as increased capacity for workload with a lower heart rate. Five years subsequent to the program, 32 percent of the 101 patients remained improved, 32 percent had died, and 36 percent were worse.

Two teams showed results in controlled studies where patients were assigned to 8-week comprehensive rehabilitative treatment or control groups.[78] Six months later rehabilitation program group members had a significant increase in exercise endurance. Ojanen[79] found after an initial 3-week program, no differences in outcome between treatment and control groups after 6 months. In a similar program evaluated by Ries,[80] benefits diminished after 12 months. Another team[81] found patients in a pulmonary rehabilitation program improved significantly over control patients on additional variables including endurance, psychological parameters, use of health care, work days, and physical activity. However, gains were no longer evident in the evaluation conducted at the end of the second year of follow-up.

In one study,[82] education without exercise training for COPD patients was compared against simply telling patients the degree of their airway obstruction. There were significant differences 1 year later in patients' perception of disease but not in respiratory symptoms, exercise tolerance, or mental health.

Sassi-Dambron[83] tried a brief pulmonary rehabilitation program focused specifically on increasing coping strategies for shortness of breath. At 6 months' follow-up, there were no significant differences on these primary outcome variables between experiment or control groups. Touguaard and coworkers,[84] however, showed education without exercise to be associated with less need for medical care. One year postprogram, hospital and physician costs for patients assigned to be educated in aspects of their COPD were significantly less than those in a physical training only control group.

Correct use of medicines poses problems for COPD patients. One study addressed incorrect metered dose inhaler (MDI) use.[85] Individuals were randomized to two conditions: (1) received verbal instructions; (2) received verbal instructions plus were taught to use automatic visual signals during respiration. Both interventions were successful, but the verbal-only condition was less time consuming. Correct use for both ways of teaching declined over time, again indicating ongoing instruction is important. Another group[86] assessed inhaler techniques after written-only, written plus verbal instruction, and demonstration at the clinic site of use of two new inhalation devices. Written instruction alone was inadequate. Verbal instruction and technique demonstrations were essential to achieve proper administration.

Rand and colleagues[87] measured use of MDI canisters at the time of clinic visits by virtue of a chronologue mechanism. A subset of patients were found to activate the device and dump the medicine just before going to see the physician where measurement of their compliance with the regimen was expected.

One team of investigators[88] examined whether the format for education influenced patients' ability to self-manage COPD, that is, group versus self-instruction. No differences were noted between the two types of programs related to acquisition of skills or management strategies either at the end of training, or at a second assessment 6 months later. Both methods appeared to be equally beneficial.

Other approaches to patient education have been explored. A taped relaxation message was tested in a small but randomly assigned group of COPD patients. Dyspnea, anxiety, and airway obstruction were reduced in patients in the relaxation group compared to controls who were simply asked to sit quietly during the relaxation period.[89]

THE SOCIAL ENVIRONMENT AND COPD

Less is known about how the social environment affects patient management of COPD compared to asthma. High stress levels and lower scores on a social assets scale have been shown to be predictive of hospitalization for persons with COPD.[90] As with asthma, caregivers may experience significant stress from their role. Cossette[91] found the more caregiving tasks a wife performed for a husband with COPD, the more negative mental health outcomes were observed for the wife.

Gender differences in COPD management by the patient have been studied by one team.[92] Self-concept after a pulmonary rehabilitation program increased for patients within 3 weeks, and were still evident 6 months after discharge. Men's self-concept was significantly higher than women's at the 3-week evaluation point, but dropped significantly by the 6-month assessment.

Cystic Fibrosis

Cystic fibrosis is a chronic, fatal disease of genetic origin which requires complex medical treatment. It is most common among white populations. Manifestations of this illness are related to an exocrine defect which leads to chronic airways obstruction and infection, abnormal pancreatic secretions, and deleterious effects on the liver, gastrointestinal tract, respiratory epithelium, reproductive system, and sweat glands.[93] Most therapy is directed at the respiratory and nutritional complications of disease and consists of time-consuming chest physical therapy, antibiotics, pancreatic enzyme supplementation, supplemental feedings, dietary restrictions, and frequent follow-up by a physician.

GOALS OF THERAPY

Goals of therapy include management of symptoms, prevention of complications, and maximum psychosocial well-be-

ing. The medical regimen for cystic fibrosis is complicated and sometimes of dubious effect, making adherence to the recommendations even more difficult to achieve as results are often not readily apparent to the patient. Short-term effects of therapy are particularly difficult to identify.[93] In the past decade, great strides have been made toward increasing the longevity of cystic fibrosis patients through the use of antipseudomonas antibiotics to the point where patients may now live beyond adolescent years and into their third or even fourth decade.[94] This provides a further challenge to patients, caregivers and health care personnel as they must attend to the various developmental tasks of teenage and young adulthood in the context of chronic illness. Tradeoffs may be necessary between optimal medical management and one's attempt to maintain a level of social normalcy.[93]

Bartholomew and coworkers[95] have developed categories of performance objectives for the management of cystic fibrosis by the patient, including: management of lower respiratory infection, respiratory obstruction, and malabsorption; maintenance of adequate nutritional status; appropriate use of health care services; engagement of developmentally appropriate activities; use of coping strategies to manage problems related to cystic fibrosis; and communicating effectively with health care providers, family, and others. Symptom presentation and disease course varies considerably between patients such that the specific management tasks required of each individual also varies.[93]

PSYCHOLOGICAL AND BEHAVIORAL FACTORS ASSOCIATED WITH DISEASE MANAGEMENT BY THE PATIENT WITH CYSTIC FIBROSIS

Virtually no rigorously evaluated disease management programs for patients with cystic fibrosis have been reported in the literature. One small study[96] examined whether a nutrition counseling program based on disease management skills had an effect on calorie intake of patients 4 to 29 years old. At the 4-year follow-up point, significant increases were noted in energy intake and body mass index values. No control group was utilized. An NHLBI Workshop Summary, published in 1987,[93] called for examination of interventions in cystic fibrosis based on models developed in asthma, COPD, and other chronic conditions.

Several studies, however, have identified potential problems associated with disease management for patients and suggested areas of emphasis for interventions. Adolescents with cystic fibrosis and their parents were studied by one team.[97] Patients described problems in self-care decision-making and carrying out home care. Another team[98] found female patients aged 18 to 50 were much less likely than a comparison group without cystic fibrosis to use contraception and more likely to believe the disease reduced fertility. A relatively high proportion of cystic fibrosis patients planned to become pregnant in the near future and were not aware of potentially negative effects of pregnancy on their condition.

THE SOCIAL ENVIRONMENT AND CYSTIC FIBROSIS

Parents of CF patients have described fear, disruption of family life, and difficulties managing at home as important problems. Maternal distress and risk for psychological stress were evident in two studies of mothers of children with cystic fibrosis.[99,100]

One research group[101] used structural modeling to show that feelings of self-efficacy of the patient and caretaker were the most important factors predicting effective monitoring and treatment of CF respiratory problems.

Fear, anxiety, and stress may be more salient for cystic fibrosis patients and families than for patients with other chronic disease,[102] and lead to differences in coping. For example, denial, which is frequently discussed as a negative response to disease, may in the case of cystic fibrosis be functional. Denying a disease for which there is no cure and no certainty about the medical regimen may enable families to carry on with some hope and optimism. Few empirical data exist to describe coping strategies of cystic fibrosis families and how those strategies change over time.

Principles of Patient Management of Lung Disease

Although asthma, COPD, and cystic fibrosis differ in terms of their physiologic presentation and their epidemiology and are unique in many respects, there are some common elements involved in successful patient management of these conditions. First, each requires patients (and/or caretakers) to engage in ongoing day by day decision making to respond to changing situations, and in order to optimally manage symptoms and minimize disruptions in social, psychological, and physical functioning. Second, family members and others close to patients inevitably play a role in either helping or hindering their management efforts to such a degree that their influence must be considered in patient education programs. Third, patients must receive comprehensive education and counseling of a type that will enable them to be effective in decision making and managing their condition. Physicians and other health care professionals play a critical role in this process to build patients' capacity by developing an effective partnership with their patients; one that demonstrates mutual respect and open communication.

Fostering adherence to the therapeutic regimen and encouraging patients to manage disease optimally, requires that the clinician consider the patients' motivations as the impetus for their behavior.

CHRONIC DISEASE MANAGEMENT BY PATIENTS

WHAT PREDISPOSES PATIENTS TO MANAGE AND WHAT IS THE GOAL OF MANAGEMENT?

To understand how to reach the goal of optimum disease management, it helps to see patient behavior in a theoretical framework based on accepted principles of learning and motivation. Several theories of human behavior apply and the model[103] in Fig. 55-1 is proposed, as an illustration, based on three ideas. First, several factors predispose or enable one to manage. Second, patient and family management is the conscious use of strategies to manipulate situations in order to reduce the impact of disease on daily life. One learns what strategies work (or do not) through processes of self-regulation. Third, management is not an end in itself but the means to other ends. These ends include: improved physiologic status; reduction of symptoms and other clinical manifestations of disease; improved functioning; reduced side effects; appropriate health care use, and perhaps the most compelling, better quality of life as perceived by the patient.

In this model, self-regulation is viewed as a means by which patients determine what they will do, given their specific goals and perceptions of their capability. They make these determinations influenced, in large part, by their social contexts and according to the resources they have available.

Articles in the literature have proposed that individuals draw from a base of knowledge about their disease and by virtue of their attitudes, beliefs, and feelings make decisions and take actions.[104] Important external factors that enhance or enable patient management of disease have also been proposed. These include role models from whom management strategies can be learned, technical professional advice and service, social support, money to obtain care and maintain an adequate physical environment. It also must be noted

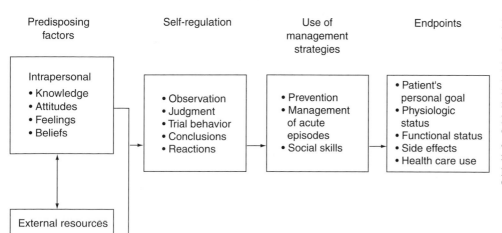

FIGURE 55-1 Patient management of chronic lung disease. Self-regulation is, in part, a function of predisposing intrapersonal and external factors. Self-regulating individuals, influenced by the factors, employ management strategies to achieve a personal goal or endpoint. Other endpoints of concern to clinicians and other health care professionals result from these efforts. (Reprinted, with permission, from Clark and Starr.[103])

that while knowledge, attitudes, and feelings are the basis for action, these can also change as a result of behavior.[105]

An individual uses his or her intrapersonal and external resources and through processes of self-regulation tries to reach a personal goal. An example would be a young man with asthma who wants to play basketball who believes he is susceptible to respiratory problems, thinks medicines will help and so uses them preventively, works out a procedure for taking a breather when active, seeks moral support from his friends and coaches, and uses other strategies that enable him to reach his personal goal. He learns which strategies are effective through self-regulation. Self-regulation may be particularly important in diseases like asthma, COPD, and cystic fibrosis where there is no sure-fire formula an individual can use to control symptoms or deal with interpersonal relationships crucial to optimum management. In these illnesses, patients (and families) must exercise a high degree of decision making usually in the absence of health professionals. The self-regulatory processes in which they engage entail observing situations where their disease contributes to problems in reaching their goals; judging what types of actions might ameliorate the situation; using management strategies, that is, trying out new behavior; and drawing conclusions or reacting to the effects of the behavior. Two important reactions are the conclusion that the behavior resulted in the desired effect, and confidence that one can effectively carry out the behavior, that is, self-efficacy (as defined by Bandura[105]). Using strategies to prevent symptoms or manage them effectively, and to maintain the interpersonal relationships needed to control disease and its effects on one's daily routine should lead to important outcomes. These likely include better quality of life for the patient, including reaching his or her personal goal, as well as improved health status as determined by the clinician, more appropriate use of health services, and so on.

Elements of this model of disease management by patients have been shown to be related to control of asthma.[106] Parents of children with asthma were studied. Those who used more asthma management strategies were also the parents who were more observant of the child's symptoms ($p = .0001$) and who felt more confident (self-efficacious) to manage them ($p = .01$). Taking more preventive actions was also associated with being more observant ($p = .001$). Taking preventive measures was associated with self-efficacy in two ways, first, with feeling confident about keeping the child out of the situation that triggered symptoms ($p = .02$) and, second, about preventing symptoms in general ($p = .001$). In this model, self-regulating individuals are viewed as consciously engaging in the cyclical process of observing, evaluating, and reacting to their own efforts to change behavior and the environment that influences it in order to achieve their personal goals. It suggests that patient education is not a matter of providing information but developing the capacity for self-regulation.

Management of disease by patients is behavior and it is the behavior that must receive our attention. We must focus primarily on what the patients or family members actually do as opposed only to what predisposes them to act: what they know, believe, or feel. Of course, it is important to understand relationships among factors such as knowledge, feelings, attitudes, and behavior. But what makes the difference in outcome is that people actually *behave* in the desired way, not that in the end they know how to behave, or hold particular attitudes. Tests of knowledge, attitudes, and feelings have sometimes been used in lung disease research as proxies for behavior, but these are not the same thing. Knowledge tests have not proven very useful in predicting health behavior. As noted, in studies of asthma among others, the link between knowing general facts about disease, for example, pathophysiology, and behaving differently is not strong.[107] The knowledge patients need is that which enables them to reach their personal goals. This information varies by individual, is very idiosyncratic, and is likely not what the health professional sees as important. Neither are attitudes very useful as predictors of health behavior. The link between general constructs of attitude and specific instances of health behavior is weak.[107] Feelings in general do not predict behavior although feeling confident appears to be very important. Feeling that one is able to carry out a management task has been shown to render people significantly more likely to try the task,[108,109] but even expressions of self-efficacy do not ensure behavior will follow.

Health beliefs have consistently been associated with behavior—especially the beliefs that one is susceptible to disease or further complications, that the consequences of disease could be serious, and that taking the recommended action produces greater benefit than cost.[110] Once again, though, the variance in behavior accounted for by health beliefs is not strong enough for belief to serve as a proxy for taking action. Intention to behave is another belief that has repeatedly been shown in the health literature to be associated with actual behavior (e.g., intending to use relaxation exercises when facing an asthma episode), but intention cannot be considered the same as behavior.[110]

There are two ways clinicians can foster patients' disease management behavior. First, is focusing on effective disease management strategies. These strategies include actions recommended by clinicians to prevent the onset of symptoms and manage episodes and those uncovered in social and behavioral research that enable patients to communicate more effectively to family, health providers, and others, and that enable them to negotiate needed relationships. Second is focusing on the behaviors that constitute self-regulation. These behaviors include patients being more observant of situations precipitating problems, trying different ways to ameliorate these situations, evaluating the efficacy of the strategies tried, reacting by feeling more confident, and refining management strategies through continuing self-regulation.

The clinician, even one with exceedingly limited time to spend with an individual, plays a critical role in enabling better disease management. An extensive amount of research, related to the relationship between health care providers and their patients, has identified ways in which professionals can foster the desired patient behavior. These clinician actions have been described as elements of provider-patient partnership.

CREATING PARTNERSHIP: CLINICIAN TEACHING AND COMMUNICATION BEHAVIOR

The importance of the clinician-patient relationship is especially salient in the management of chronic lung disease. Relationships with chronically ill patients are generally recognized in the practice of clinical medicine as differing significantly from those with acutely ill patients.[111-113] The management of chronic disease is thought to require an ongoing collaboration ("partnership") over months or years between the provider and patient. The clinician helps the patient to assume responsibility for implementing and actively monitoring the therapeutic regimen. The clinician also guides the patient when adjustments in the regimen are needed to gain optimum control over the disease.

Siminoff[114] has suggested that health professionals have four goals in communicating with patients. These are: *cognitive outcomes,* the patients' recall and understanding of what the health professional has said and why the information is important; *affective outcomes,* the reduction of patient anxiety and increasing the satisfaction of the health care provider and patient with the encounter; *behavioral outcomes,* the patient's adherence to the proposed regimen; and *clinical outcomes,* the actual prevention or control of disease or improvement in the patient's clinical condition.

A number of studies have identified factors in clinician-patient interactions beyond the technical dimensions of diagnosis and treatment that influence these four types of outcome, especially, the way patients subsequently manage their disease. Several have focused on barriers to patients trying to follow therapeutic regimens.[115-119] A synthesis of the research related to clinician actions, as well as behavior of clinical support staff, that improve relationships with the patient and augur toward better adherence to the medical regimen was provided by Becker.[120] He suggested that the clinician have a conceptual framework for thinking about patients' adherence to the therapeutic plan such as the model provided in the previous section. Understanding how the patient sees the problem can help the clinician to communicate more effectively and engender better use of medicine by patients.[121-123] Further, the clinician can have significant influence on patient behavior by addressing compliance-related beliefs during the course of the office visit. These beliefs, noted previously, are that one is susceptible to the health problem, that the situation is serious, that the benefits of the therapeutic action being recommended outweigh the costs of carrying it out, and that one has the confidence (feelings of self-efficacy) to take the recommended action.[108]

Several barriers to effective communication have been identified in studies of clinician-patient interaction.[124] It is particularly important for the clinician to recognize that patients: often feel they are wasting the clinician's valuable time; omit details they deem unimportant; are embarrassed to mention things they think will place them in an unfavorable light; do not understand medical terms; and may believe the clinician has not really listened and therefore does not have the information needed to make a good treatment decision.[111] Obviously, when patients do not fully inform clinicians both diagnosis and therapy decisions are affected. Conscious efforts on the professionals' part are needed to overcome these patient inclinations.

Desired outcomes, such as greater satisfaction of the patient with the visit, and willingness to follow the therapeutic plan,[122,125,126] are more likely to occur when the clinician follows communication and learning principles. Findings from several studies[120] suggest that certain behaviors on the part of the professional increase the amount and quality of the information the patient provides.[127] These clinician behaviors

have been identified in studies of the general population of adults and in certain cultural subgroups may not always apply. Nonetheless, they serve as useful guides for clinician behavior: (1) being attentive to the patient (signaled by cues such as using eye contact, sitting rather than standing when conversing with the patient, moving closer to the patient, and leaning slightly forward to attend to the discussion); (2) eliciting the patient's underlying concerns about the condition; (3) constructing reassuring messages that alleviate fears (reducing fear as a distraction to enable the patient to focus on what the clinician is saying); (4) addressing immediate concerns the family expresses (again, enabling patients to refocus their attention toward the information being provided); (5) engaging the patient in interactive conversation through use of open-ended questions, simple language, analogies to teach important concepts (dialogue that is interactive produces richer information); (6) tailoring the regimen by eliciting and addressing potential problems in the timing, dosage, or side effects of the medicines recommended; (7) using appropriate nonverbal encouragement (e.g., a pat on the shoulder, nodding in agreement) and verbal praise when the patient reports using correct disease management strategies; (8) eliciting the patient's immediate objective related to control of the disease and reaching agreement with the family on a short-term goal (that is, an objective that is important to the patient that both provider and patient will strive to reach between one visit and another); (9) reviewing the long-term written plan for the patient's treatment so the patient knows what to expect over time, knows the situations under which the clinician will modify treatment, and knows the criteria for judging the success of the treatment; and (10) helping the patient plan in advance for decision making about the chronic condition (e.g., using daily diary information, or guidelines for handling potential problems, or exploring contingencies in managing the disease).[127]

In one study[128] an association between clinicians' use of communication and teaching strategies and management of asthma by their patients was noted. Physicians who had a better score on a teaching and communication behavior scale were significantly more likely to have patients who were better managers of asthma, defined as their use of peak flow monitoring, a good indicator of attempts to control disease. An additional, very interesting, observation in this study is relevant to busy clinicians. Physicians who used more of the teaching and communication strategies described above spent less time with their patients than clinicians who did not use the techniques. Their patients, however, were significantly more likely to report satisfaction related to time than control group patients, that is, that the clinician had spent enough time with them during the visit. In this study, focused teaching provided via good communication strategies enabled patients to manage disease and increased their perception that the encounter with the clinician had been of the needed duration.

Although the relatively greater need for communication and education provided by clinicians treating patients with chronic compared to acute conditions has not been discussed to a great extent in the literature, it is likely that such interactions are more salient for optimum management of chronic illness where frequent fine-tuning of the treatment plan over the long term is often crucial.

Several behavioral theories support the notion that the

relationship between patient and clinician is, in fact, a significant influence on the behavior of *both*. Social cognitive theory,[105] for example, postulates that personal, social, and behavioral influences interact to cause behavior. Clinicians whose skills engender optimum responses from patients in the form of medicine taking and disease management are likely to be more motivated to continue education and counseling. Patients who feel their clinicians communicate well, and who see positive results from their own informed disease management, will likely be more satisfied with the care they receive and more motivated to take further action to control their condition. This reciprocal reinforcement, over time, may lead to stronger and stronger partnerships between clinician and patient in managing illness.

Directions for Research

Social-behavioral work to date, coupled with advancements in clinical treatment of lung disease, has led to a range of important and interesting research opportunities. A few warrant discussion here.

While we have come a distance in understanding the behavioral aspects of lung disease management by patients, we're still at a rudimentary stage. A rich range of new questions for study await, the answers to which should increase our ability to understand chronic disease management in general. Several questions cut across asthma, COPD, and cystic fibrosis, and others are particular to the given disease.

Important outcomes (e.g., using management strategies, fewer hospitalizations, less family disruption, more confidence) have resulted from patient education in lung disease. However, while the causal chain of relationships between interventions, behavior change, clinical outcome, quality of life, and health care use is implicit in these investigations, the explicit connection or sequence of impact has not been demonstrated. Exploration of these linkages is warranted to ensure causal assumptions are borne out empirically and to enable us to anticipate the relative benefit of different types of programs. For example, if programs improve the quality of life of individuals, can we assume that clinical health status or health service use also improves? At the moment, we cannot answer such questions.

The social environment, including aspects of culture, appears to be a powerful influence on disease self-management. Yet, currently we know very little about these factors. What aspects of intrafamily coping and communication are most conducive to good patient management? What patterns of social support are linked to management behavior and better health status? Do patterns of disease management differ significantly in cultural subgroups and are differences associated with clinical or quality of life outcomes? Social and cultural factors deserve more refined descriptions, and interventions appropriate to the culture of subgroups of the population deserve study.

The relative merit of self-management interventions for individuals at various stages of disease has not been examined. Studies of psychosocial factors and programs to evince change both have tended to combine populations of patients at various levels of severity. It is probable that most aspects of management by the patient differ significantly according

to his or her clinical status. With a few exceptions (for example, children with a history of hospitalization for asthma are more likely to have fewer hospitalizations subsequent to education while change is less evident in children without such a history) we cannot describe predictors or outcomes of interventions according to seriousness of disease. Effective deployment of programs necessitates understanding of which interventions work best for which populations at which stage of illness.

Few studies to date have examined the theoretical underpinnings of disease management by patients. There are several models on which to draw, for example, self-regulation, health belief models, theories of planned (reasoned) action, transtheoretical models, ecological models. Such models try to account for behavior in such a way that outcomes can be predicted. Programs or studies free of predictive theory leave us without explanations for observed results. Quite a bit of lung-related research has been conducted without attention to explicating theory and these studies have not moved us ahead as far as they should. Knowing behavioral mechanisms of effective disease management could lead to much more powerful interventions.

Similarities in management across disease entities seem probable but this assumption has not been rigorously studied. Identifying elements of problem solving and dealing with the social environment common to management of various lung diseases may enhance the efficiency of program delivery. It may be that severity of a disease, rather than which particular condition one has, is the important factor in how one manages and which tasks have to be performed.

Work is needed to examine how gains realized from interventions can be sustained over time. This would entail generating a clearer picture of when effects "kick in" subsequent to education or other ameliorative activities and when they diminish. It would also entail designing interventions with booster or follow-up events at the point of diminishing returns.

The role of health care providers in teaching and otherwise encouraging disease management by their patients is not well understood. Only one or two studies are available to describe the influence of provider actions.[129] The nature of the patient/provider partnership and ways to improve it requires further investigation, perhaps especially related to more severe forms of lung disease.

For the three conditions reviewed here there are somewhat unique research needs given the state of the science and epidemiology of the disease. For example, in asthma, work is needed to distinguish management by older and younger adult patients, men and women, different cultural groups. Studies geared to children with asthma at different age groups, especially adolescence seems warranted. In COPD it is important to understand the added value of different forms of education to exercise conditioning and how to reduce the burden on those caring for patients. In cystic fibrosis a particular challenge is to develop management models or to determine if models for other lung diseases produce desired outcomes. In several diseases (e.g., sarcoidosis) there is little or no behavioral research available.

We are only at the threshold of understanding how patients can effectively manage their lung disease. Nonetheless, it seems clear that social, psychological, and behavioral factors play a significant role.

References

1. Burrows B: The natural history of asthma. *J Allergy Clin Immunol* 80(3):373–377, 1987.
2. Burr ML: Epidemiology of asthma. *Epidemiol Clin Allergy, Monogr Allergy* 31:80–102, 1993.
3. Skobeloff EM, Spivey WH, St. Clair SS, Schoffstall JM: The influence of age and sex on asthma admission. *JAMA* 268(24):3437, 1992.
4. CDC. Asthma—United States, 1980–1987. *MMWR* 39:493, 1990.
5. Lebowitz MD, Barbee R, Burrows B: Family concordance of IgE, atopy, and disease. *J Allergy Clin Immunol* 73:259–264, 1984.
6. Weiss KB, Gergen PJ, Crain EF: Inner-city asthma: The epidemiology of an emerging US public health concern. *Chest* 101(6, suppl):362s–367s, 1992.
7. Platt-Mills TA, Ward GW Jr, Sporik R, et al: Epidemiology of the relationship between exposure to indoor allergens and asthma. *Int Arch Allergy Appl Immunol* 94:339–345, 1991.
8. Block, SH: Inner-city asthma: An allergist's perspective. *Rhode Island Med* 76:191–194, 1993.
9. Chan-Yeung M, Malo JL: Occupational asthma. *Chest* 91:130s–136s, 1987.
10. Wilson-Pessano S, Mellins RB: Summary of workshop discussion. *J Allergy Clin Immunol* 80:487, 1987.
11. Clark NM, Feldman C, Mellins R, et al: The impact of education on frequency and cost of health care utilization of low income children with asthma. *J Allergy Clin Immunol* 78(1):108–115, 1986.
12. Lewis CB, Rachelefsky G, Lewis MA, de la Sota A, Kaplan M: A randomized trial of A.C.T. (asthma care training) for kids. *Pediatrics* 74(4):478–486, 1984.
13. McNabb WL, Wilson-Pessano SR, Hughes GW, Scamagas P: Self-management education of children with asthma: AIR WISE. *Am J Pub Health* 75(10):1219–1220, 1985.
14. Mesters I, Meertens R, Kok G, Parcel GS: Effectiveness of a multidisciplinary education protocol in children with asthma (0–4 years) in primary health care. *J Asthma* 31(5):347–349, 1984.
15. Wilson SR, Mitchell JH, Rolnick S: Effective and ineffective management behaviors of parents of infants and young children with asthma. *J Pediatr Psychol* 18:63–81, 1993.
16. Evans D, Clark NM, Feldman CH, et al: A school health education program for children with asthma aged 8 to 11 years. *Health Educ Q* 14(3):267, 279, 1987.
17. Moe EL, Eisenberg JD, Vollmer WM, et al: Implementation of "Open Airways" as an educational intervention for children with asthma in an HMO. *J Pediatric Health Care* 6(6 pt 1):251–255, 1992.
18. Toelle BG, Peat JK, Salome CM, et al: Evaluation of a community-based asthma management program in a population sample of school children. *Med J Austral* 158(11):742–746, 1993.
19. Wilson SR, Scamagas P, German DF, et al: A controlled trial of two forms of self-management education for adults with asthma. *Am J Med* 94(6):564–576, 1993.
20. Kotses H, Bernstein IL, Bernstein DI, et al: A self-management program for adults with asthma. Part I: Development and evaluation. *J Allergy Clin Immunol* 95(2):529–540, 1995.
21. Bailey WC, Richards JM Jr, Brooks CM, et al: A randomized trial to improve self-management practices of adults with asthma. *Arch Intern Med* 150(80):1664–1668, 1990.
22. Pauley TR, Magee MJ, Cury JD: Pharmacist-managed, physician-directed asthma management program reduces emergency department visits. *Ann Pharmacother* 29(1):5–9, 1995.
23. Bolton MB, Tilley BC, Kuder J, et al: The cost and effectiveness of an education program for adults who have asthma. *J Gen Intern Med* 6(5):401–407, 1991.
24. Mayo PH, Richman J, Harris HW: Results of a program to reduce admissions for adult asthma. *Ann Intern Med* 112(11):864–871, 1990.
25. Yoon R, McKenzie DK, Bauman A, Miles DA: Controlled trial evaluation of an asthma education programme for adults. *Thorax* 48(11):1110–1116, 1993.
26. Kelso TM, Self TH, Rumbak MJ, et al: Educational and long-term therapeutic intervention in the ED: Effect on outcomes in adult indigent minority asthmatics. *Am J Emerg Med* 13(6):632–637, 1995.
27. Heringa P, Lawson L, Reda D: The effect of a structured education program on knowledge and psychomotor skills of patients using beclomethasone dipropionate aerosol for steroid dependent asthma. *Health Educ Q* 14(3):309–317, 1987.
28. Rubin DH, Bauman LJ, Lauby JL: The relationship between knowledge and reported behavior in childhood asthma. *J Devel Behav Pediatr* 10(6):307–312, 1989.
29. Allen RM, Jones MP, Oldenburg B: Randomized trial of an asthma self-management programme for adults. *Thorax* 50(7):731–738, 1995.
30. Trautner C, Richter B, Berger B: Cost-effectiveness of a structured treatment and teaching programme on asthma. *Eur Respir J* 6(10):1485–1491, 1993.
31. Thapar A: Educating asthmatic patients in primary care: A pilot study of small group education. *Family Prac* 11(1):39–43, 1994.
32. Beasley R, DÕSouza W, TeKaru H, et al: Trial of an asthma action plan in the Maori community of the Wairarapa. *N Zealand Med J* 106(961):336–338, 1993.
33. Osman LM, Abdalla MI, Beattie JA, et al: Reducing hospital admission through computer supported education for asthma patients. Grampian Asthma Study of Integrated Care (GRASSIC). *Br Med J* 308(6928):568–571, 1994.
34. Huss K, Squire EN Jr, Carpenter GB, et al: Effective education of adults with asthma who are allergic to dust mites. *J Allergy Clin Immunol* 89(4):836–843, 1992.
35. Harm DL, Kotses H, Creer TL: Portable peak-flow meters: Intrasubject comparisons. *J Asthma* 21(1):9–13, 1984.
36. Burdon JGW, Juniper EF, Killian KJ, et al: The perception of breathlessness in asthma. *Am Rev Respir Dis* 126:825–828, 1982.
37. McFadden ER: An analysis of exercise as a stimulus for production of airway obstruction. *Lung* 159(1):3–11, 1981.
38. Ferguson AC: Persisting airway obstruction in asymptomatic children with asthma with normal peak expiratory flow rates. *J Allergy Clin Immunol* 82:19–22, 1988.
39. Rubinfeld AR, Pain MCF: Perception of asthma. *Lancet* 1(7965):882–884, 1976.
40. Bennett E, Jayson MIV, Rubenstein D, et al: The ability of man to detect added non-elastic loads to breathing. *Clin Sci* 23:155–162, 1962.
41. Shim CS, Williams MH: Evaluation of the severity of asthma: Patients versus physicians. *Am J Med* 68:11–13, 1980.
42. Harm DL, Marion RJ, Kotses H, Creer TL: Effect of subject effort on pulmonary function measures: A preliminary investigation. *J Asthma* 21(5):295–298, 1984.
43. Hyatt RE, Black LF: The flow volume curve. *Am Rev Respir Dis* 107:191–199, 1973.
44. Malo JL, Larcheveque J, Trudeau C, et al: Should we monitor peak expiratory flow rates or record symptoms with a simple diary in the management of asthma? *J Allergy Clin Immunol* 91(3):702–709, 1993.
45. Charlton I, Charlton G, Broomfield J, Mullee MA: Evaluation of peak flow and symptoms only self-management plans for control of asthma in general practice. *Br Med J* 301(6765):1355–1359, 1990.
46. Grampian: Effectiveness of routine self-monitoring of peak flow in patients with asthma. Grampian Asthma Study of Integrated Care (GRASSIC). *Br Med J* 308(6928):564–567, 1994.
47. Jones KP, Mullee MA, Middleton M, et al: Peak flow based asthma self-management: A randomized controlled study in general practice. British Thoracic Society Research Committee. *Thorax* 50(8):851–857, 1995.

48. Ignacio-Garcia JM, Gonzalez-Santos P: Asthma self-management education program by home monitoring of peak expiratory flow. *Am J Respir Crit Care Med* 151(2 pt 1):353–359, 1995.

49. D-Souza W, Crane J, Burgess C, et al: Community-based asthma care: Trial of a "credit card" asthma self-management plan. *Eur Respir J* 7(7):1260–1265, 1994.

50. Mrazek DA, Klinnert MD, Mrazek P, Macey T: Early asthma onset: Consideration of parenting issues. *J Am Acad Child Adolesc Psychiatry* 39(2):277–282, 1991.

51. Spykerboer JE, Donnelly WJ, Thong YH: Parental knowledge and misconceptions about asthma: A controlled study. *Soc Sci Med* 22(5):553–558, 1986.

52. Miles A, Sawyer M, Kennedy D: A preliminary study of factors that influence children's sense of competence to manage their asthma. *J Asthma* 32(6):437–444, 1995.

53. Clark NM, Levison MJ, Evans D, et al: Communication within low income families and the management of asthma. *Patient Educ Couns* 15:191–210, 1990.

54. Wasilewski Y, Clark NM, Evans D, et al: The effect of paternal social support on maternal disruption caused by childhood asthma. *J Common Health* 13(1):33–42, 1988.

55. Schobinger R, Florin I, Reichbauer M, et al: Childhood asthma: Mothers' affective attitude, mother-child interaction and children's compliance with medical requirements. *J Psychosom Res* 37(7):697–707, 1993.

56. Schobinger R, Florin I, Zimmer C, et al: Childhood asthma: Paternal critical attitude and father-child interaction. *J Psychosom Res* 36(8):743–750, 1992.

57. Wilson-Pessano S, Scamagas P, Arsham GM, et al: An evaluation of approaches to asthma self-management education for adults: The AIR/Kaiser-Permanente study. *Health Educ Q* 14(3):333–343, 1987.

58. Nothwehr FK, Clark NM, Bria WF, McMorris MS: Social and behavioral factors in asthma management from the adult patient's perspective. Poster presented at the American Lung Association Conference, May 1996.

59. Janson-Bjerklie S, Ferketich S, Benner P: Predicting the outcomes of living with asthma. *Res Nurs Health* 16(4):241–250, 1993.

60. Strunk RC: Death due to asthma: New insights into sudden unexpected deaths, but the focus remains on prevention. *Am Rev Respir Dis* 148(3):550–552, 1993.

61. Sur S, Crotty TB, Kephart GM, et al: Sudden-onset fatal asthma: A distinct entity with few eosinophils and relatively more neutrophils in the airway submucosa? *Am Rev Respir Dis* 148(3):713–719, 1993.

62. Higgens MW: Chronic airways disease in the United States: Trends and determinants. *Chest* 96(3 suppl):328s–334s, 1989.

63. Dodge R, Cline MG, Burrows B: Comparisons of asthma, emphysema, and chronic bronchitis diagnoses in a general population sample. *Am Rev Respir Dis* 133:981–986, 1986.

64. DHHS: The health consequences of smoking. Chronic obstructive lung disease: A report of the Surgeon General. Rockville, MD: Department of Health and Social Services, Office on Smoking and Health, 1984.

65. Burrows B, Hasan FM, Barbee RA, et al: Epidemiologic observations on eosinophilia and its relation to respiratory disorders. *Am Rev Respir Dis* 122:709–719, 1980.

66. Becklake MR: Occupational exposures: Evidence for a causal association with chronic obstructive pulmonary disease. *Am Rev Respir Dis* 140(3, pt 2):s85–91, 1989.

67. Miedema I, Feskens EF, Heederik D, Kromhout D: Dietary determinants of long-term incidence of chronic nonspecific lung diseases: The Zutphen Study. *Am J Epidemiol* 138(1):37–45, 1993.

68. Sherrill D1, Lebowitz MD, Burrows B: Epidemiology of chronic obstructive pulmonary disease. *Clin Chest Med* 11(3):375–387, 1990.

69. Whittemore AS, Perlin SA, DiCiccio Y: Chronic obstructive pulmonary disease in lifelong nonsmokers: Results from NHANES. *Am J Publ Health* 85(5):702–706, 1995.

70. Bakke PS, Hanoa R, Gulsvik A: Educational level and obstructive lung disease given smoking habits and occupational airborne exposure: A Norwegian community study. *Am J Epidemiol* 141(11):1080–1088, 1995.

71. Di Pede C, Viegi G, Quackenboss JJ, et al: Respiratory symptoms and risk factors in an Arizona population sample of Anglo and Mexican-American whites. *Chest* 99(4):916–922, 1991.

72. Tzonou A, Maragoudakis G, Trichopoulos D, et al: Urban living, tobacco smoking, and chronic obstructive pulmonary disease: A study in Athens. *Epidemiology* 3(1):57–60, 1992.

73. Edelman NH, Cohen AB, Kleinhenz ME, Speizer FE: Chronic obstructive pulmonary disease. Executive Summary. *Chest* 102(3 suppl):243s–256s, 1992.

74. Dudley DL, Glaser EM, Jorgenson BN, et al: Psychosocial concomitants to rehabilitation in chronic obstructive pulmonary disease, Part I: Psychosocial and psychological considerations. *Chest* 77:413–420, 1980.

75. Morgan AD, Peck DF, Buchanan DH, et al: Psychological factors contributing to disproportionate disability in chronic bronchitis. *J Psychosom Res* 27:259–261, 1983.

76. Light RW, Merrill EJ, Despars JA, et al: Prevalence of depression and anxiety in patients with COPD: Relationship to functional capacity. *Chest* 87:35–38, 1985.

77. Mall TW, Medeiros M: Objective evaluation of results of a pulmonary rehabilitation program in a community hospital. *Chest* 94(6):1156–1160, 1988.

78. Toshima MT, Kaplan RM, Ries AL: Experimental evaluation of rehabilitation in chronic obstructive pulmonary disease: Short-term effects on exercise endurance and health status. *Health Psychol* 9(3):237–252, 1990.

79. Ojanen M, Lahdensuo A, Laitinen J, Karvonen J: Psychosocial changes in patients participating in a chronic obstructive pulmonary disease rehabilitation program. *Respiration* 60(2):96–102, 1993.

80. Ries AL, Kaplan RM, Limberg TM, Prewitt LM: Effects of pulmonary rehabilitation on physiologic and psychosocial outcomes in patients with chronic obstructive pulmonary disease. *Ann Intern Med* 122(11):823–832, 1995.

81. Cox NJ, Henddricks JC, Binkhorst RA, van Herwaarden CL: A pulmonary rehabilitation program for patients with asthma and mild chronic obstructive pulmonary diseases (COPD). *Lung* 171(4):235–244, 1993.

82. Howland J, Nelson EC, Barlow PB, et al: Chronic obstructive airway disease: Impact of health education. *Chest* 90(2):233–238, 1986.

83. Sassi-Dambron DE, Eakin EG, Ries AL, Kaplan RM: Treatment of dyspnea in COPD: A controlled clinical trial of dyspnea management strategies. *Chest* 107(3):724–729, 1995.

84. Tougaard L, Krone T, Sorknaes A, Ellegaard H: Economic benefits of teaching patients with chronic obstructive pulmonary disease about their illness: The PASTMA Group. *Lancet* 339(8808):1517–1520, 1992.

85. De Blaquiere P, Christensen DB, Carter WB, Martin TR: Use and misuse of metered-dose inhalers by patients with chronic lung disease: A controlled, randomized trial of two instruction methods. *Am Rev Respir Dis* 140(4):910–916, 1989.

86. Nimmo CJ, Chen DN, Martinsen SM, et al: Assessment of patient acceptance and inhalation technique of a pressurized aerosol inhaler and two breath-actuated devices. *Ann Pharmacotherapy* 27(7–8):922–927, 1993.

87. Rand CS, Mides M, Cowles MK, et al: Long-term metered-dose inhaler adherence in a clinical trial: The Lung Health Study Research Group. *Am J Respir Crit Care Med* 152(2):580–588, 1995.

88. Brough FK, Schmidt CD, Rasmussen T, Boyer M: Comparison

of two teaching methods for self-care training for patients with chronic obstructive pulmonary disease. *Patient Couns Health Educ* 492:111–116, 1982.

89. Gift AG, Moore T, Soeken K: Relaxation to reduce dyspnea and anxiety in COPD patients. *Nurs Res* 42(4):242–246, 1992.

90. Jensen PS: Risk, protective factors, and supportive interventions in chronic airway obstruction. *Arch Gen Psychiatry* 40(11):1203–1207, 1983.

91. Cossette S, Levesque L: Caregiving tasks as predictors of mental health of wife caregivers of men with chronic obstructive pulmonary disease. *Res Nurs Health* 16(4):251–263, 1993.

92. Kersten L: Changes in self-concept during pulmonary rehabilitation, Part I. *Heart Lung* 19(5 pt 1):456–462, 1990.

93. Eigen H, Clark NM, Wolle JM: Clinical-behavioral aspects of cystic fibrosis: Directions for future research. NHLBI Workshop Summary. *Am Rev Respir Dis* 136:1509–1513, 1987.

94. Matthews LW, Drotar D: Cystic fibrosis—A challenging long-term chronic disease. *Pediatr Clin North Am* 31(1):133–152, 1984.

95. Bartholomew LK, Sockrider MM, Seilheimer DK, et al: Performance objectives for the self-management of cystic fibrosis. *Patient Educ Couns* 22:15–25, 1993.

96. Luder E, Gilbride JA: Teaching self-management skills to cystic fibrosis patients and its effect on their caloric intake. *J Am Dietetic Assoc* 89(3):359–364, 1989.

97. Nuttall P, Nicholes P: Cystic fibrosis: Adolescent and maternal concerns about hospital and home care. *Issues Comprehens Pediatr Nurs* 15(3):199–213, 1992.

98. Sawyer SM, Phelan PD, Bowes G: Reproductive health in young women with cystic fibrosis: Knowledge, behavior and attitudes. *J Adolesc Health* 17(1):46–50, 1995.

99. Mullins LL, Olson RA, Reyes S, et al: Risk and resistance factors in the adaptation of mothers of children with cystic fibrosis. *J Pediatr Psychol* 16(6):701–715, 1991.

100. Walker LS, Ortiz-Valdes JA, Newbrough JR: The role of maternal employment and depression in the psychological adjustment of chronically ill, mentally retarded, and well children. *J Pediatr Psychol* 14(3):357–370, 1989.

101. Parcel GS, Swank PR, Mariotto MJ, et al: Self-management of cystic fibrosis: A structural model for educational and behavioral variables. *Soc Sci Med* 38(9):1307–1315, 1994.

102. Lawler RH, Nakielny W, Wright NA: Psychological implications of cystic fibrosis. *Can Med Assoc J* 94:1043–1046, 1966.

103. Clark NM, Starr NS: Management of asthma by patients and families. *Am J Respir Crit Care Med* 149:S54–66, 1994.

104. Clark N, Zimmerman BJ: A social cognitive view of self-regulated learning about health. *Health Educ Res* 5(3):371–379, 1990.

105. Bandura A: *Social Foundations of Thought and Action: A Social Cognitive Theory,* Englewood Cliffs, NJ, Prentice-Hall, 1986.

106. Clark NM, Evans D, Zimmerman BJ, et al: Patient and family management of asthma: Theory based techniques for the clinician. *J Asthma* 3(16):427–435, 1994.

107. Becker MH: Patient adherence to prescribed therapies. *Med Care* 23(5):539–555, 1985.

108. Clark N, Rosenstock I, Hassan H, et al: The effect of health beliefs and feelings of self-efficacy on self-management behavior of children with a chronic disease. *Patient Couns Educ* 11(2):131–139, 1988.

109. O'Leary A: Self-efficacy and health. *Behav Res Ther* 23(4):437–451, 1985.

110. Janz NK, Becker MH: The health belief model: A decade later. *Health Educ Q* 11:1–47, Spring 1984.

111. Anderson LA, Zimmerman MA: Patient and physician perceptions of their relationship and patient satisfaction: A study of chronic disease management. *Patient Couns Educ* 20:27–36, 1993.

112. Jennings B: Ethical challenges of chronic illness. *Hastings Center Rep* 18(1)Suppl:1–16, 1988.

113. Sankar A, Becker SL: The home as a site for teaching gerontology and chronic illness. *J Med Educ* 60:308–313, 1985.

114. Siminoff LA: Cancer patient and physician communications: Progress and continuing problems. *Ann Behav Med* 11(3):108–112, 1989.

115. Beckman HB, Frankel RM: The effect of physician behavior on the collection of data. *Ann Intern Med* 101:692–696, 1984.

116. Becker MH, Maiman LA: Strategies for enhancing patient compliance. *J Commun Health* 6:113–135, 1980.

117. DiMatteo MR, DiNicola DD: *Achieving Patient Compliance: The Psychology of the Practitioners Role.* New York, Pergamon Press, 1984.

118. Starfield B, Wray C, Hess K, et al: The influence of patient-practitioner agreement on outcome of care. *AJPH* 71:127–131, 1981.

119. Wasserman RC, Inui T, Barriatua R, et al: Pediatric clinicians' support for parents: An outcome-based analysis of clinician-parent interaction. *Pediatrics* 74:1047–1053, 1984.

120. Becker MH: Theoretical models of adherence and strategies for improving adherence, in Schumaker SA, Schron EG, Ockene JK (eds): *Handbook of Health Behavior Change.* New York, Springer, 1990.

121. Inui TS, Yourtee EL, Williamson JW: Improved outcomes in hypertension after physician tutorials. *Ann Intern Med* 84:646–651, 1976.

122. Maiman LA, Becker MH, Liptak GS, et al: Improving pediatricians' compliance-enhancing practices: A randomized trial. *Am J Dis Child* 142:773–779, 1988.

123. Rosenstock IM, Strecker VJ, Becker MH: Social learning theory and the health belief model. *Health Educ Q* 15:175–183, 1988.

124. Clark NM: Management of asthma by parents and children, in Kotses H, (ed): *Self Management of Asthma.* Marcel Dekker, New York, 1998.

125. Eraker SA, Becker MH: Improving compliance for the patient with diabetes. *Pract Diabetol* 3:6–11, 1984.

126. Maiman LA, Becker MH: The clinician's role in patient compliance. *Trends Pharmacol Sci* 1:457–459, 1980.

127. Clark NM, Nothwehr F, Gong M, et al: Physician-patient partnership in managing chronic illness. *Acad Med* 70(11):957–969, 1995.

128. Clark NM, Gong M, Schork MA, et al: A scale for assessing health care providers' teaching and communication behavior regarding asthma. *Health Education and Behavior* 24:245–256, 1997.

129. Clark NM, Gong M, Schork MA, et al: Impact of Education for Physicians on Patient Outcomes. *Pediatrics* 101:831–836, 1998.

Chapter 56 _____

MEDICAL ECONOMICS AND COST EFFECTIVENESS

DOUG ORENS

DEBORAH SCHNEIDER

VINOD SAHGAL

As we enter the era of managed care, the capability to allocate health care resources to members of society is becoming increasingly difficult. The cost of providing health care has become a major issue within our society. The public and private sectors continue to demand that health care expenses be curtailed and some form of coverage be accessible to all members of the society. Realization that health care expenditures have been growing at an exponential rate is common knowledge. In 1980 health care consumed 9.4 percent of the GNP; today 17 percent of the GNP is devoted to providing health care to members of our society. As we undergo the current health care revolution, the ways in which we distribute health care will be thoroughly examined. Review of the specific treatment modalities, plans, and methods will continue in order to determine the least costly means of providing care while maintaining positive outcomes. The emphasis will be placed on the prevention and maintenance by developing programs to educate and enlighten the public in various aspects of health care, which in the final analysis will reduce costs. Pulmonary rehabilitation programs are but one of many that will need to justify their existence in terms of overall benefit from a cost perspective. The primary topic of discussion of this chapter will be the analysis of pulmonary rehabilitation programs as a cost-effective method of providing debilitated pulmonary patients a means of maintaining an acceptable standard of life. Equally important is an overview of how our health care system has evolved which is essential to the understanding where programs such as pulmonary rehabilitation will fit into the health care system heading into the 21st century.

Elements of a Successful Pulmonary Rehabilitation Program

Pulmonary rehabilitation was first defined by a committee of the American College of Chest Physicians in 1974: "Pulmonary rehabilitation may be defined as an art of medical practice wherein an individually tailored multi disciplinary program is formulated which through accurate diagnosis, therapy, emotional support and education, stabilizes or reverses both the physio- and psychopathology of pulmonary disease and attempts to return the patient to the highest possible functional capacity allowed by his/her pulmonary handicap and overall life situation."[1] This statement is still valid today and is considered to be the universal definition

of pulmonary rehabilitation programs. Pulmonary rehabilitation has come to be the recognized treatment for patients with chronic obstructive pulmonary disease (COPD) and other related lung diseases. Reimbursement for pulmonary rehabilitation services however may not always be obtainable from the third-party payers. It is with this understanding that pulmonary rehabilitation programs must work to demonstrate that their outcomes help reduce the overall cost of health care. A variety of elements are available in pulmonary rehabilitation programs that allow for individually tailored treatment. Programs may vary depending on the needs of each individual patient; not all patients may require each component of pulmonary rehabilitation. The contents of a successful pulmonary rehabilitation program have been described by several authors.[1-6] Members of the rehabilitation team are listed in Table 56-1. A summary of the main components of pulmonary rehabilitation programs are as follows; education, medications, physical and occupational therapy, exercise conditioning, respiratory therapy modalities, psychosocial counseling, and vocational training.[1-3,7-11]

Education can cover a variety of topics that generally include but are not limited to an understanding of the patient's disease process, prevention of lung disease becoming a major objective of pulmonary rehabilitation programs, suitable nutrition and managing weight, smoking cessation, managing shortness of breath, environmental aspects, as well as instruction in the use and care of equipment. The goal of the educational component is to help patients get a thorough understanding of their illness and what is available in terms of helping them maintain the highest functional standard of living. Medications generally prescribed to pulmonary patients are bronchodilators, corticosteroids, cromolyn sodium, antimicrobials, diuretics, digitalis, and psychopharmacologic agents. These are used to keep the disease process under control. Physical therapy includes such measures as breathing retraining, managing dyspnea, relaxation techniques, bronchopulmonary hygiene (includes percussion, vibration, and postual drainage), as well as coughing and deep breathing exercises. The goal of physical therapy is to reduce those factors (apprehension, excessive sputum) that contribute to the patient's overall shortness of breath. Occupational therapy commonly used in conjunction with pulmonary rehabilitation programs includes work simplification, evaluation of daily activities of life, energy conservation, use of upper limb activities, and devices available to assist with daily activities of living. Exercise conditioning has been shown to improve work capacity in patients with COPD. The most common types of exercises used are walking or stair climbing. Respiratory muscle and upper and lower limb strengthening exercises are also used within exercise conditioning programs. Patients generally feel a sense of accomplishment and well-being when mastering their conditioning programs. Respiratory therapy modalities can run the gamut from oxygen therapy, aerosolized medications delivery devices, monitoring alarms, CPAP apparatus to mechanical ventilation. Proper instruction in utilization of respiratory therapy techniques and maintenance of equipment is an integral part of pulmonary rehabilitation. If there is a problem in technique or with equipment performance there is a good chance that the patient will not receive optimal care. Psychosocial counseling is another critical piece. Anxiety, depression, denial, fear, and hostility are a consequence of

665

TABLE 56-1 Pulmonary Rehabilitation Team Members

1. Physician
2. Nurse
3. Respiratory therapist
4. Physical therapist
5. Occupational therapist
6. Dietitian
7. Social worker
8. Pharmacist
9. Psychologist

COPD. These problems can be further compounded as the disease progresses, resulting in the loss of employment, decreased physical capacity, social activities, sexual vigor; all or combinations of the above lead to reduced self-esteem. All these issues should be addressed in a pulmonary rehabilitation program. Counseling is useful when dealing with stress reduction, relaxation, relieving patients fears about their disease process or death. Vocational training depends on the patient's age and the degree of severity of the disease. Many patients are unable to perform duties of their job.

Some need to be taught how to maximize their physical capacity in the work environment. Training for a new job or retraining patients in the performance of their current jobs is accomplished in the program.

These programs, thus, are based on a multispeciality approach. By "fitting each patient with his/her own individual wardrobe" (of these elements that are based on the patient's disease process) the goal is to maximize the functional outcome.

Economic Components of a Pulmonary Rehabilitation Program

A pulmonary rehabilitation program requires a number of considerations to be successful, such as strategic planning, reimbursement issues, and reporting, as well as to marketing the program.[1,3,4,7,8,12–15] This program requires a thorough assessment of the services to be provided, and the reimbursement for the rendered services.

A strategic plan should relate to the long-term goals of the institution, physician group, and/or the individual department. It should allow for an assessment of both the cost and clinical perspective of each component of the program. The payment issues are a key factor to be taken into account when assessing the external environment. A complete understanding of the reimbursement policies is a critical piece of external environmental analysis. It is essential to understand the rules and regulations of each reimbursement system. Knowing the payor mix will allow for short- and long-term planning in terms of available cash flow. Labor and equipment expenses are easily planned for by developing a business plan. Other factors of importance are the changing health care policies, the number of patients in the program, and the extent of the comprehensive services that will allow the institution or physician group to meet program goals. The business plan addresses the number of patients, patient visits, projected volume of therapies, and program outcomes.

Preparing a budget is critical to the development of a cost-effective program. The budget should include operating expenses (labor, equipment, and supplies) and proposed revenues. Expenses should take into account labor costs which include benefits and overtime, as well as any other associated employee costs. The operating costs include minor and major capital equipment required and medical supplies needed to perform services, as well as office. Travel expenses are important if home visits are part of the service package. Accounting for the physical facilities and the resources required to house the operation are required for the budgeting process. Revenues are the remaining piece of this process. Today's reimbursement policies are constantly changing and require constant review in order to assess their financial return. One must plan to provide services and receive revenues from all types of reimbursement systems, such as managed care programs, fee-for-service, Medicare, or Medicaid. Determination of collectible revenues will allow the program to be funded to provide effective care. The ability to accurately assess revenue capture is one of the most important aspects of planning. A system that easily and clearly reports all aspects of the economic components of daily operations is critical. These reporting systems can be internal, that is, monthly office supply expense reports, or external, that is, accounts receivable from patients. The point being that a distinct economic report allows operations to flow without impediment. A poor financial reporting system can cause patients and third-party payers to become dissatisfied with the program.

An effective marketing strategy is essential to promote and sell the design to prospective customers. Marketing a program that offers pulmonary rehabilitation services should be equipped to meet the needs of the population which will benefit from the program. The market segment, "those consumers who will utilize the services," should be identified and targeted as potential customers. Patients, physicians, businesses, insurance companies, HMOs, and health care institutions are some examples of potential customers. Promoting the services that are offered by a program will allow potential customers to determine if their needs will be realized. Advertising, lectures promoting pulmonary rehabilitation, providing simple tests (i.e., measuring peak flow), as a public service, and simple word of mouth are some ways to promote a new program that provides pulmonary services. Developing a brochure is an excellent way of promoting all the aspects of a program. A brochure allows for penetration into all segments of the marketplace.

Marketing a new program will benefit all involved. Understanding and implementing an effective marketing plan will ensure a successful beginning for any new program. Determining the number of patients within the local geographic area that would attend the program, and knowing what services or programs the competition is offering adds to a successful analysis. The internal environmental analysis takes into account the elements that make up the program. Consideration of what services to provide, staffing levels, schedules for implementation, equipment considerations, and contingency plans are all incorporated into this analysis. An important aspect of assessing the internal environment is to keep focused on the institution's or group's mission statement. This will keep the planning phase on target and allow the program to be assimilated into the organization's overall strategy.

TABLE 56-2 Methods of Evaluating Pulmonary Rehabilitation
Programs

**TABLE 56-2 Methods of Evaluating Pulmonary Rehabilitation
Programs**

1. Cost-benefit analysis (dollars spent/dollars saved)
2. Cost-utility (dollars spent/added useful years of life)
3. Cost-effectiveness (dollars spent/improvement in specific outcomes)
4. Cost-minimization (determine minimum dollars/for a specific outcome)

The Cost Benefit Analysis of Pulmonary Rehabilitation Programs

Most practitioners who engage in the practice of pulmonary medicine realize that there are definite enhancements both economically and in terms of quality of life issues when patients come in contact with a program tailored to meet the specific needs of their respiratory illness. The issue is to define what these advantages are and determine what impact they have in the overall allocation of health care resources. Economic evaluations include the pulmonary program itself, or various components such as health education, physical therapy (exercise programs), occupational therapy, nutrition, home care services, oxygen therapy, aerosolized medications, and instruction in various respiratory therapy modalities, such as, nasal CPAP.[16,17] Economic evaluations or analysis can be partial or full.[16] Partial economic evaluations are restricted in terms of outcomes or costs, or provide no alternatives, whereas in full economic evaluations a comparison is made between outcomes and costs for two or more alternatives. A number of authors have classified economic evaluations into one or more primary categories (see Table 56-2).

Cost benefit is defined as the traditional classification which takes into account the fiscal outcomes of a pulmonary rehabilitation program.[16,18] A number of pulmonary rehabilitation program cost-benefit studies have been identified in the literature.[16–20] The main theme of most of these studies is to show that a comprehensive program has an impact on cost reduction, or the individual components of a program can reduce health care costs. Some common examples of this show a reduction in the number of hospital admissions, length of hospital stay, or the number of outpatient or physician office visits. Kaplan and Ries summarize a number of cost-benefit studies on rehabilitation of patients with COPD.[18] In summary, cost-benefit evaluations are a way to interpret the financial impact of pulmonary rehabilitation programs or the effects of their components against the savings of health care dollars.

In a cost-utility analysis, the benefits are described as quality-adjusted life-years which are a direct result of the resources used to achieve the additional quality years.[16,18] When one examines the above definition it reflects on the purpose of providing health care to debilitated patients. Cost-utility requires the analysis of outcome data that illustrate a benefit in terms of added years. The method of cost-utility analysis is to divide the cost of a program by the amount of life-years that it produces. Review of the literature reveals that more studies need to be done to identify the cost-utility analysis of pulmonary rehabilitation in comparison to the other programs. Continued evaluation of pulmonary rehabil-

itation programs is required to determine if these are adding a cost-utility to the patients. One such study by Toves and coworkers evaluated the compliance of patients in a pulmonary rehabilitation program and determined that the program produced a "well year" at a unit cost of $24,256.[21]

Cost effectiveness can be explained as any outcome that results from some form of treatment provided by the program.[16,18,22] In cost-effectiveness analysis outcomes can be measured in quality-of-life scales, distance walked, reduction of forced expiratory volumes, or added life-years. Providing low-flow oxygen which reduces hypoxemia and dyspnea and allows a patient to perform activities of daily living and maintain employment can be classified as cost-effectiveness. Holle and associates demonstrated an example of cost-effectiveness in their report of increased muscle efficiency and sustained benefits that patients received in an outpatient community hospital–based pulmonary rehabilitation program. The issue with cost effectiveness is that it does not allow for comparisons across different treatment interventions as discussed by Kaplan and Reis.[18]

In a cost-minimization evaluation one determines how to obtain the same outcome at the lowest cost.[16] A determination of the most effective delivery device of aerosolized medications that yields the best results would be an example of a cost-minimization analysis. In most patients a metered dose inhaler (MDI) would be the effective aerosolized medication delivery device. But for those patients who cannot coordinate the MDI there would be minimal therapeutic benefit and the cost-minimization impact would be insignificant. Bach and coworkers assessed the costs of providing mechanical ventilation in an institutional versus in-home setting.[23] A cost analysis demonstrated that the in-home setting appeared to be an effective way of obtaining the same outcome at a lower cost. Cost-minimization evaluations focus on the assessment of costs and are generally used in conjuction with some other form of economic analysis.

Whichever analysis is utilized there is one common objective, that is, to determine the effectiveness of pulmonary rehabilitation programs or their components. A determination in terms of cost-benefit is required to realistically evaluate the overall positive outcome that the program or one of its components is providing to pulmonary debilitated patients.

Medical Economics of a Pulmonary Rehabilitation Program

Currently, pulmonary rehabilitation programs have not been viewed in terms of reimbursement with the same enthusiams as some established programs such as cardiac rehabilitation.[18] Reimbursement has not been easily obtained for these programs. Justification of the services administered by pulmonary rehabilitation programs require more outcome measures to be reported in order to be adequately compensated. Reimbursement for pulmonary rehabilitation services is provided via four kinds of mechanisms.[24–26] The first mechanism, which is growing in popularity in particular with the public and private sector, is managed care. This reimbursement mechanism is confusing as one explores what managed care entails. The second mechanism is fee-for-service. The third and fourth, Medicare and Medicaid, provide for reimbursement for health care services by utilizing public moneys.

Currently there is concern about maintaining the solvency of the Medicare system due to the explosion of health care costs within our society.

Perhaps the greatest confusion in understanding reimbursement issues lies in the fact that we are moving from a fee-for-service method to a truly capitated system under the managed care concept.

MANAGED CARE

Managed care is a system of health care delivery that manages the cost, quality, and access of providing health care to its members. The concept of managed care has evolved over the last 30 to 40 years and is a product that has emerged as an outgrowth of our free enterprise system. Currently, managed health care is actually a number of plans ranging from health maintenance organizations (HMOs) to preferred provider organizations (PPOs).[26-30] There are a number of hybrids of the two main types of managed care systems which tend to cloud the reimbursement picture. A brief overview of each of the primary types of managed care will be discussed.

HMOs are health care systems that assume the risk of providing the financing and the delivery of a number of broad-ranged health care services to enrolled groups of customers. HMOs can be thought of as a combination of the health insurer and delivery system. They are responsible for providing health care services by utilizing primary care physicians as gatekeepers, to members through affiliated providers who are reimbursed. HMOs have recently assumed the responsibility of assuring the quality and appropriateness of the health care provided to its members. There are five common models of HMOs: staff, network, group, direct contact, and IPA.

Physicians in a staff model are employed by the HMO. Staff models are known as closed-panel HMOs because most participating physicians are employed by the HMO and community physicians are unable to participate. Staff model HMOs usually contract with hospitals or other inpatient facilities to provide nonphysician services for their membership. The advantage of staff model HMOs appears to be that they have a greater degree of control of physician practice patterns than other HMO models. The main disadvantage of staff model HMOs is that they are quite costly to develop and operate.

Network HMOs contract with multiple group practices to provide physician services to the HMO's customers. The group is responsible for providing all physician services to the HMO's members. Network models have the advantage of providing potential customers the option of using additional services outside of many traditional HMO plans.

In a group HMO model, the HMO contracts with a multispeciality physician group practice to provide all physician services to its members. The physicians are employed by the group practice and not by the HMO. There are generally two types of group models. The first being the captive model in which the physician group provides services exclusively to the HMO's members. An example of this group is the Kaiser Foundation Health Plan, where the Permanente Medical Groups provide all physician services and the Kaiser Foundation Health Plan is the licensed HMO that is responsible for enrolling customers, collecting payments, and performing other functions required by HMOs. The second type of group model is the independent, in which the HMO contracts with an existing, independent, multispeciality physician group to provide physician services to its members. Both classifications of group models are considered to be closed-panel HMOs. Physicians must be members of the group practice to participate in the HMO. Group model HMOs provide a limited choice of physicians for their memberships which has resulted in restricting the geographic accessibility to its members. The perception of high quality associated with many of the physician group practices that are aligned with the HMO balances the disadvantages of group HMOs.

Direct contract HMO models contract directly with individual physicians to provide physician services to their customers. Direct contract model HMOs recruit community physicians. They enlist both primary care and specialist physicians while utilizing a case management approach.

With the individual practice association (IPA) model HMOs contract with an association of physicians. The physicians belong to the IPA but remain as individual practitioners. They see their own patients while maintaining their own practice. IPAs can be spread over an entire community or can be hospital based and developed so that physicians from a limited number of hospitals can participate in the model. IPA models hurdle all the disadvantages associated with the majority of the models previously described. IPA models require less capital and cash flow to start and operate. They provide a broad network of participating physicians who practice over a large portion of the community. The five models of HMOs can often overlap and add to the confusion in understanding the elements that make up the managed care climate.

Another important form of managed care is preferred provider organizations (PPOs). PPOs are organizations with which company health benefit plans and health insurance firms contract to purchase health care services for members from a selected group of participating providers. Providers who participate in the PPOs agree to accept reimbursement and payment levels, as well as utilization control and other management procedures directed by the PPO. As a result, PPOs often restrict the size of their participating providers and provide incentives for their covered members to use participating providers instead of other providers. This differs from the conventional HMO coverage as patients with PPO coverage are permitted to use non-PPO providers, although they often have higher levels of coinsurance or deductibles. PPOs contract with physicians, hospitals, and other types of health care facilities. PPOs negotiate payment rates that are competitive and provide an advantage to other types of managed care plans. Payment plans that include bundled packages of services are a common feature of PPOs. Many PPOs employ utilization controls that oversee the effectiveness and costs of services that are provided to their covered members. HMOs and PPOs and their hybrids are the components of the managed care system. Managed care and its multitude of plans have different attributes which all attempt to address cost and access to care, while maintaining quality of the provided services. Managed care continues to evolve and change as our health care system moves toward the 21st century.

MEDICARE AND MEDICAID

Medicare, Title XVIII of the Social Security Act, is a federal health insurance program for those entitled to Social Security. These individuals include those over age 65, those under age 65 who are entitled to Social Security disability benefits, and those with end stage renal disease. Medicare consists of two parts, Part A and Part B. Part A covers inpatient hospital services and other institutional health care providers. Part B, a voluntary program which requires additional premiums to be paid, covers physician services, as well as outpatient care.

In 1977, Medicare was placed under the jurisdiction of the Department of Health and Human Services, specifically the Health Care Financing Administration (HCFA). HCFA determines the policies affecting Medicare. Nationwide, there are 10 HCFA regional offices to oversee 10 geographic regions of the country. Each region is assigned a fiscal intermediary to act as a liaison between HCFA and the provider. Although HCFA determines Medicare policy, it is the intermediaries who interpret these policies. Often, it is the inconsistencies in the interpretation of the policies that lead to differences in reimbursement from region to region.

In 1982, with the passage of The Tax Equity and Fiscal Responsibility ACT (TEFRA), Medicare reimbursement for inpatient care changed from actual patient care costs for individuals, to the overall cost of care for the facility. This change was accomplished by calculating the mean cost for all discharges from the hospital during a year period, called the base year, and then paying up to that amount for each discharge. The amount set during the base year for each discharge was determined as the TEFRA limit.[31] Congress controls industry-wide annual adjustments to the TEFRA limit. The adjustments are intended to compensate for some of the changes of providing care and to provide facilities a financial incentive to provide efficient care.

In 1983, with the passage of Public Law 21 (PL-21), Congress changed the Medicare payment system to a prospective payment method called diagnosis-related groupings (DRG).[31,32] Specialized hospitals such as psychiatric, pediatric, long-term care hospitals, and free standing rehabilitation hospitals were exempt from the DRG payment system.[31] Rehabilitation and psychiatric units within an acute care hospital could also be exempted from the prospective payment system if they met the strict Prospective Payment System exclusion criteria. Most rehabilitation units within acute care hospitals, as well as free standing rehabilitation hospitals, meet the exclusion criteria and are, therefore, currently paid under the TEFRA system.

Many rehabilitation providers agree that the TEFRA system of reimbursement is grossly inadequate. As the TEFRA payment system is based on average costs during the base year, older rehabilitation hospitals and units have a significantly lower limit than newer programs which have a more recent base year.[24,32] Additionally, as the TEFRA payments system does not include any calculations for the intensity of care, there appears to be an incentive for rehabilitation

programs to provide care for less complex patients who require lower average cost of care, rather than more complex patients who would require higher resource consumption to meet their care needs.[31] Finally, as the rate of annual increase in the TEFRA limit is legislated, it has not kept pace with the increases in costs of providing care.[24]

Acute inpatient rehabilitation services are reimbursed as discussed earlier under Part A, limited to the TEFRA limit for that facility. Claims and benefit administration for Part A of Medicare are processed through the regional intermediary. The treatment covered must be determined to be medically necessary based on the patient diagnosis and condition.[24] Documentation of patient-specific goals set within a defined time frame and progress toward these goals are required to ensure reimbursement.

Outpatient services, as covered in Part B of Medicare, are processed by insurance companies called "carriers." Eligibility for Part B is based on a voluntary enrollment for those individuals who receive Part A Medicare.[33] Additional premiums paid by the beneficiary, are required for Part B coverage. Again, medical necessity or "reasonable and necessary" is the key to reimbursement. Those services which are required due to the patient diagnosis or condition can be billed under Medicare Part B. Some services which are not covered are: health promotion, routine exercise, routine screening evaluations, films and videos, and any service which is also provided by another service, such as occupational or physical therapy.[24] Reimbursement is currently at the rate of 80 percent of the Medicare approved amount for the service or item. Home health care coverage is also provided under Part B. Coverage of these services is determined on the basis of hours per week for skilled nursing, home health aids, and skilled therapy needs. To be eligible for home health care services, the patient must be homebound.

Medicaid or Title XIX of the Social Security Act is an entitlement program. Medicaid provides health insurance for low-income individuals and families. Both the federal and state level of government finance this program. The federal government reimburses sixty percent and the state government reimburses forty percent. Eligibility is based on income and expenses at a state-determined income level. The program is administered at the state level from the Department of Human Services. Medicaid provides both inpatient and outpatient care, as well as coverage for prescription medication. Physician care and long-term care are also covered services. Currently, many states are moving toward a managed care process to manage the health care needs of the Medicaid population.

FEE-FOR-SERVICE

The fee-for-service method of reimbursement emulates the way our society has blossomed from our inception into the economy we experience today.[26,34] It is a system that pays immediate rewards for the quantity of services performed. The more services that are provided the greater the reimbursement received for those services. With the fee-for-service system most physicians develop fees which are classified as usual, customary, or reasonable (UCR).[26] In general, physicians submit their bills and are reimbursed for their services. The issue with UCRs is that there is little consistency among physician fees for similar services. Today, there is a way to determine a reasonable UCR charge. Collect charges that have similar CPT codes, calculate the charge that represents the 90th percentile and call that the UCR maximum.[26] If a claim submitted is less than the 90th percentile the amount is paid in full. If it is higher than the 90th percentile it is paid at the UCR maximum. This practice is commonly used in many managed health care plans. Services are reimbursed for by Medicare by a method similar to UCR. A fee is set for a specific service or procedure and 80 percent of that fee is reimbursed by the government. This 80 percent represents the UCR fee for that particular service or procedure. By utilizing the percentage of UCR method everyone involved understands how the fee was determined and this method appears to speed up the reimbursement process. There are other forms of fee-for-service systems such as the relative value scales (RVS).[26] In this system each procedure has a relative value associated with it. The system pays on the basis of a monetary multiplier for the RVS value. A number of inequities have been identified when it comes to reimbursing for nonprocedural versus procedural services. A fee-for-service system was developed to address this issue of nonprocedural versus procedural reimbursement called the resource-based relative value scale (RBRVS).[26] It has raised the value of reimbursement for nonprocedural services and lowered the value of procedural services. This system was developed by HCFA and they have utilized it for payments of Medicare claims. The fee-for-service system is one that is dramatically changing as the movement continues toward the managed care method of providing reimbursement for medical services.

Are Pulmonary Rehabilitation Programs Cost Effective?

We will use COPD as the model. A thorough understanding of the impact of COPD is necessary in order to evaluate the efficacy of pulmonary rehabilitation programs in this disease. One must realize that full recovery from the disease is not a realistic objective of the program. Most patients that are candidates for these types of programs have irreversible lung disease. The most optimistic scenario is for these patients to improve their exercise capacity while maintaining their daily activities of life and become contributing members of society. With this in mind there are definite benefits as a result of patients participating in these types of programs.

A major impact on health care costs is a reduction in the number of repeat hospitalizations (hospital days) of patients that utilize such programs. Wright and coworkers estimated that a cost savings of $217,610 resulted due to a reduction in hospital days for a group of 57 patients in the first year following a pulmonary program.[35] Reis and associates performed a randomized comparison of rehabilitation versus education control in 119 patients.[18] The study revealed that hospital days were reduced by 2.9 in the rehabilitation group and increased by 1.6 days in the control group. Sneider and colleagues performed a very explicit study of 150 patients who self-selected themselves into various groups of a pulmonary rehabilitation program.[11] Chart review of these patients compared hospital admissions for 5 years prior to the program with those for the 5 years after the program among three different groups of patients. The first group consisted of patients who were interviewed only and did not participate in the program, the second group received only education information, and the last group participated in all the aspects of the program. In the first two groups there was a significant increase in the number of hospital days and the third group decreased by 1.53 hospital days.

Several studies have documented the advantages of exercise conditioning for patients with COPD.[10,18,36] Exercise conditioning has been shown to produce an increased exercise capacity in some patients. Cockcroft and coworkers randomly assigned 39 patients to a 6-week exercise training program or to a nontreatment group.[5] When comparing the two groups the exercise group displayed an increased walking distance in 12 min over the nontreatment group. A review done by Casaburi reviewed 37 reports of exercise training in the literature.[36] A total of 933 COPD patients had an average FEV_1 of 1.1 liters. A significant improvement in exercise conditioning was noted in the majority of these studies.

Improvement in the COPD patient's quality of life is another effect of pulmonary rehabilitation programs. A number of authors have reported evidence that components of pulmonary rehabilitation programs have a cumulative well-being effect on patients.[1-4,6,7,11,12] But there is considerable debate about the economic value of rehabilitation programs. Kaplan and Ries reported their results of a clinical trial that compared a pulmonary rehabilitation group of patients to an educational control group.[18] The pulmonary rehabilitation group did demonstrate improvement in exercise performance and relief of symptoms, but there were no significant differences between groups for measures of quality of life or lung function. An adequate number of clinical studies is lacking to determine if pulmonary rehabilitation does provide a cost-utility in terms of quality-adjusted life-years to COPD patients.

Another important aspect is a reduction in respiratory symptoms and an improved ability to carry out activities of daily living that most patients exhibit as a direct result of pulmonary rehabilitation. A number of the elements of pulmonary rehabilitation when used in conjunction can reduce respiratory symptoms and improve daily activity. As stated earlier most patients enter a program in the later stages of their disease process and reversing the disease is not a realistic goal of pulmonary rehabilitation. However, it is possible that pulmonary function may improve, or even return to normal, in those patients who have early COPD and apply the elements of a pulmonary rehabilitation program. Smoking cessation in early COPD is a chief example which has shown some positive results, contributing to saving health care dollars and reducing respiratory symptoms. The effects of pulmonary rehabilitation programs are usually evaluated in terms of improved oxygen consumption and physical measures such as a reduction in dyspnea, improved exercise capacity, and increased ambulation.[35]

There appears to be significant evidence that pulmonary rehabilitation programs can help to save health care dollars by reducing hospitalizations and emergency room and physician office visits.[21,35] More evidence is required to support the premise that pulmonary rehabilitation has impact on COPD patients in terms of improved quality of life issues from a cost perspective.

References

1. Hodgkin JE, Petty TL: *Chronic Obstructive Pulmonary Disease: Current Concepts.* Philadelphia, WB Saunders, 1987.
2. Hodgkin JE: Pulmonary rehabilitation. *Clin Chest Med* 11:447, 1990.
3. Murray E: Anyone for pulmonary rehabilitation? *Physiotherapy* 79:705, 1993.
4. Casaburi R, Petty TL (eds): *Principles and Practice of Pulmonary Rehabilitation.* Philadelphia, WB Saunders, 1993.
5. Cockcroft AE, Saunders MT, Berry G: Randomized controlled trial of rehabilitation in chronic respiratory disability. *Thorax* 36:200, 1981.
6. Ries AL, Kaplan RM, Limberg TM, Prewitt LM: Effects of pulmonary rehabilitation on physiologic and psychosocial outcomes in patients with obstruction pulmonary disease. *Ann Intern Med* 122:823, 1995.
7. Hodgkin JE: Pulmonary rehabilitation: Structure, components and benefits. *J Cardiopulmon Rehabil* 11:423, 1988.
8. Hodgkin JE: Organization of a pulmonary rehabilitation program. *Clin Chest Med* 7:541, 1986.
9. Folgering H, Rooyakkers J, Herwaarden C: Education and cost-benefit ratios in pulmonary patients. *Monaldi Arch Chest Dis* 49:166, 1994.
10. Toshima MT, Kaplan RM, Ries AL: Experimental evaluation of rehabilitation in chronic obstruction pulmonary disease: Short-term effects on exercise endurance and health status. *Health Psychol* 9:2337, 1990.
11. Sneider R, O'Malley JA, Kahn M: Trends in pulmonary rehabilitation at Eisenhower Medical Center: An 11-years experience (1976–1987) *J Cardiopulm Rehabil* 11:453, 1988.
12. Hodgkin JE, Conners GL, Bell CW (eds): *Pulmonary Rehabilitation: Guidelines to Success,* 2d ed. Philadelphia, JB Lippincott, 1993.
13. Eisenberg JM: Clinical economics: A guide to the economics analysis of clinical practices. *JAMA* 262:2879, 1989.
14. Harris JS: Watching the numbers: Basic data for health care management. *J Occup Med* 33:275, 1991.
15. Nicol J, Hodgkin JE, Connors G, et al: Strategies for developing a cost-effective pulmonary rehabilitation program. *Respir Care* 28:1451, 1983.
16. Rutten-Van Molken MPM, Van Doorslaer EICA, Rutten FFH: Economic appraisal of asthma and COPD care: A literature review 1980–1991. *Soc Sci Med* 35:161, 1992.
17. Radovich J, Hodgkin JE, Burton GG, et al: Cost-effectiveness of pulmonary rehabilitation programs, in Hodgkin JE, Connors GL, Bell CW (eds): *Pulmonary Rehabilitation: Guidelines to Success,* 2d ed. Philadelphia, JB Lippincott, 1993; p 548.
18. Kaplan RM, Ries AL: Cost-effectiveness of pulmonary rehabilitation, in Fishman A (ed): *Pulmonary Rehabilitation.* New York, Marcel Dekker 1996; p 379.
19. Guyatt G, Drummond M, Fenny D, et al: Guidelines for the clinical and economic evaluation of health care. *Soc Sci Med* 22:393, 1986.
20. Drummond MF: *Economic Appraisal of Health Technology in the European Community: Commission of the European Communities.* Oxford, Oxford University Press, 1987.
21. Toves CD, Kaplan RM, Atkins CJ: The costs and effects of behavioral programs in chronic obstructive pulmonary disease. *Med Care* 22:1088, 1984.
22. Schmidt CD, Elliott CG, Carmelli D, et al: Prolonged mechanical ventilation for respiratory failure: A cost-benefit analysis. *Crit Care Med* 11:407, 1983.
23. Bach JR, Intintola P, Alba AS, et al: The ventilator-assisted individual. Cost analysis of institutionalization vs rehabilitation and in-home management. *Chest* 101:26, 1992.
24. Connors G: Keys to the payor's vault. *J Respir Care Pract* 42:41, 1994.
25. Aitchison K: Rehabilitation at the crossroads. *Am J Phys Med Rehabil* 72:6, 1993.
26. Kongstvedt PR: *Essentials of Managed Health Care.* Gaithersburg, Aspen, 1995.
27. Bergman R: Shaping up for capitation: Managing the data. Networks retool information systems for capitation. *Hosp Health Net* 7:68, 1994.
28. Selker HP: Capitated payment for medical care and the role of the physician. *Ann Intern Med* 124:449, 1996.
29. Rahn GJ: *Hospital Sponsored Health Maintenance Organizations.* Chicago, American Hospital Publishing, 1994.
30. Mackie DL, Decker DK: *Group and IPA HMOs.* Rockville, MD, Aspen Systems, 1981.
31. Stineman M: Case-mix measurement in medical rehabilitation. *Arch Phys Med Rehabil* 76:1167, 1995.
32. Tepper S, DeJong G, Wilkerson D, et al: Criteria for selection of a payment method for inpatient medical rehabilitation. *Arch Phys Med Rehabil* 76:350, 1995.
33. Connors G, Hilling J, Morris J, et al: Obtaining third-party reimbursement for pulmonary rehabilitation. *J Cardiopulm Rehabil* 8:50, 1988.
34. Udrarhelyi IS, Jennison K, Phillips RS, et al: Comparison of the quality of ambulatory care for fee-for-service and prepaid patients. *Ann Intern Med* 115:394, 1991.
35. Wright RW, Larson DF, Mowie RG, Aldred RA: Benefits of a community-hospital pulmonary rehabilitation program. *Respir Care* 28:1474, 1983.
36. Casaburi R: Exercise training in chronic obstructive lung disease, in Casaburi R, Petty TL (eds): *Principals and Practice of Pulmonary Rehabilitation.* Philadelphia, WB Saunders, 1993; p 204.

Chapter 57

INTERDISCIPLINARY APPROACHES TO THE PATIENT WITH RESPIRATORY DISEASE

GALE BROWNING
PAM O'DELL-ROSSI
JANET BARRY
VINOD SAHGAL

Pulmonary rehabilitation teams of all sizes and in a variety of settings offer the opportunity to maximize the function and independence of the patient with respiratory disease. Table 57-1 lists the potential members of the rehabilitation team. Team composition is guided by the needs of the patient.[1] Teams may consist of a small core of professionals; for example, a physician may coordinate a home or outpatient program with a physical and an occupational therapist. Inpatient teams are more likely to include a spectrum of physicians, nurses, physical therapists, occupational therapists, social workers, respiratory therapists, and registered dietitians with consultation services available from the speech therapists, recreational therapists, vocational rehabilitation counselors, psychologists, neuropsychologists, and pharmacists. The physician may be a physiatrist (a rehabilitation specialist), pulmonologist, internist, or family practitioner, or several of these may work in collaboration.

The team approach to rehabilitation can be used in many types of pulmonary disease including chronic obstructive pulmonary disease (COPD), restrictive and interstitial lung disease, alveolar hypoventilation caused by musculoskeletal disorders, sleep apnea, ventilator weaning difficulties, and lung transplantation.[2] Patients who have undergone lung volume reduction surgery also benefit from pulmonary rehabilitation programs.

In some respiratory disease rehabilitation is the main treatment method. The benefits of pulmonary rehabilitation can extend to all patients with chronic lung disease regardless of the severity of preexisting pulmonary dysfunction.[3] Pulmonary rehabilitation has been said to be the only approach, short of lung transplantation, that improves the long-term outlook for these patients.[4] Demonstrated benefits include a decrease in respiratory symptoms, increased tolerance of dyspnea, reversal of anxiety and depression, gains in ability to perform activities of daily living, improvement in the quality of life, and a decrease in hospital admissions.[5] Pulmonary rehabilitation programs, however, have neither shown evidence of improved pulmonary function nor prolonged lifespan.[4] Ries[6] compared the outcomes of a comprehensive pulmonary rehabilitation approach with that of education alone. The comprehensive program produced a significantly greater increase in maximum exercise tolerance, maximum oxygen uptake, exercise endurance and decrease in fatigue and perceived breathlessness. All of these gains were present one year after the rehabilitation program. Cox and coworkers[7] performed a similar study following patients for 2 years with comparable findings including an increase in working days with a decrease in consumption of medical care.

Delivery of pulmonary rehabilitation can occur across the entire spectrum of care as shown in Table 57-2. Hospitalized patients who are already aware of pulmonary rehabilitation techniques can undergo a short refresher course with an occupational or respiratory therapist while being treated for their acute exacerbation. Those who are new to pulmonary rehabilitation can begin with the education portion. Once medically stabilized a patient (especially those after a lung transplant, lung volume reduction surgery, or a prolonged and difficult ventilator weaning) can begin an inpatient pulmonary rehabilitation program. This program provides multiple daily therapy sessions and offers the patient the opportunity to take advantage of the talents of many team members in a compact amount of time.

Outpatient pulmonary rehabilitation programs have the same coordinated goal-setting approach but use shorter contact times with the team members and are ongoing over several weeks to months. A patient may access this program before an acute inpatient rehabilitation stay in preparation for surgery or simply as a tool to increase endurance and quality of life. Home programs may be required by some patients who are unable to travel to the outpatient setting. These programs are important to assist in setting up small noninvasive IPPV units, monitoring oxyhemoglobin saturation, and drawing arterial blood gases.[8] The home health professionals help the patient and family engage in the rehabilitation process and assume the responsibility of providing care.[9] Wijkstra has shown that patients in home rehabilitation programs alone without inpatient or outpatient training did not improve their exercise tolerance. However, the control group that did not receive any rehabilitation demonstrated a significant deterioration in vital capacity and exercise tolerance.[10]

The Team Approach

The rehabilitation team works best when information is shared at both a formal and informal level. The patriarchal or "doctor knows best" model of medicine where the physician presides as the fountainhead of medical orders and the patient is a passive recipient of treatment has moved into the archive of the history of medicine. To achieve quality outcomes the patient, family, and the talents of a variety of medical, as well as paramedical personnel, must work together. Each team member brings unique skills to bear both in evaluation of and service to the patient. The integrative approach of the rehabilitation team transforms the medical, psychosocial, and functional needs of a patient into an achievable goal-oriented road map toward functional improvement.

There are several ways teams can be organized as shown in Table 57-3. One early attempt to place the talents of many medical professionals at the service of the patient was the multidisciplinary team. In this model, the skills of appropriate therapists and other professionals are delegated, as in consultants, to address the multifactorial needs of the respiratory compromised patient. Delegation as well

TABLE 57-1 Rehabilitation Team Members

Patient
Rehabilitation physician
Nurse
Physical therapist
Respiratory therapist
Occupational therapist
Social worker
Dietitian
Consultants such as
   Vocational rehabilitation counselors
   Recreational therapists
   Speech therapists
   Psychologists
   Pharmacists
   Physician specialists, internists, surgeons

TABLE 57-3 Types of Teams

1. Multidisciplinary: Team leader delegates aspects of patient treatment to teams' members
2. Interdisciplinary: Team develops a unified plan of therapy together considering goals of the patient and the patient's family
3. Transdisciplinary: In addition to unified planning, team members become familiar with all aspects of the treatment, and develop overlapping skills and roles

as the lack of a unified plan without communication is a shortcoming of this model. Team members also do not have the benefit of working closely with each other. The patient thus does not benefit from a true team and ultimately is underserved.

The model of the interdisciplinary team corrects the shortcomings of the multidisciplinary team approach. The interdisciplinary team works together placing the patient on the team as an important member. On the interdisciplinary team, goal setting is an important step in tailoring the rehabilitation program. This is done in conjunction with the goals of the patient and family. The flow of information (questions and concerns) is a shared responsibility. This prevents patient alienation, as well as circumventing the possibility of team splitting.

The ultimate goal of rehabilitation teams is to grow into the direction of becoming a transdisciplinary team. Here, talents are shared and information concerning all parts of the program can be competently answered by any member of the team. Overlap in roles becomes the strength of the team. This highly integrated team evolves through intense program development, continuous upgrading of communication skills, and time.

The special strengths of the rehabilitation approach are well described.[1,5,11–24] The successful interdisciplinary pulmonary rehabilitation team begins with a commitment to put the patient's needs first. The patient is an important team member. This empowers the patient and helps him or her assume a self-management role.[17] The patient remains central to the team decisions but is not making decisions for the team.[1] Each team member is responsible for their unique

TABLE 57-2 Settings for Pulmonary Rehabilitation

1. In Hospital
   During acute exacerbations
   After clinical status stabilized to maximize exercise tolerance and relieve of symptoms prior to discharge
   Perioperative
2. In Outpatient Clinic
   To improve the lifestyle
   To prevent hospitalization
3. At Home
   To improve patient independence

practice domain. Thus, each team member transforms the components of the patient's health problems into the subcategories of that discipline. All team members participate in the patient's care plan, such as education, goal setting, and team conferences.

Education

Education is an important function of the treatment plan. Patient education involves teaching the basics of respiratory pathophysiology, anxiety control, energy conservation, nutrition, and proper use of medications, as well as an exercise program. Issues of family dynamics, role changes, support systems, and sexuality are also addressed. One important purpose in this process is to allow the patient and the team to develop a reasonable expectation of the rehabilitation program outcomes and set achievable goals.

Goal Setting

Goal setting is an integral part of interdisciplinary teamwork. All team members participate in the analysis of the issues. Not only do goals require an understanding of the problem and methods with which to approach it, they must also be set in clear, concise language. Goals that have value to the patient encourage the best participation. For example, a goal of increasing shoulder flexion to full range of motion means little to most patients, while a goal of independence with styling hair or feeding her- or himself is relevant to the patient. Further, goals should be framed in positive language that will make the desired gain easy to visualize. They should be easily understood by the patient and family who are most often laypeople. Goals must be viewed as attainable in a given time span to be effective. Ultimately, goals are set to prevent or reduce handicap and to restore function. Lastly, goals should be measurable both for the use in outcome studies with which the program can be modified and more importantly for the satisfaction of the patient in appreciating undeniable and concrete gains.

The team conference is another key aspect of all rehabilitation teams. During this formally established conference, pertinent information is shared, goals are set or revised, and discussion pursued to devise the best strategy to achieve the goals. Insights into the techniques or approaches are shared. The suggestion for two therapists to treat a patient together may be made. A written record of the conference is kept for the benefit of the team and payors. The patient (if not actually attending the conference) is made aware of its outcome. The underlying impetus for the team conference is to improve communication, allowing the rehabilitation team to deliver the best program and outcome possible for each patient.

Team Members

This section will focus on the role of team members in the rehabilitation of patients with chronic obstructive lung disease.

PHYSICIAN

In many ways the role of leading the team falls to the physician. This in no way implies the physician is the most important team member. A well-integrated team will change emphasis for each patient's needs, allowing those needs to dictate which services will be given the major role in accomplishing the agreed-upon goals.

Often the physician's job begins before the patient is introduced to the team. The diagnosis must be confirmed and the patient evaluated for readiness to begin the pulmonary rehabilitation program. Patients with acute infectious exacerbations of COPD or with suboptimal management of cor pulmonale must have their clinical state improved as much as possible before initiating the rehabilitation program.[25] Exercise testing should be done to determine cardiopulmonary status and whether cardiac arrhythmias are present. The exercise test measures the patient's exercise capacity, as well as the need for supplemental oxygen (Pa_{O_2} less than 55 to 60 mmHg). Most patients cannot attain 60 to 70 percent of predicted maximum heart rate or the minute oxygen consumption necessary for an aerobic training effect.[25] Exercise ceases because of the ventilatory limitation associated with dyspnea (see Chap. 59).

The details of properly choosing bronchodilators, steroids, oxygen, antibiotics, selective beta$_2$-agonists, and diuretics, and the use of pulmonary function tests, arterial blood gases, and chest roentgenograms fall to the physician. These are discussed in other chapters and other sources.[26] Suffice it to say here that these must be optimized by the physician for a successful pulmonary rehabilitation program. Patients should be instructed to carry a list of current medications at all times. This list should be reviewed and updated with every physician visit.

The physician advises about immunizations, tobacco cessation, and avoidance of upper respiratory infections or irritants. The physician must insist on the cessation of smoking and be the patient's advocate in this process. Smoking inhibits ciliary movement in the airway; and, as a result, secretions are not cleared effectively. Smoking also inhibits alpha$_1$-antitrypsin, which allows the action of proteases, especially elastase, and possibly contributes to further lung injury. Allergens, such as dust, mold, and pet dander, should be eliminated.

Sensitivity to the signs and symptoms of depression and a willingness to open this discussion early can spare the patient undue distress. Patients may be afraid to talk about their psychological concerns because such a discussion may create emotional distress and adversely affect their breathing.[27] Anxiety and panic are intimately linked to dyspnea for the patient with respiratory disease. Further, dyspnea is viewed as so uncomfortable that to avoid it the patient chooses inactivity which can only provide for deconditioning leading to more dyspnea at a lower threshold of activity.[4,23,24,28–30] This downward spiral often leads to hospital admissions which in the end are caused by anxiety, dyspnea, and panic (see Chap. 58).

Insomnia further depletes a patient's resources for coping. Sedatives may not be an appropriate option for the patient with COPD since they depress the respiratory drive. In order to improve the patient's sleep, the physician must address the underlying physiologic issues which may include bronchospasm, congestive heart failure, poor nutrition, and lack of exercise.

Once the decision is made to have the patient admitted to a pulmonary rehabilitation program, the physician has the responsibility to write the orders or prescription for the program. This should include, at a minimum, the types of exercise (i.e., flexibility, strengthening, agility, balance, coordination, aerobics), mode, frequency, intensity, and duration.[31] A low-intensity program should be maintained until the patient can exercise for 15 to 20 min continuously. It is always wisest to slowly increase the workload. The goal is to increase the length of activity more than the intensity. Supplemental oxygen may be required with exercise. It can decrease the respiratory and heart rates, decrease minute ventilation, and increase maximal oxygen uptake and total work done. Contrary notices to the therapist, such as hold exercise for resting heart rate greater than 100, should also be included. Response to exercise including changes in breathing rate should be monitored by the therapists. Use of a target heart rate is often not practical. Usual orders for medications and laboratory work remain the responsibility of the physician. The need for special consultations, such as with other medical specialists, speech therapy, or neuropsychology, should be considered by the physician but can be suggested by any active team member.

As a team member, the physician must be available to the patient, family, and the team for education and support.

NURSE

The nurse, family members not withstanding, is clearly the team member who spends the most time with the patient in the hospital or inpatient rehabilitation setting. From this perspective, it is the nurse who will have the clearest impression of how much the patient understands and is following the pulmonary rehabilitation program. The nurse has a unique opportunity to help the patient clarify goals and identify physical and behavioral risk factors.

A significant amount of nursing time is spent on establishing and filling the education needs of the patient and family.[32] A stepwise program should be instituted to teach the patients when and how to use prescribed medications. This should begin with teaching the patients, the names, times, and expected pharmacologic action of each drug used. The patient should be taught when to ask the staff for each medication. Once successful, he or she should be advanced to having the medications at bedside and be given supervision for administration at the dispensing times. The goal is to lead the patient to complete independence with the self-medication program.

Tracheotomy care is shared between the nurse and the respiratory therapist. Both should contribute to teaching the family suctioning techniques. The nurse should also be knowledgeable of the proper technique for use of metered dose inhalers and monitor and correct the patient's technique.

Dyspnea is a major cause of disability for the patient with respiratory disease. The nurse should understand the psychological and emotional triggers for dyspnea (fear, anger, anxiety, panic), as well as the physiologic ones. The teaching task then becomes helping the patient understand that while uncomfortable, dyspnea can be managed and is not life-threatening (see Chap. 59).

A nursing staff attentive to the complex issues faced by the patient with respiratory disease can contribute to decreasing further hospitalizations.

Outpatient and home settings can offer the nurse the same opportunities for teaching and the potential to participate in case management.[33]

PHYSICAL THERAPIST

Physical therapists design exercise programs for patients with COPD. Patients with respiratory diseases do not exercise to aerobic fitness since their pulmonary pathology limits them before they reach their maximum heart rate.[34,35] These patients can make endurance gains within the limits of their pulmonary disease even though there may be little improvement in lung function. A 6- or 12-min walk test is a frequently used tool to assess and monitor endurance gains.

The effort expended in breathing in healthy individuals goes unnoticed during rest, meals, work, and exercise during normal breathing, 1 to 2 percent of inspired oxygen is used by the respiratory muscles. In contrast in a patient with COPD, the respiratory muscles may require as much as 60 percent of inspired oxygen.[4] Expiration frequently cannot be enhanced because it is limited by air trapping and airway collapsibility.[8] Therefore, a great deal of attention has been placed on inspiratory muscle training. There are currently three approaches: isocapneic hyperpnea, inspiratory resistance training, and inspiratory threshold training. These are performed for 5 to 15 min twice a day (see Chaps. 58 and 59).

Isocapneic hyperpnea involves hyperventilating into a tube that returns some of the expired carbon dioxide to the patient to prevent respiratory alkalosis. This technique is used to improve endurance in the respiratory muscles. During inspiratory resistance training, the patient inspires against specific devices, which impede airflow. This technique selectively builds strength, although it may create hypoxia. Finally, inspiratory threshold training is used to build both strength and endurance. The patient inspires against a given threshold load to release the flow of air.[36-39] Ventilatory muscle strength and endurance can be measurably increased by these exercises.

Other more familiar physical therapy techniques address correcting posture and improving flexibility, range of motion, and strength in the large muscles.[24] Once the patient can walk for 6 min without a rest, treadmill walking and stair climbing can be started.[22] These are excellent exercises since they increase mobility along with strength and endurance.

Stationary bicycling is a good alternate choice for inclement weather or for the patient whose weightbearing is limited. Pool walking or swimming is another good choice where the facilities are available (see Chap. 59).

OCCUPATIONAL THERAPIST

For the patient with respiratory disease, even the most basic daily self-care tasks can become monumental. The role of the occupational therapist is to teach the patient breathing techniques, pacing, energy conservation, and upper extremity exercises, and to help make homemaking tasks more manageable.

The first step to teaching the patient pacing and energy conservation is to make the patient aware of where and how energy is being spent. Patients are encouraged to plan their daily activities as well as scheduled rest breaks. Tasks should be broken into their separate components and the tools that they will require should be kept well organized. Activities may be modified to allow them to be accomplished from a seated position, preferably with upper extremities supported on the working surface.

Many upper extremity muscles, such as pectoralis major and minor, trapezii, latissimus dorsi, serratus anterior, and the sternocleidomastoids, are accessory muscles for breathing. Exercises for strengthening these muscles are important although patients find overhead exercises difficult to tolerate. Continual overuse of these muscles results in an increased transverse diameter of the upper rib cage.

Self-care tasks should be made easier by the use of adaptive equipment, such as raised toilet seats, grab bars, shower benches, and bedside commodes, when needed. Dressing activities should be simplified. Velcro can replace buttons; bras can be fastened in front.

Meal preparation should be performed while seated and lightweight utensils and cookware are preferred. It is important to give the patient permission to save energy for enjoyable quality of life activities and to delegate other tasks (see Chap. 58).

RESPIRATORY THERAPIST

It is in keeping with the interdisciplinary team approach that the respiratory therapist has many responsibilities in common with other disciplines already discussed, as well as those that are special. The teaching of breathing techniques, proper use of metered dose inhalers, and tracheotomy care are an important part of the interaction between the respiratory therapist and the patient.

The respiratory therapist can manage airway secretions through improving the forcefulness of the cough and by suctioning. When mucus viscosity becomes a problem, it is a signal to have humidification, hydration, and medications maximized. Postural percussion and drainage is found to be of benefit in patients who produce at least 30 mL of sputum each day. For best results, the patient should be well hydrated and bronchodilated at the time of the treatment.

Oxygen administration can be crucial in some patients. In the hypoxemic patient it has been shown to increase length and quality of life.[4] A pulse oximeter can then be employed to help the respiratory therapist determine the lowest flow of oxygen that will maintain oxygen saturations greater than 92 percent.

REGISTERED DIETITIAN

Malnutrition results in smaller muscle mass and is an enemy of the patient with respiratory disease. Weight loss is found in 10 to 26 percent of outpatients and 47 percent of inpatients with COPD.[40] Greater weight loss correlates with high death rates for the patient with COPD. The patients often complain of anorexia, increased dyspnea, and fatigue with meals and early satiety. The gastrointestinal discomfort can be secondary to medication side effects, peptic ulcer disease, or compression of the stomach from hyperinsufflation of the lungs.[41]

The type of malnutrition in COPD patients is marasmic, in which there is a preservation of visceral protein mass and a reduction in skeletal muscle mass. The skeletal muscles, which include the diaphragm and muscles of respiration, are degraded to produce energy. When this occurs in a setting of muscle atrophy from physical deconditioning, it can be life-threatening. Severe malnutrition can cause a decrease in the ventilatory response to hypoxia and hypercapnia and lead to pathologic changes in pulmonary parenchyma and decreased surfactant synthesis.[42] Hypercapneic coma can result. Nutrition is also integral to lung repair mechanisms and humeral and cellular immunity. When altered, these expose the patient to increased bacterial adhesion in the lower respiratory tract.

Early intervention by the registered dietitian is essential given the alternative. A dietary assessment should include a 24-h recall of intake, as well as a 3-day recording of actual intake for the purpose of evaluating calories and nutritional quality of meals. Anthropometric measures of body composition can help assess nutritional status.

Patients often benefit by taking multiple small meals that are high in calories and protein. They may require the use of nutritional supplements. One study showed that only patients receiving 1.5 times their basal metabolic needs developed improved respiratory muscle strength and hand grip as measured by a dynamometer.[43] Meals should be quick to prepare, appetizing, and visually pleasing.

SOCIAL WORKER

Quality of life changes are inevitably linked with chronic illnesses. Frequent exacerbations of COPD can result in patients experiencing a loss of autonomy as they increasingly depend more on others, experience social isolation, and have multiple hospital admissions. Depression is noted in 42 to 74 percent of patients.[44] As a patient advocate, it is the role of the social worker to identify and address issues of coping, role changes, family dysfunction, and loss of control. This can be done in individual or group sessions.

Psychosocial skills, such as the ability to adapt, good judgment, and good social support, improve the patient's ability to cope with chronic illness. Patients who lack social support from a spouse for instance, when stressed are more likely to seek hospitalizations.[44] The social worker can help a patient develop better coping techniques. By increasing the patient's awareness of negative feelings and substituting positive ones, the patient's self esteem can grow. Reinforcing positive lifestyle changes; for example, participating in exercise and cessation of tobacco use, the patient increases adherence to his or her medical regimen, makes both physiologic and psychological gains, and develops a new healthier coping strategy.

As the symptoms of COPD progress, the patient's role as a wage earner and as a member of the community and family begin to change.[27] Stress is felt at work when dyspnea prevents full participation or when illness impacts on attendance.

Patients become self-conscious of their need for oxygen or increased sputum production and limit their activities to their home. In the family, the presence of chronic illness can cause misunderstandings and generate tension. Dyspnea and fatigue can impact negatively on sexuality. Family members, not necessarily suited to or trained as such, become caregivers to patients as their ability to care for themselves decreases.

The patients feeling of loss of control can be manifested in sleep disturbances, anxiety, and panic. By guiding the patient in the use of the resources of the pulmonary rehabilitation team and the community and offering education and a concrete plan for behavioral changes, the social worker can turn this powerlessness into empowerment. The perception of control over one's life is essential to emotional health and successful recoveries.[9] The patient and family are given skills and information to help them see themselves as causal forces better able to adapt and self-direct.

Further, the social worker will help the patient and family interact with the medical community, especially in areas where there are gaps perceived in resources or communication. Identification of safety concerns and caregiver burdens are brought to the team's attention and addressed.

The fruits of a successful psychosocial intervention (increased autonomy, effective coping for patient and family, and compliance with the medical regimen) improve rehabilitation outcomes at all levels.

OTHER CONSULTATIVE SERVICES

Other services that may be intermittently involved on the pulmonary rehabilitation team include speech therapist, therapeutic recreation specialist, vocational rehabilitation counselor, psychologist, neuropsychologist, and pharmacist.

Patients with restrictive lung diseases caused by neuromuscular disease may be at increased risk for aspiration pneumonia because of disordered swallowing. The speech therapist can perform a bedside evaluation of swallowing to assess the aspiration risk and, if needed, a modified barium videofluoroscopy may be obtained. Oral motor and swallowing exercises should be instituted where indicated.

Safety of feeding in the presence of a tracheostomy tube can be assessed by the addition of methylene blue to the food and monitoring the tracheostomy site for the dye. Communication may be more difficult in this setting and can also be addressed by the speech therapist.[25]

The return to or modification of leisure activities is best addressed by a therapeutic recreation specialist.[22] One study found a significant increase in leisure time activities after participation in a pulmonary rehabilitation program.[7]

Modifications at the worksite or changes in work responsibilities can help the patient with COPD remain employed. The consultation of a vocational rehabilitation counselor will be beneficial to the patient and employer alike and allow for the needs of both to be addressed. A rehabilitation psychologist may be consulted to help the patient with adjustment issues and to work through the reactive depression. Techniques including biofeedback, meditation, and progressive muscle relaxation are good tools for the patient with COPD. Neuropsychological tests have shown moderately significant cognitive impairments in abstract reasoning, memory, and speed of performance to correlate to blood oxygen tension at rest.[44] Referral for formal testing may be indicated in some cases.

The pharmacist is always an excellent resource since the patient with COPD tends to be older and can have multiple cardiac, gastrointestinal, and arthritic problems in addition to their pulmonary ones. The potential for drug interactions must be vigilantly monitored.

Summary

A well-coordinated, patient-focused interdisciplinary rehabilitation team can make a positive impact on the life of the patient with respiratory disease. A number of studies have reported improvements in exercise tolerance, mobility, independence with activities of daily living, tolerance to dyspnea, health behaviors (i.e., cessation of tobacco use), return to work, increased social interactions, and a decrease in total medical costs.[2,3,35,45]

References

1. O'Toole MT: The interdisciplinary team: Research and education. *Holist Nurs Pract* 6:76–83, 1992.
2. Fishman AP: Pulmonary rehabilitation research. *Am J Respir Crit Care Med* 149:825–833, 1994.
3. Niederman MS, Clemente PH, Fein AM, et al: Benefits of a multidisciplinary pulmonary rehabilitation program. *Chest* 99:798–804, 1991.
4. Tiep BL: Reversing disability of irreversible lung disease. *West J Med* 154:591–597, 1991.
5. Hodgkin JE: Pulmonary rehabilitation. *Clin Chest Med* 11:447–454, appendix 455–460, 1990.
6. Ries AL, Kaplan RM, Limberg TM, Prewitt LM: Effects of pulmonary rehabilitation on physiologic and psychosocial outcomes in patients with chronic obstructive pulmonary disease. *Ann Intern Med* 122:823–832, 1995.
7. Cox NJM, Hendricks JC, Binkhorst RA, van Herwaarden CLA: A pulmonary rehabilitation program for patients with asthma and mild chronic obstructive pulmonary diseases (COPD). *Lung* 171:235–244, 1993.
8. Nutter PB: The role of inspiratory muscle training in a pulmonary rehabilitation program. *Phys Med Rehabil Clin North Am* 7:315–324, 1996.
9. Brown JST, Furstenberg AL: Restoring control: Empowering older patients and their families during health crisis. *Soc Work Health Care* 17:81–101, 1992.
10. Wijkstra PJ, van der Mark TW, Kraan J, et al: Long-term effects of home rehabilitation on physical performance in chronic obstructive pulmonary disease. *Am J Respir Crit Care Med* 153:1234–1241, 1996.
11. van Weel C: Teamwork. *Lancet* 344:1276–1279, 1994.
12. Rodriguez GS, Goldberg B: Rehabilitation in the outpatient setting. *Clin Geriatr Med* 9:873–881, 1993.
13. Kappeli S: Interprofessional cooperation: Why is partnership so difficult? *Patient Educ Couns* 26:251–256, 1995.
14. Schut HA, Stam HJ: Goals in rehabilitation teamwork. *Disabil Rehabil* 16:223–226, 1994.
15. Tallis R: Rehabilitation of the elderly in the 21st century. The F. E. Williams Lecture 1992. *J R Coll Physicians Lond* 26:413–422, 1992.
16. Noblitt RL, John ME, Norlund RK, et al: How to make co-management work. *Optom Clin* 4:123–130, 1994.
17. Coles C: Educating the health care team. *Patient Educ Couns* 26:239–244, 1995.
18. Lamberts H, Riphagen FE: Working together in a team for primary health care—A guide to dangerous country. *J R Coll Gen Pract* 25:745–752, 1975.
19. Vinicor F: Interdisciplinary and intersectoral approach: A challenge for integrated care. *Patient Educ Couns* 26:267–272, 1995.
20. Hockley J: Role of the hospital support team. *Br J Hosp Med* 48:250–253, 1992.
21. Rashbaum I, Whyte N: Occupational therapy in pulmonary rehabilitation. Energy conservation and work simplification techniques. *Phys Med Rehabil Clin North Am* 7:325–340, 1996.
22. Goldstein RS, Avendano MA: Model program development and outcomes in chronic obstructive pulmonary disease. *Phys Med Rehabil Clin North Am* 7:353–366, 1996.
23. Make BJ, Paine R: Pulmonary rehabilitation for COPD patients. *Hosp Pract* 22(1A):26–34, 1987.
24. Tiep BL: Inpatient pulmonary rehabilitation. A team approach to the more fragile patient. *Postgrad Med* 86:141–150, 1989.
25. Bach JR, Moldover JR: Cardiovascular, pulmonary, and cancer rehabilitation. 2. Pulmonary rehabilitation. *Arch Phys Med Rehabil* 77(3 Suppl):S45–S51, 1996.
26. Haas F, Fain R, Salazar-Schicchi J, Axen K: Pathophysiology of chronic obstructive pulmonary disease. *Phys Med Rehabil Clin North Am* 7:205–221, 1996.
27. Rabinowitz B, Florian V: Chronic obstructive pulmonary disease—Psycho-social issues and treatment goals. *Soc Work Health Care* 16:69–86, 1992.
28. Folgering H, van Herwaarden CLA: Pulmonary rehabilitation in asthma and COPD, physiological basics. *Respir Med* 87:41–44, 1993.
29. Donner CF, Howard P: Pulmonary rehabilitation in chronic obstructive pulmonary disease (COPD) with recommendations for its use. *Eur Respir J* 5:266–275, 1992.
30. Burns M: Outpatient pulmonary rehabilitation: A new lease on life. *Postgrad Med* 86:129–137, 1989.
31. Siebens H: The role of exercise in the rehabilitation of patients with chronic obstructive pulmonary disease. *Phys Med Rehabil Clin North Am* 7:299–313, 1996.
32. Gilmartin ME: Patient and family education. *Clin Chest Med* 7:619–627, 1986.
33. Spenceley SM: The CNS in multidisciplinary pulmonary rehabilitation: A nursing science perspective. *Clin Nurs Spec* 9:192–198, 1995.
34. Gosselink RIK, Troosters T, Decramer M: Peripheral muscle weakness contributes to exercise limitation in COPD. *Am J Respir Crit Care Med* 153:976–980, 1996.
35. Pashkow P: Outcomes in cardiopulmonary rehabilitation. *Phys Ther* 76:643–656, 1996.
36. Leith DE, Bradley M: Ventilatory muscle strength and endurance training. *J Appl Physiol* 41:508–516, 1976.
37. Belman MS, Mittman C: Ventilatory muscle training improves exercise capacity in COPD patients. *Am Rev Respir Dis* 121:273–280, 1980.
38. Sonne LJ, Davis JA: Increased exercise performance in patients with severe COPD following inspiratory resistive training. *Chest* 81:436–439, 1982.
39. Celli BR: Pulmonary rehabilitation in patients with COPD. *Am J Respir Crit Care Med* 152:861–864, 1995.
40. Donahoe M, Rogers R: Nutritional assessment and support in chronic obstructive pulmonary disease. *Clin Chest Med* 11:487, 1990.
41. Jardim JR, Ferreira IM, Sachs A: Nutrition, anabolic steroids, and growth hormone. *Phys Med Rehabil Clin North Am* 7:253–275, 1996.
42. Swank TM, Bach JR, Ishikawa Y, et al: Nutrition, dysphagia, and general medical considerations. *Phys Med Rehabil Clin North Am* 7:389–405, 1996.
43. Rochester DF: Nutritional repletion. *Semin Respir Med* 13:44, 1992.
44. Czajkowski SM, McSweeny AJ: The role of psychosocial factors in chronic obstructive pulmonary disease. *Phys Med Rehabil Clin North Am* 7:341–352, 1996.
45. Vale F, Reardon JZ, ZuWallack RL: The long-term benefits of outpatient pulmonary rehabilitation on exercise endurance and quality of life. *Chest* 103:42–45, 1993.

Chapter 58

OCCUPATIONAL THERAPY IN PULMONARY REHABILITATION

PAM O'DELL-ROSSI
GALE BROWNING
JANET BARRY
VINOD SAHGAL

The occupational therapist plays an integral role as a member of the pulmonary rehabilitation team. The occupational therapist's primary concern is with a patient's quality of life, and treatment plans are designed to presereve and/or restore that quality. Thus, the occupational therapist's main goal is to improve a person's functional status in all aspects of daily life and to educate both the patient and his or her family. They are educated in ways to conserve energy and simplify the daily workload to make living much less stressful and tiring.[1]

Occupational Therapy Assessment

Occupational therapy (OT) intervention should begin with a comprehensive evaluation. A careful review of the patient's medical chart and a patient and family interview are essential. During the chart review as well as in the assessment itself, the occupational therapist can determine if there are any additional or coexisting medical conditions that may influence the patient's ability to function independently in daily life tasks.[2] In addition, the therapist should gather information on all of the following:

Home and work environments
Family support
Prior self care and home-management abilities
Functional mobility status (transfers and bed mobility)
Social, vocational, and leisure interests
Primary mode of transportation
Accessibility to the community, including social events, shoping centers, municipal facilities, grocery stores, and churches

It is also beneficial to have patients, along with a family member, describe their typical day and learn from the patients how they feel their pulmonary disease has changed their daily routine. After the initial interview is complete, the occupational therapist can begin the next phase of the evaluation. During each portion of the assessment that ensues, it is vital for the occupational therapist to record all of the following about the patient being evaluated:

Level of fatigue
Degree of dyspnea
Postural habits while performing various activities
Breathing
Movement patterns
Pacing of movement
Activity tolerance
Use of pulmonary equipment such as oxygen
Heart rate
Blood pressure
Oxygen saturation rate[3,4]

The next step in the evaluation focuses on the patient's upper extremities including active and passive range of motion, sensation, strength, coordination, pain, edema, and handwriting. This is very important because the patient's arms are constantly involved in performing daily activities and patients often report that very simple tasks such as shaving or combing their hair cause extreme dyspnea and fatigue.[2,4,5]

In addition, an assessment of each daily living task both by patient report as well as actual observation is necessary.[6] Daily life tasks or activities of daily living (ADL) refer to self-care, home management, work, and leisure pursuits. Among the many ADLs that may be assessed are the following:

Feeding
Grooming (very likely to be a problem area)
Bathing
Dressing
Toileting
Functional transfers (toilet, tub, shower stall, bed, chair)
Meal preparation
Cleaning
Laundry
Work tasks
Leisure pursuits

An actual home and/or work assessment may disclose architectural barriers which can be eliminated or adapted so that a patient can function more efficiently in home and work environments.[6] These barriers may not be revealed if the assessment is only performed in the clinic. A thorough evaluation can reveal various life tasks which are important to the patient, but which may be difficult to perform due to the pulmonary disease process.

Occupational Therapy Intervention/Treatment

The first step in the treatment process involves the development of both short- and long-term goals. The therapist and patient should establish these goals together because it is essential to have the patient's willing participation in the therapeutic process in order for it to be successful. Short-term objective goals can help the client see clearly the progress and help motivate him or her to continue with the treatment program.

Once the goal-planning step has been completed the therapist can begin the treatment process. A program in upper extremity exercises should be developed to improve the patient's strength and activity tolerance.[5,6] Other upper extremity exercises and activity programs can be generated for the patient if additional problems were identified during the initial assessment, such as decreased coordination and dexterity.[2]

During ADL training a patient can learn to perform life's activities more efficiently and comfortably. Each ADL training session is completed with the following in mind:

1. Use of Assistive Equipment

   A sock-aid or long shoehorn, for example, may be helpful so bending is minimized for the patient while performing lower extremity dressing. This reduces the energy expended on this essential ADL.

2. Use of Adaptive Techniques/Economy of Motion

   Teaching a patient to use their upper extremities in a supported position versus an unsupported position can decrease oxygen utilization and therefore increase energy efficiency. If a patient is taught to keep their arms supported and within their base of support or normal work area this can significantly reduce fatigue and a patient may be able to continue the task for a longer period of time.

3. Grading the Activity

   Breaking an activity down into its component steps helps simplify the task. For example, the use of some prepared foods in the kitchen versus cooking from scratch.

4. Breathing Techniques/Control

   The physical therapist will teach the patient various breathing techniques and then the occupational therapist can teach the patient how to incorporate these learned techniques into ADLs. Proper breathing during ADL performance can dramatically increase a patient's ability to perform the task.[6]

5. Principles of Energy Conservation

   Setting priorities: Teaching a patient to set realistic daily and weekly goals and then learning to prioritize those goals can increase the efficiency with which tasks are completed, as well as helping the patient not to become overwhelmed by the amount of work he or she wishes to accomplish.

   Planning ahead: This can help a patient avoid rushing, allow sufficient time to complete a task, and eliminate unnecessary steps/tasks.

   Pacing activities: The use of slow, fluid movements expends less energy; conversely, rushing only increases energy expenditure and causes discomfort. Just by doubling work speed, two to three times more energy is depleted. Patients will find that a task they usually have difficulty performing can be done safely and without discomfort simply by lessening their pace. A slower, steady rate of work with rest breaks will get a job done without extreme fatigue or dyspnea.

6. Principles of Work Simplification

   Spreading the heavy and light tasks out throughout the day or week: For example, patients are encouraged to do their house cleaning one room per day.

   Taking rest periods: It is important for patients not to begin projects in which they are unable to stop and take rest beaks.

   Sliding objects instead of lifting them whenever possible: Slid-

ing heavy pots across a counter top or using a small utility cart saves the energy that would normally be expended by carrying the object.

   Eliminating unnecessary motions and processes: As mentioned earlier, sitting can simplify work; however, when sitting, the patient's arms should not have to extend beyond the normal work area and base of support and proper work heights which permit proper posture must be utilized.

   Duplicating supplies: If supplies are stored where they are used this eliminates having to carry them. This may mean duplicating supplies such as the cleaning supplies used in upstairs and downstairs bathrooms, but it saves on the amount of energy expended.

7. Proper Body Mechanics

   Less energy is wasted if proper body mechanics are employed and there is much less stress on the bones and muscles of the spine. The therapist should teach patients to use proper body mechanics during all ADLs, especially when lifting and bending are involved.[2,3,7]

Work and Leisure Treatment Interventions

Some patients may be able to stay in their jobs or continue their leisure interests with modifications made to various tasks they perform. Scheduling and time management techniques, along with breathing retraining methods can assist clients in meeting their return to work goals or staying in their current job. A focus on basic ergonomic principles such as prolonged or repetitive exertions, extreme ranges of motion especially with the arms overhead, static body postures, and tool designs can be reviewed and then modified to decrease the energy expenditure required. Often, simple, free, or low-cost solutions can be made that solve many work/leisure problems.[6]

When patients cannot maintain their present work or leisure pursuits it is essential to help them find another position or another interest which may be less physically demanding, but still rewarding. The occupational therapist and vocational counselor can work closely with the patient to explore options. Likewise, the occupational therapist can explore alternative leisure options with the patient through a variety of leisure inventories.[1]

Utilizing the above principles/techniques during the treatment program can increase a patient's activity tolerance during all ADLs. The primary goal throughout all of the training is to increase the patient's comfort and decrease shortness of breath and fatigue.

Although ADL training is the primary focus for the occupational therapist on the pulmonary rehabilitation team, a comprehensive program may also include relaxation, stress management, and time management training. It is often beneficial for these techniques to be taught in a group format. Problems in daily living typically encountered by persons with pulmonary disease can be explored and group problem-solving utilized so that patients can share their experiences with each other in order to reinforce what is being learned.

Relaxation training may include listening to soothing music, visualization and imagery, biofeedback, and contracting and relaxing skeletal muscle groups. In addition, relaxation training can decrease a patient's anxiety, decrease muscle tension, and decrease dyspnea.[2,3,7]

Time management techniques such as pacing, which was discussed earlier, and preplanning activities are crucial to incorporate into daily living. Becoming aware of limitations, not taking on more than can be handled comfortably, and learning to quit when feeling tired are also important aspects of time management. Finally, organizing activities and trying to do them in the same manner all the time is beneficial. Repetition of the same method makes a person more proficient and therefore saves time and energy.

Stress management training can include several of the following examples: writing down appointment times, addresses, phone numbers, and grocery lists instead of relying on memory; feeling that it is okay to say "no" and knowing that often this reduces daily demands and, therefore, reduces stress; relaxing standards in how the patient or the patient's home appears—A simple haircut that requires less time is one example; preparing for events of the next day the night before by having clothes ready and setting the alarm clock for a time where rushing will not be necessary; and, finally, finding ways to exercise that are enjoyable.[7]

The determinant to all occupational therapy interventions is the patient's ability to transfer learned techniques into his/her daily lifestyle. As with any treatment plan, it is important to monitor the patient's progress and adapt or change the goals of the program as necessary. The patient's progress can be measured by a change in work capacity, level of comfort while performing a particular task, increased activity tolerance, increased independence in ADLs, incorporation of learned techniques into daily living, and the patient's subjective report of noted progress and change. Progress can also be measured by noted changes in dyspnea, fatigue level during various ADLs, proper pacing or movement patterns that have been integrated into ADLs, improved habits of posture and breathing, use of pulmonary equipment, heart rate, blood pressure changes, and changes in the oxygen saturation rates during specific tasks.[4,5]

The occupational therapist performs an integral role within the framework of the pulmonary rehabilitation team, and good communication between all team members and with the patient can lead to a comprehensive and beneficial program from which the patient truly benefits.[7]

References

1. Hodgkin J: Pulmonary rehabilitation. *Clin Chest Med* 11:447–454, 1990.
2. Hoffman L, Berg J, Rogers R: Daily living with COPD: Self help skills to improve functional ability. *Postgrad Med* 86:153–165, 1989.
3. Tiep B: Inpatient pulmonary rehabilitation: A team approach to the more fragile patient. *Postgrad Med* 86:141–150, 189.
4. Hogan B: Pulse oximetry for an adult with a pulmonary disorder. *Am J Occupational Ther* 49:1062–1064, 1995.
5. Kelson S: Rehabilitation of patients with COPD, in Cherniak N (ed): *Chronic Obstructive Pulmonary Disease*. Philadelphia, W.B. Saunders, 1991, pp 520–531.
6. Hodgkin J: Pulmonary Rehabilitation, in Cherniak R (ed): *Current Therapy of Respiratory Disease*, vol 2. Toronto, B.C. Decker, 1986, pp 275–282.
7. Tiep B: Pulmonary rehabilitation program organization, in Casaburi R, Petty T (eds): *Principles and Practice of Pulmonary Rehabilitation*. Philadelphia, W.B. Saunders, Philadelphia, 1993, pp 302–308.

Chapter 59

PULMONARY PHYSICAL THERAPY

JANET BARRY
GALE BROWNING
PAM O'DELL-ROSSI
VINOD SAHGAL

Goals

The goals of the physical therapy program are to:

1. Improve functional mobility
2. Improve respiratory status, including improved airway clearance
3. Improve activity tolerance
4. Improve strength (extremity, trunk, and respiratory muscles) and flexibility
5. Reduce the number of emergency room visits
6. Recognize the need for medical intervention
7. Independent use of strategies to relieve shortness of breath (SOB)
8. Independent use of a home exercise program

Evaluation of the Patient

Whether the patient is hospitalized or an outpatient, the therapist must begin by evaluating the patient prior to initiating treatment; a thorough review of past medical history (and, if hospitalized, current hospital course) and current medical status is necessary. In reviewing the past medical history, special attention should be placed on: history of deep vein thrombosis (DVT), pulmonary embolism (PE), cardiopulmonary diagnosis and conditions, recent bone fractures or disease (i.e., Paget's Disease), aneurysm, recent surgical procedures, presence of cancer, presence of hemophilia, and/or recent trauma.

When available the therapist should review the physician's notes and the patient's current course (in the hospital or as an outpatient). This includes review of laboratory results, such as pulmonary function tests (PFTs), arterial blood gases (ABG), radiographs, echocardiography reports, CT scans, and MRIs. Knowledge of the patient's previous and current oxygen requirements at rest and during activity is essential. The therapist should check for any precaution and/or contraindication to chest PT.

In hospitalized patients, the therapist should carry out an examination of the patient and the patient's surroundings to determine whether the patient is on ventilatory support or being weaned. NOTE: During periods of weaning, the patient will likely be more fatigued due to the increased effort of breathing. It is important then to allow rest breaks as needed. Special attention should be directed towards emptying the water from the ventilator tubing prior to mobilizing the ventilated patient to prevent dumping water into their lungs.

The heart rate and rhythm should be checked. Is there a pacemaker and/or implanted cardiac defibrillator (ICD)? The therapist must note the location of IVs, arterial lines, intraaortic balloon pumps (IABP), Swan Ganz, urinary catheters, chest tubes, central venous pressure lines (CVP), oxygen saturation probes (O_2 sat), and determine whether there are any recent surgical incisions. The therapist should assess the patient's respiratory rate and depth, and the pattern of use of the respiratory muscles. The patient's appearance should be evaluated to answer the following questions:

Is the patient awake, alert, responsive, cooperative, etc?
Is there edema in the extremities or ascites present?
Are there pressure sores (posterior head, sacrum, heel, lateral maleoli, lateral foot at the 5th metatarsal head, greater trochanter, elbow)?
Are there obvious signs of hypoxia (cyanosis) (i.e., blue finger nail beds which indicate peripheral hypoxia versus blue lips which indicate central hypoxia)?[1]
Is there evidence of a rash, blisters, reddened skin, fragile skin?

The physical therapist should independently obtain from the patient a brief history of symptoms, particularly those that affect function. The therapist should determine the use of accessory muscles, observe the sternocleidomastoid and scalenes, and evaluate the chest wall movement.[1,2] The therapist can observe for symmetry of chest wall movement by doing the following[1]:

Upper lobe: The therapist faces the patient, places his/her thumbs at the midsternal line at the sternal notch of the patient, and wraps his/her fingers above the patient's clavicles.[1]

Middle lobe: The therapist faces the patient, places the tips of his/her thumbs at the ziphoid process, and extends his/her fingers laterally around the ribs of the patient.[1]

Lower lobe: The therapist stands behind the patient, places his/her thumbs along the spinous process of the lower thoracic vertebrae and wraps his/her fingers around the ribs of the patient.[1]

At each level the patient should be instructed to take a full breath in and out.

Vocal fremitus should be assessed during regular and deep breathing, again making sure to evaluate the upper, middle, and lower lobes.[1,2]

Breath sounds should be evaluated and cough effectiveness assessed.[1,2] Coughing should be deep and strong. If the patient has a productive cough, check the sputum for color (yellow and green indicate infection, blood streaked), consistency, and amount.[1,2]

The general strength of the patient and the flexibility and range of movement of the muscles should be determined. It is essential to measure the endurance and functional capacity.[3]

Cardiovascular functional capacity is evaluated by a graded exercise test (GXT).[3] When testing a pulmonary patient, care should be used to choose a protocol that allows for a low level to start with, followed by small incremental increases. If a GXT is unavailable, you can use a 6-min walk test to estimate the patient's current capacity.[3] (Patients are encouraged to walk as fast as they can for 6 min, resting as needed throughout.) Distances walked are used to estimate functional capacity. Borg's rating of perceived exertion scale (RPE) is used to help patients identify their level of exertion. The new scale goes from 0 to 10 and correlates to exercise-test heart rates and oxygen consumption.[3] It is easy to understand and self-monitor.

Assessment of bed mobility, transfers, and gait help determine the level of disability a patient may be experiencing. Patients are instructed in techniques which are more energy efficient to prevent dyspnea on exertion (DOE). If mobility is unsafe, appropriate assistive devices are recommended to improve safety. It has been my experience that many patients with significant COPD tend to reach for objects during ambulation, which decreases their safety. In these individuals, the use of a rolling walker has increased their ambulation distances (versus no device). However, according to Foley and coworkers, the use of a standard walker should be avoided since it significantly increases energy demand.[4]

Posture can be a good indicator of respiratory status. Patients who have elevated shoulders and are leaning forward often have obstructive lung disease. Look for the use of accessory muscles in breathing, especially the sternocleidomastoid.[2] Hypertrophy of this muscle can be expected in patients with significant obstructive lung disease. The appearance of a barrel chest is caused by hyperinflation of the chest resulting in an increased anterior-to-posterior diameter.[1] There are postural deformities and injuries that also decrease the efficiency of breathing. Examples include scoliosis, thoracic kyphosis, and thoracic spine compression fractures. In severe cases, scoliosis can lead to serious pulmonary compromise. A similar asymmetry can be observed in patients who have had thoracic surgery with a lateral incision secondary to splinting away from pain or removal of lung tissue or bone itself.[2] Thoracic kyphosis and thoracic spine compression fractures result in a shortened thoracic cavity, making deep inspiration difficult.[2]

Marked obesity and late stages of pregnancy can interfere with respiratory status by decreasing the ability of the diaphragm to move downward during deep inspiration.[2] In addition to this, the added weight on the chest wall may result in decreased motion. This results in restrictive lung volumes.

Balance and coordination may be affected by hypoxia or medication side effects. Some common side effects of pulmonary medications include nervousness, muscle tremors, and lightheadedness.

Physical Therapy Treatment

STRENGTH AND FLEXIBILITY

Patients with pulmonary compromise may have decreased range of movement in their upper extremities secondary to decreased use. Arm movement, especially shoulder flexion and abduction over 90 degrees, is associated with increased respiratory rates and may lead to dyspnea.[5-7] The forward trunk and head posture frequently used in these patients may contribute to shortened pectoralis major and tightness in triceps. The ability to expand the chest upon deep inspiration could be compromised. Use of proprioceptive neuromuscu-

lar facilitation (PNF) patterns, specifically bilateral, symmetrical D_2F pattern, can be helpful in improving trunk and shoulder range of movement.[8]

D_2F = Scapular elevation, adduction, and upward rotation
Shoulder flexion, abduction, external rotation
Forearm supination
Wrist and finger extension to radial side, thumb extension

This pattern should be timed with inspiration to achieve the greatest effects.

Increasing general flexibility, strength, and muscle endurance should be included to promote overall conditioning. In general, lower intensities with high repetitions are recommended.

CARDIOVASCULAR CONDITIONING AND AEROBIC EXERCISE

According to the American College of Sports Medicine (ACSM), aerobic capacity can be improved even in patients with lung dysfunction.[3]

INTENSITY

The intensity of exercise should be based on clinical information and graded test (GXT) results. Use of BORG's Rating of Perceived Exertion Scale (RPE) allows the patient to easily self-monitor the intensity of his/her exercise.[3] Patients should be encouraged to avoid intensities that cause excessive dyspnea. In my experience, excessive shortness of breath with exercise tends to make patients anxious, and leads to exercise dropouts.

In addition, interval training is recommended initially because it will lower oxygen debt while allowing an increase in total work. If tolerated by the patient, a progression to continuous exercise can be incorporated later.

DURATION

In the beginning, the duration of exercise may be very short, a matter of a few minutes. Gradually increase this to 20 to 30 min as the patient tolerates.[3]

FREQUENCY

The goal is to exercise 3 to 5 days per week. However, pulmonary patients tend to have lower functional capacities and may require more frequent sessions.[3]

MODE

Any form of aerobic exercise which uses large muscle groups can be utilized.[3] In my experience, walking is the optimal exercise for this population because it is functional and inexpensive. If the patient is unable to walk or does not enjoy walking, any form of aerobic exercise is fine (i.e., cycling, swimming, rowing).

BREATHING EXERCISES[1,9-12]

Breathing exercises help improve tidal volume, thoracic cage mobility, increased inspiratory capacity, and improved cough effectiveness. It is not recommended in patients who are retaining CO_2 (their muscles are already being overused) or during mechanical ventilation.

Indications:

Pneumonia
Acute respiratory distress (ARDS)
Obstructive lung disease
Pain in the thorax due to trauma or surgery
Neurologic disease or injury resulting in weak respiratory
   muscles
Chest wall and spine deformities that decrease respiratory
   function

DIAPHRAGMATIC BREATHING[1,9–12]

This technique is used to improve ventilation, oxygenation,
and excursion of the diaphragm. It is usually used with
postural drainage to assist in removal of secretions.

Technique

1. Have the patient assume a comfortable position, preferably
   in an isolated area. Use pillows for support if necessary.
2. Instruct the patient to relax. This can be observed by noting
   relaxation in the accessory muscles of the neck.
3. Place your hand on the abdomen below the rib cage.
4. Tell the patient to inhale in a slow, deep manner initiated
   by the abdomen. This can be observed by watching your
   hand slowly rise and fall. The accessory muscles of the
   shoulders and neck should not be active.
5. Have the patient repeat this three to four times before
   resting.
6. Next place the patient's hand on his/her own abdomen
   to learn how it should feel.
7. Once the technique is perfected, practice it in different positions.

SEGMENTAL BREATHING[1,11,12]

These techniques are frequently used in patients with pain
following thoracic or abdominal surgery. The purpose of this
exercise is to increase sensory awareness of movement of
the rib cage during breathing.

1. One or two hands are placed on the problem area of the
   chest. Assist the downward and inward movement of the
   ribs by gently squeezing with your palms.
2. Just before breathing in, add a quick stretch to the external
   intercostals with a quick downward and inward stretch
   to facilitate the contraction.
3. While the patient is breathing in, gently resist expansion
   of the ribs with your palms.

Techniques for different lung segments have been developed:
These techniques are described in detail elsewhere.[1]

PURSED-LIP BREATHING

This technique is most frequently taught to COPD patients
to help them deal with episodes of breathlessness. According
to Casiari and coworkers,[13] pursed lip breathing decreases
respiratory rate and increases tidal volume. Patients are instructed to breath in through their nose and passively exhale
through pursed lips.

COUGHING/SPUTUM CLEARANCE[1,9,14]

General principles to improve or teach coughing include:

1. Instruct the patient to sit with a slight forward lean

2. Say the letter *K* during exhalation
3. Instruct the patient in diaphragmatic breathing. Use the
   abdominal muscles to contract during exhalation with
   sharp cough.

Techniques:

1. *Splinting:* Splinting is typically used after thoracic or abdominal surgery. Instruct the patient to place a pillow
   firmly against the painful area while coughing.
2. *Huffing:* Instruct the patient to take a deep breath and then
   forcefully exhale with the mouth open. This is less stressful
   on the patient.
3. *Double or triple cough:* Instruct the patient to take a deep
   breath and then attempt to cough two or three times during
   the exhalation.
4. *Manual assistance:* Manual assistance is frequently used
   in spinal cord injury patients or patients with neurologic
   disease affecting the respiratory function. Place your hands
   (one hand on top of the other) below the ziphoid process
   and above the umbilicus. As the patient exhales, apply a
   quick pressure up and in.

PERCUSSION AND POSTURAL DRAINAGE (P&PD), VIBRATION[1,12,14,15]

Postural drainage is beneficial to patients with pulmonary
secretions. Gravity is used to assist in loosening secretions
from the chest wall. A detailed description of these 11 positions and procedures is described elsewhere.[1,12,15] Several
techniques are used in combination with postural drainage
to assist in this process.

PERCUSSION

Place your hands in a cupped position over the appropriate
lung segments. Move your hands in an up-and-down, rhythmic, alternating fashion while striking the chest wall. (You
should hear a dull thud versus a slapping noise if you are
doing the technique correctly.) Continue this treatment continuously for several minutes. Immediately after stopping,
have the patient sit up and use diaphragmatic breathing to
cough. Do not use over rib fractures, osteoporosis, or tumors.
Do not use in patients with pulmonary embolism, hemophilia, or low platelet count.

VIBRATION

Place your hands one over the other on the appropriate
segment. Apply pressure with vibration by tensing all the
muscles of the arm during expiration only. This technique
is frequently used after percussion to help mobilize the secretions to the proximal, larger airways.

PATIENT MOBILIZATION

Early mobilization is important for patients in the ICU; however, this is frequently limited by the medical status and
the equipment in use. Upright positioning, rolling in bed,
frequent position changes, sitting upright, transfer training,
and ambulation help loosen secretions from the chest wall
and help prevent consolidation of secretions in some areas.[9]
Deep breathing exercises and coughing can replace postural
drainage and percussion in patients who can participate.[9]

RESPIRATORY MUSCLE STRENGTH AND ENDURANCE TRAINING[1,16-18]

Training of respiratory muscle strength is described by Reid, Samrai as "high, near-maximal inspiratory or expiratory maneuvers that are usually quasi-isometric."[16] The patient is usually unable to do more than a few repetitions at a time. The purpose is to increase the amount of force produced by the respiratory muscles. However, in patients with COPD, endurance is decreased much more than strength. Respiratory muscle training is also used to improve the endurance of the inspiratory muscles. It is used in patients with COPD weaning from the ventilator and in neuromuscular weakness. In one form of endurance training, patients use a hand-held device with varying sized holes at one end to inhale through.[16,18] The smaller the hole, the more resistance there is to inhalation. However, by slowing down the speed of inspiration, patients can decrease the amount of force needed. New devices now being made have incentive spirometers attached to them so that the breathing rate and force can be consistent. Patients try to reach sessions of 20 to 30 min with this device daily. In the author's own experience, inspiratory muscle training has been as beneficial as aerobic exercise in improving functional mobility and exercise tolerance.

Some studies use weighted plungers or spring-loaded valves for threshold loading. The difference is that the patient must inhale with sufficient force to lift the plunger or open the valve.[16]

Patient and Family Education

Education is an important part of pulmonary rehabilitation. Patients and their families should learn the appropriate techniques (i.e., breathing exercises, P&PD, coughing techniques, self-monitoring of functional mobility, and aerobic exercise). The use of the Borg RPE scale is very helpful in learning to monitor the amount of activity to prevent excessive SOB from occurring. Patients should be independent with their home exercise programs prior to discharge.

References

1. Kisner C, Colby LA: *Therapeutic Exercise Foundations and Techniques.* Philadelphia, F.A. Davis, 1990.
2. Hillegass E, Sadowski HS (eds): *Essentials of Cardiopulmonary Physical Therapy.* Philadelphia, W.B. Saunders, 1994.
3. Kenny WL (ed): *ACSM's Guidelines for Exercise Testing and Prescription.* Baltimore, MD, Williams & Wilkins, 1995.
4. Foley MP, Prax B, Crowell R, Boone T: Effects of assistive devices on cardiorespiratory demands in older adults. *Phys Ther* 76:1313–1319, 1996.
5. Cousner JI, Martinez FJ, Celli BR: Pulmonary rehabilitation that includes arm exercise reduces metabolic and ventilatory requirements for simple arm elevation. *Chest* 103:34–41, 1993.
6. Celli BR, Rassulo J, Make BJ: Dyssynchronous breathing during arm but not leg exercise in patients with severe chronic airflow obstruction. *N Engl J Med* 314:1485–1490, 1986.
7. Martinez FJ, Cousner JI, Celli BR: Respiratory response to arm elevation in patients with chronic airflow obstruction. *Am Rev Respir Dis* 143:476–480, 1991.
8. Sullivan PE, Markus PD, Minor MA: *An Integrated Approach to Therapeutic Exercise Theory and Clinical Application.* Reston, VA, Reston Publishing Company, 1982.
9. Ciesla N: Chest physical therapy for patients in the intensive care unit. *Phys Ther* 76:609–625, 1996.
10. Frownfelter DL: *Chest Physical Therapy and Pulmonary Rehabilitation.* Chicago, Year Book Publishers, 1987.
11. Stiller K, Montarello J, Wallace M, et al: Efficacy of breathing and coughing exercises in prevention of pulmonary complications after coronary artery surgery. *Chest* 105:741–747, 1994.
12. Ciesla N: Postural drainage, positioning, breathing exercises, in Mackenzie CF (ed): *Chest Physiotherapy in the Intensive Care Unit.* Baltimore, MD, Williams & Wilkins, 1989, pp 97–99.
13. Casiari RJ: Effects of breathing retraining in patients with chronic obstructive pulmonary disease. *Chest* 79:393, 1981.
14. Watchie J: *Cardiopulmonary Physical Therapy: A Clinical Manual.* Philadelphia, W.B. Saunders, 1995.
15. Hilling L, Bakow E, Fink J, et al: American Association of Respiratory Care Clinical Practice Guidelines: Postural drainage therapy. *Respiratory Care* 36:1419, 1991.
16. Reid WD, Samrai B: Respiratory muscle training for patients with chronic obstructive pulmonary disease. *Phys Ther* 75:996–1005, 1995.
17. Reid WD, Dechman C: Considerations when testing the respiratory muscles. *Phys Ther* 75:971–982, 1995.
18. McCool FD, Tzelepsis GE: Inspiratory muscle training in patients with neuromuscular disease. *Phys Ther* 75:626–642, 1995.

Additional Readings

Downs AM: Physical therapy in lung transplantation. *Phys Ther* 76:626–643, 1995.

Martinez FJ, Vogel RD, Dupont DN, et al: Supported arm exercise vs unsupported arm exercise in the rehabilitation of patients with severe chronic airflow obstruction. *Chest* 103:1397–1402, 1993.

Vale F, Reardon JZ, ZuWallack RL: The long-term benefits of outpatient pulmonary rehabilitation on exercise endurance and quality of life. *Chest* 109:42–45, 1996.

Chapter 60

QUALITY OF LIFE, HEALTH STATUS, AND FUNCTIONAL IMPAIRMENT

PAUL W. JONES

Background

Impairment of respiratory function has both direct and indirect effects on the health of the patient. Direct effects are manifested through physiologic disturbances in the lungs that lead to breathlessness. Indirect physical effects include de-training, loss of lean body mass and muscle wasting resulting in weakness and fatigue. These may be as important as the direct effects, as evidenced by the observation that questionnaire items related to fatigue were judged by patients to be more important than items related to breathlessness.[1] Furthermore, it has been shown that leg fatigue is as important a determinant of exercise limitation as breathlessness.[2] Indirect psychosocial effects, such as anxiety and depression resulting from limitation of physical activity and panic due to high levels of breathlessness, also have a major impact on the patient's sense of well-being. Thus respiratory diseases may have a very broad effect on the patient's health (Fig. 60-1).

Pulmonary rehabilitation is a multidisciplinary intervention that incorporates a number of modalities discussed elsewhere in this book. A typical program will contain many components that produce a range of benefits. The relative contribution of each will vary between programs and patients. Whilst each may have a more or less specific effect, measurable using appropriate instruments, the outcome of greatest interest is the overall effect.

This chapter will focus on chronic obstructive pulmonary disease (COPD). Since COPD is a disease that causes ill health through a number of mechanisms and rehabilitation is a treatment that has a number of different outcomes, it follows that the most appropriate instrument for measuring the improvement that can be achieved through pulmonary rehabilitation will be one that can aggregate together a wide range of results into one summary measure. There are a number of measurement instruments that purport to achieve this. They fall into two main categories—those that attempt to measure the overall impact of the disease and those that restrict their focus to limitations of physical activity. The latter is not necessarily as narrow as it appears at first sight, since physical training is a fundamental component of rehabilitation, and there does appear to be a good correlation between overall health status and physical function.[3,4]

Purposes of Health Status Measurement

Before considering the types of measurement that may be made it is worth recording the reasons why we wish to make such measurements. In broad terms these are:

1. To define the health of groups of patients
2. To measure changes in the health of groups of patients
3. To predict future health resource use
4. To assess the impact of disease and treatment on an individual patient

The order in which these are presented reflects the historical development and application of these instruments. Numerous studies have addressed the validity of different types of questionnaires in patients with COPD, and several studies have attempted to measure changes with treatment. There are also some data concerning the predictive validity of some questionnaires, but there has been little work on the application of such measurements to the management of individual patients with COPD.

Since the main objectives of health measurement are to define the health status of patients and quantify the response to treatment, it is clear that standardization is required. Without this, it would be impossible to make comparisons between different patients or different treatments. Standardization imposes a number of requirements upon the design of a questionnaire (Fig. 60-2), but perhaps the most important is the choice of items that make up the questionnaire. If we wish to measure the effect of disease reliably (i.e., assess each patient in the same way using the same measurement criteria), the questionnaire should be equally relevant to all individuals who may be measured. As a result, all the items should apply potentially to all individuals who may be studied—without influence of age, gender, race, culture, or socioeconomic background. For this reason, many items may need to be excluded because of such biases.[5] The end result is often a questionnaire containing items that reflect the lowest common denominator of similarity between patients with the same disease. This practical requirement has a major effect on the design of the instrument, and clearly limits the range of effects that can be measured. That having been said, the development of the standardized tools discussed in this chapter has enabled quantification of the effects of COPD on a patient's health and their response to treatment in a way that was not hitherto possible.

Categorization of Instruments to Measure Impaired Health

A number of different terms are applied to the measurements used to quantify the impact of COPD on a patient's daily life and well-being. This can lead to confusion through overlap and differences of interpretation and definition between authors. A further problem arises in the tension generated between theoreticians who wish to analyze and define the concept of ill health due to disease, and those who wish to develop valid and practical methods for measuring ill health. To clarify these issues, the major categories of measurement will be outlined here. Where possible, overlaps between the categories will be highlighted.

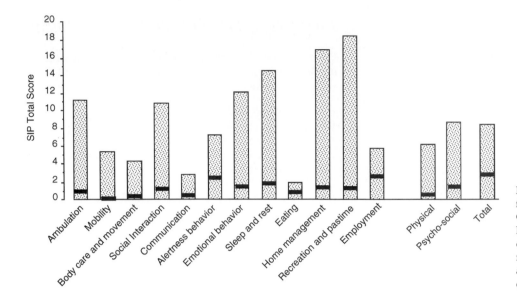

FIGURE 60-1 Sickness Impact profile (SIP) scores in patients with COPD. Their mean post-bronchodilator FEV_1 was 53 percent predicted. The thick bars indicate the normal values for patients in this age range. (Data are from reference 3.)

QUALITY OF LIFE

Quality of life (QOL) is a general term that applies to all individuals, whether diseased or healthy. It largely defies operational definition, but one useful approach is to view it as the gap between that which is desired in life and the degree to which this desire is achieved or achievable.

An alternative approach to defining QOL may be illustrated by the detailed and inclusive description of the narrower concept of health-related quality of life (HRQOL) proposed by Patrick and Erickson[6] and illustrated in Fig. 60-3. Health-related quality of life will be discussed in greater detail below, but this example is used here to illustrate the potential breadth of QOL measurement and the many ways in which interindividual variation may affect this. Whether one uses a global or detailed definition, both approaches share a common problem—the influence of individuals in setting targets for their lives. For this reason it does not appear possible to produce a practical instrument that truly measures individual quality of life in a standardized way, although a tool for the assessment of individual HRQOL has been developed.[7]

Despite the practical limitations concerning the measurability of individual QOL, the concept is immensely valuable in the context of treating individual patients. Rehabilitation is concerned with helping each patient utilize their capacities optimally. The instruments to be discussed in this chapter only reflect an individual's QOL to a certain degree. Furthermore, results of clinical trials obtained with such instruments will only indicate the average level of improved health to be expected in a typical patient. On crossing the boundary from findings obtained in groups of patients to the care of the individual, one passes from standardized measurements of health to individual QOL. In so doing, one passes from the science of health status measurement to the art and skill of the clinician.

HEALTH STATUS MEASUREMENT

The terms "Health Status," "Health Related Quality of Life," and "Functional Status" are all applied to the process of measuring the hypothetical construct of "impaired health."[8] Health status and health related quality of life will be discussed here, whilst functional status will be discussed later under its own heading.

The term "health related quality of life" (HRQOL) is often used synonymously with "health status measurement," but I will argue that it is worth drawing a distinction between these two terms. Health status measurement may be defined broadly as: quantification of the impact of disease on the patient's daily life and well being. As already discussed, Patrick and Erickson have produced a much more detailed description of the specific components of HRQOL, in which it is clear that the impact of the disease on the individual should be assessed.[6] This is, to a degree, in conflict with the objectives of the authors of standardized questionnaires who try to minimize the impact of interindividual differences on the content and structure of their questionnaires. Their approach is to produce an instrument that treats each individual as if he or she were a typical patient with the disease. Since individual quality of life components are largely absent from most of the questionnaires that have been developed, the term HRQOL would not seem to be appropriate. Health status measurement may be a better description.

In the past, health status measurement was seen to be the process of assessing the health of patients through outside observers. This was in contrast to QOL measurements which reflected the feelings of the individual sufferer. This distinction is less important now, since it is recognized that health

FIGURE 60-2 Minimum requirements for a health status questionnaire to ensure standardization of measurements.

- Same questions
- Same format
- Same instructions
- Same administration method
- Same response format
- Scored in the same way

On each occasion

OPPORTUNITY

> Social or cultural disadvantage
>
> Resilience

HEALTH PERCEPTIONS

> General
>
> Satisfaction

FUNCTIONAL STATUS

> **Social Function**
>
> > Limitations in usual roles
> >
> > Integration
> >
> > Contact
> >
> > Intimacy and sexual function
>
> **Psychological Function**
>
> > Affective
> >
> > Cognitive
>
> **Physical Function**
>
> > Activity restriction
> >
> > Fitness

IMPAIRMENT

> Symptoms
>
> Signs
>
> Self-reported disease
>
> Physiological measures
>
> Tissue alterations
>
> Diagnosis

DEATH AND DURATION OF LIFE

FIGURE 60-3 The major components of health-related quality of life as proposed by Patrick and Erickson (derived from reference 6).

status estimates can only be provided by patients themselves. It is more useful, therefore, to highlight the difference between standardized measurements of health, and individual quality of life. For this reason the term "health status" will be used throughout this chapter to describe the instruments that fall within this category of measurement. "Quality of life" will be retained for use when discussing individuals.

There are two basic types of health status instrument—generic questionnaires such as the Sickness Impact Profile (SIP), the Medical Outcomes Study Short Form 36 (SF-36), and the Nottingham Health Profile (NHP). Another generic instrument, the Quality of Well Being Scale (QWB) will be discussed under "Utility Scales." The second type of questionnaire is the disease-specific measure, the best documented of which are the Chronic Respiratory Questionnaire (CRQ) and the St. George's Respiratory Questionnaire (SGRQ). Much has been made of the differences between generic and disease-specific measures, but they are both very similar in concept. The major difference is that the content of the disease-specific measures is restricted to that known to be relevant to COPD (and asthma in the case of the SGRQ). In contrast, the generic measures are broader and designed

to cover a variety of aspects of health and be relevant to most disease states. As a result, they may contain relatively few items of direct relevance to COPD patients and many that are not.

SICKNESS IMPACT PROFILE

The Sickness Impact Profile (SIP) is a generic instrument that has been used quite widely in COPD. Its application in this setting has been reviewed at length .[9] It has 136 items that are designed to measure the impact of ill health on behavior or performance of daily life activities. Each item is a statement about aspects of dysfunction in 12 areas of activity. The items each have an empirically derived weight. The subject is asked to check each item that applies to them on that day. The categories are: ambulation, mobility, body care, and movement (these contribute to the Physical subscore); social interaction, communication, alertness behavior and emotional behavior (contributing to the Psychosocial score); sleep and rest, eating, home management, recreation and pastimes, and work (these components do not contribute to any subscore). A total score is also calculated using the responses to all 12 areas of activity. The scores range from 0 (no dysfunction) to 100 percent which indicates the worst possible score. The development and testing of the SIP has been described in detail.[10,11] There have been a number of studies describing the performance of the SIP in COPD,[3,12,13] the data in Fig. 60–1 being derived from one of these.[3] This profile of scores is quite similar to those obtained in other studies of patients with COPD of varying degrees of severity.[12,13]

The published data suggest that the SIP can discriminate between different levels of COPD, but its measurement properties warrant further discussion because they illustrate some important points concerning methods of assessing the validity of health status questionnaires. One standard approach is to relate its scores to a range of measures that are relevant to the disease in question. Figure 60-4A shows that the SIP correlates quite well with the 6-min walking distance. In fact, the correlation is as strong as that between exercise performance and the SGRQ (a disease-specific measure, to be discussed below), as shown in Fig. 60-4B. While this might suggest that the two measures behave similarly, the frequency distributions for the SIP and SGRQ scores are very different (Fig. 60-5). Scores for the disease-specific measure are normally distributed within the middle of the scoring range, but the SIP scores are highly skewed towards the mild end of the spectrum. Clearly these two questionnaires have quite different measurement properties. One conclusion to be drawn from this data is that the SIP may be more sensitive to deteriorations in health than to improvements. There have been no trials that have compared directly the performance of the SIP with disease-specific measures in COPD, so it is difficult to interpret results from studies that reported no difference between treatment and control groups in clinical trials in this condition.[14–16] Certainly, the SIP has proved to be less sensitive than disease-specific instruments in clinical trials in asthma.[17]

MEDICAL OUTCOMES STUDY SF-36

The SF-36 is a generic questionnaire that has eight component scores labeled Physical function, Physical role limitation, Emotional role limitation, Social function, Pain, Energy and vitality, General health.[18,19] These can be collapsed down to

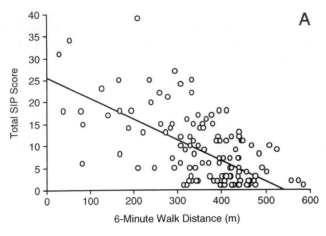

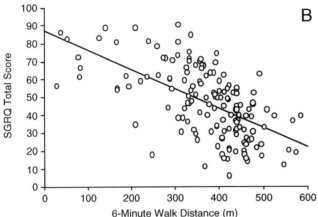

FIGURE 60-4 Correlations between exercise performance measured using a 6-min walking test and health status measured using the Sickness Impact Profile (SIP) and St. George's Respiratory Questionnaire (SGRQ) in patients with COPD. The Pearson *r* value for the correlation between walking distance and SIP was 0.64; that between SGRQ and walking distance was 0.61. (Data are from references 4 and 5.)

form a Physical component score and a Mental component score. Unlike the SIP which permits only a negative or affirmative response to each item, the SF-36 uses Lickert scales. A good correlation has been shown between dyspnea measured using the Baseline Dyspnea Index and the SF-36 scores for Physical function, Physical role limitation, Vitality, and General health.[20] Its performance in clinical trials suggests that the SF-36 may not be as sensitive as disease-specific measures. For example, in a trial of the long-acting bronchodilator, salmeterol, changes in the SF-36 scores were small and in most cases not statistically significant.[21] The Physical role limitation score achieved the greatest change, but this was markedly less than the change in the SGRQ score. Preliminary reports from two studies of pulmonary rehabilitation showed moderately large changes in SF-36 scores, but these results are currently only available in abstract form.[22,23]

NOTTINGHAM HEALTH PROFILE

The Nottingham Health Profile (NHP) is a multidimensional generic health status questionnaire.[24] It contains 38 items divided into six aspects of health (Energy, Pain, Emotional reactions, Sleep, Social isolation, and Physical mobility). A

total score is calculated as the proportion of affirmative answers and ranges from zero (no perceived distress) to 100 (maximum perceived distress). This questionnaire has been used recently, in a large study in Spanish men with COPD, to examine the relationship between health status and FEV_1.[25] The NHP showed a significant correlation with severity—assessed using the American Thoracic Society staging system, however this association was weaker than that observed in the same study between COPD severity and health status assessed using the SGRQ.

CHRONIC RESPIRATORY QUESTIONNAIRE

The Chronic Respiratory Questionnaire (CRQ) was developed specifically for use in patients with COPD.[1,26] It has 20 component items, each with a 7-point Lickert scale. These items are grouped into four components: Dyspnea, Fatigue, Mastery, and Emotion. The content of the Fatigue, Mastery, and Emotional components is fixed, but the Dyspnea component is individualized in that each patient is asked to report the five most important activities that caused them breathlessness over the previous 2 weeks. They are asked to do this by recall and by reading from a list of 26 activities. This approach was adopted to permit a degree of individualization in the questionnaire, both to measure exercise limitations that mattered to the patient and to increase the sensitivity of the questionnaire to changes in health.

FIGURE 60-5 Frequency distributions for the Sickness Impact Profile (SIP) and St. George's Respiratory Questionnaire (SGRQ) scores used for the regressions illustrated in Fig. 60-4. (Data are from references 4 and 5.)

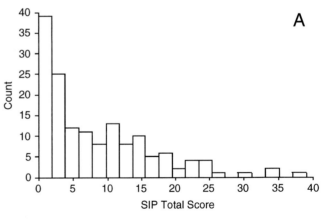

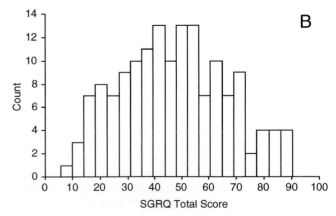

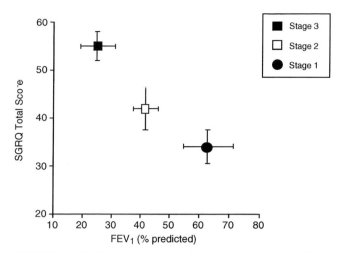

FIGURE 60-6 St. George's Respiratory Questionnaire (SGRQ) and FEV₁ data from three groups of male patients defined according to American Thoracic Society staging criteria for the severity of COPD. The error bars indicate 95 percent confidence intervals. (The data are from reference 25.)

The CRQ was developed solely as an evaluative instrument, so tests of its validity have been concerned largely with detection of changes in health. In an observational study, changes in CRQ dyspnea score correlated equally well with changes in walking distance, global dyspnea score, global fatigue, and global emotional function.[1,27] Changes in the fatigue score showed a similar pattern of correlations. The CRQ has been found to be sensitive to bronchodilator-induced changes in lung function in COPD patients.[28] Results obtained with this instrument in pulmonary rehabilitation studies will be discussed in greater depth below.

ST. GEORGE'S RESPIRATORY QUESTIONNAIRE
The SGRQ was developed for use in patients with asthma and COPD.[4,29] It has 50 items grouped into three components: Symptoms, Activity, and Impacts (the latter covering the psychosocial effects of the disease). Each item has its own empirically derived weight. These weights have been shown to be independent of age, sex, disease duration, and disease severity.[30] Furthermore they appear to be largely independent of language and culture and are not different between asthma and COPD.[29,31] A total score is also calculated. The SGRQ was subject to intensive validation.[4] In addition, it has recently been shown that the SGRQ may be a predictor of hospital readmission and nebulizer prescription in COPD.[32] In clinical trials, it has been shown to be responsive to the long-acting bronchodilator, salmeterol, and has demonstrated clear benefits from the introduction of pressure support ventilation in hypoxic hypercapnic COPD patients.[21] Whilst this questionnaire has good evaluative properties it also has discriminative properties, being able to distinguish between different levels of disease in different groups of patients[25] (Fig. 60-6). To date there have been few published studies using the SGRQ in pulmonary rehabilitation program.[33]

UTILITY SCALES

Utility scales were developed largely from a health economic perspective to quantify the utility or value placed on a health state. Methods used to obtain these utilities included techniques such as "willingness-to-pay" or trade-offs between the level and duration of health. Although these concepts are useful, the measurements are largely theoretical exercises, since the individual is not actually required to sacrifice any money or life for improved health. This problem makes the validation of such techniques very difficult. One generic health status questionnaire, the Quality of Wellbeing Scale (QWB), uses preference weights for each item in the questionnaire.[34] It also includes death as a health state, unlike other health status scales, so it can be thought of as either a generic health status instrument or a utility scale.

QUALITY OF WELLBEING SCALE
The QWB is a generic questionnaire that has utility scaling properties. An early study suggested that it does have some validity for use in patients with airways obstruction.[35] It has been used in relatively few studies in COPD. In a study of increasing doses of beta agonists, it failed to detect a benefit, despite statistically significant improvements in FEV₁.[36] In the same study, the CRQ also failed to detect a significant health status gain, so it is difficult to draw conclusions about the sensitivity of the QWB in that setting. In a more recent study of a comprehensive pulmonary rehabilitation program, the QWB failed to detect any improvement in health despite clear improvement in exercise performance and reductions in breathlessness.[37]

FUNCTIONAL STATUS

Functional status has been defined as "a multi-dimensional concept characterising the ability to perform those activities people do in the normal course of their lives to meet basic needs, fulfill usual roles and maintain their health and well-being."[38] It has been argued that functional status may be one component of health and HRQOL, but should not be considered synonymous with these concepts. The difficulty with this distinction is that Leidy, who has argued cogently for the concept of functional status in COPD, states that functional capacity includes cognitive, psychological, social, and physical functions, together with sociodemographic potential. This makes the definition of functional status very similar to that used by Patrick and Erickson for HRQOL.[6] The main difference between the two appears to lie in the emphasis placed on performance of activities in functional status measures, whereas HRQOL instruments also attempt to measure feelings.

It has been argued that functional status has four components[38]:

Functional capacity: The maximum potential to perform activities

Functional performance: The individual day-to-day level of activity

Functional reserve: The gap between functional status and functional performance that the individual can draw upon

Functional capacity utilization: The extent to which capacity is drawn upon in the selected level of performance

These constructs are valuable for their conceptual rather than their practical utility. The analogy that Leidy draws between functional capacity and the physiological measurement of the V_{O₂}max[38] illustrates the limitation of functional capacity as a practical concept. The V_{O_2}max is an end point used in a test that progressively increases the stress placed on a patient up to and beyond his or her maximum capacity to take up oxygen. There is no equivalent test that places progressively increasing demands on the functionality of the patient to the point at which their functional capacity is reached. Despite this limitation, the concept of functional reserve is useful in pulmonary rehabilitation, since it is the region in which improvements in the patient's ability to perform daily activities may be achieved.

A number of methods of measuring functional status have been described, although using Leidy's classification, these should be described as measures of functional performance. In patients with COPD, the questionnaire that has attracted most attention as a functional performance measure is the SIP, discussed above as a generic health status measure. This is because it is concerned very much with the patient's performance of a wide range of different activities. Indeed, a version produced for use in the United Kingdom was called the Functions Limitation Profile. With few exceptions, most of the instruments developed to measure functional performance in COPD have concentrated largely on physical function and mobility.

PULMONARY FUNCTIONAL STATUS AND DYSPNEA QUESTIONNAIRE

As initially developed the Pulmonary Functional Status and Dyspnoea Questionnaire (PFSDQ) had a large number of items covering activities and dyspnea.[39] It was later revised to produce the PFSDQ-M which contains 40 items and requires about 7 min to administer. It uses self-report and has been shown to require seventh-grade reading skills. The questionnaire has shown sensitivity to change in response to antidepressant therapy in COPD.[40]

PULMONARY FUNCTIONAL STATUS SCALE

In its original form, the Pulmonary Functional Status Scale (PFSS) contains 56 items covering self care, mobilization, shopping, and relationships.[41] It has been used extensively to assess the outcome of routine pulmonary rehabilitation programs, although randomized trial data using this instrument are not yet available. A 35-item version of this questionnaire contains 22 items concerned with activity and social functioning, 10 items about psychological function and three concerned with sexual function.

ACTIVITY OF DAILY LIVING SCALES

Activities of daily living (ADL) scales may be viewed as a subgroup of physical functional performance scales. They are concerned with the subject's ability to function independently in daily life. They address activities concerned with bodily needs such as dressing, eating, and bathing, but may also include activities that enable these needs to be met. Their content may overlap substantially with that of the functional performance instruments. ADL scales were developed for patients with stroke or other severe disabling conditions in the elderly, but have been applied recently in COPD. These scales may have particular application in patients who are housebound, since their content is concerned largely with activities that do not require movement outside the home. As a result, they may detect differences between levels of severe disability better than disease-specific questionnaires

such as the CRQ and SGRQ. In consequence, they may be more sensitive to changes following rehabilitation in this group of patients.

THE ACTIVITIES OF DAILY LIVING LIST

This has been used in a number of studies in COPD. Correlations have been found between ADL score and FEV_1 and dyspnea,[13,42] and with frequency of cough and wheezing.[13] In a clinical trial of respiratory muscle training on a background of pulmonary rehabilitation, the ADL scores improved in both groups whether or not they had specific inspiratory muscle training.[43] In fact there was no difference in the change in ADL between the two treatment groups.

NOTTINGHAM EXTENDED ACTIVITIES OF DAILY LIVING SCALE

The Nottingham Extended Activities of Daily Living Scale (EADL) is an instrumental ADL measure that has 22 items covering four domains of activity (Mobility, Domestic, Kitchen, and Leisure). Scores range from 0 to 22, and independent people score high. In patients with COPD on long-term oxygen therapy, EADL scores were significantly lower than in patients with equally severe airways obstruction but who were not on long-term oxygen.[44] In the same study, the SGRQ scores were not different between these two groups. The EADL scores correlated with FEV_1, SGRQ scores, and depression. In addition they correlated with Reitan Trail B—a measure of cognitive function. It appears that EADL scores may be valid instruments for use in patients with COPD, especially at the more severe end of the spectrum where other disease-specific instruments such as the SGRQ and CRQ may experience floor effects.

CLINICAL DYSPNEA RATING SCALES

These scales are included in this chapter for completeness to illustrate some of the overlaps that occur between measures that purport to measure different things. These instruments address the impact of dyspnea on daily physical activity. A number of different scales have been developed, including the British Medical Research Council Dyspnoea Scale[45] and the Oxygen Cost Diagram.[46] Another instrument, the Baseline Dyspnea Index[47] uses a similar approach, but is more sophisticated in design since it addresses both the magnitude of the task causing breathlessness and the effort involved. These instruments use self-report and rank physical activities along a continuum from very low energy expenditure to very high. In many respects they are similar to functional performance scales such as the PFSDQ and PFSS, although they are shorter and less comprehensive. They also overlap with components of some health status questionnaires, such as the Dyspnea Component of the CRQ, the Activity Component of the SGRQ, and the Physical Function component of the SF-36. These clinical rating scales will not be discussed further in this chapter since they address only a limited, albeit important, aspect of impaired health in COPD.

Health Status Measurement in Randomized Controlled Trials

There have been a number of randomized controlled trials in which health status measurements have been made. The

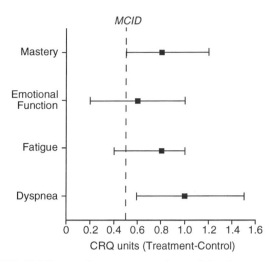

FIGURE 60-7 Results from a meta-analysis of the change in Chronic Respiratory Questionnaire scores in patients receiving pulmonary rehabilitation compared to those in the control groups. The error bars indicate 95 percent confidence intervals. MCID indicates the difference in scores between treatment groups that is considered to be the minimum clinically significant difference. The further the score lies to the left of zero, the greater the improvement in health status in the patients given rehabilitation. (The primary data for this meta-analysis are contained in references 48–52. The meta-analysis is presented in reference 53.)

majority of these have employed the CRQ.[48-52] This body of data was reviewed by Lacasse and coworkers,[53] who aggregated these results in a metaanalysis (Fig. 60-7). A picture emerged of a broad improvement in all four components of the CRQ. The metaanalysis revealed statistically significant improvements in all four components, the greatest being seen in the Dyspnea component and the least with Emotional function. For each component, the mean value for the improvement was above the threshold for a minimum clinically important difference. The improvement in Dyspnea score was twice the threshold for clinical significance and the lower 95 percent confidence interval of this estimate still lay above the threshold for improvement. The score for Mastery again showed a lower 95 percent confidence interval that lay at the threshold for a clinically significant improvement. Thus, it seems reasonable to conclude that two of the four components of impaired health addressed by this questionnaire showed an improvement following rehabilitation that was both clinically and statistically significant.

There are some interesting observations to be made about the improvements following rehabilitation as measured by the CRQ. In a recent study,[33] it was found that CRQ scores were normally distributed at baseline, but changes in CRQ score following rehabilitation showed a highly skewed distribution. No patient showed any evidence of worsening score. In contrast, the other variables measured exercise performance, SF-36 scores, SGRQ scores, and scores for anxiety and depression. All showed changes that were more normally distributed. The reason for the skewed distribution in the CRQ change scores is not entirely clear, but may be linked to the method of administration. Subjects are shown their previous scores at the time of making their follow-up estimates.[54] This lack of blinding maybe very important in a

clinical trial of pulmonary rehabilitation. The randomized controlled clinical trial design was developed to minimize systematic biases in recruitment, treatment, and outcome measurement. In a rehabilitation study it is not possible to blind the patient to the intervention since no form of sham physical training has been developed. Thus the patients are not blinded to their intervention and, when using the CRQ, they are also not blinded to their baseline scores. In other clinical trials it has been shown that lack of blinding in treatment allocation may overestimate the apparent effectiveness of a therapy by as much as 40 percent.[55] It is possible, therefore, that the CRQ may overestimate the true magnitude of benefit following rehabilitation.

Another interesting aspect of the improvement in health status following rehabilitation concerns the mechanisms by which the improvement is achieved. Physical training is one of the most important components of a rehabilitation program, so a correlation between improvement in health status and improvement in exercise performance might be expected. In fact this not always the case. Despite clinically and statistically significant improvements in CRQ scores, no correlation was found between change in any of the scores and improvement in walking distance in a study of moderately large size.[56] In a more recent randomized controlled trial of out-patient pulmonary rehabilitation,[33] significant correlations were found at baseline between exercise performance and CRQ Dyspnea and Fatigue scores (Table 60-1). These cross-sectional correlations are quite interesting, because they suggest that while the CRQ was not developed to discriminate between patients, it does have discriminant properties. The CRQ Mastery score was the strongest correlate of exercise performance, pretreatment. Following rehabilitation there were significant correlations between improvement in exercise performance and improvement in Dyspnea and Fatigue components (Table 60-1). In contrast, while the Emotion and Mastery components both improved significantly, the changes were unrelated to the improvement in exercise performance. It appears that the degree of improvement in dyspnea and fatigue following rehabilitation is quantitatively related to the improved exercise capacity, but improvement in emotional and psychological function is not. Improvements in emotions and psychological function appear to be linked to the physical component of rehabilitation, since they are not seen to the same degree in control patients who receive only education. This suggests that these improvements are either a nonspecific response to physical training or due to currently unidentified factors.

To date, there have been fewer studies using other health status measures, but a recent trial used the CRQ, the SGRQ, and the SF-36.[33] The CRQ produced statistically significant improvements in both the control and rehabilitation limbs. The improvement in the latter was significantly greater, both statistically and clinically, than in the control group. The SGRQ showed improvements that just reached the threshold for clinical and statistical significance. In the same study the SF-36 did not show statistically significant changes, although preliminary reports from two other studies using this questionnaire are encouraging.[22,23] Another generic instrument, the QWB, failed to detect any health gains from pulmonary rehabilitation in a large and comprehensive trial.[37]

It is still too soon to draw firm conclusions from differences in the size of health gain obtained with different instruments

TABLE 60-1 Correlations between Chronic Respiratory Questionnaire Scores and Exercise Performance

	Correlation between Baseline Exercise and Baseline CRQ Scores (r value)	Correlation between Change in Exercise and Change in CRQ Scores (r value)
Dyspnea	0.35*	0.43**
Fatigue	0.42**	0.38*
Emotion	0.12 N.S.	0.14 N.S.
Mastery	0.45**	0.10 N.S.

NOTE: Baseline, indicates cross-sectional comparison between patients before rehabilitation; change, indicates longitudinal comparison within patients following rehabilitation; N.S., $p > .05$; *, $p < .01$; **, $p < .001$.

following rehabilitation. Too few studies have been performed with instruments other than the CRQ to be sure that the differences that have been observed to date are real. If further studies do suggest a consistent difference in responsiveness between questionnaires, it will be necessary to test whether some of this is due to the method of administering the CRQ. If an effect of knowledge of previous scores is found, this will raise the issue of whether an improvement that is perceivable only with reference to a previous state is as important an outcome in health status measurement as an "absolute" change.

Health Status Measurement in Individual Patients

The studies discussed in this chapter are largely randomized controlled trials performed in groups of patients. They show that, on average, worthwhile improvements in health may be obtained through a pulmonary rehabilitation program. In routine practice, it would be desirable to quantify the health gain in each individual to assess whether he or she received benefit. Unfortunately, the repeatability of the health status questionnaires, although perfectly adequate for studies of groups, is too low to determine reliably whether an individual patient has had a clinically significant improvement following treatment. For this reason, the application of health status measurement to the care of individual patients must be limited. Functional performance measures such as the PFSS and PFSDQ-M have found greatest application in the evaluation of pulmonary rehabilitation programs, but they may also identify the functional needs of individual patients. This could lead to more focused and targeted objectives for each patient in a rehabilitation program.

Summary and Conclusions

The impact of COPD on the daily life and well-being of patients with this disease may be measured in a number of different ways. A range of different questionnaires are available, each purporting to measure either: health, health-related quality of life, or functional status. There is a large measure of overlap between most of these questionnaires, the chief difference between them being in the proportion of items concerned with physical function on the one hand and emotional and psychological effects of the disease on the other. The PFSDQ-M and the CRQ appear to lie at opposite ends of this spectrum. There is considerable evidence

that many of these questionnaires are valid for use in patients with COPD, but there are fewer data to show that they are responsive to pulmonary rehabilitation. The CRQ has proved to be undoubtedly the most responsive questionnaire. Its apparent sensitivity is encouraging, but the hypothesis that this might be due in part to the method of administration must be tested.

There have been relatively few programs designed specifically for patients who are too disabled to leave their home, but in them, use of instruments that measure basic activities may be more appropriate than other health status questionnaires. The use of functional performance instruments in this severe group should also be explored, because these questionnaires contain a number of items that relate to basic body care. Functional performance instruments may also have application in the initial assessment of individual patients prior to a rehabilitation program to set individualized goals for each patient. Unfortunately health status measurements do not yet appear to provide a practical method of assessing outcome in individuals.

In conclusion, the science of health status measurement has advanced greatly over the last decade. While the existing instruments all have their limitations, it is now possible to make standardized measurements of the overall impact of a rehabilitation program on the health of patients with COPD. No other single measurement can achieve this.

References

1. Guyatt GH, Berman LB, Townsend M, et al: A measure of quality of life for clinical trials in chronic lung disease. *Thorax* 42:773–778, 1987.
2. Killian KJ, Leblanc P, Martin DH, et al: Exercise capacity and ventilatory, circulatory and symptom limitation in patients with chronic airflow limitation. *Am Rev Respir Dis* 146:935–940, 1992.
3. Jones PW, Baveystock CM, Littlejohns P: Relationships between general health measured with the Sickness Impact Profile and respiratory symptoms, physiological measures and mood in patients with chronic airflow limitation. *Am Rev Respir Dis* 140:1538–1543, 1989.
4. Jones PW, Quirk FH, Baveystock CM, et al: A self-complete measure for chronic airflow limitation—the St George's Respiratory Questionnaire. *Am Rev Respir Dis* 145:1321–1327, 1992.
5. O'Leary CJ, Jones PW: The influence of decisions made by developers on health status questionnaire content. *Quality of Life Research* 7:(in press) 1998.
6. Patrick DL, Erickson P: Assessing health-related quality of life for clinical decision making, in Walker SR, Rosser RM (eds): *Quality of Life Assessment: Key Issues in the 1990s.* Hingham, MA, Kluwer Academic Publishers, 1993:11–63.

7. Hickey AM, Bury G, O'Boyle CA, et al: A new short form individual quality of life measure (SEIQoL-DW): Application in a cohort of individuals with HIV/AIDS. *BMJ* 313:29–33, 1996.

8. Guyatt GH, Feeny DH, Patrick DL: Measuring health-related quality of life. *Ann Intern Med* 118:622–629, 1993.

9. Leidy NK. Functional performance in people with chronic obstructive pulmonary disease. *Image: J Nurs Schol* 27:23–34, 1995.

10. Bergner M, Bobbitt RA, Carter WB, et al: The Sickness Impact Profile: Development and final revision of a health status measure. *Med Care* 19:787–805, 1981.

11. Bergner M: The Sickness Impact Profile, in Walker SR, Rosser RM (eds): *Quality of Life: Assessment and Application,* Boston, M.T.P., 1987:79–94.

12. McSweeny J, Grant I, Heaton RK, et al: Life quality of patients with chronic obstructive pulmonary disease. *Arch Intern Med* 142:473–478, 1982.

13. Schrier AC, Dekker FW, Kaptein AA, et al: Quality of life in elderly patients with chronic non-specific lung disease seen in family practice. *Chest* 98:894–899, 1990.

14. Nocturnal Oxygen Therapy Trial (NOTT) Group: Continuous or nocturnal oxygen therapy in hypoxemic chronic obstructive lung disease. *Ann Intern Med* 93:391–398, 1980.

15. Larson JL, Kim MJ, Sharp JT, et al: Inspiratory muscle training with a pressure threshold breathing device in patients with chronic obstructive pulmonary disease. *Am Rev Respir Dis* 138:689–696, 1988.

16. Hoffman LA, Wesmiller SW, Sciurba FC, et al: Nasal cannula and transtracheal oxygen delivery. A comparison of patient response after 6 months of each technique. *Am Rev Respir Dis* 145:827–831, 1992.

17. Jones PW, for the Nedocromil Sodium Quality of Life Study Group: Quality of Life, symptoms and pulmonary function in asthma: Long-term treatment with nedocromil sodium examined in a controlled multicentre trial. *Eur Respir J* 7:55–62, 1994.

18. Stewart AL, Hays R, Ware JE: The MOS short-form general health survey. Reliability and validity in a patient population. *Med Care* 26:724–732, 1988.

19. Ware JE, Sherbourne CA, Davies AR: *The MOS Short-Form General Health Survey,* vol Publication Number P-7444. Santa Monica, CA, Rand Corporation, 1988.

20. Mahler DA, Mackowiak JI: Evaluation of the short-form 36-item questionnaire to measure health-related quality of life in patients with COPD. *Chest* 107:1585–1589, 1995.

21. Jones PW, Bosh TK: Changes in quality of life in COPD patients treated with salmeterol. *Am J Respir Crit Care Med* 155:1283–1289, 1997.

22. Griffiths TL, Ionescu A, Mullins J, et al: Use of the SF-36 questionnaire as an outcome measure in a randomized controlled trial of pulmonary rehabilitation. *Am J Respir Crit Care Med* 157:A257, (3) 1998.

23. Benzo R, Flume P: Effect of pulmonary rehabilitation (PR) on quality of life in patients with moderate to severe dyspnea due to respiratory diseases. *Am J Respir Crit Care Med* 157:A117, (3) 1998.

24. McEwen J: The Nottingham Health Profile, in Walker RR, Rosser RM (eds): *Quality of Life Assessment: Key Issues in the 1990s.* Hingham, MA, Kluwer Academic Publishers, 1993:111–130.

25. Ferrer M, Alonso J, Morera J, et al: Chronic obstructive pulmonary disease stage and health-related quality of life. *Ann Intern Med* 127:1072–1079, 1997.

26. Guyatt GH, Townsend M, Berman LB, et al: Quality of life in patients with chronic airflow limitation. *Br J Dis Chest* 81:45–54, 1987.

27. Guyatt GH, Townsend M, Keller J, et al: Measuring functional status in chronic lung disease: Conclusions from a randomized control trial. *Respir Med* 83(4):293–297, 1989.

28. Guyatt GH, Townsend M, Pugsley SO, et al: Bronchodilators in chronic air-flow limitation. *Am Rev Respir Dis* 135:1069–1074, 1987.

29. Jones PW, Quirk FH, Baveystock CM: The St George's Respiratory Questionnaire. *Respir Med* 85(Suppl B): 25–31, 1991.

30. Quirk FH, Jones PW: Patients' perception of distress due to symptoms and effects of asthma on daily living and an investigation of possible influential factors. *Clin Sci* 79:17–21, 1990.

31. Quirk FH, Baveystock CM, Wilson RC, et al: Influence of demographic and disease related factors on the degree of distress associated with symptoms and restrictions on daily living due to asthma in six countries. *Eur Respir J* 4:167–171, 1991.

32. Osman LM, Godden DJ, Friend JAR, et al: Quality of life and hospital re-admission in patients with chronic obstructive pulmonary disease. *Thorax* 52:67–71, 1997.

33. Wedzicha JA, Bestall JC, Garrod R, et al: Randomised controlled trial of pulmonary rehabilitation in patients with severe chronic obstructive pulmonary disease, stratified for disability. *Eur Respir J* (in press) 1998.

34. Kaplan RM, Anderson JP, Ganiats TG: The Quality of Well-being Scale: Rationale for a single quality of life index, in Walker SR, Rosser RM, (eds): *Quality of Life Assessment: Key Issues in the 1990's.* Hingham, MA, Kluwer Academic Publishers, 1993:65–94.

35. Kaplan RM, Atkins CJ, Timms R: Validity of a quality of well-being scale as an outcome measure in chronic obstructive pulmonary disease. *J Chron Dis* 37:85–95, 1984.

36. Jaeschke R, Guyatt GH, Willan A, et al: Effect of increasing doses of beta agonists on spirometric parameters, exercise capacity, and quality of life in patients with chronic airflow limitation. *Thorax* 49:479–484, 1994.

37. Ries AL, Kaplan RM, Limberg TM, et al: Effects of pulmonary rehabilitation on physiologic and psychosocial outcomes in patients with chronic obstructive pulmonary disease. *Ann Intern Med* 122:823–832, 1995.

38. Leidy NK: Functional status and the forward progress of merry-go-rounds: Toward a coherent analytical framework. *Nurs Res* 43:196–202, 1994.

39. Lareau S, Carrieri-Kohlman V, Janson-Bjerklie S, et al: Development and testing of the Pulmonary Functional Status and Dyspnea Questionnaire (PFSDQ). *Heart Lung* 23:242–250, 1994.

40. Borson S, McDonald G, Gayle T, et al: Improvement in mood, physical symptoms, and function with nortryptiline for depression in patients with chronic obstructive pulmonary disease. *Psychosomatics* 33:190–201, 1992.

41. Weaver T, Narsavage G: Physiological and psychological variables related to functional staus in chronic obstructive pulmonary disease. *Nurs Res* 41:286–291, 1992.

42. Kaptein AA, Brand PLP, Dekker FW, et al: Quality-of-life in a long-term multicentre trial in chronic nonspecific lung disease: assessment at baseline. *Eur Respir J* 6:1479–1484, 1993.

43. Dekhuijzen R, Folgering H, van Herwaarden L: Target-flow inspiratory muscles training at home and during pulmonary rehabilitation in COPD patients with ventilatory limitation during exercise. *Chest* 99:128–133, 1991.

44. Okubadejo AA, O'Shea L, Jones PW, et al: Home assessment of activities of daily living in patients with severe chronic obstructive pulmonary disease on long-term oxygen. *Eur Respir J* 10:1572–1575, 1997.

45. Fletcher CM, Elmes PC, Wood CH: The significance of respiratory symptoms and the diagnosis of chronic bronchitis in a working population. *BMJ* 1:257–266, 1959.

46. McGavin CR, Artvinli M, Naoe H, et al: Dyspnoea, disability and distance walked: comparison of estimates of exercise performance in respiratory disease. *Br Med J* 2:241–243, 1978.

47. Mahler DA, Weinberg DH, Wells CK, et al: Measurements of

dyspnea. Contents, interobserver correlates of two new clinical indices. *Chest* 85:751–758, 1984.

48. Busch AJ, McClements JD: Effects of a supervised home exercise program on patients with severe chronic obstructive pulmonary disease. *Phys Ther* 68:469–474, 1988.

49. Simpson K, Killian K, McCartney N, et al: Randomised controlled trial of weightlifting exercise in patients with chronic airflow limitation. *Thorax* 47:70–75, 1992.

50. Goldstein RS, Gort EH, Stubbing D, et al: Randomised controlled trial of respiratory rehabilitaticn. *Lancet* 344:1394–1397, 1994.

51. Wijkstra PJ, Van Altena R, Kraan J, et al: Quality of life in patients with chronic obstructive pulmonary disease improves after rehabilitation at home. *Eur Respir J* 7:269–273, 1994.

52. Güell R, Morante F, Sangenis M, et al: Effects of respiratory rehabilitation on the effort capacity and on the health-related quality of life of patients with chronic obstructive pulmonary disease. *Eur Respir J* 8(suppl):356, 1995.

53. Lacasse Y, Wong E, Guyatt GH, et al: Meta-analysis of respiratory rehabilitation in chronic obstructive pulmonary disease. *Lancet* 348:1115–1119, 1996.

54. Guyatt GH, Townsend M, Keller JL, et al: Should study subjects see their previous responses: Data from a randomized control trial. *J Clin Epidemiol* 42:913–920, 1989.

55. Schulz KF, Chalmers I, Hayes RJ, et al: Empirical evidence of bias: Dimensions of methodological quality associated with estimates of treatment effects in controlled trials. *JAMA* 273:408–412, 1995.

56. Reardon J, Patel K, ZuWallack RL: Improvement in quality of life in unrelated to improvement in exercise endurance after outpatient pulmonary rehabilitation. *J Cardiopulm Rehabil* 13:51–54, 1993.

PART VII

ART AND REHABILITATION

NEIL S. CHERNIACK

Art can be used recreationally and to improve dexterity, but it can be an important tool in rehabilitation. The visual arts, drama, writing, music, and dance have been used, for example, in the treatment of emotionally disturbed patients, in the disabled, and in patients who have experienced brain injury.

Creating art allows patients to convey their feelings about their illness and also provides them with a sense of achievement. On the other hand, for the physician, the works of art of their patients open windows into feelings and emotions which would otherwise remain hidden. In a more general sense, artists can capture in their works and make real the intense swings in emotion that often accompany serious illness.

Art therapy can be therapeutic, providing an acceptable outlet for feelings and when conducted in groups can promote social interactions and communications, important steps for disabled patients. Art can also be used diagnostically to examine state of mind of the patient.

The next two chapters focus on visual art from two different perspectives. The first chapter is by a pulmonary physician and intensivist who deals on a daily basis with the crippled respiratory patient. He is also an artist and his work has appeared in shows both in the United States and abroad. His chapter is concerned with the lessons that the physician can learn from art about illness and disability and the sense of importance of life that they may engender.

The second chapter is by an artist, art teacher, and art writer who has recently been a patient and who has also provided the cover illustration for this book. He describes his ideas and experiences on how art promotes healing and feelings of well-being and achievement.

Chapter 61
ART AND REHABILITATION
The Physician's Point of View

RICHARD LEVINSON

This chapter deals with the shared experiences and fears of doctors and patients. It has to do with understanding of the spirit, both our patients' and our own. I will use art to examine spiritual, intangible issues that extend beyond the con-

fined scope of any diagnostic-related group, but which affect our patients' state of well-being as much as their physical health does. Art, even when it is not created by patients, can help physicians understand the emotional and spiritual needs of patients. Their needs are the same as our own, but their disability heightens these needs and increases their importance.

This chapter will address several such needs which can be exaggerated by disability, including feelings of mortality, isolation, inadequacy, lamentation, and the desire for freedom from the constraints imposed by illness.

Fear of Death

The fear of death is nearly universal. Consider the frightening moment of confrontation with your medical school cadaver—embalmed, abandoned, anonymous, the expressionless gape, slightly open eyes. A special light seems to have disappeared. Remember "E.T." who was thought to be dead because of his blank stare and pale color but when touched by "Elliott," the warm pink glow of life magically returns? Art is sometimes made in an effort to deal with and to control the fear of death.

Art, since prehistory, has been made by those who are compelled to document or imprint their own existence; who strive for immortality through the art object itself.

Can the fear of death be overcome by knowing more about it? The closest one can get to understanding death might be the so-called near-death experience. Patients have described a cluster of experiences which seem to be relatively uniform and independent of any particular cultural background or set of religious beliefs. These experiences involve a sense of detachment, a sense of great calm yet total awareness of the moment when death appears near. Most who have been through "near death" have subsequently lost much of their natural fear of death. Artists have tried to use "near death" in many ways. Self-mutilation has been used by some performance artists such as Chris Burden as a means of inflicting pain upon themselves and attaining a greater closeness to their own death. The German artist Rudolph Schwarzkogler fabricated situations where he appeared to be severely wounded and then subsequently photographed these scenes. Gina Pane actually engaged in self-mutilation, using her own blood as the medium of documentation.

A related feeling as seen in the works of Yves Klein, is the sense of The Void, the unknown future. We, but especially our patients, must deal with this uncertainty every day. The uncertainty which many of us feel regarding life after death will be deeply influenced by our religious and social beliefs, but also by moment to moment disturbances in our daily encounters. Artists have looked to explore the uncertainty of the future for many centuries. In this century, Yves Klein began in the 1950s to try to identify specific colors, presented in a monochromatic, nonfigurative fashion that might act as a sort of a window through which one's spirit might escape into an unbounded, unrestricted freedom of movement and existence. He described this as a new architecture of the air or "The Void." He experimented with several colors but finally settled on a deeply intense blue pigment. This was, in fact, patented and bears his name: International Klein Blue, (Fig. 61-1). It produces an extremely powerful visual field

FIGURE 61-1

when seen in color and put on rectangular wood and canvas backgrounds with no frames whatsoever. These objects, placed a few inches from the walls themselves, seem to allow you to look through them, inspiring a feeling of peering into eternity. Not infrequently when these blue monochrome paintings are displayed, people have attempted to look so closely into and through them that they have lost their equilibrium and fallen forward into the paintings themselves.

In the late 1970s James Turrell, an American artist, began to make related work using pure light installations, in galleries and museum spaces. He would arrange a series of crisply aligned lights in an empty room so that there was an appearance of a solid structure made of light itself (Fig. 61-2). The potency of these installations is quite striking. Once a visitor to the Whitney Museum attempted to lean against one of these "nonexistent" light sculptures and fell, breaking an ankle. The visitor was able to obtain an out-of-court settlement for damages from the museum.

Reaching for Immortality

Artists have looked to the skies trying to find immortality. Perhaps this is why cave dwellers painted on their ceilings rather than on the walls themselves. On the other hand, for example, certain cultures have viewed the site of immortality not as the sky but as lying beneath the surface of the earth. The Hopi use the snake dance ritual to symbolically talk to their ancestors. For the Hopi, both the snakes and their ancestors live underground together and communicate with each other. Both the underground search and the search in the heavens are attempts to reach the unknown, unreachable places, the void, in which the spirit can exist forever.

FIGURE 61-2

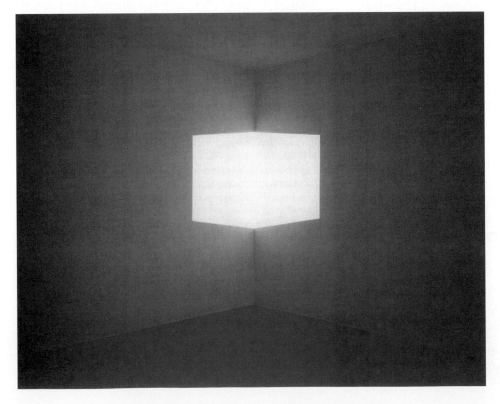

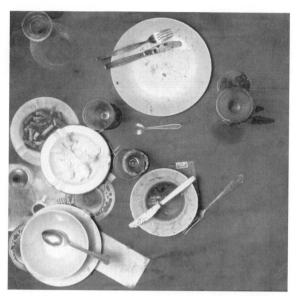

FIGURE 61-3

We, as physicians, must always try to recognize and respect the need to transcend time by leaving behind objects. We all leave things, watches, rings, musical instruments, silverware—objects that we have touched as a means of touching those who remain.

We wish to preserve the most wonderful moments of our lives in moments such as the birth of a child or grandchild,

FIGURE 61-4

a marriage, a love affair. We would like to be able to conjure them up in a nearly perfect fashion so that we can savor them repeatedly.

Daniel Spoerri is a French artist who tried to accomplish this in a most unusual way. In the 1960s he began to preserve the actual table settings which remained after he had dined with friends. At the end of a meal in a restaurant or home, he would fix each of the table items to the spot where they had been last, freezing the artifacts of that moment in perpetuity (Fig. 61-3). As strange as this idea might sound, the effect of taking these small table installations, gluing them in place right down to the last cigarette butt and empty wineglass, and standing them up on their side and attaching them behind a Plexiglas box on the wall is very compelling. In seeing these objects, we are reminded of other past moments that we wish to capture. Patients sometimes make videotapes of their last thoughts and hopes—to be seen by their families. Isn't this really motivated by the same desire as Spoerri'?

Certain artists have attempted to capture as many moments of a lifetime as possible in their work. One such artist is Roman Opalka, a Polish artist who lives in France. Many years ago he embarked on a most extraordinary project. Using a large, nearly black rectangular canvas he painted consecutive numbers, starting with the number 1. He began his numbering in a consistent fashion, with the numbers reading from left to right consecutively as if on a line. He then would drop to the next line and do the same until the entire canvas was filled with consecutive numbers (Fig. 61-4). Over the succeeding days, months, and years he has continued his pursuit of moment to moment life, and has now produced a large number of canvasses with the consecutive numbering string unbroken. With each succeeding canvas the background becomes an infinitesimally lighter shade. At the end of his journey (question end of his life) the background and the numbers will all have become nearly pure white. Associated with this have been photographs of his own face, so that the sequential passage of numbers is correlated with his own progression from youth through the aging process.

When we are well, it is easy to take health for granted. Life seems to simply go on, and it is the unusual person who is truly able to savor just a normal day. However, when illness strikes there is often an urgent need to identify and count each day to determine when the illness began and to determine the days to recover or to death. Opalka has in a way illustrated the complexity and the diligence required for us to truly savor the moments of our own lives and the passage of time.

Disparity between Inner and Outer Self

As an intensivist, I have often been struck by the custom of families placing photographs of the ill or injured on the wall adjacent to where the patient is lying. It is a striking reminder to all that the person's real life and image are so often quite different from the wounded physicality which we confront. The expressions seen in the photographs are almost universally vibrant, cheerful, full of and in context with special events of their lives.

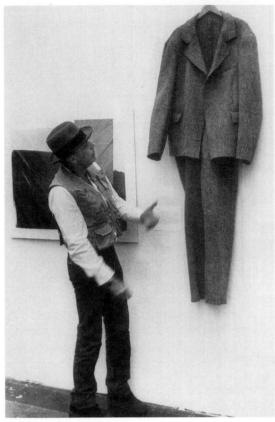

FIGURE 61-5

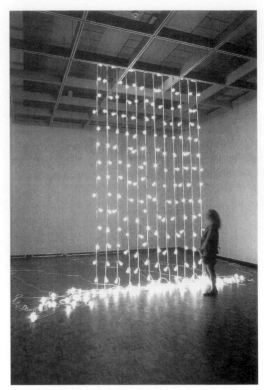

FIGURE 61-6

FIGURE 61-7

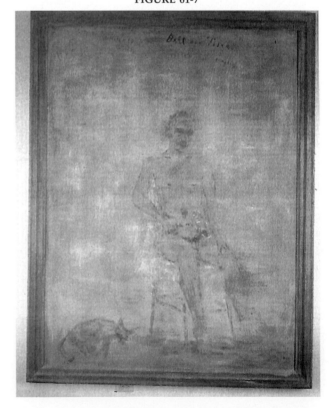

Very often, the patients themselves during their time in the Intensive Care Unit have lost most if not all of that sense of vitality in their facial expressions. They have been isolated into a sterile environment with hospital clothing which no longer distinguishes them in any way from any other patient in the hospital. Their faces often bear only the slightest resemblance to any photo taken during periods of wellness and joy.

One of my elderly patients had end-stage heart disease and severe bronchiectasis. She was oxygen-dependent and required multiple hospitalizations during her last years. She once told me that although she knew she was in her 80s, inside she truly felt as if she were no more than 35 years old. The discrepancy between the aging vessel that carries us and the ageless spiritual essence which we might feel can be great. It is important for us to recognize that patients may not see themselves as we see them. We cannot, as physicians, ignore what they say. Feelings of usefulness and vitality in the face of physical deterioration are the expressions of our patients' deepest desires for freedom not only for their bodies but perhaps from their bodies.

Artists and Their Own Illnesses

Certain artists have used their own personal experiences as a starting point for producing great work. Joseph Beuys, an important post-World War II German artist, was a pilot in the German airforce. His airplane was shot down, but his life was saved by the mountain people in Afghanistan. Beuys was severely burned in the crash of his plane. The mountain

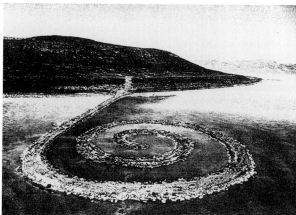

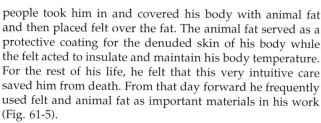

FIGURE 61-8

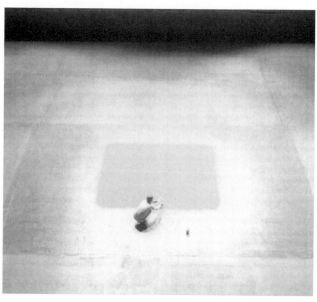

FIGURE 61-9

people took him in and covered his body with animal fat and then placed felt over the fat. The animal fat served as a protective coating for the denuded skin of his body while the felt acted to insulate and maintain his body temperature. For the rest of his life, he felt that this very intuitive care saved him from death. From that day forward he frequently used felt and animal fat as important materials in his work (Fig. 61-5).

Hannah Wilke was an accomplished artist in mid-career when she developed breast cancer. She felt compelled to document how her life had changed and was continually changing in direct relation to her physical deterioration. She documented the harshness and desperation of her medical treatment, endured in an effort to save herself. The unadorned photographs of her last months and days are singularly powerful and affecting. They are without guise or guile. They illustrate most painfully the reality of her oncoming death.

A large body of art has developed around HIV/AIDS. An extraordinary number of artists have had to confront this tragic illness and have used their personal experiences in dealing with the disease to illustrate fragility of life and the inevitability of death. Notable among these artists is the late Felix Gonzales Torres. His work is an example of remnants. His work uses the most delicate arrangements of lights, often strung in the most simple ways, expressing at once the exquisitely fragile life balance that we all strive to maintain, and life's impermanence (Fig. 61-6).

Another notable example is the work of Nicholas Africano. In the 1980s, he painted a series of portraits of a friend who had undergone colon surgery for cancer (Fig. 61-7). The paintings show an isolated figure on a very thinly painted background giving the sense that the figure, his friend, the patient, is floating in mid-air. The details of the colostomy are quite explicit as shown, and the vulnerability of the patient is without question. These paintings clearly define the isolation of the patient. At the same time the painting's format shows the patient's desire for freedom from external encumbrances,

by the figure which seems to be floating in mid-air against a blank background.

Holistic Medicine

Within the last 25 years, the issues of holistic medicine and "return to nature" have come center stage. We as physicians

FIGURE 61-10

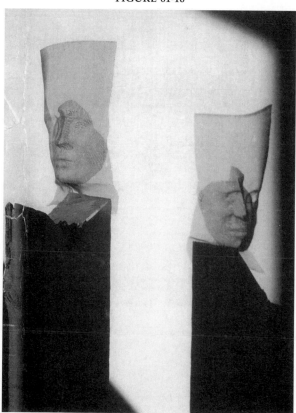

are constantly being questioned by our patients regarding nontraditional forms of therapy. In the world of art there has been a very similar intense interest shown in our natural surroundings and using them in works of art. One of the more beautiful works that have been produced is the Spiral Jetty of Robert Smithson who tragically died while in a small airplane over the artwork itself (Fig. 61-8).

Wolfgang Laib, a trained physician turned full-time artist, made his earliest artistic mark by accumulating and rearranging natural products he collected. After painstakingly gathering prodigious amounts of pollen, he installed the pollen in galleries and museums with rather astonishing ethereal effect (Fig. 6-9).

James Turrell has deeply explored the nature of light and space with respect to passage of time. In Arizona, he was given the right to manipulate the Roden Crater where a large meteorite fell to earth. He has reconfigured this site as a natural observatory after working meticulous calculations to determine when the stars, the sun, and the moon will create shadows or produce a pinhole of light within very exotic labyrinths. This is a modern example of defining infinity, resembling those carried out in Stonehenge and by the Mayans and the Incas.

On the other hand, the work of Rebecca Horn deals with the idea of impermanence of human-made objects. These are objects which are designed to deteriorate over time, perhaps illustrating our own impermanence. Anselm Keifer, a very significant contemporary German artist, has employed many materials which are already beginning to show signs of deterioration. These include mud, straw, and other very poorly preservable materials to help define our mortality.

The Intangibles of Our Patients' Lives

Over many years I have been struck, sometimes stunned, by the extraordinary differences between a person's physical and their much more potent nonphysical presence. I find it much easier, in their absence, to recall their general sense of deportment, their humor/meanness, anger, sadness, intelligence, than to be able to conjure up the details of their physi-

cal makeup. In my own art, I have tried to explore the issues of tangible and intangible reality, body, and spirit. I have done so using a technique of sculpture with wire mesh as a critical element. I have dealt much with faces. In my work, light transmits through the objects and shadows appear on adjacent walls or floors (Fig. 61-10). I found early on that the objects (mesh) and the shadows were always subtly different from each other. In many ways the sense of detail of the faces could much more easily be seen in the shadows. Moreover, and perhaps more telling, was that the shadow image, the intangible, was universally more potent than any actual, tangible, mesh face object that I produced. Once people see the shadow, they often nearly ignore the object through which it has been generated. I believe that it is never wrong for us as physicians to always strive to sense the potent intangibles of the lives of our patients.

A Kind of Summary

I am intrigued by certain phrases which relate to what we do. These include "the art of medicine," or "the healing arts." How do these phrases hold up during our increasingly technologic and computerized age? Whenever I am asked whether what I do might be replaced by a computer, I am amused. I do not believe that what we as physicians/healers do, practicing the "art of medicine," can ever be replaced by a series of ciphers. For example, when I take a history from a patient and ask him/her whether he/she has chest pain and a computer asks the same question, the computer is unable to detect a slight facial grimace or hesitancy in the voice that I will hopefully never fail to recognize. The computer will not know enough to understand all of our societal colloquialisms, based on a given patients economic or geographic background such that it can infallibly speak in the patient's own vernacular. It will never be able to look the patient in the eye to sense whether the patient is revealing all or revealing only what he/she is not afraid to reveal. Let them tell us of their tiniest steps. "I can now walk to the kitchen." "I got to the mall." "I spent two hours without any oxygen." "I slept all night and I had a wonderful dream." "I dreamed I could run."

Even if they can never run again, let us remember that they can still fly.

Chapter 62

ART AND REHABILITATION
The Patient's Point of View

CHARLES DUNN

The first thing I saw after my open heart surgery was a particularly gory medical illustration, a whole lot of blood amid a network of green, snaky things. The picture looked as if it had been lifted from an outdated medical text on what to avoid in surgery. It struck me as a strange choice for a cardiac recovery unit but I was still under the effects of the anesthesia so I didn't give it much thought; I just rolled over and went back to sleep. Later, after the anesthesia wore off, I realized the picture on my wall was a pleasant, rather innocuous watercolor depicting red flowers and green leaves.

Whoever selected the art for that cardiac care unit was on the right track; after all, florals make sense as decorations in a unit like the one I was in. What he or she didn't think about—or know (and how could they unless they had come out of deep anesthesia themselves and been confronted by that picture?)—was the effect that painting's colors and shapes would have on a heavily sedated patient who was just glad to be alive and was wondering how long, or even if, he would continue to live?

In my neck of the woods, hospitals advertise for cardiac care patients much the same as automobile dealers advertise for car buyers. The hospital's advertising doesn't engender a whole lot of confidence on the part of prospective patients like me because they boast of 98 percent (more or less) survival rates. And, if you read the small print, that's the percentage that get out of the hospital alive. Well, that's a step in the right direction. Fifty to one in my favor are odds I'd settle for most anytime but I want better odds if my life is on the line. So even though I was awake after a "successful" surgery, doped up as I was I still knew I wasn't out of the woods yet and those bloody veins or whatever they were on my wall didn't exactly engender confidence on my part about my recovery.

So, I think art, even the art on the patient's hospital walls, plays a part in recuperation. In fairness, however, I must admit the art on hospital walls seems to me very much better than anything I've ever seen in a hotel or motel room. I think the Hiltons, Sheratons, and Holiday Inns select paintings for their rooms on the basis of how ugly they are. That way the canny hoteliers avoid folks stealing the paintings right off their walls. They're so ugly, who'd want them?

Perhaps my experience in recuperating—and recuperating fast—from major surgery has some application to other forms of surgery and to rehabilitation in general.

Will Dwiggins, a premier graphic designer of the 1920s to 1940s, wrote, "I can only get at my own mind." True. So perhaps my experiences in recuperating from major surgery will give you some insight into how some of your patients may be able to speed their recoveries.

I entered New York-Cornell Hospital on November 19th for what was supposed to be a routine angiogram. As I understood it, the whole procedure should have taken no more than an hour or so unless there were unforseen complications. There were. Fifteen days later I was discharged with four new arteries and a pacemaker.

Less than 3 months later I was at my full-time day job, as well as actively pursuing my night- and spare-time careers as a painter, educator, and writer at age 66.

My doctors and knowledgeable friends are amazed that less than 90 days after my surgery I'm carrying a full schedule, I'm as strong as or stronger than I was before I went into the hospital with no special therapy, perhaps because of my age (I became 66 during those 90 days).

Mainly, I think the secret is that I've been busy and not with busy work. I suspect my recovery was speeded because I had pictures to paint. For example, each year I paint all our Christmas cards. The year of my bypass surgery was no exception. I had everything figured out so that I would have at least most of them completed by December 1st. Well, that sure didn't happen. In fact, from December 3d to, as I recall, about December 23d I spent 3 h or more every day painting so everyone on our Christmas list would get their annual original.

By January 2d I started work on a one-person show for late April which meant more than 40 new paintings. Later that month I resumed my full teaching load. The following month I went back to my day job.

So the prescription for a speedy recovery is to find something that's important to you and get busy doing it. For me it was painting transparent watercolors.

In the end, it really is a matter of passion. For instance, my brother-in-law's art and passion is cooking. Give him a dinner party to prepare and watch how fast he recuperates. Although most people seem to be primarily visually oriented, there are those whose orientation is auditory and for whom things heard mean more than things seen, and still others, those who are kinetically orientated, dancers and the like. But, at a guess there are more would be painters than musicians, dancers, or mimes, so I'll restrict myself to painting (more or less).

Winston Churchill wrote with his usual eloquence on behalf of painting, "Many men have found great advantage in practicing a handicraft for pleasure. Joinery, chemistry, bookbinding, even bricklaying—if one were interested in them and skillful at them—would give a real relief to the overtired brain. But, best of all and easiest to procure are sketching and painting in all their forms. I consider myself very lucky that late in life I have been able to develop this new taste and pastime. Painting came to my rescue in a most trying time."

Before I left for my book tour, my publisher's publicity agent briefed me and suggested I drop the names of a few famous people who paint.[1] I suggested Churchill and she told me that no one watching television would know who Churchill was. She told me I'd do better by dropping the name of an actress, Jane Seymour. There are some things that just don't get better with age.

Anyway, the kind of interest I'm talking about here is not the passing or casual interest the words *hobby* or *avocation* suggest. It is a second vocation, all absorbing in whatever time you have to spend practicing it, as Churchill points out.

Incidentally, Churchill found time to paint while he was conducting World War II. And you're too busy to paint or learn to paint—even though you'd like to. Whether it's painting, cooking, or carpentry, you have to take it seriously. It must absorb you at the time you're doing it. (It's the kind of passion my friend Marge Soroka had for watercolor painting; she just couldn't wait to retire to devote all her time to the one thing she wanted to do.)

Just what is art? What is it that makes one person an artist and not another? Can your patients make art? Can you be an artist even though you can't draw a straight line? The once familiar aesthetic ground is shifting under our feet even as we speak. These days it seems anything can be art as long as somebody, anybody, says it is. You don't have to be able to draw any more. Jackson Pollack took care of that for you back in the 1940s and 1950s. How do you become an artist today? Apparently the same way Mel Brooks's, Docker Haldanish (Oh, that's a "k," not a "t'") became a psychiatrist. "I went out into the desert and put my hand on a rock and said, 'I *am* a psychiatrist,'" So maybe whatever you do, I guess, it's art if you call it art, and you're an artist if you say so. Just put your hand on a rock.

These days, you don't even have to be a human to be an artist. Catalogs offer, and apparently, successfully sell the work of elephants, chimpanzees, and bottle-nosed dolphins at higher prices than paintings by good painters command.

"Art" today is photography, video, performance art including self-mutilation, installation art often with a political edge, and sometimes, even what was once called pornography. Nothing deserves disdain more than recognizable images like trees, people, and boats.

Where does that leave those of us who try to paint pretty pictures of the people, places, and things around us?

Well, we're in trouble. But, we're not completely alone. We have an articulate spokesperson in Alexandre Solzhenitsyn.

For several decades now (Solzhenitsyn writes) world literature, music, painting and sculpture have exhibited a stubborn tendency to grow not higher but to the side, not toward the highest achievements of craftsmanship and the human spirit but toward their disintegration into a frantic and insidious novelty. To decorate public spaces we put up sculptures that aestheticize pure ugliness—but we no longer register surprise. And if visitors from outer space were to pick up our music over the airwaves, how could they ever guess that earthlings once had a Bach, a Beethoven, a Schubert, now abandoned as out of date and obsolete?

New York Times Book Review (2/7/93)

Some things are better and more directly stated in visual terms just as others are best expressed in mathematical terms. (Can you think of a better way to say two plus two equals four than $2 + 2 = 4$?) We find painting gives us another way to express ourselves in addition to speech, writing, and gesture. Somehow the attempt to make beautiful images gives us joy. We respect and admire the skills of predecessors. We honor our artistic mothers and fathers.

There are those who hold us in disdain as "Sunday painters" because we put supporting our families ahead of making "art." We, however, are in the company of such "part-timers" as T. S. Eliot, Josef Albers, William Carlos Williams, and Wallace Stevens (to name a few who come readily to mind).

About 20 years ago there was an Australian girl, Janice, in one of my classes. I've changed the names of the innocent to protect their privacy. Any resemblance to persons living or dead, however, is the result of very hard work. Janice studied with me for a couple of years and despite being one of the hardest, most dedicated workers I've ever seen, she showed absolutely no improvement.

I found myself on the horns of a moral dilemma. Should I have her give up painting, or keep on taking her money and hope for a miracle? It seemed to me that telling her to quit would be the kind thing to do. But, for some reason, I never got around to it, and then, one day, Janice didn't come to class. She'd been diagnosed with a tubal pregnancy and was near death in a New York hospital.

It wasn't until many months later that a pale Janice came back to class. She took me aside to tell me that only the thought of coming back to class had kept her alive during her months in the hospital. That was very gratifying. Trouble was her painting was still terrible, but how could I tell her to give up now? So I didn't.

There is a happy ending to this. A month or so later, she came into class, glowing. She had exhibited at one of the local malls and taken first prize. She offered her painting for criticism and it was a knockout. She had outpainted us all, including art teachers, fine and commercial artists, and the holders of advanced degrees in fine art. From that day on, Janice never looked back.

I heard from Janice years later. She had returned to Australia where her husband abandoned her and the kids for another woman. Mercifully, painting was still her salvation. She was teaching, selling, and winning awards.

Even at its worst, Janice's work was far better than anything I've ever seen painted by an elephant, a chimpanzee, or a bottle-nosed porpoise. Hers was an honest attempt by a sensitive, sentient human being to communicate some of the beauty and joy she found in the world with others.

It might be fair to say that art helped Janice survive and, in turn, Janice became a successful artist (at least on her terms and mine).

What art did for Janice it can do for you and your patients—if you'll let it.

No time for shuffleboard? I see them now those great geriatric cases: Renoir crippled with arthritis, his brushes strapped to his hands, still creating those uniquely sensuous surfaces, Leonardo working to the day of his death at 67. Frank Lloyd Wright designing his masterful Guggenheim when he was in his 90s. My most influential teacher, Ed Whitney, taught watercolor painting up to the day he died at 96.

Hokusai always encourages me. "From the age of six, I was in the habit of drawing all kinds of things. Although I had produced many designs by my fiftieth year, nothing that I did before my seventieth is worth considering. Now 73, I have come to understand the true form of animals, insects and fish, and the nature of plants and trees. By the age of 86 I shall have made more and more progress, and at 90 I shall have got closer to the essence of art. At the age of 100 I shall have reached a magnificent level; at 110 each dot and line will be alive. I would like to ask those who outlive me to observe that I have not spoken without reason."

Since he died at 84 we'll never know just how good Hokusai might have become. We do know, however, that most critics agree his best work came after 70. So maybe there's hope for youngsters like us.

For 25 years I've taught what has become a master class. Many of us in the group have grown older together; older, not old together. As we've aged we've grown and become better painters; exactly how much better in direct proportion to the time we were able to devote to improving our craft skills.

Janet, a hospice nurse who never painted or drew before, came to one of my workshops the week after her fiftieth birthday. She told me in her work the only regret people had was for the things they hadn't done. She said, painting was something she had always wanted to do and she wasn't going to die without having at least tried it.

In my annual Elderhostel workshops I see folks looking to capture something they feel they missed along the way, looking for something that art and creativity offer them.

Somehow the attempt to make art or, perhaps better, to improve one's craft skills seems intrinsic to the human soul and it affirms the best in us.

Our working careers are not always satisfactory. Even the best doctors eventually lose their patients; generals win wars at the expense of young lives; as for the clergy, no wars have ever been more horrible or condoned worse atrocities than religious wars. All political systems eventually crumble. Where would the lawyers be if we all followed the Golden Rule? The essential nature of commerce is duplicity.

Despite a general lack of financial support, artists have always plied their craft and somehow the art endures. Although Rembrandt and Vermeer are both today still unreleased bankrupts, they continue to endure because they stand for something more than mere self-satisfaction or self-mutilation. When we look at their painting we feel better about ourselves. (They have also made a significant contribution to the Dutch Tourism Board's efforts to attract free-spending visitors to the Netherlands.)

Who knows why some of us, including many doctors, choose to pursue second careers as artists? For example, Dr. Neal is good enough that if a major gallery or museum discovered him, his paintings would sell for thousands of dollars. Meanwhile, his home is a spectacular gallery featuring a one-person show unlike any I've ever seen anywhere.

Then there was the late Dr. Ed who spent his spare time making museum quality doll houses and furnishings for his grandchildren. Those dollhouses have outlived his patients and perhaps provided Ed with some measure of immortality.

As the saying goes, the coin outlasts Tiberius.

Dr. Lewis may be as successful an artist as he is a physician.

The good doctor embraces the latest trends and views art from the modernist point of view and he knows how to create things that please the folks who count in the art world.

I wonder if maybe doctors aren't attracted to the certainties of art. For instance, in over 3000 years no one's yet come up with a better way to divide space than the Golden Section. On the other hand, a doctor must continually replace his knowledge and update his skills. He or she continually needs to be recertified. That expensive medical education is pretty quickly outdated. On the other hand, the artist continually adds to his knowledge because the arts are based on absolutes like the Golden Section.

Maybe that's why so many doctors paint, sculpt, or play musical instruments? Maybe it's because of some half-formed hope for immortality. Maybe it's simply because they love doing it and that's reason enough.

Maybe it's as Ed Whitney said, "All you need to keep sane is a craft activity and someone who loves you. Craft gives back in direct proportion to your investment. It's the only component of your life that's fair, you get what you earn." As for someone who loves you, "There's always mommy."

There will be future editions of this book. Advances in technology alone insure that. This chapter, however, will not be outdated or need to be rewritten. If it is rewritten it will be because it can be better expressed, not because the fundamental truths in it became obsolete. The writer's ability to make art may improve but the bedrock upon which art exists remains solid.

Should your patients take up art to speed their recuperations? Should you start attending art classes? Answer: It's never too late as long as it's something you or they want to do badly enough to do it.

My own mind is still the only one I can get at and I know painting has seen me through the rough times, both physically and psychologically, and, if you will let it, painting or the art or craft of your choice will see you and your patients through, too.

If you want, you too can enjoy the consolation of craft—the more you practice the better you'll become. Maybe you'll even get to Carnegie Hall someday but, meanwhile, it's a great trip. Hop aboard and enjoy the scenery as it passes.

Reference

1. Dunn C: *Conversations in Paint.* Workman, NY 1995.

INDEX

Page numbers in *italics* refer to illustrations; those ending in the letter "t" refer to tables.

707

ISBN 0-07-011649-0

90000>